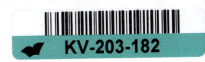

Food Toxicology

PART A: PRINCIPLES AND CONCEPTS

FOOD SCIENCE AND TECHNOLOGY

A Series of Monographs, Textbooks, and Reference Books

1. Flavor Research: Principles and Techniques, *R. Teranishi, I. Hornstein, P. Issenberg, and E. L. Wick (out of print)*

2. Principles of Enzymology for the Food Sciences, *John R. Whitaker*

3. Low-Temperature Preservation of Foods and Living Matter, *Owen R. Fennema, William D. Powrie, and Elmer H. Marth*

4. Principles of Food Science
    Part I: Food Chemistry, *edited by Owen R. Fennema*
    Part II: Physical Methods of Food Preservation, *Marcus Karel, Owen R. Fennema, and Daryl B. Lund*

5. Food Emulsions, *edited by Stig Friberg*

6. Nutritional and Safety Aspects of Food Processing, *edited by Steven R. Tannenbaum*

7. Flavor Research: Recent Advances, *edited by R. Teranishi, Robert A. Flath, and Hiroshi Sugisawa*

8. Computer-Aided Techniques in Food Technology, *edited by Israel Saguy*

9. Handbook of Tropical Foods, *edited by Harvey T. Chan*

10. Antimicrobials in Foods, *edited by Alfred Larry Branen and P. Michael Davidson*

11. Food Constituents and Food Residues: Their Chromatographic Determination, *edited by James F. Lawrence*

Other Volumes in Preparation

Food Toxicology

(in two parts)

PART A: PRINCIPLES AND CONCEPTS

Jose M. Concon

University of Kentucky
Lexington, Kentucky

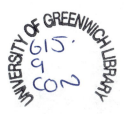

MARCEL DEKKER, INC.   New York and Basel

Concon, Jose M.
    Food and technology.

    (Food science and technology ; 26-27)
    Includes bibliographies and index.
    Contents: part A. Principles and concepts -- part B.
Contaminants and additives.
    1. Food poisoning. 2. Food contamination. I. Title.
II. Series: Food science and technology (Marcel Dekker,
Inc.) ; 26-27.
RA1258.C66   1988   615.9'54   87-22231
ISBN 0-8247-7736-0 (part A)
ISBN 0-8247-7737-9 (part B)

MARCEL DEKKER, INC.
270 Madison Avenue, New York, New York 10016

Current printing (last digit):
10 9 8 7 6 5 4 3 2 1

PRINTED IN THE UNITED STATES OF AMERICA

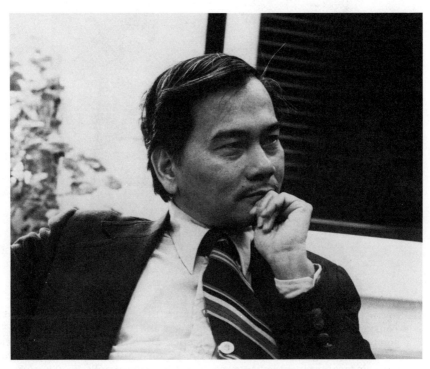

Jose M. Concon (1932–1984)

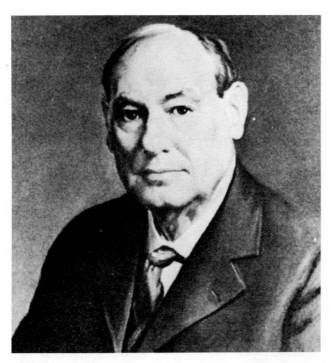

Dr. Harvey W. Wiley, head of the first Food and Drug Agency of the United States, 1907, is considered the "Father of the Pure Food and Drug Act," which marked a turning point in his untiring fight for protection of consumers. As consumers, we owe a sincere debt of gratitude to Dr. Wiley, because without such legislation many of the toxins and contaminants discussed in these books would be far more numerous in our nation's food supply and the nation would not have the degree of good health that it enjoys.

To my wife, Jayne,
whose untiring effort, love, and dedication
have made this book possible

Preface

At a meeting of the American College of Nutrition, the nutrition curricula in medical schools were being discussed. I asked one of the speakers why the subject of food toxicology was not included in any of the curricula. I added that it was unfortunate that the study of nutrition ignored the subject of food toxicants—or, at the most, treated it superficially. "Do you know of any comprehensive book on the subject?" he asked. I answered that there were only a number of books on scattered subjects in the field and that there is no single book that treats the subject of food toxicology as a unit as there is in most other disciplines. "Why don't you write one?" he challenged. Thus, the idea of initiating this project was nurtured during that conversation.

The subject of food toxicology is complex, and at the same time intriguing and challenging. Consider just the endogenous components. Thousands of compounds have already been identified; and by the time food has reached the table, the number of substances in it that nature has not intended has already increased to a staggering proportion. Many of the substances are introduced by manufacturers (given the impetus of progress) influenced by such factors as technology, leisure and convenience, profit motive, the pressure of overpopulation, and the insatiable human desire and penchant to improve on nature. Many are in foods as contaminants because of ignorance, apathy, carelessness, and neglect. A large number of new compounds are produced in the food because of chemical reactions within and between individual food components, aided no doubt by human activity.

Most of these substances have no known nutritional value, and because they are reactive compounds they can be expected to have some effects. The questions to be asked are: What are these substances and what are their effects? What conditions or factors influence these effects?

Research in the past several decades, and especially the last decade, has provided some of the answers. A tremendous amount of information has accrued since the biblical account of the poisoning of the Hebrews with normally nontoxic quails. A majority of the information developed piecemeal, and not as a result of systematic inquiry. There has been little attempt at formalization of the discipline. Therefore, practitioners in the health field, especially the physicians, nutritionists, and public health professionals, are often uninformed or have scattered knowledge in an area of tremendous importance to health.

This lack of formalization explains why the subject of food toxicants is often superficially treated, if not left out, in many nutrition curricula. These two volumes represent an attempt at such formalization.

Inevitably, the subject matter that can be dealt with within the confines of two volumes will be limited. Thus, the materials I have chosen are, in my opinion, sufficient to give the reader a cohesive perspective on the subject. Chapters 1-7 deal with toxicological principles relevant to the question of toxicants in foods. The subjects covered in these first seven chapters are intended to give the reader a balanced view of the toxic phenomena as circumscribed by the factors and conditions affecting the toxicological response.

Chapters 8-11 cover a whole range of endogenous toxicants as defined in Chapter 1. However, for the sake of completeness and relevance, some subjects that appropriately belong under a different heading are included, such as ciguatera and paralytic shellfish toxins.

Chapters 13-17 cover the subject of micro- and macrobiological contaminants. The inclusion of bacterial pathogens as food toxicants may foment some controversy. However, this is hardly the space to indulge in apologia, except to say that the action of the pathogens involved in "food poisoning" are mediated by means of toxins. Thus, the phenomenon of bacterial action in this case is truly toxicological.

Chapter 19 covers the subject of manmade chemical contaminants. The so-called "incidental" or "unintentional food additives" are also included as contaminants. The reason for considering these substances as contaminants is discussed in the chapter. Naturally occurring radionuclides are also included here for the sake of completeness and relevance (Ch. 20).

Chapters 12 and 21 include "intentional" food additives and derived toxicants. The latter term is used for the first time to designate those toxic compounds formed by chemical reactions occurring in the food during processing, preparation, or storage.

The two volumes do not cover methodologies. For example, little discussion is devoted to risk-benefit estimation—a subject of considerable controversy.

I want to thank sincerely the individuals who were helpful in the preparation and writing of *Food Toxicology, Parts A and B*, particularly the following: E. P. Baxter, J. M. Lane, A. P. Powell, A. M. Bushnell, J. C. Gilmore, and E. R. Pray.

My special thanks to Dr. Donald Tressler, whose interest in this project allowed the glow of my efforts to remain undiminished in spite of the many problems and frustrations encountered during its writing.

Above all, my heartfelt gratitude to my wife, Jayne, for her most valued assistance in preparing, typing, and editing the manuscript, and especially for her understanding and encouragement.

Jose M. Concon

Acknowledgments

When my husband passed away suddenly after completing the manuscripts for Parts A and B, there was still quite a bit of work left to be done. There were references that still needed to be checked and completed, to name just one of the remaining tasks.

Since I had worked with my husband on his project since 1975 (mainly typing and helping to locate and check references), it seemed only natural that I finish the basically clerical work that remained to be done. I was prepared to work long hours for many months, but I wasn't prepared for the outpouring of love and help from some very special people. Without their support, I couldn't have completed such a large volume of work under such difficult circumstances.

I wasn't prepared to redraw all the chemical structures in India ink either, but a former student of my husband's was. To Carol Charles, the commercial artist whose expertise in drawing the chemical structures was crucial to getting the manuscript in a form acceptable for publication, go my heartfelt thanks. I also wish to thank Dr. David Newburg for initially contacting Carol and securing her participation.

For adding to the already heavy demands on their time and their thoroughness when helping me crosscheck the hundreds of references in the text, I want to express my deep appreciation to Carol "Robin" Luger, Linda Smith, Joan Williams, and Mildred Yates.

For their consistent resourcefulness in helping me find information, journals, books, and locating and checking references, I want the following librarians to know that their expertise created a sense of security that enabled me to continue working when I often felt like quitting—Stephanie Allen, Peter Costich, Jane Lane, Kerry Kressie, Tony Powell, Joyce Gilmore, Diane Brunn, Barbara Hahn, and Sara Bushnell.

For all her help, encouragement, and interest, plus the time she gave to me on the manuscript to ensure its accuracy, I am most indebted to Dr. Linda Chen, Chairman of the Department of Nutrition and Food Science, College of Home Economics, University of Kentucky.

And a very special word of thanks to Creed and Elsa Black, who provided the kind of environment and steadfast support required for the written manuscript to develop into a document suitable to be submitted for publication.

Jayne W. Concon

Contents of Part A

Contents of Part B

Food Toxicology

PART A: PRINCIPLES AND CONCEPTS

1

General Toxicological Principles Applicable to Foods and Food Toxicants

DEFINITION OF TOXICOLOGICAL CONCEPTS

Food toxicology is a science which deals with the nature, sources, and formation of toxic substances in foods, their deleterious effects, the manifestations and mechanisms of these effects, and the identification of the limits of the safety of these substances. Food in this sense includes all substances or mixtures of substances, both solid and liquid, which are intended for human ingestion for their nutritional and/or pleasurable benefits. This definition includes not only natural solid and liquid foods but also drinking water and synthetic or manufactured products, such as formulated or engineered products and alcoholic and other beverages.

A substance is toxic when it causes cellular or tissue injury by mechanisms other than physical trauma. Such substances are said to possess toxicity, which is defined as the capacity to produce toxic injury to cells or tissues. Toxic injury in this sense refers to an actual or potentially harmful alteration of cellular or tissue constituents and processes, which may or may not be manifested by clear clinical symptoms.

A substance may not be actually toxic but the conditions are such that it presents a hazard (the probability that a toxic substance will cause toxic injury under the conditions of use). Thus, hazard is a relative term, dependent on various exogenous and endogenous factors. Toxicity is similarly dependent on these factors.

A substance is deemed safe when it is practically certain that under the conditions of use, no toxic injury will result. The safety of any substance is dependent similarly on exogenous and endogenous factors. The safety, hazard and toxicity of a substance are relative properties which depend on various factors and conditions. Without the proper reference to these factors, they are meaningless by themselves.

SCOPE OF (TOOD) TOXICOLOGY

The scope of food toxicology comprises the factors and conditions which define toxicity, the hazard and safety of various substances found in foods, and the nature of the response of the host to these substances. These factors are varied and complex. Endogenous factors arise from the complexities of the biochemistry and physiology of the host and its interaction with the environment. Exogenous factors are determined by the nature of the toxic compounds, their chemical and biological relationships with other components in the food, and chemicals in the environment.

A primary objective of food toxicology is the understanding of the nature and properties of all toxic substances in foods and the nature and magnitude of the hazard

they present under various conditions. Such an understanding results in a clear delineation of the safety limits. A specification of the safety limits presupposes knowledge of the underlying toxicological mechanisms associated with each toxicant. While
such knowledge is incomplete (e.g., in carcinogenesis), an unambiguous definition of
safety will not be possible and can only be specified tentatively and relatively.

Principal concern is the toxicological interaction of food components and environmental chemicals. This is an area where information is minimal and vigorous research
is needed.

Toxic compounds occurring in foodstuffs present a far more complex toxicological
dimension than isolated compounds. In many instances, food toxicants incite the entire
spectrum of human concern. These substances, being a part of foods, present not
only health implications but also involve economic, social and political factors. Modern
technology has made the concern for food safety more urgent and profound and the
field of food toxicology more relevant.

It is also the aim of the study of food toxicology to put food toxicants in perspective so that hysteria or apathy arising from ignorance will give way to rational assessment. Rationality can only be accomplished when accompanied by scientific judgment.
Because many food toxicants occur in foods in minute quantities, a rational assessment
of their hazard or safety can only be made by studying their toxicological effects and
the body.s response to their presence in tissues. For example, one may contend that
the small amounts of cyanogen in lima beans (Chap. 8) present no hazard. However,
this will be pure speculation if we do not have knowledge of how the body responds
to traces of cyanide. Fortunately, such information is available (Chap. 4), and the
contention regarding the safety of small amounts of cyanogen in lima beans has a scientific basis.

Food Toxicology and Nutritional Science

Food toxicology is indeed a part of the discipline of nutritional science. A study of
toxic substances in foods should be as much a concern of nutritional and medical scientists as the nutrients themselves. One can view food toxicants as counteracting the
beneficial effects of nutrients as a whole, although in many cases, one-to-one,
nutrient-toxicant interactions are evident. Clearly, a study of nutritonal science without food toxicants is incomplete and inappropriate. Such a narrow view, which has
persisted for decades up until a few years ago, may account in part for the lack of a
systematic approach to the study of food toxicants.

TOXIC POTENTIAL OF FOOD

Paradoxical as it may seem, food whose principal function is the maintenance of life
and well-being is also the source or cause of toxic injury, which in many cases is devastating and fatal. This has been known through the centuries. The Bible describes
an incident of nonbacterial acute mass food poisonings among the early Hebrews.
During the wanderings of the Hebrews in the desert after their exodus from Egypt,
quails descended on their campsite in large numbers. The Hebrews, who had hungered
and complained for meat, greedily ate large numbers of the birds and "while the flesh
was yet between their teeth, ere it was chewed, . . . The Lord smote the people with
a very great plague." The Bible narrative suggests that many of the Hebrews died of
this poisoning (Numbers 11:31−34). Quail poisonings, in fact, have been described by
ancient writers, and Sergent (1941) suggested that the quails mentioned in the biblical
incident had become poisonous by feeding on hemlock seeds (Conium maculatum), to
which most quails are resistant.

During the Middle Ages, an epidemic of ergotism, a convulsive and gangrenous
mycotoxicosis, plagued many countries in Europe. The disease was caused by the

consumption of grains contaminated with ergot derived from the fungus *Claviceps purpurea* which infected the cereal plants in the field (p. 727).

Food derived from the sea has also been implicated in countless incidences of food poisonings. Islanders, in fact, know this only too well, and navigators to the New World in the eighteenth and nineteenth centuries described many instances of sailors who had fallen victims of fatal poisonings from toxic clams and fish (Chap. 11).

In the United States in the 1800s or earlier, settlements were dissipated into ghost towns following an epidemic of the so-called "milk sickness." The disease was later shown to be caused by the toxic alcohol trimetol, derived from white snakeroot, growing on the edges of meadows and eaten by dairy cattle (Chap. 17).

Over time, the contamination of the food supply with toxic chemicals has increased steadily, so that at the present time it is difficult to find a food product which does not contain one or more kinds of contaminants. Furthermore, the increased activity of the processed food industries has resulted in the presence of an increasing number of synthetic or foreign chemicals in the food supply in the form of food additives. Some of these compounds have not been thoroughly tested for safety. Indeed, the growing realization in many countries of the toxic potentials of these contaminants and food additives has prompted the enactment of laws and regulations aimed at protecting public health. Indeed, some of these additives which have been considered safe for centuries have been implicated in the causation of modern epidemic diseases. A case in point is common table salt, which is now considered to be the principal cause of the prevailing pandemic of hypertension (p. 1294).

The world's scientific literature since the turn of this century contains descriptions of countless incidences of illnesses and poisonings caused by the consumption of specific foods. In the United States alone, it is estimated that more than a million cases of foodborne bacterial infections and intoxications occur each year (Brachmann et al. 1972). Foodborne and waterborne transmission of such diseases as cholera and shigellosis still occur in some parts of the world.

No doubt, toxic injury caused by eating specific foods will continue to occur, in part owing to ignorance. Thus, a systematic study of toxicants in food or the toxic potential of food, the conditions and factors affecting the presence of these factors in food and the response of the body to these factors, and the means of prevention or minimization of these effects are of profound significance and relevance to food safety, especially at the present time.

CLASSIFICATION OF FOOD TOXICANTS ACCORDING TO SOURCE

According to their sources, food components may be classified into four types: naturally occurring constituents, biological and chemical contaminants, food additives, and derived substances. Each of these may be assigned to one of three toxicological categories in the concentrations present in specific food products: inactive or inert; active but nontoxic; and toxic. These are relative properties which can be influenced in one or more ways by several factors.

Naturally Occurring Toxicants

Naturally occurring toxicants are products of the metabolic processes of animals, plants, and microorganisms from which the food products are derived. It seems strange that these harmful substances are also produced together with the nutrients. The teleological reasons for their presence in the food sources can only be surmised. For example, what is the purpose, biological or otherwise, of linamarin, a cyanogenic glycoside in casava?

Primitive man probably learned by trial and error, and by observations of either humans or animals, which natural products must be avoided as poisonous, or at least eaten with caution. Many naturally occurring substances in food products are potent poisons which produce, under certain conditions, severe if not fatal symptoms. As expected, those products which produce immediate adverse effects are promptly avoided except in those cases in which the toxic materials can be easily removed, for example, by washing with water. Unfortunately, there are naturally occurring substances in food products which have delayed toxicity, and the recognition of their presence in food as well as the cause and effect relationships between the observed poisoning and the food is often slow in coming.

Biological and Chemical Contaminants

It can be said that in their living state food sources are products of their environment. As such, our food sources therefore are easy targets for contamination. Contamination of foodstuffs may come from all directions — from the air, soil, and water, and from other plants or animals. To this list must be added a most important source of contamination, human beings themselves.

Food products may be contaminated by the natural inorganic constituents in the soil and water. Many toxic chemicals present in the soil and water are absorbed by plants and by land and marine animals themselves. For example, selenium (Rosenfeld and Beath 1964) and nitrates (Barker et al. 1971) may accumulate in plants to toxic levels. Toxic levels of other metallic elements have also been reported to accumulate in plants and animals (Underwood 1973).

Indirect contamination of meats, milk, or eggs may occur as a result of ingestion of contaminated foodstuffs by animals. Likewise, land and marine animals may ingest toxic substances, so that their flesh, milk, or eggs become contaminated.

Microorganisms abound in the soil, water, and air, and may infect the growing plant and stored products and produce toxic metabolites. Typical examples are various fungi which appear to have strong affinities for living or dead plant tissues. Under the right temperature and moisture content, stored food products contaminated by various microorganisms may become toxic from the growth of the infecting microorganisms. Indeed, these types of contaminated foodstuffs have been the cause of many serious, severe, and fatal poisonings in man and animals. Certain types of microorganisms may also proliferate on entering the gastrointestinal tract where the conditions may be conducive for their growth. Exotoxins excreted by the microorganisms or endotoxins released upon disintegration or death of bacterial cells may be absorbed into the circulatory system and produce the specific toxic effects in specific tissues or in the entire organ system.

Contamination may also occur during the gathering or harvesting of food products. For example, certain toxic plants may be harvested with the edible species unintentionally. Likewise, contaminated foodstuffs may be mixed with the wholesome products.

Finally, a major source of contamination from nonbiological sources are the products of a fast-growing modern technology. The increasing world population as well as the mass migration into the cities demands a massive and rapid increase in our food supply. Increased agricultural productivity required constant large-scale application of fertilizers, insecticides, herbicides, fungicides and other pesticides, growth stimulants, and antibiotics. Residues, sometimes at toxic levels, from most of these products end up in the food supply via the soil, air, and water. It can be assumed at present that the bodies of most human beings contain one or more pesticides in detectable amounts.

Technological contaminants also come from other sources besides agriculture. Modernization of the population's lifestyles also has resulted in the proliferative production of synthetic chemicals for use in all aspects of modern life — in industry, transportation, housing, household activities, entertainment, leisure activities, education, and research. The control of diseases and various human complaints, real or imagined, also has resulted in the ever-expanding arsenal of drugs and medicines. A significant number of these chemicals ultimately, one way or another, end up in our food and water supply.

Contaminants may also be derived during storage from packaging and canning materials in contact with the foodstuffs. Such contaminants as plasticizers may be leached out of plastic materials. In the case of metallic cans, acidic conditions in the stored products may cause the surface layer of the cans to dissolve into the food products. Aluminum containers, which can also be slowly dissolved under acidic conditions, are more rapidly corroded under more alkaline conditions. Another source of chemical contaminants is vessels and utensils used in cooking, food preparation, and short-term household storage of prepared foods and beverages.

Unfortunately, the manifestation of toxic effects from chemical contaminants may be delayed in view of the small quantities ingested over a period of time. Thus, the cause and effect relationship cannot be easily demonstrated. This is complicated further by the multiplicity of chemical contaminants that may be ingested at any given time.

Presently, there is a growing awareness and alarm regarding the ever-increasing number of toxic substances that are being spewed into our environment by modern technology. This awareness was probably ushered into our era by Rachel Carson (1962) in her book, *Silent Spring*, in which she decried the excessive and rampant use of pesticides with seeming disregard for the ecological system.

This awareness has spurred and prompted more stringent and stricter regulatory actions in many countries. Indeed, an apparent by-product of this public awareness is the growing and more widespread public concern and alarm regarding another source of toxicants, the food additives, which are also a result of modern technology.

Food Additives

Food additives are used for many purposes, such as food preservation. The large amounts of products produced cannot be immediately consumed or transported into the population centers far removed from the place of production. Therefore, these products must be preserved and stored. The use of chemical preservatives is one of the most popular and economical methods of food preservation. Unfortunately, many chemical preservatives may have delayed toxicity, as demonstrated in animal tests, but so far, cause and effect relationships of human toxicity have not been easily demonstrated with respect to many of these substances. Meanwhile, they may remain in our food supply for economic reasons until convincing proof of their toxicity in humans has been demonstrated.

Food additives are also used in food processing to impart many supposedly desirable physical, functional, organoleptic, and nutritional properties to food. Chemicals such as food colorants and flavorings are added simply for esthetic purposes. Justification for their use has become even more difficult as more and more of these types of additives have been demonstrated to be carcinogenic in animals.

The number of food additives has increased significantly since the beginning of this century. The toxicological properties of many compounds in this category have not been thoroughly investigated. There are many additives that have been used for many years without apparent or demonstrated ill effects, and therefore are considered and generally recognized as safe (GRAS). Such an arbitrary criterion immediately suggests to the concerned student of food toxicology an item-by-item examination of the toxicological properties of these substances in view of the increasing knowledge in this field. This, in fact, is the case. The GRAS list is now being re-evaluated (Federation of American Societies for Experimental Biology 1977; Hall 1975).

A more detailed discussion of food additives is given in Chapter 19.

Derived Toxic Substances in Foods

Naturally occurring and other food components, being reactive chemicals, can be expected to react with one another. Such reactions may either diminish the toxic potentials of specific compounds or produce additional toxic materials. These reactions may be brought about or hastened by heat, as in cooking and processing. The presence of specific substances may have catalytic effects; for example, acids and metals which catalyze hydrolysis and oxidation, respectively. Slower reactions may produce an increasing number of toxic products during storage. In addition, food constituents may also react with contaminants during processing, and especially during storage. Such reactions may be influenced by light and moisture or concomitant heating effects occurring during storage. The products of these reactions in situ are aptly called derived substances.

Derived substances are also produced by the action of contaminating microorganisms or those intentionally inoculated in food products. Such is the case with many fermented foods in which the action of microorganisms on food components may produce toxic substances. For example, bacterial decarboxylases and deaminases may produce toxic amino acid derivatives. Bacteria may also convert nitrates to nitrites by the action of reductases (Phillips 1971).

Thus, the type of toxicants to which modern human beings may be exposed are varied and numerous. To what extent this increasing load contributes to many human infirmities and degenerative diseases in modern times cannot be ascertained at the present time. Analyses of human tissues have revealed the presence of significant amounts of specific toxicants, such as DDT (dichlorodiphenyltrichloroethane) (Hoffmann et al. 1964), PCB (polychlorinated biphenyls) (Hammond 1972), and metals (Engel et al. 1971; Minst. Agric. Fish Food 1971, 1972).

It can only be said with almost a sense of helplessness that while we are on the verge of eliminating most microbial diseases that have ravaged mankind in centuries past, we are nowhere in sight of the control of degenerative diseases involving the central nervous system, the cardiovascular and circulatory system, birth defects, endocrine diseases, and above all, the malignant diseases. The control of microbial diseases was partly accomplished through sanitation. By the same token, it is not too farfetched and unreasonable to suggest that the control of modern diseases may also be accomplished partly by stringent control of human exposure to potential toxicants in food, water, air, and other vehicles of exposure.

FACTORS AFFECTING TOXICITY OF COMPOUNDS

Many exogenous and endogenous factors affect the toxicity of compounds. Among the exogenous factors are the nature of the compound, the dose, the frequency of exposure, the route of exposure, the presence of other compounds, and various environmental factors. Among endogenous factors are the physiology and morphology of the gastrointestinal tract, the nature of intestinal bacteria, and the metabolic activity of the body.

Exogenous Factors

Nature of the Compound

As we shall see, the chemical and physical properties of a compound can affect its toxic potential. To be toxic, most substances must be absorbed, although this is not always applicable. The absorption of a compound in the gastrointestinal (GI) tract is dependent on its molecular size, its solubility in aqueous or lipid medium, and its electrical charge or polarity. Unabsorbed toxic substances can damage the intestinal tract by transforming the intestinal mucosa such that nutrients are not absorbed, or by allowing water to leak into the intestinal lumen. Substances that are not absorbed can also manifest their toxicity by changing the osmotic equilibrium between the blood and the fluid of the intestinal lumen. Nonabsorbable substances can also become toxic or nontoxic after being metabolized by intestinal bacteria. These substances may also prevent the absorption of nutrients by chemically or physically combining with them.

As shown in the next section, the most important property that governs the toxicity of a compound is its chemical reactivity. Such highly reactive substances can combine with enzymes, nucleic acids, hormones, nerve cells, cell membranes, and other target molecules or sites in the body and interfere with their activities. Substances that are subject to metabolic transformation or conjugation can cause their toxicological properties to be significantly changed, for better or for worse.

In addition, a substance which chemically resembles a vital metabolite or nutrient in all probability will have toxic effects (Chapt. 9).

Chemical Structure and Toxicity

The chemical structure of any compound determines its chemical reactivity, biological activity, rate of gastrointestinal absorption and entry to the tissues and cells, biotransformation, and excretion. The chemical structure also influences the metabolism of the compound by intestinal bacteria. Therefore, the toxicity of any compound is a function of its structure.

Derivatives of ethane are examples of the influence of structure on toxicity (Table 1). This gas is narcotic only at high concentration (Stecher et al. 1960), and thus, is relatively nontoxic.

Note that with the ethanol derivatives the toxicity is enhanced if a hydrogen of the second carbon is substituted, in increasing order, with hydroxyl, amino, and chloride groups, the latter substituent producing the greatest toxicity.

The differences in toxicity can be accounted for primarily by the manner of their metabolism. Ethanol is oxidized initially to ethanal (Hawkins and Kalant 1972; Russell and Van Bruggen 1964). The aldehyde is seven times more toxic than the alcohol, owing to the greater reactivity of the former. The aldehyde can react with amino

$$CH_3CH_2OH \xrightarrow{(O)} CH_3-\overset{\overset{\text{H}}{|}}{\underset{\delta+}{C}}=\overset{..}{\underset{}{O}}:\delta-$$

groups of proteins to form imines or Schiff bases by nucleophilic addition to the carbonyl carbon.

$$CH_3-\overset{\overset{\text{H}}{|}}{C}=O \;+\; \overset{..}{N}H_2- \;\text{Protein} \longrightarrow CH_3\overset{\overset{\text{H}}{|}}{C}=\overset{..}{N}- \;\text{Protein} \;+\; H_2O$$

Such a reaction may result in enzyme inhibition, for example, of acetaldehyde dehydrogenase (AD) (Majchrowicz 1973) and the monoamine oxidases (MAO); the inhibition of MAO may account in part for the elevation of neuroamines in the blood following ethanol ingestion (Davis et al. 1970; Garlind et al. 1960; Perman 1958; Walsh et al. 1970; Yamanaka and Kono 1974); the inhibition of AD and MAO provides ample opportunity for reaction of acetaldehyde with various biological amines. Thus, psychoactive morphine-like alkaloids (e.g., tetrahydropapaveroline) have been detected following incubation of rat brain with either ethanol or acetaldehyde in the presence of dopamine (Cohen and Collins 1970; Davis et al. 1970). Therefore, it was postulated that alcohol addiction may be related to this phenomenon (Davis et al. 1970).

In the case of 1,2-ethanediol (ethylene glycol) (ED), the principal toxic metabolites are glyoxylic (CHOCOOH) and oxalic (HOOC-COOH) acids. The principal toxic

Table 1. Relationship of the Actute Toxicities and Chemical Structures of Derivatives of Ethane

Compound	Structure	LD$_{50}$ (Rat, oral, g/kg)[a,b]
Ethanol	CH_3CH_2OH	13.7
1,2-Ethanediol	$HOCH_2CH_2OH$	6.1
2-Aminoethanol	$H_2NCH_2CH_2OH$	2.1
2-Chloroethanol	$ClCH_2CH_2OH$	0.095
Ethylamine	$CH_3CH_2NH_2$	0.40
1,2-Diaminoethane	$H_2NCH_2CH_2NH_2$	1.16
Diethylamine	$(C_2H_5)_2NH$	0.54
Ethyleneimine	$CH_2\!-\!CH_2$ over NH (triangle)	
1,2-Dichloroethane	$Cl\!-\!CH_2\!-\!CH_2\!-\!Cl$	0.77
Ethanal	$Cl_3C\!-\!COOH$	1.93
Ethanoic acid (Acetic)	$ClCH_2COOH$	3.3-3.5
Monochloroethanoic acid (Monochloroacetic)	$CL_2CHCOOH$	0.076
Dichloroethanoic acid (Dichloroacetic)	$CL_3C\text{-}COOH$	4.5
Trichloroethanoic acid		3.3
Acetamide		30.0

[a] Spector (1956).

[b] Stecher et al. (1960).

effect of ED is renal damage. This effect has been related to the formation of oxalic acid, which in turn can form insoluble calcium oxalate salts in the renal tubules (Gessner et al. 1961; Roberts and Seibold 1969). Susceptibility to renal damage has been correlated with the degree of oxalate conversion of ED (Gessner et al. 1961).

Glyoxylic acid toxicity follows from its inhibitory effects on mitochondrial function (Bachmann and Goldberg 1971), and a decrease in liver function (e.g., following partial hepatectomy) increases glyoxylic acid toxicity (Richardson 1973).

The amino substituent in 2-aminoethanol (ethanolamine) increases toxicity more than sixfold in relation to ethanol. Again, this can be accounted for by its metabolism. This amine can be transmethylated to choline ($HOCH_2CH_2^+[CH_3]_3$) (Williams 1959), which is definitely more toxic than ethanol. In addition, toxicity can arise as a result of the effects of the competition for methyl groups by various biochemical processes. For example, many detoxification mechanisms, particularly of endogenous amines, depend on methylation reactions. Failure to detoxify these amines will result in increased amine toxicity.

As seen in Table 1, 2-chloroethanol is extremely toxic. This degree of toxicity follows from its conversion to chloroacetaldehyde (CH_2CLCHO) (Johnson 1967) and thence to monochloroacetic acid ($CH_2CLCOOH$); the latter is thought to act as a metabolic poison (Williams 1959).

$$CICH_2CH_2OH \longrightarrow CICH_2CHO \longrightarrow CICH_2COOH$$

The mechanism of toxicity of $CLCH_2COOH$ is thought to be different from 2-fluoroacetic acid (CH_2FCOOH). The latter inhibits the enzyme aconitase of the Kreb's cycle (Hayes et al. 1973), since it is converted to fluoronitrate, the actual aconitase inhibitor (Peters 1953, 1963). Monochloroacetic

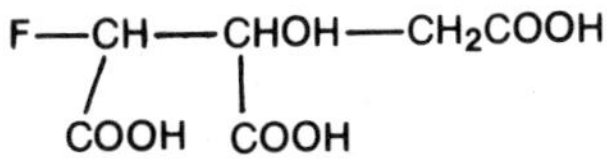

$$F-CH-CHOH-CH_2COOH$$
$$\underset{COOH}{|} \quad \underset{COOH}{|}$$

Fluorocitric acid

acid conjugates with glutathione to form S-(carboxymethyl) glutathione, and thus provokes a rapid drop in hepatic gluthathione (Johnson 1967). This could account partly for its toxicity, owing to the importance of glutathione in many biochemical processes. The extreme toxicity of monochloroacetic acid is in remarkable contrast to that of acetic, dichloroacetic, and trichloroacetic acids (Woodward et al. 1941).

$$CCl_3-COOH > CHCl_2COOH > CH_2ClCOOH > CH_3COOH$$

The inductive effects of the chlorine substituents enhance the acidity of the acids as indicated by their dissociation constants, as shown above. It follows from this fact also that their lipid solubility will decrease with increasing ionizability. Likewise, the chlorine substituents enhance the positive character of the carboxyl carbon. This would be susceptible to attack by nucleophilic reagents. However, this reaction will produce an unstable product because with the types of nucleophiles in the tissues, stabilization energy of the carbonyl group will be markedly diminished.

The chlorine atom in monochloroacetic acid is readily substituted by nucleophils. In this case, the positive character of the alpha-carbon is due to the electron-withdrawing character of the carbonyl function. The substitution of the halogens in

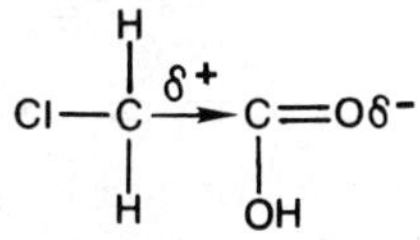

$$Cl-\underset{\underset{H}{|}}{\overset{\overset{H}{|}}{C}} \xrightarrow{\delta+} \underset{OH}{\overset{}{C}}=O\delta-$$

Monochloroacetic acid

dichloro- and trichloroacetic acids will not be as facile owing to the greater total negative inductive effects of the halogens in these acids compared to the monochloro derivative. This can more than offset the inductive effects of the carbonyl function. Therefore, the approach of a nucleophile will, in this case, be less favored so that the

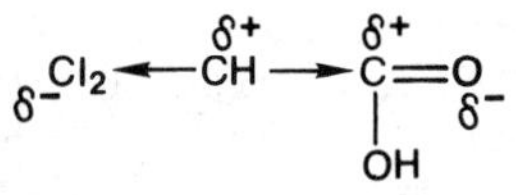

$$\delta-Cl_2 \leftarrow \overset{\delta+}{CH} \rightarrow \underset{OH}{\overset{\delta+}{C}}=\underset{\delta-}{O}$$

Chloroacetic acid

alpha-carbon atom of dichloro- and trichloroacetic acids are expected to be less reactive. These differences in reactivity, then, may largely explain why monochloroacetic acid is 59 and 43 times more toxic than dichloro and trichloro acids, respectively.

Dichloro- and tricholoroacetic acids, as strong organic acids, belong to a group of compounds known as alkaloidal reagents. These compounds bind to proteins by forming ionic bonds so that precipitation of the proteins results. Thus, in the gastrointestinal tract, these acids can react with the proteins of the gastrointestinal mucosa, so that their absorption can be markedly reduced. Thus, the differences between the degree of absorption of monochloroacetic acid and the dichloro or trichloro acids also account for the differences in toxicities.

Further examples of the effect of the nature of functional groups are seen in the case of the amines. The amino group, as in ethylamine, confers greater toxicity to the compound compared to the hydroxyl groups. This has been already seen in the case of 2-aminoethanol as compared to 1,2-ethanediol. In human subjects, ethylamine has been shown to be excreted largely unchanged (Rechenberger 1940), but a fraction of a given dose of the amine may be oxidized to acetaldehyde and ammonia (Parke 1968), both of which can contribute to the greater toxicity of ethylamine.

Substitution of a hydrogen in the second carbon by another amino group, as in 1,2-diaminoethane, reduces acute toxicity lower than that of ethylamine, but not quite approaching 2-aminoethanol. Diamines are metabolically oxidized in the presence of diamine oxidases, possibly in stepwise fashion to aminoaldehydes, and finally to di-aldehydes and ammonia (Williams 1959).

$$NH_2CH_2CH_2-NH_2 \xrightarrow{DAO} NH_2CH_2CHO \xrightarrow{DAO} OHC-CHO + NH_3$$
$$+ NH_3 \qquad\qquad Glyoxal$$

$$HOOC-COOH$$
DAO = Diamino oxidase   Oxalic acid

The bifunctional glyoxal is very reactive and will bind to proteins through cross-linking of amino groups by imine formation (Roberts and Caserio 1965). Its high re-activity is also shown by its explosive reaction with air and in the presence of water

$$Protein -NH=\overset{H}{\underset{}{C}}-\overset{H}{\underset{}{C}}=N- Protein$$

(Stecher et al. 1960). Such reactivity can be expected from its structure. It can be seen that the condensation reaction with amino groups to form an imino bond will be

$$\overset{\delta^-}{O}=\overset{\overset{H}{|}}{\underset{\delta^+}{C}}-\overset{\overset{H}{|}}{\underset{\delta^+}{C}}=\overset{\delta^-}{O}$$
Glyoxal

facilitated by the adjacent δ^+ carbons. The oral LD$_{50}$ in rats of glyoxal is 2 g/kg (Stecher et al. 1960), indicating a lower toxicity than 1,2-diaminoethane (Table 1). This is to be expected since it probably has lower GI absorption because of its re-action with the proteins of the GI mucosa. Nevertheless, it may have other toxic ef-fects, since similar compounds, e.g., malonaldehyde (OHC-CH$_2$-CHO) was shown to be carcinogenic (Chap. 12).

Diethylamine is comparable in acute toxicity to the primary amine as shown in Table 1. A significant fraction of this secondary amine is excreted unchanged in the human subjects tested (Rechenberger 1940). However, secondary amines may be de-alkylated by oxidation of the alkyl substituents (Norton 1975; Williams 1970); in this case, the ethyl group may be oxidized to acetaldehyde. Thus, it is to be expected that the toxicity of diethylamine is comparable to that of ethylamine.

$$(CH_3CH_2)_2NH \xrightarrow{\{O\}} CH_3CH_2\overset{H}{\underset{}{N}}-CH_3CH_2OH \xrightarrow{\{O\}} CH_3CH_2NH_2 + CH_3CHO$$
$$\downarrow \{O\}$$
$$CH_3CHO + NH_3$$

More importantly as a consequence of their structure, secondary amines are toxi-cologically more interesting on account of their ability to form more stable N-nitrosamine derivatives compared to primary and tertiary amines. Nitrosoamines are metabolized to alkylating species as discussed in Chap. 12.

Ethyleneimine (aziridine) in Table 1 represents a class of highly strained cyclic compounds whose extreme toxicity can be correlated to its high reactivity and alkylating ability. Note that its acute oral toxicity is about 27, 36, and 77 times greater than those of ethylamine, diethylamine, and 1,2-diaminoethane, respectively. The high reactivity of this amine stems from its highly strained three-membered configuration. In vivo, this compound is transformed into an immonium ion by gaining a proton. This electrophil can attack strong nucleophilic centers such as the N-7 of guanine of nucleic acids:

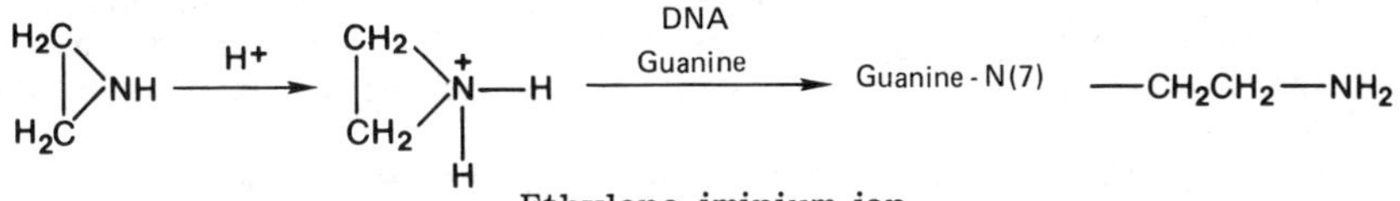

Ethylene-iminium ion

This position of guanine appears to be highly favored by many alkylating agents (Brookes and Lawley 1961; Colburn and Boutwell 1968; Lawley et al. 1974; Swann and Magee 1968).

The effectiveness of the aziridines as oncogenic agents appears to be increased by the substitution of the hydrogen on the nitrogen by an alkyl, acyl, or certain aromatic substituents (Walpole et al. 1954). Several other highly strained cyclic compounds are also very reactive, and thus are highly toxic. Among these are the various cyclic ethers, also known as oxiranes or epoxides. The simplest compound among these is ethylene oxide

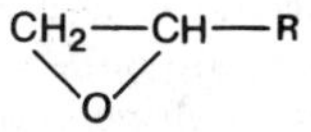

Monofunctional epoxide

(R=H in the above formula), which is an irritating, toxic gas. Other monofunctional epoxides are similarly highly toxic. A number are carcinogens and mutagens (Lawley 1976). The carcinogenic monofunctional epoxides have substituents (R in the above formula) which may be an aromatic amine derivative, a phenyl, a glycidyl ester of fatty acids, an aldehyde, methyl groups, or another epoxide ring system (Lawley, 1976; Van Duuren et al. 1963, 1966; Walpole 1958).

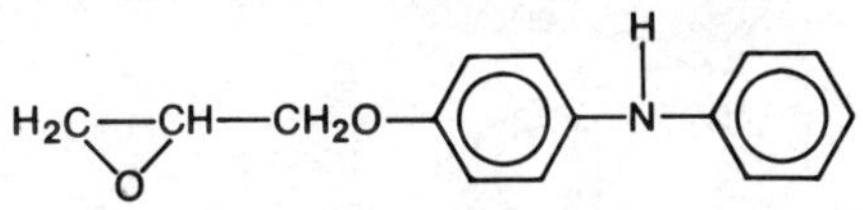

p-Hydroxydiphenylamineglycidyl ether

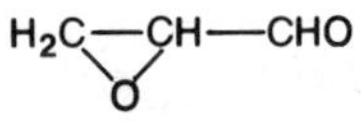

Glycidaldehyde

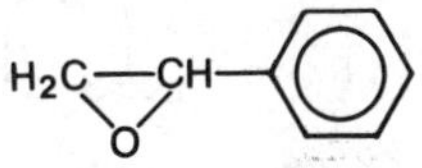

Styrene oxide

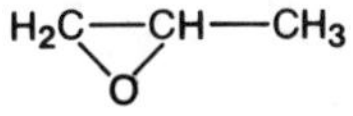

Propylene oxide

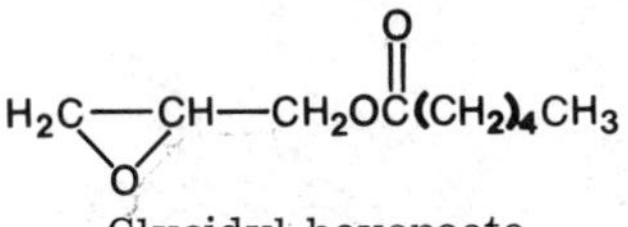

Glycidyl hexanoate

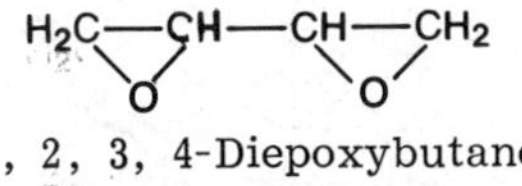

1, 2, 3, 4-Diepoxybutane

These substituents may modify the reactivity or enhance lipid solubility in the case of hydrophobic groups. Indeed, all the above compounds can be expected to have greater lipid solubility than the simpler epoxides. The opening of the ring occurs readily under mild conditions. The initial reaction is protonation of the oxygen, followed by the formation of a carbonium ion intermediate and then a nucleophilic attack on the secondary carbon. The alkylation reaction is a unimolecular nucleophilic substitution (S_N1).

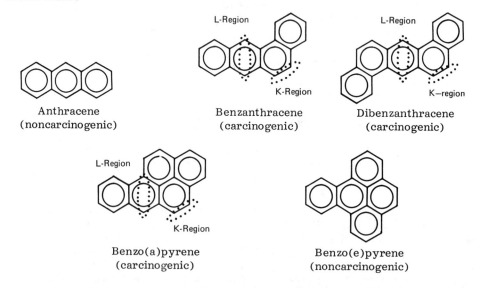

Where Nu = nucleophilic substituent

The electrophilicity of the intermediate will obviously be modified by the inductive effect of R. An electron-attracting group, such as carbonyl, halogen, methoxyl, and similar nitrogen or oxygen groups will enhance the positive character of the carbonium ion. Electron-donating groups, such as alkyl groups, will obviously have the opposite effects.

Many carcinogenic compounds are metabolically activated by epoxidation. Examples of these are the polycyclic aromatic hydrocarbons and aflatoxins. These types of activation by epoxidation are discussed in Chapter 6. The effect of this epoxidation is the formation of alkylating agents. As shown in Chapter 6, many other types of carcinogens are metabolically activated to form highly reactive alkylating agents.

However, the formation of such alkylating intermediates does not necessarily confer carcinogenicity and similar biological activity (e.g., mutagenicity). Certain structural features must be fulfilled for compounds to possess such activities. This is exemplified by the polycyclic aromatic hydrocarbons (Dipple 1976).

This group of compounds has been more intensively studied than any other class regarding the relationship between chemical structure and carcinogenic activity (Arcos and Argus 1968; Bergmann and Pullman 1969; Coulson 1953; Dipple 1976; Herndon 1974; Jones and Matthews 1974; Miller and Miller 1963; Pullman and Pullman 1955). However, the mechanisms underlying such relationships are only partially understood, consequently, so far, no acceptable generalized expression of this relationship has been proposed to encompass all classes of polycyclic aromatic hydrocarbons (PAH). This is perhaps to be expected because of the many different types of compounds of varying complexities as well as the lack of a clear understanding of the mechanism of carcinogenesis.

Nevertheless, the connection between structure and carcinogenicity is seen in many classes of PAH. Among these classes of compounds are the various derivatives of anthracene. The structures of some of the principal compounds in this group are shown below:

Anthracene
(noncarcinogenic)

Benzanthracene
(carcinogenic)

Dibenzanthracene
(carcinogenic)

Benzo(a)pyrene
(carcinogenic)

Benzo(e)pyrene
(noncarcinogenic)

In the preceding structures, anthracene is noncarcinogenic. Addition of a benzene ring at a specific strategic position confers some carcinogenicity. We see this in benz-(a)anthracene, a weak carcinogen. However, carcinogenicity is markedly enhanced when a fifth benzene ring is added at some other strategic positions, as in dibenz-(a,h)anthracene and benzo(a)pyrene, but not in benzo(e)pyrene (Dipple 1976). Similarly, electron-donating or withdrawing substituents can affect carcinogenicity depending on the position. Thus, methyl substitution in benz(a)anthracene at the 6, 7, 8, or 12 position produces high activity, but at the 1, 2, 3, 4, 5, 9, 10, or 11 position inactive or slightly active compounds are obtained. But many of these substituents, particularly electron-withdrawing groups (e.g., -OH, NO_2, -Cl, -COCl, $-CH_2Cl$), at position 7 also result in inactive or slightly or moderately active compounds. Thus, the precise effects of substitutents in these positions are not immediately evident as there is a lack of consistency in this respect (Dipple 1976).

With respect to the dimethyl substitutions in benz(a)anthracene, the location of these groups at strategic positions can either result in inactivated or greatly activated derivatives. Thus, inactive compounds are produced when the pair of methyl groups are located, for example, at positions 1.7; 1,12; 2,9; 2,10; 3,9; 3,10; 12,4; 12,5; 4,7; or 8,11. Highly active derivatives are produced when the pair of methyls are located at positions 7,12; 7,11; 7,6; 7,8; 12,6; 12,8; 4,5; or 8,9.

In order to correlate carcinogenic activity with chemical structure, such as the relationships shown above, several hypotheses were proposed (Coulson 1953; Dipple 1976). One of these is that proposed by Pullman (1945). This hypothesis proposes to explain carcinogenic activity in terms of the chemical reactivity of the so-called K- and L-regions in the molecule. In the case of benz(a)anthracene, these positions are bound by carbons 5 and 6, and 7 and 12, respectively, as indicated in the preceding structures. The hypothesis specifies that carcinogenic potency is a function of the reactivity of the K-region (which is related to the total charge of the region; i.e., the pi electron density) provided the L-region is unreactive (Pullman 1954; Pullman and Pullman 1955). Thus, if the two carbons of the L-region are substituted with methyl groups, as in 7.12-dimethylbenz(a)anthracene, the carcinogenic potency is increased.

The K- and L-region hypothesis appears to apply in many cases (Flurry 1964; Mainster and Memory 1967; Scribner 1969), but there are also many exceptions. For example, substitution of ethyl groups on carbons 7 and 12 results in inactivation (Pataki et al. 1971). Whereas the replacement of $-CH_3$ on carbon-7, with $-CH_2OH$ does not inactivate the compound (Flesher and Sydnor 1971), the more bulky $-CH_2-CH_2-OH$ results in inactivation (Pataki and Huggins 1967). The hypothesis also does not seem to apply to carcinogenic compounds like dibenz[a,c]anthracene, which according to the hypothesis will be inactive. It cannot account for the fact that substituents on benz(a)-anthracene,

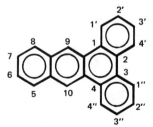

Dibenz{a,c}anthracene
(1,2:3,4-Dibenzanthracene)

like $-CH_2OH$ on carbon-12 and a $-CH_3$ group on carbon-7, results in inactivation (Boyland et al. 1965), but not when these groups are located in the reverse positions (Flesher and Sydnor 1971).

It is evident that the complexities of the structure-carcinogenic activity relationship cannot be satisfactorily explained by Pullman's (1945) hypothesis, but it is obvious that certain structural features of these hydrocarbons determine their activity. In this connection, it is certainly true that these structural features have profound influences on the metabolitic transformation of these compounds and subsequent reaction of these metabolites with critical molecular groups in the cells—reactions which are mandatory for carcinogenic initiation.

Another class of compounds that provides an interesting study regarding the relationship of structure and toxicity is the alkaloids. Many types of alkaloids are found in foods (Concon 1977), and several are discussed throughout this book. The structures of these compounds vary in complexity and all involve a characteristic nitrogen atom. Although the term alkaloid implies a basic property, this is not true in many cases. Many alkaloids contain heterocyclic rings involving the nitrogen; all such compounds whose biological activities have been studied possess high toxicity. However, heterocyclic involvement of the nitrogen is not a prerequisite for biological activity.

For many types of alkaloids, however, biological activity can be related to the similarity of their structures to endogenous compound of animal tissues. For example, the neurological activity of muscarine (Chap. 10) can be related to the similarity of its structure to acetylcholine, an important neurotransmitter.

Muscarine   Acetylcholine

Muscarine is toxic because it can mimic the function of acetylcholine and resist enzymatic degradation longer than acetylcholine (Chap. 10)

Many other alkaloids have central nervous system (CNS) effects because of the similarity of their structures to various neurotransmitters. For example, psilocybin and similar indole alkaloids structurally resemble serotonin (see structures in Chap. 10, p. 000). Amphetamines and mescaline, both potent neurological poisons resemble norepinephrine or epinephrine.

Amphetamine   Mescaline

Norepinephrine   Epinephrine

Note that above physiological levels, both norepinephrine and epinephrine are highly toxic and safeguards against dangerous accumulations are provided by the monoamine oxidases, and possibly by some nonenzymatic process (Montgomery et al. 1974). Unlike norepinephrine and epinephrine, amphetamine (Beckett 1969; Dring et al. 1966) and mescaline (Charalampous et al. 1964) are oxidized only to a lesser extent. Most are excreted unchanged in humans.

Another classic example of the relationship between structure and toxicity is that seen in the organophosphate insecticides. In this group of chemically interesting compounds are the phosphorothionates and their oxygenated analogs, which are represented by the general formulas:

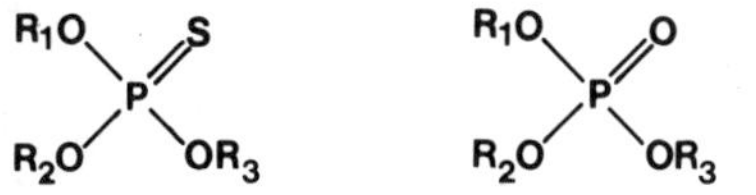

Alkyl (or aryl)   Alkyl (or aryl)
phosphorothionate   phosphonate

Where R_1 and R_2 represent either alkyl, aryl, or amino groups. R_3 represents various displaceable groups.

These compounds are acetylcholinesterase inhibitors by phosphorylation of serine at the active center of the enzyme (Aldridge 1971; O'Brien 1969A). Even though these insecticides have other effects, this inhibitory action is essential to their toxicity (DuBois 1971; Durham and Hayes 1962).

The reactivity of these compounds, and thus their toxicity, is influenced by their structures. Thus, substitution of the sulfur in the above structure with oxygen by oxidation greatly increases the toxicity. For example, in vivo, parathion is desulfurated to the more toxic paraoxon.

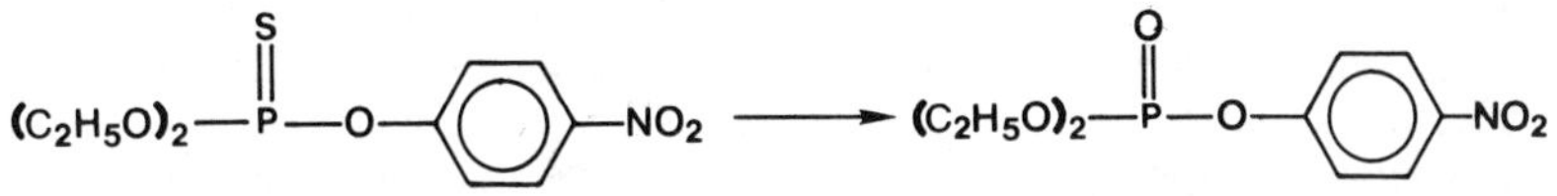

Parathion   Paraoxon

Oxygen is more electronegative than sulfur, so that the phosphorus atom in paraoxon is more electrophilic than in parathion. Therefore, reaction with the nucleophilic esteratic site of acetylcholine esterase can occur more readily, and the alkyl(aryl) phosphate group will be more firmly bound. Furthermore, the thionophosphoryl group (P=S), compared to the oxophosphoryl group (P=O), lends greater stability to the compound against nonenzymatic hydrolysis which may occur before the insecticide reaches the target sites.

The magnitude of the toxicity of many organophosphate insecticides is also a function of their lipid solubility (Reiffe et al. 1971). For example, tetraethylpyrophosphate (TEPP) (Reiffe et al. 1971) and Schradan (DuBois et al. 1953; Frawley et al. 1952) have low lipid/water partition coefficient so that poisoning of the nerve axon or the CNS are unaffected.

The duration or intensity of toxic effects of these insecticides is also influenced by the rate the phosphate-serine bond in the inhibited enzyme is hydrolyzed. The rate of hydrolysis is also a function of the structure. In the case of the dialkyl phosphates, the rate of hydrolysis decreases according to the following order: $(CH_3O)_2 - > (C_2H_5O)_2 - > (C_3H_7O)_2 - > iso - (C_3H_7O)_2 -$. In other words, the stability of the enzyme-inhibitor complex increases with the degree of steric hindrance (Blaber and Crasey 1960; Burgen and Hobbiger 1951; Friedman et al. 1949; Hobbiger 1951).

Isomerism is also an important aspect of the structure-toxicity relationship. This is exemplified by the various isomers of hexachlorocyclohexane (HCH). There are eight possible isomers. The most toxic is the γ isomer or lindane (LD_{50} = 125–200 mg/kg rat oral) (Spector 1956). Reportedly, both the ε and η isomers are inactive. The α and γ isomers are convulsants, whereas the β and δ isomers are CNS depressants (O'Brien 1967). The α and γ isomers are more rapidly metabolized; the β-isomers appear to remain in the tissues much longer, accounting for 90% of the total residue of the total HCH residue in human tissues (Abbott et al. 1968; Egan et al. 1965;

Hays 1966). The mechanism for these differences in toxic effects is not known, but as
O'Brien (1967) suggested, these differences may be due to the stereochemical relationships between the various HCH isomers and the specific target sites or molecules in
the nervous system. In other words, the activity of each isomer depends on how well
the molecules bind or fit into the target sites.

Numerous other examples can be cited with respect to the relationships of toxicity
and chemical structures. In succeeding chapters, examples of these relationships can
be deduced from the activities of various compounds.

The preceding examples illustrate very well the significance of chemical structure
in determining toxicity. Recently, statistical models based on published data have
been devised in order to predict specific toxicity endpoints (e.g., acute toxicities,
carcinogenicity) of untested compounds. Parameters used in this prediction include
the structural features of specific molecules, molecular weights, and so forth (Enslein and Craig 1979, 1978). Using a carcinogenesis statistical model Enslein (1979) predicted that piperine, the main alkaloid of black pepper (Chap. 8), has a very high
probability of being a carcinogen. Preliminary data suggest that piperine may indeed
be a strong carcinogen (Concon et al. 1981).

Dose

The Latin expression *dosis sola facit venenum* (the dose makes the poison), attributable to the ancient Romans, is a fundamental principle in classic toxicology. When the
dose is related to the response, this principle applies to all types of toxicants. A cor-
ollary to this principle is that expressed by the microbiologist Emil Mrak of the Commission on Pesticides: "There are no harmless substances, there are only harmless
ways of using substances." One of these ways is the amount of substance to which one
is exposed. For many types of substances, a toxicological spectrum can be constructed
showing the transition of the biological effects as a function of dose. There are two
types of substances based on the transition of the types of biological effects on the
host with increasing dose:

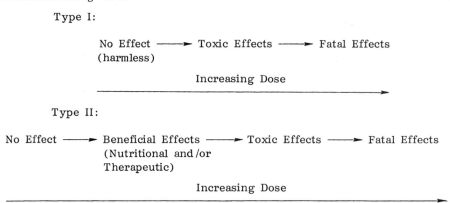

Type II may be subdivided into three types, of which the beneficial effects are (1)
only nutritional; (2) only therapeutic; and (3) nutritional and therapeutic, for which
there may be a transition from the nutritional to the therapeutic effects with increasing dose. The first and third types are clearly limited to that group of compounds
which comprises the nutrients. The second type consists primarily of the various
drugs, medicines, and antibiotics in the medical armamentarium as well as many nonnutritive compounds present in foodstuffs (e.g., various xanthines — caffeine, theobromine, theophylline).

Type I consists primarily of most types of toxicants, as classified in the foregoing
section. These compounds, which clearly present no known beneficial effects, are the
focus of this book.

For a specific substance, the dose at which a particular effect may be observed will depend on the particular subject; there is a certain threshold for that subject above which a beneficial or deleterious effect may be detected. This threshold may differ from one group of subjects to another. In addition, the threshold can also be influenced by several other factors, as we shall see later. However, the level of a chemical to which a given population is exposed may be increased until an increasing number of individuals will show one or more deleterious responses. A dose will be attained above which all subjects will respond with varying degrees of severity. Finally, there is a dose lethal to all subjects.

Lethal Dose Toxicologists have used the LD_{50} (lethal dose$_{50}$) to characterize the toxic potency of a compound. This is defined as that dose which produces a 50% mortality in a given test population. This term is useful insofar as it gives an indication of the magnitude of the toxicity of one compound compared to another. Other criteria may be used to define the toxicity of a compound. Thus, if tumor production is sought, a TD_{50} (tumor dose$_{50}$) can similarly be defined. The significance of these indices with respect to different groups may be subject to considerable uncertainty, since here again, various factors can modify various toxicological responses.

For a given large population, the responses to a given dose of a particular compound may follow a normal distribution pattern (Gaussian). This immediately presents difficulty in predicting the response of a specific individual, since response to a given dose may be unique and fall anywhere along the normal dis tribution curve, or even outside it.

Experimentally, a dose-response curve may be plotted, using any one of toxic symptoms elicited by a chemical compound. Examples of dose-response curves based on lethality are shown in Figure 1A – C. Several properties of these curves are immediately apparent. Note that in Figure 1A, several compounds share the same 50% lethality, yet each compound is not equally toxic. Some compounds shown a 100% lethality at a much lower dose than others. This fact is probably indicated by the slopes of each curve. Thus, the magnitude of the slope reveals how quickly a particular compound may attain toxic levels.

No Effect Dose Of great public health interest is the no effect dose (NED) or level (NEL), the points where the curves in Figures 1A – C bisect the abscissa. In Figure 1A the compounds are shown to have equal LD_{50}s but different NEDs. There are also compounds with equal NEDs but different LD_{50}s, as shown in Figure 1B. Figure 1C shows the dose-response curves of compounds which have different NEDs and LD_{50}s. Thus, LD_{50} alone is a poor indication of the toxicity of a compound. Perhaps a two-point index which indicates both the NED and the LD_{50} will be more meaningful. Obviously, such an index will need more refinement as our knowledge of the toxicological properties of compounds becomes more definite.

The NED shows more appropriately the safety of a compound than any other index. However for many compounds, the determination of such a value is replete with difficulties. Foremost among these is the time factor involved in the production of specific toxic responses (p. 33). Whereas some compounds may produce immediate effects, others have delayed responses. Some of these compounds, such as the carcinogens, have long "latency" periods lasting several months or, in the case of humans, years. The NED for a particular compound also may vary from one subject to another, within or between species. This difficulty is magnified considerably when translating the observed effects in animals to man.

It should be borne in mind that a NED may apply only to a specific response in an acute test and may not reflect the highly delayed effects. It is in the delayed effects that the problem regarding the NED becomes difficult to resolve, especially if extremely small amounts of a compound are adequate to produce a toxic effect. Examples of such very low dose levels that are effective may be cited. A diet containing as low as 1 ppb of aflatoxin fed to Fischer rats over a lifetime was sufficient to induce cancer in

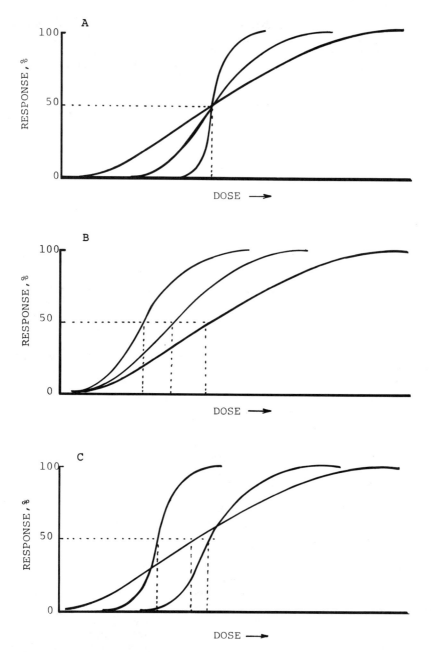

Figure 1   A, dose-response curves representing three compounds with the same LD_{50} but different no-effect doses and LD_{100}. B, Dose-response curves representing three compounds with different LD_{50} but the same no-effect dose. C, Dose-response curves representing three compounds with different LD_{50}, LD_{100} and no-effect doses.

some animals as compared to controls which did not [Wogan et al. 1974]. In mice, a NED of 4 µg was found for the carcinogen 3-methylcholanthrene [Bryan and Shimkin 1943]. Similarly, for butter yellow (dimethylaminoazobenzene), the NED for the rats is 0.3 mg per day [Druckrey 1959]. If these extremely low levels are effective in animals, are they also effective at such levels in humans, or should they be lower or higher? There are no satisfactory methods to answer these questions experimentally.

The variability of the NED for a particular compound is illustrated by aflatoxin carcinogenesis. Thus, whereas in one study as cited above, 1 ppb resulted in the production of tumors, in another, as high as 80 ppb did not [Alfin-Slater et al. 1969]. The difference here may be explained by the strain of rat used and the nature of the diet as well as the number of animals tested. Thus, in the case of the latter study, 10 animals were used against 22 animals in the former. Critics to the NED concept with regard to the carcinogens contend that the NED obtained from a few animals is not sufficient to establish the value for 100,000 or 1 million individuals, assuming such values can be extrapolated to man. The uncertainty of the NED has led to the establishment of the zero tolerance for chemical carcinogens (National Cancer Institute 1971).

Other indexes were proposed, apparently attempting to arrive at some more appropriate approach to a safe dose for man. Mantel and Bryan (1961) suggested what they called the virtually safe dose (VSD) for such carcinogens as 3-methylcholanthrene. This is the exposure level which will produce only one tumor in 100 million persons. The VSD is obtained by means of a probit curve utilizing a 99% confidence limit. For methylcholanthrene, the VSD on this basis for the mouse is 9×10^{-5} µg or 90 pg. An even more stringent safety index was proposed by Schneiderman (1970), who used a one-particle curve to arrive at an acceptable risk dose (ARD). This is equivalent to an exposure level which will produce only one tumor in 100,000 persons. A safety factor of 1×10^{-6} was suggested when applying to man the ARD value from animal tests to allow for species differences, interaction with other carcinogens, and possible error in extrapolating animal weight or surface area to that of man. The ARD of Schneiderman (1970) is 0.33×10^{-7} of the VSD of Mantel and Bryan (1961) when applied to 3-methylcholanthrene, or 3.2×10^{-6} pg. The Food and Drug Administration (FDA) (1973) proposed a simpler method for determining the socially acceptable dose (SAD). This value is obtained by linear extrapolation from the observable range from animal studies to the 1 tumor/100 million people risk dose by changing the slope in the lower part of the curve somewhat to allow for sampling errors.

None of the above indexes has any valid scientific basis. In the long run, all the proposed indexes are variations of the zero tolerance, and may not be easy to justify. For example, Claus et al. (1974) calculated that the VSD of Mantel and Bryan is equivalent to an exposure level of one molecule of 3-methylcholanthrene per 700 of the approximately 140 trillion cells in an average human body. The same VSD dose, if confined exclusively to the human liver, would be equivalent to two molecules of 3-methylcholanthrene per five of the approximately 500 billion human liver cells. With the same carcinogen, Schneiderman's ARD is equivalent to one molecule per 20 billion human body cells, or one molecule per 25 liver cells; and for the FDAs SAD, one molecule per 16 human body cells, or 175 molecules per 10 liver cells.

It might be asked, how many molecules entering a cell are sufficient to initiate carcinogenesis or any toxic episode? Dinman (1972) and Hutchinson (1964) agree that no biological activity for any single substance can occur in a single cell below 10,000 molecules. From various considerations, the threshold value for many substances is above 10,000 molecules [Claus et al. 1974]. Many target-specific substances may require less in terms of total body cells. When considered only in relation to their target cells, these substances will require for biological activity a number of molecules well above 10,000. For example, 2 µg or 8×10^{12} molecules of the botulinum exotoxin (mol. wt. = 150,000) [Das Gupta et al. 1970] are sufficient to produce lethal effects in man [Lamanna 1959]. When considered in terms of total body cells, this toxic dose is less than the 10^4-molecule threshold. This value is exceeded when the dose is based on the specific target of the poison, the neuromuscular junctions.

This threshold of 10^4 molecules appears reasonable in view of the many interferences within the cell. At any rate, poisoning is a physicochemical reaction and the rate of reaction is rightly dependent on the concentration of reactants.

There are also other factors to consider with respect to the NED of food toxicants. One is the interaction with other components in the food which could lead to large diminution of the amounts absorbed. Another is the intestinal barrier which may exclude many substances from being absorbed. Factors in the blood, such as proteins and lipids, may also bind these toxicants, further reducing their effectiveness. Compartmentalization within the cell with membrane barrier is another. Finally, there are competing metabolic reactions and excretory and storage mechanisms which tend to diminish the biological activity of toxic compounds. However, a major task lies ahead of the toxicologist in the identification and quantification of the various factors that tend to reduce the toxicity of compounds.

It may be valid to speak of NED or threshold when referring to acute effects or other toxicological endpoints for which the mechanism of action is known. But as Brown (1976) has stated, it will be fruitless to attempt to determine the NED for substances such as carcinogens for which the mechanism is still unclear. Furthermore, multiple exposures to carcinogens of various types and promoting agents (Chap. 6) are probably the norm rather than the exception. Thus, any additional introduction of carcinogens in the body, no matter how small, will only serve to increase the probability of cancer induction. There are, of course, substances that are carcinogenesis inhibitors which further complicate the issue. Many other factors affect this process (Chaps. 6 and 7), so thus predicting the existence of a NED or the minimum effective dose for the human population will be impossible.

Therefore, in view of the impossibility of determining such a threshold, a zerc tolerance level has been established for carcinogens in the food supply in the United States and elsewhere (Chaps. 18 and 19). This zero threshold was affirmed by the National Cancer Institute (1971). Its Ad Hoc Committee on the Evaluation of Low Levels of Environmental Chemical Carcinogens concluded:

> It is impossible to establish any absolutely safe level of exposure to a carcinogen for man. The concept of "toxicologically insignificant" levels (as advanced by the Food Protection Committee of the NAS/NRC in 1959), of dubious merit in any life science, has *absolutely no validity in the field of carcinogenesis* [author's italics]. Society must be willing to accept some finite risk as the price of using any carcinogenic material in whatever quantity. The best that science can do is to estimate the upper probable limit of that risk. For this reason, the concept of safe level for man, as applied to carcinogenic agents should be replaced by that of a socially acceptable risk.

Zero threshold is, of course, only a theoretical concept dependent on the sensitivity of analytical methods used in detecting carcinogenic residues. Thus, for practical and regulatory purposes, this concept is replaced by an operational or practical zero which logically is equivalent to the legal requirement of "no residue" of the carcinogenic compound used in food. This practical zero, as set by the FDA, is consistent with the acceptable dose that would present a degree of lifetime risk equivalent to one in one million persons — a risk which is believed not to increase significantly the human risk for cancer; in other words, below this value, no further protection from cancer can be realized. This risk is also consistent with the acceptable level of risk for other substances already considered safe [Food and Drug Administration 1979].

The determination of the concentration of carcinogenic residue equivalent to this risk level is based on linear extrapolation of the dose-response curve obtained in animal tests. Response in this case is the tumor incidence; i.e., the percent of animals

having tumors. Comparisons between the results of animal tests and human epidemiological studies for a few carcinogens have indicated that the lifetime human cancer
incidence from chronic exposure to these carcinogens can be acceptably approximated
with the lifetime cancer incidence in similarly exposed experimental animals [Mantel and
Schniderman 1975; Saffiotti 1978].

From statistical consideration, a zero response in a limited number of experimental
animals at a certain dose level is not actually zero. For an experimental population of
N subjects, a zero response is consistent at the 5% significance level. This means that
there is a probability that the response is actually between zero and 3/N [Brown
1976]. The smaller the total number of experimental animals, the higher the number of
animals that will probably give a positive response if the test were repeated a number
of times. Thus, if 50 animals were used, a zero response at the 5% significance level
may actually mean a response between 0 and 6%. Thus, to obtain a value approaching
the actual zero, a large number of animals needs to be used.

Frequency of Exposure

The frequency of exposure factor is related to the dose. It should be stated that for
some toxicants such as carcinogens, a single exposure may be all that is necessary for
cancer induction. Nevertheless, some carcinogens are more effective with multiple exposure at smaller doses over a long period of time. This is particularly true with the
potent carcinogens, the nitrosamines [Lijinsky 1976].

Multiple exposure ensures continued toxic insult, which may have cumulative
effects. Multiple exposures, therefore, result in a relatively large total dose. This
situation is encountered in actual life; human beings are continuously exposed to deleterious substances over their lifetime.

Therefore, any assessment of safety of a food substance must consider the probability of multiple exposure.

Route of Exposure

The toxicity of a compound differs with the route of exposure. A few examples of these
differences in toxicity are shown in Table 2.

Note that with few exceptions the oral route renders the compound less toxic.
Except for DDT, the parenteral route makes the compounds more toxic. Exceptions are
those compounds which are transformed and activated in the GI tract by digestive and
other tissue enzymes or by intestinal bacteria. Examples of compounds activated by
intestinal bacteria are cycasin and the cyanogenic glycosides (Chaps. 3 and 8).

There are, of course, several reasons why the oral route renders most compounds
less toxic. Among these are the possible decreased rate of absorption; proximity to
the liver, so that biotransformation-detoxication can take place before the compound is
distributed throughout the body; action of digestive and other enzymes of the GI mucosa; action of intestinal bacteria; and interaction and dilution with GI content (i.e.,
digesta and intestinal secretions). As discussed in Chapter 2, the GI tract provides a
formidable barrier to the absorption of many toxicants. In additon, in spite of the
large surface area, many compounds that depend on the passive absorption process
may be absorbed only very slowly. Gradual absorption ensures that the toxicant
reaches the target tissues in smaller amounts such that to a large degree the law of
mass action influences the degree of toxic injury. In other words, the amounts of toxicants reaching the target site may be insufficient to cause toxic injury and there are
no cumulative effects.

Dietary Factors

A distinction should be made between (1) dietary factors which interact with toxicants
so as to modify their toxic properties or interfere in their absorption, and (2) those

Table 2. Differences of Toxicities of Compounds as a Function of Route of Exposure

| Toxicant | Animal | Parameter | LD_{50} (mg/kg body weight) | | | |
			Oral	s.c.	i.v.	i.p.
KCN	Rat	MLD	10-15	17	2.5	
Sodium salicylate	Mouse	LD_{50}	900	520		
	Rat		1600	650		
Caffeine	Rat	LD_{50}	233 ± 14		104.8 ± 1.87	
$NaNO_2$	Dog	MLD	330	50-70		
Myristicin	Cat	LD	570	4000^a		
Malathion	Rat	LD_{50}	1400		50	750
Furfural	Dog	LD	2318		166	
Formaldehyde	Rat	LD_{50}	800	420		
Ethanol	Rat	LD_{50}	13,000			5000
	Mouse	LD_{50}	9488	8285	1973	
DDT	Rat	LD_{50}	200-800	1500	40-50	

Abbreviations: s.c., subcutaneous; i.v., intravenous; i.p., intraperitoneal; MLD, minimum lethal dose; LD, lethal dose.

[a]Compound suspended in gum acacia solution.
Source: Spector (1956).

factors which change the nutritional state of the host. The latter factors may not have any effect on the toxicological property of the compound until the nutritional status of the host is sufficiently changed. Examples of the first type are long chain fatty acids of the diet which render many toxic metals less absorbable by forming metallic soaps. Phosphates and similar ions may form insoluble salts. Sugars and other carbonyls may react with amines and amino acids by the Amadori reaction, resulting in less absorbable complexes (Chap. 21). Ascorbic acid may prevent the nitrosation reaction in the GI tract (Chaps. 7 and 12).

Dietary factors may delay, prevent, or enhance absorption. For example, fats may enhance or delay absorption of fat soluble compounds. Because fats are emptied slowly into the small intestines, toxic substances dissolved in fat may be absorbed more slowly. Similarly, acids will also delay gastric emptying [Hunt and Knox 1961]. Acids may also alter the stability or promote chemical changes (e.g., hydrolysis) of specific compounds. Food additives such as ethylenediamine tetraacetic acid (EDTA) may increase the absorption of many types of compounds by chelation and other non-specific effects (Levine and Pelikan 1964). Those toxicants which share an active transport system with vital nutrients or other biological compounds may be displaced, and are therefore prevented from being absorbed by their nutritive competitor. For example, calcium may interfere in the absorption of lead [Sobel et al. 1938]; or iron in the absorption of thallium [Leopold et al. 1969]. Many more examples can be cited.

Other Exogenous Factors

Other factors, such as light, environmental temperature, and atmospheric pressure, may affect compound toxicity. The effect of light is seen in the case of photodynamic action (p. 30).

The effects of temperature [Cremer and Blight 1969; Doull 1972; Weihe 1973] and pressure [Doull 1972] are well known to pharmacologists. For example, cold exposure increases the toxicity of the insecticides malathion and Sarin; on the other hand, hyperthermia increases the effects of parathion. These effects may be related to the influence of external temperature on various physiological processes, such as excretory processes and blood flow.

Temperature may also influence gastric emptying. For example, it was shown in experiments in rats and dogs [Erni and Ritschel 1977; Gorisch 1967] and humans [James 1957; Ritschel and Erni 1977] that cold solutions are emptied more quickly into the intestines than warm solutions. Therefore, the absorption of cold solutions of toxicants will occur more rapidly, and thus will become more toxic. This effect was observed in the case of various cold, as contrasted to warm, liquids [Erni and Ritschel 1977; Gorisch 1967] and meals [James 1957], and insoluble capsules administered with water at 4 to 45°C [Ritschel and Erni 1977].

The effect of atmospheric pressure on the toxicity of compounds was observed in rats. For example, Doull (1972) reported that psychoactive drugs were less toxic when rats were exposed to reduced atmospheric pressure even though the oxygen partial pressure was normal.

Endogenous Factors

Because toxic reactions are initiated at the molecular level, biochemical and physiological variability explain the differences in response among individuals to toxic substances. Genetics, age, sex, immune competence, and the nutritional and physiological states have significant effects on the toxic response. Furthermore, the ability of the body to metabolize foreign compounds certainly determines to a large extent the toxicity of compounds. These factors are discussed in Chapter 4. Chapter 6 also examines the influence of these factors on carcinogenesis. Chapter 7 considers the effect of nutritonal factors and status on carcinogenesis.

The biochemistry, physiology, histology, and morphology of the gastrointestinal tract regulate the toxicity of most compounds. For ingested compounds, this organ system is the first protective mechanism against toxic injury. This aspect is discussed in Chapter 2.

Intestinal bacteria also play a significant role in regulating the toxicological potentials of many compounds. Their activities can diminish or exacerbate the toxicity of various compounds (Chap. 3).

In the following sections, other physiological factors which can influence toxic injury are discussed.

Binding of Toxicants to Plasma Proteins and Tissues

Plasma proteins and certain tissues are known to bind effectively many types of toxicants. Obviously, the binding of toxicants in these cases affects the toxic response of the host by modifying the effective dose. Toxic compounds have different affinities to plasma proteins [Goldstein et al 1968], and their displacement from plasma proteins by compounds with greater affinity for them will obviously increase the effective dose and consequently their toxicity [Davidson 1971]. An example of this phenomenon is the displacement of bilirubin from plasma albumin by DDE (dichlorodiphenyldichloroethylene) and certain drugs [Schoor 1973; Silverman et al. 1956]. The free bilirubin becomes more toxic to neonates, since a larger dose of this toxic substance can diffuse into the brain. The resulting disease syndrome, kernicterus, can produce a severe form of brain damage [Silverman et al. 1956].

Many compounds have a propensity for binding in specific tissues, such as adipose tissues, bone, kidney, and liver.

Binding of fat-soluble toxicants obviously takes place very readily in adipose tissues. Thus various pesticides, such as DDT and its metabolites, have been found to accumulate in these tissues (Wooley and Talens 1971; Chaps. 4 and 18). Clearly, toxicants that are so deposited will have diminished effects, at least in their acute effects. However, when these compounds eventually are released into the blood, increased toxicity may be expected.

Heavy metals such as lead and cadmium may be bound in the bones, and therefore may have diminished toxic effects (Chaps. 5 and 18). However, greater toxicity may result when the accumulated toxic metal is released in larger amounts into the bloodstream.

Similarly, the liver has a great ability to bind foreign compounds so that their concentrations in the blood are diminished rapidly. A liver protein known as *ligandin* has been observed to bind many organic compounds; e.g., organic acids or other anions [Levi et al. 1969], azo dyes, steroids, bilirubin, and other compounds [Litwack et al. 1971]. The liver also has the ability to bind toxic heavy metals such as lead [Klaassen and Shoemann 1972].

This affinity of the liver for foreign compounds is consistent with its primary role in the process of biotransformation of these compounds. This affinity also explains in part why the liver is highly vulnerable to toxic injury from many compounds.

The kidneys are also efficient in binding certain types of toxicants. For example, these organs tend to accumulate cadmium (Chap. 18). Indeed, a cadmium-binding protein has been isolated from the kidneys [Margoshes and Vallee 1957].

Membrane Barrier

The tissues also may be protected from toxic injury by the so-called membrane barrier. This barrier appears to function similarly to that in the gastrointestinal tract. The barrier to the brain known as the blood-brain barrier excludes many toxicants more effectively than other tissues; nevertheless, many toxic compounds can pass through this barrier. Its effectiveness varies in different areas of the brain. For example, the lateral nuclei of the hypothalamus and the area postrema, the posterior lobe of the pituitary gland, and the cortex have greater permeability than other areas [Goldstein et al. 1968]. Thus some of these areas are more easily subject to toxic injury. Brain damage as a result of exposure to high levels of glutamate or aspartate occurs predominantly in some of these areas (Chap. 21).

The blood-brain barrier in the newborn [Pentschew and Garro 1966] is less developed than that of adults. Therefore, as demonstrated in rats, toxicants can be more damaging to the neonates than to the adules [Kupferberg and Way 1963; Pentschew and Garrow 1966]. For example, the glutamate damage mentioned above occurs more readily and severely in neonates.

The so-called placental barrier also operates by the law of membrane diffusion, as in the case of the gastrointestinal tract (Chap. 2). Therefore, many essential substances pass this barrier by active transport [Ginsburg 1971; Gurtner and Burns 1972; Young 1969], since their chemical and physical properties will not permit them to pass by simple diffusion. Substances with properties in accord with the laws of membrane diffusion will pass the placental barrier. Thus, the placenta cannot be considered a highly effective barrier; many toxic substances, including viruses and microorganisms, can cross it [Goldstein et al. 1968].

Excretory Processes

The major excretory routes of absorbed toxicants are through the urine and the bile.

Urinary Excretion   The mechanism of elimination of absorbed toxicants through the urine is by passive glomerular filtration and tubular diffusion as well as by active tubular transport. Glomerular filtration and active tubular transport account for most of the excretion of toxic and other compounds. The compounds in the kidney tubules may be reabsorbed by passive diffusion depending on the pH of the urine. Therefore, depending on whether a toxicant is basic or acidic, the pH of the urine may hasten or retard its urinary excretion. Thus, an alkaline urine will hasten the excretion of acidic compounds, and vice versa [Weiner and Madge 1964].

Urinary excretion by active transport also controls the elimination of acidic and basic substances; each type is actively excreted by separate processes, so that compounds in each type may compete with each other for the active transport system [Cafruny 1971]. Therefore, the presence of a toxicant may delay the excretion of another by preventing it from being carried by the common transport system, or by displacing it from the carrier system. The active transport system is particularly necessary for the excretion of those compounds that are bound to plasma proteins.

Obviously, effects of toxicants are increased when they are not easily eliminated, such as in kidney failure or in the case of the newborns whose urinary excretory processes are not yet fully developed [Barnett et al. 1949; Hirsch and Hook 1970].

Biliary Excretion Many toxic compounds which are removed by the liver from the blood may be excreted directly through the bile; this route is necessary for those compounds requiring the detergent action of the bile for effective solubilization. The liver is particularly well suited for excretory function, being the major site for the biotransformation as well as conjugation of most toxic substances. In this way, a major fraction of the amount of absorbed toxicant is not distributed throughout the body because the blood from the GI tract passes through the liver first.

However, in several cases, the biliary excretory route is largely ineffective because many biotransformed substances are sufficiently lipid soluble for repeated absorption. This process, known as enterohepatic circulation, ensures the continued exposure of the body to toxicants and even at increasing doses when toxic substances are repeatedly ingested. Nevertheless, biliary excretion prevents or minimizes the toxicity of many compounds, again, by reducing the effective dose. The importance of biliary excretion in decreasing toxicity has been demonstrated in rats with ligated bile ducts exposed to toxic substances [Klaassen 1973]. For example, diethylstilbestrol (DES), which is essentially eliminated only through the bile, becomes 130 times more toxic in the ligated rodents as compared to sham-operated animals. Diethylstibestrol in this case remained elevated in the body and became highly toxic; the LD_{50} decreased from 100 to 0.75 mg/kg [Klaassen 1973]. Furthermore, it has also been shown that when bile secretion was stimulated (e.g., by certain steroids), the toxicity of many compounds was also decreased [Selye 1971]. The toxicity of mercury reportedly also diminished with increased biliary excretion [Haddow and Marshall 1972; Selye 1972].

Because the newborn does not have a fully developed biliary excretory mechanism, many compounds are more toxic in the newborn than in the adult [Klaassen 1973, 1972].

Therefore, liver injury which causes the biliary excretory process to fail will result in greater toxicity for specific compounds as a consequence. One of the diagnostic signs of liver injury is jaundice (Chap. 5). This symptom may be accompanied by other toxic manifestations owing to unexcreted substances. This was demonstrated in sheep poisoned with photodynamic substances when these animals suffered biliary failure following ingestion of icterogenic plants (pp. 30-32).

Other Excretory Routes Excretory routes, e.g., lungs, sweat, saliva, and milk, may also aid in the elimination of toxic substances. However, these routes are of minor importance compared to the urine and bile for ingested substances. In the case of milk, however, the level of toxicant may be sufficiently high to pose a hazard to the milk-drinking populations, especially infants and children. Various drugs and toxic compounds are eliminated through the milk [Howard and Herbold 1979], and the tragic epidemic of nonbacterial milk poisoning in the nineteenth century in certain parts of the United States is another grim ecample of the hazard of drinking milk from unknown sources.

THE BIOCHEMICAL BASIS OF THE TOXICITY OF COMPOUNDS

Requirements and Limitations of Cellular Operations

The fundamental unit of life, the cell, is engaged in multifarious activities, including series of intricate sequential chemical reactions. These reactions occur at precise rates and are interrelated with other metabolic pathways. Some means of coordination, integration, and control are necessary. The cell operates primarily to produce energy and for the biosynthesis of its components or those of other cells requiring specific compounds. Thus, there is an interdependence among chemical reaction pathways. There is also an interdependence among cells and consequently among tissues and organs. Thus, the living system is an ordered, coordinated, and harmonious system, in functional equilibrium.

The cell's operation is mediated by specific enzymes, and as a means of coordination and control, these enzymes are compartmentalized in the cell. This requires a membrane system to control the passage of substances entering and leaving the cells or its organelles. In this way, the internal and external environments of the cell are regulated.

The cell operates within qualitative, quantitative, and time limitations. In other words, the required precise types of compounds, in the proper amounts, must be present at the proper time. Any deviation, within certain limits, from these precise operational specifications of the cell will naturally result in a disturbance which, if magnified to a certain percentage of the total functional cells of an organ or tissue, will result in a detectable functional aberration. The functional disturbance may or may not be indicated by a grossly observable structural damage to the tissues, depending on the relative reserve capacity of those tissues or organs.

Qualitative Requirements of Cellular Operation

The stringent qualitative requirements of the cells follow from the involvement of specific enzymes which can utilize only specific compounds or structurally related compounds. Many of these compounds must be biosynthesized by the cell itself, thus affording it some safeguards. To the extent that these compounds can be synthesized, the intricate biochemical pathways can proceed smoothly. In humans and other animals, however, several of the cell's required compounds cannot be biosynthesized, so these must be provided from external sources. These exogenous compounds are known collectively as the nutrients. In higher forms of life, there is a complex and intricate system for delivering these nutrients to the cell. Some of the most essential compounds, especially those required for energy, are stored in the body to provide for those occasions when they are temporarily unavailable from external sources.

Quantitative Requirements of Cellular Operation

The quantitative requirements of the cell arise not only from the inherent continuous need of a dynamic system to have a definite quantity of specific compounds, but also from the nature of the macromolecules synthesized. The proteins and nucleic acids are formed by repeating units of smaller compounds. Because of this, it is obvious that a definite quantity of raw materials must be present in order to build bigger molecules.

The quantitative requirements also have a negative aspect in that the cell cannot tolerate an excess of all its necessary compounds. The limit of tolerance for some of these compounds is rather narrow and, therefore, they are promptly excreted or excluded from the cell. An excess also may interfere in the cell's operation, since one means of control is feedback inhibition; that is, an excess of a product may inhibit the activity of the enzyme regulating the pathway. An excess also may speed up a certain reaction or biochemical pathway beyond the capacity of the cell. Obviously, if for no other reason, a confined structure has quantitative limits.

Time Limits of Cellular Operation

The time limits required in the operation of the cell obviously follow from the dynamic nature of its processes. The limits in the energy-yielding process in some specialized cells are rather narrow. For example, the brain cells cannot be deprived of oxygen for more than a few minutes.

Coordination of the Activities of Cells and Tissues

The functions of various cells and tissues must be synchronized and coordinated among themselves because of their interdependence. Thus, the synthesis of hemoglobin and other blood components by specialized cells must be coordinated in response to the nutritive need of all cells in the body. The entire organ systems must also be coordinated and harmonized with the external environment. Thus, it is evident that some form of extracellular master control must be present to coordinate internal activities and to regulate the system's responses to the external environment. This control resides in the nervous and hormonal systems. The nervous system is electrochemical, the hormonal system, chemical. These two systems themselves are coordinated.

Interference of Cellular Functions by Various Compounds

Because the cell's components are reactive chemicals, it is obvious that many foreign compounds can react with its components and interfere in its operation. The foreign substances which interfere in the cell's activity are called intrinsic toxicants. Those compounds native or familiar to the cell and are toxic when present in excess are called relative toxicants. Many of the latter compounds are in fact necessary for the normal operation of the cell; others are metabolic by-products.

There are safeguards against the intrusion of unwanted chemicals. However, these safeguards, which we shall discuss later, are imperfect. When these safeguards fail, toxic effects result.

Biochemical Effects Resulting in Toxic Injury

From the above discussion, toxic effects eventually indicated by gross functional disturbances must necessarily initiate injury at the molecular level. Although the biochemical mechanisms of toxicity of a large number of compounds are still unknown, the biochemical bases of their toxicities may include one or more of the following general types.

Deficiency of Essential Compounds It has been mentioned that the nutrients which cannot be synthesized by higher living forms necessarily must be supplied from external sources. The urgency of delivering these compounds to the cell depends on their rate of usage and degradation, the extent of cell storage, and the magnitude of their involvement in energy production, the cell's primary need. Nutrient deficiencies in cells can occur either through the absence of nutrients in food, a primary deficiency, or the failure or interference in their delivery or metabolism. Such an internal obstruction is termed a secondary deficiency. One of the following mechanisms may be responsible for such a failure:

Inhibition of digestive enzymes or other digestive factors: Numerous examples of these will be evident in the succeeding chapters.

Absence of digestive enzymes or other digestive factors: A familiar example is the toxicity of lactose on account of the absence of lactase. Similar problems have arisen with the other disaccharides because of the absence of the corresponding digestive enzymes.

Interference in the absorption of essential compounds: Interference may be accomplished as follows: (1) Chemical or physical combination of one compound with another, resulting in the formation of a nonabsorbable complex. (2) Absence of the compound necessary for the absorption of the compound; for example, the vitamin cobalamin is not effectively absorbed in the absence of the intrinsic factor. (3) Interaction or modification of the gastrointestinal mucosa. An example of this is the group of compounds known as lectins (Chap. 8), which bind on the absorptive surface of the intestinal mucosa. (4) Inhibition of enzymes involved in absorption. For example, the antibiotic actinomycin D, which inhibits ribonucleic acid (RNA) and protein synthesis, including presumably, enzymes necessary for the absorption of amino acids [Yamada et al. 1967]. (5) Solubilization of essential compounds in solvents that are non-absorbable. This factor may fall under item 1 but deserves emphasis. An example of this is mineral oil, which may dissolve the lipid vitamins and prevent their absorption. (6) Increased motility of the gastrointestinal tract. Many factors can affect this motility. Certain factors in foodstuffs may cause diarrhea and similar rapid evacuation of intestinal contents, resulting in poor absorption of essential compounds.

Interference of the transport of essential compounds to the cells: For example, nitrite ions interfere in the transport of oxygen by hemoglobin.

Degradation of essential compounds: Nutrients may be destroyed even before they are absorbed. For example, there are factors in foods which destroy thiamin (thiaminases [Fujita, 1954]); retinol and carotenoids may be destroyed by oxidizing agents and ascorbic acid, by ascorbic acid oxidase (Chap. 9).

Inactivation of essential compounds: Certain substances may react with some of the nutrients without degradation rendering them inactive. For example, cyanide may interact with cobalamin to form cyanocobalamin, which is biologically inactive. It is believed that chronic cyanide intoxication may be the cause of tropical amblyopia as a result of cyanide inactivation of cobalamin (Chap. 8).

Interference of the uptake of essential compounds in the cells or tissues: For example, thiocyanate inhibits the iodine uptake of thyroid cells (Langer and Stolc 1964); glucose and amino acid uptake of muscle cells does not occur in the absence of insulin.

Antagonism between essential compounds: An antagonism exists between leucine, isoleucine, and valine when one of these is present in relatively large excess over another [Harper et al. 1970]; Beta-carotene and cholecalciferol are also antagonistic [Weits 1964].

Inhibition of Metabolic and Other Nondigestive Enzymes There are many examples of poisons which inhibit the activity of metabolic and other nondigestive enzymes. Carbamates and organophosphates, for example, are potent inhibitors of acetylcholine esterase, an enzyme necessary for neurotransmission [Aldridge and Reiner 1969; O'Brien 1969a,b]. The inhibition of monoamine oxidases by antidepressant drugs has been shown to increase the biological activity of pressor amines found in several foods [Vettorazzi 1974].

Interference with Neurotransmission It was stated previously (p. 45) that the nervous system may be considered one of the coordinators of the activities of organs and tissues. Many elegant works in past decades have elucidated some of the electro-chemical mechanisms underlying nervous function. In order to understand better how toxicants affect the nervous system, the mechanism of neurotransmission [O'Brien 1969b] will be summarized here.

The propagation of a nervous impulse may be looked upon as a wave of depolarization along an axon. The latter contains pores or gates through which Na^+ and K^+ ions pass, Na^+ from the extra-axonal fluids and K^+ from the intra-axonal compartment. (There is evidence to indicate that the gates through which Na^+ and K^+ pass are shut or opened by some mechanism which is still not understood.) Normally, the axon membrane is polarized, the interior surface negative by 50 to 100 mV relative to the exterior surface. On application of a stimulus to the surface, polarization reverses in the region of stimulation owing to the inward flow of Na^+ followed by an outward flow of K^+. The current flow in the stimulated region causes partial depolarization of the adjacent region, and likewise, the opposite flow of Na^+ and K^+ occurs, resulting in a reversal of polarity in that adjacent region. Meanwhile, the preceding region regains its original polarity. In this way, the nervous impulse is propagated region-by-region along the membrane of the axon until the nerve terminal is reached.

The impulse or action potential is propagated to the next nerve, or to a muscle cell through a gap or synapse. Located at the surface of the presynaptic terminal are small granules (boutons) which secrete a chemical, the neurotransmitter. Upon arrival of the impulse, the neurotransmitter is released to diffuse across the synaptic gap and combine at a specific site on the surface of the postsynaptic terminal. The transmitter is believed to change the surface of the postsynaptic unit so that the flow of ions is permitted. The impulse-receiving neuron may have several synapses, many of which may be "firing" at the same time. These impulses may be inhibitory (hyperpolarizing) or excitatory (depolarizing).

These miniature hyperpolarized or depolarized charges spread through the cell surface by electrical conduction (electrotonic spread), as in any electrical conducting surface. The algebraic sum of these opposite charges produces an area known as an axon hillock. If the axon hillock is depolarized sufficiently, for example, by 40 mV, the influx of Na^+ occurs, propagating the impulse down the new axon as before. The receptor neuron is said to have fired.

This simplified description of neurotransmission suggests several aspects of this complex process which may be susceptible to the action of various toxicants. The propagation of the nervous impulse is a rapid process, and obviously an energy-requiring process. The complexity and rapidity of neurotransmission also lay the bases for its vulnerability. Thus, many substances may interfere in this process.

The interference of many of these substances on neurotransmission, as experience has shown, is usually quite serious and often fatal. For example, the deadly poisons tetrodotoxin, from the puffer fish, and saxitoxin, from shellfish and clams, derive their lethality from their capacity to block specifically the sodium gates [Kao 1972; Narahashi 1972]. DDT, on the other hand, acts opposite to these poisons by keeping the sodium channel open but partially blocking the potassium channel [Narahashi and Haas 1967].

The synaptic mechanism appears to be the specific target of many potent poisons. The release of the neurotransmitter acetylcholine can be blocked by the botulinum toxin [Burgen et al. 1949; Brooks 1956] (Chap. 14). The binding of the same transmitter on the receptor is blocked by curare or succinylcholine. The enzyme choline acetyltransferase, required for the synthesis of acetylcholine, can be inhibited by the hemicholiniums [Schueler 1961]. Acetylcholine, after performing its role in facilitating the transfer of impulses, is hydrolyzed by acetylcholine esterase. This enzyme can be the target of many poisons, such as organophosphates [O'Brien 1969a,b], and the cholinesterase inhibitors in the potato, eggplant, tomato, and sugar beets [Orgell 1963].

The checks and balances of the nervous system involve also an inhibitory transmission by inhibitory neurons. Their activities can also be blocked by a substance such as strychnine, which interferes with the binding of the neurotransmitter to the postsynaptic neuron [Curtis 1962], or by possibly blocking the release of the neurotransmitter at the presynaptic junction by substances such as picrotoxinin [Eccles et al. 1963], obtained from the berries of the East Indian shrub *Anamirta cocculus*. Both strychnine and picrotoxinin are convulsants.

Many other food poisons show similar symptoms as those given by the toxins mentioned above. Although their actual mechanism of toxicity has not been studied, the symptoms elicited will give a clue to the possible target cells or molecules.

Other neurotransmitter substances are known. This is especially true of the central nervous system. In addition to acetylcholine [De Robertis 1964; Whittaker 1964], there are the monoamines — the cathecholamines, norepinephrine and 3,4-dihydroxyphenylethylamine (dopamine), and 5-hydroxytryptamine (serotonin [De Robertis 1964; Vogt 1954]. The amino acids, glutamate [Krnjevic and Straughan 1964], γ-aminobutyric

acid (GABA) [Krnjevic and Schwarz 1966] and β-alanine are also possible neurotransmitters. Histamine [Gaddum 1963] has also been considered to be a transmitter.
Another powerful group of substances, the prostaglandins, also appear to have effects
given by neurotransmitters [Avanzino et al. 1966; Horton and Main 1966]. Knowledge
of the substances functioning as neurotransmitters may help elucidate how an exogenous compound causes toxic injury. Many exogenous substances can mimic the effects of neurotransmitters. Muscarine, the toxic alkaloid from the mushroom Amanita
muscaria, behaves like acetylcholine [Bradley et al. 1966]. Its extreme toxicity may be
the result of its resistance to degradation in the tissues [Waser 1960].

Furthermore, these neurotransmitters, having powerful effects on the nervous
system, could be highly deleterious if their concentrations in the body exceeded that
required for their activity. Severe acute symptoms, depending of course on the dose,
can result from such excesses. Almost all of the aforementioned neurotransmitters are
found in many food products, sometimes in significant amounts.

The preceding mechanisms explain in part why toxic reactions directly involving
the nervous system are generally more severe, with an almost immediate appearance of
symptoms. Furthermore, other toxicity mechanisms, such as interference in the transport of nutrients, protein synthesis, energy metabolism, and respiration, will indirectly affect the nervous system. This vulnerability of the nervous system is, of course,
predicated on the assumption that the toxicants reach the target site. Toxic injury to
the nervous system is indicated by unmistakable clinical signs. These aspects are discussed in Chapter 5.

Phototoxic Reaction   Certain exogenous and endogenous compounds in skin cells,
when sufficiently illuminated, may become highly reactive with cellular components,
resulting in extensive damage or death of the cell. This process by which light damages tissues, in the presence of a photosensitive substance, is called phototoxic reaction. Two types of phototoxic reactions are recognized: (1) photoautoreaction, and
(2) photoheteroreaction [Ippen 1969]. In the first type, the photosensitive substance
merely induces the normal photochemical reaction of the cell, such as in sunburn
formation. In other words, in the presence of the phototoxic compound, skin may become more easily susceptible to the deleterious effects of sunlight. Most phototoxic reactions, such as those caused by the furocoumarins (see below), are of this type. In
the second type, a toxic product is formed from the photochemical reaction of the
photoactive substance. This toxic derivative may be formed independent of the tissues.
Chlorpromazine and sulfanilamide are examples of compounds which are involved in
phototoxic reaction of the second type. Photoallergic reaction is a form of photoheteroreaction. It is obvious in this case that the photochemical reaction produces an
allergen.

Phototoxic reaction is variously known as photosensitization or photodynamic
action. The latter term was coined by Tappeiner and Jodlbauer (1904) to distinguish
this effect from nonbiological phenomena, such as the effect of light on photographic
plates. Blum (1941) suggested that the term photodynamic action be restricted to reactions involving both a photosensitive substance and molecular oxygen; that is, a
photoauto-oxidation. The more general term phototoxic reaction, as proposed by Ippen
(1969), is preferred.

In order to distinguish a true phototoxic reaction from say, ordinary sunburn,
Blum (1941) suggested certain criteria which must be met:

1. Light at wavelengths greater than 320 nm should produce the symptoms in the
    presence of the suspected phototoxic compound.
2. The phototoxic substance must be isolable from the tissues of the affected sub-
    ject and must reproduce the symptoms when the subject is exposed to it and
    illuminated.

3. There must be a reasonable agreement between the action spectrum (i.e.,
    wavelength producing the injury) of the phototoxic reaction and the absorp-
    tion spectrum (a photochemical property) of the purified phototoxic compound.

Concerning the first criterion, it should be pointed out that sunburn is produced
by light at wavelengths between 280 and 320 nm, and that the penetration of the skin
layers by light at wavelengths above 320 nm extends beyond the Malpighian layer and
capilliary network [Fitzpatrick et al. 1963]. The second criterion, together with the
first, should demonstrate conclusively the presence of a phototoxic compound. The
third criterion may not always be true, since the chemical environment in which the
absorption and action spectra are obtained may not be the same. For example, as reported by Pathak (1969), the action and absorption spectra of the furocoumarins are
quite different. This investigator suggested that the absorption spectra of these compounds bound to the cellular materials in the skin may be different from those in pure
solutions.

The classes of phototoxic compounds include both natural and synthetic compounds.
The natural compounds include the hypericins [Blum 1964], the furocoumarins (psoralens) [Pathak 1969], porphyrins [Clare 1956; Rimington et al. 1967], steroids, essential oils [Spikes 1968], and riboflavin [Fowlks 1959; Spikes and Glad 1964] and flavin
mononucleotide (FMN) [Frisell et al. 1959]. The natural source of a number of these
compounds are discussed in Chapter 8 of this book.

The synthetic phototoxic compounds include many drugs prescribed routinely,
such as anesthetics, antibiotics, antidiabetics, antihistamines, diuretics, barbiturates,
sulfonamides, phenothiazines, dyes and other coal tar and petroleum products, and
perfumes and colognes [Spikes 1968].

The porphyrins are present in all aerobic organisms in the form of heme, cytochromes, various enzymes, chlorophyll, and derivatives of those compounds. Obviously, the porphyrins are present in many types of food products, notably in certain
fruits, vegetables, and meats. These foods pose no phototoxic hazard unless there is
damage to the biliary excretion mechanism. Such is the case in sheep afflicted by the
disease, geeldikkop (Dutch, "yellow, thickhead") following the consumption of icterogenic forage plants such as those belonging to the genus *Tribulus* (e.g., *T. terrestis*
and *T. ovis*). The obstruction of the biliary excretion by icterogenic compounds in
these plants causes jaundice and the accumulation of the phototoxin phylloerythrin in
the skin, which becomes damaged on exposure to light [Clare 1956; Rimington and
Quin 1934].

Likewise, various forms of porphyrias, which are hereditary or congenital diseases
in man, are also characterized by toxic reactions in the skin following exposure to light
and accumulation of heme-derived photosensitive porphyrins [Burnham 1969; Peterka
et al. 1965; Rimington et al. 1967].

Damage to the cell due to the phototoxic reaction might result in part from the
aerobic photodegradation of free or protein-bound tryptophan, histidine, tyrosine,
methionine, and cysteine [Spikes and Livingston 1969]. The effect on proteins does
not necessarily involve rupture of the peptide bond [Ghiron and Spikes 1965a,b;
Weil et al. 1953]. Phototoxicity may also arise from damage to nucleic acids, nucleosides, and nucleotides. In particular, the photoreaction may involve guanine and
thymine residues [Spikes 1968; Zenda et al. 1965]. The photosensitizing compound in
this case may involve riboflavin.

It has been observed that deoxyribonucleic acid (DNA) becomes more resistant to
enzyme hydrolysis following photodynamic reaction [Dellweg and Opree 1966]. Deoxyribonucleic acid also binds covalently with the carcinogen 3,4-benzpyrene when appropriately illuminated [Reske and Staueff 1965]. Depolymerization of hyaluronic acid can
result following a photoreaction with riboflavin [Matsumura 1966] or the hematoporphyrin [Castellani 1954].

Various dyes appear to require ascorbic acid and oxygen for photodynamic activity [Sundblad and Balazs 1966]. In addition, the photo-oxidation of ascorbic acid can be photosensitized by riboflavin [Pirie 1965].

A proposed mechanism [Spikes and Glad 1964] for the photochemical reactions leading to phototoxicity is described below:

Initially, the sensitive material (PS) in the ground state captures a photon (hv), transforming the molecule to the first excited singlet state (^{1}PS), followed by the singlet-to-triplet state (^{3}PS) transition:

$$PS + hv \text{ (photons)} \longrightarrow {}^1PS \longrightarrow {}^3PS$$

The triplet state of the photosensitizer has a relatively greater half-life, so that a photoreaction has a greater chance of occurring. The photosensitive compound in the triplet state may react with the substrates (amino acids, purines, and so forth), as in any of the possible schemes shown below:

1. $\quad {}^3PS + AH_2 \text{ (substrate)} \longrightarrow AH_2^* + PS \xrightarrow{O_2} \text{degradation products;}$

   $\quad \text{or, } {}^3PS + AH_2 \longrightarrow PSH_2 + A \xrightarrow{O_2} PS + H_2O_2$

2. $\quad {}^3PS + O_2 \longrightarrow O_2^* + PS \xrightarrow{AH_2} \text{degradation products;}$

   $\quad \text{or, } {}^3PS + O_2 \longrightarrow PSOO \longrightarrow \text{degradation} + PS.$
   $\qquad\qquad\qquad\quad \text{"moloxide"} \qquad\ \ \text{products}$

3. $\quad PS + AH_2 \xrightarrow{hv} PSAH_2 \longrightarrow PSAH_2^* \longrightarrow {}^3PSAH_2$

   $\qquad \xrightarrow{O_2} PS + \text{degradation products}$

The molecules in activated state are asterisked.

Any of the above mechanisms may be involved in the formation of cholesterol α-oxide by the photochemical reaction of cholesterol and other sterols. This powerful carcinogen [Bischoff et al. 1955] has been observed to be formed in human skin irradiated in vitro [Black and Lo 1971] and in mouse skin irradiated in vivo [Black and Douglas 1972]. In the case of the latter, the amount of carcinogen remained constant during the first 6 weeks of ultraviolet (mercury lamp) irradiation in the range of 0.3 to 1.0 μg/g skin or around 2 μg/mouse. This value peaked to 16 μg/mouse in 10 weeks, and the first squamous cell carcinoma developed after the level of the carcinogen began to drop with a 90% incidence by the twenty-fourth week [Black and Douglas 1973]. The formation of this carcinogen, characterized by a rapid increase after a protracted lag period, may reflect a breakdown of some detoxification mechanism on continuous irradiation so that the photochemically induced autooxidation can proceed to its natural course.

It is highly probable that other carcinogens are formed by photochemical reactions in the skin, since a previous result with cholesterol α-oxide produced only a 20 to 50% tumor incidence with a subcutaneous dose of 20 mg [Bischoff 1969]. This dose is much higher than that obtained by photo-oxidation of the skin and found to induce a 90% tumor incidence by Black and Douglas (1973). More of these will be discussed in the chapter on carcinogenesis (Chap. 6).

Interference with DNA and RNA Synthesis and Function Aside from the inhibition of enzyme action involved in DNA and RNA synthesis, toxic compounds may also affect DNA and RNA formation and function, by reacting with the macromolecules themselves. For example, DNA replication, RNA translation, and consequently protein synthesis may be interfered with by alkylation of the DNA or RNA purine and pyrimidine bases by N-nitroso compounds, such as the nitrosamines (Chap. 12). It has been reported that mitochondrial DNA is more easily alkylated than the nuclear variety [Wunderlich 1971; Wunderlich and Tetzlaff 1970; Wunderlich et al. 1972].

Deoxyribonucleic acid function may also be interfered with by intercalation of the toxic compound between the DNA double strand, so that its replication is prevented [Scholtissek 1965]. The acridines were reported to behave in this manner.

Another form of nonspecific binding of toxic compounds on DNA was also observed in the case of the carcinogenic and hepatotoxic pigment luteoskyrin (Chap. 13) from *Penicillium islandicum* which infects rice grains. This compound binds without intercalation parallel to the DNA axis and perpendicular to the plane of the bases [Uraguchi 1971]. This bound luteoskyrin blocks RNA polymerase, which must combine with DNA for the transcription of RNA [Lill et al. 1969].

There is ample evidence which shows that interference of DNA or RNA activity may result in mutagenic transformation. This effect is considered by many investigators as an important event in the initiation of carcinogenesis (Chap. 5). Mutagenic effects involving the germinal cells have the potential for hereditary transmission. Therefore, the damage of these effects can extend beyond one generation and across pedigrees and population groups.

The Time Factor in the Toxicity of Compounds

The toxic manifestations of various substances appear at different rates. In general, the rate of appearance and the nature of symptoms are functions of the type of compound, dose, receptor cell, tissue or organ, rate of absorption, and biological peculiarity of the subject. Toxic effects may manifest in terms of functional disturbances, biochemical abnormality, and structural cell or tissue damage.

Acute and Chronic Poisonings or Effects

We should distinguish here the difference between acute and chronic poisonings or exposures, on one hand, and acute and chronic effects or symptoms on the other. Acute and chronic poisonings differ in the number and duration of exposures to the toxicant. Generally, the former is a single exposure, and the latter is a protracted or multiple exposure over a period of time. Usually, the term chronic poisoning is reserved to cases occurring for periods lasting several months, while acute poisoning involves contact with the toxicant over a period of 24 hr. However, it is possible that an acute poisoning may result in chronic symptoms. Thus, a single exposure to nitrosamines may result in the chronic symptoms of cancer, whereas a chronic exposure to cyanide in sufficient dose will result always in acute symptoms. Therefore, the terms acute and chronic when used to describe symptoms, refer to the duration and reversibility of the symptoms. An acute symptom is of short duration, usually severe and generally reversible after removal of the toxicant. Chronic symptoms, on the other hand, are prolonged and persist even after removal of the toxicant. For example, some organophosphates produce chronic paralysis [Hays 1972]. Liver carcinogens in small doses may result in hepatic cancer but acute hepatic damage in large doses. Exposures to toxicants between 24 hr and 90 days are usually referred to as prolonged intoxication.

Depending on several factors, such as dose, type of compound, and route of contact, symptoms may be immediate or delayed. Toxic compounds which produce immediate symptoms may easily be identified as the cause of intoxication and therefore can be avoided. In contrast, those with delayed symptoms, especially if the effects do not appear until after several months or years, are not easily identified. Many food poisons fall under the highly delayed category. These compounds, therefore, are of profound concern because of their possible role in modern epidemic diseases whose etiologies have been difficult to establish. Furthermore, when symptoms are delayed, antidotal therapy, assuming that it is known, may be difficult to administer unless the symptoms have been clearly correlated with those of a particular compound. Even so, antidotes are of no value when the appearance of symptoms is markedly delayed; e.g., cancer and other effects indicating structural tissue damage.

Although chronic symptoms are not necessarily due to the accumulation of the poison in the tissues, there are toxicants which accumulate in the tissues to toxic levels, resulting in chronic delayed toxic symptoms. Examples of these are lead, mercury, and DDT (Chaps. 18 and 19).

Toxic compounds may or may not have the property of eliciting chronic poisoning. For example, many of the neurotoxicants, such as the botulinum exotoxin, which are extremely powerful poisons, may progress from the no effect to the lethal level without passing the chronic range. On the other hand, many carcinogens at the lower doses will initiate carcinogenesis but produce acute hepatic or renal damage at higher doses.

Chronicity

Because the problem of chronicity has significant bearing on public health, it is essential that those compounds having this property be identified and their other toxicological properties established. Therefore, some quantitative measure of the chronicity of a compound is important. However, the determination of chronicity has the inherent weakness in that it is based on data obtained from experimental animals with short lifespans. The major problem of validly extrapolating the data to man remains. Nevertheless, such indexes of chronicity may be potentially useful in serving as a guide in identifying those compounds which may behave similarly in man.

Usually, chronicity studies are conducted over one-tenth of the lifespan of the experimental animals. In the case of the rat, this is about 90 to 100 days. The test substance is mixed with the diet at different concentrations. A 90-dose LD_{50}, expressed as mg/kg/day, is calculated based on the dose giving 50% mortality over one-tenth of the lifespan of the rat. This is calculated from the feed consumption for 90 days. Usually, the surviving animals are fed a normal diet for 2 additional weeks to observe further effects.

By comparing the 90-dose LD_{50}, the chronic dose, with the single dose LD_{50}, the acute dose, it becomes apparent that many compounds when given in small doses over prolonged periods take much less to produce a 50% mortality compared to the acute dose. In these compounds, the toxicity is enhanced by feeding over a period of time. However, in some cases, the chronic dose is much higher than the acute dose.

REFERENCES

Abbott, D. C., Goulding, R., and Tatton, J. O'G. 1968. Organochlorine pesticide residues in human fat in Great Britain. *Br. Med. J. 3:* 146−149.
Aldridge, W. N. 1971. The nature of the reaction of organophosphorus compounds and carbamates with esterases. *Bull. W.H.O.* 44: 25−30.
Aldridge, W. N. and Reiner, E. 1969. Acetylcholinesterase. Two types of inhibition by an organophosphorus compound: One the formation of phosphorylatedenzyme and the other analogous to inhibition by substrate. *Biochem. J.* 115: 147−162.
Alfin-Slater, R. B., et al. 1969. Studies of long term administration of aflatoxin to rats as a natural food contaminant. *J. Am. Oil Chem. Soc. 46:* 493.
Arcos, J. C. and Argus, M. F. 1968. Molecular geometry and carcinogenic activity of aromatic compounds: New perspectives. *Adv. Cancer Res. 11:* 305−471.

Avanzino, G. L., Bradley, P. B. and Wolstencroft, J. H. 1966. Actions of prostaglandins E_1, E_2, F_{22} on brain stem neurons. *Br. J. Pharmacol. Chemother. 27:*
157–163.

Bachmann, E. and Goldberg, L. 1971. Reappraisal of the toxicology of ethylene glycol.
III. Mitochondrial affects. *Food Cosmet. Toxicol. 9:* 39–55.

Barker, A. V., Peck, N. H. and MacDonald, G. E. 1971. Nitrate accumulation in
vegetables. I. Spinach grown in upland soils. *Agron. J. 63:* 126.

Barnett, H. L., McNamara, H., Schults, S. and Tampselt, R. 1949. Renal clearance
of sodium penicillin G, procaine penicillin G, and insulin in infants and children.
Pediatrics 3: 418–422.

Beckett, A. H. 1969. Kinetics of the absorption and elimination of "amphetamines" in
normal humans. In: Abuse of Central Stimulants. F. Sjoqvist and M. Tottie
(eds.). Almquist and Wiksell, Stockholm.

Bergmann, E. D. and Pullman, B. 1969. *Physico-Chemical Mechanisms of Carcinogenesis.* Israel Academy of Sciences and Humanities, Jerusalem.

Bergmann, E. D.; Blum, J. and Haddow, A. 1963. Carcinogenic activity of some
fluorinated polycyclics. *Nature 200:* 480.

Bischoff, F. 1969. Carcinogenic effects of steroids. *Adv. Lipid Res. 7:* 161–244.

Bischoff, F., Lopez, G., Ruff, J. J. and Gray, C. L. 1955. Carcinogenic activity of
cholesterol degradation products. *Proc. Fed. Am. Soc. Exp. Biol. 14:* 183.

Blaber, L. C. and Crasey, N. H. 1960. The mode of recovery of cholinesterase activity in vivo after organophosphorus poisoning. 2. Brain cholinesterase. *Biochem.
J. 77:* 591–597.

Black, H. S. and Lo, W. 1971. Formation of a carcinogen in human skin irradiated with
ultraviolet light. *Nature 234:* 306–308.

Black, H. S. and Douglas, D. R. 1972. A model system for the evaluation of the role
of cholesterol α-oxide in ultraviolet carcinogenesis. *Cancer Res. 32:* 2630–2632.

Black, H. S. and Douglas, D. R. 1973. Formation of a carcinogen of natural origin in
the etiology of ultraviolet light-induced carcinogenesis. *Cancer Res. 33:* 2094–
2096.

Blum, H. F. 1941. *Photodynamic Action and Diseases Caused by Light.* Reinhold,
New York.

Blum, H. F. 1964. *Photodynamic Action and Diseases Caused by Light.* Hafner, New
York.

Boyland, E., Sims, P. and Huggins, C. 1965. Induction of adrenal damage and cancer
with metabolites of 7,12-dimethylbenz(a)anthracene. *Nature 207:* 816–817.

Brachmann, P. S., Taylor, A., Gangarosa, E. J., Merson, M. H. and Barker, W. H.
1973. Food poisoning in the U.S.A. In: *The Microbiological Safety of Food.*
B. C. Hobbs and J. H. B. Christian (eds.). Academic Press, New York.

Bradley, P. B., Dhawar, B. N. and Wolstencroft, J. H. 1966. Pharmacological properties of cholinoceptive neurons in the medulla and pons of the cat. *J. Physiol.
(Lond.) 183:* 658–674.

Brookes, P. and Lawley, P. D. 1961. The reaction of mono- and di-functional alkylating agents with nucleic acids. *Biochem. J. 80:* 496–503.

Brooks, V. B. 1956. An intracellular study of the action of repetitive nerve valleys
and of botulinum toxin on miniature end-plate potentials. *J. Physiol. (Lond.) 134:*
264–277.

Brown, A. L. 1976. Evaluation of environmental carcinogens for cancer in man.
Oncology 33: 58–60.

Bryan, W. R. and Shimkin, M. B. 1943. Quantitative analysis of dose-response data
obtained with three carcinogenic hydrocarbons in strain C3H male mice. *J. Natl.
Cancer Inst. 3:* 503–531.

Burgen, A. S. V. and Hobbiger, F. 1951. The inhibition of cholinesterases by alkyl-
phosphates and alkylphenol-phosphates. *Br. J. Pharmacol. Chemother. 6:*
593–605.

Burgen, A. S. V., Dickins, F. and Zatman, L. J. 1949. The action of botulinum toxin on the neuromuscular junction. *J. Physiol. (Lond.) 109:* 10–24.

Burnham, B. F. 1969. Metabolism of porphyrins and corrinoids. In: *Metabolic Pathways.* 3rd ed. Vol. 3. D. M. Greenberg (ed.). Academic Press, New York.

Cafruny, E. J. 1971. Renal excretion of drugs. In: *Fundamentals of Drug Metabolism and Drug Disposition.* B. N. LaDu, H. G. Mandel, and E. L. Way (eds.). Williams & Wilkins, Baltimore.

Carson, R. L. 1962. *Silent Spring.* Houghton Mifflin, Boston.

Castellani, A. 1954. Photodynamic depolymerization of hyaluronic acid by hematoporphyrin. *Giorn. Biochim. 3:* 19–28.

Charalampous, K. D., Orengo, A., Walker, K. E. and Kinross-Wright, J. 1964. Metabolic fate of β-(3,4,5-trimethoxyphenyl) ethylamine (mescaline) in humans: Isolation and identification of 3,4,5-trimethoxyphenyl acetic acid. *J. Pharmacol. Exp. Ther. 145:* 242–246.

Clare, N. T. 1956. Photodynamic action and its pathological effects. *Radiation Biol. 3:* 693–723.

Claus, G., Krisko, I. L. and Bolander, K. 1974. Chemical carcinogens in the environment and in the human diet: Can a threshold be established. *Food Cosmet. Toxicol. 12:* 737–746.

Cohen, G. and Collins, M. 1970. Alkaloids from catecholamines in adrenal tissue: Possible role in alcoholism. *Science 167:* 1749–1751.

Colburn, N. H. and Boutwell, R. K. 1968. The in vivo binding of β-propiolactone to mouse skin DNA, RNA, and protein. *Cancer Res. 28:* 642–652.

Concon, J. M. 1977. Alkaloids. In: *Encyclopedia of Food Science.* M. S. Peterson and A. H. Johnson (eds.). AVI Publishing, Westport, Connecticut.

Concon, J. M., Swerczek, T. W. and Newburg, D. S. 1981. Potential carcinogenicity of black pepper (Piper nigrum). In: *Antinutrients and Natural Toxicants in Foods.* Food and Nutrition Press, Westport, Connecticut.

Coulson, C. A. 1953. Electronic configuration and carcinogenesis. *Adv. Cancer Res. 1:* 1–56.

Cremer, J. E. and Bligh, J. 1969. Body-temperature and responses to drugs. *Br. Med. Bull. 25:* 299–306.

Curtis, D. R. 1962. The depression of spinal inhibition by electrophoretically administered strychnine. *Int. J. Neuropharmacol. 1:* 239–250.

Das Gupta, B. R., Berry, L. J. and Daniel, A. 1970. Purification of clostridium botulinum Type A toxin. *Biochim. Biophys. Acta 214:* 343–349.

Davidson, C. 1971. Protein binding. In: *Fundamentals of Drug Metabolism and Drug Action.* B. N. LaDu, H. G. Mandel, and E. L. Way (eds.). William & Wilkins, Baltimore.

Davis, V. E., Walsh, M. J. and Yamanaka, Y. 1970. Augmentation of alkaloid formation from dopamine by alcohol and acetaldehyde in vitro. *J. Pharmacol. Exp. Ther. 174:* 401–412.

Dellweg, H. and Opree, W. 1966. The photodynamic effect of thiopyronin on nucleic acid. *Biophysik 3:* 241–248. (German)

De Robertis, D. A. 1964. Electron microscope and chemical study of binding sites of brain biogenic amines. *Prog. Brain Res. 8:* 118–136.

Dinman, B. D. 1972. "Non-concept" of "no-threshold": chemicals in the environment. Stochastic determination impose a lower limit on the dose-response relationship between cells and chemicals. *Science 175:* 495–497.

Dipple, A. 1976. Polynuclear aromatic carcinogens. In: *Chemical Carcinogens.* C. E. Searle (ed.). American Chemical Society, Washington, D. C.

Doull, J. 1972. The effect of environmental factors on drug response. In: *Essays in Toxicology.* W. I. Hays (ed.). Academic Press, New York.

Dring, L. G., Smith, R. L. and Williams, R. T. 1966. The fate of amphetamine in man and other mammals. *J. Pharm. Pharmacol. 18:* 402–404.

Druckrey, H. 1959. Pharmacological approach to carcinogenesis. In: *Ciba Foundation Symposium on Carcinogenesis: Mechanism of Action.* E. E. W. Wulstenholme and M. O'Conner (eds.). Little Brown, Boston.

Dubois, K. P. 1971. The toxicity of organophosphorus compounds to mammals. *Bull. W.H.O. 44:* 233–240.

Dubois, K. P., Doull, K., Okinaka, A. J. and Coon, J. M. 1953. Studies on the toxicity and pharmacological actions of symmetrical and unsymmetrical diethyl bis(dimethylamido)pyrophosphate. *J. Pharmacol. Exp. Ther. 107:* 464–477.

Durham, W. F. and Hayes, W. J. 1962. Organic phosphorus poisoning and its therapy. *Arch. Environ. Health 5:* 21–47.

Eccles, J. C., Schmidt, R. F. and Willis, W. D. 1963. Pharmacological studies of pre-synaptic inhibition. *J. Physiol. (Lond.) 168:* 500–530.

Egan, H., Goulding, R., Roburn, J. and Tatton, J. O'G. 1965. Organo-chlorine residues in human fat and human milk. *Br. Med. J. 2:* 66–69.

Engel, R. E. et al. 1971. Environmental lead and public health. Air Pollution Control Office (U.S.) Publ. AP-90.

Enslein, K. 1979. Personal Communication. Rochester, New York.

Enslein, K. and Craig, P. N. 1978. A toxicity estimation model. *J. Environ. Pathol. Toxicol. 2:* 115–132.

Enslein, K. and Craig, P. N. 1979. Status report on development of predictive models in toxicological endpoints. Genesee Computer Center, Rochester, NY.

Erni, W., and Ritschel, W. A. 1977. Effect of temperature of perorally administered phenol red solution on gastric emptying in the rat. *Arzneimittelforsch. 27:* 1043–1045.

Federation of American Societies for Experimental Biology. 1977. Evaluation of health aspects of GRAS food ingredients: Lessons learned and questions unanswered. *Fed. Proc. 36:* 2519.

Fitzpatrick, T. B, Pathak, M. A., Magnus, I. A. and Curwen, W. L. 1963. Abnormal reactions of man to light. *Annu. Rev. Med. 14:* 195–214.

Flesher, J. W. and Sydnor, K. L. 1971. Carcinogenicity of derivatives of 7,12-dimethylbenz(a)anthracene. *Cancer Res. 31:* 1951–1954.

Flurry, R. L. 1964. A simple method for predicting the carcinogenic properties of polycyclic aromatic molecules. *J. Med. Chem. 7:* 668–670.

Food and Drug Administration. 1973. FDA introduction to total drug quality. U. S. Department of Health, Education, and Welfare. Public Health Service. Food and Drug Administration. Rockville, Maryland. DHEW Publ. No. (FDA) 74-3006.

Food and Drug Administration. 1979. Chemical compounds in food-producing animals. *Fed. Regist. 44:* 17070–17114.

Fowlks, W. L. 1959. The mechanism of photodynamic effect. *J. Invest. Dermatol. 32:* 233–247.

Frawley, J. P., Hagan, E. C. and Fitzhugh, O. G. 1952. A comparative pharmacological and toxicological study of organic phosphate-anticholinesterase compounds. *J. Pharmacol. Exp. Ther. 105:* 156–165.

Friedman, A. M., Willis, A. and Himwich, H. E. 1949. Correlation between signs of toxicity and cholinesterase level of brain and blood during recovery from di-isopropyl fluorophosphate (DFP) poisoning. *Am. J. Physiol. 157:* 80–87.

Frisell, W. R., Chung, C. W. and Mackenzie, C. G. 1959. Catalysis of oxidation of nitrogen compounds by flavin coenzymes in the presence of light. *J. Biol. Chem. 234:* 1297–1302.

Fujita, A. 1954. Thiaminase. *Adv. Enzymol. 15:* 389–421.

Gaddum, J. H. 1963. Substances released in nervous activity. Proc. 1st Int. Pharmacol. Meeting, 8. Stockholm, 1961.

Garlind, T. et al. 1960. Effect of ethanol on circulatory, metabolic and neurohormonal function during muscular work in men. *Acta Pharmacol. Toxicol. 17:* 106–114.

Gessner, P. K., Parke, D. V. and Williams, R. T. 1961. Studies in detoxication. The metabolism of ^{14}C-labelled ethylene glycol. *Biochem. J. 79:* 482–489.

Ghiron, C. A. and Spikes, J. D. 1965. The flavin-sensitized photoinactivation of trypsin. *Photochem. Photobiol. 4:* 901–905.

Ghiron, C. A., and Spikes, J. D. 1965. The photoinactivation of trypsin as sensitized by methylene blue and eosin y. *Photochem. Photobiol. 4:* 13–26.

Ginsburg, J. 1971. Placenta drug transfer. *Annu. Rev. Pharmacol. 11:* 387–408.

Goldstein, A., Aronow, L. and Kalman, S. H. 1968. *Principle of Drug Action.* Harper & Row, New York.

Gorisch, V. 1967. Influence of temperature on stomach-emptying. *Ost. Apoth. Zty. 21:* 20–22. (German)

Gurtner, G. H. and Burns, B. 1972. Possible facilitated transport of oxygen across the placenta. *Nature. 240:* 473–475.

Haddow, J. E. and Marshall, P. 1972. Increased stool mercury excretion in the rat: The effect of spironolactone. *Proc. Soc. Exp. Biol. Med. 140:* 707–709.

Hall, R. L. 1975. GRAS—Concept and application. *Food Technol. 29:* 48–53.

Hammond, A. L. 1972. Chemical pollution. Polychlorinated biphenyls. *Science 175:* 155–156.

Harper, A. E., Benevenga, N. J. and Wohlhueter, R. M. 1970. Effects of disproportionate amounts of amino acids. *Physiol. Rev. 50:* 428–558.

Hawkins, R. D. and Kalant, H. 1972. The metabolism of ethanol and its metabolic effects. *Pharmacol. Rev. 24:* 67–157.

Hayes, F., Short, R. and Gibson, J. 1973. Differential toxicity of monochloroacetate, monofluoroacetate and monoidoacetate in rats. *Toxicol. Appl. Pharmacol. 26:* 93–102.

Hays, W. B., Jr. 1966. Monitoring food and people for pesticide content. In: *Scientific Aspects of Pest Control.* National Academy of Sciences National Research Council, Washington, D.C.

Hays, W. J. 1972. Tests for detecting and measuring long-term toxicity. *Essays Toxicol. 3:* 65–77.

Herndon, W. C. 1974. Theory of carcinogenic activity of aromatic hydrocarbons. *Trans. N.Y. Acad. Sci. 36:* 200–217.

Hirsch, G. H. and Hook, J. B. 1970. Maturation of renal organic transport: Substrate stimulation by penicillin and p-aminohippurate (PAH). *J. Pharmacol. Exp. Ther. 171:* 103–108.

Hobbiger, F. 1951. Inhibition of cholinesterases by irreversible inhibitors in vitro and in vivo. *Br. J. Pharmacol. 6:* 21–30.

Hoffmann, W. S., Feshbein, W. I. and Andelman, M. B. 1964. Pesticide storage in human fat tissue. *J.A.M.A. 188:* 819.

Horton, E. W. and Main, I. H. M. 1966. Relation between the chemical structure of prostaglandins and their biological activity. *Mem. Soc. Endocrinol. 14:* 29–36.

Howard, R. B. and Herbold, N. H. 1979. *Nutrition in Clinical Care.* McGraw-Hill, New York.

Hunt, J. N. and Knox, M. T. 1961. The slowing of gastric emptying by nine acids. *J. Physiol. (Lond.) 201:* 161–179.

Hutchinson, G. E. 1964. The influence of the environment. *Proc. Natl. Acad. Sci. 51:* 930.

Ippen, H. 1969. Mechanisms of photopathological reactions. In: *Biological Effects of U.V. Radiation.* F. Urbach (ed.), Pergamon Press, Oxford, England.

James, A. H. 1957. *The Physiology of Gastric Digestion.* Edward Arnold, London.

Johnson, M. K. 1967. Metabolism of chloroethanol in the rat. Biochem. Pharmacol. 16, 185–199.

Jones, D. W. and Matthews, R. S. 1974. Carcinogenicity and structure in polycyclic hydrocarbons. *Prog. Med. Chem. 10:* 159–203.

Kao, C. Y. 1972. Pharmacology of tetrodotoxin and saxitoxin. *Fed. Proc. Fed. Am. Soc. Exp. Biol. 31:* 1117–1123.

Kimura, R. 1965. Thiamine decomposing bacteria. In: *Review of Japanese Literature on Beriberi and Thiamine.* N. Shimazono and E. Katsura (eds.). Vitamin B Research Committee of Japan Clinical Nutrition, Faculty of Medicine, Kyoto University, Kyoto, Japan.

Klaassen, C. D. 1972. Immaturity of the newborn rats hepatic excretory function for ouabain. *J. Pharmacol. Exp. Ther. 183:* 520–526.

Klaassen, C. D. 1973a. Comparison of the toxicity of chemicals in newborn rats to bile duct-ligated and sham-operated rats and mice. *Toxicol. Appl. Pharmacol. 24:* 37–44.

Klaassen, C. D. 1973b. The effect of altered hepatic function on the toxicity, plasma disappearance and biliary excretion of diethylstilbestrol. *Toxicol. Appl. Pharmacol. 24:* 142–149.

Klaassen, C. D. and Shoemann, D. W. 1972. Biliary excretion of lead. Proc. 5th Int. Congr. Pharmacol. 757. (abstract)

Krnjevic, K. and Schwarz, S. 1966. λ-Aminobutyric acid an inhibitory transmitter? *Nature 211:* 1372–1374.

Krnjevic, K. and Straughan, D. W. 1964. The release of acetylcholine from the denervated rat diaphragm. *J. Physiol. (Lond.) 170:* 371–378.

Kupferberg, H. J. and Way, E. L. 1963. Pharmacologic basis for the increased sensitivity of the newborn rat to morphine. *J. Pharmacol. Exp. Ther. 141:* 105–112.

Lamanna, C. 1959. Botulinal toxin. *Scientia (Milan) 94:* 135–138.

Langer, P. and Stolc, V. 1964. Relations between thiocyanate formation and goitrogenic effect of foods. V. Comparison of the effect of white cabbage and thiocyanate on the rat thyroid gland. *Physiol. Chem. 335:* 216–220.

Lawley, P. D. 1976. Carcinogenesis by alkylating agents. In: *Chemical Carcinogens.* C. E. Searle (ed.). American Chemical Society, Washington, D.C.

Lawley, P. D., Shah, S. A. and Orr, D. J. 1974. Methylation of nucleic acid by 2,2-dichlorovinyl dimethylphosphate (dichlorvas, DDVP). *Chem. Biol. Interact. 8:* 171–182.

Leopold, G., Furukawa, E., Forth, W. and Rummel, W. 1969. Comparative studies of absorption of heavy metals in vivo and in vitro. *Arch. Pharmacol. Exp. Pathol. 263:* 275–276.

Levi, A. J., Gatmaitan, Z. and Arias, I. M. 1969. Two hepatic cytoplasmic protein fractions Y and Z and their possible role in hepatic uptake of bilirubin, sulfobromophthalein, and other anions. *J. Clin. Invest. 48:* 2156–2167.

Levine, R. R. and Pelikan, E. W. 1964. Mechanisms of drug absorption and excretion. *Annu. Rev. Pharmacol. 4:* 69–84.

Lijinsky, W. 1976. Interaction with nucleic acids of carcinogenic and mutagenic N-nitroso compounds. *Prog. Nucleic Acid Res. Mol. Biol. 17:* 247–269.

Lill, U., Santo, R., Sippel, A. and Hartmann, G. 1969. Inhibitors of RNA polymerase reaction. In: *Inhibitors, Tools in Cell Research,* Proc. 20th Mosbach Colloq. T. Buecher (ed.). Springer-Verlag, Berlin.

Litwack, G., Ketterer, B. and Arias, I. M. 1971. Ligandin: A hepatic protein which binds steroids, bilirubin, carcinogens, and a number of exogenous organic anions. *Nature 234:* 466–467.

Mainster, M. A. and Memory, J. D. 1967. Superdelocalizability indices and the Pullman theory of chemical carcinogenesis. *Biochim. Biophys. Acta 148:* 605–608.

Majchrowicz, E. 1973. Alcohol, aldehydes, and biogenic amines. *Ann. N.Y. Acad. Sci. 215:* 84–88.

Mantel, N. and Bryan, W. R. 1961. "Safety" testing of carcinogenic agents. *J. Natl. Cancer Inst. 27:* 455–470.

Mantel, N. and Schneiderman, M. 1975. Estimating safe levels, a hazardous undertaking. *Cancer Res. 35:* 1379–1386.

Margoshes, M. and Vallee, B. L. 1957. A cadmium protein from equine kidney cortex. *J. Am. Chem. Soc. 79:* 4813–4814.

Matsumura, G. 1966. Depolymerization of hyaluronic acid by autoxidants and radiations. *Radiat. Res. 28:* 735–752.

Miller, J. A. and Miller, E. C. 1963. The carcinogenicities of fluoroderivatives of 10-methyl-1,2-benzanthracene. II. Substitution of the K region and 3'-, 6-, and 7-positions. *Cancer Res. 23:* 229–239.

Ministry of Agriculture, Fisheries and Food. 1971. Survey of mercury in foods. 1st Rep. The Working Party on the Monitoring of Foodstuffs for Mercury and other Heavy Metals. Ministry of Agriculture, Fisheries and Food, Her Majesty's Stationary Office, London.

Ministry of Agriculture, Fisheries and Food. 1972. Survey of lead in food. 2nd Rep. The Working Party on the Monitoring of Foodstuffs for Heavy Metals. Ministry of Agriculture, Fisheries and Food. Her Majesty's Stationary Office, London.

Montgomery, R., Dryer, R. L., Conway, T. W. and Spector, A. A. 1974. Biochemistry. A Care-Oriented Approach. Mosby, St. Louis.

Narahashi, T. 1972. Mechanism of action of tetrodotoxin and saxitoxin on excitable membranes. *Fed. Proc. Fed. Am. Soc. Exp. Biol. 31:* 1124–1132.

Narahashi, T. and Haas, H. G. 1967. DDT: Interaction with nerve membrane conductance changes. *Science 157:* 1438–1440.

National Cancer Institute. 1971. *Evaluation of Environmental Carcinogens.* Report to the Surgeon General, USPHS, April 22, 1970. Ad Hoc Committee on the Evaluation of Low Levels of Environmental Chemical Carcinogens, National Cancer Institute, Bethesda, Maryland.

Norton, T. R. 1975. Metabolism of toxic substances. In: *Toxicology. The Basic Science of Poisons.* L. J. Casarett and J. Doull (eds.). Macmillan, New York.

O'Brien, R. D. 1967. *Insecticides, Action and Metabolism.* Academic Press. New York.

O'Brien, R. D. 1969a. Biochemical effects. Phosphorylation and carbamylation of cholinesterase. *Ann. N.Y. Acad. Sci. 160:* 204–214.

O'Brien, R. D. 1969b. Poisons as tools in studying the nervous system. In: *Essays in Toxicology.* Vol. 1. F. R. Blood (ed.). Academic Press. New York.

Orgell, w. H. 1963. Inhibition of human plasma cholinesterase in vitro by alkaloids, glycosides, and other natural substances. *Lloydia 11:* 36–43.

Parke, D. V. 1968. *The Biochemistry of Foreign Compounds.* Pergamon Press, London.

Pataki, J. and Huggins, C. B. 1967. Adrenal destruction and cancer induced by droxyalkyl derivatives of 7,12-dimethylbenz(a)anthracene. *Biochem. Pharmacol. 16:* 607–612.

Pataki, J. et al. 1971. Carcinogenic and adrenocorticolytic derivatives of benz(a)-anthracene. *J. Med. Chem. 14:* 940–945.

Pathak, M. A. 1969. Basic aspects of cutaneous photosensitization. In: *Biological Effects of U. V. Radiation.* F. Urbach (ed.). Pergamon Press, Oxford, England.

Pentschew, A. and Garro, F. 1966. Lead encephalo-myelopathy of the suckling rat and its implications on the porphyrinopathic nervous diseases. *Acta Neuropathol. 6:* 266–278.

Perman, E. S. 1958. The effect of ethyl alcohol on the secretion from the adrenal medulla in man. *Acta Physiol. Scand. 44:* 241–247.

Peterka, E. S. et al. 1965. Erythropoietic protoporphyria. I. Clinical and laboratory features in seven new cases. *J.A.M.A. 193:* 1036–1042.

Peters, R. A. 1953. Significance of biochemical lesions in the pyruvate oxidase system. *Br. Med. Bull 9:* 116–122.

Peters, R. A. 1963. *Biochemical Lesions and Lethal Synthesis.* Pergamon Press, Oxford, England.

Phillips, W. E. J. 1971. Naturally-occurring nitrate and nitrite in foods in relation to infant methaemoglobinaemia. *Food Cosmet. Toxicol. 9:* 219–228.

Pirie, A. 1965. A light-catalysed reaction in the aqueous humour of the eye. *Nature 205:* 500–501.

Pullman, A. 1945. A relation between the distribution of electronic charges and the carcinogenic potency of a certain class of hydrocarbons. *Acad. Sci. (Paris) 221:* 140–142.

Pullman, A. 1954. Electronic structure and carcinogenic activity of aromatic hydro-carbons. *Bull. Soc. Chim. (France) 1954:* 595–603.

Pullman, A. and Pullman B. 1955. Electronic structure and carcinogenic activity of aromatic molecules. *New Dev. Adv. Cancer Res. 3:* 117–169.

Rechenberger, J. 1940. Volatile alkylamine in human metabolism. *Z. Physiol. Chem. 265:* 222–232.

Reiffe, B., Lambert, S. M. and Natoff, I. L. 1971. Inhibition of brain cholinesterase by organophosphorus compounds in rats. *Arch. Int. Pharmacodyn. Ther. 192:* 48–60.

Reske, G. and Staueff, J. 1965. Photoreactions and spectral changes of 3,4-benzy-pyrene in aqueous protein and DNA solutions. *Z. Naturforsch. 206:* 15–20.

Richardson, K. E. 1973. The effect of partial hepatectomy on the toxicity of ethylene glycol, glycolic acid, glyoxylic acid and glycine. *Toxicol. Appl. Pharmacol. 24:* 530–538.

Rimington, C. and Quin, J. I. 1934. The photosensitization of animals in South Africa. VII. The nature of the photosensitizing agent in geeldikkop. *J. Vet. Sci. 3:* 137–157.

Rimington, C., Magnus, I. A., Ryan, E. A. and Cripps, D. J. 1967. Phorphyria and photosensitivity. *J. Med. 36:* 29–57.

Ritschel, W. A., and Erni, W. 1977. Influence of temperature of ingested fluid in stomach emptying time. *Int. J. Clin. Pharmacol. Biopharm. 15:* 172–175.

Roberts, J. D. and Caserio, M. C. 1965. *Basic Principles of Organic Chemistry.* W.A. Benjamin. New York.

Roberts, J. A. and Seibold, H. R. 1969. Ethylene glycol toxicity in the monkey. *Toxicol. Appl. Pharmacol. 15:* 624–631.

Rosenfeld, I. and Beath, O. A. 1964. The influence of protein diets on selenium poisoning. *Am. J. Vet. Res. 7:* 52.

Russell, P. T. and Van Bruggen, J. T. 1964. Ethanol metabolism in the intact rat. *J. Biol. Chem. 239:* 719–725.

Saffiotti, U. 1978. Experimental identification of chemical carcinogens, risk evaluation, and animal to human correlations. *Environ. Health 22:* 107–113.

Schantz, E. J. and Sugiyama, H. 1974. The toxins of Clostridium botulinum. In: *Essays in Toxicology.* Vol. 5. W. J. Hays, Jr. (ed.). Academic Press, New York.

Schneiderman, M. A. 1970. A method for determining the dose compatible with some "acceptable" level of risk. In: *Report to the Surgeon General by the Ad Hoc Committee on the Evaluation of Low Levels of Environmental Chemical Carcinogenesis.* U.S. Department of Health, Education and Welfare, Washington, D.C.

Scholtissek, C. 1965. Synthesis of an abnormal ribonucleic acid in the presence of proflavin. *Biochim. Biophys. Acta 103:* 146–159.

Schoor, W. P. 1973. In vivo binding of p,p'-DDE to human serum proteins. *Bull. Environ. Contam. Toxicol. 9:* 70–74.

Schueler, F. W. 1961. The hemicholiniums. *Fed. Am. Soc. Exp. Biol. 20:* 561–599.

Scribner, J. D. 1969. Formation of a sigma complex on a hypothetical rate-determining step in the carcinogenic action of unsubstituted polycyclic aromatic hydrocarbons. *Cancer Res. 29:* 2120–2126.

Selye, H. 1971. Hormones and resistance. *J. Pharm. Sci. 60:* 1–28.

Selye, H. 1972. Mercury poisoning: Prevention by spironolactone. *Science 169:* 775–776.

Sergent, E. 1941. The quail poisonings in the Bible and in present-day Algeria. *Arch. Inst. Pasteur Alger. 19:* 161. (French)

Silverman, W. A., Anderson, D. H., Blanc, W. A. and Crozier, D. N. 1956. A difference in mortality rate and incidence of kernicterus among premature infants allotted to two prophylactic antibacterial regimens. *Pediatrics 18:* 614–625.

Sobel, A. E., Gawron, O. and Kramer, B. 1938. Influence of vitamin D in experimental lead poisoning. *Proc. Soc. Exp. Biol. Med. 38:* 433–437.

Spector, W. S. 1956. *Handbook of Toxicology*. Vol. I. Saunders, Philadelphia.

Spikes, J. D. 1968. Photodynamic action. In: *Photophysiology. Current Topics.* Vol. III. A. C. Giese (ed.). Academic Press, New York.

Spikes, J. D. and Glad, B. W. 1964. Photodynamic action. *Photochem. Photobiol. 3:* 471–487.

Spikes, J. D. and Livingston, R. 1969. The molecular biology of photodynamic action: Sensitized photoautoxidations in biological systems. *Adv. Radiat. Biol. 3:* 29–121.

Stecher, P. G., Finkel, M. J., Siegmund, O. H. and Szafranski, B. M. 1960. *The Merck Index of Chemicals and Drugs*. 7th ed. Merck, Rahway, New Jersey.

Sundblad, L. and Balazs, E. A. 1966. Chemical and physical changes of glycosamino-glycans and glycoproteins caused by oxidation-reduction systems and radiations. In: *The Amino Sugars*. Vol. IIB. E. A. Balazs and R. W. Jeanlog (eds). Academic Press, New York.

Swann, P. F. and Magee, P. N. 1968. Nitrosoamine-induced carcinogenesis. The alkylation of nucleic acids of the rat by N-methyl-N-nitrosourea, dimethylnitro-soamine, dimethyl sulphate and methyl methanesulphonate. *Biochem. J. 110:* 39–47.

Tappeiner, H. V. and Jodlbauer, A. 1904. Cited by Spikes, J. D. 1968. Photodynamic action. In: *Photophysiology. Current Topics.* Vol. III. A. C. Giese (ed.), Academic Press, New York.

Underwood, E. J. 1973. Trace elements. In: *Toxicants Occurring Naturally in Foods*. Committee on Food Protection. National Academy of Sciences, Washington, D.C.

Uraguchi, K. 1971. Pharmacology of Mycotoxins. Pharmacology and Toxicology of Naturally Occurring Toxins, Section 71, 2: 143–299. H. Raskova (ed.). In: *International Encyclopedia of Pharmacology and Therapeutics*. Pergamon, Oxford, England.

Van Duuren, B. L. et al. 1963. Carcinogenicity of epoxides, lactones, and peroxy compounds. *J. Natl. Cancer Inst. 31:* 41–55.

Van Duuren, B. L. et al. 1966. Carcinogenicity of epoxides, lactones, and peroxy compounds. IV. Tumor response in epithelial and connective tissue in mice and rats. *J. Natl. Cancer Inst. 37:* 825–838.

Vettorazzi, G. 1974. 5-Hydroxytryptamine content of bananas and banana products. *Food. Cosmet. Toxicol. 12:* 107–113.

Vogt, W. 1954. Identity of substance DS and 5-hydroxytryptamine. *Arch. Exp. Pathol. Pharmakol. 222:* 427–430. (German)

Vogt, M. 1959. Catecholamines in brain. *Pharmacol. Rev. 11:* 483–489.

Walpole, A. L. 1958. Carcinogenic action of alkylating agents. *Ann. N.Y. Acad. Sci. 68:* 750–761.

Walpole, A. L. et al. 1954. Cytotoxic agents. IV. The carcinogenic actions of some monofunctional ethyleneimine derivatives. *Br. J. Pharmacol. Chemother. 9:* 306–323.

Walsh, M. J., Truitt, E. B., Jr. and Davis, V. E. 1970. Acetaldehyde mediation in the mechanism of ethanol-induced changes in norepinephrine metabolism. *Molec. Pharmacol. 6:* 416–424.

Waser, P. G. 1960. The cholinergic receptor. *J. Pharm. Pharmacol. 12:* 577–594.

Weithe, W. H. 1973. The effect of temperature on the action of drugs. *Annu. Rev. Pharmacol. 13:* 409–425.

Weil, L., James, S. and Buchert, A. R. 1953. Photooxidation of crystalline chymo-trypsin in the presence of methylene blue. *Arch. Biochem. Biophys. 46:* 143–299.

Weiner, I. M. and Madge, G. H. 1964. Renal tubular mechanisms for excretion of organic acids and bases. *Am. J. Med. 36:* 743–762.

Weits, J. 1964. The antagonism between vitamin A and vitamin D. *Voeding 25:* 486–493. (Dutch)

Whittaker, V. P. 1964. Investigations in the storage sites of biogenic amines in the central nervous system. *Prog. Brain Res. 8:* 90–117.

Williams, R. T. 1959. *Detoxication Mechanisms*. 2nd ed. Chapman and Hall, London.

Williams, R. T. 1970. The metabolic pathways of exogenous substances. In: *Metabolic Aspects of Food Safety.* F. J. C. Roe (ed.). Academic Press, New York.

Wogan, G. N., Paglialunga, S. and Newberne, P. M. 1974. Carcinogenic effects of low dietary levels of aflatoxin B_1 in rats. *Food Cosmet. Cosmetol. 12:* 681–685.

Woodward, G., Lange, S. W., Nelson, K. W. and Calvery, H. O. 1941. The acute oral toxicity of acetic, chloracetic, dichloroacetic and trichloroacetic acids. *J. Ind. Hyg. Toxicol. 23:* 78–82.

Wooley, D. E. and Talens, G. M. 1971. Distributions of DDT, DDD, and DDE in tissues of neonatal rats and in milk and other tissues of mother rats chronically exposed to DDT. *Toxicol. Appl. Pharmacol. 18:* 907–916.

Wunderlich, V. 1971. Mechanism of chemical carcinogenesis. Advances and problems. *Arch. Geschwulstforsch. 38:* 310–326. (German)

Wunderlich, V. and Tetzlaff, I. 1970. Alkylation of nuclear DNA of various organs of the rat by nitrosomethyl urea in vivo. *Arch. Geschwulstforch. 35:* 251–258. (German)

Wunderlich, V., Tetzlaff, I., and Graffi, A. 1972. Studies on nitrosodimethylamine: preferential methylation of mitochondrial DNA in rats and hamsters. *Chem. Biol. Interact. 4:* 81–89.

Yamada, C., Clark, A. J. and Swendseid, M. 1967. Actinomycin D effect on amino acid absorption from rat jejunal loops. *Science 158:* 129–130.

Yamanka, Y. and Kono, S. 1974. Brain serotonine turnover in alcoholic mice. *Jpn. J. Pharmacol. 24:* 247–252.

Young, M. 1969. Three topics in placental transport: Placental function during labour. In: Foetus and Placenta. A. Klopper and E. Dicgfalusy (eds). Blackwell, Oxford, England.

Zenda, K., Saneyoshi, M. and Chihara, G. 1965. Biological photochemistry. I. Correlation between the photodynamic behavior and the chemical structure of nucleic acid bases, nucleotides and related compounds in the presence of methylene blue. *Chem. Pharm. Bull. (Tokyo) 13:* 1108–1113.

2

The Toxicological Role of the Gastrointestinal Tract

The gastrointestinal (GI) tract has a major and fundamental influence on the oral toxicity of compounds. The rate of emptying or passage of food through the GI tract, the mechanism by which the compounds are absorbed or excluded by the GI mucosa, and the activities of digestive enzymes and those of the intestinal microflora (Chap. 3) are factors that can affect significantly the toxicity of any compound. These factors individually or collectively can either exacerbate or diminish the toxicity of most compounds.

BASIC PRINCIPLES OF ABSORPTION

The Small Intestines as Main Organ of Absorption

The principal site or organ of absorption of ingested compounds is the small intestine. However, in many cases, the stomach and the colon as well as the oral cavity may also be significant routes for absorption.

The morphology of the small intestine makes it well suited for the absorption of compounds. It is about 3 m long with three distinct functional anatomical parts: the duodenum, the jejunum, and the ileum. The system of folds (folds of Kerkring) in its mucosa is lined with finger- or leaflike projections called villi (0.5–1.5 mm long), which are in turn covered with microvilli about 1 μm long and 0.1 μm wide. The total number of villi in the human small intestine has been estimated at approximately 25 million (Crane 1979). This system gives the small intestine an enormously large absorptive surface. Various estimates of the total absorptive surface area of the human small intestines vary from 200 m^2 (Wilson 1962) to 4500 m^2 (Texter et al. 1968). The microvilli are located on the luminal border of the columnar, absorbing cells lining each villus. In the mouse, there may be as many as 600 microvilli per cell, or 50 million microvilli per mm^2 of mucosal surface.

In the center of each villus is the *lamina propria*, through which a well-developed network of blood and lymphatic capillaries is dispersed. The blood capillaries are lined with a monolayer of endothelial cells. The walls of these capillaries are perforated with fenestrae, which are 20 to 50 nm wide (Bennett et al. 1959). The lacteals can be distinguished from the blood capillaries by having no perforations or basement membrane, and having walls five to six times thicker than those of the blood capillaries. The walls of the lacteals are also lined with endothelial cells, which may be noncontiguous at certain points. It is believed that the gaps in the walls of the lacteals provide for the passage of interstitial fluids and lymph (Palay and Karlin 1959a, b).

These two drainage systems are the major routes for the transport of absorbed substances into the systemic circulation. The gastrointestinal capillaries drain ultimately into the portal vein; the lacteals empty ultimately into the left subclavian vein at the base of the neck through the thoracic duct. The gastrointestinal blood capillaries are the principal conduits for the transport of nutrients other than the lipids (except fatty acids smaller than decanoic acid). The lipids are transported through the lymphatics, which are also important routes for the absorption of certain proteins and fat-soluble xenobiotics (Kamp and Neumann 1975; Sieber 1974, 1976). Thus, as demonstrated in rabbits, the botulinum toxin enters the blood stream via the lymph (May and Whaler 1958). Minerals, electrolytes, and most absorbed organic compounds are transported by way of the gastrointestinal blood capillaries into the portal vein.

The Mechanisms of Intestinal Absorption

Absorption into the intestinal mucosa is a complex process involving: (1) passive diffusion; (2) active transport; (3) mediated or facilitated transport, and (4) pinocytosis. In spite of these processes, the intestinal mucosae are relatively impermeable tissues to many substances, including various electrolytes, many organic compounds, and water-soluble macromolecules such as starches, pectins, and other heteropolysaccharides and hydrocarbons (Crane 1979; Henning 1979; Schanker 1971; Texter et al. 1968).

Passive Diffusion

The nature of the mucosal membrane is such that even passive diffusion of compounds is selective. Five factors govern the passive diffusion of substances: (1) Fick's law; (2) molecular size; (3) lipid solubility; (4) the degree of ionization; (5) the "drag" effect or bulk flow of the absorption of water; and (6) the Donnan distribution effect.

Fick's Law   Many substances may undergo simple diffusion through the water-filled channels in the cell membrane. The average diameter of these pores is estimated by Lindemann and Solomon (1962) to be about 8 Å. Thus, for those molecules that can easily pass through these pores, their rate of diffusion can be predicted by Fick's law

$$J = KA (C_e - C_i)/h \tag{1}$$

$$= PA (C_e - C_i)$$

where

J	=	the rate of diffusion
K	=	the diffusion coefficient
A	=	area of surface of diffusion
h	=	the membrane thickness
C_e and C_i	=	the concentrations of the solute outside and inside the cell, respectively and
P	=	K/h, the permeability coefficient

Fick's law holds quite well for nonelectrolytes such as urea (Lathe 1943). However, an additional mechanism is also operative with substances such as fructose (Riklis and Quastel 1958; Texter et al. 1968) and mannose and xylose (Texter et al. 1968; Verzar 1935), even though their absorption also appears to follow Fick's law. These sugars appear to be absorbed by facilitated diffusion. Simple diffusion through the cell membrane obeying Fick's law generally cannot take place against a concentration gradient, and is not inhibited by substances as dinitrophenol and phlorizin.

Furthermore, there is no competitive absorption with other substances (Friedhandler and Quastel 1955; Levine 1970; Schanker 1961).

Effect of Molecular Size   Figure 1A and B show the influence of molecular size on the absorption of amides and various sugars, respectively, by the intestinal epithelium. In the case of the amides, a steep inverse linear relationship is observed between increasing molecular weights and decreasing rates of absorption (Höber and Höber 1937). This inverse relationship, in the case of the sugars, is less abrupt, probably because the sugars are already poorly absorbed. In this case, even the smallest member of this class of substances already has a high molecular weight. It should also be pointed out that other factors are expected to influence the effect of molecular size on the absorption of these compounds. As discussed in the next sections, lipid solubility and ionization effects may be more important in regulating the passive absorption of compounds through the intestinal tract.

Effect of Lipid Solubility   There are substances which seem to be absorbed through the intestinal tract by passive diffusion even though their molecular size greatly exceeds the postulated average pore size of the intestinal epithelium. It follows that a route of entry through the cell membrane other than through the pores must be available to these molecules. Evidence indicates that these substances enter the cell by "dissolving" into the cellular membrane material, which is highly lipidic in nature (Schanker 1961). Thus, their rate of absorption can be correlated by their solubility in oil or lipid solvents. This fact is illustrated in Table 1, in which the partition coefficients of these substances in heptane or chloroform are compared with their percentage absorption in the gastrointestinal tract (Höber and Höber 1937; Schanker 1959). In general, a direct relationship between lipid solubility and absorbability can be shown, especially with compounds with similar chemical properties, as with barbital and its homologs. Understandably, the correlation is poor when compounds with dissimilar chemical properties, such as aniline and benzoic acid, are compared. Note that these compounds have the same percentage absorption even though aniline is more than 5 times more soluble in heptane and almost 10 times more soluble in chloroform than benzoic acid. The lack of correlation in this case may be due to the fact that in addition to their lipid solubility characteristics, these compounds also behave like weak electrolytes in aqueous medium, and as explained in the next section, the rate of absorption of weak electrolytes through the cell membrane can be markedly affected by a change in pH.

Effect of the Degree of Ionization   As a rule, the cell membrane is also more easily penetrable by uncharged molecules, particularly if they are also more lipid soluble. This phenomenon was observed with a wide range of substances, including weak acids and ammonium salts (Jacobs 1920a, b 1922, 1950), and dyes (Höber 1945). This is particularly true of substances whose absorption is not also mediated by mechanisms (see following) other than simple diffusion. This ability of the cell membrane to regulate in this manner the types of molecules that can enter the cell has been observed repeatedly in the case of the gastrointestinal epithelium (Hogben et al. 1957, 1959; Schanker 1959; 1961; Schanker et al. 1958). Therefore, for many weak electrolytes, which include many natural and synthetic food substances, the pH of the gastrointestinal lumen determines whether or not significant absorption of these substances can occur. In the human being, the gastrointestinal PH varies from pH 2 in the stomach to pH 5.5 to 6.0 in the duodenum, pH 6.0 to 6.5 in the jejunum, pH 6.0 to 6.5 in the ileum, and around pH 8 in the colon.

Thus, the absorbability of weal electrolytes can be roughly predicted from their acid-base properties or their pK values. Figure 2 demonstrates rather dramatically the influence of pH on the absorption of a weak acid and a weak base. Note that in the case of the weak base quinine, the absorption increases as the pH approaches pH 8.4, the pK_b of quinine. It can also be seen that the weak acid 5-nitrosalicylic acid will be

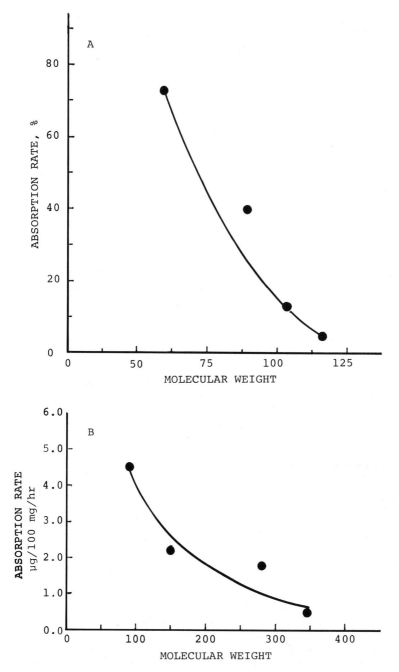

Figure 1. Effect of molecular size on the rate of intestinal absorption. A. Amides. In decreasing rates of absorption: acetamide > lactamide > malonamide > succinamide (Höber and Höber 1937). B. Sugars. In decreasing rates of absorption: glyceraldedyde > arabinose > mannose > lactose (Wilson and Vincent 1955).

Table 1. Correlation Between the Gastrointestinal Absorption Rate and the Partition Coefficient in Oil or Lipid Solvent

Compound	Partition coefficient		Percentage absorbed	Ref.
	Oil/water	Chloroform/water		
Malonamide	0.00008		13	Höber and Höber (1937)
Lactamide	0.00058		67	Höber and Höber (1937)
Succinamide	0.00490		82	Höber and Höber (1937)
Barbital		0.70	12	Schanker (1959)
Butethal		11.70	24	Schanker (1959)
Hexethal		> 100.00	44	Schanker (1959)

poorly absorbed in the intestine where the pH departs considerably from the pK_a of of this compound ($pK_a = 2.3$). However, a different situation may be observed for the same compound in the stomach where the pH is much lower.

Studies with different compounds by Schanker et al. (1958) show that the absorption of weak acids and bases drops significantly for those with pK_a below 2, and pK_b above 9, respectively.

The ratio of ionized and unionized species (A^-/HA) can be calculated from the Henderson-Hasselbalch equation,

$$pH = pK + \log (A^-/HA)$$

where A^- and HA are the ionized and unionized species, respectively. Thus, weak acids with pK values of around 2 will be ionized in the small intestine at pH 6 to the extent of around 10,000:1; and with weak bases with pK_a of around 9, the degree of dissociation will be around 1000:1. It was postulated by Schanker et al. (1958) that the effective mucosal cell pH is around 5; thus, for weak acids, with a pK_a of 2, the degree of dissociation in the cell is around 1000:1 whereas that of weak bases with pK_a values around 9, the degree of dissociation will be around 10,000:1. Therefore, these values appear to be the minimum ratios that must be present for effective absorption of these compounds in the gastrointestinal tract.

Thus, on the basis of the effect of pH in the absorption of compounds, it seems that the degree of toxicity of a weak acid or base may be predicted from the pH of the gastrointestinal tract. This was dramatically demonstrated by Travell (1940) with strychnine. A solution containing 5 mg of this poison at different pH values was injected into the stomach of a cat which was tied to prevent emptying. At pH 8, strychnine is 54% dissociated (uncharged form) and the animal survived for only 24 min; at pH 6 with 1.2% dissociation, the survival time was 89 min. At pH 3, only 0.001% of the poison is dissociated, and in this case the animal survived the otherwise lethal dose.

However, when the total area of absorptive surface and the rate of passage are considered, the pH effect may not have a significant influence on the total amount absorbed. For example, the absorption of a weakly acidic substance may be highly favored in the stomach as the pH of its contents decreases, but more of the substance may be absorbed in the intestines, assuming a normal rate of emptying occurs. This is because even though greater dissociation occurs in the intestines, the pH here permits the existence of a significant proportion of undissociated species, and the large surface area compared to that of stomach results in greater total absorption. The experiments of Magnussen (1968) demonstrate this effect in the case of the weak acids

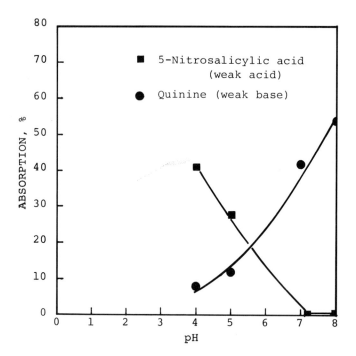

Figure 2. Effect of pH on the absorption of a weak acid and a weak base (Hogben et al. 1959).

phenobarbital and pentobarbital, whereby the intestines absorbed, in 10 min, two to three times the amount absorbed in the stomach in 1 hr. Even though the rate of absorption in the intestines per unit area may be less than that in the stomach, the greater surface area of the former results in greater total absorption.

Now, if attempts are made to diminish absorption of a weak acid by increasing the pH of the stomach (e.g., by use of antacids), such a goal may not be realized because the increased alkalinity hastens stomach emptying into the intestines where greater total absorption occurs as discussed previously (Levine and Walsh 1975).

Therefore, the large surface area of the intestines may obviate any advantage or disadvantage that the dissociation effect may have in the absorption of substances. However, this effect can still have a significant modulating influence in the absorption of compounds, more so when other factors are considered, as discussed elsewhere in the following sections.

The ionization effects explain the poor absorbability by passive diffusion in the small intestines of salts, strong acids, bases, and organic and essential cations such as Fe^{2+}, Fe^{3+}, Mg^{2+}, Ca^{2+}, Zn^{2+}, Mn^{2+}, Co^{2+}, and other trace metallic ions, and the anions, such as PO_4^{3-} and Cl^-. Examples of organic anions that are poorly absorbed are citrates, lactates, and tartrates. The poor absorbability of these substances, in fact, form the physiological basis for their cathartic effects. Similarly, nonabsorbable sulfates and phosphates are cathartics.

Therefore, for nutritionally essential minerals, special mechanisms are necessary for their absorption in order to provide adequate amounts for the animal's nutritional requirements. Those mechanisms have, in fact, been demonstrated for several essential minerals (Texter et al. 1968; Wilson 1962).

However, even with these special mechanisms, absorption of these minerals is limited and is controlled by the body's physiological requirements. These limitations afford a measure of protection for the organism because above a certain level, these substances are quite toxic (Ulmer 1977). These mechanisms involving active or carrier-mediated transport are discussed in the next section.

"Drag" Effect and Bulk Flow of the Absorption of Water   When water and a solution are separated by a semipermeable membrane, water from the compartment with higher activity, that is, with lower solute concentration, will diffuse to the solution of lower water activity (higher solute concentration). If there are pores across the membrane, the tendency of water to flow to the more solute-concentrated solution will produce a hydrostatic flow of water through the pores. This flow roughly follows Poiseuille's law

$$V = 8\pi r^4 P \eta l \qquad\qquad (2)$$

where

V = rate of flow
r = radius of the pore
P = hydrostatic pressure or the osmotic pressure
η = viscosity of solution flowing through the pore
l = length of the pore.

The extent of hydrodynamic flow across the membrane of intestinal epithelium differs from what can result from the osmotic gradients across the membrane of the small intestines (Visscher et al. 1944 a, b). This difference is explained on the basis of the concept of bulk flow (Ussing and Andersen 1956).

The bulk flow can increase transport of solutes through the pore by "dragging" the molecules in the moving stream. Such drag effect was observed, for instance, in the case of urea, mannitol, or creatinine (Fisher 1955) across the intestinal wall in the rat; or in the case of chloride, in the epithelium of the colon of a dog (Cooperstein and Brockman 1959).

The dragging effect may be expected to be greater at the time when absorption by the various mechanisms is at full capacity, so much so that the total osmolar concentration in the plasma is much greater than that in the intestinal lumen. In this case, the greater the total rate of absorption, the higher the total osmolar concentration of the plasma. Consequently, the dragging effect will also be greater. The dragging effect will obviously be expected to be greatly increased when the amount of fluid ingested is large, since, in addition to osmotic effects, the hydrostatic pressure will also be greater.

However, by its very nature, the contribution of the dragging phenomenon to the total absorption of substances is probably much less than those from other mechanisms, e.g., active transport.

Donnan Distribution Effect   This phenomenon will be observed if a pH differential is present on opposite sides of a membrane, which allows only undissociated particles to diffuse out. The process by which this effect causes a net transfer of a substance to another compartment is visualized as follows: A dissociable substance which is free to diffuse through a membrane will ionize in the compartment where this dissociation is favored. This dissociation reduces the concentration of the diffusible substance so that a concentration differential is established. More of the diffusible substance migrates to the other compartment where it can be ionized more favorably until equilibrium between the two compartments with respect to this substance is attained.

The Donnan distribution effect may be a significant factor governing the flow of a weak acid (HA) from the stomach (pH 2 to 4) or the small intestines (pH 4.5 to 6.5) to the blood (pH 7.35 to 7.45). For example, assume a weak acid has a pK of 4. At an intestinal pH of 5, it can be shown from the Henderson-Hasselbalch equation,

$pH = pK + \log(A^-/HA)$, that at equilibrium, $A^-/HA = 10$. If, for the sake of argument, the blood pH is assumed to be 7, in this medium, $A^-/HA = 1000$. It follows that more of HA will diffuse into the blood, and at equilibrium the total amount of (HA + A^-) in the blood will be more than a hundred times the amount remaining in the intestines, assuming no other factors are in effect.

The degree to which this effect will enhance the net transfer of a substance across the gastrointestinal mucosa is highly dependent on the pH differential between the intestinal medium and the blood and the pK of the substance. An example of this type of distribution as shown by the study of Shore et al. (1957), who injected acidic and basic drugs intravenously in dogs. In the gastric juice, where their ionization is favored, the concentration of basic drugs at equilibrium increased to as much as 40 times those in the plasma, whereas acidic drugs, whose ionization is not favored, either were absent or increased in concentrations to no more than six-tenths of those in the plasma. And as shown by Zawoiski et al. (1958), the concentration in the gastric juice of an organic base injected in the dog increased as the pH decreased.

The Donnan distribution effect is apparently less effective in the transfer of weak bases such as some alkaloids from the GI tract to the blood. The reason is that in the blood ionization will be less favorable, so that the concentration differential will be comparatively small, if any.

The Donnan distribution will also occur if one of the charged components in one compartment is a macromolecule too large to diffuse through the membrane. When this molecule dissociates, and one of the particles so formed is freely diffusible, the movement of this particle to the opposite side must be accompanied by a movement in the opposite direction of a particle of the same charge to maintain electrical neutrality. Thus, this may cause the transfer of a different substance to the compartment containing the macromolecule. If, on the other hand, the compartment opposite that containing the macromolecule has freely diffusible positive and negative ions, and the ions are the same as those associated with the macromolecule, then at equilibrium a net increase of these ions will be found in the macromolecule compartment. This type of transfer of charged particle, to a large extent, may not be applicable in the case of the gastrointestinal tract because charged particles are not freely diffusible across the gastrointestinal mucosal membrane. Thus, it becomes necessary that charged substances that are important to life are transported by special mechanisms, as discussed in the next sections.

A net transfer of a substance can also result from the Donnan distribution effect, if in one compartment, a nondiffusible substance, for example a protein, can bind the diffusible molecule. The movement of the diffusible substance bound by the protein will follow Fick's law, since in effect, a large concentration gradient will be present as long as the binding capacity of the protein is not exhausted.

Active Transport

If the gastrointestinal absorption were to rely solely on passive diffusion, the limitations imposed on this process would exclude many compounds, even those essential for the survival of the organism. Those compounds which meet the conditions necessary for passive absorption, in many cases, cannot be absorbed at a rate commensurate with the needs of the body. Furthermore, the requirement of these substances by the body may be such that their concentration in the lumen of the gastrointestinal tract may be lower than that in the blood. Therefore, even though the gastrointestinal epithelium is an "open" membrane, absorption under these conditions would be thermodynamically impossible. Instead of absorption, leakage into the gastrointestinal lumen would result. For many essential substances, the gastrointestinal epithelium is equipped with an active transport process, ensuring adequate absorption of otherwise unabsorbable compounds. Active transport permits the absorption of the compound even against a concentration gradient. This process requires the expenditure of energy.

Exactly how this process is accomplished is still subject to much research. However, certain facts with respect to this process have emerged. Among these is the
existence of a carrier system, possibly proteins which have specificities for certain
kinds of chemical groups and configurations (Crane 1979). This system can also be inhibited by a variety of compounds. For example, the transport of sugars and amino
acids can be inhibited by cyanide, dinitrophenol, malonate, fluoroacetate, arsenate,
copper, acid, and so forth. (Ther and Winne 1971). The carrier system can also be
saturated, and this fact can impose a limit on the rate of absorption, even though the
amount absorbed generally is a function of the dose (Ther and Winne 1971). Many
similar compounds will compete with a carrier system. For example, amino acids will
compete with each other (Lin, et al. 1961; Paine et al. 1960; Pinsky and Geiger 1952;
Spencer and Samiy 1961; Wiseman 1955). Foreign compounds will also compete with the
carrier systems of essential nutrients. This is especially true of substances which
structurally resemble the nutrients, and other endogenous physiologically essential
compounds. Some compounds are inhibitory because their structures contain critical
groups which are necessary for absorption as found in corresponding essential compounds. For example, those resembling the pyrimidines are transported also by the
pyrimidine system (Schanker 1961; Schanker and Tocco 1960; Shanker et al. 1958);
3-O-methylglucose is transported by the glucose transport system (Kimmich 1979;
Texter et al. 1968; Wilson and Vincent 1955). The absorbability of nitrogen mustard—
type drugs is increased when these contain amino acid groups (Bergel 1958).

It has also been shown that the active transport of organic chemicals appears to be
closely associated with the sodium transport. Thus, compounds which inhibit the sodium transport will also inhibit the transport of the organic compounds (Ther and Winne
1971). In this connection, cathartics which also inhibit sodium transport produce diarrhea, partly by the resulting accumulation of sodium salts (Phillips et al. 1965).

This energy-requiring mechanism can be inhibited by interference in the metabolic
source of energy. Thus, cyanides (Agar et al. 1954), dinitrophenol (Friedhandler and
Quastel 1955; Agar et al. 1953), and fluoroacetate (Winter 1953) are inhibitors of
amino acid transport because they, too, are inhibitors of oxidative phosphorylation.
It follows from these results that removal of oxygen will inhibit amino acid transport
(Friedhandler and Quastel 1955) except perhaps in the newborn (Wilson and Lin
1960).

Various sections of the gastrointestinal tract seem to have specific preference for
the active absorption of a compound or groups of compounds. The sugars (Fisher and
Parsons 1949, 1953 a, b) as well as the neutral amino acids (Wiseman 1953) are largely
absorbed in the middle portion of the small intestine, whereas the basic amino acids
are absorbed equally in all parts of the small intestines (Hagihira et al. 1961). Bile
salts (Lack and Weiner 1961) and cobalamin (Booth et al. 1957; Reynell et al. 1957) are
absorbed mostly in the ileum; Ca^{2+} (Schacter and Rosen 1959), Fe^{2+} (Dowdle et al.
1960) and Cl^- (Parsons 1956) are absorbed mostly in the upper small intestines. In
contrast, Na^+ appears to be equally absorbed in all parts of the small intestines and
colon (Curran and Solomon 1957; Parsons 1956; Visscher et al. 1944b); H^+ is absorbed
mostly in the ileum and colon (D'Agostino et al. 1953; Parsons 1956; Wilson and Kazyak
1957).

The active absorption process is of fundamental toxicological interest not only because it is a device for excluding many toxic compounds, even though imperfect, but
also because it is potentially a target of many poisonous substances which are inhibitors of the process in one way or another. From the nutritional standpoint, active
transport being subject to competitive inhibition even among the nutrients is also relevant to the toxic effects of nutrient excesses.

Facilitated Transport

There are transport mechanisms which have the characteristics of active transport
except that the process cannot take place against a concentration gradient. For this

process, the term facilitated diffusion was coined by Danielli (1954). Thus, facilitated diffusion is subject to the saturation phenomena, competitive inhibition of similar compounds, stimulation by sodium ions, and a temperature effect. Some examples of facilitated transport by the intestinal epithelium are D-xylose (Salomon et al. 1961) and 6-deoxy-1,5-anhydro-D-glucitol (Crane et al. 1961). Some workers found that chloride is absorbed by facilitated transport in the frog colon (Cooperstein and Hogben 1959). There are results which suggest that glutamic and aspartic acids are also transported across the intestinal epithelium by facilitated diffusions (Wiseman 1953). The significance of facilitated transport in the absorption of toxic materials in food deserves further investigations. There is evidence which indicates that facilitated transport may also apply to xenobiotics (Fiese and Perrin 1969).

Pinocytosis

Several studies have demonstrated that this absorption process, which was presumed to be confined to lower forms of life, is in fact present in higher forms, especially in the newborn. Clark (1959) demonstrated the ability of suckling animals to absorb whole proteins by phagocytosis during the first 8 postnatal days. This ability completely disappears afterward. The lower segments of the small intestine appear to be the area most associated with this process. The absorption of macromolecules in the form of antibodies, which are essential in producing and enhancing acquired passive immunity, was demonstrated by serological tests in nursing human infants (Ogra et al. 1977). The presence of foreign antigens have been found in the blood of bottle-fed infants (Walker and Isselbacher 1974). Absorption in the rat by pinocytosis of insoluble dye particles (Barnett 1959), triglycerides (Palay and Karlin 1959b), and latex spheres 1000 to 2000 Å in diameter in mice have also been reported.

In adult rats, highly sensitive techniques demonstrated the pinocytosis of trace amounts of foreign proteins (Walker and Isselbacher 1974). Using a precipitin test, Alexander et al. (1936) demonstrated the presence of egg white proteins in the systemic circulation of dogs fed the proteins by stomach tube. These investigators showed conclusively that the route of absorption was via the lymph, through the thoracic duct.

A defect in the intestinal epithelium may also enhance the pinocytosis of macromolecules. Thus, endotoxins from the enteropathogenic *Escherichia coli* (Chap. 15) were found to be pinocytosized by the immature intestinal epithelia of neonatal pigs (Crawford and Leece 1979).

Certainly, this process may explain the absorption of protein toxins and other toxic materials which otherwise would be excluded from the intestinal epithelium for reasons of molecular size alone. Since many toxic substances in foods are macromolecules, their toxicity is related to the ability of the small intestine to absorb them.

Other Sites of Absorption in the Alimentary Canal

Even though the small intestine is the major site of absorption because of its vast absorptive surface, other parts in the alimentary canal may be important sites of absorption for many substances. These other sites are the mouth, the stomach, and the colon.

The Mouth

Experiments with dogs have shown that the mucosa of the oral cavity behaves just like other membranes; their lipid character prevents absorption of many substances. Thus, in the case of several alkaloids, it has been shown that the rate of absorption is roughly proportional to the oil-water partition coeffieients of these substances (Walton 1935, 1944). It also has been shown that lipid-soluble compounds, such as antipyrine, are absorbed to the extent of 30 to 40% in 20 min in the human mouth, whereas lipid-insoluble compounds such as N^1-methylnicotinamide are scarcely absorbed (Schanker 1964).

Because a compound's residence time in the mouth is very short, the toxicological significance of absorption in the mouth may be inconsequential.

The Stomach

Although the area of the mucosal surface of the stomach is much less than that of the small intestine, this organ becomes toxicologically important for substances that are rapidly absorbed. The gastric epithelium allows for rapid absorption of lipid-soluble materials, such as ethanol (Berggren and Goldberg 1940), whereas this lipid membrane rarely permits the absorption of charged particles. Because of the highly acidic nature of its secretion, only weak acids are significantly absorbed and most weak bases are virtually excluded. Thus, such weak acids as barbiturates, salicylates, and phenolics are readily absorbed in the human stomach (Hogben et al. 1957). The pH effect, in the case of weak bases, has already been mentioned in connection with the poisonous effects of strychnine in the experiments of Travell (1940). Other weak bases are also poorly absorbed in the stomach (Schanker 1964). It follows, therefore, that if the gastric secretion were made alkaline by simultaneous intake of, for example, sodium bicarbonate, the absorption of weak bases will be markedly enhanced. This, in fact, was the case in Travell's experiment. This effect was also shown by the works of Hogben et al. (1957) and Schanker et al. (1957).

Because of the large pH differential between the stomach fluids and the plasma, the Donnan distribution effect (pp. 51—52) would probably be highly operative for the absorption of weak acids from the stomach. There is a large pH differential between the stomach content (pH 1—5) and that of plasma (pH 7.2—7.4). The experiment of Shore et al. (1957) demonstrated the partitioning of substances between the gastric juice and the plasma. This partitioning of compounds appears to be a function of their pK_a values. The basic compounds tend to concentrate in the gastric juice rather than in the plasma, whereas the acidic compounds have the opposite tendency.

Since with increasing acidity the rate of emptying from the stomach diminishes (Hunt and Knox 1969), it follows that this organ becomes a major site of absorption of acids as the secretion of HCl from the parietal cells is increased; similarly, substances taken in an acid solution or ingested simultaneously with stronger acids may be absorbed increasingly in the stomach.

The Colon

It has been stated previously that there is significant absorption of compounds in the colon. The epithelium of the colonal lumen behaves much like the small intestines, but unlike the latter, active transport has been demonstrated only with a few substances (Visscher et al. 1944b); for example, sodium and hydrogen ions (D'Agostino et al. 1953).

The colon is also the major site of water absorption. Thus, the dragging effect is probably highly operative in this tissue.

The metabolic activity of the colon microflora may change the absorbability as well as the toxicological properties of a compound. Their effects in transforming the acidity of this organ's secretion as well as the acid-base and lipid solubility properties of the compound itself by metabolic degradation may transform the toxicological characteristics of the food altogether. The subject of the effect of intestinal microflora is discussed in Chapter 3.

FACTORS AFFECTING GASTROINTESTINAL ABSORPTION

It is obvious from the preceding discussion that the various absorption processes can modify the toxicological properties of a compound. Each of these processes may increase or decrease the toxicity. In many instances, the toxicity of compounds absorbed through the intestinal tract is much less than when compounds gain entry through other routes. This is because the gastrointestinal tract imposes certain limitations on their rates of absorption. Most substances absorbed in the alimentary canal must pass through the liver where they can be metabolized to derivatives of lesser or greater toxicity. (It is, therefore, to be expected that the liver, in many instances, is subject to greater toxic injury. The role of the liver with respect to the toxicity of a compound is discussed in Chapter 4.)

Many other factors can influence the absorption of a compound. A number of these will be discussed in the following paragraphs.

Effect of Blood Flow

Obviously, the draining effect of blood will increase the rate of absorption simply from a consideration of Fick's law, since the removal of absorbed substances in the serosal side of the gastrointestinal epithelium will maintain a large concentration gradient. Normally, the rate of blood flow in the portal vein is around 1.2 L/hr/kg (Bradley et al. 1945), and after a meal there is a 30% increase in blood flow through the splanchnic area (Brandt et al. 1955). Therefore, an increased absorption of a toxic compound may result if it is ingested during a meal, assuming that the pH is favorable, and the compound is not bound to other components in the food, preventing its effective absorption. The increase in the absorption of various compounds with increased blood flow is clearly shown in Fig. 3. Note, however, that the rate of absorption as influenced by changes in blood flow rates varies with the nature of the compound. For many compounds, small or moderate changes in blood flow rates, especially in the small intestine, may have little effect on the absorption rate. In part, this is due to the already substantial diversion of the total blood supply to this organ, estimated at 17 to 60% (Levine 1970).

Compounds that have effects on blood flow will generally increase or decrease the absorption rate. Thus, the vasoconstrictive compounds, serotonin, norepinephrine, or vasopressin (Ochsenfahrt et al. 1966; Winne 1966), diminish blood flow, and consequently the absorption of water. This was demonstrated by use of tritiated water. Such a decrease in absorption was observed both in the small intestine (Lembeck et al. 1964) and colon (Sewing et al. 1965) of the rat.

In contrast, ethanol, which increases the blood flow rate, has been shown to increase significantly its absorption in the stomach as well as those of such drugs as phenobarbital or pentobarbital (Magnussen 1968). But the increase in blood flow rate was not large enough to make a significant difference in the rate of absorption of these drugs in the small intestine, which is already highly perfused with blood as noted previously.

However, it was also shown that an increased intestinal blood flow does not necessarily always enhance the absorption of a compound. For example, while epinephrine infused intra-arterially increased the blood flow, it caused a simultaneous decrease in the rate of absorption of glucose and acetylcholine from the intestines (Varro et al. 1967). The reason for these results is not immediately evident.

Blood flow can also influence absorption by its effect on the supply of oxygen and other nutrients. This follows from the fact that active transport requires oxygen. Indeed, there appears to be a critical blood flow rate through the splanchnic area below which active transport ceases (Guthrie and Quastel 1956; Robinson et al. 1964, 1966). The loss of active transport capacity of the intestinal epithelium was also confirmed in intestinal ischemia (Robinson et al. 1965, 1966); such loss of active transport capacity can be prevented by perfusion of the ischemic tissues with solution saturated with oxygen (Guthrie and Quastel 1956; Robinson et al. 1964).

The decrease in blood flow rate by 20 to 30% of normal flow rate for a certain period of time may cause morphological alteration of the intestinal epithelium, resulting

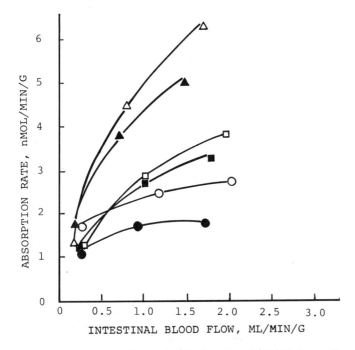

Figure 3. Effect of intestinal blood flow on the absorption of various compounds. (Ther and Winne 1971). ● Urea; ○ Ethylene glycol; ■ Glycerol; □ Methanol; ▲ Aniline; △ ^3H_2O.

in a decrease in intestinal absorption (Ochsenfahrt and Winne 1968, 1969; Winne 1970). The morphological changes of the intestinal epithelium can be detected by the decrease in the active transport of glucose even though normal blood rate is resumed (Winne 1970).

It is clear from the preceding discussion that a normal blood flow rate must be maintained in the intestinal epithelium in order to maintain normal rates of absorption. From the toxicological standpoint, any compound which also increases the blood flow rate may also have an enhanced toxicity. This hypothesis may have some relation to the toxicity of histamine which can cause a short rise in blood flow rate (Winne 1966). It should be expected that the absorption and toxicity of some compounds may decrease in certain disease states accompanied by a decrease in blood flow rate through the intestines. The opposite case may also be true; that is, increased toxicity from increased absorption and flow rates.

Effect of Lymph Flow Rate

The lymph flow rate is about 1 to 2 ml/hr/kg in man, or one-six hundredth to one-thousandth of that of the blood (Bollman et al. 1948; Forth et al. 1969; Reininger and Sapirstein 1957; Yoffey and Courtice 1956). Bulk flow may appear unimportant for those compounds that are transported mostly by way of the blood. However, for highly toxic substances, such as the botulinum toxin, that are transported by this route, the increase or decrease in the lymphatic flow rate may be significant. It has been shown that tripalmitin doubles the lymph flow rate, thus increasing the lymphatic concentration of tetracycline, which normally is absorbed only slightly by the lymph (De Marco and Levine 1969). Does a high fat diet increase the rate of appearance of symptoms in case of botulinum poisoning? Unfortunately, this question remains unanswered.

Gut Motility and Emptying Time

It can be inferred from the preceding discussion that gut motility and the rate of passage and elimination of food from the gastrointestinal tract can influence the rate of absorption of a compound. It is obvious that charged or uncharged substances will be absorbed faster in the stomach or intestines if the residence time in these organs is increased. The opposite effect is equally true with a decrease in residence time (Levine 1970; Levine and Walsh 1975). Therefore, any conditions which decrease or increase gut motility and emptying or passage time will have a corresponding effect on the toxicity of compounds.

The toxicological importance of the rate of emptying may be viewed in another way. As discussed earlier in this chapter, there are mechanisms which will reduce or enhance the toxicity of a compound upon absorption. The final toxicological effect is the algebraic sum of each of these separate effects. For example, a substance may be metabolized in the liver and other tissues to derivatives with lesser or greater toxicity (p. 56); it would also be excreted by the different routes, bound on plasma proteins, or stored in the adipose tissues. It is also possible that metabolism of the substance occurs in the intestines (Chabra 1979; Hoensch et al. 1979). However, toxicity will still occur if, in spite of all these minimizing effects, a sufficient dose of its metabolite(s) reaches and interacts with toxicologically sensitive cell receptors.

If smaller amounts of these substances are presented slowly for absorption in the intestines, there may be sufficient time and several ways to dispose of the undesirable substance. Consequently, a toxicologically insignificant amount, if any, will ultimately reach the receptors. For example, it has been reported that a cold neostigmine hydrobromide solution is significantly more toxic than a warm solution (Ther and Winne 1971). This may be explained by the observation of Gorisch (1967) and by Ritschell and Erni (1977) that cold solutions empty more rapidly from the stomach of rats or dogs than warm solutions. It is obvious that assuming neostigmine hydrobromide is not destroyed in the stomach, as lower emptying time will allow for disposal of a limited load, thus diminishing its toxicity. Substances which delay stomach emptying may have significant effects on the absorption of compounds. For example, the absorption of the weak acid p-aminosalicylic acid (PAS) has been shown to be delayed in human subjects by pretreatment with the antihistamine diphenhydramine (Benadryl), which inhibits stomach emptying (Lavigne and Marchand 1973). Anticholinergic compounds have similar inhibitory effects on stomach emptying (Levine 1970).

The emptying or passage time in the GI tract may present other consequences with respect to the toxicity of compounds. For example, a substance which is made toxic by action of the intestinal microflora may show no toxic effects if it moves slowly through the intestinal tract. The reason is that only small amounts unabsorbed by the intestines would reach the colon where microflora are most abundant. On the other hand, a substance may move rapidly in the gastrointestinal tract for various reasons (e.g., stimulation by cathartics), so that a fraction of the toxic dose is absorbed. The same reasoning applies to stomach emptying for those compounds absorbed in the ileum or colon. The rate of appearance of substances in the colon will also regulate their metabolism by the microflora, influencing their absorption and toxicity.

For substances that are metabolized by intestinal microflora, stagnation of their metabolites may be responsible for damage to the intestinal epithelium. It has been suggested that the lack of colon cancer among the Bantu is due to their propensity for frequent bowel movements, sometimes three or four times per day. The Bantu have a bulky and fibrous diet (Ackerman 1972) and tests have shown that Bantu intestinal transit time for food residues are almost three times as fast as that of the English (Burkitt 1971).

The gastric emptying time may be influenced by the type (Grossman 1950) and volume of the meal (Hunt and MacDonald 1954); the acidity of the gastric content (Hunt and Knox 1969); the neutralization process in the duodenum (Lagerlof et al. 1960); and drugs (Holz 1968) such as the pressor amines, norepinephrine, histamine, and tyramine, and other factors (Levine 1970; Levine and Walsh 1975). These drugs are found in many types of food products (Chaps. 8 and 19) even though their concentrations are often too low to affect intestinal function. They also have potent effects on the motility of the intestines and colon (Holz 1968). Microbial infections of the intestinal wall and other disease syndromes may also affect the intestinal motility. Such diseases produce a rapid transit time of intestinal contents, as in diarrhea, or the opposite effect, as in constipation. These conditions are extreme examples of contrasting effects of gut motility and transit time.

Pathological conditions in the GI tract may affect the integrity of the intestinal mucosa as to influence absorption; for example, lipid absorption (Kowlessar 1975). Because many toxic substances are lipid soluble and are absorbed and transported in association with lipids via the lymphatic system, malabsorption of fats may have far-reaching toxicological implication other than those involving these substances directly.

Diarrhea

Several causes of diarrhea are shown in Table 2. It can originate in either the small intestines or the colon. In most cases, the listed causes result in either malabsorption of the components of the diet owing to damage to the intestinal mucosa, or in defects in the digestive process, particularly when the specific enzymes are missing or less active.

Thus, inflammatory diseases (Aune and White 1951), celiac diseases, gluten-induced enteropathy (Zollinger-Ellison syndrome) (Fordtran et al. 1967), occlusion of the major arteries of the stomach and intestines (Reiner 1964), and stasis in the venous supply (Williams 1971) all result in diarrhea. Excessive amounts of HCl in the intestines (Fordtran 1967), and *congenital alkalosis*, the absence of the usual exchange mechanism between chloride and bicarbonate, also result in malabsorption, and rapid transit of intestinal content (Bieberdorf et al. 1972). In E. coli and *Vibrio cholerae* infections, the diarrhea follows from excessive leakage of fluids into the intestinal lumen; and in the case of cholera, the volume of the stool may be as much as 17 L/day (Watten et al. 1959). The diarrhea in Salmonella infection seems to involve both excessive fluid secretion and malabsorption (Rout et al. 1973). Tumors affecting the acinar cells of the pancreas (Cerda et al. 1970) and the thyroid glands (Berneir et al. 1969) are accompanied by diarrhea. Certain tumors which produce excessive prostaglandins (Williams et al. 1968) or cathecholamines (Rosenstein and Engleman 1963) are accompanied by episodes of diarrhea. There is also diarrhea in diabetes mellitus, which may indicate a degeneration of the sympathetic afferent nerves (Whalen et al. 1969).

Fatty diarrhea (steatorrhea) results when there is a deficiency in bile secretion into the intestinal lumen. This deficiency may result from interference in bile synthesis, blockage of bile flow by gallstones or tumors, or interferences in the enterohepatic circulation of bile (Williams and Sidorov 1971).

Psychological or emotional stresses may be translated into physiological responses, one of which is diarrhea. This is understandable from the involvement of pressor amines (p. 58) in gastrointestinal motility.

Similar general causes mentioned may also apply to colonic diarrhea. Thus, all factors which interfere with the absorptive function of the colon will precipitate diarrhea. Saline cathartics and colon bacterial metabolites of substances undigested in the small intestines may cause hypertonicity of the colon fluids and, consequently, osmotic type diarrhea.

The so-called nervous diarrhea is observed in persons with irritable colon. In this case, emotional stress may affect colon motility, often distinguished by a reduction in contractile activity of the distal colon (Connell 1962). Contractile activity in persons afflicted with diarrhea can be increased by physical activity after a meal, or with certain drugs such as prostigmine (Misiewicz et al. 1966). The effect of food in increasing colonic activity may be hormonally mediated (Haldstock and Misiewicz 1970; Connell and McKelvy 1970).

Table 2. Selected Causes of Diarrhea Involving Food and Drinking Water

Type	Example of causation	Food involved	Ref.
Parasitic diseases			
Amebiasis	Entamoeba histolytica	Infected food and water	Craig (1944)
Schistosomiasis	Schistosoma mansoni	Infected water	Bockus (1944)
Tape worm infestation	Diphyllobothrium-latum	Raw fish	Belding (1952)
	Taenia saginata	Undercooked beef	Belding (1952)
	Taenia solium	Undercooked pork	Augustine and Neva (1958)
Liver Fluke Infestation	Fasciola spp.	Raw liver and infected vegetables; raw fish	Craig (1944)
	Fasciolopsis buski	Raw water plants	Belding (1952)
Trichinosis	Trichinella spiralis	Undercooked pork	Freies (1951)
Enteric bacterial diseases	See Chaps. 12-14		
Mycetism	See Chap. 10		
Metal poisoning	See Chap. 16		
Food allergy	Various foods See Chap. 5		Freies (1951), Ingelfinger et al. (1949), Johnstone (1954)
Malabsorption syndrome			
Disaccharide intolerance	Absent or inactive disaccharides	Disaccharides	Holzel et al. (1959), Weijers et al. (1960)
Steatorrhea	Impaired fat absorption from various causes	Fatty foods	
Gluten-gliadin induced enteropathy	Gluten or gliadin	Wheat, rye, oats, barley	Bayless et al. (1964), Frazer et al. (1959), Sleisenger et al. (1953), Weijers and Van de Kamer (1960), Weijers et al. (1960)
Milk sensitivity	β-Globulin fraction of milk	Milk and milk products	Davidson (1958)

Constipation

The opposite of rapid transit of intestinal content is constipation. This condition is identified by infrequent defecation, hard fecal matter with straining at defecation, or with the feeling of incompleteness of bowel movement. Children and the elderly are the frequent victims of constipation. A sampling of the elderly in one study showed a 17 to 22% incidence of constipation (Avery-Jones and Godding 1972). Constipation may result from personal habits such as dietary faddism, lack of exercise, and avoidance of bowel movements. External conditions which interfere with normal defecation may also lead to constipation.

There is evidence which suggests that the increased incidence of constipation in Western society may be related to the low fiber diets in these populations (Cummings 1973). The results reported by Burkitt (1971) show that low fiber diets diminish intestinal transit time compared to high fiber diets. These low fiber diets have been implicated in the high incidence of diverticulitis, appendicitis, and colon cancer in Western societies (Bralow and Brooks 1974). In this respect, the genetic basis for these maladies is discounted by the observation that black Africans living in the United States have the same incidence of colon cancer as the Caucasians (Bralow and Brooks 1974). Diseases of the colon and rectum as well as those of neurological, endocrine, and metabolic origin (Avery-Jones and Godding 1972) may cause constipation. Strangely enough, diabetes and irritable colon disease can cause diarrhea in some cases and constipation in others.

Just as emotions can induce diarrhea, depression and chronic psychoses may result in constipation. It is obvious that psychological conditions leading to decreased food intake may produce constipation.

Certain forms of poisoning, such as lead poisoning, and medications, such as antacids and opiates, can also cause constipation.

It is also strange that some diseases caused by opposing mechanisms, for example, hypothyroidism and hyperthyroidism, both lead to constipative defects in the colon. It is understandable that metabolic disturbances leading to dehydration and debility, and iatrogenic causes, such as immobilization following surgery, anesthesia, and other nonsurgical illnesses may result in constipation (Levine 1978).

Whatever the cause may be in constipation, toxic food substances, especially if they are absorbed slowly in the colon, may reside in this organ longer with toxicological consequences. This is particularly true if such substances are metabolized by gastrointestinal microorganisms. The role of intestinal microflora in the toxicity of compounds is discussed in Chapter 3.

Chemical Factors Affecting Absorption

Chemicals may affect the absorption of compounds by (1) formation of insoluble precipitates, or complexes with specific substances, or formation of chelates which facilitate or inhibit absorption and solubilization; (2) competition for binding or carrier proteins involved in absorption; and (3) modification of the motility or absorptive capacity of the gastrointestinal mucosa.

Examples of the formation of insoluble precipitates are given in Chapter 11 in the case of phytates and oxalates reacting with bivalent metals and in Chapter 8, in the case of nonabsorbable complexes as exemplified by gossypol, which reacts with iron, amino acids, and proteins. Insoluble precipitates may also be formed by phosphates, fatty acids, and alkalis (e.g., antacids) reacting with polyvalent metals. Phosvitin in egg yolks inhibits iron absorption by complexation (Moore and Dubach 1951).

Chelation appears to increase absorption of certain substances. For example, citric acid has been shown to increase the absorption of lead (Graber and Wei 1974). The absorption of dicoumarol is enhanced by chelation with magnesium (Ambre and Fischer 1973). Similarly, in addition to its reducing effect, ascorbic acid has been shown to enhance the absorption of iron by chelation (Cook and Monsen 1977). In contrast, ethylenediaminetetraacetic acid (EDTA) can inhibit iron absorption significantly, especially with an EDTA to iron ratio of 1:1 or higher (Cook and Monsen 1976). This inhibition can counteract even the positive effect of ascorbic acid (Monsen and Page 1978). This may be related to the modification of the absorptive capacity of the GI mucosa, as discussed elsewhere in this section. The formation of insoluble chelates such as those formed between tetracyclines and polyvalent metals (Kunin and Finland 1961) would naturally diminish absorption not only of the metal but also of the chelator as well. Removal of the metal by other means, say, by soap formation, should then enhance the absorption of the chelator. For example, tripalmitin, which can form soaps with calcium following lipase digestion, enhances the absorption of tetracyclines (De Marco and Levine 1969).

Thus, these interactions (i.e., precipitation and chelation) have immediate influence on the absorption of two substances. It can be presumed that the coprecipitation phenomenon, which is well known to the analytical chemists, may increase the range of substances whose absorption may be influenced by the occurrence of the precipitation process. The amount of substances coprecipitated, of course, depends on the volume and nature of the precipitates as well as the nature of the substances being coprecipitated.

Solubilization in a nonabsorbable medium such as mineral oil may also diminish absorption of the dissolved substances. Poorly absorbed surfactants were observed to inhibit or retard absorption of dissolved substances (Hurwitz et al. 1963).

Competition for carrier proteins is discussed in connection with active transport of compounds (discussed later in this chapter). In this connection, similarity in general structure may be sufficient to influence absorption, as exemplified by the competition between pyrimidines (Schanker and Tocco 1962) and steroids such as hydrocortisone and the convallotoxin (Lauterbach 1967). Such competition is evident, for example, in the absorption of trace metals such as lead and cadmium (Sandstead 1977). Thus, the intestinal absorption of lead and cadmium is inhibited by high levels of calcium and zinc and possibly by other metals as well. Iron (Seely et al. 1972) and zinc (Evans 1973) can depress copper absorption; the latter, in turn, has an inhibiting effect on the absorption of zinc (Evans 1973). Similarly, cobalt interferes in the absorption of iron (Thompson et al. 1971).

Many chemicals can modify gut motility as discussed previously in connection with diarrhea, constipation, and stomach emptying. In so doing, these chemicals influence gastrointestinal absorption.

Chemicals can also modify the absorptive capacity of the intestinal mucosa by interaction with its structural constituents. Such modification is indicated by the effects of lectins in the intestinal absorption of various substances, as discussed in Chapter 9. Lectins have been shown to bind strongly with specific receptors in cell membranes. There is evidence that these receptors may involve the sialic acid-containing components of the cell membrane, such as the mucoproteins (Jaffe 1969).

The aforementioned chelator, EDTA, has been shown to increase the absorption of a wide range of substances such as mannitol, sulfanilic acid, and decamethonium (a quarternary ammonium compound) (Schanker and Johnson 1961), phenol red (Tidball 1964), salicylic acid (Shrewsbury 1977), and even macromolecules such as inulin (Schanker and Johnson 1961) and heparin and other heparinoids (Windsor and Cronheim 1961). This effect apparently occurs only at lower concentrations (e.g., at 5 mg/ml) and shorter exposure time of the intestinal mucosa because at higher levels (e.g., over 10 mg/ml) absorption is decreased (Shrewsbury 1977). It appears that EDTA causes changes in epithelial structure (presumably by chelation of calcium or magnesium), consequently, as observed by electron microscopy, there is a loosening of the intercellular binding between the epithelial cells of the intestinal mucosa (Shrewsbury 1977). This creates a wider channel so as to admit various substances (Cassidy and Tidball 1967) and even macromolecules, as mentioned earlier. At higher concentrations, the intercellular binding substance is greatly weakened; as a result the mucosal barrier is disrupted and the villi are damaged. Consequently the net absorptive area and the degree of absorption of compounds are decreased (Shrewsbury 1977).

The absorptive capacity of the intestinal mucosa may be affected by changes in the acidity of the intestinal mucosa. Thus, compounds (e.g., certain sulfonamides) which inhibit carbonic anhydrase will result in a decrease in intestinal pH. In this case, the absorption of weakly acidic compounds may be increased and that of the basic ones decreased (Schnell and Miya 1970). Carbonic anhydrase (CA), it should be recalled, catalyzes the rapid decomposition of carbonic acid (H_2CO_3) or bicarbonate anion (HCO_3^-) to CO_2 and water:

$$H^+ + HCO_3^- \overset{CA}{\rightleftharpoons} H_2CO_3 \overset{CA}{\rightleftharpoons} CO_2 + H_2O$$

Thus, its inhibition can, understandably, cause an increase in tissue pH.

Metabolism of compounds in the intestinal mucosa has been mentioned earlier. This metabolic activity may have a large influence on the amount of compound reaching the systemic circulation when only small doses are internalized into the mucosal cells, commensurate with the activity of the metabolizing enzymes. Those substances, therefore, which inhibit or stimulate the activity of enzymes, or induce their biosynthesis must necessarily influence the rate at which compounds react with target sites in the body.

The general metabolic integrity of the GI mucosal tissues is essential to their structural and functional status. Any substance or condition which destroys the metabolic integrity of these tissues will have an adverse effect on their function and structure. Thus, benzmalecene, which inhibits enzymes of the Krebs cycle has been shown to inhibit absorption of various compounds (Lack and Weiner 1961). Inhibition of protein synthesis can similarly retard the absorption of many substances requiring protein carriers.

This process alone with its attendant modifiers may explain partly the variability and complexity of toxicological response. Nevertheless, unraveling the factors involved in gastrointestinal absorption provides a sound basis for assessing the toxic potential of any given compound, particularly if its properties are known.

REFERENCES

Ackerman, L. V. 1972. Some thoughts on food and cancer. *Nutr. Today* 7: 2−9.

Agar, W. T., Hird, F. J. R. and Sidhu, G. S. 1953. The active absorption of amino acids by the intestine. *J. Physiol.* (London) 121: 255−263.

Agar, W. T., Hird, F. J. R. and Sidhu, G. S. 1954. The uptake of amino acids by the intestine. Biochim. *Biophys. Acta* 14: 80−84.

Alexander, H. L., Shirley, K. and Allen, D. 1936. Route of ingested egg white to systemic circulation. *J. Clin. Invest.* 15: 163−167.

Ambre, J. J. and Fischer, L. J. 1973. Effect of coadministration of aluminum and magnesium hydroxides on absorption of anticoagulants in man. *Clin. Pharmacol. Ther.* 14: 231−237.

Augustine, D. L. and Neva, F. A. 1958. The diagnosis and treatment of intestinal parasitism. *Med. Clin. North Am.* 42: 1387−1399.

Aune, E. F. and White, B. V. 1951. Gastrointestinal complications of irradiation for carcinoma of the uterine cervix. *J. A. M. A.* 147: 831−834.

Avery-Jones, F. A. and Godding, E. W. 1972. *Management of Constipation*. Blackwell, Oxford, England.

Barnett, R. J. 1959. The demonstration with the electron microscope of the end-products of histochemical reactions in relation to the fine structure of cells. *Exp. Cell Res.* (Suppl) 7: 65−89.

Bayless, T. W., Walter, W. and Barber, R. 1964. Disaccharidase deficiencies in tropical sprue. *Clin. Res.* 12: 445.

Belding, D. L. 1952. *Textbook of Clinical Parasitology.* 2nd Ed. Appleton-Century-Crofts, New York.

Bennett, H. S., Luft, J. H. and Hampton, J. C. 1959. Morphological classifications of vertebrate blood capillaries. *Am. J. Physiol.* 196: 381–390.

Bergel, F. 1958. Design of alkylating agents for selectivity of action. *Ann. N.Y. Acad. Sci.* 68: 1238–1245.

Berggren, S. M. and Goldberg, L. 1940. Absorption of ethyl alcohol from the gastrointestinal tract as a diffusion process. *Acta Physiol. Scand.* 1: 246–270.

Berneir, J. J., Ramband, J. C., Cattan, D. and Prost, A. 1969. Diarrhoea associated with medullary carcinoma of the thyroid. *Gut* 10: 980–985.

Bieberdorf, F. A., Gorden, P. and Fordtran, J. S. 1972. Pathogenesis of congenital alkalosis and diarrhea. *J. Clin. Invest.* 51: 1958–1968.

Bockus, H. L. 1944. *Gastroenterology.* 1st Ed. Saunders, Philadelphia.

Bollman, J. L., Cain, J. C. and Grindlay, J. H. 1948. Techniques for the collection of lymph from the liver, small intestines, or thoracic duct of the rat. *J. Lab. Clin. Med.* 33: 1349–1352.

Booth, C. C., Chanarin, L., Anderson, B. B. and Mollin, D. L. 1957. The site of absorption and tissue distribution of orally administered Co^{56}-labelled vitamin B_{12} in the rat. *Br. J. Haematol.* 3: 253–261.

Bradley, S. E. Ingelfinger, F. J., Bradley, G. P. and Curry, J. J. 1945. The estimation of hepatic blood flow in man. *J. Clin. Invest.* 24: 890–897.

Bralow, S. P. and Brooks, F. P. 1974. Gastrointestinal cancer. In: *Gastrointestinal pathophysiology.* F. P. Brooks (ed.). Oxford Univ. Press, London.

Brandt, J. L. et al. 1955. The effect of oral protein and glucose feeding on splanchnic blood flow and oxygen utilization in normal and cirrhotic subjects. *J. Clin. Invest.* 34: 1017–1025.

Burkitt, D. P. 1971. Epidemiology of the colon and rectum. *Cancer* 28: 3–13.

Cassidy, M. M. and Tidball, C. S. 1967. Cellular mechanism of intestinal permeability alterations produced by chelation depletion. *J. Cell Biol.* 32: 685–698.

Cerda, J. J. Raffensperger, E. C. and Rawnsley, H. M. 1970. Choleralike syndrome and pancreatic islet cell tumors. *Med. Clin. North Am.* 54: 567–575.

Chabra, R. S. 1979. Intestinal absorption and metabolism of xenobiotics. *Environ. Health Perspect.* 33: 61–69.

Clark, S. L., Jr. 1959. The ingestion of proteins and colloidal materials by columnar absorptive cells of the small intestine in suckling rats and mice. *J. Biophys. Biochem. Cytol.* 5: 41–50.

Connell, A. M. 1962. The motility of the pelvic colon. Part II. Paradoxical motility in diarrhoea and constipation. *Gut* 3: 342–348.

Connell, A. M. and McKelvy, S. T. D. 1970. The influence of vagotomy on the colon. *Proc. R. Soc. Med.* (Suppl.) 63: 7–9.

Cook, J. D. and Monsen, E. R. 1976. Food iron absorption in human subjects. II. The effect of EDTA on the absorption of dietary non-heme iron. *Am. J. Clin. Nutr.* 29: 614–620.

Cook. J. D. and Monsen, E. R. 1977. Vitamin C, the common cold, and iron absorption. *Am. J. Clin. Nutr.* 30: 235–241.

Cooperstein, I. L. and Brockman, S. K. 1959. The electrical potential difference generated by the large intestines. The relation to electrolyte and water transfer. *J. Clin. Invest.* 38: 435–442.

Cooperstein, I. L. and Hogben, C. A. M. 1959. Ionic transfer across the isolated frog large intestine. *J. Gen. Physiol.* 42: 461–473.

Craig, C. F. 1944. *The Etiology, Diagnosis and Treatment of Amebiasis.* Williams & Wilkins, Baltimore.

Crane, R. K. 1979. Intestinal structure and function related to toxicology. *Environ. Health Perspect.* 33: 3–8.

Crane, R. K., Miller, D. and Bihler, L. 1961. The restriction on possible mechanisms of intestinal active transport of sugars. In: *Membrane Transport and Metabolism Symposium*. A. Kleinzeller and A. Kotyk (eds.). Publishing House of the Czechoslovak Academy of Science, Prague.

Crawford, P. C. and Leece, J. G. 1979. Internalization of endotoxin (CPS) by Enterocytes of neonatal pigs inoculated with Eserichia coli. Abst. Proc. 79th Ann. Meet. Am. Soc. Microbiol.

Cummings, J. H. 1973. Dietary fibre. *Gut* 14: 69–81.

Curran, P. F. and Solomon, A. K. 1957. Ion and water fluxes in the ileum of rats. *J. Gen. Physiol.* 41: 143–168.

D'Agostino, A., Leadbetter, W. F. and Schwartz, W. B. 1953. Alterations in the ionic composition of isotonic saline solutions instilled into the colon. *J. Clin. Invest.* 32: 444–448.

Danielli, J. F. 1954. Present position in the field of facilitated diffusion and selective active transport. In: *Recent Developments in Cell Physiology*. Proc. 7th Symposium Colston, Research Soc. University of Bristol. J. A. Kitching (ed.), Academic Press, New York.

Davidson, J. 1958. Clinical conference: The celiac syndrome. *Pediatrics* 21: 508–511.

DeMarco, T. J. and Levine, R. R. 1969. The role of the lymphatics in the intestinal absorption and distribution of drugs. *J. Pharmacol. Exp. Ther.* 169: 142–151.

Dowdle, E. B., Schachter, D. and Schenker, H. 1960. Active transport of Fe^{59} by everted segments of rat duodenum. *Am. J. Physiol.* 198: 609–613.

Evans, G. W. 1973. Copper homeostasis in the mammalian system. *Physiol. Rev.* 53: 535–570.

Fiese, G. and Perrin, J. H. 1969. Further investigations into the absorption of dextromethorphan from the rat stomach. *J. Pharm. Sci.* 58: 599–601.

Finch, L. R. and Hird, F. J. R. 1962. The uptake of amino acids by isolated segments of rat intestine. II. A survey of affinity for uptake from rates of uptake and competition for uptake. *Biochim. Biophys. Acta* 43: 278–287.

Fisher, R. B. and Parsons, D. S. 1953a. Glucose movements across the wall of the rat small intestine. *J. Physiol.* (London) 119: 210–223.

Fisher, R. B. and Parsons, D. S. 1953b. Galactose absorption from the surviving small intestine of the rat. *J. Physiol.* (London) 119: 224–232.

Fisher, R. B. 1955. The absorption of water and of some small solute molecules from the isolated small intestine of the rat. *J. Physiol.* (London) 130: 655–664.

Fisher, R. B. and Parsons, D. S. 1949. Glucose absorption from surviving rat small intestine. *J. Physiol.* (London) 110: 281–293.

Fordtran, J. S. 1967. Speculations on the pathogenesis of diarrhea. *Fed. Proc. Fed. Am. Soc. Exp. Biol.* 26: 1405–1414.

Fordtran, J. S. Rector, F. C., Locklear, T. W. and Ewton, M. F. 1967. Water and solute movement in the small intestine. *J. Clin. Invest.* 47: 884–900.

Forth, W., Furukawa, E. and Rummel, W. 1969. Comparative studies of the absorption and elimination of tritium-labelled cardiac glycosides. *Arch. Pharmakol. Exp. Pathol.* 263: 206–208.

Frazer, A. C. et al. 1959. Gluten-induced enteropathy. The effect of partially digested gluten. *Lancet* 2: 252–255.

Freies, J. H. 1951. Factors influencing clinical evaluation of food allergy. *Pediatr. Clin. North Am.* 6: 867.

Friedhandler, L. and Quastel, J. H. 1955. Absorption of sugars from isolating surviving intestine. *Arch. Biochem.* 56: 412–423.

Gorisch, V. 1967. The influence of temperature on stomach emptying. Ost. Apoth. Ztg. 21: 20–22. (German)

Gould, S. E. 1945. *Trichinosis*. Thomas, Springfield, Illinois.

Graber, B. T. and Wei, E. 1974. Influence of dietary factors on the gastrointestinal absorption of lead. *Toxicol. Appl. Pharmacol.* 21: 685–691.

Granger, D. N. et al. 1980. Role of the intestinal matrix during intestinal volume absorption. *Am. J. Physiol.* 238: G183—189.

Grossman, M. I. 1950. Gastrointestinal hormones. *Physiol. Rev.* 30: 33—90.

Guthrie, J. E. and Quastel, J. H. 1956. Absorption of sugars and amino acids from isolated surviving intestine after experimental shock. *Arch. Biochem.* 62: 485—496.

Hagihira, H., Lin, E. C. C. and Wilson, T. H. 1961. Active transport of lysine, ornithine, arginine, and cystine by the intestine. *Biochem. Biophys. Res. Commun.* 4: 478—481.

Haldstock, D. J. and Misiewicz, J. J. 1970. Factors controlling colonic motility. Colonic pressures and transit after meals in patients with total gastrectomy, pernicious anemia or duodenal ulcer. *Gut* 11: 100—110.

Henning, S. J. 1979. Biochemistry of intestinal development. *Environ. Health Perspect.* 33: 9—16.

Höber, R. 1945. *Physical Chemistry of Cells and Tissues.* Blakiston, Philadelphia.

Höber, R. and Höber, J. 1937. Experiments on the absorption of organic solutes in the small intestine of rats. *J. Cell Comp. Physiol.* 10: 401—422.

Hoensch, H. P., Hutt, R. and Hartmann, F. 1979. Biotransformation of xenobiotics in human intestinal mucosa. *Environ. Health Perspect.* 33: 71—78.

Hogben, C. A. M., Schanker, L. S., Tocco, D. J. and Brodie, B. B. 1957. Absorption of drugs from the stomach. II. The human. *J. Pharmacol. Exper. Ther.* 120: 540—545.

Hogben, C. A. M., Tocco, D. J., Brodie, B. B. and Schanker, L. S. 1959. On the mechanism of intestinal absorption of drugs. *J. Pharmacol. Exper. Ther.* 125: 275—282.

Holdstock, D. J. and Misiewicz, J. J. 1970. Factors controlling colonic motility: Colonic pressures and transit after meals in patients with total gastrectomy, pernicious anemia or duodenal ulcer. *Gut* 11: 100—110.

Holz, S. 1968. Drug action on the digestive system. *Annu. Rev. Pharmacol.* 8: 171—186.

Holzel, A., Schwarz, V. and Sutcliffe, K. W. 1959. Defective lactose absorption causing malnutrition in infants. *Lancet* 1: 1126—1128.

Hunt, J. N. and Knox, M. T. 1969. The slowing of gastric emptying by nine acids. *J. Physiol. (Lond.)* 201: 161—179.

Hunt, J. N. and MacDonald, I. 1954. The influence of volume on gastric emptying. *J. Physiol.* (London) 126: 459—474.

Hurwitz, A. R., DeLuca, P. P. and Kostenbauder, H. B. 1963. Binding of organic electrolytes by a nonionic surface active agent. *J. Pharm. Sci.* 52: 893.

Ingelfinger, J. F., Lowell, F. C. and Franklin, W. 1949. Gastrointestinal allergy. *N. Engl. J. Med.* 241: 303—308.

Jacobs, M. H. 1920a. To what extent are the physiological effects of carbon dioxide due to hydrogen ions? *Am. J. Physiol.* 51: 321—331.

Jacobs, M. H. 1920b. The production of intracellular acidity by neutral and alkaline solutions containing carbon dioxide. *Am. J. Physiol.* 53: 457—463.

Jacobs, M. H. 1922. The influence of ammonium salts on cell reaction. *J. Gen. Physiol.* 5: 181—188.

Jacobs, M. H. 1950. Surface properties of the erythrocyte. *Ann. New York Acad. Sci.* 50: 824—834.

Jaffe, W. G. 1969. Hemagglutinins. In: *Toxic Constituents of Plant Foodstuffs.* J. E. Liener (ed.), Academic Press, New York.

Johnstone, D. E. 1954. Symposium on pediatric allergy: Allergic celiac syndrome. *Pediatr. Clin. North Am.* 1: 1007-1016.

Kamp, J. P. and Neumann, H. G. 1975. Absorption of carcinogens into the thoracic duct lymph of the rat: Aminostilbene derivatives and 3-methylcholanthrene. *Xenobiotica* 5: 717—727.

Kimmich, G. A. 1979. Intestinal transport: Studies with isolated epithelial cells. *Envir. Health Perspect.* 33: 37–44.

Kowlessar, O. D. 1975. Intestinal malabsorption. In: *Functions of the Stomach and Intestine.* M. H. F. Friedman (ed.), University Park Press, Baltimore.

Kunin, C. M. and Finland, M. 1961. Clinical pharmacology of the tetracycline antibiotics. *Clin. Pharmacol. Ther.* 2: 51–69.

Lack, L. and Weiner, L. M. 1961. In vitro absorption of bile salts by small intestine of rats and guinea pigs. *Am. J. Physiol.* 200: 313–317.

Lagerlöf, H. O. et al. 1960. The neutralization process in duodenum and its influence on the gastric emptying in man. *Acta Med. Scand.* 168: 269–284.

Lathe, G. H. 1943. The effect of the concentration of different substances in the intestinal contents on their absorption from the small intestines. *Rev. Canad. Biol.* 2: 134–142.

Lauterbach, F. 1967. On the differences in mechanisms of the enteric absorption of cardiotonic steroids and other drugs. *Arch. Pharmakol. Exp. Pathol.* 257: 432–457. (German)

Lavigne, J.-G. and Marchand, C. 1973. Inhibition of the gastrointestinal absorption of p-aminosalicylate (PAS) in rats and humans by diphenhydramine. *Clin. Pharmacol. Ther.* 14: 404.

Lembeck, F., Sewing, K.-Fr. and Winne, D. 1964. The influence of 5-hydroxytryptamine on the resorption of tritium-water (HTO) from rat colon in vivo. *Arch. Exp. Pathol. Pharmakol.* 252: 286–290. (German)

Levine, R. R. 1970. Factors affecting gastrointestinal absorption of drugs. *Am. J. Digest. Dis.* 15: 171–188.

Levine, R. R. and Walsh, C. T. 1975. Drug interactions in the gastrointestinal tract. In: *Functions of the Stomach and Intestines.* M. H. F. Friedman (ed.), University Park Press, Baltimore.

Lin, E. C. C., Hagihira, H. and Wilson, T. H. 1961. Active transport of amino acids by hamster intestines. *Fed. Proc. Fed. Am. Soc. Exp. Biol.* 20: 243.

Lindemann, B. and Solomon, A. K. 1962. Permeability of luminal surface of intestinal mucosal cells. *J. Gen. Physiol.* 45: 801–810.

Magnussen, M. P. 1968. The effect of ethanol on the gastrointestinal absorption of drugs in the rat. *Acta Pharmacol. Toxicol.* 26: 130–144.

May, A. J. and Whaler, B. C. 1958. The absorption of Clostridium botulinum type A toxin from the alimentary canal. *Br. J. Exp. Pathol.* 39: 307–316.

Misiewicz, J. J., Connell, A. M. and Pontes, F. A. 1966. Comparison of the effect of meals and prostigmine on the proximal and distal colon in patients with and without diarrhea. *Gut* 7: 468–473.

Monsen, E. R. and Page, J. F. 1978. Effects of EDTA and ascorbic acid on absorption of iron from an isolated rat intestinal loop. *J. Agric. Food Chem.* 26: 223–226.

Moore, C. V. and Dubach, R. 1951. Observations on the absorption of iron from foods tagged with radio iron. *Trans. Assoc. Am. Physicians* 64: 245–256.

Ochsenfahrt, H. and Winne, D. 1968. Intestinal blood flow and drug absorption from the rat jejunum. *Life Sci.* 7: 493–498.

Ochsenfahrt, H. and Winne, D. 1969. Influence of blood flow on the absorption of drugs from the jejunum of the rat. *Arch. Pharmakol. Exp. Pathol.* 264: 55–75.

Ochsenfahrt, H., Winne, D., Sewing K.-Fr. and Lembeck, F. 1966. Secretion of tritiated water in jejunal loops of rats under the influence of 5-HT and noradrenaline. *Arch. Pharmakol. Exp. Pathol.* 254, 461–469.

Ogra, S. S., Weintraub, D. and Ogra, P. L. 1977. Immunological aspects of human colustreum and milk. III. Fate and absorption of cellular and soluble components in the gastrointestinal tract of the newborn. *J. Immunol.* 119: 205–248.

Osterhout, W. J. V. 1925. Is living protoplasm permeable to ions? *J. Gen. Physiol.* 8: 131–146.

Paine, C. M., Newman, H. J. and Taylor, M. W. 1959. Intestinal absorption of methionine and histidine by the chicken. *Am. J. Physiol.* 197: 9–12.

Palay, S. L. and Karlin, L. J. 1959b. An electron microscopic study of the intestinal villus. II. The pathway of fat absorption. *J. Biophys. Biochem. Cytol.* 5: 373–384.

Parsons, D. S. 1956. The absorption of bicarbonate-saline solutions by the small intestine and colon of the white rat. *Q. J. Exp. Physiol.* 41: 410–420.

Phillips, R. A., Love, A. H. G., Mitchell, T. G. and Neptune, E. M. 1965. Cathartics and the sodium pump. *Nature* 206: 1367–1368.

Pinsky, J. and Geiger, E. 1952. Intestinal absorption of histidine as influenced by tryptophan in the rat. *Proc. Soc. Exp. Biol. Med.* 81: 55–57.

Pratt, E. L. 1958. Food allergy and food intolerance in relation to the development of good eating habits. *Pediatrics* 21: 642–648.

Reiner, L. 1964. Mesenteric arterial insufficiency and abdominal angina. *Arch. Intern. Med.* 114: 765–772.

Reininger, R. J. and Sapirstein, L. A. 1957. Effect of digestion on distribution of blood flow in the rat. *Science* 126: 1176.

Reynell, P. C., Spray, G. H. and Taylor, K. B. 1957. The site of absorption of vitamin B_{12} in the rat. *Clin. Sci.* 16: 663–667.

Riklis, E. and Quastel, J. H. 1958. Effects of cations on sugar absorption by isolated surviving guinea pig intestine. *Can. J. Biochem. Physiol.* 36: 347–362.

Ritschel, W. A. and Erni, W. 1977. Influence of temperature of ingested fluids in stomach emptying time. *Int. J. Clin. Pharmacol. Biopharm.* 15: 172–175.

Robinson, J. W. L., Jequier, J. Cl. and Taminelli, F. 1964. The measurement of amino-acid absorption in vitro. *Gastroenterologia* 102: 292–299.

Robinson, J. W. L., Jequier, J. Cl., Felber, J. P. and Mirkovitch, V. 1965. Amino acid absorption by the intestinal mucosa. *J. Surg. Res.* 5: 150–152.

Robinson, J. W. L., Antonioli, J. A. and Mirkovitch, V. 1966. The intestinal response to ischaemia. *Arch. Pharmakol. Exp. Pathol.* 255: 178–191.

Rosenstein, B. J. and Engleman, K. 1963. Diarrhea in a child with a catecholamine-secreting ganglioneuroma. *J. Pediatr.* 63: 217–226.

Rout, R., Giannella, R., Formal, S. and Dammin, G. 1973. The pathophysiology of Salmonella diarrhea in Rhesus monkey. *Gastroenterology* 64: 793.

Salomon, L. L. et al. 1961. Possible carrier mechanism for the intestinal transport of D-xylose. *Biochem. Biophys. Res. Commun.* 4(2): 123–126.

Sandstead, H. H. 1977. Nutrient interaction with toxic elements. In: *Toxicology of Trace Elements*. R. A. Goyer and M. A. Mehlman (ed.). Hemisphere, Washington, D.C.

Schacter, D. and Rosen, S. M. 1959. Active transport of Ca^{45} by the small intestine and its dependence on vitamin D. *Am. J. Physiol.* 196: 357–362.

Schanker, L. S. 1959. Absorption of drugs from the rat colon. *J. Pharmacol. Exp. Ther.* 126: 283–290.

Schanker, L. S. 1961. Mechanism of drug absorption and distribution. *Ann. Rev. Pharmacol.* 1: 29–44.

Schanker, L. S. 1964. Passage of drugs across body membranes. *Pharmacol. Rev.* 14: 501–530.

Schanker, L. S. 1971. Drug absorption. In: *Fundamentals of Drug Metabolism and Drug Disposition*. B. N. LaDu, H. Mandel and E. L. Way (eds.), Williams & Wilkins, Baltimore.

Schanker, L. S. and Johnson, J. M. 1961. Increased intestinal absorption of foreign organic compounds in the presence of ethylenediaminetetracetic acid (EDTA). *Biochem. Pharmacol.* 8: 421–422.

Schanker, L. S. and Tocco, D. J. 1960. Active transport of some pyrimidines across the rat intestinal epithelium. *J. Pharmacol. Exp. Ther.* 128: 115–121.

Schanker, L. S. and Tocco, D. J. 1962. Some characteristics of the pyrimidine trans-
    port process of the small intestines. *Biochim. Biophys. Acta* 56: 469–473.
Schanker, L. S., Shore, P. A., Brodie, B. B. and Hogben, C. A. M. 1957. Absorp-
    tion of drugs from the stomach. I. The rat. *J. Pharmacol. Exp. Ther.* 120:
    528–539.
Schanker, L. S., Tocco, D. J., Brodie, B. B. and Hogben, C. A. M. 1958. Absorp-
    tion of drugs from the rat small intestines. *J. Pharmacol. Exp. Ther.* 123: 81–88.
Schnell, R. C. and Miya, T. S. 1970. Increased ileal absorption of salicylic acid in-
    duced by carbonic anhydrase inhibition. *Biochem. Pharmacol.* 19: 303–305.
Seely, J. R., Humphrey, G. B. and Matter, B. J. 1972. Copper deficiency in a pre-
    mature infant fed an iron-fortified formula. *N. Engl. J. Med.* 286: 109–170.
Sewing, K.-F., Winne, D. and Lembeck, F. 1965. The influence of 5-hydroxytryptam-
    ine on the resorption of tritium-water (HTO) in the colon of the rat in vivo. *Arch.
    Pharmakol. Exp. Pathol.* 252: 286–290. (German)
Sieber, S. M. 1974. The entry of foreign compounds into the thoracic duct lymph of
    the rat. *Xenobiotica* 4: 265–284.
Sieber, S. M. 1976. The lymphatic absorption of pp[1]-DDT and some structurally relat-
    ed compounds in the rat. *Pharmacology* 14: 443–454.
Shore, P. A., Brodie, B. B. and Hogben, C. A. M. 1957. The gastric secretion of
    drugs: A pH partition hypothesis. *J. Pharmacol. Exp. Ther.* 119: 361–369.
Shrewsbury, R. P. 1977. "Some factors influencing drug absorption through biologic
    membranes: Percutaneous and intestinal administration." Ph.D. Thesis. Univer-
    sity of Kentucky, Lexington.
Sleisenger, M. H., Almy, T. P. and Barr, D. P. 1953. The sprue syndrome secondary
    to lymphoma of the small bowel. *Am. J. Med.* 15: 666–674.
Spencer, R. P. and Samiy, A. H. 1961. Intestinal absorption of L-phenylalanine in
    vitro. *Am. J. Physiol.* 200: 501–504.
Texter, E. C., Ching-Chung, C., Laureta, H. C. and Vantrappen, G. R. 1968.
    Physiology of the *Gastrointestinal Tract*. Mosby, St. Louis.
Ther, L. and Winne, D. 1971. Drug absorption. *Annu. Rev. Pharmacol.* 11: 57–70.
Thompson, A. B. R., Valberg, L. S. and Sinclair, D. G. 1971. Competitive nature of
    intestinal transport mechanisms for cobalt and iron in the rat. *J. Clin. Invest.*
    50: 2384–2394.
Tidball, G. S. 1964. Magnesium and calcium as regulators of intestinal permeability.
    Am. J. Physiol. 206: 243–246.
Travell, J. 1940. The influence of the hydrogen ion concentration on the absorption of
    alkaloids from the stomach. *J. Pharmacol. Exp. Ther.* 69: 21–33.
Ulmer, D. D. 1977. Trace elements. *N. Engl. J. Med.* 297: 318–319.
Ussing, H. H. and Andersen, B. 1956. The relation between solvent drag and active
    transport of ions. In: *Proceedings of the 3rd International Congress on Bio-
    chemistry*. Brussels, 1955. Liebecq, C. (ed.). Academic Press, New York.
Varro, V., Blako, G., Csernay, L., Jung, and Szarvas, p. 1965. Effect of decreased
    local circulation on the absorptive capacity of a small intestinal loop in the dog.
    Am. J. Digest Dis. 10: 170–177.
Varró, V., Blabo, G., Csernay, L., Jung, I. and Szarvas, F. 1965. Effect of de-
    creased local circulation on the absorptive capacity of a small intestinal loop in the
    dog. *Am. J. Digest Dis.* 10: 170–177.
Verzar, F. 1935. The role of diffusion and the activity of the mucous membrane in the
    absorption of various sugars from the intestines. *Biochem. Z.* 276: 17–27.
    (German)
Visscher, M. B. et al. 1944a. Isotopic tracer studies on the movement of water and
    ions between intestinal lumen and blood. *Am. J. Physiol.* 142: 550–575.
Visscher, M. B. et al. 1944b. Sodium movement between the intestinal lumen and the
    blood. *Am. J. Physiol.* 141: 488–505.
Walker, W. A. and Isselbacher, K. J. 1974. Uptake and transport of macromole by the
    intestine. Possible role in clinical disorders. *Gastroenterology* 67: 531–550.

Walton, R. P. 1935. Absorption of drugs through the oral mucosa. III. Fat-water solubility coefficient of alkaloids. *Proc. Soc. Exp. Biol. Med.* 32: 1488−1492.

Walton, R. P. 1944. Recent advances in drug therapy. A review of outstanding developments during 1943. *Rev. Argent. Norteam. Cien. Med. (Buenos Aires)* 1: 782−788. (Spanish & English)

Watten, R. H. et al. 1959. Water and electrolyte studies in cholera. *J. Clin. Invest.* 38: 1879−1889.

Weijers, H. A. and Van De Kamer, J. H. 1960. Celiac disease and wheat sensitivity. *Pediatrics* 25: 127−134.

Weijers, H. A., Van De Kamer, J. H. and Dicke, W. K. 1957. Celiac disease. *Adv. Pediatr.* 9: 277−318.

Weijers, H. A., Van De Kamer, J. H., Mossel, D. A. A. and Dicke, W. K. 1960. Diarrhea caused by deficiency of sugar-splitting enzymes. *Lancet* 2: 296−297.

Whalen, G. E., Soergel, K. H. and Geenen, J. E. 1969. Diabetic diarrhea. A clinical and pathophysiological study. *Gastroenterology* 56: 1021−1032.

Williams, L. F., Jr. 1971. Vascular insufficiency of the intestines. *Gastroenterology* 61: 757−777.

Williams, C. N. and Sidorov, J. J. 1971. Steatorrhea in patients with liver disease. *Can. Med. Assoc. J.* 105: 1143−1146.

Williams, E. D., Karim, S. M. M. and Sandler, M. 1968. Prostaglandin secretion by medullary carcinoma of the thyroid. A possible cause of the associated diarrhoea. *Lancet* 1: 22−23.

Wilson, T. H. 1962. *Intestinal Absorption*. Saunders, Philadelphia.

Wilson, T. H. and Kazyak, L. 1957. Acid-base changes across the wall of hamster and rat intestine. *Biochim. Biophys. Acta* 24: 124−132.

Wilson, T. H. and Lin, E. C. C. 1960. Active transport by intestines of fetal and newborn rabbits. *Am. J. Physiol.* 199: 1030−1032.

Wilson, T. H. and Vincent, T. N. 1955. Absorption of sugars in vitro by the intestine of the golden hamster. *J. Biol. Chem.* 216: 851−866.

Windsor, E. and Cronheim, G. E. 1961. Gastrointestinal absorption of heparin and synthetic heparinoids. *Nature* 190: 263−264.

Winne, D. 1966. Influence of various drugs on intestinal bleeding and resorption of tritiated water in the small intestines of the rat. *Arch. Pharmakol. Exp. Pathol.* 254: 199−224. (German)

Winne, D. 1970. Formal kinetics of water and solute absorption with regard to intestinal blood flow. *J. Theor. Biol.* 27: 1−18.

Winne, D. 1980. Influence of blood flow on intestinal absorption of xenobiotics. *Pharmacology* 21: 1−15.

Winter, M. 1953. Effect of monofluoroacetic acid on the intestinal absorption of glucose and glycine. *Acta Physiol. Acad. Sci. Hung.* 4: 91−95.

Wiseman, G. 1953. Absorption of amino acids using an in vitro technique. *J. Physiol.* 120: 63−72.

Wiseman, G. 1955. Preferential transference of amino acids from amino acid mixtures by sacs of everted small intestines of the golden hamster (Mesocricetus auratus). *J. Physiol.* (London) 127: 414−422.

Yoffey, J. M. and Courtice, F. C. 1956. *Lymphatics, Lymph and Lymphoid Tissue*. Harvard University Press, Cambridge, Massachusetts.

Zawoiski, E. J., Baer, J. E., Braunschweig, L. W., Paulson, S. F., Shermer, A. and Beyer, K. H. 1958. Gastrointestinal secretion and absorption of 3-methylaminoisocamphane hydrochloride (mecamylamine). *J. Pharmacol. Exp. Ther.* 122: 442−448.

3

The Role of Intestinal Microflora in the Toxicity of Food Components

Undoubtedly, the microflora inhabiting the gastrointestinal (GI) tract plays a role in modifying the toxicological properties of food compounds.

Table 1 shows the distribution, number, and predominant genera of intestinal microorganisms found in sampling healthy human volunteers. The samples were obtained by intubation (Drasar et al. 1970). Note that the dominant varieties belong to the genera Bacteroides and the Bifidobacterium. Both are nonsporeforming anaerobes. The species commonly encountered include *Bacteroides fragilis, B. melaninogenicus,* and *Bifidobacterium adolescentis* (Williams and Drasar 1972). The aerobic microorganisms found in the GI tract belong to the genera of the family (e.g., *Klebsiella aerogenes, Proteus mirabilis,* and mostly, *Escherichia coli*); *Streptococcus (S. viridans [mitior]* and *S. faecalis)* and *Lactobacillus (L. acidophilus* and *L. casei)*. *Clostridium* (e.g, *C. perfringens* and *C. sporogenes)* and *Veillonella* (e.g., *V. parvula* and *V. alcalescens*) are also constant anaerobic inhabitants of the gastrointestinal tract in many persons. There are, however, individuals who do not harbor these organisms. Sometimes, the aerobes *Staphylococcus aureus* and *Pseudomonas aeruginosa* are detected in the colon or rectum of certain individuals.

Of special interest is the presence in certain populations of thiamin-destroying microorganisms. Japanese workers have identified these three species of thiamin-degrading microorganisms in Japanese fecal matter (Kimura 1965): *Bacillus thiaminolyticus* and *Bacillus aneurinolyticus*, both aerobes, and *Clostridium thiaminolyticus*, an anaerobe. The growth of *B. thiaminolyticus* appears to be controlled by the concentration of bile acids in the gastrointestinal tract (Hamada 1954).

Table 1 shows the increase in density of microbial populations toward the distal segments of the gastrointestinal tract. The stomach is generally sterile when no food is present, or when the acidity falls below pH 3 (Drasar et al. 1969). The bacterial count in this organ may increase to 10^5 bacteria/ml of gastric content. After eating most of these are derived from the mouth and the food, and include species of Streptococci, Enterobacteria, Bacteroides, and Bifidobacteria. This bacterial population drops drastically toward the latter part of gastric digestion when the pH of the stomach content drops significantly.

Bacterial density begins to increase in the small intestines, but in the proximal part of the organ, including the proximal ileum, each particular species rarely exceeds 10^5 microorganisms present (Drasar et al. 1969). The distal ileum is more heavily laden with microorganisms. Both aerobes and anaerobes are represented in the bacterial populations. Like the stomach, the bacterial populations of the small intestines, particularly the proximal sections, also increase after a meal and may be as high as 10^5 microorganisms/ml of intestinal content (Gorbach et al. 1967).

Table 1. Microflora of the Gastrointestinal Tract of Man

Type of Organism	Number of Viable Organisms per Gram of Wet Sample				
	Stomach	Duodenum-jejunum	Ileum	Colon	Rectum-feces
Streptococci	$0-10^5$	$0-10^5$	10^3-10^4	—	10^2-10^6
Lactobacilli	$0-10^4$	$0-10^2$	10^3-10^6	10^4-10^9	10^2-10^9
Bacteroides	$0-10^4$	$0-10^5$	10^5-10^7	10^6-10^{10}	10^9-10^{11}
Bifidobacteria	$0-10^3$	$0-10^4$	10^5-10^7	10^4-10^8	10^9-10^{11}
Enterobacteria	0	0	10^3-10^4	10^6-10^8	10^4-10^8
Clostridia	0	0	0	—	$0-10^5$
Veillonellae	0	0	$0-10^3$	$0-10^4$	$0-10^6$
Staphylococci	0	0	0	—	—
Yeasts	0	0	0	—	$0-10^4$

Source: Drasar et al. (1970)

As expected, the bacterial count in the large intestines and rectum is much great-er than that of the small intestines. The colonal and rectal bacterial count can be as high as 10^9 bacteria/g of sample (Gorbach et al. 1967). In the feces, the total viable bacterial count can be as high as 10^{11} bacteria/g of sample (Moore et al. 1969).

FACTORS REGULATING GASTROINTESTINAL BACTERIAL POPULATIONS

We have already indicated that gastric acidity controls the bacterial population in the stomach. It is therefore understandable that in people with achlorhydria, increased bacterial counts as high as 10^6/ml of gastric content have been reported (Drasar et al. 1969), Escherichia coli being the principal species. Indirect evidence suggests that bile will actually stimulate bacterial growth. Thus, it has been found that people on Western diets, who have relatively high concentrations of bile salts and their deriva-tives in the feces, also have high counts of Bacteroides (Hill et al. 1971).

The normal motility of the gastrointestinal tract appears to control the bacterial populations. When the normal peristaltic activity is impaired, there is an increase in the bacterial population, particularly in the ileum (Gorbach 1971). Thus, in the "stag-nant loop" syndrome, a wide variety of fecal microorganisms can accumulate in the upper intestines, resulting in undesirable effects described below.

TOXICOLOGICAL EFFECTS OF INTESTINAL BACTERIA

Interference in the Absorption of Various Compounds

In the blind loop syndrome, there is malabsorption of essential nutrients, particularly cobalamin, fatty acids, cholecalciferol, and sugars, resulting in malnutrition (Dyer and Hawkins 1972). Specific signs of nutrient deficiencies are evident in patients with this syndrome. Thus, anemia due to cobalamine deficiency is quite common (Mollin and Ross 1954). Osteomalacia is an occasional complication (Cooke et al. 1963) owing to either impaired cholecalciferol absorption (Tabaqchali and Booth 1970) or bile salt deficiency. The defect in fat absorption, owing in part to the deconjugation of the bile salt by the intestinal bacteria (Tabaqchali et al. 1968), results in steatorrhea. This occurs in about one-third of the patients with the blind loop syndrome, according to Donaldson (1968). Transport of water, sodium, and potassium is interfered with by the deconjugated bile. This fact may explain the presence of diarrhea in the blind loop syndrome, which occurs more frequently than steatorrhea. Sometimes severe portein-calorie malnutrition occurs in these patients (Krikler and Schrire 1958). This suggests that protein digestion or amino acid absorption is also impaired.

Defect in the Mucosal Structure

When the germ-free and normal animals are compared, it becomes evident that somehow the intestinal microflora influences the mucosal structure (Abrams et al. 1963). The germ-free animals lack the usual histological features of the gastrointestinal mucosa found in the normal animals. However, markedly increased bacterial populations in the gastrointestinal tract of normal animals cause significant structural changes in the gastrointestinal mucosa, for example, flattening of the mucosal surface (Cavallaro and Rosenweig 1971) and inflammatory patches (Paulley 1969; Anent et al. 1971). More mucosal lesions are revealed in these cases with the electron microscope.

Metabolic Transformation of Various Compounds

The toxicological properties of compounds may be modified considerably by the metabolic activity of these organisms. Most reactions are degradative in nature and thus the products have smaller molecular weights. The ability of these organisms to ferment changes the reaction milieu, often toward greater acidity. An acid environment can promote certain types of reactions with great toxicological significance; e.g., nitrosamine formation.

METABOLISM OF FOOD COMPONENTS BY INTESTINAL BACTERIA

We note from Table 1 that bacterial populations increase in density in the distal ileum and more so in the colon and rectum. The microbial species found in this part of the gastrointestinal tract have high metabolic activity. Thus, compounds which are not absorbed in the small intestines may be degraded by these microorganisms to products of lesser or greater toxicity than the parent compounds, if for no other reason than their conversion to more absorbable derivatives.

Most of our data on the metabolism of nonnutrient food compounds are derived from animal studies. It is debatable whether these results can be extrapolated to man. However, since similar microbial species are demonstrable in both man and such experimental animals as the rat, mouse, dog, and rabbit, it is likely that results from animal studies may be applicable to man. Exceptions to this conclusion are perhaps the differences in the rate of breakdown of these compounds by human intestinal bacteria and those of the experimental animals. Of course, the toxicological properties of these metabolites may be quantitatively different in man than in animals.

Several types of reactions have been demonstrated with these intestinal microorganisms. These include (1) hydrolysis, (2) decarboxylation, (3) deamination, (4) O-demethylation, (5) ring opening of heterocyclic compounds, (6) reduction, (7) dehydroxylation, (8) aromatization, and (9) dehalogenation. Very often reaction types are degradative.

Hydrolysis

Glycosides

Many toxicologically important, naturally occurring substances in plants are present as glycosides. Generally, they are not readily absorbed and are therefore less toxic. However, they are hydrolyzed by intestinal bacterial to the aglycone and the corresponding sugar. The aglycone may, in fact, be responsible for the observed toxicity. For example, cycasin, the glucoside of methylazoxymethanol, is nontoxic, but upon hydrolysis by intestinal bacteria, manifests potent hepatotoxicity and carcinogenicity (Spatz et al. 1967).

Cycasin ⟶ β-Glucosidase (Bacteria) ⟶ Methylazoxymethanol

$CH_3^+ + N_2 + OH^- \longleftarrow CH_2-N=N-OH \longleftarrow CH_3N=NH$

The methyl carbonium ion is believed to be the alkylating species and to be responsible for the toxic effects (Matsumoto and Higa 1966; Shank and Magee 1967).

The aglycone in this case is absorbed and metabolized in the tissues to azoxymethane and diazomethane. The latter compounds most likely are responsible for the hepatotoxicity and carcinogenicity of cycasin, since these are potent alkylating agents to nucleic acids and proteins.

Cyanogenic glycosides are rendered toxic by intestinal microbial hydrolysis. Thus, amygdalin (found in almonds), the gentiobioside of benzaldehyde cyanohydrin, is degraded to mandelonitrile, which breaks down to benzaldehyde and hydrogen cyanide (Williams 1970).

HNL = Hydroxynitrile lyase

Similar reactions may be expected of the other cyanogenic glycosides found in other food products. (It should be pointed out that the tissues of the plants may themselves produce the enzyme for the hydrolysis of the cyanogen, as has been reported in a number of cases [Conn 1969].

The potato alkaloid, solanine, can be rendered less toxic by intestinal microbial hydrolysis to solanidine, which is less toxic and even less absorbable (Nishie et al. 1971).

$$C_6H_{11}O_4-O-C_6H_{10}O_4-O-C_6H_{10}O_4-O-C_{27}H_{42}N$$

Rhamnose   Galactose   Glucose   Solanidine

Solanine

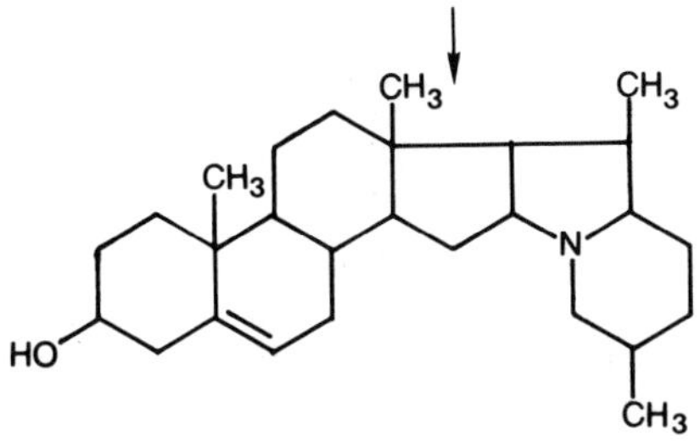

Solanidine

The initial degradation reaction of flavonoid glycosides by intestinal bacteria is hydrolysis. Thus, hesperidine, a rhamnoglucoside found in grapefruit (Higby 1941), is first hydrolyzed to hesperitin and phenyl-β-D-glucoside. Further microbial degradation yields phenol (Scheline 1968b). The aglycone, hesperitin, is more fat soluble than the parent compound.

$$C_6H_{11}O_4-O-C_6H_{10}O_4-O-C_{16}H_{14}O_6$$

Rhamnose   Glucose   Hesperetin

Hesperidin

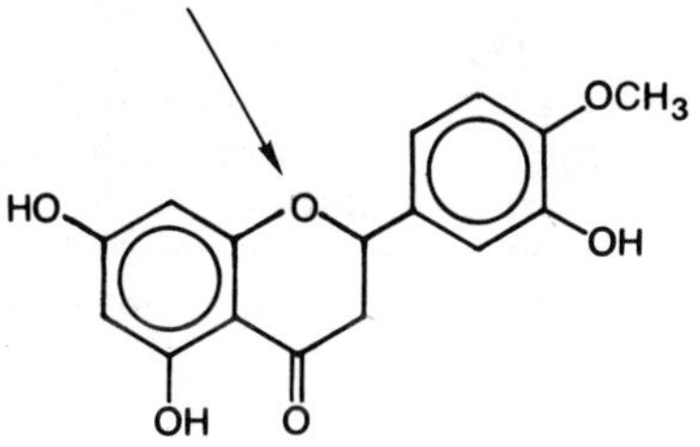

Hesperetin

A similar situation is encountered with naringin (Booth et al. 1958), also found in grapefruit (Pulley and von Loesecke 1939; Zoller 1917) and rutin (Booth and Williams 1963b; Booth et al. 1956), which is presently in relatively large amounts in buckwheat and other plants (Eskew et al. 1946).

Conjugates

Compounds that are absorbed may be conjugated with glucuronic acid, glycine, taurine, and other compounds. The conjugates may be excreted in the bile and then hydrolyzed by intestinal microorganisms. The free compounds can then be reabsorbed. Thus, by means of the enterohepatic circulation, the compound is recirculated in the body. In this way, the toxicity of a compound may be enhanced, since the exposure of the body to the compound is prolonged.

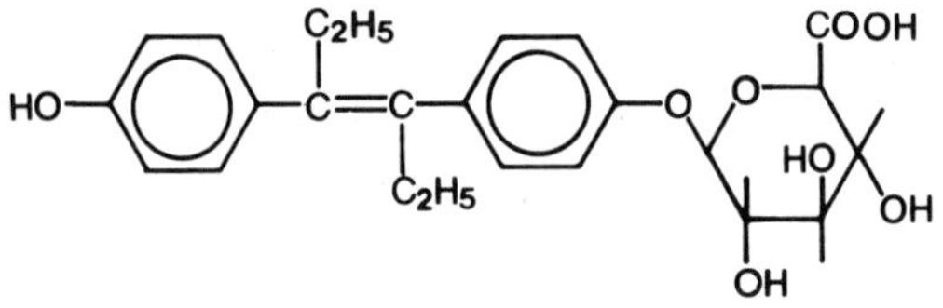

DES   β-glucuronide

β-glucuronidase
(bacteria)

DES + Glucuronic acid

Examples of glucuronide hydrolysis by intestinal bacteria are diethylstilbestrol (DES) (Milburn et al. 1967) and di-*tert*-butylhydroxybenzoate from BHT (Daniel et al. 1968). The enterohepatic circulation of the aglycones of DES-glucuronide (Hanahan et al. 1953; Williams 1970) and BHT-glucuronide (Daniel et al. 1968) has been demonstrated in rats.

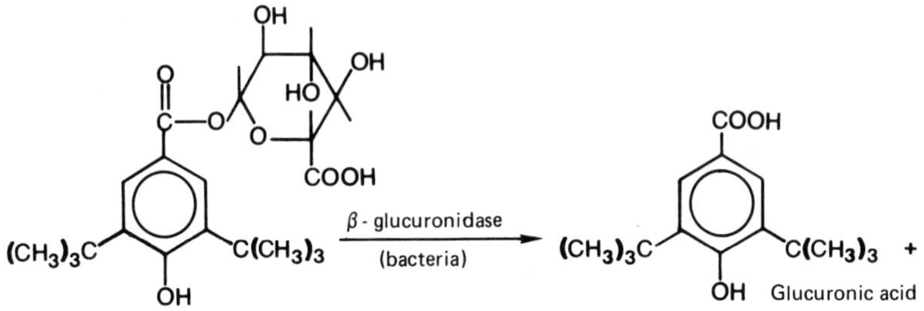

Di-tert-butylhydroxybenzoate
β-glucuronide

β-glucuronidase
(bacteria)

Glucuronic acid

Plant phenolics are probably excreted as glucuronide conjugates in the bile. Similarly, these glucuronides are subject to intestinal microbial hydrolysis prior to other microbial degradation. Thus, the glucuronide of ferulic acid (3-methoxy-r-hydroxy cinnamic acid) is hydrolyzed by intestinal bacteria. The free acid is then reduced at the double bond, demethylated, and dehydroxylated. The final product of these reactions, *m*-hydroxyphenylpropionic acid, is absorbed and excreted in the urine (Scheline 1968a).

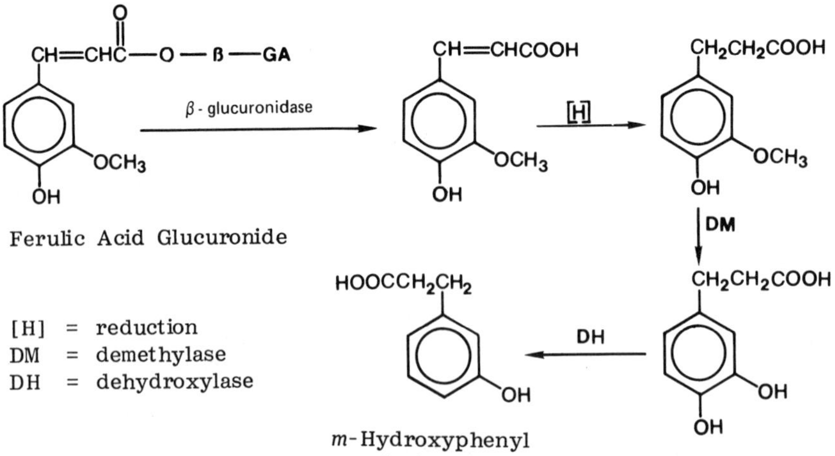

Ferulic Acid Glucuronide

β-glucuronidase

[H]

DM

DH

[H] = reduction
DM = demethylase
DH = dehydroxylase

m-Hydroxyphenyl
propionic acid

The hydrolysis of the glucuronide releases a more polar compound, in this case, ferulic acid, which will have a decreased rate of absorbability in the intestines. Demethylation further increases polarity of the compound, but the dissociation of the phenolic hydroxy groups is expected to be insignificant. The formation of a o-dihydroxyphenol may result in some antithiamine activity, as discussed in Chapter 9. However, the subsequent dehydroxylation should abolish this effect, assuming no substantial absorption of the o-dihydroxyphenol has occurred.

The enzyme, β-glucuronidase, is found in many species of intestinal bacteria, particularly *E. coli* (Buehler et al. 1951; Glazko et al. 1952). The high degree of β-glucuronidase activity in the colon and cecum correlates well with the high microbial density in these parts on the GI tract (Table 1).

Hippuric acid, a glycine conjugate of benzoate is also hydrolyzed by intestinal bacteria, particularly by species of Enterococci (Norman and Grubb 1955). The benzoates produced, being ionized at alkaline pH, may be poorly absorbed owing to the slightly alkaline pH of the colon where significant hydrolysis of hippuric acid takes place.

Hippuric acid   Benzoic acid   Glycine

Esters

Examples of intestinal microbial hydrolysis of esters are those of glycyrrhetinic acid hemisuccinate (Iveson et al. 1966), methyl gallate, an antioxidant (Scheline 1968b), and chlorogenic acid (Booth et al. 1957) an ester of caffeic and quinic acids. Glycyrrhetinic acid is lipid soluble and may be absorbed easily in the GI tract. Licorice contains the glucuronide form, glycyrrhizic acid.

$RO-COCH_2CH_2COOH \longrightarrow ROH + HOOCCH_2CH_2COOH$

Glycyrrhetinic acid hemisuccinate   Glycyrrhetinic acid   Succinic acid

Methyl gallate   Gallic acid

Chlorogenic acid   Caffeic acid   Quinic acid

Glycyrrhizic acid produces effects similar to deoxycorticosterone, so that when it is taken in sufficiently high amounts, salt retention, hypertension, and heart enlargement may result (Chamberlain 1970; Conn et al. 1968; Koster and David 1968).

Gallic acid is sufficiently soluble in lipids, so that it may be absorbed to a significant extent in the colon. Since it is methylated in the tissues, it may compete for essential methyl groups (Potter and Fuller 1968; Rayudu et al. 1970). Weakness and other neurological disorders in animals have been demonstrated with gallic acid (Stecher et al. 1960). As shown in the next section, intestinal bacteria can metabolize gallic acid to more toxic derivatives.

One of the products of the microbial hydrolysis of chlorogenic acid is caffeic acid. This degradation product may produce a sensitization-type of dermatitis (Stecher et al. 1960). However, as shown in the next section (p. 80), further degradation products of caffeic acid may have greater toxicological importance than caffeic acid itself.

Sulfamate Hydrolysis

Sodium and calcium cyclohexane sulfamate (cyclamate) is a sweetening agent (Chap. 21). Intestinal bacteria degrade it to cyclohexylamine and sulfate (Williams 1971), probably by hydrolysis.

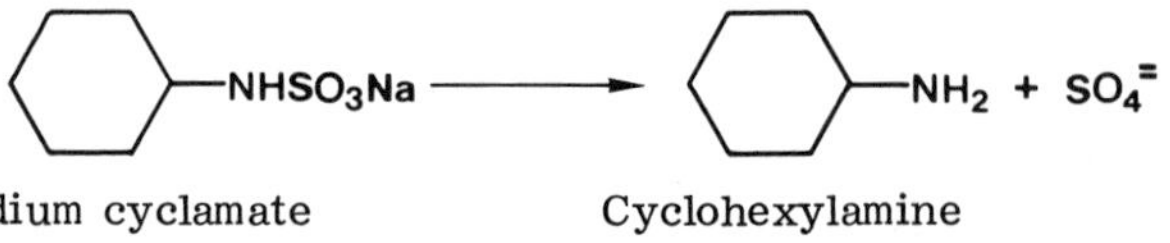

$$\text{Sodium cyclamate} \qquad \qquad \text{Cyclohexylamine}$$

Considerable prior exposure to cyclamate is required to break down the compound. Even then, Williams (1971) reported that not all humans are capable of breaking down this compound extensively to cyclohexylamine. Most Wistar rats are able to break down the sweetener. The rabbit behaves like humans in that the ability to metabolize the compound extensively is not a general phenomenon. Thus, it appears that induction of the specific metabolic enzymes is necessary in this case. The bacteria responsible appear to be Enterococci. Note that cyclohexylamine will be less ionized in the intestines and therefore more absorbable.

Hydrolysis of Thiamin

Many species of intestinal bacteria have been shown to decompose thiamin (Murata 1965). Three in particular were isolated from the fecal matter of a patient with persistent thiamindeficiency, healthy individuals, and hospitalized patients. The organisms are *Bacillus thiaminolyticus, Bacillus aneurinolyticus,* and *Clostridium thiaminolyticum* (Kimura 1965). The first two are spore-forming aerobes, the latter is an anaerobe. *B. thiaminolyticus* and *C. thiaminolyticum* produce the enzyme thiaminase I, and *B. aneurinolyticus,* thiaminase II. These two enzymes differ in their mode of action. Thiaminase I promotes exchange reactions with various compounds for the thiazole moiety following hydrolysis. Thus, aniline, cysteine, nicotinic acid, and others can be exchanged for the thiazole moiety (Murata 1965).

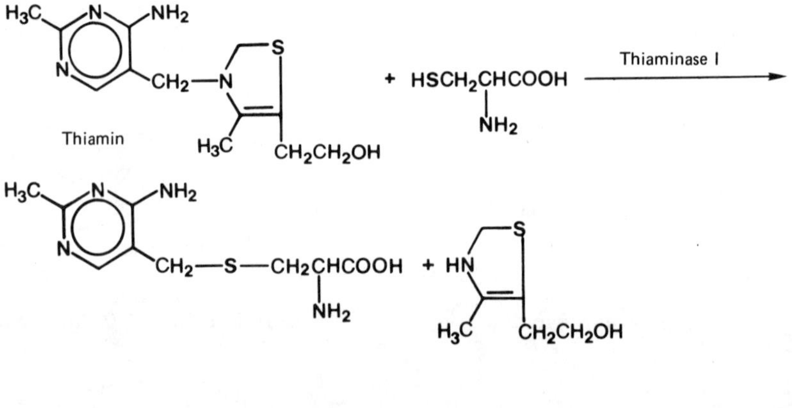

Thiaminase II catalyzes straight hydrolysis of the CH_2-N- bond between the pyrimidine and thiazole moieties (Murata 1965).

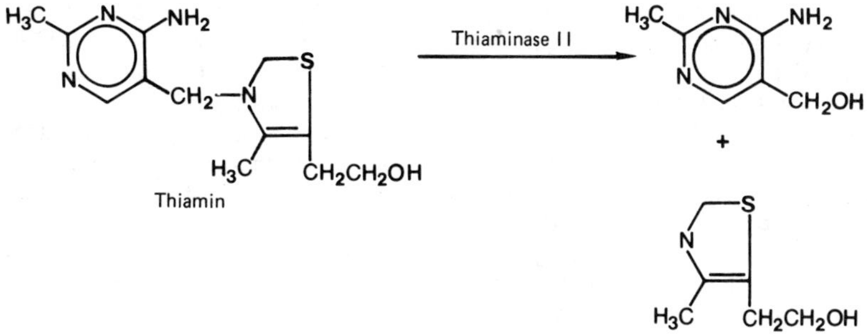

Thiamin

Thiaminase II

Decarboxylation

The intestinal microbial decarboxylation of phenolic acids may produce products of greater toxicity than the parent compound. The following examples will illustrate this point.

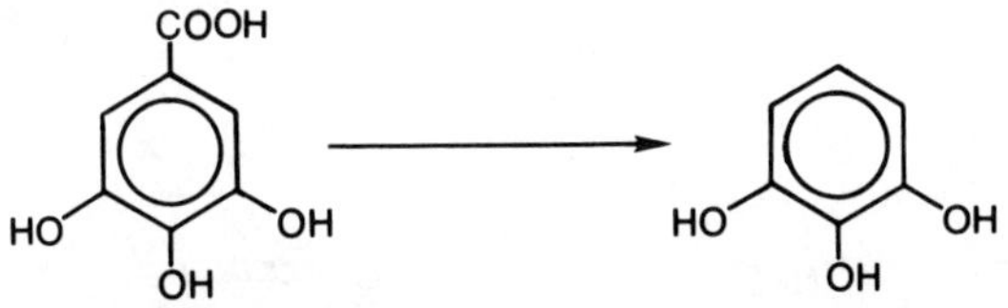

Gallic acid

Pyrogallol

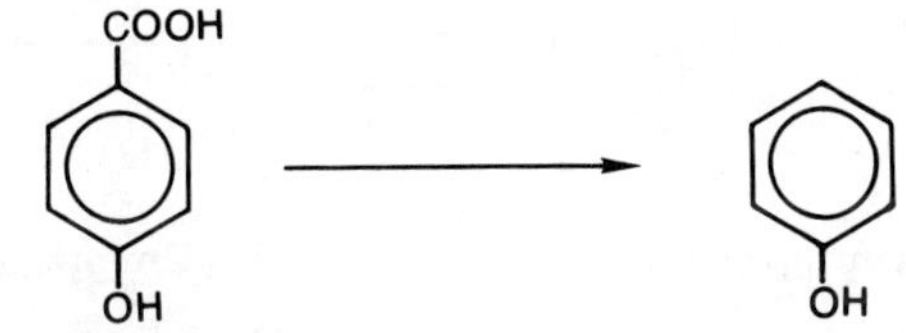

p-Hydroxy-
benzoic acid

Phenol

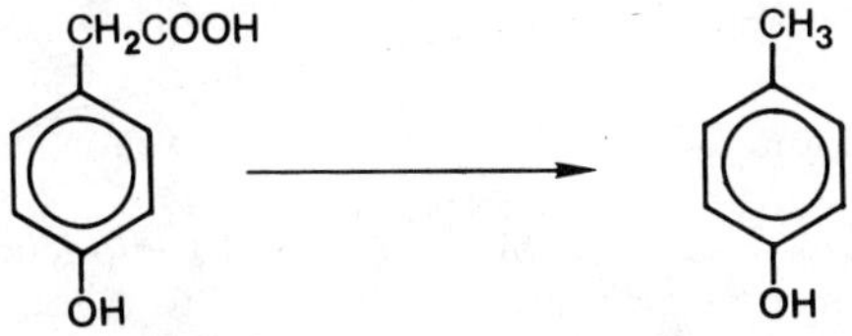

p-Hydroxyphenyl-
acetic acid

p-Hydroxytoluene

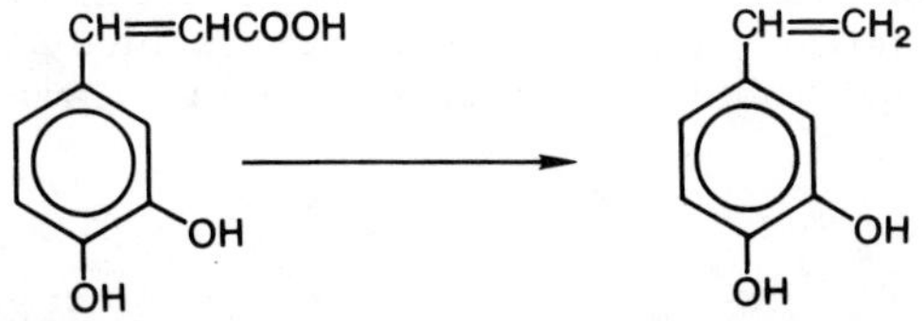

Caffeic acid

4-Vinylcatechol

Note that all the above examples have the *para*-hydroxy group. From decarboxylation studies with a large number of phenolic benzoic acids with rat cecal microorganisms, it has been demonstrated that the hydroxyl group in the *para* position is necessary for the decarboxylation reaction to occur (Scheline 1966a, b; 1967; 1968a). The products of decarboxylation are frequently absorbed and can be detected in the urine. Tompsett (1958) isolated pyrogallol in human urine and pointed to the decarboxylation of gallic acid by intestinal bacteria as the possible source. Of concern is the formation of vinyl-catechol by intestinal microbial decarboxylation of caffeic acid (Scheline 1968a,b), as demonstrated in the rat. The carcinogenicity of vinyl compounds has been demonstrated (Wagoner and Infante 1977). The phenolic products are certainly more lipid soluble, and thus are more easily absorbed than the parent phenolic acids. Pyrogallol (MLD = rats, 700 mg/kg, s.c.; dogs, 25 mg/kg, oral) is more toxic than gallic acid (LD = rats, 4 g/kg, s.c.). The toxicity of phenol is well known. However, in this case, a more significant toxicological property of phenols is their possible role as cancer promoters (Boutwell and Bosch 1959; Kaiser 1967; Van Duuren et al. 1968).

A source of amino acids in the colon is undigested proteins, dead bacteria, and cellular detritus, which are hydrolyzed by bacterial proteases to component amino acids. These together with amino acids leaking from the blood into the lumen and the unabsorbed amino acids from intestinal digestion of proteins comprise the amino acid pool which serves as substrate for bacterial decarboxylation and deamination. The products of these reactions possess varying degrees of toxicity. A number of these products have pressor activity. Thus, decarboxylation of tyrosine, tryptophan, phenylalanine, histidine, cysteine, and lysine produces tyramine, tryptamine, phenylethylamine, histimine, and cysteamine (aminoethyl mercaptan) and cadaverine, respectively). The first three amines are hypertensive compounds; the last three amines are hypotensives.

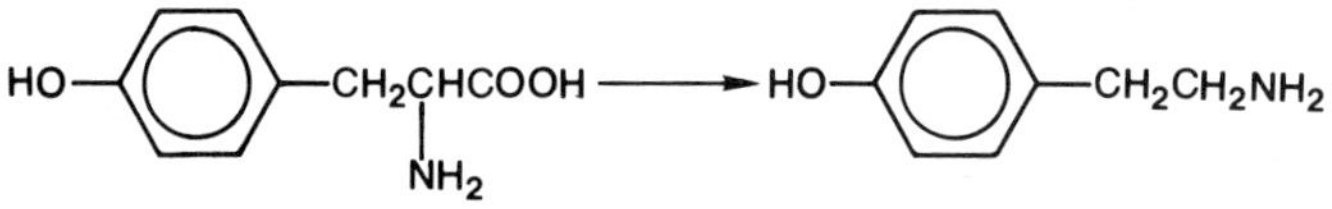

Tyrosine   Tyramine

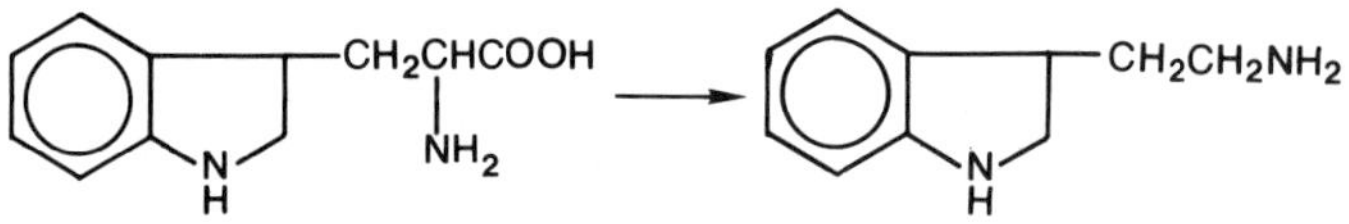

Tryptophan   Tryptamine

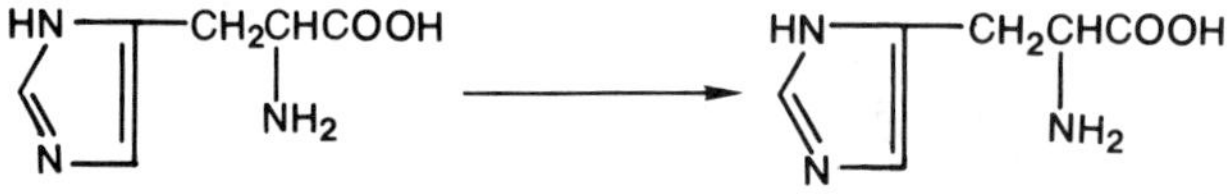

Histidine   Histamine

Again, both the increased absorbability of dihydroxyphenols and their anti-thiamin effects as mentioned previously may contribute significantly to their increased toxicity.

The decarboxylation of arginine by intestinal bacteria proceeds first by elimination of a formamidine group (HN=C—NH$_2$) to produce ornithine. Further decarboxylation and deamination of subsequent derivatives by bacteria produce Δ'-pyrroline, which is reduced to pyrrolidine as shown in the following scheme (Drasar and Hill 1974).

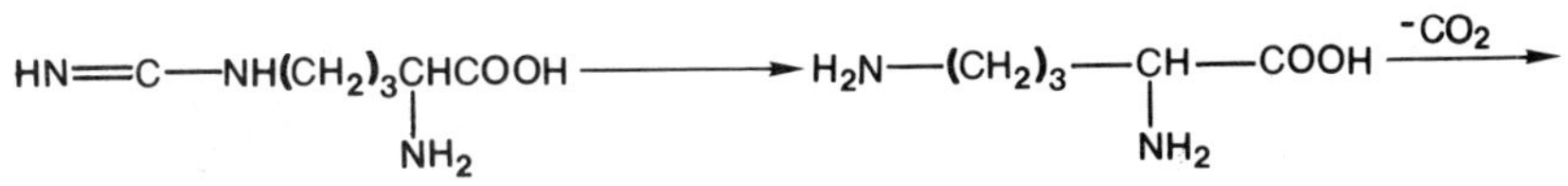

$$HN\!=\!\!C\!-\!NH(CH_2)_3CHCOOH \longrightarrow H_2N\!-\!(CH_2)_3\!-\!CH\!-\!COOH \xrightarrow{-CO_2}$$

with NH_2 groups below, labeled:

Arginine   Ornithine

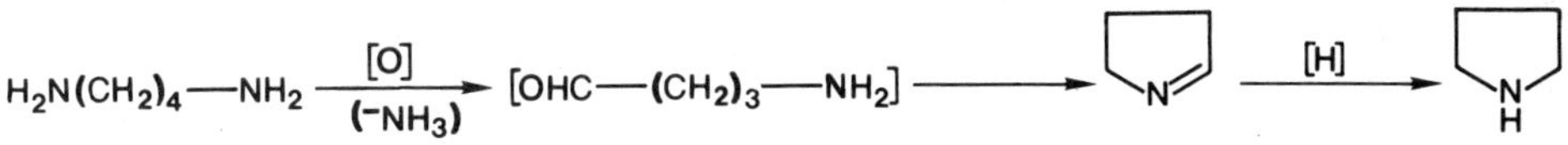

$$H_2N(CH_2)_4\!-\!NH_2 \xrightarrow[(-NH_3)]{[O]} [OHC\!-\!(CH_2)_3\!-\!NH_2] \longrightarrow \text{(1-pyrroline)} \xrightarrow{[H]} \text{(pyrrolidine)}$$

Putrescine   Pyrrolidine

Pyrrolidine can also be produced by decarboxylation of proline by intestinal bacteria (Asatoor and Kerr 1961).

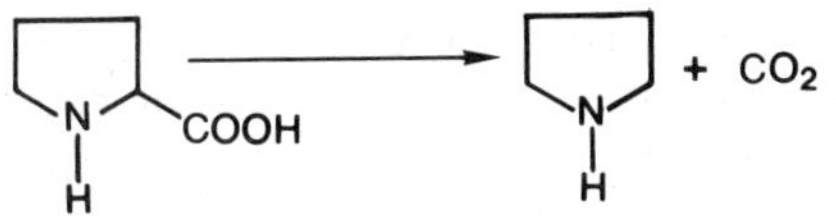

$$\text{Proline} \longrightarrow \text{Pyrrolidine} + CO_2$$

Proline   Pyrrolidine

Similarly cadaverine from the bacterial decarboxylation of lysine undergoes cyclization reaction to form piperidine (Drasar and Hill 1974).

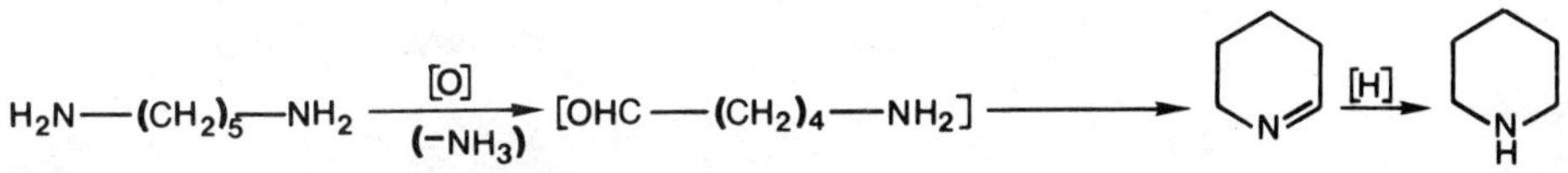

$$H_2N\!-\!(CH_2)_5\!-\!NH_2 \xrightarrow[(-NH_3)]{[O]} [OHC\!-\!(CH_2)_4\!-\!NH_2] \longrightarrow \text{(tetrahydropyridine)} \xrightarrow{[H]} \text{(piperidine)}$$

Cadaverine   Piperidine

The formation of pyrrolidine and piperidine by intestinal bacteria is perhaps of greater toxicological significance than that of the diamines because the amount formed of the latter is usually insufficient to produce significant toxic effects. In contrast, intestinal bacteria, e.g., E. coli, may promote the formation of nitrosamines from these cyclic secondary amines (Hawksworth and Hill 1971a,b; Hill and Hawksworth 1972). Nitrosopiperidine and nitrosopyrrolidine are relatively potent carcinogens.

Piperidine and pyrrolidine were excreted in the urine in human subjects that were studied at the rate of 0.8 and 0.4 mg/day (Drasar and Hill 1974). These amounts will, of course, vary with the diet and other sources. Thus, these two amines may have to be considered in the etiology of bladder and gastrointestinal cancers, especially under conditions of high intakes of nitrates in the diet and drinking water. In this case, nitrate is reduced to nitrite by intestinal bacteria, as discussed previously.

Deamination

Products of amino acid decarboxylation may further undergo deamination, or the amino acids may be deaminated first before decarboxylation (Melnykowycz and Johansson 1955; Orten and Neuhaus 1975). For example, tyrosine may undergo the following reaction:

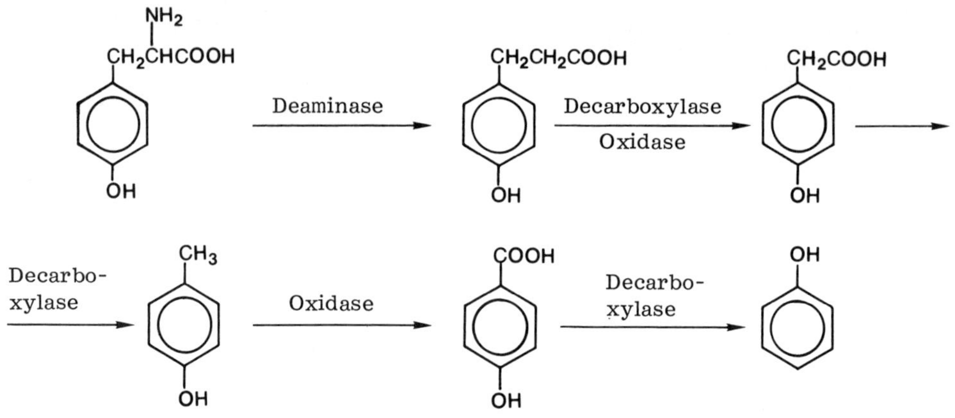

Similarly, cysteine may be degraded by both pathways, producing ethyl mercaptan, which is degraded further to methyl mercaptan and ultimately to H_2S:

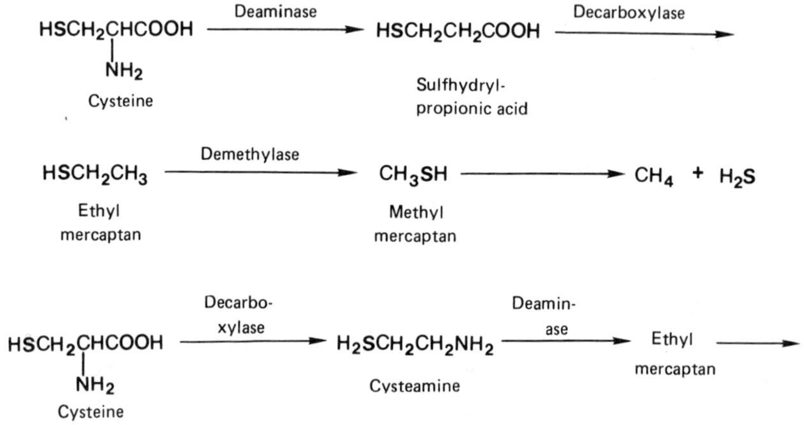

H_2S is, of course, an extremely poisonous gas, death occurring in a few seconds when a lethal level is inhaled (lowest lethal concentration [LC low] in rats = 1500 mg/m^3 of air; lowest toxic concentration [TC low] = 14 ppm) (Christensen 1973). However, the amount produced from proteins will rarely attain toxic levels, and will not produce significant toxic hazards. Ethyl mercaptan is toxic and may produce toxic (narcotic) effects in man if inhaled at 4 ppm. The LD_{50} of CH_3-SH in the mouse is 2.4 mg/kg, and the lowest lethal concentration by inhalation for the rat is 1000 ppm (Christensen 1973).

Tryptophan following bacterial deamination to indole propionic acid is further degraded to indoleacetic acid and finally to skatole and indole; the latter two substances give the characteristic foul odor of feces.

Indole has an oral LD_{50} for the rat of 1g/kg (Christensen 1973). LD_{50} i.v. for the dog is 60 mg/kg (Stecher et al. 1960). Bladder tumors developed in rats fed 2-acetylaminofluorene in the diet with tryptophan (1.4 or 4.9%), indole (0.8 or 1.6%), or indole acetic acid (1.0%). 2-Acetylaminofluorene alone did not (Dunning et al. 1950, 1958). Indole is easily fat soluble and should be readily absorbed. The absorbability of indole is indicated by the presence in the urine of indoxyl sulfate (indican)—a detoxification product of indole. Normally from 4 to 20 mg indoxyl sulfate may be

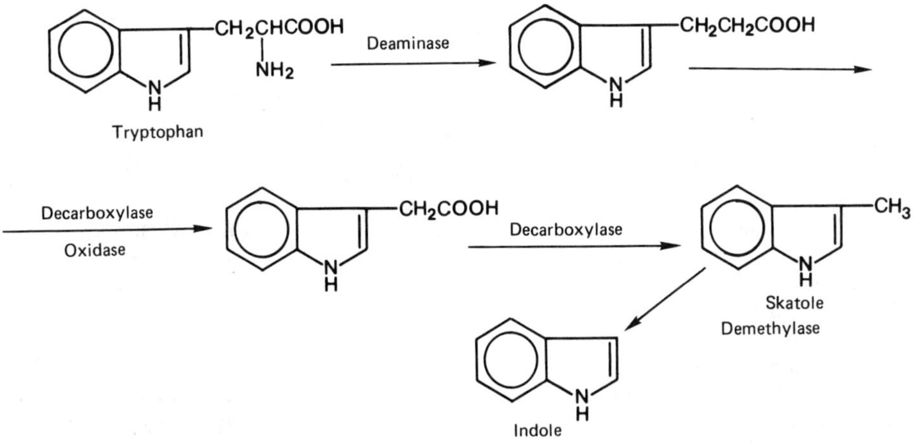

Tryptophan

Indole

excreted (Orten and Neuhaus 1975). In disease conditions such as hypochlorhydria, obstructive jaundice, and various diarrheas, relatively large amounts of indoxyl sulfate may be excreted. Thus, this detoxication product of indole (Chap. 4) is an index of the absorption of putrefactive products of intestinal bacteria.

Like indole, skatole is also easily fat soluble. The subcutaneous MLD in frogs is 1 g/kg (Stecher et al. 1960); however, because of easy conversion to indole, it poses little toxicological significance.

Dehydroxylation

Certain species of anaerobic bacteria belonging to the genera Bacteroides, Clostridium, and Veillonella and the species *Streptococcus faecalis,* which inhabits the mammalian GI tracts, are able to dehydroxlate cholic acid to deoxycholic acid (Hill and Drasar 1967; Norman and Sjövall 1958a,b).

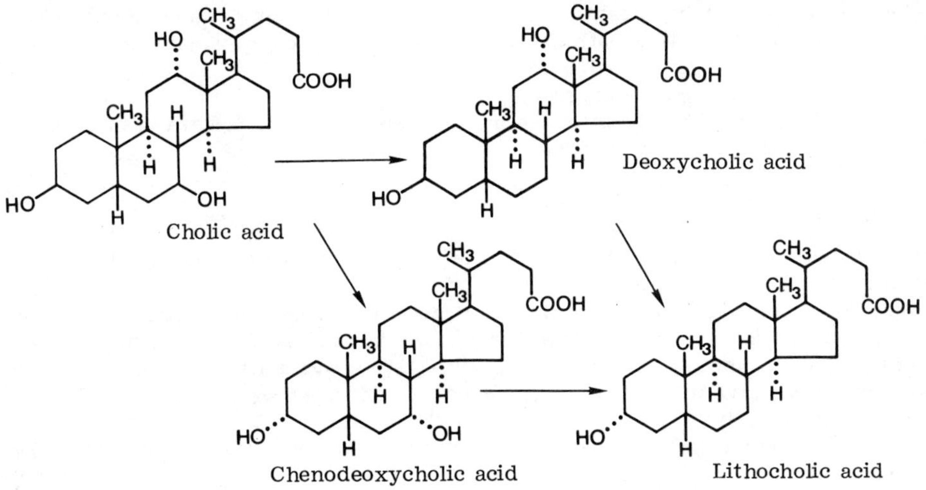

Cholic acid

Deoxycholic acid

Chenodeoxycholic acid

Lithocholic acid

Certain strains are also able to dehydroxylate at the 12 position of cholic acid to produce chenodeoxycholic acid; removal of the OH⁻ at the 12 position by intestinal bacteria produces lithocholic acid. As already mentioned, cholic acid is a product of the deconjugation of bile salts. Deoxycholic acid has been shown to induce local sarcomas

following subcutaneous injection in rats or mice (Hartwell 1951). In the mouse, a minimum tumorigenic dose of this carcinogen has been found to be 2700 mg/kg (Salaman
and Roe 1956).

Dehydroxylation in these cases, of homoprotocatechuic acid (3.4-dihydroxypheny-
lacetic acid) (Scheline et al. 1960), caffeic acid (3,4-dihydroxycinnamic acid), and
3,4-dihydroxyphenylalanine (DOPA) (Booth and Williams 1963a,b) phenylpropionic
acid have been reported. The first and third compounds dehydroxylated to *m*-
hydroxyphenylacetic acid with L-DOPA deaminating; caffeic acid dehydroxylated to
m-hydroxycinnamic acid. The actual bacterial species responsible for dehydroxylation
have not been identified. A strain of Pseudomonas from rat feces was found to dehydroxylate caffeic acid (Perez-Silva et al. 1966).

It seems that the carboxyl group of the above compounds is not necessary for dehydroxylation, since pyrogallol can be dehydroxylated by intestinal bacteria to resorcinol (Scheline 1966a).

Metabolities of tryptophan have been shown to be dehydroxylated by intestinal
bacteria. Thus, kynurenic and xanthurenic acids are dehydroxylated to quinaldic and
8-hydroxyquinaldic acid (Takahashi and Price 1958; Takahashi et al. 1956).

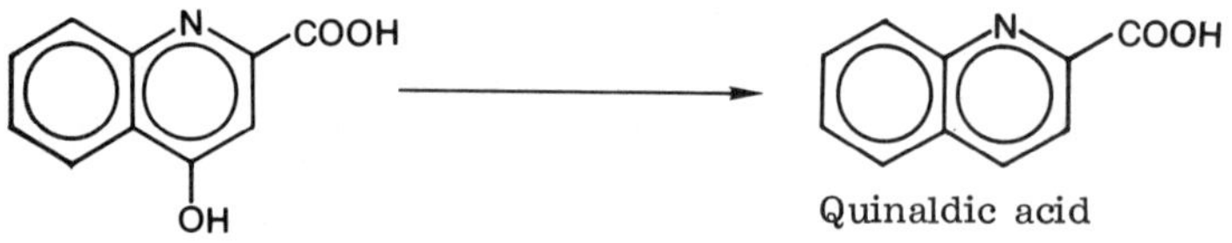

Kynurenic acid

Quinaldic acid

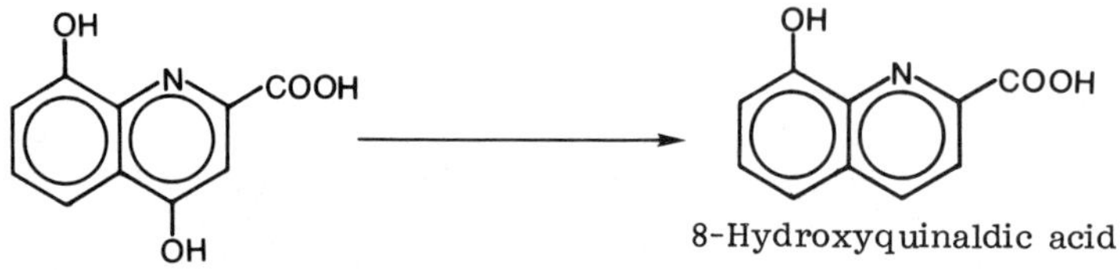

Xanthurenic acid

8-Hydroxyquinaldic acid

The role of intestinal bacteria in promoting dehydroxylation has been confirmed by the
use of antibiotics which prevent such reactions from occurring (Kaihara and Price
1963). It is interesting that both xanthurenic and 8-hydroxyquinaldic acids have been
reported to be tumorigenic, inducing bladder tumors in mice, as have other metabolites
of tryptophan (Bryan and Springberg 1966).

Many other dehydroxylation reactions by intestinal bacteria have been reported
(Scott et al. 1964; Smith et al. 1964).

Demethylation

Some examples of demethylation reactions promoted by intestinal bacteria have been
given in connection with other reactions. Additional types of demethylation reactions
induced by intestinal bacteria are O- and N-demethylations. Some compounds degraded
by O-demethylation are flavonoids and methoxy derivatives of benzoic, phenylacetic,
phenylpropionic, and cinnamic acids (Scheline 1966b; 1968a,b). *o*-Demethylation results in the formation of *o*-dihydroxyphenols, which may have antithiamin effects, as
discussed previously.

N-demethylation is also accomplished by intestinal bacteria. Free choline and
lecithin derivatives following hydrolysis can be N-demethylated to give a tertiary
dimethylamine (Asatoor and Simenhoff 1965). The action of enterobacterial phospholipase and phosphatase on lecithin produces choline (Asatoor and Simenhoff 1965),
which in turn is degraded to trimethylamine by strains of Bacillus spp. and Clostridium
spp. (Cohen et al. 1947). N-Demethylation of trimethylamine by *E. coli, Bacteroides*

fragilis, Bifidobacterium spp., and Clostridium spp. (Asatoor and Simenhoff 1965), such as *C. bifermetans* (Hawksworth and Hill 1971a) produces dimethylamine. Bacte-

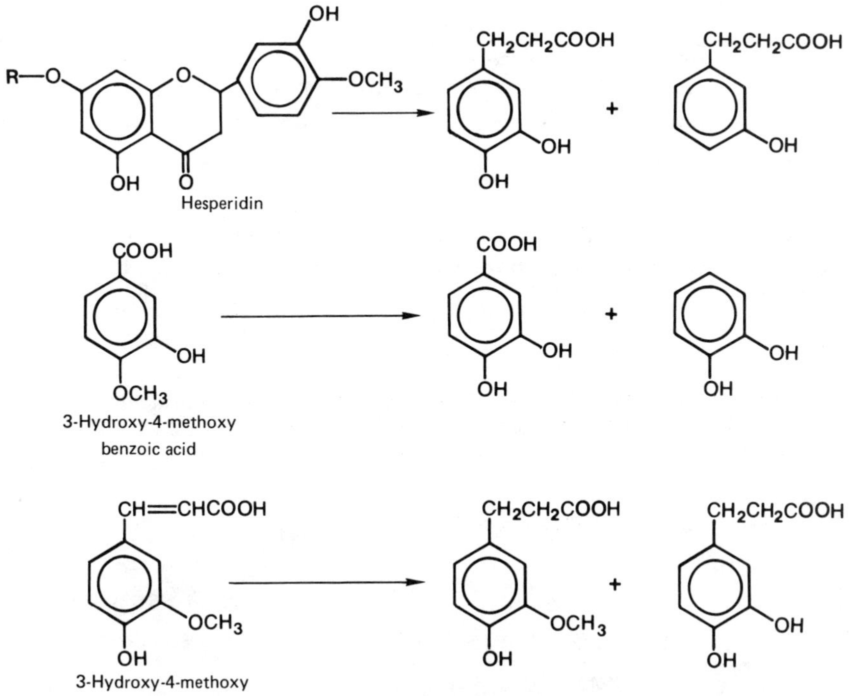

OH

R—O ... OCH$_3$ ... CH_2CH_2COOH ... OH ... + ... CH_2CH_2COOH ... OH

OH   O
Hesperidin

OH   OH

COOH ... COOH ... + ... COOH

OH ... OH ... OH

OCH$_3$ ... OH ... OH
3-Hydroxy-4-methoxy
benzoic acid

CH=CHCOOH ... CH_2CH_2COOH ... + ... CH_2CH_2COOH

OCH$_3$ ... OCH$_3$ ... OH

OH ... OH ... OH
3-Hydroxy-4-methoxy

roides, bifidobacteria, and clostridia as well as *E. coli* and *S. faecalis* can promote the nitrosation of dimethylamine to dimethylnitrosamine (Hawksworth and Hill 1971a,b; Hill and Hawksworth 1972). (See also Chap. 12.)

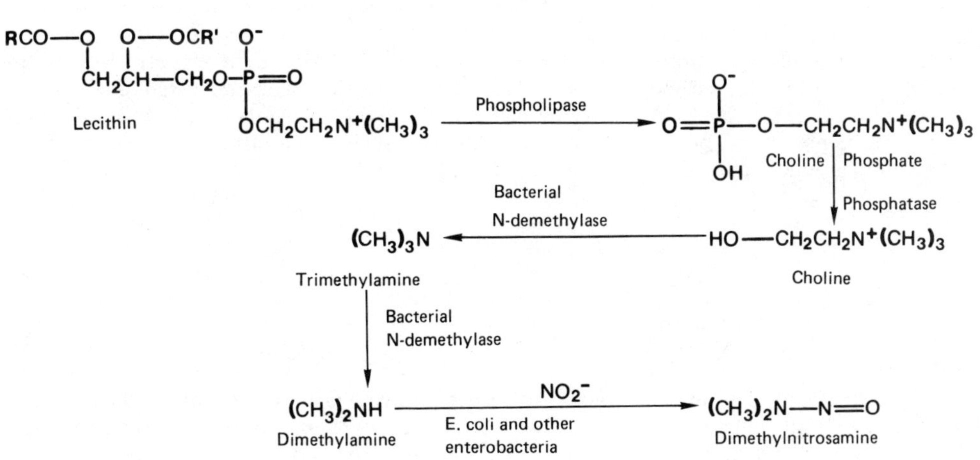

RCO—O O—OCR' O$^-$
        | | |
CH$_2$CH—CH$_2$O—P=O
                    |
Lecithin   OCH$_2$CH$_2$N$^+$(CH$_3$)$_3$

Phospholipase → O=P—O—CH$_2$CH$_2$N$^+$(CH$_3$)$_3$
                     |
                    OH   Choline | Phosphate

Bacterial
N-demethylase   Phosphatase

(CH$_3$)$_3$N ← HO—CH$_2$CH$_2$N$^+$(CH$_3$)$_3$

Trimethylamine   Choline

Bacterial
N-demethylase

NO$_2^-$
(CH$_3$)$_2$NH ————————→ (CH$_3$)$_2$N—N=O

Dimethylamine   E. coli and other   Dimethylnitrosamine
                 enterobacteria

Dimethylamines may be significant in nitrosamine formation (Chap. 21).

Dehalogenation

A good example of a dehalogenation reaction carried out by intestinal bacteria is the reductive dechlorination of DDT (Mendel and Walton 1966).

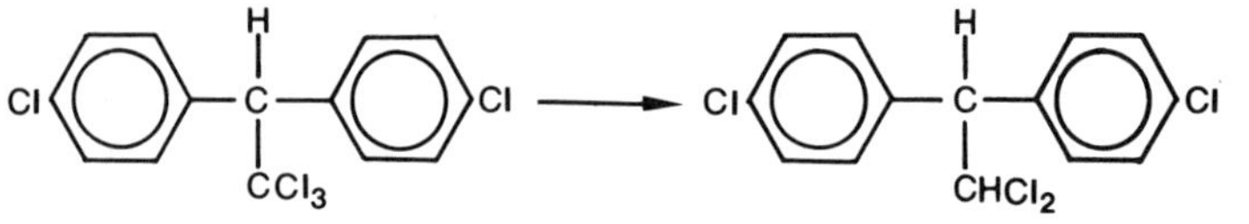

DDT   DDD

Aerobacter aerogenes and *E. coli* isolated from rat intestines appear to readily dechlorinate DDT. *A. aerogenes*, however, can degrade DDT further to several metabolites (Wedemeyer 1966, 1968).

Reduction

Hydrogenation of unsaturated fatty acids and other unsaturated acids, nitro compounds, and azo groups is one form of reduction. The reduction of the unsaturated fatty acids, linolenic and linoleic acids, occurs in the human intestine.

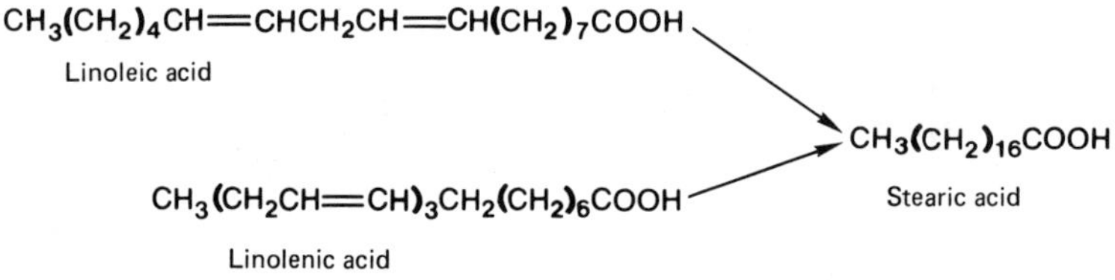

$$CH_3(CH_2)_4CH=CHCH_2CH=CH(CH_2)_7COOH$$

Linoleic acid

$$CH_3(CH_2)_{16}COOH$$

Stearic acid

$$CH_3(CH_2CH=CH)_3CH_2(CH_2)_6COOH$$

Linolenic acid

Common intestinal bacterial species, Clostridium perfringens, Streptococcus faecalis, *E. coli* and others, only in a mixed culture, were observed to hydrogenate linolenic and oleic acids (Wilde and Dawson 1966).

Intestinal bacteria also hydrogenate caffeic acid (Booth and Williams 1963a; Scheline 1968a) and other phenolic unsaturated acids (Scheline 1968a).

Nitro compounds are reduced to the corresponding amines by intestinal bacteria. Proteus vulgaris and *E. coli* reduce chloramphenicol and other organic nitro compounds to the corresponding aryl amines (Saz and Slie 1954a,b; Smith and Worrell 1950, 1949). Aromatic nitro compounds, 2,3,4,5-tetrachloronitrobenzene, nitrobenzene, o-, m-, and p-nitrobenzoic acid and their amides, m- and p-nitrophenol, and o- and p-nitrotoluene can all be reduced by intestinal bacteria. The latter three compounds are reduced much more slowly (Bray et al. 1953).

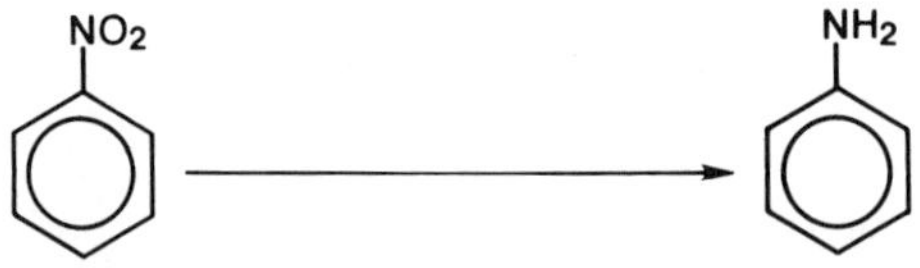

Nitrobenzene   Aniline

The herbicide trifluralin is also reduced to its monoamino derivative. The herbicide is poorly absorbed in rat intestine (approximately 20%). However, the amino derivative appears to be more readily absorbed and depropylated in vivo.

Trifluralin

Many species of intestinal bacteria reduce nitrate to nitrite by means of nitrate reductase, aerobically and anaerobically (Drasar and Hill 1974). One of the most active among these is *E. coli*, one of the most abundant microbial species in the GI tract. This reductive activity of enterobacteria apparently is closely associated with the nitrosation reaction mentioned earlier. However, the same bacterial species may also cause the reduction of nitrite to either N_2 or ammonia. Azo reduction by intestinal bacteria has incurred much attention in recent years, since azo dyes are used as food coloring agents. Breakdown of the azo linkage produces various types of aromatic amines. Many of these products have not been toxicologically evaluated. Nevertheless, breakdown of the azo link has been shown to reduce the carcinogenicity of certain azo dyes. Azo reduction of azo dyes is represented by amaranth (FD&C Red 2), trisodium 1-(4-sulfo-1-naphthylazo)-2-naphthol-3,6-disulfonate) (Radoms and Mellingen 1962), a common food coloring.

Amaranth	1-Amino-2-hydroxy	1-Amino-2-naphthalene
(FD and C Red No. 2)	-3,6-naphthalene	sulfonic acid
	disulfonic acid	

Other azo dyes such as tartrazine (Jones et al. 1964) and acid yellow (4-aminoazobenzene-3,4'-sodium sulfonate) (Scheline and Longberg 1965) also undergo reductive cleavage of the azo bond.

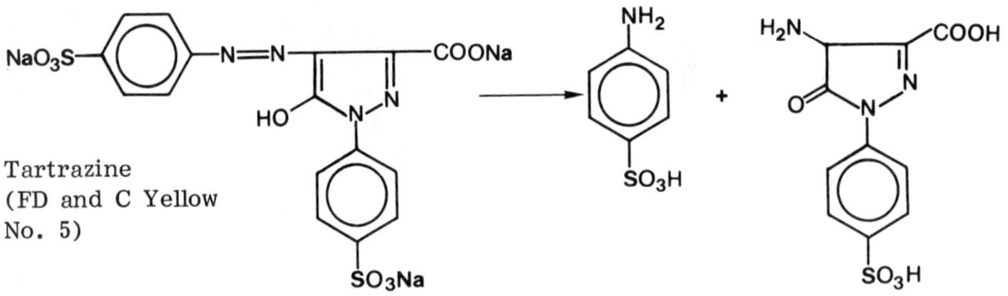

Tartrazine
(FD and C Yellow
No. 5)

It appears that *S. faecalis* has been implicated in a number of bacterial azo reductions Roxon et al. 1966; Scheline 1968b; Scheline and Longberg 1965). *E. coli, A. aerogenes,* and Bacillus proteus have been implicated in the azo reduction of oil-soluble dyes such as 1-phenylazo-2-naphthol and methyl red (4-dimethylaminoazobenzene-2'-carboxylic acid) (Childs et al. 1967; Scheline 1968b). As represented by the reduction of amaranth and tartrazine, products of azo reduction are aromatic amines. Azo reduction may cause reduction of the carcinogenicity of these compounds. However, some of these amines have been found to be carcinogenic, and the toxicological properties of other known products of bacterial reduction have not been determined. Many products of bacterial action on exogenous compounds have not been identified or characterized.

Aromatization

Aromatization carried out by intestinal bacteria is illustrated by the dehydroxylation of quinic acid (Asatoor 1965; Cotran et al. 1960) or shikimic acid, producing benzoic and vanillic acids.

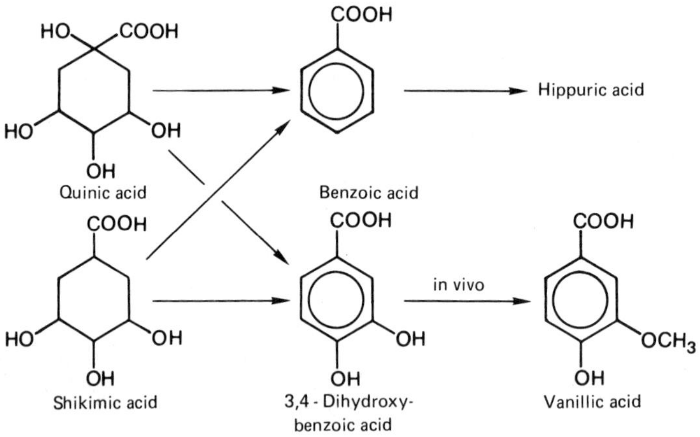

The methylation of 3,4-dihydroxybenzoic acid to form vanillic acid probably does not occur in the presence of bacteria but in the liver. Benzoic and protocatechuic acids are absorbed and conjugated as hippuric acids. Protocatechuic acid may be trans-methylated to vanillic acid and possibly conjugated with glycine to form a hippuric acid derivative. The involvement of intestinal bacteria was suspected when neomycin prevented the formation of hippuric acids from quinic (Cotran et al. 1960) and shikimic acids (Asatoor 1965).

Scission of the Heterocyclic Ring

Scission of the heterocyclic ring by intestinal bacteria has been shown to occur with flavonoids. Rutin, a common flavonoid (Booth and Williams 1963a), is converted to m-hydroxyphenylpropionic acid and m-hydroxyphenylacetic acid (Scheline 1968b).

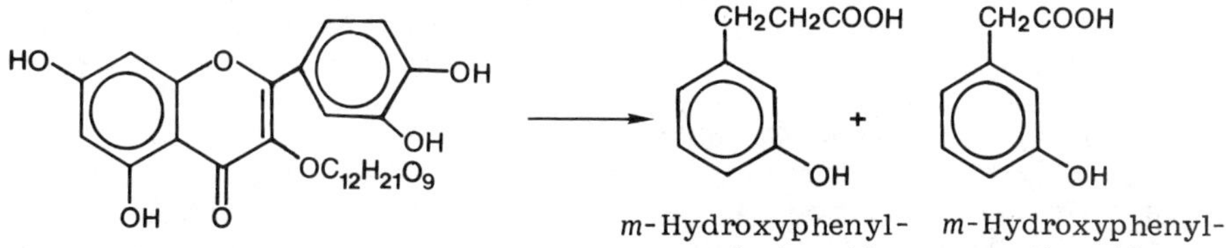

Rutin

m-Hydroxyphenyl-
propionic acid

m-Hydroxyphenyl-
acetic acid

A similar observation has been reported for another flavonoid, hesperidine, which produces similar metabolites to rutin (Booth et al. 1958; Scheline 1968b). The hydroxy groups appear essential to this ring scission, since flavone appears to be cleaved only to a limited extent by intestinal bacteria (Das and Griffiths 1966).

Coumarin is also cleaved to produce melilotic acid by rat cecal microorganisms (Scheline 1968a). The heterocyclic ring is hydrogenated before the cyclic ester bond is broken.

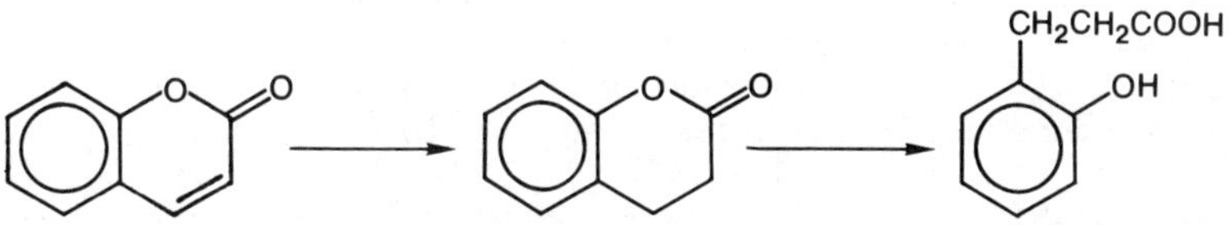

Coumarin   Dihydrocoumarin   Melilotic acid

Intestinal bacteria also cleave the heterocyclic rings of indigo carmine (Lethco and Webb 1966) and tartrazine dyes (Roxon et al. 1967).

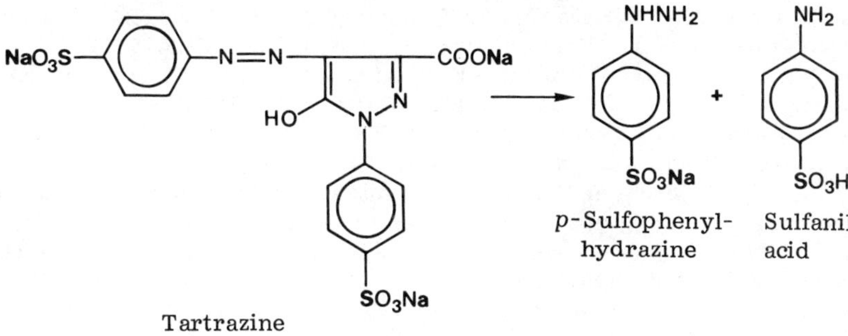

Tartrazine

p-Sulfophenyl-
hydrazine

Sulfanilic
acid

Synthetic Reactions

Intestinal bacteria can acetylate histamine (Sjaastad 1966) and amino sulfonic acid derivatives of azo dyes, such as acid yellow as well as sulfanilic acid and p-phenylenediamine (Scheline and Longberg 1965).

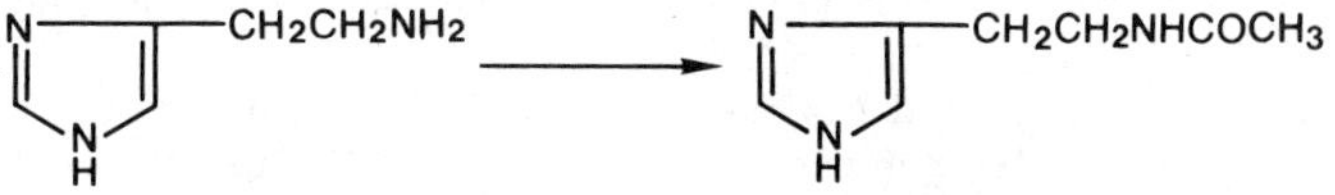

Histamine   N-Acetylhistamine

Esterification of coprosterol and cholesterol has also been observed (Rosenfeld et al. 1967).

Nitrosamine formation at near neutral pH in the gastrointestinal tract is mediated by several species of intestinal bacteria as discussed previously. This topic is treated at length in Chapter 2.

It is obvious from the preceding discussion that the intestinal bacteria must be included in the assessment of the toxicological properties of exogenous compounds. The variety of reactions that intestinal bacteria are capable of presents a formidable problem for the food toxicologists. It is possible that certain diseases, particularly cancer of the GI tract, must involve the activity of intestinal bacteria in their etiologies (Hill 1977; Hill et al. 1971). Evaluating the role of intestinal bacteria in the etiology of a disease is difficult considering the vast number of exogenous and endogenous compounds modified by them. More staggering still is the number of possible metabolites that can be produced by the bacterial reactions in the gastrointestinal tract.

REFERENCES

Abrams, G. D., Bauer, H. and Sprinz, H. 1963. Influence of the normal flora on mucosal morphology and cellular renewal in the ileum. A comparison of germ-free and conventional mice. *Lab. Invest.* 12: 355–364.

Anent, M. E, Shimoda, S. S., Saunders, D. R. and Rubin, C. E. 1971. The pathogenesis of steatorrhea in stasis syndrome. *Gastroenterology* 60: 637.

Asatoor, A. M. 1965. Aromatization of guinic acid and shikimic acid by bacteria and the production of urinary hippurate. *Biochim. Biophys. Acta* 100: 290–292.

Asatoor, A. M. and Kerr, D. N. S. 1961. Amines in blood and urine in relation to liver disease. *Clin. Chim Acta* 6: 149–156.

Asatoor, A. M. and Simenhoff, M. L. 1965. The origin of urinary dimethylamine. *Biochim. Biophys. Acta* 111: 384–392.

Booth, A. N. and Williams, R. T. 1963a. Dehydroxylation of caffeic acid by rat and rabbit caecol contents and sheep rumen liquor. *Nature* 198: 684–685.

Booth, A. N. and Williams, R. T. 1963b. Dehydroxylation of catechol acids by intestinal contents. *Biochem. J.* 88: 66.

Booth, A. N. Murray, C. W., Jones, F. T. and DeEds, F. 1956. The metabolic fate of rutin and quercetin in the animal body. *J. Biol. Chem.* 223: 251–257.

Booth, A. N., Emerson, O. H., Jones, F. J. and DeEds, F. 1957. Urinary metabolites of caffeic and chlorogenic acids. *J. Biol. Chem.* 229: 51–59.

Booth, A. N., Jones, F. T. and De Eds, F. 1958. Metabolic fate of hesperidin, eriodictyol, and diosmin. *J. Biol. Chem.* 230: 661–668.

Boutwell, R. K. and Bosch, D. K. 1959. The tumor-promoting action of phenols and related compounds for mouse skin. *Cancer Res.* 19: 413–424.

Bray, H. G., Hybs, Z., James, S. P. and Thorpe, W. V. 1953. The metabolism of 2:3:5:6- and 2:3:4:5-tetrachloronitrobenzenes in the rabbit and the reduction of aromatic nitro compounds in the intestine. *Biochem. J.* 53: 266–273.

Bryan, G. T. and Springberg, P. D. 1966. The role of the vehicle in the genesis of bladder carcinomas in mice by the pellet implantation technic. *Cancer Res.* 26: 105–109.

Buehler, H. J., Katzman, P. A. and Doisy, E. A. 1951. Studies on β-glucuronidase from E. coli (18591). *Proc. Soc. Exp. Biol. Med.* 76: 672–676.

Cavallaro, J. B. and Rosenweig, N. S. 1971. Chronic afferent loop syndrome with malabsorption "sprue-like" mucosa and mid-loop stenosis. *Gastroenterology* 60: 646.

Chamberlain, T. J. 1970. Licorice poisoning, pseudoaldosteronism, and heart failure. *J.A.M.A.* 213: 1343.

Childs, J. J., Nakajima, C. and Clayson, D. B. 1967. The metabolism of 1-phenylazo-2-napthol in the rat with reference to the action of the intestinal flora. *Biochem. Pharmacol.* 16: 1555–1561.

Christensen, H. E. 1972. Toxic substances list. United States National Technical Information PB Rep. No. 213613/3. Service. Publications Board Report.

Christensen, H. E. (ed.). 1973. *The Toxic Substances List.* 1973 ed. U.S. Department Health Education, Welfare, Rockville, Maryland.

Cohen, G. N., Nisman, S. and Raynaud, M. 1947. Bacterial degradation of choline and ethanolamine. C. R. Hebd. Seances Acad. Sci. (Paris) 225: 647–650. (French)

Conn, E. E. 1969. Cyanogenic glycosides. *J. Agr. Food Chem.* 17: 519–526.

Conn, J. W., Rovner, D. R. and Cohen, E. L. 1968. Licorice-induced pseudoaldosteronism. Hypertension, hypokalemia, aldosteronopenia, and suppressed plasma renin activity. *J.A.M.A.* 205: 492–496.

Cooke, W. T. et al. 1963. The clinical and metabolic significance of jejunal diverticula. *Gut* 4: 115–131.

Cotran, R., Kendrick, M. E. and Kass, E. H. 1960. Role of intestinal bacteria in aromatization of quinic acid in man and guinea pig. *Proc. Soc. Exp. Biol. Med.* 104: 424–425.

Daniel, J. W., Gage, J. C. and Jones, D. L. 1968. The metabolism of 3,5-ditert-butyl-4-hydroxytoluene in the rat and in man. *Biochem. J.* 106: 783–790.

Das, N. P. and Griffiths, L. A. 1966. Studies on flavonoid metabolism. Metabolism of flavone in the guinea pig. *Biochem. J.* 98: 488–492.

Donaldson, R. M. 1968. Role of indigenous enteric bacteria in intestinal function and disease. In: *Handbook of Physiology.* Sect. 6.5 C. F. Code (ed.) American Physiological Society, Washington, D.C.

Drasar, B. S. and Hill, M. J. 1974. *Human Intestinal Flora.* Academic Press, London.

Drasar, B. S., Shiner, M. and McLeod, G. M. 1969. Studies on the intestinal flora. 1. The bacterial flora of the gastrointestinal tract of healthy and achlorhydric persons. *Gastroenterology* 56: 71–79.

Drasar, B. S., Hill, M. J. and Williams, R. E. O. 1970. The significance of the gut flora in safety testing of food additives. In: *Metabolic Aspects of Food Safety.* F. J. C. Roe (ed.). Academic Press, New York.

Dunning, W. F. and Curtis, M. R. 1958. The role of indole in incidence of 2-acetylaminofluorene-induced bladder cancer in rats. *Proc. Soc. Exp. Biol. Med. N.Y.* 99: 91–95.

Dunning, W. F., Curtis, M. R. and Maun, M. E. 1950. The effect of added dietary tryptophane on the occurrence of 2-acetylaminofluorene-induced liver and bladder cancer in rats. *Cancer Res.* 10: 454–459.

Dyer, N. H. and Hawkins, C. 1972. Blind loop syndrome. In: *Recent Advances in Gastroenterology.* J. Badenoch and B. N. Brooke (eds.). Williams & Wilkins, Baltimore.

Eskew, K., MacPherson Phillips, G. W., Griffin, E. L. and Edwards, P. W. 1946. Production of rutin from buckwheat-leaf meal. United States Department of Agriculture. Bureau of Agricultural and Industrial Chemistry. AIC-114.

Glazko, A. J., Dill, W. A. and Wolf, L. M. 1952. Observations on the metabolic disposition of chloramphenicol (chloromycetin) in rat. *J. Pharmacol. Exp. Ther.* 104: 452–458.

Gorbach, S. L. 1971. Intestinal microflora. *Gastroenterology* 60: 1110–1129.

Gorbach, S. L., Nahas, L., Lerner, P. I. and Weinstein, L. 1967. Studies of intestinal microflora. I. Effect of diet, age, and periodic sampling on numbers of fecal microorganisms in man. *Gastroenterology* 53: 845–855.

Hamada, K. 1954. Studies on disposition of carriers of Bacillus thiaminolyticus Matsukawa et Misawa in the intestinal canal. (IV). Action of bile and bile acids of various animals on B. thiaminolyticus Matsukawa et Misawa. *Vitamins* 7: 70–72.

Hanahan, D. J., Daskalakis, E. G., Edwards, T. and Dauben, H. J., Jr. 1953. Metabolic pattern of C^{14}-diethylstilbestrol. *Endocrinology* 53: 163–170.

Hartwell, J. L. 1951. Survey of compounds which have been tested for carcinogenic activity. U.S. Public Health Service Publication No. 149. 2nd ed. U.S. Government Printing Office, Washington, D.C.

Hawksworth, G. M. and Hill, M. J. 1971a. Bacteria and the N-nitrosation of secondary amines. *Br. J. Cancer* 25: 520-526.

Hawksworth, G. M. and Hill, M. J. 1971b. The formation of nitrosamines by human intestinal bacteria. *Biochem. J.* 122: 288.

Higby, R. H. 1941. The chemical nature of hesperidin and its experimental medical use as a source of vitamin P. A review. *J. Am. Pharm. Assoc.* 30: 629–635.

Hill, M. J. 1977. The role of unsaturated bile acids in the etiology of large bowel cancer. In: *Origins of Human Cancer,* Book C. H. H. Hiatt, J. D. Watson and J. A. Winsten (eds.). Cold Spring Harbor Laboratory, New York.

Hill, M. J. and Drasar, B. S. 1967. Bacterial degradation of bile salts. *Biochem. J.* 104: 55.

Hill, M. J. and Hawksworth G. M. 1972. Bacterial production of nitrosamines in vitro and in vivo. In: *N-Nitroso Compounds: Analysis and Formation.* Proc. Working Conf. 1971. P. Bogovski, R. Preussmann, E. A. Walker (eds.), IARC Scientific Publication 3: 116–121.

Hill, M. J., Crowther, J. S. and Drasar, B. S., 1971. Bacteria and the aetiology of cancer of the large bowel. *Lancet* 1: 95–100.

Iveson, P., Parke, D. J. and Williams, R. T. 1966. The metabolic fate of [^{H}C]carbenoxolone in the rat. *Biochem. J.* 100: 28.

Jones, R., Ryan, A. J. and Wright, S. E. 1964. The metabolism and excretion of tartrazine in the rat, rabbit, and man. *Food Cosmet. Toxicol.* 2: 447–452.

Kaihara, M. and Price, J. M. 1963. The effect of feeding neomycin on the dehydroxylation of xanthurenic acid to 8-hydroxyquinaldic acid by the rabbit. *J. Biol. Chem.* 238: 4082–4084.

Kaiser, H. E. 1967. Cancer-promoting effects of phenols in tea. *Cancer* 20: 614–616.

Kimura, R. 1965. Thiamine decomposing Bacteria. In: *Review of Japanese Literature on Beriberi and Thiamine.* N. Shimazono and E. Katsura (eds.). Vitamin B Research Committee of Japan, Kyoto University, Japan.

Koster, M. and David, G. K. 1968. Reversible severe hypertension due to licorice ingestion. *N. Engl. J. Med.* 278: 1381–1383.

Krikler, D. M. and Schrire, V. 1958. "Kwashiorkor" in an adult due to an intestinal blind loop. *Lancet* 1: 510-512.

Lethco, E. J. and Webb, J. M. 1966. The fate of FD&C Blue No. 2 in rats. *J. Pharmacol. Exp. Ther.* 154: 304–389.

Matsumoto, H. and Higa, H. H. 1966. Studies on methylazoxymethanol, the aglycone of cycasin. Methylation of nucleic acids in vitro. *Biochem. J.* 98: 20C.

Melnykowycz, J. and Johansson, K. R. 1955. Formation of amines by intestinal microorganisms and the influence of chlortetracycline. *J. Exp. Med.* 101: 507–517.

Mendel, J. L. and Walton, M. S. 1966. Conversion of p,p,'-DDT to p,p'-DDD by intestinal flora of the rat. *Science* 151: 1527–1528.

Milburn, P., Smith, R. L. and Williams, R. T. 1967. Biphenyl, stilbesterol and phenolphthalein in the rat. Molecular weight, polarity and metabolism as factors in biliary excretion. *Biochem. J.* 105: 1275–1281.

Mollin, M. L. and Ross, G. I. M. 1954. Vitamin B_{12} deficiency in the megaloblastic anaemias. *Proc. Soc. Med.* 47: 428–431.

Moore, W. E. C., Cato, E. P. and Haldeman, L. V. 1969. Anaerobic bacteria of the gastrointestinal flora and their occurrence in clinical infections. *J. Infect. Dis.* 119: 641–649.

Murata, K. 1965. Thiaminase. In: *Review of Japanese Literature on Beriberi and Thiamine.* N. Shimazono and E. Katsura (eds.). Vitamin B Research Committee of Japan, Kyoto University, Japan.

Nishie, K., Gumbmann, M. R. and Keyl, A. C. 1971. Pharmacology of selanine. *Toxicol. Appl. Pharmacol.* 19: 81–92.

Norman, A. and Grubb, R. 1955. Hydrolysis of conjugated bile acids by clostridia and enterococci. *Acta Pathol. Microbiol. Scand.* 36: 537–547.

Norman, A. and Sjövall, J. 1958a. Microbial transformation products of cholic acid in the rat bile acids and steroids. *Biochem. Biophys. Acta* 29: 467—468.

Norman, A. and Sjövall, J. 1958b. On the transformation and enterohepatic circulation of cholic acid in the rat. *J. Biol. Chem.* 233: 872—885.

Orten, J. M. and Neuhaus, O. W. 1975. *Human Biochemistry*. Mosby, St. Louis.

Paulley, J. W. 1969. The jejunal mucosa in malabsorption states with high bacterial counts. In: *Malabsorption*. R. H. Girdwood and A. N. Smith (eds.). University Press, Edinburgh.

Perez-Silva, G., Rodriguez, D. and Perez-Silva, J. 1966. Dehydroxylation of caffeic acid by bacterium isolated from rat feces. *Nature* 212: 303—304.

Potter, D. K. and Fuller, H. L. 1968. Metabolic fate of dietary tannins in chickens. *J. Nutr.* 96: 187—191.

Pulley, G. N. and Von Loesecke, H. W. 1939. Preparation of rhamnose from naringin. *J. Am. Chem. Soc.* 61: 175—176.

Radomski, J. L. and Mellingen, T. J. 1962. The absorption, fate and excretion in rats of the water-soluble azo dyes, FD&C Red No. 2, FD&C Red No. 4 and FD&C Yellow No. 6. *J. Pharmacol. Exp. Ther.* 136: 259—266.

Rayudu, G. V. N., Kadirvel, R., Vohra, P. and Kratzer, F. H. 1970. Toxicity of tannic acid and its metabolites for chicken. *Poult. Sci.* 49: 957—960.

Rosenfeld, R. S., Paul, I. and Yamauchi, T. 1967. Sterol esterification in feces. *Arch. Biochem. Biophys.* 122: 653-657.

Roxon, J. J., Ryan, A. J. and Wright, S. E. 1966. Reduction of tartrazine by a Proteus species isolated from rats. *Food Cosmet. Toxicol.* 4: 419—426.

Roxon, J. J., Ryan, A. J., Welling, P. G. and Wright, S. E. 1967. Origin of urinary sulphanic acid from tartrazine. *Food Cosmet. Toxicol.* 5: 447—449.

Salaman, M. H. and Roe, F. J. C. 1956. Further tests for tumor initiating activity: N,N-di(2-chloroethyl)-p-aminophenylbutyric acid (CB1348) as initiator of skin tumor formation in mouse. *Br. J. Cancer* 10: 363—378.

Saz, A. K. and Slie, R. B. 1954a. The inhibition of organic nitro reductase by aureomycin in cell-free extracts. II. Co-factor requirements for the nitro reductase enzyme complex. *Arch. Biochem. Biophys.* 51: 5—16.

Saz, A. K. and Slie, R. B. 1954b. Reversal of aureomycin inhibition of bacterial cell-free nitro reductase by manganase. *J. Biol. Chem.* 210: 407—412.

Scheline, R. R. 1966a. The decarboxylation of some phenolic acids by the rat. *Acta Pharmacol. Toxicol.* 24: 275—285.

Scheline, R. R. 1966b. Decarboxylation and dimethylation of some phenolic benzoic acid derivatives by rat cecal contents. *J. Pharm. Pharmacol.* 18: 664—669.

Scheline, R. R. 1967. 4-Methylcatechol, a metabolite of homoprotocatechuic acid. *Experientia* 23: 493-494.

Scheline, R. R. 1968a. Metabolism of phenolic acids by the rat intestinal microflora. *Acta Pharmacol. Toxicol.* 26: 189—205.

Scheline, R. R. 1968b. The metabolism of drugs and other organic compounds by intestinal microflora. *Acta Pharmacol. Toxicol.* 26: 332—342.

Scheline, R. R. and Longberg, B. 1965. The absorption, metabolism, and excretion of the sulphonated azo dye, acid yellow, by rats. *Acta Pharmacol. Toxicol.* 23: 1—14.

Scheline, R. R., Williams, R. T. and Wit, J. G. 1960. Biological dehydroxylation. *Nature* 188: 849—850.

Scott, T. W., Ward, P. F. V. and Dawson, R. M. C. 1964. The formation and metabolism of phenyl-substituted fatty acids in the ruminant. *Biochem. J.* 90: 12—24.

Shank, R. C. and Magee, P. N. 1967. Similarities between the biochemical actions of cycasin and dimethylnitrosamine. *Biochem. J.* 105: 521—527.

Sjaastad, O. 1966. Histamine formation and catabolism in the faeces with special reference to dystrophia myotonica. *Scand. J. Gastroenterol.* 1: 173—187.

Smith, A. A., Fabrykant, M., Kaplan, M. and Gavitt, J. 1964. Dehydroxylation of some catecholamines and their products. *Biochem. Biophys. Acta* 86: 429–437.

Smith, G. N. and Worrell, C. S. 1949. Enzymatic reduction of chloramphenicol (chloromycetin). *Arch. Biochem. Biophys.* 24: 216–223.

Smith, G. N. and Worrell, C. S. 1950. The decomposition of chloromycetin (chloramphenicol) by microorganisms. *Arch. Biochem. Biophys.* 28: 232–241.

Spatz, M., Smith, D. W. E., McDaniel, E. G. and Laquer, G. L. 1967. Role of intestinal microorganisms in determining cycasin toxicity. *Proc. Soc. Exp. Biol. Med.* 124: 691–697.

Stecher, P. G., Finkel, M. J., Siegmund, O. H. and Szafranski, B. M. 1960. Merck Index of Chemicals and Drugs. 7th Edition. Merck & Co., Rahway, N.J.

Tabaqchali, S. and Booth, C. C. 1970. Bacteria and the small intestines. In: *Modern Trends in Gastroenterology*. W. I. Card and B. Creamer (eds.). Butterworth, London.

Tabaqchali, S., Hatzioannou, J. and Booth, C. C. 1968. Bile salt deconjugation and steatorrhea in patients with the stagnant loop syndrome. *Lancet* 2: 12–16.

Takahashi, H. and Price, J. M. 1958. Dehydroxylation of xanthurenic acid to 8-hydroxyquinaldic acid. *J. Biol. Chem.* 233: 150–153.

Takahashi, H., Kaihara, M. and Price, J. M. 1956. The conversion of kynurenic acid to quinaldic acid by humans and rats. *J. Biol. Chem.* 223: 705–708.

Tompsett, S. L. 1958. The determination and excretion of polyhydroxy (catecholic) phenolic acid in urine. *J. Pharm. Pharmacol.* 10: 157–161.

Van Duuren, B. L. et al. 1968. Initiators and promoters in tobacco carcinogenesis. *Natl. Cancer Inst. Monogr.* 28: 173–180.

Wagoner, J. K. and Infante, P. F. 1977. Vinyl chloride: A case for the use of laboratory bioassay in the regulatory control procedure. In: *Origins of Human Cancer*. Book C. H. H. Hiatt, J. D. Watson and J. A. Winsten (eds.). Cold Spring Harbor Laboratory, New York.

Wedemeyer, G. 1966. Dechlorination of DDT by Aerobacter aerogenes. *Science* 152: 647.

Wedemeyer, G. 1968. Role of intestinal microflora in the degradation of DDT by rainbow trout (Salmo gairdneri). *Life Sci.* 7: 219–223.

Wilde, P. F. and Dawson, R. M. C. 1966. The biohydrogenation of α-linoleic acid and oleic acid by rumen micro-organism. *Biochem. J.* 98: 469–475.

Williams, R. T. 1959. *Detoxication Mechanisms*. 2nd ed. Chapman and Hall, London.

Williams, R. T. 1970. Discussion in Drasar, B.S. et al. 1970. The significance of the gut flora in safety testing of food additives. In: *Metabolic Aspects of Food Safety*. F. J. C. Roe (ed.), Academic Press, New York.

Williams, R. T. 1971. The metabolism of certain drugs and food chemicals in man. *Ann. New York Acad. Sci.* 179: 141–153.

Williams, R. E. O. and Drasar, B. S. 1972. Alterations in gut bacterial flora in disease. In: *Recent Advances in Gastroenterology*. 2nd ed. J. Badenoch and B. N. Brooke, Churchill-Livingston, London.

Zoller, H. F. 1917. Some constituents of American grapefruit (Citrus decumana). *J. Ind. Eng. Chem.* 10: 364–373.

4

Metabolism of Nonnutritive Components in Foods and Related Compounds

Mammalian cells of specific organs possess enzymes which transform nonnutritive food compounds and other exogenous substances into more water-soluble derivatives, thus facilitating their elimination through the bile or urine. These enzymes are strategically located in cells of tissues through which foreign compounds can be absorbed into the body—namely, the skin, the gastrointestinal tract, liver, lungs and kidneys. The liver is the organ where the bulk of xenobiotic metabolism occurs.

While it may be contended that the principal result of the activity of these enzymes is to render these compounds less toxic, the facts argue against this, for there are many cases where metabolism enhances the toxic potentials of compounds.

Following absorption, a compound passes through the liver and is metabolized to an extent depending on the dose and the condition of this organ. Those escaping metabolism are dispersed through other tissues by the blood or lymph and act on specific target receptors in specific cells, thus causing their toxic effects. The compounds may then be metabolized in the extrahepatic cells or be exuded back into the circulation, and to pass through the liver once more. This time, they do not escape biotransformation into more excretable by-products.

Some substances may be taken out of the circulation and rendered less active for a time by being stored in the fatty deposits of cells, or in the tissues of the bone or hair. These stored substances, except those in the hair, may be readmitted into the circulation under certain conditions. For example, substances stored in the adipose tissues may again be found in the general circulation following loss of fat in the body (Conney et al. 1967; Dale et al. 1962).

The enzymes involved in the metabolism of exogenous nonnutritive compounds are located in the endoplasmic reticulum; they are generally referred to as microsomal enzymes following their isolation in vitro from microsomes. The microsomes are fragments of the endoplasmic reticulum mechanically disrupted from the cell.

The compounds that enter the body can be classified into two major groups based on (1) water or (2) lipid solubility. Water-soluble compounds are promptly eliminated without being metabolized by the microsomal enzymes. The lipid-soluble compounds may react with a specific group of enzymes in two phases (Williams 1970).

In Phase I, the compounds are degraded into more polar derivatives by oxidation, reduction, hydrolysis, and other degradative reactions. These products have reduced molecular weights and are still too nonpolar for excretion. Occasionally, the derivatives are more toxic than the parent compounds.

In Phase II reactions detoxify the metabolites, often through conjugation with polar moieties. These synthetic processes produce higher molecular weight compounds excretable in the bile or urine.

PHASE I REACTIONS

In Phase I, polar reactive groups such as $-OH$, $-NH_2$, $-SH$, $-COOH$, and similar polar groups are introduced or unmasked by any one of the following:

Oxidation

Microsomal Oxidation

The oxidation of foreign compounds in the liver, according to Holtzman and coworkers (1968), involves at least four factors, namely, nicotinamide adenine dinucleotide phosphate (NADPH), cytochrome reductase (flavoprotein [FAD]), and cytochrome P-450, and O_2. A fifth factor which appears to be a nonheme sulfur iron protein (adrenodoxin) (Orten and Neuhaus 1975) is required in the adrenal mitochondria but possibly not in the liver microsomes. The oxidation of compounds with the above factors is shown in the following scheme with the fifth factor (X) included.

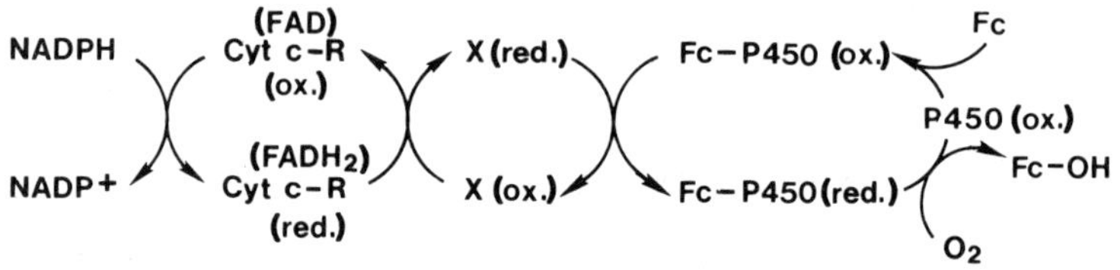

Cyt c-R = cytochrome c reductase flavoprotein (FAD)
P450   = cytochrome P-450
X   = Nonheme si (e.g., adrenodoxin or testodoxin in
ox.   = oxidize the adrenal or testicular mitochondria,
red.   = reduce, respectively [Orten and Neuhaus 1975]
Fc   = foreign compound
Fc-OH   = oxidized foreign compound

The above system of enzymes is often referred to as the "mixed function oxidase system." The foreign compound binds firmly to cytochrome P-450 until it is oxidized. This mechanism can be inhibited by carbon monoxide or cyanide which also binds firmly with cytochrome P-450. Cytochrome P-450 is called a terminal oxidase. In the case of polycyclic aromatic hydrocarbons and polychlorinatedbiphenyls (PCB), the terminal oxidase is cytochrome P-448 (Kappas and Alvares 1975). The mixed function oxidase system for the polycyclic aromatic hydrocarbons is called aryl hydrocarbon hydroxylase.

The types of oxidation-reduction reactions carried out by the mixed function oxidase system include the following (Norton 1975; Williams 1970).

Aromatic Oxidation In this case an $-OH$ is introduced into the aromatic ring.

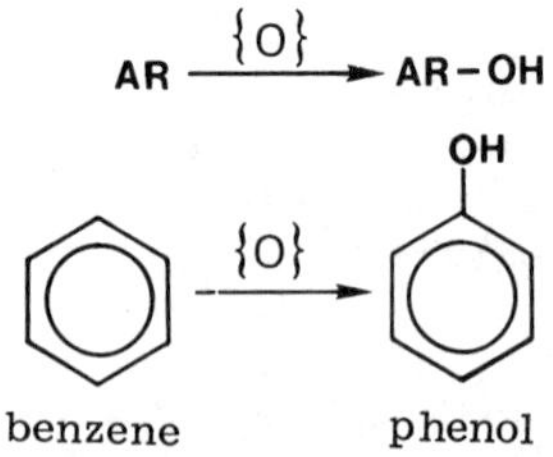

(O) = mixed function oxidase system—
        cytochrome P-450 or P-448
AR = aromatic ring

The aromatic compounds may contain substituents. In this case, the —OH may be introduced o- or p- to the substituents.

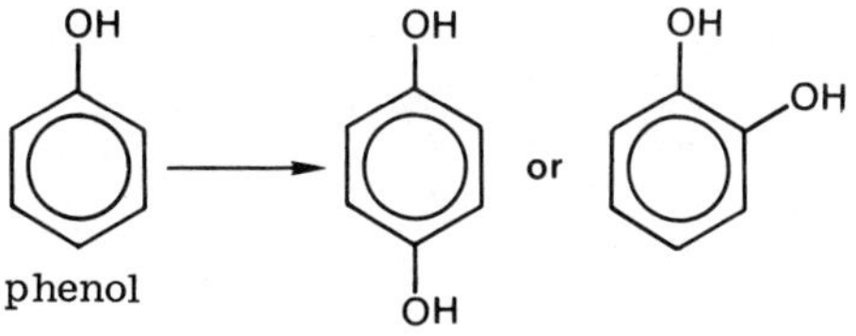

OH

phenol

hydroquinone pyrocatechol

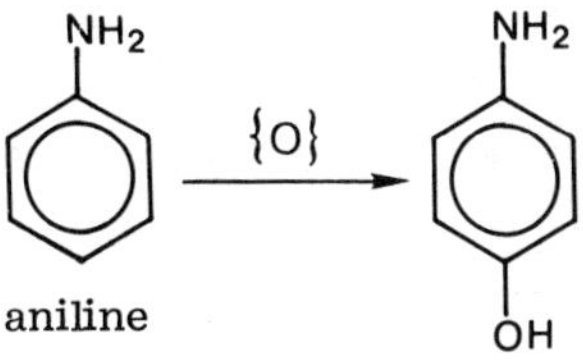

aniline

p-aminophenol

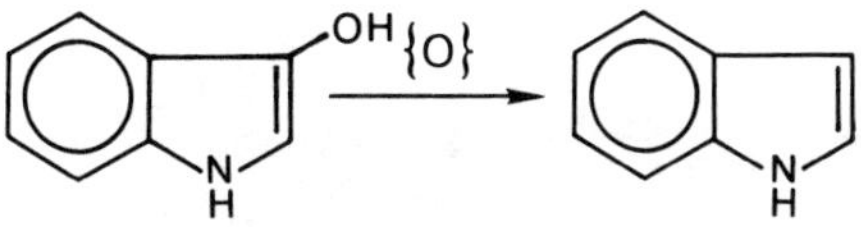

indole

indoxyl

Aliphatic Oxidation For aliphatic hydrocarbons, the initial oxidation product is an alcohol which is oxidized further to a carboxylic acid.

$$CH_3CH_2CH_2CH_2CH_2CH_3 \xrightarrow{\{O\}} CH_3(CH_2)_5OH \xrightarrow{\{O\}} CH_3(CH_2)_4COOH$$

The carboxylic acid (a fatty acid) is oxidized further by β-oxidation:

$$CH_3(CH_2)_4COOH \xrightarrow[\text{thiokinase}]{\text{ATP, CoA}} CH_3(CH_2)_4COSCoA \xrightarrow[\text{dehydrogenase}]{\text{FAD}}$$

$$CH_3(CH_2)_2CH=CHCOSCoA \xrightarrow[\text{hydrase}]{H_2O} CH_3(CH_2)_2\overset{OH}{\underset{|}{C}}HCH_2COSCoA$$

$$\xrightarrow[\text{dehydrogenase}]{\text{NAD}} CH_3(CH_2)_2\overset{O}{\overset{\|}{C}}CH_2COSCoA \xrightarrow[\text{thiolase}]{\text{CoA}} CH_3(CH_2)_2COSCoA +$$

$$CH_3COSCoA$$

$$CH_3(CH_2)_2COSCoA \xrightarrow[\text{dehydrogenase}]{\text{FAD}} \beta\text{-Oxidation} \rightarrow CH_3COSCoA \rightarrow \text{Krebs cycle}$$

A comparison between aliphatic and aromatic oxidation shows that the latter can take place much less easily as exemplified by n-propylbenzene (Parke 1968).

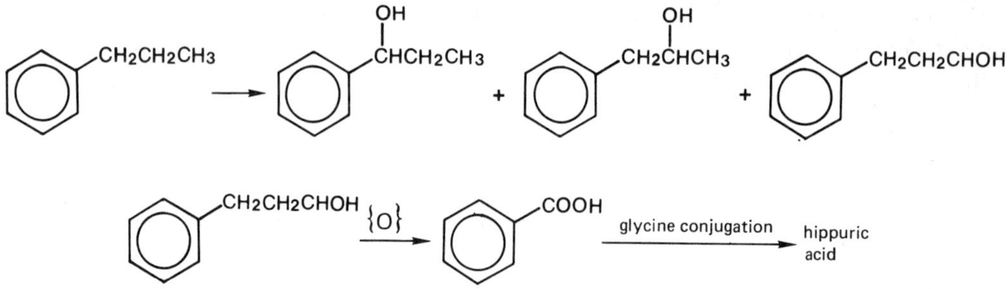

$$\text{C}_6\text{H}_5\text{-CH}_2\text{CH}_2\text{CH}_3 \longrightarrow \text{C}_6\text{H}_5\text{-}\underset{\text{OH}}{\text{CHCH}_2\text{CH}_3} + \text{C}_6\text{H}_5\text{-}\text{CH}_2\underset{\text{OH}}{\text{CHCH}_3} + \text{C}_6\text{H}_5\text{-CH}_2\text{CH}_2\text{CHOH}$$

$$\text{C}_6\text{H}_5\text{-CH}_2\text{CH}_2\text{CHOH} \xrightarrow{\{O\}} \text{C}_6\text{H}_5\text{-COOH} \xrightarrow{\text{glycine conjugation}} \text{hippuric acid}$$

Dealkylation This reaction may proceed, presumably, by initial introduction of —OH to the alkyl group forming an unstable hemiacetal which decomposes to an alcohol and an aldehyde.

$$\text{R}-\text{O}-\text{CH}_2\text{R}' \longrightarrow \text{R}-\text{O}-\underset{\text{OH}}{\text{CH}}-\text{R}' \longrightarrow \text{ROH} + \text{R}'\text{CH=O} \longrightarrow \text{R}'\text{COOH} \longrightarrow$$

$$\text{CO}_2 + \text{H}_2\text{O} \qquad \text{hemiacetal}$$

A specific example is butylatedhydroxyanisole (BHA) (Astill et al. 1960, 1962).

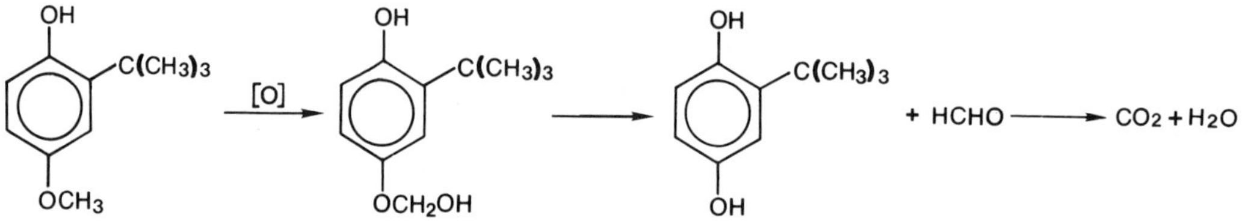

BHA: $\text{OH, } \text{C(CH}_3)_3\text{, OCH}_3$ ring $\xrightarrow{[O]}$ $\text{OH, C(CH}_3)_3\text{, OCH}_2\text{OH}$ ring $\longrightarrow$ $\text{OH, C(CH}_3)_3\text{, OH}$ ring $+ \text{HCHO} \longrightarrow \text{CO}_2 + \text{H}_2\text{O}$

BHA

Demethylation of BHA, however, is accomplished by rats and dogs; human subjects tested by Astill et al. (1960) were unable to O-demethylate this compound.

N-Dealkylation Cleavage of the $-\overset{|}{\text{N}}-\overset{|}{\text{C}}-$ bond can lead to the formation of a free amino group. Like O-dealkylation, an unstable hydroxyl intermediate (aldehyde-amine) is presumed to be formed.

$$\text{R}-\text{NHCH}_2-\text{R}' \longrightarrow \text{R}-\text{NH}\underset{\text{OH}}{\text{CH}}-\text{R}' \longrightarrow \text{RNH}_2 + \text{R}'\text{CHO}$$

Specific examples of N-dealkylation reactions are the herbicide trifluralin (Emmerson and Anderson 1966) and the azo dye 4-dimethylaminoazobenzene (Miller and Bauman 1945; Stevenson et al. 1942).

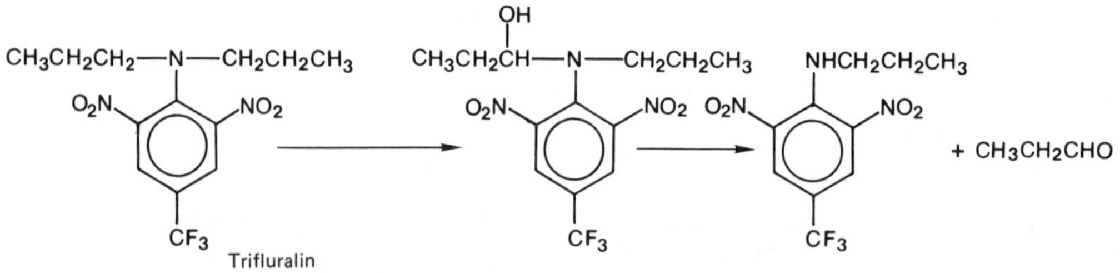

$$\text{CH}_3\text{CH}_2\text{CH}_2\text{-N-CH}_2\text{CH}_2\text{CH}_3 \longrightarrow \text{CH}_3\text{CH}_2\underset{\text{OH}}{\text{CH}}\text{-N-CH}_2\text{CH}_2\text{CH}_3 \longrightarrow \text{NHCH}_2\text{CH}_2\text{CH}_3 + \text{CH}_3\text{CH}_2\text{CHO}$$

(ring substituents: O_2N, NO_2, CF_3)

Trifluralin

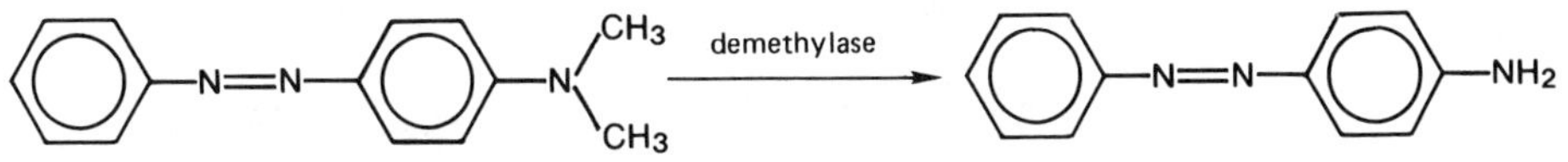

4-Dimethylaminoazobenzene

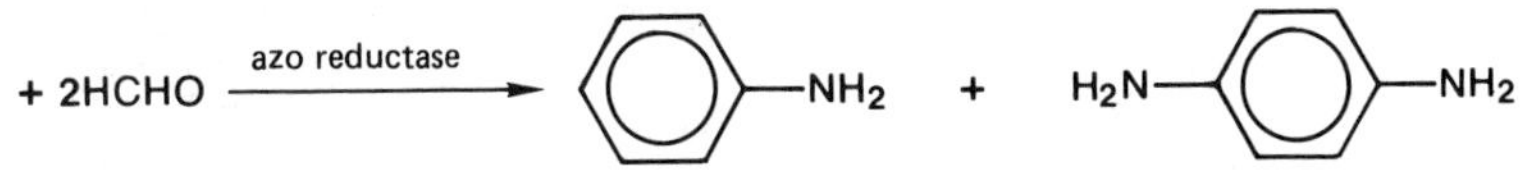

S-Dealkylation

$$R-S-CH_3 \xrightarrow{[O]} R-S-CH_2OH \longrightarrow RSH + HCOH$$

An example of S-dealkylation reaction is the herbicide prometryne. The resulting mercaptan is oxidized to the disulfide (Boehme and Baer 1967). The herbicide can also be N-dealkylated to an aminotriazine, and the resulting amino groups are oxidized to −OH (Knuesli et al. 1969). In the above reaction, for prometryne,

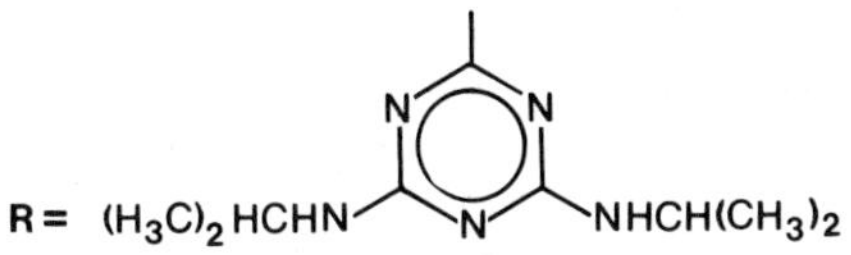

$$R = (H_3C)_2 HCHN \quad \cdots \quad NHCH(CH_3)_2$$

The N-dealkylation of prometryne is shown as follows:

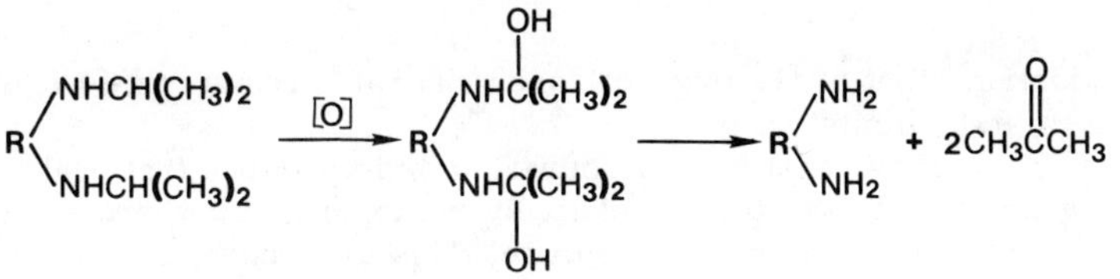

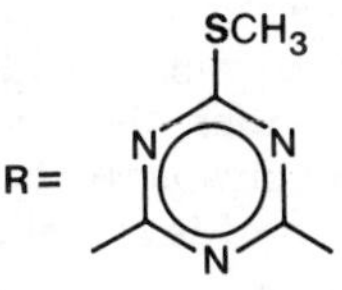

N-Oxidation   A specific example of this type of reaction is the oxidation of 2-aminoacetylfluorene (Grantham et al. 1968); this reaction is an activation step.

The introduction of −OH to the nitrogen renders this compound carcinogenic. The metabolism of this compound is discussed further in Chapter 6.

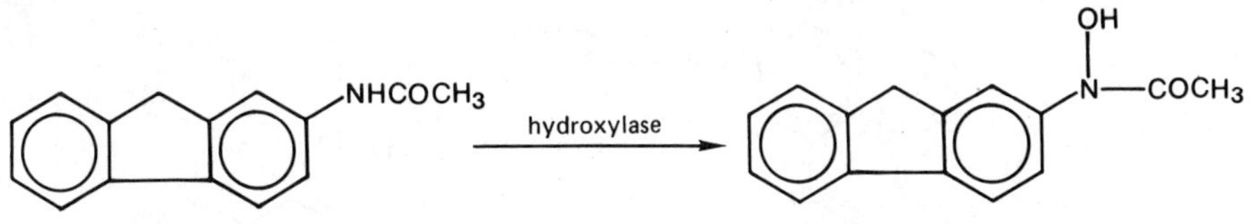

2-Aminoacetylfluorene

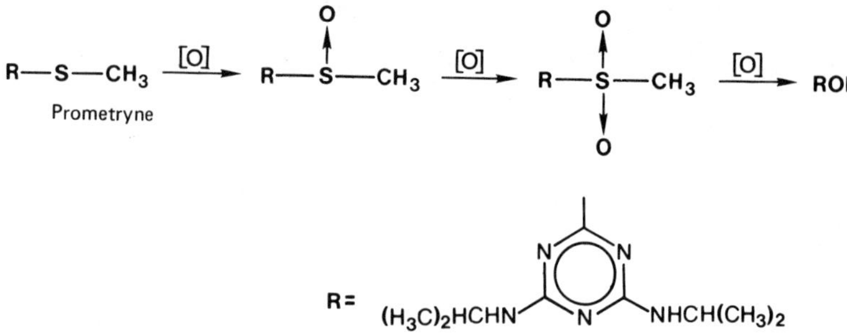

$$R—S—CH_3 \xrightarrow{[O]} R—\overset{\displaystyle O}{\underset{}{S}}—CH_3 \xrightarrow{[O]} R—\overset{\displaystyle O}{\underset{\displaystyle O}{S}}—CH_3 \xrightarrow{[O]} ROH$$

Prometryne

R= (H₃C)₂HCHN—(triazine ring)—NHCH(CH₃)₂

$R=$ $(H_3C)_2HCHN$ —(triazine)— $NHCH(CH_3)_2$

S-Oxidation   Two types of S-oxidation reactions may occur depending on the nature of the sulfur atom in the molecule. As shown in the following reactions, where the bonds of the divalent sulfide atom are saturated, sulfoxide and sulfone formation result. A specific example is the oxidation of herbicide prometryne (Boehme and Baer 1967). In another case, the thionosulfur is removed, replaced by oxygen, and oxidized to sulfate. An example is the oxidation of thioureas (Williams 1959) and organothiophosphates (O'Brien 1967).

$$(NH_2)_2—C{=}S \longrightarrow (NH_2)_2—C{=}O + SO_4^{=}$$

Thiourea   Urea

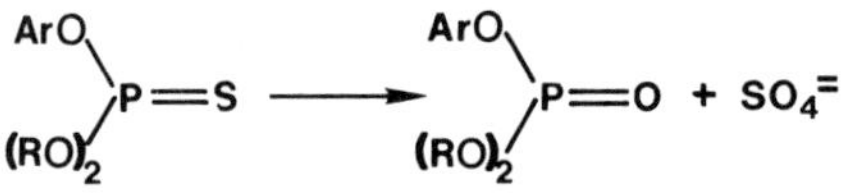

$$\begin{matrix} ArO \\ \diagdown \\ \diagup \\ (RO)_2 \end{matrix} P{=}S \longrightarrow \begin{matrix} ArO \\ \diagdown \\ \diagup \\ (RO)_2 \end{matrix} P{=}O + SO_4^{=}$$

Organothionophosphate

The latter oxidation, that of the organothionophosphate, results in a more potent acetylcholine esterase inhibitor.

Note that in the above examples, thiourea, a toxic product (rat oral LD_{50} = 125 to 1830 mg/kg) is oxidized to the relatively nontoxic urea, whereas the opposite is seen in the case of the organothionophosphate. This difference in toxicity is not due to the differences in the effects associated with the $=C{=}O$ or the $=P{=}O$ function, but rather to the other groups in the molecule. Thus, the carbamate insecticides, e.g., carbaryl, which are potent acetylcholinesterase inhibitors, contain the $=C{=}O$ function. They are direct inhibitors of this enzyme and thus do not require activation (Campbell et al. 1963). Thiourea is toxic because only a small proportion of it is metabolized to urea (Williams 1959).

Epoxidation   Polar hydroxy groups may be introduced into aromatic hydrocarbons such as benzene (Udenfriend et al. 1969) and polycyclic aromatic hydrocarbons (Grover et al. 1971). The epoxidation of benzo(a)pyrene results in an active metabolite, which is detoxified subsequently by hydrolysis and then by appropriate conjugation of the phenolic derivatives.

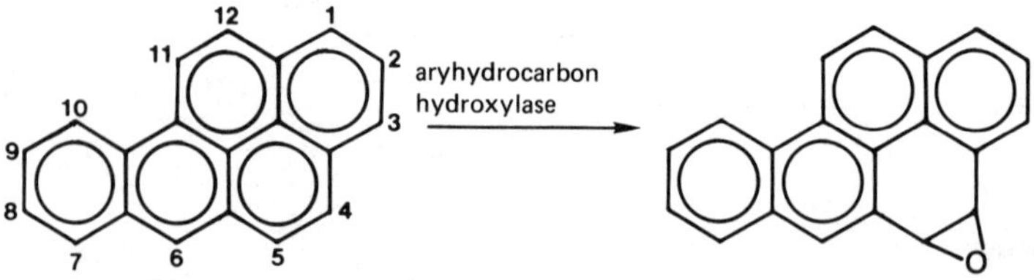

aryhydrocarbon hydroxylase

3,4-Benzpyrene   3,4-Benzpyrene-4-epoxide

Epoxidation at strategic positions in the molecule such as the 4-5 position shown above confers carcinogenic activity on this compound. This aspect is discussed further in Chapter 6. Epoxidation of this compound also occurs at other positions in the molecule; e.g., at the 7,8-, and 9,10-positions (Dipple 1976).

Nonmicrosomal Oxidation

Oxidation of compounds also occurs in the mitochondria and cytoplasm. This generally involves primary amines, alcohols, and aldehydes (Parke 1968).

Amine Oxidations   For amines, two types of amine oxidases are present, the diamine and monoamine oxidases. Primary amines, represented by tyramine, are de-aminated with monoamine oxidases (MAO). These enzymes provide an essential and effective control of both biogenic and exogenous primary amines which have profound biological effects (Chaps. 8 and 12).

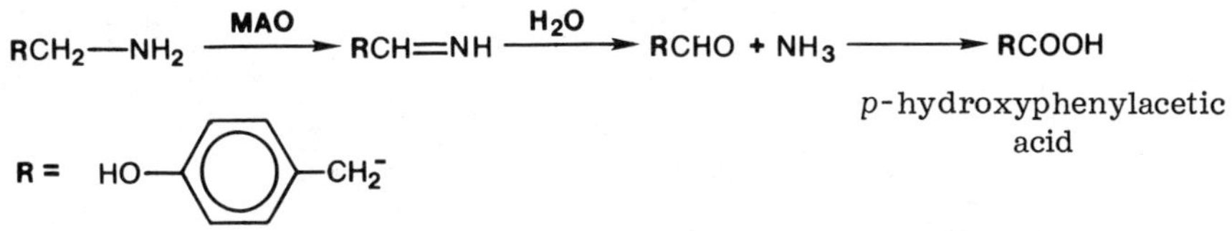

$$RCH_2-NH_2 \xrightarrow{\textbf{MAO}} RCH=NH \xrightarrow{H_2O} RCHO + NH_3 \longrightarrow RCOOH$$

p-hydroxyphenylacetic
acid

R =   HO—⟨○⟩—CH$_2^-$

Diamines represented by putrescine and histamine may be deaminated by diamine oxidases (DAO), which catalyze the removal of only one of the amino groups. This enzyme effectively controls the levels of diamines which may be derived from intestinal bacterial decarboxylation of basic amino acids (Chap. 3).

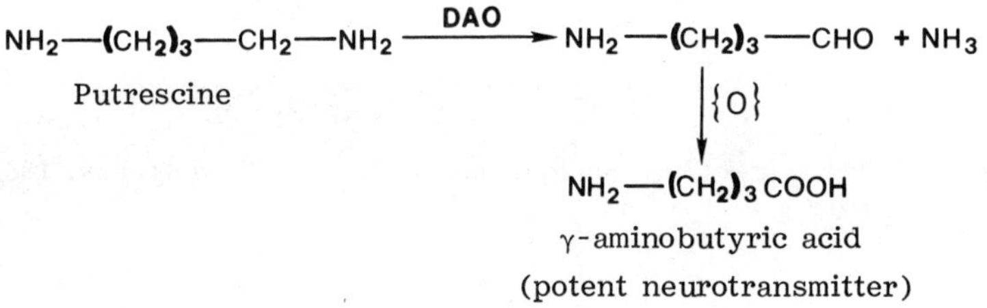

$$NH_2-(CH_2)_3-CH_2-NH_2 \xrightarrow{\textbf{DAO}} NH_2-(CH_2)_3-CHO + NH_3$$

Putrescine

$$\downarrow \{O\}$$

$$NH_2-(CH_2)_3 COOH$$

γ-aminobutyric acid

(potent neurotransmitter)

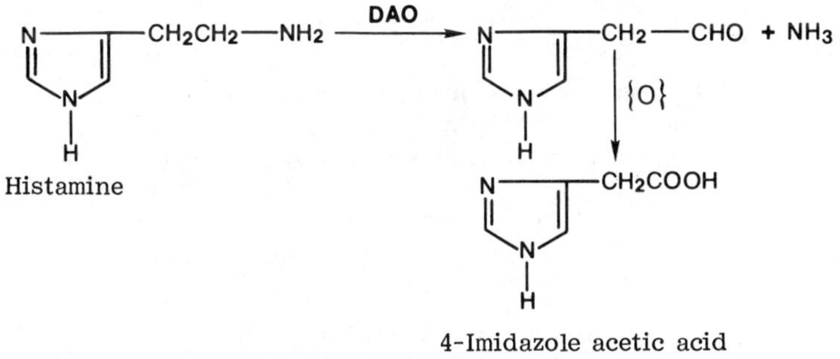

Histamine

4-Imidazole acetic acid

Alcohol and Aldehyde Oxidations   Alcohol oxidation by alcohol dehydrogenases is limited to primary and secondary alcohols. Tertiary alcohols are conjugated instead (Norton 1975).

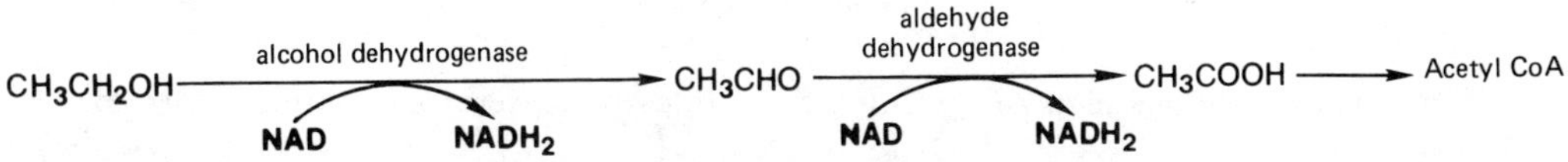

$$CH_3CH_2OH \xrightarrow[\substack{\text{NAD} \quad \text{NADH}_2}]{\text{alcohol dehydrogenase}} CH_3CHO \xrightarrow[\substack{\text{NAD} \quad \text{NADH}_2}]{\substack{\text{aldehyde}\\\text{dehydrogenase}}} CH_3COOH \longrightarrow \text{Acetyl CoA}$$

Reduction

Two examples of microsomal reduction follow.

Nitrate reduction

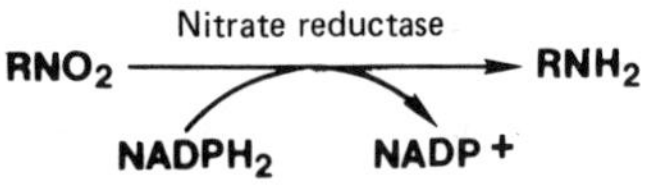

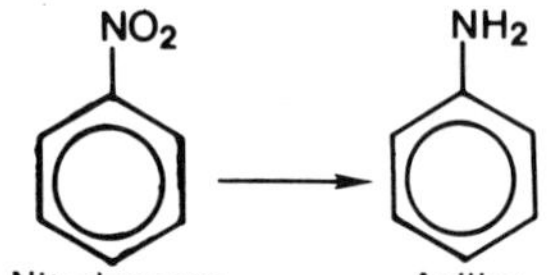

Nitrobenzene Aniline

Azo Reduction

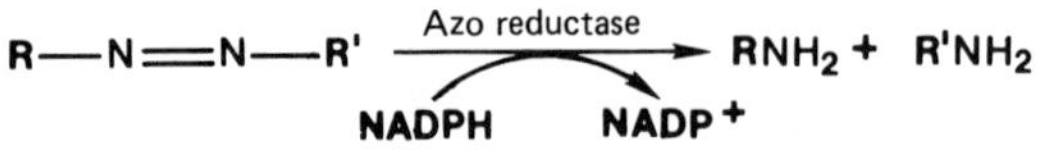

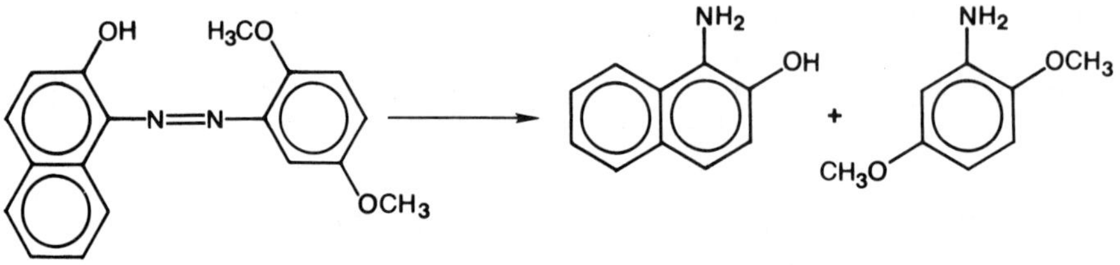

Citrus Red No. 2 1-Amino-2-naphthol

Note that 1-amino-2-naphthol is a bladder carcinogen in mice (Boyland 1963; Clayson et al. 1968; Dacre 1965).

Hydrolysis

Esters.

$$RCOOR' \xrightarrow[\text{Hydrolase}]{H_2O} RCOOH + R'OH$$

$$CH_3—CH_2COOH \longrightarrow CH_3CH_2OH + HCOOH$$

Ethyl formate

Amides.

$$RCONHR' \xrightarrow[\text{Hydrolase}]{H_2O} RCOOH + R'NH_2$$

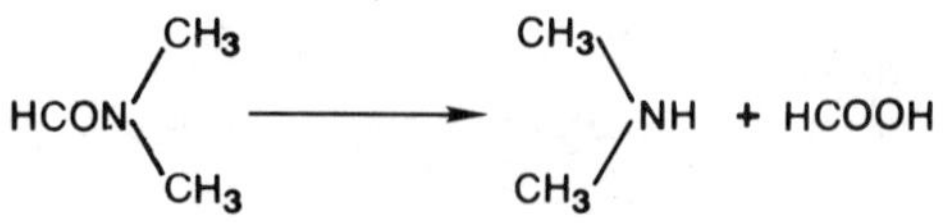

N,N-Dimethyl formamide

Various glycosides may be hydrolyzed by intestinal bacteria or after absorption.

Other Biotransformation Reactions

Increasingly, research on microsomal reactions reveals that biotransformation reactions are not confined to the major reactions just discussed. In addition to the preceding reactions, others which have been demonstrated include the following.

Dehydroxylation

Both aromatic and aliphatic dehydroxylations have been demonstrated in mammalian systems. Dehydroxylation of meta or para hydroxyl groups of protocatechuic acid has been reported in rabbits (Scheline et al. 1960).

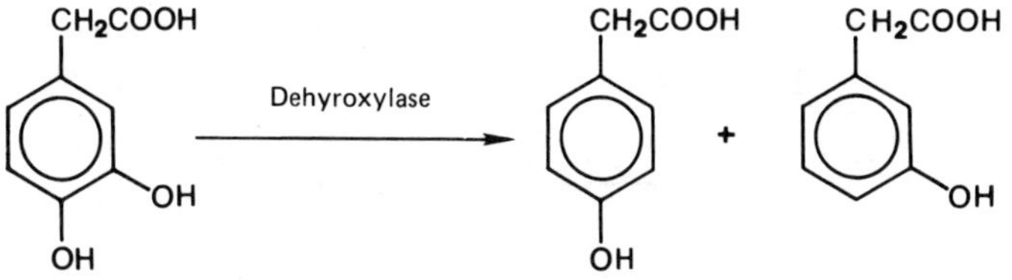

Protocatechuic acid

Similarly, dehydroxylation of catecholamines involving the aliphatic hydroxy group can also occur. For norepinephrine, dehydroxylation follows transmethylation and oxidative deamination (Smith et al. 1964).

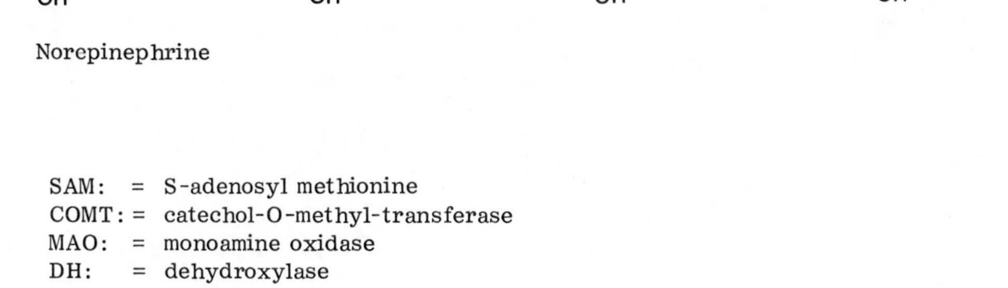

Norepinephrine

SAM: = S-adenosyl methionine
COMT: = catechol-O-methyl-transferase
MAO: = monoamine oxidase
DH: = dehydroxylase

Dehalogenation

An example of dehalogenation is the dechlorination of DDT. In humans, DDT is dechlorinated to DDE (1,1-dichloro-2,2-bis(p-chlorophenyl)ethylene), DDD (1,1-dichloro-2,2-bis(p-chlorophenyl)ethane) and ultimately to DDA (2,2-bis [p-chlorophenyl] acetic acid) (Ottoboni et al. 1968; Peterson and Robison 1964).

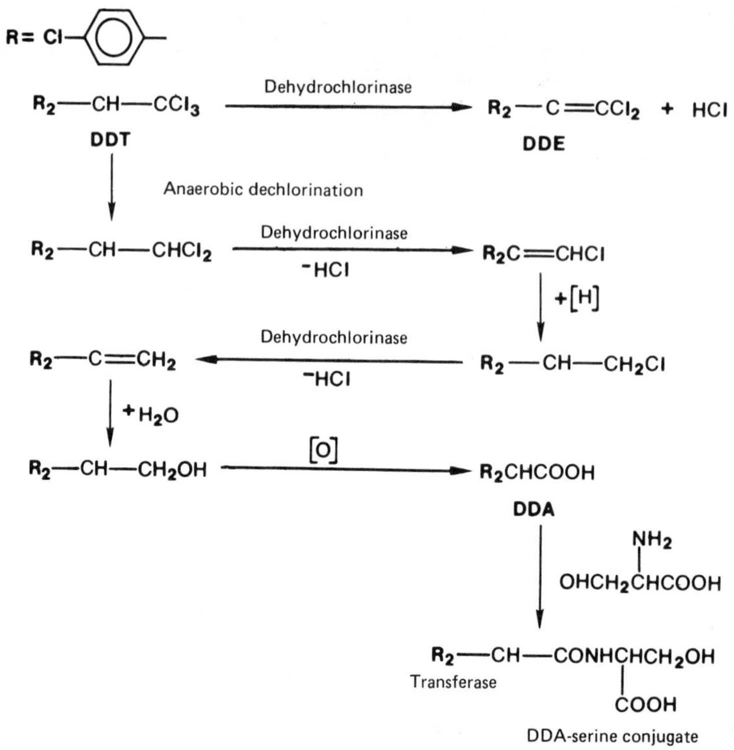

$$R = Cl - \bigcirc -$$

$$R_2-CH-CCl_3 \xrightarrow{\text{Dehydrochlorinase}} R_2-C=CCl_2 \; + \; HCl$$

$$\text{DDT} \qquad\qquad\qquad\qquad\qquad\qquad\qquad \text{DDE}$$

↓ Anaerobic dechlorination

$$R_2-CH-CHCl_2 \xrightarrow[-HCl]{\text{Dehydrochlorinase}} R_2C=CHCl$$

↓ +[H]

$$R_2-C=CH_2 \xleftarrow[-HCl]{\text{Dehydrochlorinase}} R_2-CH-CH_2Cl$$

↓ +H_2O

$$R_2-CH-CH_2OH \xrightarrow{[O]} R_2CHCOOH$$

$$\text{DDA}$$

↓ $\overset{NH_2}{OHCH_2CHCOOH}$

$$R_2-CH-CONHCHCH_2OH$$
$$\text{Transferase} \qquad\qquad\qquad |$$
$$COOH$$

DDA-serine conjugate

DDA conjugated to serine or aspartic acid is the principal DDT metabolite excreted in mammalian urine (Pinto et al. 1965).

Dehalogenation may also occur by initial displacement by mercapturic conjugation, the acetylcysteine moiety being eliminated by hydrolysis. This process is illustrated by the dechlorination of trichloroaniline (Parke 1968).

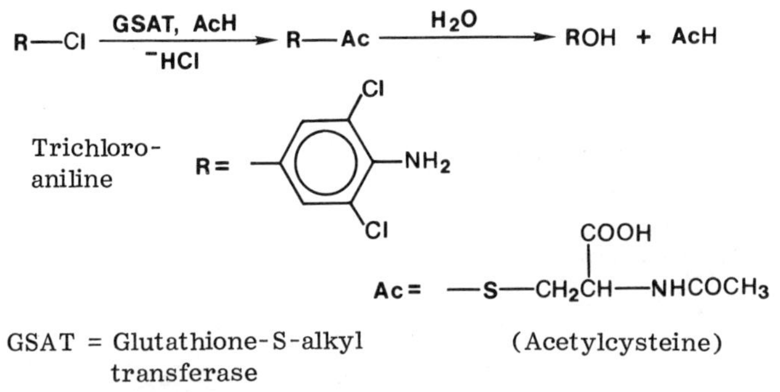

$$R-Cl \xrightarrow[-HCl]{\text{GSAT, AcH}} R-Ac \xrightarrow{H_2O} ROH \; + \; AcH$$

Trichloro-
aniline $\quad R=$

$$Ac= \quad -S-CH_2\overset{COOH}{CH}-NHCOCH_3$$

GSAT = Glutathione-S-alkyl   (Acetylcysteine)
        transferase

Oxidative dehalogenation has been postulated as another mechanism for removing halogens from organic compounds. This is particularly the case with aliphatics. Thus, conceivably, finding high levels of carboxymethemoglobin following exposure to methylene chloride may be due to the breakdown of this compound to CO and HCl (Stewart et al. 1972).

Ring Opening

Microsomal oxidation may also open rings in cyclic compounds. The result of ring opening is the formation of polar groups (Parke 1968). Thus, opening the pyrrole ring in an indole following oxidation and hydrolysis leads to the formation of anthranilate containing both carboxyl and amino groups. The oxidation and hydrolysis of the lactone ring in coumarin produce both —OH and —COOH in the product 2-hyroxyphenylacetic acid. The oxidative cleavage of benzene produces the dicarboxylic, trans-muconic acid.

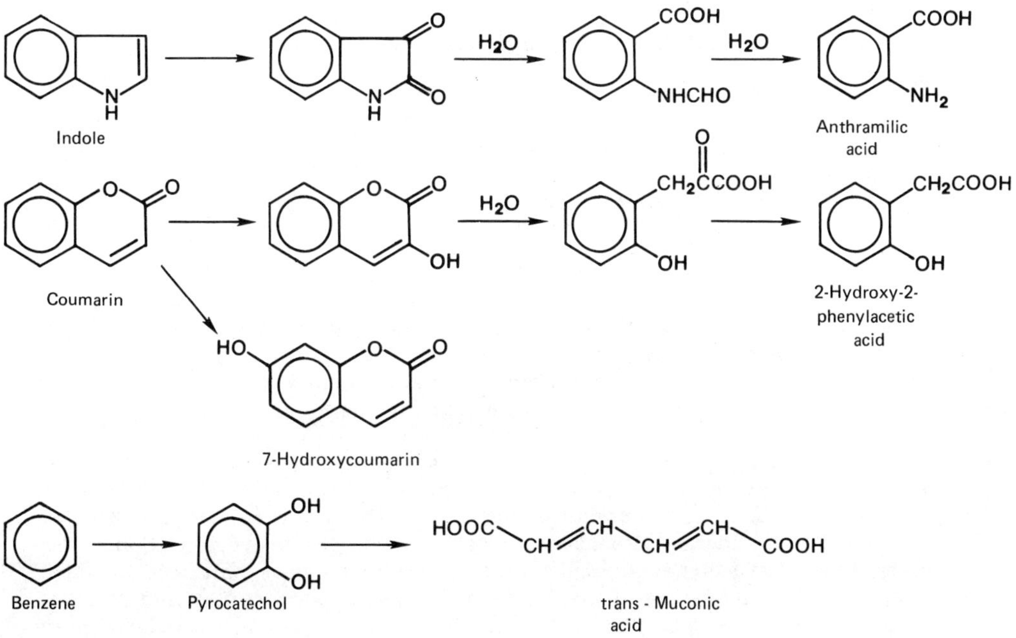

Cyclization

The opposite of ring opening, cyclization, has also been observed in rare instances. Thus, following exposure to 2-hydroxyethyl aniline, increased excretion of indican is noted (Parke 1968).

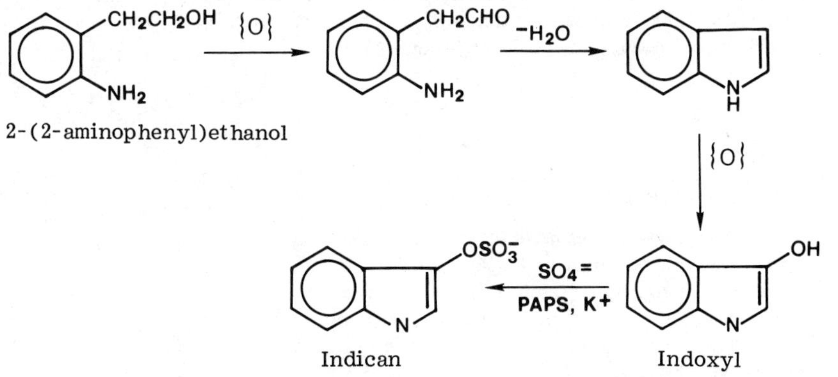

PAMS = 3'-Phosphoadenosine-5'-phosphosulfate

Lethal Synthesis

Several examples of Phase I reactions have resulted in products which are more toxic than the parent compounds. Sometimes, a very toxic product is produced when the metabolite resembles an essential normal metabolic product. Thus, nontoxic fluoroethanol is converted into an extremely toxic metabolite, fluorocitrate, which interferes in the function of the tricarboxylic acid cycle by inhibiting the enzyme aconitase (Peters 1963).

$$F-CH_2CH_2OH \xrightarrow{\{O\}} F-CH_2COOH \xrightarrow[Thiolase]{CoA} F-CH_2CO-SCoA \longrightarrow$$

Fluoroethanol   Fluoroacetate

$$\underset{\underset{Fluorocitrate}{HOOC \quad\quad OH \quad COOH}}{F-CH-\overset{\overset{COOH}{|}}{C}-CH_2}$$

A reaction, such as the preceding example, producing a very toxic metabolite from a less toxic precursor was termed "lethal synthesis" by Peters (1963).

Thus, Phase I reactions are not primarily detoxification reactions. The apparent result of these reactions is polarization, thus increasing the water solubility and therefore the excretability of the compound. However, the process of introducing polar groups by oxidation or by unmasking by such means as hydrolysis or dealkylation may produce reactive intermediate products. Such reactive derivatives may indeed account for the observed toxicity of the parent compounds. Thus, the epoxidation of 3,4-benzpyrene and the oxidation of benzene and ethanol and the N-hydroxylation of 2-aminoacetylfluorene are further examples of reactions which cause enhanced toxicity. Thus, depending on the nature of the compound, Phase I reactions may increase rather than decrease toxicity. The relationship between the nature of a compound and its toxicity is discussed in Chapter 1. In general, any compound that is metabolized to intermediate(s) which can react unhindered with vital components of the cells, e.g., nutrients, hormones, enzymes, nucleic acids, and membranes, so as to interfere with their function will show enhanced toxicity. Note that the principal requirement of toxic activity is reactivity, and Phase I reactions introduce or produce reactive groups.

Detoxification is accomplished in most cases by Phase II reactions while further enhancing the solubility of the metabolites. For example, the Phase I reaction product of benzene is phenol, which has a pK_a of 10 and is about 0.25% dissociated at the pH of blood (pH 7 to 7.3). Following Phase II reaction, the product, phenylglucuronide, is almost 100% dissociated (pK_a 3.4) (Williams 1970).

PHASE II REACTIONS

Glucuronide Conjugation

One of the most important detoxification reactions is glucuronide conjugation. This process increases the solubility of glucuronide by introducing a highly polar sugar moiety and a free carboxylic group. These have a lower dissociation constant (pK_a) than the free toxicant. Thus, products of glucuronide conjugation are easily eliminated in the urine or in the bile. Glucuronide conjugation also reduces the potential toxicity of compounds.

Glucuronic acid (GA) is formed from glucose by way of glucose-1-phosphate.

G   = glucose;
P   = $-PO_4^{3-}$
UTP   = uridine triphosphate;
P_i = inorganic phosphate
UDPG   = uridine diphosphate glucose
X   = foreign compound
X–GA   = glucuronide of X

Compounds containing $-OH$, $-COOH$, $-NH_2$, and $-SH$ may be conjugated with glucuronic acid. These groups react with the α-1-hydroxyl group of GA. But the glucuronide has a β-configuration following Walden inversion (Dutton 1966). Phenolics, alcohols, amino alcohols, or enols (ketones) may be conjugated with GA, forming an ether or an acetal.

In the case of aliphatic alcohols and enols (ketones), GA conjugation appears to be confined to higher alcohols. Among lower alcohols, the capability for glucuronide conjugation is confined to branched, secondary, and tertiary alcohols. Thus, n-hexanol and isobutyl and isopropyl alcohols are conjugated in the rabbit and many other species (Williams 1959), whereas n-butyl and n-propyl alcohols, ethanol, and methanol are ultimately oxidized to CO_2 and H_2O, —the first two, through the usual metabolic pathways for fatty acids.

RCOOH is conjugated with GA forming esters or hemiacetals. These substrates are mainly aromatic acids.

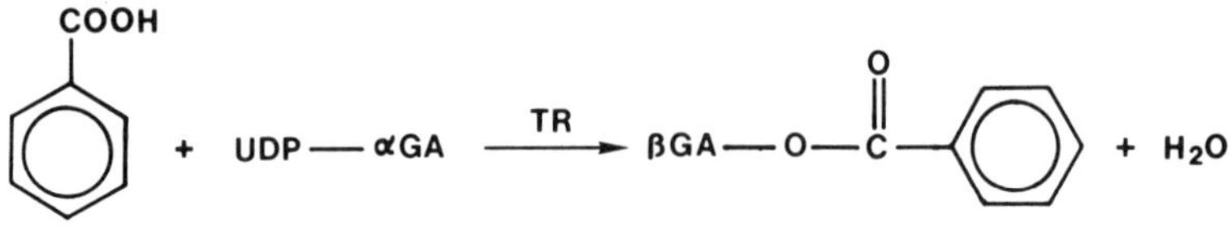

Benzoic acid

Some substituted benzoic acids such as the berbicide D icamba (2-methyl-3,6-dichlorobenzoic acid) are promptly eliminated, mostly unchanged, in the rat (Tye and Engel 1967) and cow (St. John and Lisk 1969). However, at least 20% of a dose may be GA conjugated in these species.

Amines and amides including sulfonamides form amino ethers. For example:

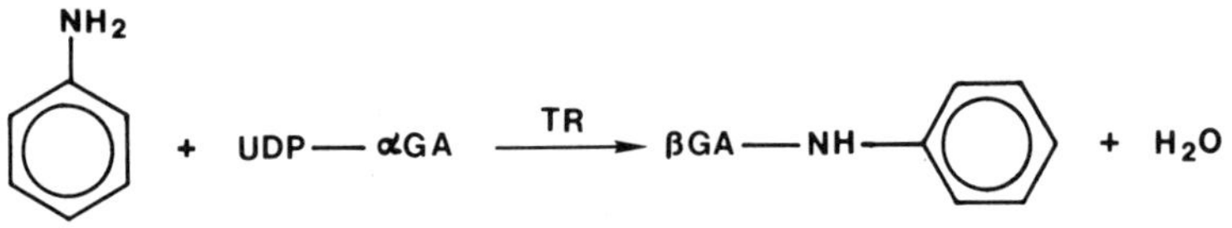

Aniline

However, where both −OH and −NH$_2$ exist in the same molecule, the conjugation in rabbits occurs preferentially with the −OH as in p-aminophenol (Parke and Williams 1956). A similar situation is encountered with the metabolic reduction product of Citrus Red No. 2 and presumably other azo dye food colors. Thus, 1-amino-2-naphthol is conjugated at the −OH rather than the −NH$_2$ group (Radomski 1961, 1962).

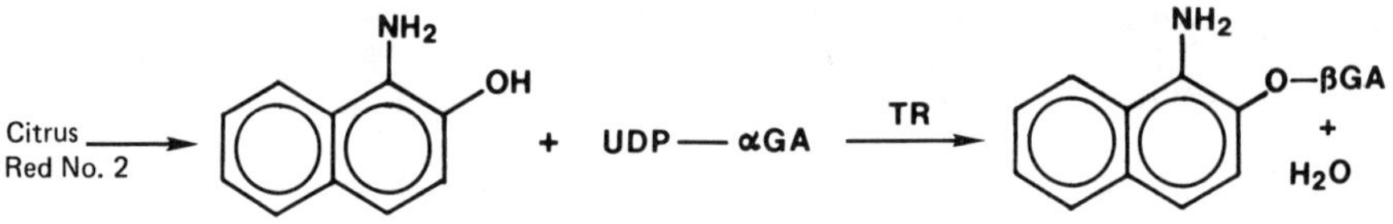

1-Amino-2-naphthol

Thiol groups are conjugated with GA forming thioacetal compounds.

$$RSH \ + \ UDP—\alpha GA \ \xrightarrow{TR} \ \beta GA—SR \ + \ H_2O$$

Hippuric Acid Synthesis

Conjugation of aromatic acids with glycine produces hippuric acid.

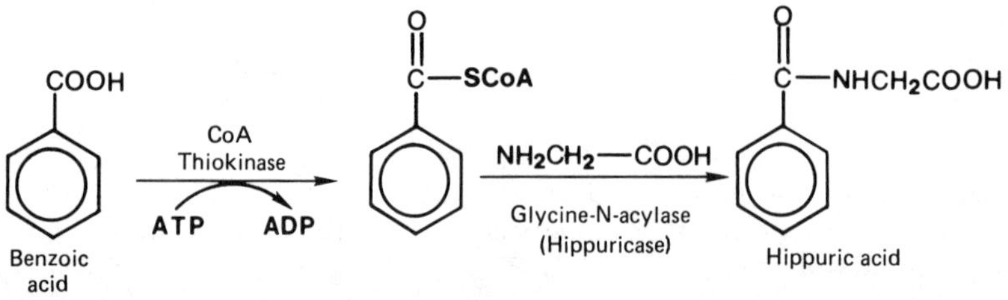

Benzoates are present in cranberries to the extent of 50 to 90 mg/100 g. One-tenth percent sodium benzoate is permitted by law in catsup, other food and beverages as a preservative.

The excretion of hippuric acid is often used as a test for liver function. Normally, for 5 to 9 g of sodium benzoate, 3-5 g of hippuric acid should be excreted in 4 hr (Orten and Neuhaus 1975).

Mercapturic Acid Synthesis

The reaction of foreign compounds with glutathione and acetic acid produces a conjugation product with N-acetylcysteine. The types of compounds detoxified and excreted as mercapturic acid conjugates are even more varied than those excreted as glucuronides. The classes of compounds reported by Boyland and Chasseaud (1969) are listed in Table 1. Note that aromatic hydrocarbons, cycloalkenes, and arylketides

Table 1. Classes of Compounds Metabolized to Mercapturates

Compound class	Example	Thiol-reacting group
Aromatic hydrocarbon	Benzene, naphthalene, anthracene, benz(a)-anthracene	Epoxide intermediates
Arylamine	Aniline, 2-naphthylamine	Hydroxylamine intermediates
Arylhalide	Chlorobenzene, 1,2-dichlorobenzene, 1-choloronaphthalene	Epoxide intermediates
Halogenonitrobenzene	1,2-Dichloro-4-nitrobenzene, pentachloronitrobenzene	Cl NO_2
Aralkyl ester	Benzyl acetate	$OCOCH_3$
Aralkyl halide	Benzyl chloride	Cl
Alkyl halide	Allyl chloride, bromomethane	Cl Br
Alkyl phenol	3,5-di-tert-butyl-4-hydroxytoluene	H of tolueyl CH_3
Nitroalkane	1-Nitropropane	NO_2
Halogenocycloalkane	Bromocyclohexane	Br
Carboxylic acid	Maleic acid	α, β=Double bond
Ester	Ethyl methanesulphonate, urethane	CH_3SO_3 $OCONH_2$
Sulfonamide	Benzothiazolesulfonamide	SO_2NH_2
Sulfur mustard	Bis-β-chloroethyl sulfide	Cl
α, β-Unsaturated compound	Arecoline, ethacrynic acid	α, β=Double bond

Source: Boyland and Chasseaud (1969).

may undergo the Phase I reaction of epoxidation before these compounds are conjugated as mercapturates. Other compounds appear to react directly without further activation. Thus, the thiol group in glutathione displaces the halogens in arylalkyl halides
and halonitrobenzenes.

The source of cysteine is gluthathione, and conjugation is catalyzed by
glutathione-S-transferases. Three other enzymes are involved in the pathway toward
mercapturate formation. These enzymes trim down the glutathione moiety after reaction
with the active foreign compound (Boyland and Chasseaud 1969).

The sequence of reactions leading to the mercapturate excretion product is illustrated by the conjugation of the insecticide lindane or γ-benzenehexachloride (BCH).
Initially, a dehydrochlorination resulting in aromatization takes place prior to mercapturate formation.

γ-Benzene
hexachloride

BHC-DC = γ-BHC dehydrochlorinase
                          CONHCH$_2$COOH
                          |
SCys-Gly = HSCH$_2$CH
                          |
                          NH$_2$
                          Cysteinyl glycine

GSH-SAT = glutathione S-aryltransferase
GT = γ-glutamyl transferase

                                              CONHCH$_2$COOH
                                              |
GSH (reduced glutathione) = HS–CH$_2$CH
                                              |
                                              NHCOCH$_2$CH$_2$CHOOH

The aryl halides and aromatic hydrocarbons appear to be oxidized first to phenols
probably by prior epoxidation. However, experiments using ^{14}C-labeled benzene cast
some doubt on the existence of such epoxide intermediates (Udenfriend et al. 1969).
Rather, a phenolic carbonium ion intermediate is postulated.

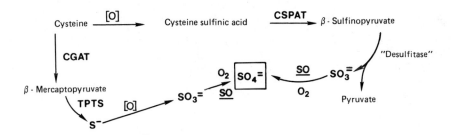

Similarly,

GSH = Reduced glutathione

Mercapturate formation increases the water solubility of an otherwise lipid-soluble compound, owing to the introduction of an ionizable carboxyl group.

Sulfate ("Ethereal") Conjugation

In general, sulfate conjugation probably ranks with glucuronic and mercapturic acid conjugation as the most commonly occurring excretory biotransformation process for phenols, alcohols, and aryl amines. The sulfated compounds become salts of strong acids and are therefore highly ionized at the pH of the body; consequently, the sulfate conjugates are very soluble and promptly eliminated in the urine. The sulfate ion is derived from methionine via cysteine. Several mechanisms have been postulated (Orten and Neuhaus 1975).

CSPAT = cysteine sulfinic acid pyruvate aminotransferase
CGAT   = cysteine glutamate aminotransferase
TPTS   = thiol pyruvate transsulfinase
SO   = sulfite oxidase

SO_4^{2-} is activated in a pathway involving ATP, Mg^{2+}, adenosine phosphosulfate pyrophosphorylase (APSPP), and adenosine-5'-phosphosulfate-3'-phosphokinase (APPSP), forming adenosine-5'-phosphosulfate (APS) and 3'-phosphoadenosine-5'-phosphosulfate (PAPS) (Orten and Neuhaus 1975).

PP_i = Pyrophosphate

The conjugation of phenols, alcohols, and arylamines with PAPS results in the formation of aryl and alkyl acid sulfates for the first two types of compounds, respectively, and N-aryl sulfamates for the amines.

$$ROH \longrightarrow ROSO_3^- \; ; \quad \text{where } R = \text{—⬡ or an alkyl group}$$

$$Ar\!-\!NH_2 \longrightarrow ArNHSO_3^- ; \quad \text{where } Ar = \text{—⬡}$$

Thus, phenol undergoes both glucuronide and sulfate conjugation (Parke and Williams 1953).

The sulfonate conjugation of an arylamine is exemplified by aniline. Note that phenyl acid sulfate as well as the sulfamate would be highly ionized at physiological pH.

Glutamine Conjugation

So far, this mechanism is exclusively found in man and other primates (Williams 1970). The steps involved are similar to glycine conjugation. Activation of the aromatic acid with ATP and coenzyme A is required before glutamine-N-acylase can conjugate it with glutamine.

Gln = Glutamine   Gln-NA = Glutamine-N-acylase

Transmethylation

The introduction of a methyl group to $-NH_2$, $-NH$, $-N=$, $-OH$, $-SH$ groups of specific compounds is an example of a metabolic process whose primary purpose is detoxification rather than excretion. In this case, the methylated compound may show decreased toxicity and, simultaneously, diminished polarity. Therefore, the methylated products have diminished solubility in waters.

The methylated species in these reactions is "active methionine," S-adenosylmethionine (SAM), which is formed by methyladenosyl transferase in the presence of adenosine triphosphate (ATP).

S-Adenosyl methionine
(SAM)

Examples of transmethylation of $-\overset{\|}{N}$ group are pyridine and its naturally occurring analog, nicotinamide.

Examples of transmethylation involving $-OH$ are epinephrine and norepinephrine, which are powerful pressor amines occurring endogenously in both plant and animal tissues (Chap. 8). The reaction is catalyzed by catechol-O-methyl transferase (COMT) (Orten and Neuhaus 1975).

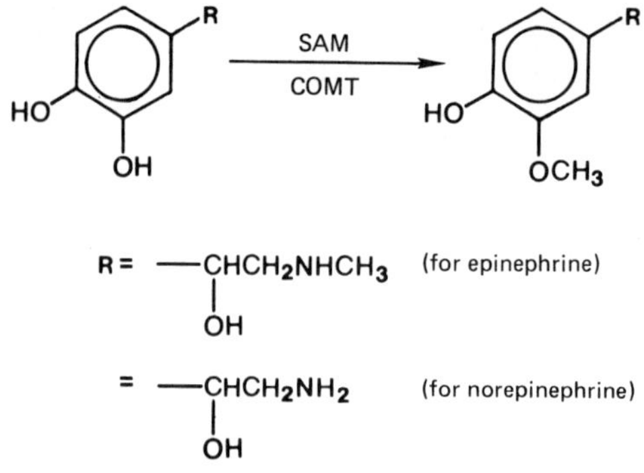

R = —CHCH$_2$NHCH$_3$ (for epinephrine)
     |
     OH

= —CHCH$_2$NH$_2$ (for norepinephrine)
   |
   OH

Acetylation

Acetylation involves reacting acetate with $-NH_2$ groups, particularly in amines, hydrazines, and sulfonamines. Acetate is donated from the substituted nucleotide acetyl-CoA. Like transmethylation, acetylation results primarily in detoxification rather than increased water solubility, by masking a reactive amino group. The resulting amide is less water soluble than the parent compound. An example is the acetylation of nitroaniline following prior reduction of the nitro group (Williams 1959).

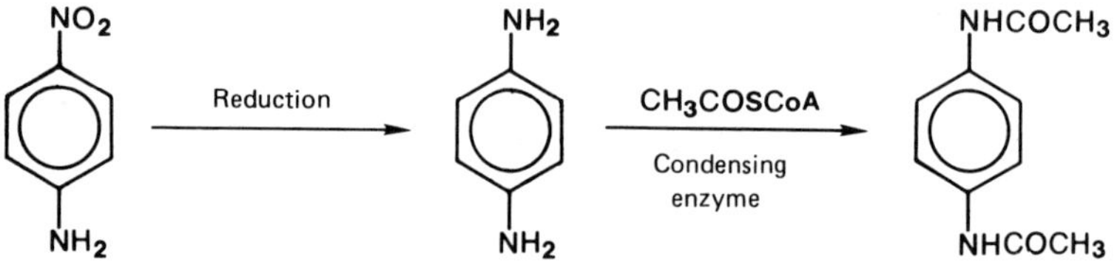

p-Nitroaniline

Hydrazine is detoxified in a similar manner.

The increased tendency of sulfonamide drugs to crystallize in the urinary system follows from the decreased solubility of the acetylated product. This was a major problem in sulfa drug therapy.

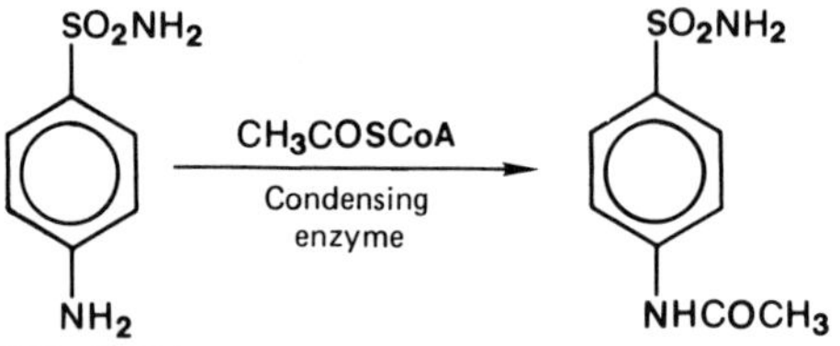

Sulfanilamide

The problems associated with sulfa drug precipitation with consequent renal damage is minimized or eliminated by use of the types of sulfa drugs that are more soluble at urinary pH, with consideration for their therapeutic effectiveness toward certain pathogens. Precipitation of the drug occurs most readily at acidic pH, so that even those relatively soluble sulfa drugs, such as sulfisoxazole, may crystallize in the kidneys in the presence of acidic urine. However, alkalinization of the urine with the proper dose of sodium bicarbonate will reduce the risk of crystallization considerably.

Adequate intake of water to produce a urine output in adults of at least 1200 ml/day is sufficient by itself to reduce the risk of crystallization in most cases (Weinstein 1970).

Thiocyanate Synthesis

Thiocyanate synthesis is a specific for cyanide detoxification. The enzyme rhodanase catalyzes the formation of thiocyanate. It is widely distributed in tissues, but the liver is the principal cyanide detoxification site.

$$CN^- + S^0 \xrightarrow[\text{(Rhodanase)}]{\text{Sulfur transferase}} CNS^-$$

While exogenous thiosulfate ($S_2O_3^{2-}$) can be the source of the sulfur atom, it can also be derived from the oxidation of sulfide, produced from the desulfuration of cysteine. However, $S_2O_3^{2-}$ can be produced from the reduction of SO_3^{2-} by β-mercaptopyruvic acid (β-MPA), resulting from the transamination of cysteine with α-ketogluturate (p. 111) (Norton 1975).

$$SO_3^{==} + HS-CH_2\overset{\overset{\text{O}}{\|}}{C}-COOH \longrightarrow S_2O_3^{==} + CH_2\overset{\overset{\text{O}}{\|}}{C}-COOH$$
β-MPA

Alternatively, β-MPA may react directly with cyanide in the presence of a specific sulfur transferase.

$$CN^- + HS-CH_2\overset{\overset{\text{O}}{\|}}{C}-COOH \longrightarrow CNS^- + CH_2\overset{\overset{\text{O}}{\|}}{C}-COOH$$

The preceding discussion illustrates the apparent versatility of the microsomal enzyme system in the detoxification of foreign compounds. Nevertheless, mammalian species, including man, differ in their capability to metabolize these compounds. Similarly, there is also variability within species. This capability obviously is genetically determined. Other factors modify this capability and are discussed in the next section.

FACTORS AFFECTING THE METABOLIC TRANSFORMATION OF EXOGENOUS COMPOUNDS

The toxicological response following ingestion or other forms of exposure to a foreign compound will vary from subject-to-subject, not only between species but also within a species. In addition to the genetic factors in the species, strain and sex of the host, age, disease, stress, frequency of exposure, diet and nutritional status, presence of other foreign compounds, and intestinal microorganisms can also influence the fate of these substances in the body. Obviously, the complex interplay of these factors determines the final response. It is impossible at this stage of our knowledge to predict accurately the response of an individual to a given exogenous compound when these factors are considered, particularly at relatively low levels of exposure. Nevertheless, an understanding of the role of these factors will provide essential guidelines in the assessment of toxic hazards of specific compounds.

Effect of Species and Strain — Metabolic Differences

Species respond differently when challenged with a given dose of a toxicant. This fact creates a serious difficulty in extrapolating the effect of a compound to man and remains a fundamental problem in toxicology. These species differences in the metabolism of a compound depend on qualitative as well as quantitative variation in the enzymes involved (Smith 1968; Williams 1967). For example, the dog, cat, rabbit, mouse, rat, and hamster can N-hydroxylate the carcinogen 2-acetamidofluorene, and all respond to its carcinogenic action; on the other hand, the steppe lemming and the guinea pig, which do not N-hydroxylate this compound, are not susceptible. Humans can N-hydroxylate this compound, and thus it is highly possible that it is also a human carcinogen (Weisburger et al. 1964).

Species differences are immediately evident from LD$_{50}$ values, even though such differences may not necessarily be due to variations in enzyme activity. This is because the rate of absorption, manner of administration even through the same route of entry, and so forth, can make a difference. However, an examination of the types of metabolites produced from a compound will unequivocally demonstrate species differences. For example, humans, rats, and rabbits all form ether glucuronides of butyl hydroxytoluene, but in different proportions — man, forming almost twice as much of the ether glucuronide as the other species. Humans do not form the mercapturate conjugate, whereas the rat has the ability to form this compound (Daniel and Gage 1965; Daniel et al. 1967; Tye et al. 1965). The human being, rabbit, dog, and rat are all able to excrete BHA as the glucuronide, but the dog excretes BHA in this form only to a minor extent (Astill et al. 1960, 1962; Dacre 1960; Dacre et al. 1956). Demethylation of BHA also occurs in both the rat and the dog but humans and rabbits are unable to do so.

Intraspecific differences in metabolism are perhaps best illustrated by differences in the percentage of DDE to total DDT in adipose tissues of different populations (Table 2). Note that Czechoslovakians, Hungarians, Spaniards, Asian Indians, Israelies, and Australians metabolize DDT to DDE to a significantly lesser extent than northern Europeans and United States caucasians.

Several studies on drug metabolism in humans also show considerable variability in individual responses. For example, such drugs as isoniazid and sulfadimidine are detoxified by acetylation at different rates by human subjects. In this case, there are slow and fast detoxifiers among individuals, the former group experiencing greater benefits or toxic side effects than the latter group (Evans 1965). A similar observation has been reported regarding the activity of plasma "pseudocholinesterase," which hydrolyzes esters such as the muscle relaxant succinylcholine (Evans 1965). Certain individuals are also deficient in glucose-6-phosphate dehydrogenase, and thus are susceptible to hemolytic anemia from such pyrimidines as divicine and isouramil, present in broad (fava) beans (Majer et al. 1965) (Chap. 8).

Studies using several strains of rabbits show considerable variation in the ability of their livers to detoxify various compounds (Cram et al. 1965).

Effect of Sex

There are male and female differences among individuals in their metabolism of foreign compounds. For example, female rats appear to be more susceptible to a number of toxicants such as those listed in Table 3. Note, however, that the insecticide Schradan (octamethylprophosphoramide) is more toxic to the male than the female.

The greater toxicity of certain substances in females may be explained by the rates of transformation to more or less toxic metabolites. For example, strychnine is more toxic to female rats because it is metabolized slowly to less toxic metabolites (Kato et al. 1962a). In the case of parathion, females are more susceptible to this insecticide because they can metabolize it more rapidly to the more toxic compound,

Table 2. DDE Levels as Percentage of Total DDT in Adipose Tissues of Different Populations

Country	Year	DDE as Percentage of Total DDT
Holland	—	85.4
Denmark	1965	84.5
England	1963–1967	67.6–74.3
Belgium	—	64.2
France	1961	68.6
Italy	1965–1966	64.0–76.3
Spain	1966	56.0
Czechoslovakia	1963–1964	43.0
India	1964	34.5–42.8
Israel	1963–1966	54.6–55.7
Australia	1965–1966	55.4–70.6
New Zealand	1963[a]	62.2–73.0
Canada	1959–1960, 1966	66.0–68.6
United States	1964–1967	67.1–80.4

[a]Not available.
Source: Hayes (1965).

Table 3. Sexual Differences in LD_{50} Values of Various Toxicants in the Rat

Toxicant	Route	LD_{50}, mg/kg body weight Male	Female	Reference
Parathion	oral	15	6	DuBois et al. (1949); Davison (1955)
Warfarin	oral	323	58	Hagan and Radomski (1953)
Schradan	i.p.	7	27	Davison (1955)
Strychnine	s.c.	4.01	1.81	Kato et al. (1962a,b)
	i.p.	2.82	1.62	

Abbreviations: i.p. = intraperitoneal; s.c. = subcutaneous

paraoxon than males can (Davison 1955; DuBois et al. 1949). The breakdown of paraoxon to p-nitrophenol is not sex dependent.

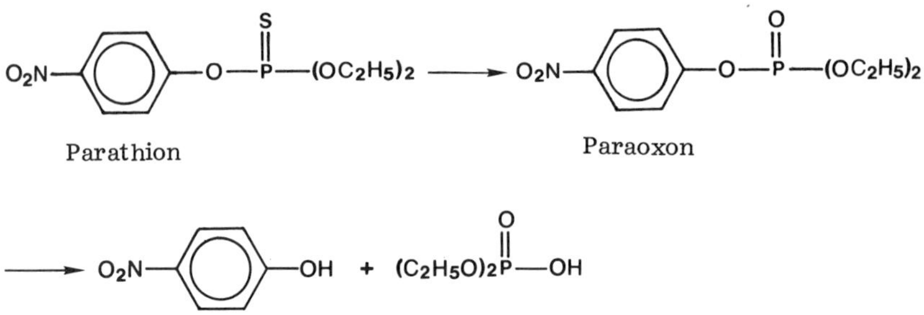

In contrast, Schradan is more toxic to males who can metabolize this compound more rapidly to a toxic metabolite than females (Davison 1955; Spencer et al. 1957).

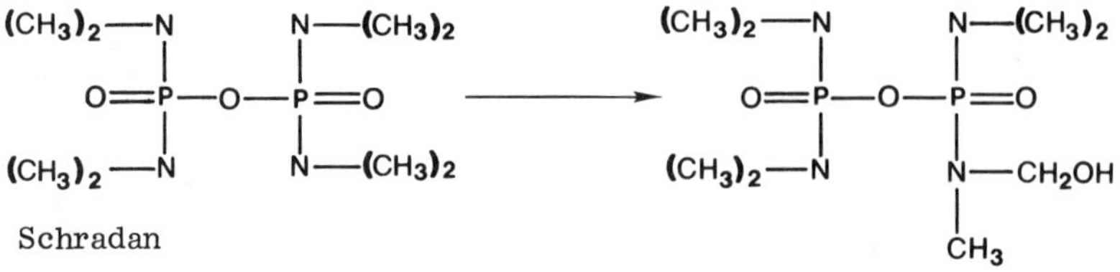

Schradan

Hydroxyschradan
(more toxic)

Other examples from animal studies indicating sexual differences in the metabolism of foreign compounds include the metabolism of hexobarbitone and amidopyrine or ethylmorphine. Greater activity of enzymes metabolizing these compounds has been observed in male rats (Quinn et al. 1958). Thus, in males, these compounds have a shorter duration of activity. Kinetics studies suggest that the differences are not only due to the quantity of enzymes but also the affinity of the enzymes for substrates. Thus, both the level of microsomal enzymes metabolizing amidopyrine and ethylmorphine, and their affinity for these substrates is greater in males than in females (Davies et al. 1968; Schenkman et al. 1967).

Sexual differences in toxicities of compounds have also been demonstrated in human beings. Females are more susceptible to the toxic effects of benzene and amidopyrene than males (Hurst 1958). Similarly, men can metabolize nicotine to cotinine to a greater extent (Beckett et al. 1971). This sex difference is seen only in nonsmokers. Among smokers these differences tend to disappear except that there appears to be a group of male smokers who metabolize nicotine to a large extent by pathways other than the cotinine route. The increased conversion of nicotine to cotinine among female smokers compared to nonsmokers underscores the importance of previous exposure in the metabolism of foreign compounds.

Hormones seem to be involved, since sexual differences in the toxicity of many of these compounds seem to manifest themselves only after puberty (Davies et al. 1968; Davison 1955; Gram et al. 1969). The influence of male hormones is verified by the decrease, for example, of N-demethylase activity for ethylmorphin by castration (Davies et al. 1968). The rate of metabolism of this compound in castrated individuals is increased by the administration of methyltestosterone (Green et al. 1968). Similarly, the activity of microsomal enzymes in female rats is stimulated to activity by androgens (Booth and Gillette 1962).

Effect of Age

There is a remarkable difference in the capability of the young and newborn as compared to adults in the detoxification of foreign compounds. For example, most drugs are two to 10 times more toxic in a newborn rat than in an adult (Yeary et al. 1966). This is because the newborn and fetus metabolize foreign substances more slowly (Parke 1968). Enzymes involved in Phase I reactions (Fouts 1965; Fouts and Adamson 1959) as well as most Phase II conjugating enzymes are either absent or present at low concentrations. Exceptions among the Phase II enzymes are the sulfokinase and acetyl condensing enzymes which are present at normal levels in some species. In the case of glucuronyl transferase, newborn rats and humans have low levels in the liver, and the former attain adult levels by about 30 days (Dutton 1964); humans attain adult levels in about 8 weeks (Nyham 1961). Human infants have the ability to hydroxylate acetanilide but appear poorly equipped for glucuronyl conjugation (Vest 1959).

However, whether or not newborns are more susceptible to toxic effects of foreign compounds cannot be generalized. The reason is that the toxic effects of the three insecticides shown in Table 4 are variable in the newborn, more resistant in some, and highly sensitive in others.

Note that the newborn (less than 24 hr old) is more sensitive to malathion compared to the older animals. The newborn, however, is more resistant to dieldrin, and highly so to DDT as compared to the older animals. The samer pattern is seen with preweaning animals (14 to 16 days old) as compared to adults (3 to 4 months). Note, however, that there is a marked change in either resistance or susceptibility to compounds in just 2 weeks after birth, as shown by a comparison of the LD_{50} values for newborn and preweaning rats.

The smaller values for the cumulative LD_{50} in contrast to the acute LD_{50} values in the preweaning animals may be attributable to differences in the efficiency of absorption—that is, greater efficiency can occur when the dose is given in smaller amounts over a given period. In adults, the cumulative LD_{50}s are greater than the acute dosages. This may be a manifestation of the saturation effect. As explained previously, only a fraction of a given dose above a certain level may be metabolized or detoxified per unit time as a toxicant passes through the liver. Therefore, the smaller the given dose per unit time, the greater the efficiency of detoxification and, consequently, the less the toxicity.

There are other examples of differences in toxicity between young and adult animals. In most of these cases, young animals seem more susceptible to toxic effects.

Table 4. Comparative Sensitivity to Insecticides of Newborn, Preweanling, and Adult Rats

Age (days)	Oral LD_{50} (mg/kg) Malathion	Dieldrin	DDT	Cumulative Oral LD_{50} (Mean) (mg/kg)[a] Malathion	Dieldrin	DDT
1	124.1	167.8	4000+	—	—	—
14−16	386.8	24.9	437.8	331.2	9.04	279.2
90−120	925.4	37.0	194.5	1559.0	54.8	285.6

[a]Daily dose for 4 consecutive days.
Source: Lu et al. (1965).

Thus, intraperitoneal injections in rats of various pesticides show that the suckling rats are e.g., about four times more susceptible than adults to EPN (ethyl-p-nitrophenyl thionobenzene phosphate) and trithion (carbophenothion); about twice as susceptible to parathion, Delnav (dioxathion), Di-Syston (disulfoton), and methyl parathion; one to one and a half times more susceptible to Systox (Demeton-S), Phosdrin (Mevinophos), Guthion (azinphosmethyl), Co-Ral (coumaphos), Sevin (carbaryl), and Dipterex (trichlorfon) (Brodeur and DuBois 1963). As with Schradan, the weanling rats show remarkable resistance to a number of insecticides (Brodeur and DuBois 1963) such as DDT and dieldrin (Lu et al. 1965).

The newborn and young animals generally exhibit greater susceptibility to toxic compounds than adults, but there are examples showing greater resistance. Thus, 1.5 to 4.5-month-old rats are less sensitive to caffeine than 12-month-old-rats (Peters and Boyd 1967). Histamine dihydrochloride is less toxic to 10-day-old guinea pigs than older animals (Chen and Robbins 1944b). Young mice tolerate ethanol better than older ones (Chen and Robbins 1944a). On a body weight basis, children require 50% more digitalis than adults (Mathes et al. 1952). Newborn rats are shown to be less susceptible to the effects of convulsants than older animals (Setnikar and Magistretti 1964). Notwithstanding these observations, there are many compounds to which there are only slight differences between the young and adult animals (Done 1964, 1966).

In aged animals, there appears to be a reversal toward greater susceptibility to toxic effects of compounds. For example, myocardial necrosis following acetylcholine treatment was more severe in older dogs than the younger animals (Hall et al. 1936); a similar effect has been observed in older rats following isoproterenol administrations (Rona et al. 1959). Many other examples appear to indicate the increased susceptibility of old rats to various drugs compared to young adults (Chen and Robbins 1944b). However, this is not always the case, as some substances, such as amphetamines, may actually be less active in old rats than the young adults (Farner and Verzar 1961).

It should be mentioned that the differences in susceptibility between the immature, adult, and old animals may be due to factors other than qualitative and quantitative differences in enzyme systems. For example, there may be a difference in the distribution of a compound in tissues. In particular, the blood-brain barrier in younger animals may not be as well developed as in adults. This has been observed with tryphan blue in mice, with phosphate, chloride, and potassium ions in newborn rabbits, rats, and chicks (Waelsch 1955), and with morphine in 16-day-old, in contrast to 32-day-old, rats (Kupferberg and Way 1963).

There may also be differences in renal clearance between the young and adult. For example, the clearance of newborn infants for a tetracycline derivative has been reported to be 11% of that found in older children (Sereni et al. 1965).

Effect of Nutrition and Diet

Because toxic effects depend to a large extent on the ability of the cell to respond to a foreign compound, any factor which can modify this response must also modify the toxic effects. There is ample evidence to indicate alteration in body composition and biochemical and physiological activities resulting from changes in diet or nutritional status (Jost et al. 1968; Munro 1964; Williams et al. 1966). For example, on a low protein-high carbohydrate diet, the acute toxicity of CCl_4 in male rats is quite low ($LD_{50} = 14.7$ ml CCl_4/kg body weight), whereas with standard diets, high in protein, CCl_4 is quite toxic ($LD_{50} = 6.4$ ml/kg body weight) (McLean and McLean 1969). Low protein-high carbohydrate diets offer protection against CCl_4 and $CHCl_5$ poisoning as opposed to high fat or high protein diets (Campbell and Kosterlitz 1948; Opie and Alford 1915). The toxicity is enhanced by fasting or by prior administration of DDT or phenobarbital, since $CHCl_4$ toxicity depends on its metabolism by microsomal hydroxylating enzymes. The activity of these enzymes is depressed by protein deficiency (Marshall and McLean 1969). DDT and phenobarbital induce synthesis of these enzymes

(Conney et al. 1956), but induction of these enzymes is inhibited in protein deficiency (McLean and McLean 1966). The enhanced toxic effects of CCl_4 on fasted animals previously fed either low protein or standard diets most likely suggests the protective effect of liver glycogen. It is increased even with low protein-high carbohydrate diets and reserves are easily depleted by fasting (McLean and McLean 1969).

A similar protective effect of protein deficiency has been reported for dimethylnitrosamine poisoning in rats (McLean and Verschuuren 1969). In this case, the LD_{50} is increased and liver damage is minimized (Swann and McLean 1968). However, while liver carcinogenesis is prevented by low protein diets, kidney tumor formation is enhanced. This is because its metabolism in the kidneys is unaffected and more of the toxicant reaches this organ as a result of decreased metabolism in the liver.

The opposite observation was reported in acute aflatoxin B_1 poisonings (Madhavan and Gopalan 1965). In this case, protein deficiency in rats enhances its acute effects. This is also reversed by DDT and phenobarbital, which apparently induce enzymes rendering aflatoxin B_1 less poisonous (Chap. 6).

On a very high protein diet (80% casein), 66mM glycine/kg body weight injected into rats after fasting overnight was highly poisonous (Wergedal and Harper 1964). Apparently, when on an extremely high protein diet, rats deaminate glycine rapidly and fasting depletes the liver of the metabolic intermediates required for urea synthesis. Thus, the rats died of hyperammonemia, which can be prevented by feeding or injecting arginine.

The effect of diet and nutritional factors on carcinogenesis is discussed in Chapter 7.

Effect of Liver Diseases

Decreased ability to detoxify compounds is to be expected in subjects with liver diseases. Thus, impaired ability for glucuronide and sulfate conjugation has been observed in patients with liver cirrhosis, hepatitis, and obstructive jaundice (Muting 1963). In rabbits, experimental obstructive jaundice produced by bile duct ligation caused diminished activity of Phase I liver enzymes (Mcluen and Fouts 1961); liver damage, similarly, causes greater formation of N-hydroxyacetylaminofluorene, a carcinogenic metabolite, than C- or ring-hydroxylated metabolites which are non- or less carcinogenic (Margreth et al. 1964).

Effect of Temperature and Other Stress Factors

The metabolism of a compound may be modified by cold temperature exposures or excessive noise. This modification may be the result of a response to stress hormones, the corticoids, that are increased following stress. These hormones apparently increase the activity of microsomal enzymes. For example, hydroxylation of acetanilide and 2-naphthylamine is doubled in rats and mice, respectively, following exposure to cold temperatures (Dewhurst 1963). Conversion of 2-naphthylamine to 2-amino-1-naphthol is increased more than 100% if the mice are exposed to both cold temperature and excessive noise (Dewhurst 1963).

Effect of Simultaneous or Prior Exposure to Other Foreign Compounds

The activity of hepatic enzymes can increase two to 10 times by prior treatment of foreign compounds. This phenomenon is observed with various drugs, steroids, many food additives, pesticides, aromatic hydrocarbons, aromatic amines, and naturally occurring nonnutritive substances such as β-ionone derivatives, safrole (Parke and Rahman 1969), and bioflavonoids (Chap. 6).

Pretreatment of a given substance or chronic exposure to these substances may also result in enhanced activity of enzymes metabolizing these substances. For

example, phenobarbital pretreatment will enhance the rate of detoxification of dicoumarol, and thus reduce its effectiveness. Tolerance to drugs such as barbiturates is the
result of enhanced activity of enzymes metabolizing them (Conney 1967).

In rats, the metabolism of drugs like phenacetin by O-dealkylation is enhanced by
pretreatment with cigarette smoke (Pantuck et al. 1974a; Welch et al. 1972), 3-methyl-
cholanthrene (Welch et al. 1972), and 3,4-benzpyrene (Pantuck et al. 1974b). The
metabolism of the latter and phenacetin is stimulated by polycyclic aromatic hydrocarbons (Conney et al. 1966; Watenberg et al. 1962). Thus, broiled beef cooked
directly over burning charcoal, containing the aromatic hydrocarbon 3,4-benzpyrene
(Lijinsky and Shubik 1964), also enhances the metabolism of the same compound (Harrison and West 1971) as well as phenacetin (Pantuck et al. 1975). Studies with nonsmoking human volunteers, who were also nonheavy drinkers of alcohol, tea, or coffee, showed a similar enhanced metabolism of phenacetin following a 4-day diet of
broiled beef directly exposed to burning charcoal. This is compared to the control diet
whose beef was cooked on aluminum foil, thus separating it from the charcoal (Pantuck
et al. 1976). Presumably, the aluminum foil prevented significant formation of aromatic
hydrocarbons (Lijinsky and Shubik 1964). Thus, with the test beef diet, the ratio of
plasma concentration of the metabolite N-acetyl-p-aminophenol to phenacetin its precursor was consistently higher than the control diet — reaching a value of over 500
mg after 7 hr as compared to about 200 mg for the control diet.

When there are competing pathways for the metabolism of a foreign compound,
another compound may increase the rate of one pathway over others. For example,
pretreatment with 3-methylcholanthrene (3-MC) diverts the hydroxylation of dimethylbenzanthracene preferentially from the methyl groups to the aromatic ring. This shift
results in less production of the adrenocorticolytic 7-hydroxymethyl derivatives.
Thus, 3-MC pretreatment prevents adrenal necrosis (Boyland and Sims 1967). Phenobarbital pretreatment also prevents adrenal necrosis by promoting further hydroxylation of the 12-methyl group following hydroxylation of the 7-methyl group (Boyland
and Sims 1967).

4-Hydroxy DMBA
(noncarcinogenic)

7,12-Dimethyl-
benzanthracene (DMBA)

7,12-Dihydroxy DMBA
(weakly carcinogenic)

7-Hydroxy DMBA (carcinogenic)
(Dipple 1976)

Preferential N-hydroxylation of 2-acetylaminofluorene occurs following repeated exposure to the carcinogen (Grantham et al. 1968). Otherwise, ring-hydroxylated derivatives are also formed in relative abundance. In this case, the carcinogenicity of the compound is diminished, since less N—hydroxy metabolite is formed. The sulfate-conjugate of this N-hydroxy metabolite has been shown to be the primary carcinogen (De Baum et al. 1970; Weisburger et al. 1972).

The effect of other foreign compounds in modifying toxic effects is discussed in more detail in the chapter on carcinogenesis (Chap. 6). The principles and examples discussed in that chapter also apply in regard to toxicants in general.

REFERENCES

Astill, B. D., Fassett, D. W. and Roudabush, R. L. 1960. The metabolism of phenolic antioxidants. 2. The metabolism of butylated hydroxyanisole in man and dog. *J. Agr. Food Chem.* 75: 543—551.

Astill, B. D. et al. 1962. Food additive metabolism: Fate of butylated hydroxyanisole in man and dog. *J. Agr. Food Chem.* 10: 315—319.

Beckett, A. H. Gurrod, J. W. and Jenner, P. 1971. The effect of smoking on nicotine metabolism in vivo in man. *J. Pharm.* 23: 625—675.

Boehme, C. and Baer, F. 1967. The transformation of triazine herbicides in the animal. *Food Cosmet. Toxicol.* 5: 23—28.

Booth, J. and Gillette, J. R. 1962. The effect of anabolic steroids on drug metabolism by microsomal enzymes in rat liver. *J. Pharmacol. Exp. Ther.* 137: 374—379.

Boyland, E. 1963. *The Biochemistry of Bladder Cancer*. Charles C Thomas, Springfield, Illinois.

Boyland, E. and Chasseaud, L. F. 1969. The role of glutathione and glutathione s-transferases in mercapturic acid biosynthesis. *Adv. Enzymol.* 32: 173—219.

Boyland, E. and Sims, P. 1967. The effect of pretreatment with adrenal-protecting compounds on the metabolism of 7,12-dimethylbenz(a)anthracene and related compounds by rat liver homogenates. *Biochem. J.* 104: 394—403.

Brodeur, J. and DuBois, K. B. 1963. Comparison of acute toxicity of anti-cholinesterase insecticides to weaning and adult male rats. *Proc. Soc. Exp. Biol. Med.* 114: 509—511.

Campbell, R. M. And Kosterlitz, H. W. 1948. The effects of short-term changes in dietary protein on the response of the liver to carbon tetrachloride injuries. *Br. J. Exp. Pathol.* 29: 149—158.

Casida, J. E. 1963. Mode of action of carbamates. *Ann. Rev. Entomol.* 8: 39—58.

Chen, K. K. and Robbins, E. B. 1944a. Influence of age of mice on the toxicity of alcohol. *J. Am. Pharm. Assoc. Sci. Ed.* 33: 62—63.

Chen, K. K. and Robbins, E. B. 1944b. Age of animals and drug action. *J. Am. Pharm. Assoc. Sci. Ed.* 33: 80—82.

Clayson, D. B., Pringle, J. A. S., Bonser, G. M. and Wood, M. 1968. The technique of bladder implantation: Further results and an assessment. *Br. J. Cancer* 22: 825—832.

Conney, A. H. 1967. Pharmacological implications of microsomal enzyme induction. *Pharmacol. Rev.* 19: 317—366.

Conney, A. H., Miller, E. C. and Miller, J. A. 1956. The metabolism of methylated aminoazo dyes. V. Evidence for induction of enzyme synthesis in the rat by 3-methylcholanthrene. *Cancer Res.* 16: 450—459.

Conney, A. H. et al. 1966. Enzyme induction and inhibition in studies on the pharmacological actions of acetophenetidin. *J. Pharmacol. Exp. Ther.* 151: 133—138.

Conney, A. H., Welch, R. M., Kuntzman, R. and Burns, J. J. 1967. Effects of pesticides on drug and steroid metabolism. *Clin. Pharmacol. Ther.* 8: 2—10.

Cram, R. L., Juchan, M. R. and Fonts, J. R. 1965. Differences in hepatic drug metabolism in various rabbit strains before and after pretreatment with phenobarbital. *Proc. Soc. Exp. Biol. Med.* 118: 872—875.

Dacre, J. C. 1960. Metabolic pathways of the phenolic antioxidants. *N.Z. Inst. Chem.* 24: 161—171.

Dacre, J. C. 1965. Chronic toxicity and carcinogenicity studies on citrus red No. 2. *Proc. Univ. Otago Med. Sch.* 43: 31–33.

Dacre, J. C., Denz, F. A. and Kennedy, T. H. 1956. The metabolism of butylated hydroxyanisole in the rabbit. *Biochem. J.* 64: 777–782.

Dale, W. E., Gaines, T. B. and Hayes, W. J., Jr. 1962. Storage and excretion of DDT in starved rats. *Toxicol. Appl. Pharmacol.* 4: 89–106.

Daniel, J. W. and Gage, J. C. 1965. The absorption and excretion of butylated hydroxytoluene (BHT) in the rat. *Food Cosmet. Toxicol.* 3: 405–415.

Daniel, J. W., Gage, J. C., Jones, D. I. and Stevens, M. A. 1967. Excretion of butylated hydroxytoluene (BHT) and butylated hydroxyanisole (BHA) in man. *Food. Cosmet. Toxicol.* 5: 475–479.

Davies, D. S., Gigon, P. S. and Gillette, J. R. 1968. Sex differences in the kinetic constants for the N-demethylation of ethylmorphine by rat liver microsomes. *Biochem. Pharmacol.* 17: 1865–1872.

Davison, A. N. 1955. The conversion of Schradan (OMPA) and parathion into inhibitors of cholinesterase by mammalian liver. *Biochem. J.* 61: 203–209.

De Baum, J. R., Smith, J. Y. R., Miller, E. C. and Miller, J. A. 1970. Reactivity in vivo of the carcinogen N-hydroxy-2-acetylaminofluorene: Increase by sulfate ion. *Science* 167: 184–186.

Dewhurst, F. 1963. The effect of stress upon the metabolism of 2-naphthylamine in mice. *Experientia* 19: 646–647.

Dipple, A. 1976. Polynuclear aromatic carinogens. In: *Chemical Carcinogens.* C. E. Searle (ed.). American Chemical Society, Washington, D. C.

Done, A. K. 1964. Developmental pharmacology. *Clin. Pharmacol. Ther.* 5: 432–479.

Done, A. K. 1966. Perinatal pharmacology. *Annu. Rev. Pharmacol.* 6: 189–208.

DuBois, K. B., Doull, J., Salerno, P. R. and Coon, J. M. 1949. Studies on the toxicity and mechanism of action of p-nitrophenyl diethylthionophosphate (parathion). *J. Pharmacol. Exp. Ther.* 95: 79–91.

Dutton, J. G. 1964. Neonatal drug toxicity caused by defective glucuronide synthesis: Unsuitability of the rat as a test animal: *Proc. Eur. Soc. Study Drug Toxic.* IV: 121–129.

Dutton, G. J. 1966. *Glucuronic Acid, Free and Combined. Chemistry, Biochemistry, Pharmacology and Medicine.* Academic Press, New York.

Emmerson, J. L. and Anderson, R. C. 1966. Metabolism of trifluralin in the rat and dog. *Toxicol. Appl. Pharmacol.* 9: 84–97.

Evans, D. A. P. 1965. Individual variations of drug metabolism as a factor in drug toxicity. *Ann. N.Y. Acad. Sci.* 123: 178–187.

Farner, D. and Verzar, F. 1961. The age parameter of pharmacological activity. *Experientia* 17: 421–422.

Fouts, J. R. 1965. The metabolism of drugs by the foetus. In: *Embryopathic Activity of Drugs.* J. M. Robson, F. Sullivan, and R. L. Smith (eds.). Churchill, London.

Fouts, J. R. and Adamson, R. H. 1959. Drug metabolism in the newborn rabbit. *Science* 129: 897–898.

Gram, T. E., Guarino, A. M., Schroeder, D. H. and Gillette, J. R. 1969. Changes in certain kinetic properties of hepatic microsomal aniline hydroxylase and ethylmorphine demethylase associated with post-natal development and maturation in male rats. *Biochem. J.* 113: 681–686.

Grantham, P. H. et al. 1968. Alteration of the metabolism of the carcinogen N-2-fluorenylacetamide by acetanilide. *Toxicol. Appl. Pharmacol.* 13: 118–130.

Green, F. E., Stripp, B. and Gillette, J. R. 1968. Cited by Gillette, J.R. and Brodie, B.B. 1970. Enzyme induction in laboratory animals and its relevance to food additive investigations. In: *Metabolic Aspects of Food Safety.* F.J.C. Roe (ed.). Academic Press, New York.

Grover, P. L., Hewer, A. and Sims, P. 1971. Epoxides as microsomal metabolites of polycyclic hydrocarbons. *Fed. Eur. Biochem. Soc. Lett.* 18: 76–80.

Hagan, E. C. and Radomski, J. L. 1953. The toxicity of 3-(acetonyl benzyl)-4-hydroxycoumarin (Warfarin) to laboratory animals. *J. Am. Pharm. Assoc.* 42: 379–382.

Hall, G. E., Ettinger, G. H. and Banting, F. G. 1936. Experimental production of coronary thrombosis and myocardial failure. *Can. Med. Assoc. J.* 34: 9–15.

Harrison, Y. E. and West, W. L. 1971. Stimulatory effect of charcoal-broiled ground beef on the hydroxylation of 3,4-benzpyrene by enzymes in rat liver and placenta. *Biochem. Pharmacol.* 20: 2105–2108.

Holtzman, J. L., Gram, T. E., Gigon, P. L. and Gillette, J. R. 1968. The distribution of the components of mixed-function oxidase between the rough and the smooth endoplasmic reticulum of liver cells. *Biochem. J.* 110: 407–412.

Hurst, E. W. 1958. Sexual differences in the toxicity and therapeutic action of chemical substances. In: *The Evaluation of Drug Toxicity*. A.L. Walpole and A. Spinks (eds.). Little Brown, Boston.

Jost, J. P., Khairallah, E. A. and Pitot, H. C. 1968. Studies on the induction and repression of enzymes in rat liver. V. Regulation of the rate of synthesis and degradation of serine dehydratase by dietary amino acids and glucose. *J. Biol. Chem.* 243: 3057–3066.

Kappas, A. and Alvares, A. P. 1975. How the liver metabolizes foreign substances. *Sci. Am.* 232(6): 22–31.

Kato, R., Chiesara, E. and Vassanelli, P. 1962a. Increased activity of microsomal strychnine-metabolizing enzyme induced by phenobarbital and other drugs. *Biochem. Pharmacol.* 11: 913–922.

Kato, R., Chiesara, E. and Vassanelli, P. 1962b. Metabolic differences of strychnine in the rat in relation to sex. *Japn. J. Pharmacol.* 12: 26–33.

Knuesli, E., Berrer, D., Dupuis, G. and Esser, H. 1969. S-triazines. In: *Degradation of Herbicides*. P.C. Kearney and D.D. Kaufman (eds.). Marcel Dekker, New York.

Kupferberg, H. J. and Way, E. L. 1963. Pharmacologic basis for the increased sensivity of the newborn rat to morphine. *J. Pharmacol. Exp. Ther.* 141: 105–112.

Lijinsky, W. and Shubik, P. 1964. Benzo(a)pyrene and other polynuclear hydrocarbons in charcoal-broiled meat. *Science* 145: 53–55.

Lu, F. C., Jessup, D. C. and Lavallee, A. 1965. Toxicity of pesticides in young versus adult rats. *Food Cosmet. Toxicol.* 3: 591–596.

Madhavan, T. V. and Gopalan, C. 1965. Effect of dietary protein on aflatoxin liver injury in weanling rats. *Arch. Pathol.* 80: 123–126.

Majer, J. et al. 1965. Metabolic effects of pyrimidines derived from fava bean glycosides on human erythrocytes deficient in glucose-6-phosphate dehydrogenase. *Biochem. Biophys. Res. Commun.* 20: 235–240.

Margreth, A., Lotlikar, P. D., Miller, E. C. and Miller, J. A. 1964. The effect of hepatotoxic agents and of liver growth on the urinary excretion of N-hydroxy metabolite of 2-acetylaminofluorene by rats. *Cancer Res.* 24: 920–925.

Marshall, W. J. and McLean, A. E. M. 1969. The effect of oral phenobarbitone on hepatic microsomal cytochrome P-450 and demethylation activity in rats fed normal and low protein diets. *Biochem. Pharmacol.* 18: 153–157.

Mathes, S. et al. 1952. Comparison of the tolerance of adults and children to digitoxin. *J.A.M.A.* 150: 191–194.

McLean, A. E. M. and McLean, E. K. 1966. The effect of diet and 1,1,1-trichloro-2,2-bis-(p-chlorophenyl)ethane (DDT) in microsomal hydroxylating enzymes and on sensitivity of rats to carbon tetrachloride poisoning. *Biochem. J.* 100: 566–571.

McLean, A. E. M. and McLean, E. K. 1969. Diet and toxicity. *Br. Med. Bull.* 25: 278–281.

McLean, A. E. M. and Verschuuren, H. G. 1969. Effects of diet and microsomal enzyme induction on the toxicity of dimethylnitrosamine. *Br. J. Exp. Pathol.* 50: 22–25.

McLuen, E. F. and Fouts, J. R. 1961. The effect of obstructive jaundice in drug metabolism in rabbits. *J. Pharmacol. Exp. Ther.* 131: 7—11.

Miller, J. A. and Bauman, C. A. 1945. The determination of p-dimethylaminoazobenzene, p-monomethylaminoazobenzene, and p-aminoazobenzene in tissue. *Cancer Res.* 5: 157.

Munro, H. N. 1964. General aspects of the regulation of protein metabolism by diet and by hormones. In: *Mammalian Protein Metabolism*. Vol. I. H.N. Munro and J.B. Allison (eds.). Academic Press, New York.

Muting, D. 1963. Detoxication capacity of the diseased liver. *Ger. Med. Monogr.* 8: 198—202.

Norton, T. R. 1975. Metabolism of toxic substances. In: *Toxicology. The Basic Science of Poisons*. L.J. Casarett and J. Doull (eds.). MacMillan, New York.

Nyham, W. L. 1961. Toxicity of drugs in the neonatal period. *J. Pediatr.* 59: 1—20.

O'Brien, R. D. 1967. *Insecticides, Action and Metabolism*. Academic Press, New York.

Opie, E. L. and Alford, L. B. 1915. The influence of diet upon necrosis caused by hepatic and renal poisons. *J. Exp. Med.* 21: 1—37.

Orten, J. M. and Neuhaus, O. W. 1975. *Human Biochemistry*. Mosby, St. Louis.

Ottoboni, A., Gee, R., Stanley, R. L. and Goetz, M. E. 1968. Evidence for conversion of DDT to TDE in rat liver. II. Conversion of p,p'-DDT to p,p' TDE in axenic rats. *Bull. Environ. Contam. Toxicol.* 3: 302—308.

Pantuck, E. J. et al. 1974a. Effects of enzyme induction on intestinal phenacetin metabolism in the rat. *J. Pharmacol. Exp. Ther.* 191: 45—52.

Pantuck, E. J. et al. 1974b. Effect of cigarette smoking on phenacetin metabolism. *Clin. Pharmacol. Ther.* 15: 9—17.

Pantuck, E. J., Hsiao, K. C., Kuntzman, R. and Conney, A. H. 1975. Intestinal metabolism of phenacetin in the rat: Effect of charcoal-broiled beef and rat chow. *Science* 187: 744—746.

Pantuck, E. J. et al. 1976. Effect of charcoal-broiled beef on phenacetin metabolism in man. *Science* 194: 1055—1057.

Parke, D. V. 1968. *The Biochemistry of Foreign Compounds*. Pergamon Press, London.

Parke, D. V. and Rahman, H. 1969. The effects of some terpenoids and other dietary nutrients on hepatic drug metabolizing enzymes. *Biochem. J.* 113: 12P

Parke, D. V. and Williams, R. T. 1953. Studies in detoxication. 54. The metabolism of benzene...the metabolism of C^{14}-phenol. *Biochem. J.* 55: 337—340.

Parke, D. V. and Williams, R. T. 1956. Species differences in the o- and p-hydroxylation of aniline. *Biochem. J.* 63: 12P

Peters, R. A. 1963. *Biochemical Lesions and Lethal Synthesis*. Pergamon Press, Oxford.

Peters, J. M. and Boyd, E. M. 1967. The influence of sex and age in albino rats given a daily oral dose of caffeine at a high dose level. *Can. J. Physiol. Pharmacol.* 45: 305—311.

Peterson, J. E. and Robison, W. H. 1964. Metabolic products of p,p'-DDT in the rat. *Toxicol. Appl. Pharmacol.* 6: 321—327.

Pinto, J. D., Camiem, M. N. and Dunn, M. S. 1965. Metabolic fate of p,p'-DDT [1,1,1-trichloro-2,2-bis(p-chlorophenyl)ethane] in rats. *J. Biol. Chem.* 240: 3148—3154.

Quinn, G. P., Axelrod, J. and Brodie, B. B. 1958. Species, strain and sex differences in metabolism of hexobarbitone, amidopyrene, and aniline. *Biochem. Pharmacol.* 1: 152—159.

Radomski, J. L. 1961. The absorption and fate and excretion of Citrus Red No. 2 (2,5-dimethoxyphenylazo-2-naphthol) and Ext. D and C Red No. 14 (1-xylylazo-2-naphthol). *J. Pharmacol. Exp. Ther.* 134: 100—109.

Radomski, J. L. 1962. 1-Amino-2-naphthyl glucuronide, a metabolite of 2,5-dimethoxyphenylazo-2-naphthol and 1-xylylazo-2-naphthol *J. Pharmacol. Exp. Ther.* 136: 378—385.

Rona, G., Chappel, G. I., Balazs, T. and Gandry, R. 1959. The effect of breed, age, sex on myocardial necrosis produced by isoproterenol in the rat. *J. Geron-tol.* 14: 169–173.

St. John, L. E. and Lisk, D. J. 1969. Metabolism of Banvel D herbicide in a dairy cow. *J. Dairy Sci.* 42: 392–393.

Scheline, R. R., Williams, R. T. and Wit, J. G. 1960. Biological dehydroxylation. *Nature* 188: 849–850.

Schenkman, J. B., Frey, I., Remmer, H. and Estabrook, R. W. 1967. Sex differ-ences in drug metabolism by rat liver microsomes. *Mol. Pharmacol.* 3: 516–525.

Sereni, F., Perletti, L., Manfredi, N. and Marina, A. 1965. Tissue distribution and urinary excretion of a tetracycline derivative in newborn and older infants. *J. Pediatr.* 67: 299–305.

Setnikar, I. and Magistretti, M. J. 1964. The toxicity of central nervous system stimulants in rats of different ages. In: *Some Factors Affecting Drug Toxicity.* Int. Congr. Ser. Excerpts Medica, Amsterdam, Holland.

Smith, A. A., Fabrykant, M., Kaplan, M. and Gavitt, J. 1964. Dehydroxylation of some catecholamines and their products. *Biochim. Biophys. Acta* 86: 429–437.

Smith, J. M. 1968. The comparative metabolism of xenobiotics. *Adv. Comp. Physiol. Biochem.* 3: 173–232.

Spencer, E. Y., O'Brien, R. D. and White, R. W. 1957. Permanganate oxidation products of schradan. *J. Agr. Food Chem.* 5: 123–127.

Stevenson, E. S., Dobriner, K. and Rhoads, C. P. 1942. The metabolism of dimethylaminoazobenzene (butter yellow) in rats. *Cancer Res.* 2: 160–167.

Stewart, R. D. et al. 1972. Carboxyhemoglobin elevation after exposure to dichloromethane. *Science* 176: 295–296.

Swann, P. F. and McLean, A. E. M. 1968. The effect of diet on the toxic and car-cinogenic action of dimethylnitrosamine. *Biochem. J.* 107: 14P–15P.

Tye, R. and Engel, J. D. 1967. Distribution and excretion of Dicamba by rats as determined by radiotracer technique. *J. Agr. Food Chem.* 15: 837–840.

Tye, R., Engel, J. D. and Rapien, I. 1965. Disposition of butylated hydroxytoluene (BHT) in the rat. *Food Cosmet. Toxicol.* 3: 547–551.

Udenfriend, S. et al. 1969. Significance of the NIH shift with respect to liver microsome hydroxylations. In: *Microsomes and Drug Oxidations.* J.R. Gillette, A.H. Conney, G.J. Cosmides, R.W. Estabrook, J.R. Fouts and G. J. Mannering (eds.). Academic Press, New York.

Vest, M. 1959. Studies on the development of glucuronide conjugating capacity of the liver of the newborn. *Schweiz. Med. Wochenschr.* 89: 102–105.

Waelsch, H. 1955. The turnover of components of the developing brain; the blood barrier. In: *Biochemistry of the Developing Nervous System.* H. Waelsch (ed.). Academic Press, London.

Watenberg, L. W., Leong, J. L. and Strand, P. J. 1962. 3,4-Benzpyrene hydroxy-lase activity in the gastrointestinal tract. *Cancer Res.* 22: 1120–1125.

Weinstein, L. 1970. The sulfonamides. In: *The Pharmacological Basis of Therapeu-tics.* 4th ed. L.S. Goodman and A. Gilman (eds.). Macmillan, New York.

Weisburger, J. H. et al. 1964. Activation and detoxification of N-2-fluorenylacet-amide in man. *Cancer Res.* 24: 475–479.

Weisburger, J. H. et al. 1972. On the sulfate ester of N-hydroxy-N-2-fluorenylacetamide as a key ultimate hepatocarcinogen. *Cancer Res.* 32: 491–500.

Welch, R. M. Cavallito, J. and Loh, A. 1972. Effect of exposure to cigarette smoke on the metabolism of benzo(a)pyrene and acetophenetidin by lung and intestine of rat. *Toxicol. Appl. Pharmacol.* 23: 749–758.

Wergedal, J. E. and Harper, a. E. 1964. Metabolic adaptations in higher animals. IX. Effect of high protein intake on amino nitrogen catabolism in vivo. *J. Biol. Chem.* 239: 1156–1163.

Williams, R. T. 1959. *Detoxication Mechanisms*. 2nd ed. Chapman & Hall, London.

Williams, R. T. 1967. Comparative patterns of drug metabolism. *Fed. Proc. Fed. Am. Soc. Exp. Biol.* 26: 1029–1039.

Williams, R. T. 1970. The metabolic pathways of exogenous substances. In: *Metabolic Aspects of Food Safety*. F.J.C. Roe (ed.), Academic Press, New York.

Williams, J. N., Jr., Jacobs, R. M. and Hurlebaus, A. J. 1966. Changes in rat liver cytochromes b, c_1, and c and mitochondrial protein in prolonged protein deficiency. *J. Nutr.* 90: 400–404.

Yeary, R. A., Benish, R. A. and Finkelstein, M. 1966. Acute toxicity of drugs in newborn animals. *J. Pediatr.* 69: 663–667.

5

Manifestations of Toxic Effects

The biochemical events following exposure to a toxic agent generally result in clinical manifestations or symptoms. The symptoms may be characteristic of the particular physiological process or organ system thus affected. Often multiple symptoms associated with the toxicological events indicate that more than one system is affected. Virtually all physiologies or organ systems in the body are subject to toxic effects; and it should be emphasized that all these systems are interrelated, so that toxic injury to the primary target may have repercussions in other systems. This is particularly true of damage to the central nervous and the hematopoietic systems.

The symptoms or effects of poisoning associated with food toxicants are discussed in succeeding chapters. However, several important manifestations of toxicity are briefly discussed in this chapter. These include neurotoxicity, hepatotoxicity, nephrotoxicity, and hematopoietic, skeletal, and reproductive toxicity. The toxic effects most relevant to food toxicants are allergenicity, mutagenicity, teratogenicity, and carcinogenicity. This is because these effects, in many cases, may be induced by toxicants at the very low levels that are found in food. This does not mean that the other aforementioned toxic effects may not be induced by small quantities of toxicants, for example, neurotoxicity. allergenicity, mutagenicity, and teratogenicity are also discussed in this section. Carcinogenicity, which is believed to be the most common and the most controversial consequence of many food toxicants, is discussed in Chapters 6 and 7.

NEUROTOXICITY

The brain is susceptible to the toxic effects of substances, in spite of the blood—brain barrier. This barrier, which normally protects the brain from substances that can damage other soft tissues, does not exclude all toxic substances.

The brain may be damaged by a lack of oxygen, diminished respiration, or by direct damage to the neuronal and other tissues, structures, and enzymes in the brain (Norton 1975).

The lack of oxygen may result from a decreased blood supply, failure in blood oxygenation, or interference in oxygen transport, cellular metabolism, or respiration. The decrease or lack in blood supply may occur following cardiac arrest or rupture of critical blood vessels in the brain, resulting in hemorrhage or thrombosis. Severe hypertension can rupture blood vessels in the brain. Pressor amines in the presence of monoamine oxidase inhibitors may precipitate a severe hypertensive crisis (Chap. 8).

Severe hypotension also can diminish the brain's blood supply considerably, as in the effect of cyanide poisoning on the heart (Norton 1975). Failure in blood oxygenation may follow from respiratory paralysis by paralytic agents such as botulinum exotoxin and saxitoxin.

Interference in oxygen transport may be brought about by oxidants such as the nitrites. Nitrites oxidize Fe^{2+} to Fe^{3+} in hemoglobin, resulting in methemoglobinemia.

Metabolic inhibitors can interfere with cellular metabolism or respiration. Examples of this type of inhibitor are cyanide and methionine sulfoximine. It follows that hypoglycemic agents such as hypoglycin A, from the akee fruit, are also metabolic or respiratory inhibitors of brain cells.

Direct effects on neuronal structures producing brain lesions may be caused by mercury, lead, excessive glutamate and aspartate intake, and certain nutrient antagonists. Such antinutritives are antimetabolites, antiniacinamides, (acetyl pyridine), and antithiamin factors.

Interference in neurotransmission, either in the central or peripheral nervous system, is another manifestation of neurotoxicity. Several examples will be evident in other chapters; e.g., DDT (dichlorodiphenyltrichlorothane), organophosphates and carbamates, and various seafood toxicants.

The damage to the central nervous system (CNS) by toxicants may be manifested by diminished or absent sensory and motor functions, and various integrative functions of the brain (Norton 1975). Sensory loss is exemplified by blindness, deafness, and loss of the sensation to touch, temperature, pressure, and pain, and paresthesia.

Loss of motor functions is associated with general paralysis or paresis and muscle incoordination (ataxia).

Neurotoxicity is also associated with signs suggesting loss of integrative functions such as loss of memory and learning ability, seizures, convulsions, excitation, hyperkinetic behavior, depression, and coma. Many types of behavior (Chapman and Wolff 1959), emotional alterations, and mental retardation are also manifestations which definitely are associated with neurotoxic effects (Chisholm and Kaplan 1968; Wiener 1970). An example of these effects are those associated with lead poisoning (Chap. 18).

HEPATOTOXICITY

As already stated, compounds absorbed in the gastrointestinal (GI) tract must then pass through the liver, where, in the case of toxicants, they are biotransformed into more or less toxic derivatives. Thus, the liver may bear the brunt of the toxic effects of compounds. With sufficient dose, liver damage ensues.

Liver damage may be manifested by hepatomegaly, inflammation, necrosis, venoocclusive lesions, cellular degeneration, fatty accumulations, cessation of bile flow (cholestasis), bile duct proliferation, and tumor formation. However, liver enlargement does not always signify a pathological effect (Wilson et al. 1970).

Histologically, chemically induced liver injury is associated with damage or changes in various organelles — the nucleus, endoplasmic reticulum, mitochondria, and lysosomes (Plaa 1975). Many hepatotoxins affect all of these organelles: CCl_4 Dianzani 1963; Rechnagel 1967), dimethylnitrosamines (DMN) (Emmelot and Benedetti 1960; Rouiller 1964), and the pyrrolizidine alkaloids (Mclean 1970). Aflatoxin (Wogan 1969), DMN (Emmelot and Benedetti 1960), and cyclopeptidic mycotoxins (Chap. 10) affect only the nucleus. The cyclic peptides can also affect other organelles.

Clinically, liver injury may be indicated, among other signs, by jaundice, hyperbilirubinemia, abdominal pain, and gastrointestinal symptoms (e.g., vomiting, diarrhea, and coma). Because of the liver's ability to repair itself following injury, the clinical signs, other than tumor formation, may not be observable immediately unless a significant portion of the liver is damaged beyond its capacity for rapid repair. Delay in the appearance of symptoms may also be a function of the rate of biotransformation, biliary or urinary excretion, adipose tissue storage or release, enterohepatic circulation, or a combination of all these factors.

Prime examples of very potent hepatotoxins with delayed clinical manifestations are the amanita toxins and other mycotoxins.

Several biochemical factors in the blood can indicate liver injury: ammonia, plasma proteins, enzymes (e.g., transaminases), bile pigments, organic acids, and steroids.) Aberration in liver function can be detected by the ability of the liver to clear certain dyes (e.g., Bromsulphalein [sulfobromophthalein]) from the blood (Oser 1965).

NEPHROTOXICITY

The kidneys, more than any other organ in the body, have a greater chance for toxic injury from ingested substances (Foulkes and Hammond 1975). This is because from 20 to 25% of the resting blood output of the heart passes through them. This large volume of blood—more than 400 ml/100 g of kidney cortex per min—indicates that a large amount of circulating toxic substances will come in contact with kidney tissues. In addition, the kidney, fulfilling its excretory function, accumulates toxic substances within its parenchyma, either through active transport (Foulkes 1963; Kessler et al. 1959), special binding proteins, e.g., Cd-binding metallothionein (Pulido et al. 1966; Chap. 18), or through the sodium ion and water reabsorption mechanism (Kriz and Lever 1969). Furthermore, shifts in the pH of nephrons responding to similar shifts in the systemic circulation can promote changes in the chemical and physical properties, leading to increased toxicity (Foulkes and Hammond 1975).

Nephrotoxic compounds may lead to chronic or acute renal failure, which is manifested by the uremic syndrome. Uremia is characterized by oliguria and increases in blood nitrogen, mostly in the form of urea, and other substances normally excreted in the urine. Renal failure may be complete, in which case, anuria occurs, resulting in a fatal prognosis unless there is prompt medical intervention.

Kidney damage by toxicants may be assessed by an evaluation of its function. Basically, the concentration of normal urine consitituents are measured. For example, the concentration of NaCl in the urine may indicate a failure to concentrate urine or reabsorb water and sodium. Also, an abnormal excretion of glucose in the absence of hyperglycemia, high urinary amino acid—creatine ratio (amino aciduria), proteins and sediments, and urinary enzymes, such as glutamic oxalacetate transaminase (Prescott and Ansari 1969) and alkaline and acid phosphatases (Nomiyama et al. 1973) are all indicative of renal failure. Also, clearance of specific substances, e.g., p-aminohippurate (PAH) (McCurdy et al. 1968) may also indicate renal damage.

While these signs are associated with renal damage, these symptoms may not be visible in mild cases or the early development of kidney damage (Sharratt and Frazer 1963). In animal experiments, histological evaluation of renal tissues may give more reliable information regarding early kidney injury.

The kidney's role in cholecalciferol metabolism may be reflected by abnormalities in calcium metabolism. In addition, anemia may suggest damage to the kidneys because of the role of these organs in erythropoiesis.

Many substances which can damage the liver may also damage the kidneys. Thus, both kidney and liver damage can occur in CCl_4 and mushroom poisoning. Renal damage may also be induced by hypertension which may be related to excessive NaCl consumption.

A discussion of the mechanisms of renal injury caused by toxic substances is beyond the scope of this book. The reader is referred to the review of Foulkes and Hammond (1975) for a discussion of this subject.

HEMATOTOXICITY

Toxic injury to the blood cells and blood-forming tissues is known as hematotoxicity. In humans, the bone marrow constitutes the principal blood-forming tissue. The bone marrow produces stem cells which are precursors of the red blood cells (erythrocytes), white blood cells (leukocytes), and platelets (thrombocytes). The red blood cells primarily deliver oxygen to all cells in the body and remove CO_2 from these cells. They contain hemoglobin, the iron-containing heme-protein which is responsible for their respiratory function. Injury to the red blood cells or hemoglobin can result in impairment of oxygen transport, and consequently peripheral hypoxia. The symptoms associated with this condition reflect the damage to the CNS and/or heart, which are most sensitive to oxygen deprivation.

Hematoxicity is manifested by anemia, agranulocytosis, methemoglobinemia, polycythemia, leukemia, thrombocytopenia and other blood-clotting disorders, and defects in the immune system.

Anemias

The anemias are characterized by a reduction in the number of circulating red blood cells (RBCs), in the volume of packed red cells per unit volume of blood (hematocrit), in hemoglobin concentration per 100 ml of blood, or a combination of two or all these factors.

There are an average of 5.5 million RBCs mm^3 in human males and 4.5 million/ mm^3 in females. Infants have higher RBC concentrations. Persons living at altitudes of 3000 m or higher may have an RBC concentration of 8 million/mm^3. The RBC has a normal lifespan of 120 days, and in order to maintain the normal RBC concentration, about 2.2 and 2.7 million RBCs/sec must be produced in adult females and males, respectively.

The normal hematocrit values in men at sea level are between 40 and 54%, average, 47%; in women, the range is 37 to 47%, average 42%; children, 31 to 49% depending on the age; and newborns, 49 to 54%. The normal hemoglobin values average 14 to 18 g/100 ml in males, 12 to 16 g/100 ml in females, and 10 to 12 g/100 ml in children. In pregnancy, the normal hemoglobin values decrease to about 11 g/100 ml, and the hematocrit to 34%; the latter is due to hemodilution.

Anemia can result from damage to the bone marrow and other erythropoietin-producing tissues, particularly the kidneys; increased rate of destruction over rate of production of RBCs; decreased nucleic acid synthesis; deficiency of iron and other minerals; vitamin deficiencies; and excessive hemorrhage.

Damage to the bone marrow by toxic agents results not only in anemia, but also leukemia, polycythemia, thrombocytopenia, and other blood-clotting disorders.

Damage to the erythropoietin-producing tissues can result in a failure in the production of RBCs in erythroid tissues, i.e., bone marrow and spleen. Erythropoietin is a hormone produced by the kidneys and other tissues. As stated previously, renal disease is commonly associated with anemia.

An increased rate of destruction of RBCs over the rate of production will obviously lead to anemia. This condition occurs when the RBCs are unusually fragile and are easily hemolyzed. The factors associated with hemolytic anemias are discussed in a later section.

The production of RBCs is highly dependent on many nutrients, especially iron, folic acid, cobalamin, and other vitamins and minerals. Thus, substances which interfere in the availability of these nutrients will cause anemia.

Because cellular formation is primarily dependent on nucleic acid synthesis, it is obvious that any substance interfering in this process will also induce anemias. Both folic acid and cobalamin as well as other nutrients influence this process. Therefore, their unavailability can be expected to cause anemia.

Hemorrhage occurs as a result of clotting disorders such as in thrombocytopenia and other conditions where the myriads of clotting factors are either absent or nonfunctional. One clotting factor is methylnaphthoquinone (vitamin K), which is essential in the biosynthesis of prothrombin. Prothrombin is converted to thrombin in the presence of thrombokinase and other factors. Thrombin promotes the formation of fibrin (blood clot) from fibrinogen. Hemorrhages, especially internal ones, will occur in the presence of the methylnaphthoquinone antagonists, such as bishydroxycoumarin, and large doses of salicylates (Orten and Neuhaus 1975). Antinapthoquinones are discussed in Chapter 9.

In addition, conditions which interfere with the absorption of vitamin K will also increase the hazard of hemorrhage. These conditions include biliary insufficiency, high fat diets coupled with poor fat absorption, fatty diarrheas, and the ingestion of mineral oils, drugs, and other substances that destroy intestinal bacteria (Orten and Neuhaus 1975).

Other hemorrhagic conditions include gastric and intestinal ulcers, scurvy, and capilliary fragility. These conditions may be induced by toxicants, such as ulcerogenic irritants (certain spices) and antiascorbates.

Examples of anemias due to defective formation of red blood cells include hypochromic, aplastic, macrocystic/megaloblastic, and pernicious anemias.

Hypochromic anemia

Hypochromic anemia is generally associated with iron deficiency, and is therefore called iron-deficiency anemia. Hemoglobin cannot be synthesized without iron, and thus under this condition, the red cells are deficient in hemoglobin and appear pale under the microscope (hypochromia). Normal hemoglobin concentrations in humans have already been mentioned.

Factors interfering in the absorption or availability of iron will induce hypochromic anemia. This includes high fat diets and other substances which form insoluble iron soaps and salts, respectively. In order to be absorbed easily, ferrous iron (Fe^{2+}) must be reduced to ferric iron (Fe^{3+}). Ascorbic acid, which is necessary for this reduction is also necessary in iron transport and utilization because Fe^{3+} must be reduced to Fe^{2+} in order to be retrieved from its storage form. Therefore, factors causing a persistent destruction of ascorbic acid in the diet may induce hypochromic anemia, in addition to other abnormalities. Toxicants which interfere in the utilization and transport of iron will also induce hypochromic anemia.

Copper appears to be required in the incorporation of iron into hemoglobin (Cummings and Earl 1960). In the form of ceruloplasmin, a ferroxidase, copper promotes the oxidation of $Fe^{2+} \longrightarrow Fe^{3+}$; Fe^{3+} can then combine with apotransferrin to form transferrin, the transport form of iron (Peisach et al. 1966). Therefore, substances interfering in the availability of copper may also induce hypochromic anemia; e.g., those forming unabsorbable complexes with copper.

Toxic substances may also interfere in the biosynthesis of heme. Lead-induced anemia may be the result of lead interfering in the metabolism of δ-aminolevulinic acid, a heme precursor (Haeger-Aronsen 1960; Orten and Neuhaus 1975).

Aplastic Anemia

When the bone marrow is severely damaged by toxic substances, aplastic anemia can develop. In this case, the marrow fails to proliferate and produce the cells of the blood. Benzene and a number of pesticides have been implicated in aplastic anemia.

Megaloblastic and Macrocystic Anemia

The maturation of the RBCs may be hampered by deficiencies in cobalamin and folic acid. Under these conditions, megaloblastic and/or macrocystic anemia may develop.

Megaloblastic anemia is characterized by large numbers of immature forms of RBCs—the erythroblast or megaloblast, which are nucleated, oval or slightly irregular red blood cells, 11 to 20 μm in diameter. Macrocystic anemia, on the other hand, is marked by the presence of relatively large numbers of macrocytes, large RBCs 10 μm or more in diameter. Both types of cells may be present simultaneously as in pernicious anemia (see below).

In addition to dietary deficiency of these vitamins (primary deficiency), secondary deficiencies can occur in the presence of antimetabolites or antagonists to these vitamins. Anticobalamin and antifolacin factors are discussed in Chapter 9.

Pernicious Anemia A deficiency of cobalamin causes pernicious anemia, a condition marked by the presence of both macrocytes and megaloblasts in the blood. This form of anemia is characterized not only by an abnormal blood picture but also by neuro- logical damage. Usually, pernicious anemia develops in persons over 35 years old who cannot produce the intrinsic factor because of atrophic fundal gastric mucosa. This intrinsic factor is required for the absorption of cobalamin. It is not known whether pernicious anemia can be induced directly by toxic agents, although one can assume that toxic injury to the stomach glandular mucosa may inhibit intrinsic factor synthesis.

Clinical Signs of Anemia

An excessive rate of destruction of the RBCs over the rate of RBC biosynthesis is one cause of hemolytic anemia. The RBC is readily ruptured or hemolyzed, allowing hemo- globin to leak into the plasma. Many food toxicants may induce this unusual fragility of the erythrocyte membrane.

An hereditary condition known as favism, induced by the ingestion of fava beans, is characterized by hemolytic anemia. The basic defect is postulated to be a deficiency in glucose-6-phosphate dehydrogenase. This enzyme is required in the reduction of NADP (nicotinamide adenine dinucleotide phosphate) to NADPH (the reduced form) during the conversion of glucose-6-Phosphate to gluconolactone 6-Phosphate. NADPH is needed in the reduction of oxidized glutathion (GSSG) to the reduced form (GSH) in the presence of GSSG reductase. GSH is required for the decomposition of H_2O_2 in the presence of glutathion peroxidase. H_2O_2 may damage the cell membrane, rendering it susceptible to hemolysis. Nitrite, an oxidant, can promote the formation of the superoxide radical, O_2^-, which combines with H^+ in the presence of the enzyme superoxide dismutase to form H_2O_2. Such a radical is formed in the oxidation of hemo- globin to methemoglobin. The latter, although present in small quantities (0.3 g/100 ml blood) (Orten and Neuhaus 1975) in normal human blood, may increase markedly in the presence of oxidants. A hematotoxic condition known as methemoglobinemia is a manifestation of nitrite poisoning (Chap. 18).

Hemolytic Anemias

Anemia is generally recognized by weakness, vertigo, headache, sore tongue, drowsi- ness, general malaise, dyspnea, tachycardia, palpitation, angina pectoris, gastro- intestinal disturbances, amenorrhea, lack of libido, slight fever, and pallor of the skin, fingernail beds, and mucous membranes. The basal metabolic rate (BMR) may be increased in severe cases (Thomas 1977).

In pernicious anemia, in addition to the aforementioned symptoms, neurological signs such as paresthesias of the extremities may also be observed. In severe cases, these symptoms may be accompanied by signs of cardiac failure (Thomas 1977).

Other Blood Abnormalities

Several other blood abnormalities can be caused by toxic substances. One is polycythemia, a condition marked by abnormal proliferation of red blood cells. This condition, it seems, may be induced by the ingestion of large amounts of cobalt. For example, beer once contained cobalt salts to enhance foaming (Anon 1968). In animal
tests, the level of cobalt necessary to induce polycythemia has been shown to be approximately 200 to 250 ppm in the diet (Grant and Root 1952). Since the beer contained
only 1.2 to 1.5 ppm of cobalt, other factors such as species sensitivity, alcoholic content, low protein diets (Alexander 1969), and thiamin deficiency (Grinvalsky and Fitch
1969) have been suggested as possibly having synergistic or additive effects to cobalt
in inducing polycythemia and cardiomyopathy in beer drinkers.

Pancytopenia, a condition marked by decreased formation of all three major types
of blood cells is another blood abnormality. Many types of toxicants, such as benzene
and arsenic, can promote this blood abnormality (Harris and Kellermeyer 1970).

Agranulocytosis can also be induced by toxic chemicals (Pisciotta 1971) having
cytotoxic effects on bone marrow.

Leukemia is discussed under carcinogenesis in Chapter 6.

Immunological defects due to cytotoxic agents are discussed in connection with
carcinogenesis and organic chemical contaminants.

SKELETAL TOXICITY

Toxic injury to the bones may arise from interference in bone metabolism and deposition of radioactive and other toxic metals.

Interference in Regulatory Factors in Bone Metabolism

Bone metabolism is under the influence of hormones: growth, thyroid, sex, adrenocorticotropic hormones (ACTH), adrenocorticoids, and parathormone (Budy 1975).
Thus, any substance adversely affecting the function of these factors may indirectly
have deleterious effects on bones. For instance, if the secretion of a growth hormone
is diminished, growth and development of bones will be retarded. Overproduction of
growth hormones will cause an enlargement of bones, resulting in a grotesque condition known as acromegaly. This may occur, for example, if a tumor, i.e., an eosino-
philic adenoma, develops in the pituitary gland. While thyroid hormones are essential
for the normal development of the bones, excessive production or administration of
them will, in fact, lead to retardation of bone growth. Excess production or administration of adrenocorticoids will cause osteoporosis (loss of bone mineral). Parathormone
regulates the mobilization of calcium in bone, so that excessive secretion of this hormone will lead to excessive calcium loss.

Vitamin D₃

Cholecalciferol (vitamin D$_3$) in the form of its active derivative 1,25-dihydroxychole-
calciferol regulates the mineralization of bone. Excessive doses of this vitamin will
cause the resorption of bones, poor calcification, and formation of a matrix that is un-
calcifiable. In other words, an overdose will lead to a form of rickets as does cholecalciferol deficiency. Hypervitaminosis D, in this case, occurs at doses of 50,000 IU or
more per day. The toxic threshold, however, is 20,000 to 25,000 IU/kg of body weight
per day.

The toxic symptoms associated with cholecalciferol poisoning also include headache,
nausea, anorexia, weakness, digestive disturbances, irreversible kidney damage, excessive urination (polyurea), and calcification of the soft tissues (Orten and Neuhaus
1975).

Deficiency of the vitamin produces rickets in children, even among early adolescents. In adults, deficiency results in a condition known as osteomalacia. Rickets is associated with defective ossification (mineralization), so that the bones become soft and pliable. Pressure on the bones results in clinical deformities; e.g., bowlegs, knock-knees, enlargement of the ends of bones, swelling at the rib junction ("rachitic rosary"), contraction of pelvis, and bossing of the temporal bones.

In osteomalacia, as in rickets, there is demineralization of the bones, but the latter become softer than rachitic bones. Deformities are also observed. Serum calcium may also diminish markedly, so that tetany ensues (Orten and Neuhaus 1975). In this condition, there is an increased proportion of collagen over mineral content. Osteomalacia should be distinguished from osteoporosis in that the ratio of the organic and inorganic content in the bone in the latter condition is generally normal, but the total mass of the bone is considerably decreased. This decreased mass results in increased porosity. The bone, although normal in size, becomes increasingly fragile. Osteoporosis, which is commonly found in women after menopause, appears to be induced by decreased estrogen, fluoride (Marx 1980), and 1,25-dihydroxycholecalciferol (DHC) secretion, and increased parathormone (PTH) production. Therefore, any substance which causes a decrease in estrogen, DHC, and fluoride, or a marked increase in PTH secretion will promote osteoporosis.

Cholecalciferol deficiency can result from defective absorption. Absorption is inhibited when there is interference in bile secretion, when high fat diets are consumed, and when fat-soluble laxatives, such as mineral oil, are used. Many toxic substances causing liver damage may interfere in biliary secretion.

Fatty diarrheal diseases, such as celiac disease, will also lead to the demineralization of bone owing to insufficient absorption of cholecalciferol and calcium. The latter forms insoluble soaps with fatty acids.

Vitamin A

Both excesses and deficiencies of retinoids (vitamin A) can lead to toxic injury to bones. Excessive ingestion of this vitamin causes bone fragility and fractures of the long bones as well as other symptoms: anorexia, irritability, fissures at the corner of the mouth, cracking and bleeding of lips, loss of hair, liver enlargement, and pain in the joints and bones.

Deficiency of this vitamin will lead to retardation of bone growth, especially the formation of endochondral bone. In animals, this retardation of bone growth results in paralysis and nerve degeneration because of the failure of the cranium to grow commensurate with the growth of the brain (Orten and Neuhaus 1975).

Any factor which retards the absorption of cholecalciferol will also retard the absorption of retinoids.

Vitamin C

Ascorbic acid is essential for the formation and maintenance of the intercellular ground substance, collagen. A deficiency of this vitamin will hinder its formation or result in the production of a defective protein. This defective collagen cannot be calcified (Budy 1975). Of course, ascorbic acid deficiency will also affect other tissues besides the bone.

Ascorbic acid deficiency can be produced by substances which cause its destruction or prevent its absorption. Some of these degradatory substances are discussed in Chapter 9. Factors or conditions interfering in the absorption of most nutrients can also be expected to interfere in the utilization of the vitamin.

Deposition of Radioactive Metals, Other Toxic Minerals, and Organic Toxicants

Many metals tend to concentrate in the bone. Some of them will replace calcium in the crystal lattice. Others are bound to specific bone proteins such as the sialoproteins. Those metals that tend to replace calcium include strontium (Sr), barium (Ba), radium (Ra) (Vaughn 1971), lead (Goyer and Mushak 1977), vanadium (Waters 1977), and cadmium (Itokawa et al. 1973, 1974; Pond and Walker 1975). Others like beryllium, will deposit on the crystal surfaces (Mclean and Budy 1964). Metals that bind to bone proteins include lanthanum, thorium, and plutonium.

Toxic injury to the bones occurs when radioactive metals are deposited therein. From the food toxicology perspective, the main toxic effects that can be related to chronic ingestion of radioactive "bone-seeking" elements are bone cancers. This has been clearly established in the case of radium-226 involving watch dial workers (Evans et al. 1969; Finkel et al. 1969), and in the case of strontium-90 in animals (Goldman and Bustad 1972; McClellan and Jones 1969).

Another type of toxic injury associated with the deposition of toxic metals in bones is exemplified by the effects of cadmium. In an organism deficient in calcium, the deposition of cadmium in bones and soft tissues is enhanced (Itokawa et al. 1974; Larsson and Piscator 1971; Pond and Walker 1975). Cadmium also strongly inhibits calcium deposition in the bones of pigs with adequate dietary calcium (Hennig and Anke 1964); a similar observation has been reported in chicks (Stancer and Dardzonov 1967). This effect is partly due to interference in intestinal calcium absorption and inhibition of 1,25-dihydroxycholecalciferol synthesis in the kidney (Suda et al. 1974). Thus, the inhibitory effects of cadmium on bone calcification may be responsible for the painful osteomalacia associated with cadmium poisoning in humans (Itokawa et al. 1973).

There are, of course, other effects on bones. But in these cases, the role of toxic substances are less clear.

REPRODUCTIVE TOXICITY

The reproductive system is sensitive to many toxic substances. Toxicants can have direct and indirect effects on the reproductive system: indirectly, by affecting hormones originating outside the reproductive organs; directly, by affecting the egg, sperm, and supporting structures or tissues. The main clinical manifestation of reproductive toxicity is infertility or sterility.

Many types of steroids with hormonal activity have been found to prevent ovulation, so a number of these substances are used as oral contraceptives (Diczfalusy 1969). These substances, however, should be considered toxic because of their effects on normal reproductive processes. Indeed, aside from their reproductive toxicity, these substances have other toxic effects, e.g., carcinogenicity and hematotoxicity.

Apparently, these steroids inhibit ovulation by suppressing the follicle-stimulating hormone (FSH), in the case of estrogenic steroids, and luteinizing hormones (LH), in the case of the progesteronic steroids in the hypothalamus and pituitary gland (Diczfalusy 1969; Emmens 1970). In addition, these substances also change the responsiveness of the ovaries to gonadotropin stimulation in the biosynthesis and degradation of FSH and LH. These steroids inhibit the capacitation of sperm and interfere with the implantation of the egg.

Estrogenic compounds are present in food in the form of naturally occurring compounds, additives, or food contaminants. Beer contains estrogenic bitter acids derived from hops (*Humulus lupulus*) used during brewing to impart the bitter taste. Other naturally occurring estrogens found in forage plants have been implicated in causing sterility in livestock. Diethylstilbestrol (DES), a contraceptive, which was formerly used as a growth-promoting implant in beef cattle is now prohibited for use in the

United States; it has been shown to cause cancer in the female offspring of women administered a therapeutic dose of DES (Chap. 19).

A number of steroids also inhibit spermatogenesis (Emmens 1970). Diethylstilbestrol may interfere in the development of the spermatocyte (Jackson and Schnieden 1968; Lacy and Lofts 1965).

Central nervous system depressants, such as epinephrine, norepinephrine, and serotonin, depress ovulation in rabbits (Curie et al. 1969) and in mice (Pushottam et al. 1961). Their effects, however, depend on the precise time of exposure after mating. Thus, complete inhibition has been observed 1 min after exposure with epinephrine at 300 μ g/kg; serotonin produces similar effect at 5 mg/kg after 5 min (Curie et al. 1969).

Certain insecticides and toxic metals have direct toxic effects on reproductive cells. In sheep, hexachlorophene has been shown to degenerate spermatogenic cells and cause extensive damage to the germ cells at the spermatogonium stage. These effects have been induced at a dose of 2.5 g/kg, followed by 50 mg/kg 2 days later; after 21 days following the last treatment, neither sperm in the epididymis nor spermatogenesis has been observed (Thorpe 1969). Dieldrin administered at doses of 1.25—5 mg/kg for up to 10 days causes a decrease in the uptake of testosterone in the prostate in mice, but an acute dose causes the opposite effect. DDT appears to have a similar effect (Thomas 1972). Sevin affected spermatogenesis in the white rat, especially at the spermatid and spermatogonium stage, at doses above 0.5 mg/kg; this threshold dose affecting sperm production is much lower than the dose (4 mg/kg) producing general toxic effects in this animal (Vashakidze 1971).

It has been demonstrated that cadmium administered as a single subcutaneous dose of 0.5 mol/kg in rabbits causes atrophy of the testes and aspermia for several weeks (Paufler 1969). In rats, this metal causes hemorrhagic necrosis in the testes and caput epididymis within 24—40 hr, and the consequent reduction in testosterone secretion causes atrophy in accessory glands, cauda epididymis, and vas deferens, and degeneration of the spermatozoa (Gunn et al. 1970). It has been shown that Cd has a direct effect on DNA (deoxyribonucleic acid) synthesis. It interferes in the incorporation of thymidine into spermatogonia without affecting the incorporation of uridine and leucine.

Alkylating agents, such as triethylenephosphoramide (Joshi et al. 1970) and many other carcinogens, can be expected to be toxic to the reproductive system because of their effects on DNA.

ALLERGENICITY

An allergic reaction, or allergy, is a condition whereby body tissues of sensitive persons react to allergens which have no effect on nonsensitive persons similarly exposed. It is essentially an antigen—antibody reaction triggering the release of histamine or similar compounds from injured cells. An allergic reaction differs from other toxic reactions in that (1) virtually all types of substances that can be absorbed in the body may cause an allergy, and (2) the reaction is highly subjective, manifesting only in sensitive individuals. Thus, unlike other toxic substances, the effect of an allergen on subjects chosen at random, even among those who may be sensitive, cannot be predicted.

No doubt an allergic reaction is a toxic reaction, producing toxic symptoms, including urticaria (angioedema), eczema, rash, asthma, hay fever, headache (including migraine), hemorrhage, and gastrointestinal disturbances. Other signs of allergic reaction are labyrinthitis, conjunctivitis, nausea, and vomiting. In rare cases, allergenicity may be manifested by generalized systemic reaction, circulatory collapse, shock, and death (Burton 1976). These symptoms indicate that the so-called shock organs frequently involved are the skin, respiratory organs, and the gastrointestinal tract.

The central nervous system and the eyes are also usually affected. However, almost all body tissues may be affected (Perlman 1964).

An allergic reaction may be immediate or delayed. The immediate symptoms may be quite violent and may cause death from shock and spasm of bronchiole muscles. This type is observed in anaphylactic reactions. In this case, the subject is hypersensitized from prior exposure to an antigen. In penicillin anaphylaxis, a patient may be hypersensitized to penicillin from previous consumption of bread infected by molds of the genus Penicillium. However, symptoms of anaphylaxis may be mild, occurring in the form of slight fever, erythema, itching, and urticaria.

It has been demonstrated that certain cases of the sudden death syndrome (SDS) in infants may be caused by an allergy to cow's milk (Parish et al. 1960). It has been shown that infants may have antibodies to cow's milk at moderate levels. When 0.25 ml cow's milk or the stomach content of SDS victims was introduced into the trachea of guinea pigs sensitized to cow's milk, these animals also died suddenly. Thus, it has been postulated that death was due to anaphylaxis from the lungs following regurgitation and aspiration of the stomach content into the lung during sleep.

In delayed allergic reaction, the symptoms may not be observed for several hours or a few days. Such is the case with mango dermatitis and other types of anacardiaceous dermatitis. In many cases, the delayed appearance of symptoms makes identification of the allergenic substance difficult.

Allergenicity is an overreaction of the tissues to foreign proteins or conjugates of exogenous or endogenous proteins and nonproteins known as haptens. The protein or the protein-nonprotein conjugate is called the antigen or allergen. The body attempts to neutralize or eliminate the allergen by conjugating or binding with antibodies.

The humoral antibodies associated with skin reactions are called skin sensitizing or reaginic antibodies, or simply reagins. These are thermolabile proteins and may remain for many years, even throughout a lifespan. On the other hand, the humoral antibodies responsible for anaphylaxis lasts for only a few weeks. They are also thermolabile (Perlman 1964).

The antibodies associated with delayed hypersensitivity reactions are noncirculating cellular antibodies. These are the antibodies associated with homograph rejection or the tuberculin reaction. It has been postulated that these antibodies may be dislodged from the cells and become free, circulating antibodies (Perlman 1964).

Prolonged exposure to an allergenic substance may enhance sensitization instead of desensitization. On the other hand, sensitive persons may "outgrow" their allergy by abstention from offending foods. This has been clearly demonstrated in a patient who was allergic to eggs but lost his sensitivity to this food by abstention for several years. This patient became sensitive again and developed severe urticaria following repeated administration of large amounts of eggs by stomach tube (Perlman 1964).

Allergens are generally high molecular weight proteins which contain specific reactive groups. One such group may be the sulfhydryl group. Thus, a nonallergenic gelatin is devoid of cysteine or cystine. Low molecular weight organic compounds (haptens) may derive their allergenicity from their binding with endogenous proteins, causing changes in their structures so as to become "foreign" proteins subject to antibody attack. This concept explains in part the allergenicity of many low molecular weight compounds. Examples of such haptens are nordihydroguaiuretic acid, a food antioxidant (Griepentrog 1961), and chlorogenic acid, from green coffee and other sources (Freedman et al. 1962). Examples of allergenic low molecular weight compounds are certain pesticides, food additives, and many plant metabolites.

The allergenicity of food proteins must be predicated with the assumption that these food proteins escape digestion and are absorbed. That this can occur has been, in fact, demonstrated by Walzer (1927); thus, the high incidence of food allergy among children is a consequence of the greater permeability of the intestinal mucosa to proteins and the incomplete development of digestive processes in this population group (Strauss 1964).

The most common allergenic food products are also proteinaceous food. These include cow's and human milk, eggs, seafood, chicken, pork, and beef. However, several others are frequent offenders: wheat, nuts, chocolate, corn, other cereals except rice, strawberries, tomatoes, legumes, potatoes, mustard, cucumbers, squash, melons, watermelon, citrus fruits, garlic, and cottonseed (Burton 1976). Note that much of this food is not high in protein. It should be emphasized that a cross-reaction can occur, not only within a botanical family but also between families. This suggests that similar antigens are found in these families.

 Since many nonprotein substances can induce allergic reactions, possibly contaminants are responsible for the toxic properties of some food. For example, dates and figs become allergenic when fumigated with methyl bromide. In addition, peaches untreated with pesticides are nonallergenic but are not tolerated by patients when so treated (Randolph et al. 1950).

The fact that allergenicity is manifested in cooked food suggests that antigenic substances may be thermostable (Malkin and Markow 1939; Saperstein and Anderson 1962). This should be expected for the low molecular weight substances. However, for some protein antigens, there is evidence that heat denaturation can abolish or diminish allergenicity (Saperstein and Anderson 1962). In others, such as casein, cooking does not eliminate allergenicity.

MUTAGENICITY

As discussed in Chapter 1, one of the fundamental biochemical mechanisms underlying toxic injury is interference in DNA (deoxyribonucleic acid) or RNA (ribonucleic acid) function. Toxicants can interfere directly by chemical reaction with any of the several reactive groups present in DNA or RNA purine and pyrimidine bases and phosphate groups (e.g., $-NH_2$, $-NH-$, $-N=$, $-\overset{\overset{O}{\|}}{C}-$, $-OH$, $-CH_3$). Indirectly, these substances can interfere by inhibiting specific enzymes involved in DNA and RNA synthesis, or by obstructing the synthesis of enzymes not involved in DNA or RNA formation. Interference in the availability of nutrients and necessary hormonal factors may also lead to an aberration in DNA or RNA synthesis and function.

Types of Mutations

In general, chemical interference in cellular function can lead to mutation, especially when the compounds react directly with DNA. Mutation is defined as a hereditable change or changes in the gene or chromosome, resulting in a deviation of specific phenotypic makeup of the progeny. From the standpoint of the DNA or chromosomes, several types of mutations exist (Rohrborn 1970).

Point Mutation

In a strict sense, point mutation is an alteration of a specific locus on the DNA double helix (Vogel 1970). It consists of base pair exchanges on DNA; i.e., the so-called (1) transitions — substitution of a purine with another purine, or pyrimidine with another pyrimidine, and vice versa; (2) deletions or insertions of single bases; (3) all other changes in DNA which are not manifested as microscopically visible changes.

Without knowing the actual base or codon sequences, point mutation may be suspected or possibly identified by the number of functions or proteins altered owing to changes in amino acid sequence of a specific protein. For example, several variants in the hemoglobin amino acid sequence in humans have been identified as an alteration in a single amino acid. Thus, in sickle cell anemia, the β-chain of hemoglobin has valine substituted for glutamic acid. Indeed, about 100 hemoglobin variants in humans have been identified (Lehmann and Carrell 1969; Vogel 1969).

Chromosome Mutation

Chromosome mutation consists of any structural changes involving the loss or reorganization of chromosomal segments. These changes may be intrachromosomal, such as segmental deletions and inversions, or interchromosomal, such as duplications or translocations. The latter changes also may be intrachromosomal. Deletion consists of absence of terminal or intercalary segments of the chromosomes. Duplication consists of the presence of several identical genes within the genome. In chromosome inversion, a segment is inverted and replaced in its original location; in translocation, a chromosome segment is displaced either within the same chromosomes or to other chromosomes.

Genome Mutation

Genome mutation consists of a change in ploidy, or the number of chromosomes per cell. These changes can result in polyploidy, in which more than one set of chromosomes is present, or in aneuploidy, in which there are either missing or extra chromosomes in a set. However, the extra chromosomes are not sufficient to make an entire additional set of chromosomes. An example of an aneuploid condition with an extra chromosome is trisomy in mongolism.

Mutation can occur in both somatic and germinal cells. However, because of the transmissibility of the mutated traits to several generations, deleterious mutations in the germinal cells have far-reaching implications to future generations. In these cases, based on present knowledge, a cure for an inherited disease is impossible. Of course, germinal mutation may be lethal to the cell; in which case, hereditary transmission of a deleterious mutation is averted.

Somatic mutation, on the other hand, cannot be transmitted and the mutated cells die with the host. It is theorized that somatic mutation is an underlying mechanism in carcinogenesis.

Mutagenic Agents

The human population is exposed to many chemical mutagens present in food, drugs, and the environment (Barthelmess 1970). Most of these chemical mutagens can be grouped into seven general chemical classes of compounds (Freese 1971): (1) alkylating agents, (2) free radical-forming agents, (3) purine and pyrimidine analogs, (4) oxidizing agents, (5) DNA synthesis inhibitors, (6) intercalating agents, and (7) metals. Alkylating agents, free radical-forming agents, oxidizing agents, and metals are widespread in food. The other classes have more or less limited distribution.

Alkylating Agents

The alkylating agents are exemplified by various chemical carcinogens, most of which are metabolized to active forms. Examples are cycasin, nitrosamines, epoxides, which are the metabolic intermediates of the polycyclic aromatic hydrocarbons, reactive acetones (aflatoxin and other mycotoxins), and organic residues such as the pesticides endrin, dieldrin, ethylene dibromide, and Aramite.

An alkylating agent reacts readily with nucleophilic groups: amino, sulfhydryl, thio ester, and ionized acids. However, it is contended that their alkylation of phosphate groups and ring nitrogens in the purine and pyrimidine bases is the basis for their mutagenic effects. The N-7 position of guanine in double-stranded DNA, or the N-1 of adenine in single-stranded or denatured DNA, appears to be the principal target (Lawley and Brookes 1963). Following alkylation, guanine or adenine is hydrolyzed off, thus destabilizing the DNA backbone and breaking the macromolecule. Alkylation of phosphate groups also causes the DNA backbone to break (Rhaese and Freese 1969). Therefore, alkylating agents cause point mutations (mainly transitions), chromosome breaks, and chromosome mutations. These substances, therefore, are extremely toxic and have been implicated as teratogens and carcinogens.

Free Radical Formers

Free radical formation is the basis of the DNA alkylation reaction; thus, other forms of free radicals would be expected to cause DNA damage. Peroxides, aldehydes, phenols, and azo compounds are free radical formers that may be found in food. Peroxides and aldehydes may be derived substances from peroxidation of unsaturated fatty acids or other compounds. Peroxidation may also occur in animals (Tappel 1970). Phenols are abundant and endogenous in plant-derived food and are metabolites in animal-derived food. The toxic azo compounds are exemplified in food colors, cycasin in cycad nuts, hydrazine in certain species of mushrooms, and the herbicide maleic hydrazide.

Free radical formation can be catalyzed by the transition metals Fe^{2+}, Fe^{3+}, and Cu^{2+}. Free radicals can damage DNA directly and indirectly. The direct reaction is probably remote because this is possible only when the free radicals are formed adjacent to the DNA (Freese 1971) and protective mechanisms cannot interfere (e.g., catalase and peroxidases, tocopherols, and other free radical "traps" or scavengers). Indirect damage is more likely because of less interference. It can occur following formation of reactive compounds. Free radicals can react with each other and produce reactive compounds that then can diffuse to DNA and react with reactive groups.

Free radical formation in the body is dependent on oxygen, and thus is affected by reducing agents which can either diminish or enhance the process — weak reducing agents, such as cysteine, suppress free radical formation; strong ones, such as ascorbic acid, enhance it (Freese 1971).

Ionizing radiation, e.g., x-, α-, β-, and γ-rays, generally affect chromosomes by forming free radicals, but seldom by a direct hit. This is because the chromosomes are in an aqueous medium which shields against ionizing radiation. When the radiation hits a molecule, it could knock out a single electron or excite the molecule, which then decomposes into a free radical. The electron may be captured by a water molecule, which also becomes a free radical, the so-called "hydrated electron" (Sussman and Halvorson 1966).

The effect of x-rays is generally greater in the presence of oxygen. This is because peroxy radical $(R-OO)$ formation is catalyzed by x-rays. That is, hydroxyperoxy bases are formed, resulting in a breakdown of these bases or the DNA backbone (Freese 1971).

Similarly, ultraviolet (uv) light catalyzes the formation of free radicals. In the presence of uv light, hydroperoxides produce greater mutagenic effects in fruit flies of the genus Drosophila (Altenburg 1955). The photochemical decomposition of DNA in the presence of hydroperoxides has been reported (Butler and Conway 1953). The pyrimidine ring appears to be more easily affected than the purine ring.

Purine and Pyrimidine Analogs

Freeze (1959a,b; 1963) has experimentally verified, using bacterial systems, that certain types of bases that are not normal constituents of DNA and RNA can be incorporated into nucleic acids. Such an incorporation results in a transition error or point mutation; in other words, a substitution of an adenine—thymine pair for a guanine—cytosine pair happens in the next replication (Howard and Tessman 1964; Tessman et al. 1964).

These base analogs also cause chromatid and chromosome breakage (Dubinin and Soyfer 1969).

Thus, the purines, theophylline and theobromine (Barthelmess 1970), xanthines and especially caffeine have been shown to induce mutagenic effects in both bacterial and human cells in vitro (Novick 1956; Wragg et al. 1967). However, by the dominant lethal assay in which fetal deaths or preimplantation losses have been determined in female mice mated with caffeine-treated males, caffeine failed to induce mutagenic effects or to synergize the effects of known mutagens (Epstein 1970). However, in the same experiments, the incidence of pregancy was definitely reduced even though there

was no consistency over dose. Further discussion on the potential mutagenicity of caffeine can be found in Chapter 8.

Oxidizing Agents

The most notable oxidizing agent to cause mutation is nitrous acid. This compound can
deaminate cytosine to uracil, adenine to hypoxanthine, and guanine to xanthine.
These deaminations are mutagenic, resulting in base-pair transitions. Xanthine cannot pair with either thymine or cytosine, and this inability to pair bases inactivates
the DNA (Freese 1971).

The mutagenicity of nitrites and their nitrate precursors is especially relevant
because of their prevalence in food. Results showing their potential carcinogenicity in
animals suggest that nitrites may be mutagenic even in vivo.

Other mutagenic oxidizing agents, the peroxides, are discussed in connection with
free radical formation.

DNA Synthesis Inhibitors

DNA synthesis inhibitors are compounds which antagonize the incorporation of specific
groups into DNA. Most noteworthy are the folic and glutamic acid antagonists used in
cancer chemotherapy. In foodstuffs, similar antagonists are rare. Antifolacins are discussed in Chapter 9.

DNA Intercalating Agents

Intercalators may cause frameshift point mutations, which are deletions or insertions
of one or more bases (Freese 1971).

Metals

Some heavy metals, such as Co, Ni, Cr, Zn (Glass 1956), Mn (Orgel and Orgel 1965),
and mercurials (Ramel 1969) can produce mutations in DNA. The mechanism of their
effects is not known, although some of these may catalyze free radical formation from
peroxides (Freese 1971).

The preceding discussion indicates that there are a large number of potential
mutagens, both natural and man-made, that may be found in food. Their identification
and evaluation is of urgent importance because it is assumed that genetic alteration by
chemicals is always harmful.

Significance of Mutagenesis

Undoubtedly, mutations in the germ cells may lead to cell death. If not, the abnormal
cell may replicate and create deleterious effects in the progeny. Cell death early in
the differentiation process may result in teratogenic effects (see next section). Repli-
cated mutated cells may produce abnormal fetal development, resulting in abortion,
stillbirth, or teratogenic defects. The mutagenic effects, expressed as inborn errors
of metabolism, may be delayed in their appearance, until puberty or adulthood.

Somatic mutation in the fetus may lead to teratogenic effects and cancer.
Warburton and Fraser (1964) reported that in their study, at least 15% of all con-
ceptions were spontaneously aborted. Also, in a study by Mellin (1963), 7% of full-
term children exhibited congenital malformations. In a report by Stevenson et al.
(1966), of 426,932 infants born after the week 27, the rates of major and minor malformations were 12.7 and 4.6 per 1000, respectively. These incidences obviously did
not reflect anomalies that were not immediately apparent (e.g., allergy predisposition,
immunological abnormalities, subtle muscular and skeletal abnormalities, and other
somatic defects, not to mention those that do not develop until later in life.) Therefore, higher incidences must be assumed. It also has been reported that among spontaneously aborted babies, 20% had visible chromosome defects (Carr 1967; World

Health Organization 1966). Again, the frequency of genetic abnormalities in this case must be assumed to be much higher because the incidence of point mutation is usually much higher (Freese 1971). To what extent these effects are due to toxicants in food and the environment is not known.

TERATOGENIC EFFECTS

A teratogen is a compound that causes malformation in an unborn animal or human. The teratogen may be a chemical, physical, nutritional, or hormonal factor. These factors may initiate teratogenic effects in two ways: (1) through gene or chromosome mutation in germinal cells, and (2) through alterations or interference with the normal processes of the developing embryo (Kalter 1971). As stated in the preceding section, nonlethal gene or chromosome mutations are hereditary, and therefore malformation initiated in this manner may become a permanent feature of succeeding progenies. Teratogenic changes occurring during embryonic differentiation and organogenesis are, of course, nontransmissible.

Becker (1975) states that no teratogenic effects can occur after the end of organogenesis. Chemical teratogens can initiate these changes only during the formation of tissues, cells, and physiological and biochemical systems. This conclusion is based on the observation that no major congenital malformation is evident after the completion of organogenesis, especially the last trimester of intrauterine life. Therefore, this phase of gestation is considered immune from teratogenic effects, and in the past has been ignored by teratologists (Langman et al. 1975). However, in recent years, the effect of teratogens during this period is gradually being appreciated. Teratogens can, in fact, cause damage even though gross malformations are not observed. During the late period of fetal development, teratogens may interfere with cellular proliferation; cellular differentiation and/or cell migration may also be adversely affected so that minute cell anomalies and dystopia, respectively, may occur. These defects may only be recognized by the appearance of functional abnormalities after birth (Langman et al. 1975).

The central nervous system is particularly vulnerable to the effects of teratogens because its development continues throughout gestation. Certain regions of the CNS continuously show marked cellular proliferation even up to shortly before birth. Cellular migration and neuronal differentiation continue to occur throughout the late stages of prenatal life. The effects of teratogens on these cells may not be morphologically discernible, but they may be manifested as behavioral abnormalities after birth.

Abnormalities caused by teratogenic action late in fetal life may also be reflected by functional deficiencies in the endocrine, immunological, hematopoietic, and other systems (Langman et al. 1975).

Fetal death is not always associated with teratogenic effects (Becker 1975; Kalter 1971). Such deaths may be due to toxic effects other than teratogenesis.

There is evidence of a genetic susceptibility to teratogenic effects (Carter 1965, 1969; Edwards 1969). It was hypothesized that the combined effects of several genes produce a condition whereby teratogens are more effective, and that a genetic predisposition to teratogens, statistically speaking, is normally distributed in the human population. As observed in humans (Fraser and Pashayan 1970) and in mice (Trasler 1968), the facial shape, which is genetically determined, appears to have some influence on cleft palate formation.

Teratogenic effects include not only physical or anatomical defects but also biochemical, physiological, organic and mental defects. The latter may be expressed as behavioral defects (Barlow and Sullivan 1975). External anatomical defects are easily discernible at birth, but other types may not be so readily apparent, unless some functional disturbance becomes evident. Mental and behavioral defects may not become evident until the individual reaches adolescence. Certain types of tissue anomalies may not be evident without tissue dissection.

Factors Affecting the Teratogenicity of Compounds

Aside from the nature of the compound, other factors influence chemical teratogenesis. These are (1) the dose and duration of exposure; (2) maternal and fetal regulatory factors; (3) transport and access to the developing embryo (4) time of exposure during embryonal development; and (5) individual susceptibility.

Dose and Duration of Treatment

The existence of a teratogenic threshold or no effect level is accepted by most teratologists (Wilson 1974, 1973). Such a threshold is probably valid in the case of embryonic developmental teratogenesis because of the regulatory factors present in the mother and embryo. However, as in carcinogenesis, one may question the presence of such a threshold in mutagenic teratogenesis. Experimentally at least, the presence of such a threshold may be difficult to validate with the small number of experimental animals used.

Animal experiments have shown that a single dose of a teratogen is more effective in inducing teratogenic changes than multiple exposures (King et al. 1965; Robens 1969). A possible explanation for this observation is that the effective dose is probably decreased because repeated exposures may induce specific metabolic enzymes. This reduction is probably attained during the critical period in the development of the embryo.

However, repeated exposure may cause liver and kidney damage, so that metabolic detoxication and excretion of the compound or its metabolites may be inhibited.

Maternal and Fetal Regulatory Factors

The ultimate concentration of a teratogen reaching the target embryonic tissue or cells obviously will be a function of the physiological mechanisms which tend to reduce this concentration. Thus, the rates of absorption in the gastrointestinal tract, excretion in the urine and bile, protein binding, and tissue storage (e.g., adipose tissue) are factors that tend to dissipate the concentration of a teratogen before reaching the embryo (Wilson 1973). Furthermore, the maternal and fetal metabolic processes (Rane et al. 1973a), including the placenta (Juchau et al. 1973a,b; Kyegombe and Franklin 1973), may diminish the dose of a teratogen reaching target embryonic tissues. However, it must be recognized that such metabolic transformations may produce more toxic substances than their precursors, as discussed in Chapter 4. Furthermore, the capacity of fetal tissues for detoxication is quite limited (Rane et al. 1973b). Therefore, the initial dose entering the maternal bloodstream and the effectiveness of the metabolic processes of the mother to detoxify the teratogen will determine to a large extent the occurrence of teratogenic injury.

Transport and Access to the Developing Embryo

The concentration of a substance reaching the embryo is regulated by the placenta. The mechanics of simple diffusion, as discussed for the GI tract, also operate in this case. Thus, the concentrations of many substances in the fetal fluids and tissues may be lower than those in the maternal plasma (Idänpään-Heikkilä et al. 1971; Nishimura 1973). However, as in the rat, there are instances in which the opposite is true (Dagg et al. 1966; Scott et al. 1971). Therefore, the placenta, which was once considered being an effective barrier to many toxic substances, does not in fact exclude many types of toxicants (Adamson 1965; Horning et al. 1973; Mirkin 1973). Nevertheless, this tissue does bar certain compounds, such as molecules with molecular weights greater than 600 and those that are highly polar (Wilson 1973). These compounds traverse the placenta at a slower rate, so that dispersal mechanisms in the maternal body have adequate time to decrease the amount of toxic material crossing the placenta.

Time of Exposure During Fetal Development

Embryonic tissues and organs develop at varying rates, and thus, at different times. It follows that the timing of exposure to a teratogen will have a critical influence in the development of malformation. In humans, susceptibility to teratogenic effects appears to be highest between day 17 and day 50 following fertilization, after which susceptibility gradually diminishes (Wilson 1973). Thus, in the case of the thalidomide teratogenesis, malformations (phocomelia) occurred when the drug was administered between days 35 and 50 of pregnancy. No malformations occurred outside this period (Lenz 1962; Taussig 1962). Experiments in rats with overdoses of retinol have shown that different developing tissues may be affected by exposure at different times during the critical period. Thus, when 15,000 IU/kg were given to rats on day 8 of gestation, skeletal malformation occurred; when given on day 12, cleft palate resulted (Becker 1975). The time of exposure may be very critical, so that even a difference of half a day of exposure time may produce marked differences in the type of fetal damage. For example, when lead nitrate at 25 mg/kg was injected iv into rats on day 9.5 of gestation, malformations were confined to the posterior parts of the fetus; on day 10, fetal death was observed. This was explained by the presence of a functioning fetal circulation which encompassed the entire fetal body by day 10; thus, lead was distributed throughout the body. The general circulation is not fully developed even until day 9.5 of gestation; only the vitelline vessels serve the posterior position of the embryo up to this period (Gibson and Becker 1968).

When proliferation and differentiation of tissues and organs are virtually completed, exposure to teratogens may have little effect on the occurrence of gross malformation or embryonic death. At this period of development, toxic compounds may produce growth and functional retardation. However, high dosages may still cause malformations (Wilson 1974).

In the case of the human brain, the effects of teratogens may extend beyond birth because this organ continues to develop throughout infancy and childhood. Maximum brain growth occurs around the seventh and eighth month of gestation and continues up to the fifth month after birth (Dobbing 1974). Thus, the brain is much more vulnerable to toxic effects throughout the gestation period and even postnatally compared to other organs. Such effects may manifest in degenerative neurological disorders, cerebral palsy (Miller 1974), abnormal motor development (Brazelton 1970), and behavioral and learning anomalies (Butcher et al. 1972; Desmond et al. 1969). An example of a substance causing damage to fetal and neonatal brains of rodents and primates is monosodium glutamate (Nagasawa et al. 1974; Olney and Sharpe 1969).

Individual Susceptibility

A fetus may inherit anatomical, physioloical, and biochemical characters which predispose it to teratogenic effects. For example, the absence of critical detoxication enzymes, such as conjugases, may prevent effective elimination of a teratogen. Another genetic characteristic, the shape of the face, may predispose one to certain facial abnormalities, e.g., cleft palate. The so-called polygenic or multifactorial inheritance may provide the necessary characteristics which increase the predisposition toward a specific toxin-induced teratogenic defect (Carter 1969; Edwards 1969; Falconer 1967).

Teratogenic Compounds

Many teratogenic compounds are also carcinogenic. These include aflatoxins, the aminoazobenzenes, 3,4-benzopyrene, cycasin, CCl_4, pyrrolizidine alkaloids, podophyllotoxin, caffeine (Connors 1975), methylmercury (Miller 1974; Spyker et al. 1972),

2,4,5-tricholorophenoxyacetic acid (2,4,5-T) (Sjoden and Soderberg 1972), ethylene
thiourea, a decomposition product of the fungicide bisdithiocarbamate, retinol (Hale
1937; Warkany and Schraffenberger 1946), and cholecalciferol. The latter is, of
course, a known human teratogen (Becker 1975). Retinol teratogenicity has been
demonstrated in pigs (Hale 1937). Methylmercury is teratogenic in humans; this toxicant has been implicated in the occurrence of cerebral palsy among children whose
mothers ingested mercury-contaminated fish (Miller 1974). The powerful carcinogens
such as aflatoxin (Elis and DiPaolo 1967) and cycasin (Spatz et al. 1967) produce CNS
abnormalities in guinea pigs in addition to other defects. Caffeine produces limb and
palate abnormalities in rodents (Nishimura and Nakai 1960). In the case of 2,4,5,-T,
the factor responsible for its teratogenic effects is its contaminant, the dioxins.

It may be safely stated that mutagens and/or carcinogens may also be considered
as potential teratogens (Connors 1975).

CARCINOGENIC EFFECTS

Carcinogenic effects are probably most commonly associated with food toxicants. Already, many food toxicants have been strongly implicated as human carcinogens (e.g.,
aflatoxin, cycasin, 3,4-benzopyrene). Others are so potent, producing tumors in many
animal tissues, that many consider them to be also human carcinogens; e.g., the
nitrosamines.

Because of their broad food toxicological, public health, and social implications,
the subject of carcinogenic effects of food toxicants is discussed separately in Chapters 6 and 7.

MISCELLANEOUS TOXIC EFFECTS

No doubt many other toxic effects can be induced by food toxicants. These other effects involve other parts of the endocrine system (e.g., thyroids, adrenals, pancreas); the skin and other sensory organs, the heart and blood vessels, and the
gastrointestinal tract.

The latter deserves special mention here, for indeed, these are the organs that
are first affected by food toxicants. Bacterial toxins induce abdominal pain and massive, sometimes bloody, painful diarrhea; ulcerogenic compounds (e.g., capsicums);
gossypol, and lectins interfere in the absorption of nutrients in the GI mucosa. Other
gastrointerotoxic effects in connection with specific food toxicants will be discussed in
succeeding chapters.

Phototoxicity is another important toxic manifestation that may be associated with
food toxicants. Toxicants possessing photodynamic activity can be found in both
animal- and plant-derived foodstuffs. The phototoxic reaction may manifest in the form
of dermal lesions and skin cancers.

REFERENCES

Adamson, K. 1965. *Symposium on the Placenta*. D. Bergsma (ed.). National Founda-
    tion — March of Dimes 1: 27–34.
Alexander, C. S. 1969. Cobalt and the heart. *Ann. Intern. Med.* 79: 411.
Altenburg, L. S. 1955. The synergism between ultraviolet light and tertrarybutyl
    hydroperoxide in their mutagenic effectiveness in *Drosophilia*. *Proc. Natl. Acad.
    Sci. U.S.A.* 41: 624–628.
Anon. 1968. Epidemic cardiac failure in beer drinkers. *Nutr. Rev.* 26: 173.

Barlow, S. M. and Sullivan, F. M. 1975. Behavioral teratology. In: *Teratology Trends and Applications*. C.L. Berry and D.E. Poswillo (eds.), Springer-Verlag, New York.

Barthelmess, A. 1970. Mutagenic substances in the human environment. In: *Chemical Mutagenesis in Mammals and Man*. F. Vogel (ed.), Springer-Verlag, New York.

Becker, B. A. 1975. Teratogens. In: *Toxicology. The Basic Science of Poisons*. L.J. Casarett and J. Doull (eds.). Macmillan, New York.

Brazelton, T. B. 1970. Effect of prenatal drugs on the behavior of the neonate. *Am. J. Psychiatry* 126: 1261–1266.

Budy, A. 1975. Toxicology of the skeletal system. In: *Toxicology — The Basic Science of Poisons*. L.J. Casarette and J. Doull (eds.). Macmillan, New York.

Burton, B. T. 1976. *Human Nutrition*. McGraw-Hill, New York.

Butcher, R. E., Brunner, R. L., Roth, T. and Kimmel, C. A. 1972. A learning impairment associated with maternal hypervitaminosis-A in rats. *Life Sci.* 11: 141–145.

Butler, J. A. V. and Conway, B. E. 1953. The action of photochemically generated radicals from hydrogen peroxide on deoxyribonucleic acid and model substances. *Proc. R. Soc. Lond. (Biol).* 141: 562–580.

Carr, D. H. 1967. Chromosome anomalies as a cause of spontaneous abortion. *Am. J. Obstet. Gynecol.* 97: 283–293.

Carter, C. O. 1965. The inheritance of common congenital malformations. *Prog. Med. Genet.* 4: 59–84.

Carter, C. O. 1969. Genetics of common disorders. *Br. Med. Bull.* 25: 52–57.

Chapman, L. F. and Wolff, H. G. 1959. The cerebral hemispheres and the highest integrative functions of man. *Arch. Neurol.* 1: 357–424.

Chisholm, J. J. and Kaplan, E. 1968. Lead poisoning in childhood — Comprehensive management and prevention. *J. Pediatr.* 73: 942–950.

Connors, T. A. 1975. Cytotoxic agents in teratogenic research. In: *Teratology. Trends and Applications*. C.L. Berry and D.E. Poswillo (eds.). Springer-Verlag, New York.

Cummings, J. M. and Earl, C. J. 1960. Caeruloplasmin as demonstrated by starch gel electrophoresis. *J. Clin. Pathol.* 13: 69–71.

Curie, G. N., Black, D. L., Armstrong, D. T. and Greep, R. O. 1969. Blockade of ovulation in the rabbit with catecholamines and sympathomimetics. *Proc. Soc. Exp. Biol. Med.* 130: 598–602.

Dagg, C. P., Schlager, G. and Doerr, A. 1966. Polygenic control of teratogenicity of 5-fluorouracil in mice. *Genetics* 53: 1101–1117.

Desmond, M. M. et al. 1969. Behavioural alterations in infants born to mothers in psychoactive medication during pregnancy. In: *Congenital Mental Retardation*. G. Farrell (ed.). University of Texas Press, Austin.

Dianzani, M. U. 1963. Lysosome changes in liver injury. In: *Ciba Foundation Symposium on Lysosomes*. A.V.S. deReuck and M.P. Cameron (eds.). Little Brown, Boston.

Diczfalusy, E. 1969. Mode of action of contraceptive drugs. *Am. J. Obstet. Gynecol.* 100: 136–161.

Dobbing, J. 1974. Later development of the brain and its vulnerability. In: *Scientific Foundations of Paediatrics*. J.A. Davis and J. Dobbing (eds.). Heinemann, London.

Dubinin, N. P. and Soyfer, V. N. 1969. Chromosome breakage and complete gene mutation production in molecular terms. *Mutat. Res.* 8: 353–365.

Edwards, J. H. 1969. Familial predisposition in man. *Br. Med. Bull.* 25: 58–64.

Elis, J. and DiPaolo, J. A. 1967. Aflatoxin B_1. Induction of malformations. *Arch. Pathol.* 83: 53–57.

Emmelot, P. and Benedetti, E. L. 1960. Changes in the fine structure of rat liver brought about by dimethylnitrosamine. *J. Biophys. Biochem. Cytol.* 7: 393–396.

Emmens, E. W. 1970. Antifertility agents. *Annu. Rev. Pharmacol.* 10:   237—254.

Epstein, S. 1970. The failure of caffeine to induce mutagenic effects or to synergize the effects of known mutagens in mice. In: *Chemical Mutagenesis in Mammals and Man.* I. Vogel and G. Rohrborn (eds.). Springer-Verlag, New York.

Evans, R. O. et al. 1969. Radiogenic tumors in the radium and mesothorium cases studied at M.I.T. In: *Delayed Effects of Bone-seeking Radionuclides.* C.W. Mays et al. (eds.). University of Utah Press, Salt Lake City.

Falconer, D. S. 1967. The inheritance of liability to diseases with variable age of onset with particular reference to diabetes mellitus. *Ann. Hum. Genet.* 31: 1—20.

Finkel, A. J., Miller, C. E. and Hasterlik, R. J. 1969. Radium-induced malignant tumors in man. In: *Delayed Effects of Bone-seeking Radionuclides.* C.W. Mays et al. (eds.). University of Utah Press, Salt Lake City.

Foulkes, E. C. 1963. Kinetics of p-aminohippurate secretion in rabbits. *Am. J. Physiol.* 205: 1019—1024.

Foulkes, E. C. and Hammond, P. B. 1975. Toxicology of the kidney. In: *Toxicology — The Basic Science of Poisons.* L.J. Casarett and J. Doull (eds.). Macmillan, New York.

Fraser, F. C. and Pashayan, H. 1970. Relation of face shape to susceptibility to congenital cleft lip. *J. Med. Genet.* 7: 112—117.

Freedman, S. O., Krupey, J. and Schon, A. H. 1961. Chlorogenic acid: An allergen in green coffee bean. *Nature* 192: 241—243.

Freese, E. 1959a. The specific mutagenic effect of base analogues on phage T-4. *J. Mol. Biol.* 1: 87—105.

Freese, E. 1959b. The difference between spontaneous and base-analogue induced mutations of phage T4. *Proc. Natl. Acad. Sci. U.S.A.* 45: 622—633.

Freese, E. 1963. Molecular mechanisms of mutations. In: *Molecular Genetics.* J.H. Taylor, (ed.). Academic Press, New York.

Freese, E. 1971. Molecular mechanisms of mutations. In: *Chemical Mutagens. Principles and Methods for their Detection.* Vol. 1. A. Hollaender (ed.). Plenum Press, New York.

Gibson, J. E. and Becker, B. A. 1968. The teratogenicity of cyclophosphamide in mice. *Cancer Res.* 28: 475—480.

Glass, E. 1956. The distribution of breaks and achromatic regions in the chromosomes of Vicia faba after treatment with heavy metal salts. *Chromosoma* 8: 260—284.

Goldman, M. and Bustad, L. K. (eds.). 1972. *Biomedical Implications and Radiostrontium Exposure.* AEC Symp. Ser. 25, Atomic Energy Commission, Office of Information Services, Springfield, Virginia.

Goyer, R. A. and Mushak, P. 1977. Lead toxicity. Laboratory aspects. In: *Toxicology of Trace Elements.* R.A. Goyer and M.A. Mehlman (eds.). Hemisphere, Washington, D.C.

Grant, W. C. and Root, W. S. 1952. Fundamental stimulus for erythropoiesis. *Physiol. Rev.* 32: 449—498.

Griepentrog, F. 1961. Allergy studies with simple chemical compounds. VII. Nordihydroguairetic acid. *Arzneimittelforsch.* 11: 920—922.

Grinvalsky, H. T. and Fitch, D. M. 1969. A distinctive myocardiopathy occurring in Omaha, Nebraska. Pathological aspects. *Ann. N.Y. Acad. Sci.* 156: 544—565.

Gunn, S. A., Gould, T. C. and Anderson, W. A. D. 1970. Maintenance of structure and function of the cauda epididymis and contained spermatozoa by testosterone following cadmium-induced testicular necrosis in the rat. *J. Reprod. Fertil.* 24: 443—448.

Haeger-Aronsen, B. 1960. Studies on urinary excretion of δ-aminolaevulinic acid and other haem precursors in lead workers and in lead-intoxicated rabbits. *Scand. J. Clin. Lab. Invest.* (Suppl. 47) 12: 1—128.

Hale, F. 1937. The relation of maternal vitamin A deficiency to microophthalmia in pigs. *Tex. J. Med.* 33: 288.

Harris, J. W. and Kellermeyer, R. W. 1970. *The Red Cell, Production, Metabolism, Destruction: Normal and Abnormal.* Rev. ed. Harvard University Press, Cambridge, Massachusetts.

Hennig, A. and Anke, M. 1964. Cadmium; an antimetabolite of iron and zinc. *Arch. Tierernaehr.* 14: 55–57.

Horning, M. G. et al. 1973. In: *Fetal Pharmacology.* L.O. Boreus (ed.). Raven Press, New York.

Howard, B. D. and Tessman, J. 1964. Identification of the altered bases in mutated single-stranded DNA. II. In vivo mutagenesis by 5-bromodeoxyuridine and 2-aminopurine. *J. Mol. Biol.* 9: 364–371.

Idäpään-Heikkilä, J. E., Jouppila, J. E., Poulakka, J. O. and Vorne, M. S. 1971. A placental transfer and fetal metabolism of diazepam in early human pregnancy. *Am. J. Obstet. Gynecol.* 109: 1011–1016.

Itokawa, Y., Abe, T. and Tanaka, S. 1973. Bone changes in experimental chronic cadmium poisoning: Radiological and biological approaches. *Arch. Environ. Health* 26: 241–244.

Itokawa, Y., Abe, T., Tabei, R. and Tanaka, S. 1974. Renal and skeletal lesions in experimental cadmium poisoning. *Environ. Health* 28: 149–154.

Jackson, M. and Schnieden, A. 1968. Pharmacology of reproduction and fertility. *Annu. Rev. Pharmacol.* 8: 467–490.

Joshi, S. R. et al. 1970. Fertilization and early embryonic development subsequent to mating with TEPA (triethylene phosphoramide)-treated male mice. *Genetics* 65: 483–494.

Juchau, M. R., Pedersen, M. G., Fantal, A. G. and Shepard, T. H. 1973a. Drug metabolism by placenta. *Clin. Pharmacol. Ther.* 14: 673–679.

Juchau, M. R. et al. 1973b. Oxidation and reduction of foreign compounds in the human placenta and fetus. In: *Fetal Pharmacology.* L. Boreus (ed.). Raven Press, New York.

Kalter, H. 1971. Correlation between teratogenic and mutagenic effects of chemicals in mammals. In: *Chemical Mutagens. Principles and Methods for their Detection.* A. Hollaender, (ed.), Plenum Press, New York.

Kessler, P. H., Hierholzer, K., Gurb, R. S. and Pitts, R. F. 1959. Localization of action of chlorothiazide in the nephrone of the dog. *Am. J. Physiol.* 196: 1346–1351.

King, C. T. G., Weaver, S. A. and Narrod, S. A. 1965. Antihistamines and teratogenicity in the rat. *J. Pharmacol. Exp. Ther.* 147: 391–398.

Kriz, W. and Lever, A. F. 1969. Renal counter current mechanisms: Structure and function. *Am. Heart J.* 78: 101–118.

Kyegombe, D. and Franklin C. 1973. Drug-metabolizing enzymes in the human placenta, their induction and repression. *Lancet* 1: 405–406.

Lacy, D. and Lofts, B. 1965. Studies on the structure and function of the mammalian testes. *Proc. R. Soc. Lond. (Biol.)* 162: 188–197.

Langman, J., Webster, W. and Rodier, P. 1975. Morphological and behavioral abnormalities caused by insults to the CNS in the perinatal period. In: *Teratology Trends and Applications.* C.L. Berry and D.E. Poswillo (eds.), Springer-Verlag, New York.

Larsson, S. E. and Piscator, M. 1971. Effect of cadmium on skeletal tissue in normal and calcium-deficient rats. *Isr. J. Med. Sci.* 7: 495–498.

Lawley, P. D. and Brookes, D. 1963. Further studies on the alkylation of nucleic acids and their constituent nucleotides. *Biochem. J.* 89: 127–138.

Lehmann, H. and Carrell, R. W. 1968. Differences between α- and β-chain mutants of human hemoglobin and between α- and β-thalassemia. Possible duplication of the α-chain gene. *Br. Med. J.* 4: 748–750.

Lehmann, H. and Carrell, R. W. 1969. Variations in the structure of human haemo-globin. *Br. Med. Bull.* 25: 14–23.

Lenz, W. 1962. Thalidomides and congenital abnormalities. *Lancet* 2: 1332.

Malkin, J. I. and Markow, H. 1939. Analysis of the comparative results of skin testing with cooked and uncooked foods. *J. Allergy* 10: 337–341.

Marx, J. L. 1980. Osteoporosis: New help for thinning bones. *Science* 207: 628–630.

McClellan, R. O. and Jones, R. K. 1969. Sr-induced neoplasia: A selective review. In: *Delayed Effects of Bone-Seeking Radionuclides.* C. W. Mays et al. (eds.). University of Utah Press, Salt Lake City.

McCurdy, D. K., Frederick, M. and Elkinton, J. R. 1968. Renal tubular acidosis due to amphotericin B. *N. Engl. J. Med.* 278: 124–131.

McLean, A. E. M. 1970. The effect of protein deficiency and microsomal enzyme in-duction by DDT and phenobarbitone on the acute toxicity of chloroform and pyrrolizidine alkaloid, retrorsine. *Br. J. Exp. Pathol.* 51: 317–321.

McLean, F. C. and Budy, A. M. 1964. *Radiation, Isotopes, and Bone.* Academic Press, New York.

Mellin, G. W. 1963. The frequency of birth defects. In: *Birth Defects.* M. Fishbein (ed.). Lippincott, Philadelphia.

Miller, R. W. 1974. How environmental effects in child health are recognized. *Pediatrics* 53: 792–796.

Mirkin, B. L. 1973. Maternal and fetal distribution of drugs in pregnancy. *Clin. Pharmacol. Ther.* 14: 643–647.

Nagasawa, H. Yanai, R and Kikuyama, S. 1974. Irreversible inhibition of pituitary prolactin and growth hormone secretion and of mammary gland development in mice by monosodium glutamate administered neonatally. *Acta Endocrinal.* (Copen-hagen) 75: 249–259.

Nishimura, H. 1973. Comparative study on maternal embryonic transfer of drugs in man and laboratory animals. In: *Fetal Pharmacology.* L.O. Borens (ed.). Raven Press, New York.

Nishimura, H. and Nakai, K. 1960. Congenital malformations in offsprings treated with caffeine. *Proc. Soc. Exp. Biol.* 104: 140–142.

Nomiyama, K., Sato, C. and Yamamoto, A. 1973. Early signs of cadmium intoxication in rabbits. *Toxicol. Appl. Pharmacol.* 24: 625–635.

Norton, S. 1975. Toxicology of the central nervous system. In: *Toxicology — the Basic Science of Poisons.* L.J. Casarett and J. Doull (eds.). Macmillan, New York.

Novick, A. 1956. Mutagens and antimutagens. *Brookhaven Symp. Biol.* 8: 201.

Olney, J. W. and Sharpe, L. G. 1969. Brain lesions in an infant rhesus monkey treated with monosodium glutamate. *Science* 166: 386–388.

Orgel, A. and Orgel, L. E. 1965. Induction of mutations in bacteriophage T4 with divalent manganese. *J. Mol. Biol.* 14: 453–457.

Orten, J. M. and Neuhaus, O. W. 1975. *Human Biochemistry.* Mosby, St. Louis.

Oser, B. L. 1965. *Hawk's Physiological Chemistry.* 14th ed. McGraw-Hill, New York.

Parish, W. E., Barrett, A. M. and Coombs, R. R. A. 1960. Hypersensitivity to milk and sudden death in infancy. *Lancet* 2: 1106–1110.

Paufler, S. K. 1969. Effect of triethylenemelamine (TEM) and cadmium chloride on spermatogenesis in rabbits. *J. Reprod. Fertil.* 19: 309–319.

Peisach, J., Aisen, P. and Blumberg, W. E. (eds.). 1966. *The Biochemistry of Cop-per. Proc. Symp. Copper in Biological System.* Academic Press, New York.

Perlman, F. 1964. Immunochemistry. In: *Symposium on Foods.* 3rd ed. H.W. Schultz (ed.). AVI Publishing, Westport, Connecticut.

Pisciotta, A. V. 1971. Drug-induced leukopenia and aplastic anemia. *Clin. Pharmacol. Ther.* 12: 13–43.

Plaa, G. L. 1975. Toxicology of the liver. In: *Toxicology — The Basic Science of Poisons.* L.J. Casarett and J. Doull (eds.). Macmillan, New York.

Pond, W. G. and Walker, E. F., Jr. 1975. Effect of dietary Ca and Cd level of pregnant rats on reproduction and on dam and progeny tissue mineral concentrations. *Proc. Soc. Exp. Biol. Med.* 148: 665–668.

Prescott, L. F. and Ansari, S. 1969. The effects of repeated administration of mercuric chloride on exfoliation of renal tubular cells and urinary glutamic-oxaloacetic transaminase activity in the rat. *Toxicol. Appl. Pharmacol.* 14: 97–107.

Pulido, P., Kagi, J. H. R. and Vallee, B. L. 1966. Isolation and some properties of human metallothionein. *Biochemistry* 5: 1768-1777.

Pushottam, N., Mason, M. and Pincus, G. 1961. Induced ovulation in the mouse and the measurement of its inhibition. *Fertil. Steril.* 12: 346–352.

Ramel, C. 1969. Genetic effects of organic mercury compounds. I. Cytological investigations on Allium roots. *Hereditas* 61: 208.

Randolph, T. G. 1948. Corn starch as an allergen. Sources of contact in food containers. *J. Am. Diet. Assoc.* 24: 841–846.

Randolph, T. G., Rollins, J. P. and Walker, C. K. 1950. Allergic reactions following intravenous injection of corn sugar. *Arch. Surg.* 61: 554–564.

Rane, A., Berggren, M., Yaffe, S. J. and Erisson, J. L. E. 1973a. Oxidative drug metabolism in the perinatal rabbit liver and placenta. *Xenobiotica* 3: 37–48.

Rane, A., Jjoqvist, F. and Orrenius, S. 1973b. Drugs and fetal metabolism. *Clin. Pharmacol. Ther.* 14: 666–672.

Rechnagel, R. O. 1967. Carbon tetrachloride hepatotoxicity. *Pharmacol. Rev.* 19: 145–208.

Rhaese, H. J. and Freese, E. 1969. Chemical analysis of DNA alterations. IV. Reactions of oligodeoxynucleotides with monofunctional alkylating agents leading to backbone breakage. *Biochem. Biophys. Acta* 190: 418–433.

Robens, J. F. 1969. Teratologic studies of carbaryl, diazinon, norea, disulfiram and thiram in small laboratory animals. *Toxicol. Appl. Pharmacol.* 15: 152–163.

Rohrborn, G. 1970. Biochemical mechanisms of mutation. In: *Chemical Mutagenesis in Mammals and Man.* F. Vogel and G. Rohrborn (eds.). Springer-Verlag, New York.

Rouiller, C. 1964. (ed.) Experimental toxic injury to the liver. In: *The Liver.* Vol. 2. Academic Press, New York.

Saperstein, S. and Anderson, D. W. 1962. Antigenicity of milk proteins of prepared formulas measured by precipitin ring test and passive cutaneous anaphylaxis in the guinea pig. *J. Pediatr.* 61: 196–204.

Scott, W. J., Ritter, E. J. and Wilson, J. G. 1971. DNA synthesis inhibition and cell death associated with hydroxyurea teratogenesis in rat embryos. *Dev. Biol.* 26: 306–315.

Sharratt, M. and Frazer, A. C. 1963. The sensitivity of function tests in detecting renal damage in the rat. *Toxicol. Appl. Pharmacol.* 5: 36–48.

Sjoden, P. and Soderberg, U. 1972. Sex-dependent effects of prenatal 2-4-5-trichlorophenoxyacetic acid on rats' open field behavior. *Physiol. Behav.* 9: 357–360.

Spatz, M. Dougherty, W. J. and Smith, D. W. E. 1967. Teratogenic effects of methylazoxymethanol. *Proc. Soc. Exp. Biol.* 124: 476–478.

Spyker, S. M. Sparber, S. B. and Goldberg, A. M. 1972. Subtle consequences of methyl mercury exposure. Behavioral deviations in offspring of treated mothers. *Science* 177: 621–623.

Stancer, H. and Dardzonov, T. 1967. *Cited by* Sandstead, H.H. 1977. Nutrient interactions with toxic elements. In: *Toxicology of Trace Elements.* R.A. Goyer and M.A. Mehlman (eds.). Hemisphere, Washington, D.C.

Stevenson, A. C., Johnston, H. A. Stewart, M. I. P. and Golding, D. R. 1966. Congenital malformations: A report of a study of series of consecutive births in 24 centres. *Bull. W.H.O. (Suppl.)* 34: 9–127.

Strauss, M. B. 1964. Food allergens. In: *Symposium on Foods*. 3rd. H.W. Schultz (ed.). AVI Publishing, Westport, Connecticut.

Suda, T. et al. 1974. Prevention of metallothionein of cadmium-induced inhibition of vitamin D activation reaction in kidney. *FEBS Lett*. 42: 23–26.

Sussman, A. S. and Halvorson, H. O. 1966. Spores, their dormancy and germination. Harper & Row, New York.

Tappel, A. L. and Caldwell, K. A. 1967. Redox properties of selenium compounds related to biochemical function. *Proceedings of the 1st Int. Symp. Selenium Biomed*. Oregon State University 1966.

Taussig, H. 1962. The study of the German outbreak of phocomelia. *J.A.M.A*. 180: 1106–1114.

Tessman, J., Poddar, R. K. and Kumar, S. 1964. Identification of altered bases in mutated single-stranded DNA. I. In vitro mutagenesis by hydroxylamine, ethyl methanesulphonate and nitrous acid. *J. Mol. Biol*. 9: 352–363.

Thomas, C. L. (ed.). 1977. *Taber's Cyclopedic Medical Dictionary*. 13th ed. F.A. Davis, Philadelphia.

Thomas, J. A. et al. 1972. Actions of dieldrin on the uptake of testosterone-1,2-H^3 by prostate glands of the male mouse. Abstr. Eleventh Annual Meeting, Society of Toxicology. *Toxicol. Appl. Pharmacol*. 22: 326–327.

Thorpe, E. 1969. Some toxic effects of hexachlorophene in sheep. *J. Comp. Pathol*. 79: 167–171.

Trasler, D. G. 1968. Pathogenesis of cleft lip and its relation to embryonic face shape in A/J and C57BL mice. *Teratology* 1: 33–50.

Vashakidze, V. I. 1971. The effect of sevin on spermatogenesis in the white rat. *Biol. Abstr*. 52: 46271.

Vaughn, J. M. 1971. The effect of radiation on bone. In: *Biochemistry and Physiology of Bone*. Vol. 3. G.H. Bourne (ed.), Academic Press, New York.

Vogel, F. 1969. Point mutations and human hemoglobin variants. *Humangenetik* 1: 253–263.

Vogel, F. 1970. Spontaneous mutation in man. In: *Chemical Mutagenesis in Mammals and Man*. F. Vogel and G. Rohrborn (eds.). Springer-Verlag, New York.

Walzer, M. 1927. Studies in absorption of undigested proteins in human beings. I. A simple direct method of studying absorption of undigested protein. *J. Immunol*. 14: 143–174.

Warburton, D. and Fraser, F. C. 1964. Spontaneous abortion risks in man: Data from reproductive histories collected in a medical genetics unit. *Am. J. Hum. Genet*. 16: 1–25.

Warkany, J. and Schraffenberger, E. 1946. Congenital malformations induced in rats by maternal vitamin A deficiency. I. Defects of the eye. *Arch. Ophthalmol*. 35: 150.

Waters, M. D. 1977. Toxicology of vanadium. In: *Toxicology of Trace Elements*. R.A. Goyer and M.A. Mehlman (eds.). Hemisphere, Washington, D.C.

Wiener, G. 1970. Varying psychological sequelae of lead ingestion in children. *Public Health Rep*. 85: 19–24.

Wilson, J. G. 1973. *Environment and Birth Defects*. Academic Press, New York.

Wilson, J. G. 1974. Factors determining the teratogenicity of drugs. *Annu. Rev. Pharmacol. Toxicol*. 14: 205–217.

Wilson, R., Doell, B. H., Groger, W., Hope, J. and Gellatly, J. B. M. 1970. The physiology of liver enlargement. In: *Metabolic Aspects of Food Safety*. Roe, F. J. C. (ed.). Blackwell Scientific, Oxford, England. 363–418.

Wogan, G. N. 1969. Metabolism and biochemical effects of aflatoxins. In: *Aflatoxins*. L.A. Goldblatt (ed.). Academic Press, New York.

World Health Organization. *W.H.O. Bull. Memo*. 34: 765.

Wragg, J. B., Carr, J. V. and Roos, V. 1967. Inhibition of DNA polymerase activity by caffeine in a mammalian cell line. *J. Cell Biol*. 35: 146A–147A.

6

Carcinogenesis

WHAT IS CANCER?

Cellular proliferation following physical injury or hormonal stimulation to a tissue is a phenomenon known as hyperplasia. Hyperplasia is characterized by an observable accumulation of cells ultimately producing a visible change in the appearance of the tissue; i.e., a lesion, inflammation, lump, or tumor. This proliferation subsides when the cause for the increased cellular activity is removed. Henceforth, a homeostatic situation resumes, wherein the rate of cell division balances the rate of cell death, so that the tissues concerned appear to be normal with no apparent increase in volume or weight. In this case, the hyperplasia is said to be reversible. However, when the rate of cellular activity diminishes, as when the tissues begin to age, the opposite effect, hypoplasia or hypotrophy or shrinkage, may be observed. Thus, it appears that some unknown mechanism determines and controls the extent of cell proliferation, and the normal number of cells for a given tissue is maintained within a definite range for most of the adult life of the organism.

Sometimes a situation arises whereby the action of certain factors (which will be discussed later) causes the control of cell proliferation to fail. This failure results in an unregulated cell division even after removing the factor which incited the change. Ultimately this proliferation is manifested by an abnormal mass of tissue called a tumor or neoplasm. This mass of tissue appears to be morphologically different from the host tissue, although it may retain many of the normal biochemical and physiological characteristics of the cells of that tissue. Thus, this abnormal mass of cells is said to have undergone dedifferentiation.

However, if this abnormal mass remains confined to that tissue, or a portion of it, the tumor characterized by a certain boundary or territorality is said to be benign. This type of tumor is usually enclosed by connective tissues which define the territory of the tumor mass.

In other cases, the proliferative process is not strictly limited to a particular location in the tissue. The abnormal mass of cells escapes its boundary and invades and disrupts surrounding areas. Such abnormal cells are usually carried by the blood or the lymph and establish colonies in distant and unrelated tissues. Such a process is known as metastasis. These abnormally proliferating cells, which are invasive and/or metastatic, produce a neoplasm or tumor which is referred to as malignant or cancerous. Thus, the disease characterized by such types of tumors is known as cancer.

One significant characteristic of malignant tumors is their apparent autonomy. The tumors appear to grow unrestrained and uncoordinated, seemingly independent of general somatic control. This characterization, however, must be viewed in a limited sense.

The growth of tumors, at least in the early stages of development, can be affected by hormones and nutrients (Arcos et al. 1968).

Benign and malignant tumors, then, differ from simple hyperplasia in that tumors continue to grow unrestrained even after removal of the stimulus.

Cancer formation is a multistep process (Farber and Cameron 1980). It involves both initiation into the preneoplastic state and promotion into the neoplastic progression. The process of initiation and promotion are not yet understood. However, results indicate that cancerous transformations of cells involve certain genes, termed proto-oncogens (Cairns and Logan 1983). In order that these genes can direct the carcinogenic process, they must be activated or mutated. Evidently, from cell culture experiments, their ability to transform a cell into the neoplastic step requires that the cell may have already been somehow initiated into a preneoplastic state by a carcinogen (Newbold and Overell 1983), or that the cell is transfected with complementary oncogens from tumor viruses (Land et al. 1983; Ruley 1983) or other specific virally transformed genes (Land et al. 1983).

Thus, the multistep process in carcinogenesis appears to have a genetic basis.

Cancer is really a collective name for a group of 100 or more related diseases, all of which have features in common. A malignant tumor can occur in virtually all tissues and organs, and at any age. However, some tissues and organs are more susceptible than others, and cancer is more common in older people.

Of particular interest in food toxicology is the incidence of cancer of the gastro-intestinal tract.

There are also different susceptibilities to certain forms of cancer based on race, sex, national origin, and geography.

CANCER INCIDENCE

Cancer incidence and mortality is increasing at an alarming rate. Figure 1 shows the increase in cancer mortality from 1950 to 1970 in the United States. At present, the disease is the second leading cause of death in the United States, and accounts for about 20% of the total deaths. Similar trends are being recognized in other parts of the world.

The Third National Cancer Survey (TNCS) for the period 1969 to 1971 and the Surveillance, Epidemiology and End Results (SEER) program for the period 1973 to 1976 has provided data showing a trend toward significantly increasing cancer incidence for the white population* in the United States for the period 1969 to 1976 (Pollack and Horn 1980). Over the 7-year period, the data show an increase in cancer incidence by approximately 9 and 14% among white males and females, respectively. Table 1 shows the annual and total percentage change in cancer incidence per 100,000 population during the 7-year period based on the data compiled by Pollack and Horn (1980). An average annual increase in the incidence rate of 1.3 and 2.0% for all sites combined among white males and females, respectively, was observed. This is equivalent to a 9.1 and 14.0% increase, respectively, for the entire 7-year period. Table 2 shows a similar trend in increased mortality over the same 7-year period involving cancer of all sites combined. The trends in mortality involving selected sites, which are the more common forms of cancer, are also shown. Similar trends have been recognized in other industrialized countries (National Cancer Institute 1974).

---

*The available data for the black population could not be used for determining a similar trend that is statistically sound because of changes in the black population base during the SEER survey period; i.e., two areas with large black populations were added during 1974 and 1976. Thus, a more accurate analysis of the trend among the black population can be made only with data beginning in 1976. Nevertheless, inspection of the data for 1969 to 1976 also shows an increasing trend in cancer incidence for specific sites (Pollack and Horn 1980).

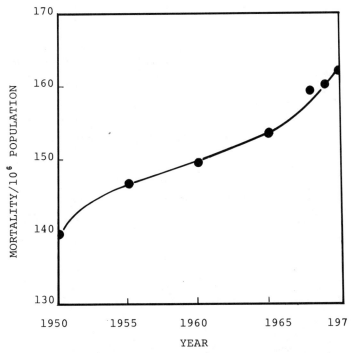

Figure 1. U.S. mortality from cancer from 1950 to 1970 (Statistical Abstract of the United States 1972).

Although the incidence of some cancer sites is drastically decreasing, for a majority of sites the incidence is increasing. Nevertheless, improvements in mortality rates are evident in Table 2, especially among females. Improvement in mortality rates, however, has no significance in terms of causation as long as there is no corresponding improvement in cancer incidence.

A large proportion of these increases is due to the staggering increase in lung cancer incidence, as seen in Table 1. Thus, the increased rate of cigarette smoking among the population registered in the past 20 to 30 years undoubtedly contributed to this large increase in cancer incidence, particularly among women. According to Schneiderman (1980), however, less than half of this increase is due to cigarette smoking, whereas exposure to chemicals may be responsible for a major part of the increase. The large increases in cancer of colon, rectum, skin (melanoma), bladder, kidney, and breast are consistent with this hypothesis. However, the role of environmental chemicals in these increases can be assessed better by use of epidemiological data, as in the case of many substances identified as carcinogenic to humans.

Although there are 100 or more distinct kinds of cancer, based on the tissue or organ of occurrence and the kind of cells that are involved, most forms are rare. The cancers of three organs — lung, large intestine, and breast — are the most common and therefore account for about 50% of all cancer deaths. (Of interest to food toxicologists are cancers of the large intestine and breast because some correlation between diet and cancer in these organs has been observed [Cairnes 1975; Zippin and Petrakis 1971]). Liver and bladder cancer also have a strong association with dietary factors.

Table 1. Annual and Total Percentage Change of Age-Adjusted Cancer Incidence Rates[a] for All and Selected Sites During a 7-Year Period, 1969-1976, for the U.S. White Population in Participating Areas Surveyed in the TNCS and SEER Programs

Sites	Male	(95% C.I.[c])		Female	(95% C.I.[c])		Total % Change[b] Male	Female
		Average Annual Percentage Change						
All sites	1.3	(0.74	1.86)	2.0	(1.28	2.72)	9.1	14.0
Stomach	-2.3	(-3.34	-1.26)	3.7	(-4.70	-2.70)	-16.1	-25.9
Colon only	1.5	(0.29	2.71)	0.7	(-0.22	1.62)	10.5	4.9
Rectum	1.3	(0.6	2.00)	1.2	(0.18	2.22)	9.1	5.8
Pancreas	-0.5	(-1.96	0.96)	0.9	(-0.61	2.41)	-3.5	6.3
Lung	1.4	(0.87	9.14)	8.6	(8.06	9.14)	9.8	60.2
Melanoma	6.8	(5.32	7.08)	6.2	(5.32	7.08)	47.6	43.4
Bladder	2.3	(1.31	3.29)	2.5	(1.01	3.99)	16.1	17.5
Kidney	1.2	(-2.20	2.60)	1.3	(-1.09	3.69)	8.4	9.1
Leukemia	-0.2	(-1.51	1.11)	-1.0	(-2.14	0.14)	-1.4	-7.0
Prostate	2.3	(1.27	3.33)				16.1	
Breasts				1.8	(1.17	2.43)		12.6
Cervix				-5.9	(-6.67	-5.13)		-41.3
Corpus + uterus[d]				5.9	(4.48	7.32)		41.3
Ovary				-0.4	(-1.61	0.81)		-2.8

[a]Cancer incidence rates per 100,000 population.
[b]Over 7-year period, i.e., average annual percentage change x 7.
[c]Confidence interval for percentage change.
[d]Not otherwise specified.
Source: Pollack and Horn (1980), used with permission.

ENVIRONMENTAL ASPECTS OF CARCINOGENESIS

An examination of the occurrence of cancer in man reveals some interesting observations: (1) Roughly 90% of adult human cancers occur in epithelial tissues, in spite of the fact that mesenchymal tissues comprise the bulk of the body tissues (Miller and Miller 1974). (2) Approximately half of all epithelial cancers occur in tissues that are directly exposed to the environment — skin, gastrointestinal, and bronchial epithelia. (3) A study of the cancer incidence among migrants and selected ethnic groups reveals an environmental component. For example, Japanese migrants in the United States show a decline in stomach cancer incidence compared to that in Japan, which is the highest in the world (Haenszel and Kurihara 1968). On the other hand, these migrants show an increased incidence of colon cancer approaching that of the white population in the United States. The sons of these migrants approach that incidence even more closely (Cairns 1975). In Figure 2 the bar graph illustrates the change of incidence of stomach, liver, colon, and prostate cancer of Japanese migrants and their sons in California as compared to those of the Japanese in Japan and United States whites in California.

Table 2. Annual and Total Percentage Change of Cancer Mortality Rates[a] for All
and Selected Sites During a 7-Year Period, 1969-1976, for the U.S. White Population in Participating Areas Surveyed in the TNCS and SEER Programs

Sites	Average Annual Percentage Change				Total % Change[b]	
	Male	(95% C.I.[c])	Female	(95% C.I.[c])	Male	Female
All sites	0.9	(0.60 1.20)	0.2	(-0.20 0.60)	6.3	1.4
Stomach	-2.9	(-3.13 -2.67)	-3.6	(-3.95 -3.25)	-20.3	-25.2
Colon only	1.3	(0.90 1.70)	0.0	(-0.47 0.47)	9.1	0.0
Rectum	-3.0	(-3.37 -2.63)	-3.1	(-3.75 -2.45)	-21.0	-21.7
Pancreas	0.2	(-0.14 0.54)	0.3	(-0.03 0.63)	1.4	2.1
Lung	2.6	(2.20 3.00)	7.1	(6.60 7.60)	18.2	49.7
Melanoma	4.0	(2.94 5.06)	0.8	(-0.84 2.44)	28.0	56.6
Bladder	0.6	(0.05 1.15)	-1.4	(-2.53 -3.27)	4.2	-9.8
Kidney	0.6	(0.06 1.14)	0.7	(0.17 1.23)	4.2	4.9
Leukemia	-0.4	(-0.82 0.02)	-1.7	(-2.24 -1.16)	-2.8	-11.9
Prostate	1.2	(0.77 1.63)			8.4	
Breasts			0.3	(0.09 0.69)		2.1
Cervix			-4.9	(-5.56 -4.24)		-34.3
Corpus + uterus[d]			-1.7	(-2.26 -1.14)		-11.9
Ovary			-0.3	(-0.79 0.19)		-2.1

[a]Cancer mortality rates per 100,000 population.
[b]Over 7-year period, i.e., average annual percent change x 7.
[c]Confidence interval for percentage change.
[d]Not otherwise specified.
Source: Pollack and Horn (1980), used with permission.

Similarly, data on the overall cancer incidence of Jewish immigrants to Israel from
Western Europe or the United States compared to native-born Jews or non-Jewish
Israelis, also show a trend similar to that of the Japanese immigrants. The bar graph
in Figure 3 illustrates the influence of environment on the overall cancer incidence of
an ethnic group. In this case, Jews who have immigrated to Israel from the United
States or Europe show a much higher cancer incidence than compared to those born in
Israel or to those immigrants born in Asia or Africa. The cancer incidence of Israeli
immigrants from Europe or the United States approaches that of the United States
population.

In the data cited for both the Japanese and the Jews, genetic factors or change in
intensity of ultraviolet (uv) radiation has been ruled out. In the first case, the
change incidence occurred much earlier for genetics to account for the difference. The
difference in uv radiation is insignificant among the different locations.

Other examples of the variation of cancer incidence from country-to-country (Segi
et al. 1969) or within regions in a country (Kmet and Mahboubi 1972; Wynder and
Mabuchi 1972) lead to the conclusion that there is an environmental element in the
etiology of cancer. The suspicion points to chemicals and viruses in the environment

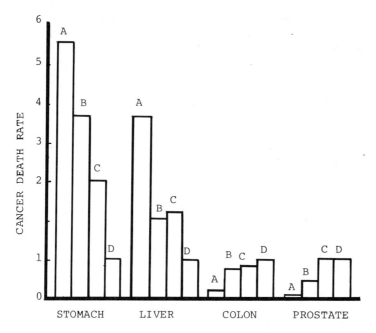

Figure 2. Changes in incidence of cancer of the stomach, liver, colon, and prostate of Japanese immigrants to California (column B) and their sons (column C) compared to those in Japan (column A) and among white Californians (column D). (From Cairns 1975, used with permission.)

as the two factors responsible in the causation of cancer. However, since the role of viruses has not been confirmed in human cancer, their implication in these cancers is a weak one, in spite of the fact that some types of cancers have been experimentally induced by viruses in animals. Thus, it is now highly suspected that possibly as much as 90% of all human cancers are caused by environmental chemicals principally in food, water, air, drugs, and other vehicles by which these chemicals enter the body (Boyland 1967; Higginson 1969, 1976).

These chemicals include both naturally occurring as well as man-made substances. The latter have proliferated with the advances in modern technology. Such chemicals found their way into our food and water supply either as contaminants or additives for one reason or another. Other chemicals are generated in situ by reactions occurring between food components during food processing, preparation, and storage.

Many naturally occurring carcinogenic compounds (Weisburger 1975; Wogan 1974) have been discovered during the past decades. Many of these are contaminants of food products or are endogenous metabolites of the plant or animal from which the food is processed.

TYPES OF CHEMICAL CARCINOGENS ACCORDING TO BIOLOGICAL ACTIVITY

While chemical carcinogens (henceforth referred to simply as carcinogens) may be classified in the same way as toxicants in general (endogenous, derived, contaminants, and so forth), these substances may be further classified as: (1) primary; (2) secondary carcinogens (procarcinogens); and (3) carcinogenic promoters and cocarcinogens.

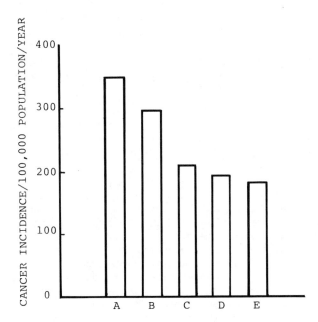

Figure 3.   Cancer incidence of Jewish immigrants to Israel from the United States and Western Europe compared to native born Jews or non-Jewish Israelis. Column A, U.S. population; B, American- or European-born Israeli immigrants; C, Asian- or African-born Israeli immigrants; D, native Israeli Jews; E, other Israelis (predominantly Arabs). (From Cairns 1975, used with permission.)

Primary Carcinogens

Primary carcinogens are inherently biologically active, and they initiate carcinogenesis directly without metabolic activation. Thus, many of these compounds act at the point of initial contact even though they may also induce cancer in remote tissues.

A fundamental property of primary carcinogens is their high chemical reactivity which is inherent in their structures. These substances include a number of alkylating agents such as dimethyl sulfate and lactones, β-propionolactone and propane sulfone. These carcinogens are electrophilic substances, and therefore react with nucleophilic receptors in the cell. A number of these receptors have been identified and consist mainly of amino acid, purine, and pyrimidine residues (Miller and Miller 1974). Precisely which of these receptors are the critical targets essential to carcinogenic processes has not been determined. There have been correlations of the binding of carcinogens to DNA (deoxyribonucleic acid), RNA (ribonucleic acid), or proteins in the cell (Boutwell et al. 1969; Brookes and Lawley 1964b; Kriek 1969, 1970). In studies with alkylating agents, however, no definite association between the extent of binding and carcinogenicity can be established (Swan and Magee 1968, 1971).

Metal and Solid-State Carcinogenesis

Excluding certain metals which are carcinogenic because of their radioactivity, i.e., uranium[236], radium, strontium[90], certain types of inorganic chemicals induce cancer in animals, sometimes at the site of injection (Maenza et al. 1971). This is exemplified by tumor formation in animals following the subcutaneous injection of nickel (Furst and Haro 1969; Sunderman 1971; Weisburger 1973). Among the metallic elements only titanium, nickel, chromium, cobalt, lead, manganese, beryllium and arsenic are carcinogenic. Nickel and titanium salts seem to be the more potent. It has been reported that selenium is also carcinogenic (Muth 1967); nevertheless, other evidence indicates that selenium is noncarcinogenic (Sunderman 1971). These metals are potential contaminants in food and water (World Health Organization 1972).

Little work has been done on metallic carcinogenesis. Thus, hardly anything is known regarding the carcinogenic mechanisms of metals. Their carcinogenic activity may follow from their electrophilic nature. Thus, metals can react with nucleophilic parts of macromolecules (Miller 197a). The binding of metals to purine and pyrimidine bases (Fuwa et al. 1960; Shapiro 1968) or phosphate groups of DNA (Eichhorn et al. 1966) has been noted. The binding of metals to amino groups may lead to the instability of the duplex structure of these macromolecules (Furst and Haro 1969), or even lead to depolymerization of the polynucleotides, as in the case of Ni^{2+} (Butzow and Eichhorn 1965).

Solid-state or foreign-body carcinogenesis is associated with the presence of films or discs of plastic or metals lodged in tissues. In general, the neoplastic process is independent of the chemical nature of the film or disc, since both plastic or chemically inert metallic foils or films can induce sarcomas (Bischoff 1972; Bischoff and Bryson 1964; Klarner 1962; Northdurft 1955). As a rule, foreign-body carcinogenesis has no food toxicological significance, except possibly in the case of asbestos. However, the association between exposure to asbestos and cancer of the gastrointestinal (GI) tract, indicating food and water as vectors, is still inconclusive (Martin 1970; Wagner et al. 1971). Nevertheless, asbestos has been associated with bronchogenic cancer and mesothelioma (a rare form of cancer of the pleura and peritoneum). The fact that it may be a contaminant in water and food makes it a potential food- or waterborne carcinogen. Small amounts of asbestos have been universally detected in river waters (Wright 1969), and it appears that it takes only a few asbestos fibers to induce a mesothelioma (Martin 1970). Because it is an air pollutant (Selikoff et al. 1971; U.S. Environmental Protection Agency 1971) and has been used extensively (Hendry 1965; Wagner et al. 1971), its presence in food and water is very likely.

Although the primary carcinogens provide only academic interest to the food toxicologist, studies of their mechanisms of action or the mode of biological activity provide useful information toward understanding the mode of action of the most common types of carcinogens, the secondary carcinogens.

Secondary Carcinogens

Most recognized carcinogens such as those likely to be found in food, belong to this type (Miller 1971a; Miller and Miller 1971a; Weisburger 1973). These substances, also known as procarcinogens, require metabolic transformation to active forms. The metabolic derivatives thus become the primary carcinogens. Several examples of secondary carcinogens that have been detected in food are listed in Table 3, classified according to their source. Note that several types of chemical forms are represented, and like the primary carcinogens, their derivatives are also strong electrophiles. Even though metabolic activation is a prerequisite to carcinogenicity, this does not diminish the potency of many carcinogens; on a mole-to-mole basis, many secondary carcinogens are just as potent as the direct-acting carcinogens.

Metabolic activation of these compounds implies the presence of enzyme systems whose main function is to promote their excretion by increasing their water solubility. This process results in decreased chemical reactivity and, for certain compounds, carcinogenicity as well. Thus, metabolic transformation may result in either activation or deactivation (detoxification).

Examples of metabolic activation reactions involving carcinogens are the following:

Epoxidation

Epoxidation can be illustrated by the metabolic transformation of the strong carcinogen, benzo(a)pyrene, commonly found in smoked food (Howard and Fazio 1969;

Table 3. Secondary Carcinogens in Foods

Carcinogen	Food
Polycyclic aromatic hydrocarbon	Smoked and broiled products, vegetable oils, margarine, mayonnaise, tea and coffee, cereals, and shellfish
Nitrosamines	Fried bacon; fried, salted, and fresh fish; cheese; mushrooms; luncheon meat; Danish pork, and Hungarian salami
Cycasin	Cycad products
Pyrrolizidine alkaloids	Cereal flour contaminants
Aflatoxins	Peanuts and other agricultural products
Sterigmatocystin	Cereals, flour, and legumes
Luteoskyrin	Rice
Pesticide residues	All types of foodstuffs
Saccharin	Diet beverages and other products
Safrole	Sassafras tea and various spices
Estragole	Certain spices and flavorings
Tannins	Tea, wine, and other products
Psoralens	Parsnip, citrus fruits, spices, and flavors

See text for a discussion of secondary carcinogens in food as well as other examples of these compounds and the products in which they can be found.

Malanoski et al. 1968). Thus, as shown in the following reaction, this hydrocarbon is first oxidized to an epoxide (Daly 1971; Grover et al. 1972).

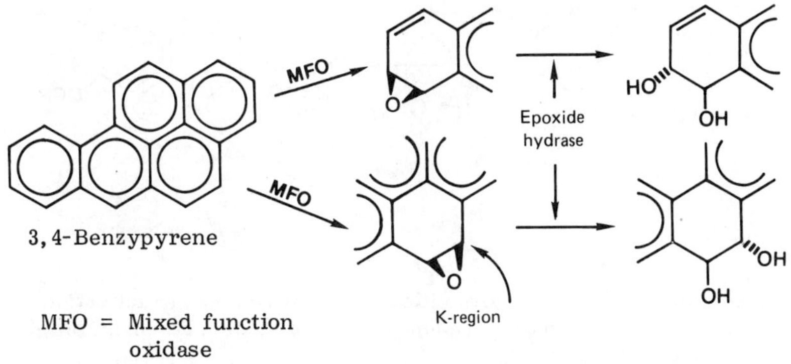

3,4-Benzypyrene

MFO = Mixed function oxidase

K-region

Epoxide hydrase

The conversion of the hydrocarbon to an active form, the epoxide, requires an enzyme comples (mixed function oxidase) located in the endoplasmic reticulum or microsomes (Gelboin et al. 1974). The enzyme complex consists of three components, a mono-oxygenase, a cytochrome reductase, and a lipid component (Lu et al. 1972). Cytochromes P-450 and P-448 are two known forms of the oxygenases. All three components are necessary for activity of the enzyme complex. The enzyme complex is closely linked to a hydrase, the so-called epoxide hydrase (Oesch et al. 1972). The enzyme complex for the oxidation of aromatic hydrocarbons, including the hydrase, is often referred to as aryl hydrocarbon hydroxylase (AHH). For example, the enzyme for benz(a)pyrene is called benzo(a)pyrene hydroxylase. The enzyme complex is found in most tissues of most animal species studied so far (Nebert and Gelboin 1969; Nebert et al. 1969; Wattenberg and Leong 1962; Whitlock et al. 1972). Liver contains the largest amount relative to other tissues.

The enzyme complex is inducible by polycyclic aromatic hydrocarbons (PAH), drugs, and other foreign compounds (xenobiotics). It appears that induction of the enzyme complex is necessary for the reaction of benz(a)pyrene with DNA and protein (Gelboin 1969). The susceptibility of cells in tissue culture to the toxicity of hydrocarbons has been correlated with the level of this enzyme complex (Gelboin et al. 1969; Nebert and Gelboin 1968).

When tested in cell cultures, the K-region epoxides, as indicated in the preceding reaction scheme for benz(a)pyrene, are generally more reactive in producing malignancy than the parent hydrocarbon or the dihydrodiols (Grover et al. 1971; Huberman et al. 1971). Such epoxides are also mutagenic to mammalian cells (Huberman et al. 1971), and this mutagenicity produced by the K-region epoxides correlates highly to the in vivo carcinogenicity of the parent hydrocarbon (Ames et al. 1972; Cookson et al. 1971).

The phenols formed by the AHH are also further rendered innocuous and excretable by conjugation with a number of factors, notably glutathione (Boyland and Williams 1965) (p. 210).

The K-region epoxides are not the only products of aromatic hydrocarbon oxidation (Selkirk et al. 1972). Non-K region epoxides are also produced which may not be as stable as the K-region epoxides, and thus generally escape detection.

Epoxidation appears to be a major metabolic activation reaction for procarcinogens. Aflatoxins B_1 and G_1, which are powerful mycocarcinogens from *Aspergillus flavus* and similar molds, appear to be activated by epoxidation at the 2,3-position of the furane ring (Swenson et al. 1973, 1974; Patterson 1973).

Aflatoxin B_1

Hydroxylation–Esterification

This activation process may be exemplified by the carcinogenic activation of safrole (Borchert et al. 1973a,b), an endogenous flavoring agent present in oil of sassafras.

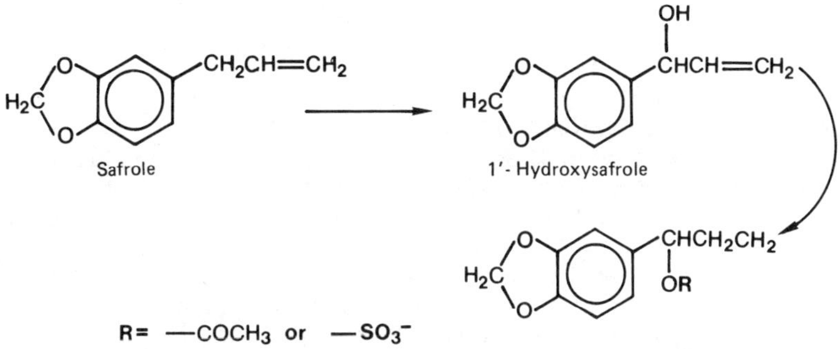

Safrole   1'- Hydroxysafrole

R = —COCH$_3$ or —SO$_3^-$

The carcinogenic activation of this compound occurs when the allyl group is hydroxylated at the 1'-position. 1'-Hydroxy safrole causes tumors more rapidly at lower doses than safrole. Often, however, the final oncogenic species is the ester, since the hydroxyl group fails to react in vitro with model receptors, unlike the ester form, acetoxy-1'-hydroxysafrole.

Many other types of hydroxylation-esterification activation reactions have been noted with different types of procarcinogens. Such is the case of carcinogenic aromatic amines where N-hydroxylation followed by sulfate (Miller and Miller 1971a; Weisberger and Weisberger 1973), or acyl (Bartsch et al. 1973) conjugation appears to be the principal activation steps.

Oxidation and Carbonium Ion Formation

The formation of carbonium ions during the activation of a number of procarcinogens has been postulated. This process is preceded by an oxidation step. An example would be the activation of nitrosamines (Druckrey et al. 1967; Magee and Schoental 1964). Some forms of these carcinogenic substances have been detected in a variety of smoked food and dried fish (Fong and Walsh 1971) (Chap. 12). In the case of dimethylnitrosamines, as proposed by Druckrey (1973a), the initial step appears to be oxidation of one of the alkyl carbons (α-position) to form the hydroxyalkyl derivative. On rearrangement and in the presence of H$^+$, the hydroxymethyl derivative breaks down to yield the CH$_3^+$.

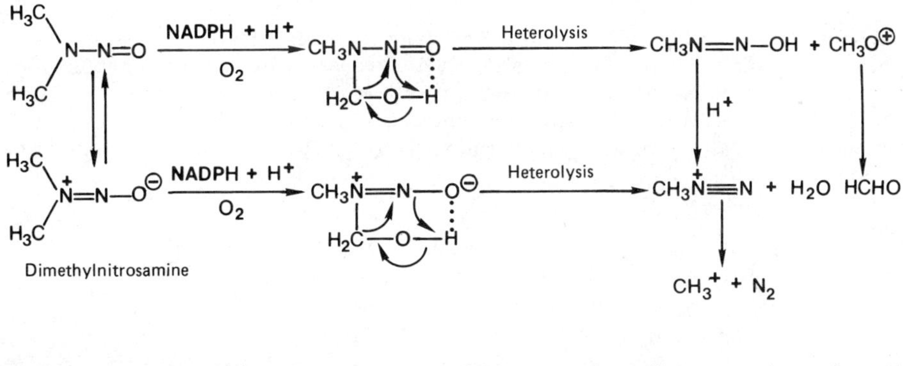

Dimethylnitrosamine

The above mechanism presupposes that CH$_3$ has an immediate receptor, since these species are highly reactive and unstable. Indeed, alkylated nucleic acids have been detected after treatment with these alkylating agents (Lawley et al. 1968; Lawley et al. 1973; Lijinsky et al. 1968; O'Connor et al. 1973). The major target of alkylating agents appears to be the N-7 position of guanine, although these agents also attack to a lesser degree other positions in guanine as well as other nucleic acid bases.

The higher homologues of the alkylamines appear to undergo metabolic β-oxidation, yielding the simpler homolog, so that the final methylating agent is dimethylnitrosamine. Thus, dipropyl and dibutylnitrosamine, such as β-hydroxypropylpropylnitrosamine, 2-oxopropylpropylnitrosamine, and methylpropylnitrosamine, yield 7-methyl guanine (Kruger 1973; Kruger and Bertram 1973).

Some evidence indicates that cyclic nitrosamines may undergo ring opening (Kruger 1972; Stewart and Magee 1972). For instance, it has been reported that nitrosopyrrolidine produces 7-methyl guanine (Lee and Lijinsky 1966). More work is needed regarding the metabolic activation of cyclic nitrosamines.

Other examples of carbonium ion formation producing active metabolites are the pyrrolizidine (Senecio) alkaloids and halogenated hydrocarbons. These pyrrolizidine alkaloids, which are potent hepatotoxins and hepatocarcinogens, are naturally occurring contaminants of some foods. These compounds, of which several types are known (Bull et al. 1968; Culvenor et al. 1971), appear to be metabolically activated by dehydrogenation to pyrrole derivatives. The distribution of charges results in highly reactive allylic ester metabolites; carbonium ions (Hsu et al. 1973; Mattocks and White 1973) are formed upon cleavage of an acid group.

Pyrrolizidine
alkaloid

The resulting carbonium ion is a potent alkylating agent (Mattocks 1968, 1969; White and Mattocks 1972).

The halogenated hydrocarbons are more or less potent carcinogens depending on their structure. These compounds undergo metabolic activation by dehalogenation (Fowler 1969; Gandolfi and Van Dyke 1973; Uehleke et al. 1973), resulting in carbonium ions which are also alkylating agents. These compounds are mostly contaminants in food.

The insecticide DDT (dichlorodiphenyltrichloroethane) has been found to be hepatotumorigenic in mice (Innes et al. 1969). Several dechlorinated metabolites of DDT have been isolated in human tissues as well as in experimental animals (Dacre 1970; Ottoboni et al. 1968; Peterson and Robison 1964). A carbonium ion is postulated to be an intermediate during the conversion of DDT to DDE (dichlorodiphenyldichloroethylene).

[1,1-Dichloro-2,2-bis
(p-chlorophenyl)ethylene]

[1,1-Dichloro-2,2-bis
(p-chlorophenyl)ethane]

Chlorinated hydrocarbons such as chloroform have been detected in the drinking water of certain communities in the United States (see Chap. 19).

Hydrolysis by Intestinal Microorganisms

The role of intestinal microorganisms in the activation or inactivation of toxicants has been amply discussed in Chapter 3. However, we need to stress in this discussion that the activity of intestinal microflora is, in some cases, essential to the activation of certain procarcinogens. An excellent example is the activation of cycasin, a procarcinogen endogenous to cycad seeds. The activity of this compound requires the release of the active aglycone, methylazoxymethanol, by action of bacterial β-glucosidase (Lacquer and Spatz 1968; Mickelson 1972).

The role of intestinal microflora in the activation of cycasin was ascertained only when given orally to normal rats, but not to germ-free animals or when injected intraperitoneally or subcutaneously. However, it appears that the tissues of newborn animals contain the required β-glucosidase, since subcutaneous injection in these animals resulted in cancer (Magee et al. 1976).

Cocarcinogens or Carcinogenic Promoters

There are noncarcinogenic or, at most, weakly carcinogenic substances which produce greater carcinogenic response when applied along with or following a trace amount of a carcinogen (Hecker 1971; Salaman and Roe 1964; Van Duuren 1976). The substance which is applied along with the carcinogen is called the cocarcinogen; that which is applied subsequently is known as the tumor promoter. Presently, this distinction is mainly operational. It is not possible to distinguish between cocarcinogens and tumor promoters based on mechanism of action because our knowledge of the carcinogenic process is incomplete. As a matter of fact, the relationships between cocarcinogens and tumor promoters appear to be quite complex. Thus, there are substances which have both cocarcinogenic and tumor-promoting activity (e.g., phorbol myristate acetate, anthralin, and n-dodecane [Van Duuren 1976]); and similar substances may show different effects. Thus, phenol has a tumor-promoting activity, whereas catechol (o-hydroxyphenol) and pyrogallol (2,3-dihydroxyphenol) have cocarcinogenic effects (Van Duuren 1976).

The significance of these cocarcinogenic or promoting substances is that tumor growth may not occur with trace amounts of carcinogens unless contact with these substances also occurs. In this case, contact with the promoters may be as essential to carcinogenesis as the carcinogens themselves. Thus, as observed in experimental animals, even though the interval between exposures to a carcinogen and the promoting substance may be prolonged — weeks or months — a tumor may still appear (Bates et al. 1968; Segal et al. 1972).

The discovery of the tumor-promoting ability of substances supported previous observations. These concluded that latent cells, previously induced into malignancy, can be promoted into activity by non-specific stimuli. The range of such a stimuli is wide: from punching holes in rabbits' ears to the application of turpentine or chloroform (Fridewald and Rous 1944, 1950; Rous and Kidd 1941). These observations lead to the hypothesis of the two-stage or sequential mechanism of carcinogenesis. This hypothesis proposes that the induction of tumorigenesis and the promotion of tumor growth depend on different stimuli and different mechanisms.

One of the earliest known chemical cocarcinogens and tumor promoters is croton oil, from the seeds of the plant *Croton tiglium*. The oil is a highly poisonous irritant. Its most active components are the ester derivatives of a complex tetracyclic alcohol, phorbol: 13-myristyl- and the 12-myristyl-13-acetyl-phorbol ester (Hecker 1968).

Phorbol ester

Monoester: $R_1 = H$

$R_2 = CH_3-(CH_2)_{12}-\overset{\displaystyle O}{\overset{\|}{C}}-$

Diester: $R_1 = CH_3-(CH_2)_{12}-\overset{\displaystyle O}{\overset{\|}{C}}-$

$R_2 = CH_3-\overset{\displaystyle}{\underset{\displaystyle O}{\overset{\|}{C}}}-$

Some naturally occurring tumor promoters in food include citrus oils, particularly D-limonene, a component of these oils (Homburger and Boger 1968; Roe and Pierce 1960). Sterculic and malvolic acids, the cyclopropenoid fatty acids from cottonseed, are cocarcinogens or tumor promoters for aflatoxin B_1 (Lee et al. 1968).

A number of surface active agents, such as polysorbate (Tween) or sorbitan (Span) have also bee found to be cocarcinogenic or tumor promoters (Setälä et al. 1954, 1957). Likewise phenol and a number of its derivatives (Boutwell and Bosch 1959, Rusch et al. 1955), n-dodecane (Saffioti and Shubik 1956; Shubik et al. 1956), and other alkanes and 1-alkyl alcohols (Sice 1966).

The varied chemical nature of cocarcinogens and tumor promoters known so far indicates that, like the carcinogens, there are probably many more compounds yet to be identified. The number of known food-related cocarcinogens and tumor promoters is limited. Nevertheless, it is very likely that several of these yet unidentified substances may be present in food in the form of naturally occurring substances, derived compounds, or contaminants. Unfortunately, it is still not known whether these substances when occurring simultaneously will have greater or lesser effects in proportion to the number of compounds present.

FACTORS AFFECTING CARCINOGENESIS

The extrinsic and intrinsic factors affecting the carcinogenic response to a particular compound are: (1) dose, including frequency of exposure; (2) age; (3) sex; (4) hormonal status; (5) genetic background; (6) immunological factors; (7) specific chemical modifiers other than cocarcinogens and promoters; (8) nutritional factors; and (9) route of bodily entry of the carcinogen. In the case of the last factor, only the oral route is of principal interest in food toxicology. Thus, a discussion of other routes of entry is beyond the scope of this book. However, other routes of entry, particularly in the case of multiple exposures, may have an important impact on the total cancer induction process. This will become evident in the discussion on specific chemical modifiers (pp. 202–215).

Because the subject of carcinogenesis is one of the major thrusts in food toxicology, a detailed treatment of the factors affecting carcinogenesis is presented here and in the next chapter. A number of other factors may also influence the carcinogenic process; e.g., physical and emotional or psychological stresses; light; bacterial or viral diseases; and solid particles. Some of these factors have been briefly mentioned in other sections or chapters. However, as firm evidence in most cases has not yet been obtained supporting such alleged effects, these other factors are not discussed here.

Effect of Dose

A carcinogen, like other types of toxicants, possesses dual toxic responses depending on the dose: the immediate or acute response, and the chronic or delayed, the carcinogenic response. Thus, one may administer an increasing dose of a carcinogen from a virtually "no effect dose," progressing to a range of carcinogenic doses, thence to a range of sublethal toxic doses, and finally, to lethal doses. In this section, we will be concerned exclusively with the carcinogenic dose.

Two observed properties of the carcinogenic response that are dependent on the dose are latency and tumor incidence. Latency, also known as specific tumor induction time, is defined as that period of time from the initial exposure to the carcinogen to the appearance of the first tumor in the exposed population. Latency is sometimes expressed by some investigators as the median latent period, which is the time after exposure when 50% of a given population develop tumors. Others prefer to use the term mean latency, which is the arithmetic average of the individual latencies. The latency may vary from a few weeks to several years; the latter is seen in animals with long lifespan; e.g., humans. Within certain limits, latency is an inverse logarithmic function of the dose.

Tumor incidence is defined as that part or percentage of the surviving exposed population which develop tumors at a predetermined time period or age. In experimental oncology, the effective group is defined by many investigators as the number of surviving animals at the time the first tumor appears, or the number of animals surviving up to the time of the mean latent period.

Latency

Figure 4 shows double logarithmic plots (log-log) of latency as a function of daily dose of the carcinogens, 4-dimethylaminoazobenzene (4-DAB) (Druckrey 1954; Druckrey and Kupfmuller 1948) and diethylnitrosamines (DENA) (Druckrey et al. 1963). Many other examples showing similar relationships have also been reported (Druckrey 1975; Rajewsky et al. 1966). There have been criticisms (Arcos et al. 1968; Druckrey 1959) regarding the manner in which the data on induction time were obtained for these carcinogens. However, the data obtained with 4-DAB and DENA, showing the mathematical relationships between latency and dose, can be considered valid as a first approximation. Because of the difficulty and the large expenditure in time, effort, and resources needed in these types of experiments, accurate assessment of tumor latency by periodic sacrifice of a significant number of animals was not done. The values were determined by sampling "a few" of the experimental animals or by gross observation of tumors; e.g., by palpation. Thus, the points in the curves should be regarded as reasonable estimates. The general shape of the curves would probably not change if the actual points were determined.

The logarithmic relationships between dose and latency shown in Figure 4 are given in Equation 1.

$$\text{Log } t = -m\log d + \log k \tag{1}$$

By taking antilogarithms, Equation 1 reduces to

$$t\, d^{-m} = k; \quad t = k/d^m \tag{2}$$

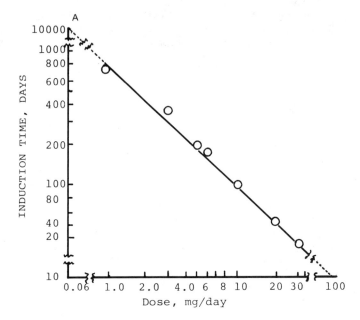

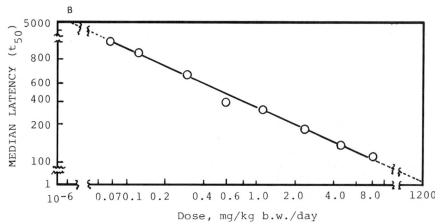

Figure 4. Log-Log plot of latency as a function of the daily doses for: A, 4-Dimethylaminoazobenzene. (From Druckrey 1954, used with permission.) B, Diethylnitrosamine. (From Druckrey et al. 1963, used with permission.)

where t = latency; d = dose; m = slope of the curve and k = the intercept on the axis of the ordinate, the latency. k represents the latency at any chosen unit dose.

In Equation 2, the slope m, according to Druckrey et al. (1963) is a characteristic of the particular carcinogen. For 4-DAB, m is almost equal to unity, so that the product dt = t, being almost a constant, is essentially equal to the minimum total dose necessary for maximum tumor induction. Equation 2 shows the inverse relationship between the latency and the dose and that the magnitude of m determines the degree of acceleration of the carcinogenic process.

Figure 4 is extrapolated beyond the lifespan of the rat on the assumption that Equation 2 can also apply to animals with longer lifespan; e.g., humans. It is clear that in carcinogenicity testing, the dose used may be too small to demonstrate this effect in animals with a short lifespan. This is especially true when m in Equation 2 is less than unity. The implications with regard to the human situation are obvious. Therefore, investigators have found it advantageous to use larger doses of suspected carcinogens in order to detect carcinogenicity potentials which would otherwise go undetected. An excellent example in this case is saccharin. Of course, many factors can increase or decrease the latency at any given dose.

The doses used in the experiments depicted in Figure 4 were designed to produce maximum tumor development with varying latency. These doses may be considered as "saturation doses." Animals in these experiments were exposed to the carcinogens continuously until the appearance of tumors. However, as in the case of 4-DAB, the effective doses below saturation level were inversely proportional to the latency. At lower doses, the longest latency also produced the lowest tumor incidence. Continuous exposure, therefore, is not an absolute requirement in the induction of cancer. This fact is illustrated in Figure 5: A single dose of ethyl nitrosourea is sufficient to induce cancer in nervous tissues (Druckrey et al. 1970a). In this case, the saturation dose appears to be 10 mg/kg.

It can be deduced from Figure 6 that Equation 2 also applies to a single exposure to a carcinogen. This observation demonstrates the independence of the carcinogenic process from the inducing agent after initiation has occurred. Figure 5 also provides evidence that the carcinogen triggers an irreversible change in some cellular function(s) or target site which causes the cell to digress to the neoplastic state.

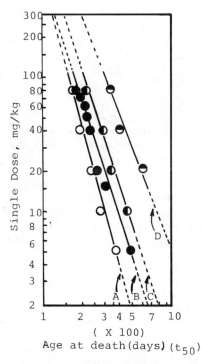

Figure 5. Semilogarithmic plot of the relationship between the dose of ethylnitrosourea and tumor incidence "Age of exposure to ENU: A, Postnatal day 1; B, transplacental, on day 13 to 18 of gestation; C, postnatal day 10; D, postnatal day 30. (From Druckrey et al. 1970; Ivankovic and Druckrey 1968, used with permission.)

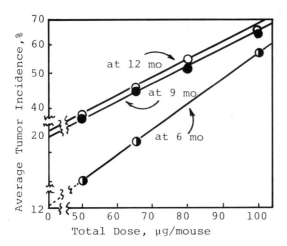

Figure 6. Semilogarithmic plot of the relationship between the dose of 3,4-benzpyrene and tumor incidence. (From Leiter and Shear 1942-1943, used with permission.)

Equation 2 appears to be valid for a number of carcinogens even with different chemical and physical properties (Druckrey 1959). This equation, if proven to be generally valid, would be useful in predicting the carcinogenic response in the case of low doses. However, its applicability to all types of carcinogens remains to be ascertained. Nevertheless, in the absence of firm evidence to the contrary and if it is assumed that all carcinogenic inductions have the same underlying mechanism(s), then Equation 2 may be considered valid for most chemical carcinogens. In fact, the annual death rate from cancer in the United States as a function of age shows similar logarithmic relationship as Equation 2 (Cairns 1975).

Tumor Incidence

Figures 6 and 7 show the semilogarithmic relationship between dose and tumor incidence. The logarithm of the cancer incidence due to 3,4-benzypyrene or 4-DAB, respectively, is directly proportional to the dose up to a certain value. For 4-DAB, no further increase in tumor incidence has been observed above a maximum dose of 700 mg (Druckrey 1959).

In Figure 6, the average tumor incidence as observed after 6, 9, and 12 months is plotted against the dose of benz(a)pyrene. A linear semilogarithmic relationship is observed. Actually, the dosage was not extended beyond 100 µg/mouse, so that the saturation dose is not readily apparent from the available data. These results are from the experiments of Leiter and Shear (1942-1943). Benz(a)pyrene was dissolved in tricaprylin and injected subcutaneously into strain A mice.

In both Figures 6 and 7, there appears to be a maximum tumor incidence for each specific dose. In the case of benz(a)pyrene, the slope of the 6-month curve indicates an acceleration of the tumor development with increasing doses. Projection of this curve to values over 100 µg/mice indicates that the same tumor incidence at 9 or 12 months, induced with approximately 125 µg of benz(a)pyrene, can be attained at 6 months with the same amount of carcinogen.

The results of a similar study with the same carcinogen under slightly different experimental conditions are shown in Figure 8 (Payne and Hueper 1960). The tumor incidence induced with different doses of carcinogen, applied singly, or once each month until the specified end period (i.e., 6, 12, 18, and 24 months) was recorded. Note that at 6 months (Fig. 8A, curve I), the monthly injections produced fewer tumors than single injections, even though mice were exposed to greater total doses

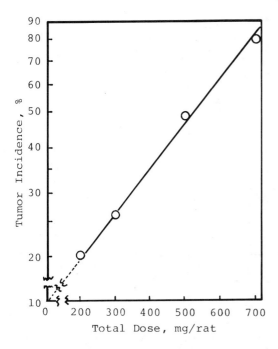

Figure 7. Semilogarithmic plot of the relationship between the dose of 4-dimethyl-aminoazobenzene and tumor incidence. (From Druckrey 1959, used with permission.)

with the monthly injections. At 12 months (Fig. 8A, curve IV), the tumor incidence at doses lower than 200 μg injected monthly was less than those produced by a single injection (Fig. 8A, curve III) of the same dose. As with the 6-month end period, a maximum saturation dose with single injections appears to be attained, above which no further increase in tumor incidence is observed. This maximum dose appears to be around 300 μg for the 6-month period and approximately 150 μg for the 12-month period. The full expression of carcinogenicity seems to be attained with approximately 150 μg benz(a)pyrene administered in single injections, since no further increase in tumor incidence is obtained even after 24 months with the higher doses (Fig. 8B, curve V).

Expression of carcinogenicity seems to be suppressed even after 6 months with repeated monthly injections, as shown by the lower incidences with this regimen (Fig. 8A, curves I and IV) compared to single injections (Fig. 8A, curves II and III). The suppression still occurs even at the lower doses given in the monthly injections over a period of 12 months. This suppression seems to be only a temporary occurrence, the multiple exposure producing a delayed response, since after 18 or 24 months, the tumor incidence with the multiple injections is significantly higher than in those given single injections (Fig. 8B, curve VI).

Some of the conclusions that may be drawn from Figure 8, at least with benz(a)-pyrene, are as follows: (1) A single exposure is sufficient to induce cancer in a significant number of subjects. (2) With single exposures, there is a dose threshold above which no greater increase in tumor incidence can be expected even with higher doses of this carcinogen. Multiple exposure may delay the expression of carcinogenicity and longer delay is observed at lower doses.

The dose-response behavior of benz(a)pyrene in this experiment is peculiar, in view of the dose threshold observed with single injections and progressively increased response with multiple injections. A reference to Figure 8A, curve II, with respect to

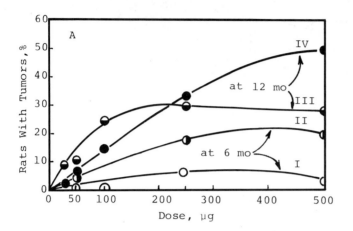

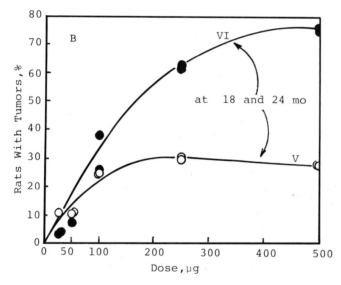

Figure 8. Tumor incidence induced by 3,4-benzpyrene at different doses for:
A, 6 and 12 months (curves I and IV) monthly injections; (curves II and III) single
injection. B, 18 and 24 months (curve V) monthly injections; (curve VI) single injection. (From Hueper 1960, used with permission.)

the response after 6 months, clearly demonstrates this peculiarity. Note that a single
injection of 250 μg of carcinogen produced a tumor incidence greater than 15% (Fig.
8A, curve I). A monthly dose of the same amount, giving a total dose of 150 μg, produced only about 6% tumor incidence. After 12 months, the single injection of 250 μg
produced a 30% tumor incidence. However, 12 monthly injections of the same dose,
giving a total dose of 250 μg, produced 32% tumor incidence. After 18 and 24 months
(Fig. 8B), this dose administered as a single injection did not produce any increase in
tumor incidence over that observed after 12 months. The tumor incidence of 60% following monthly injections for 18 months appears to be maximum, since no more increase
was observed after 24 months.

No factual explanation has been offered for the cellular events leading to the observed results. However, the data once again demonstrate that a single exposure is

sufficient to induce carcinogenesis, and that the hazard and intensity of effect are increased with multiple exposure to a potential carcinogen.

Other examples of dose-tumor incidence relationships can be cited (Saffioti et al. 1972; Truhaut and Dechambre 1972; Turusov et al. 1971; Weil 1972).

Carcinogens may be said to be unique toxicants because of their generally long latency before manifestation of the toxic effects to an apparently nontoxic dose. With most common toxicants, the effects are immediate, or at most, manifest in a few hours or days. In addition, the effects of most toxicants in sublethal doses wear off and disappear, so that the affected tissues resume their normal pattern or function. Subsequent exposure or contact with the same toxicant is a new episode; the physiological or pharmacological effects may have little or no bearing on the previous exposures.

The above statements, of course, apply to toxicants which are not physically accumulated in the tissues. Accumulated toxicants manifest their toxicity above a critical tissue level. One should also distinguish here those toxicants which do permanent damage to the nerve or brain tissues, whose effects in most cases are immediate.

With carcinogens, even exposure to vanishingly low levels may leave long-lasting effects on specific cell receptors. Certain cells are apparently permanently changed following initial exposure to a given dose of carcinogen. The changes becomes more aggravated with subsequent exposures. A series of cellular events are set in motion by the carcinogen, and evidence based on chromosomal studies suggests that a full blown cancer can arise from a single affected cell or, at most, a very few affected cells (Atkin 1970; Fialkow 1970). Once set in motion, this single neoplastic cell will be autonomous, and will thrive in the absence of the initiating carcinogen or its derivatives. The transformation is irreversible under physiological conditions. Unless destroyed, the autonomous neoplastic cells will undergo repeated cell division, producing a clone of cells. Such clones may still be vulnerable to the body's natural destructive or defense systems. However, a critical clonal size can be attained beyond the body's ability to destroy these cells without the assistance of external factors in the form of drugs, radiation, surgery, or a combination of these.

While the dose-latency and dose-tumor incidence phenomena have been demonstrated mostly with experimental animals, similar observations have been reported from epidemiological studies involving human beings. Unlike animals with short lifespans, the reported latency in human beings induced by occupational carcinogens ranges from a short 10 months for epithelioma formation from pitch, to as long as 50 to 60 years for the less carcinogenic shale and mineral oils (Henry 1947). A latency of 11 to 16 years have been estimated for bladder cancer among dye factory workers induced by 2-naphthylamine and benzidine (Goldblatt 1947), and 5 to 19 years for bladder tumors induced by 4-aminobiphenyl in similar types of subjects (Melick et al. 1955). The latency of tobacco-induced lung cancer has been estimated at 20 or more years (Cairns 1975).

The dose-tumor incidence phenomenon in humans has been more thoroughly studied for tobacco-induced cancers. This dose effect has been clearly demonstrated in the results of prospective and retrospective studies; i.e., the greater the number of cigarettes smoked, the greater the risk for lung cancer (U.S. Public Health Service 1964, 1971-1973).

Effect of Age

There are three aspects regarding the effect of age on the carcinogenic process. There are the: (1) specific sensitivity of the young to a carcinogen, especially the fetus and neonate; (2) decreased sensitivity of older persons; and (3) age-related prevalence or increase in tumor incidence among older persons. The latter is, of course, related to the latency. As discussed in the previous section, latency is dependent on the age when initial exposure to the carcinogen occurred as well as the intensity and frequency of exposure to specific carcinogens.

Juvenile Sensitivity to Carcinogenic Induction

Sensitivity of the very young to a carcinogen, especially the unborn organism and neonate, has been well documented in experimental animals (Della Porta and Terracini 1969; Toth 1968). For example, polycyclic aromatic hydrocarbons produce liver tumors when administered to newborn mice or rats, but do not affect the same organs when administered to young adult animals (Della Porta and Terracini 1969; Toth 1968). A similar observation was noted in mice administered aflatoxin B_1. Liver tumors are induced when the carcinogen is given after birth but not after weaning (Vesselinovitch et al. 1972). Similarly, newborn hamsters show similar susceptibility to aflatoxin-induced liver tumors compared to weaned animals (Homburger 1972), even though this difference in susceptibility is not as pronounced as those in rats (Weisburger et al. 1972). The age-related sensitivity of rats to ethylnitrosourea (ENU) neurocarcinogenesis is illustrated in Fig. 5 (Druckrey et al. 1970a). For example, a 10-day difference in the administration of 4 mg ENU/kg body weight soon after birth resulted in a 100-day difference in the median age mortality (t_{50}) from neurogenic tumors. This difference is more pronounced at lower doses, judging from the slopes of each curve. A 30-day difference in the administration of the carcinogen doubles the median age of death. The t_{50} is increased from 300 to 700 days when 10 mg/kg body weight is administered 30 days after birth, rather than 1 day after.

Transplacental Exposure to Carcinogens

The results of transplacental exposure to carcinogens as plotted in Figure 5, curve B, show t_{50} values intermediate between values corresponding to day 1 (curve A) and day 10 (curve C) of postnatal administration. This fact probably reflects a difference in the doses that finally come in contact with the fetus. Since some of the administered carcinogen will be taken up and metabolized by the mother's tissues, as well as the placenta, the carcinogenic dose in the fetus will be significantly reduced.

The fetal brain of rats is about 60 times more sensitive to carcinogens than that of the adult (Druckrey et al. 1967; Ivankovic and Druckrey 1968). The median carcinogenic dose for the fetal brain is 3 mg/kg compared to 180 mg/kg for the adult rat. There is also a fetal age element in the carcinogenic susceptibility of the fetus to various carcinogens (Druckrey 1973b; Druckrey et al. 1970a). For example, administration of even a high dose of 60 mg/kg ethylnitrosurea to BD-IX rats before the twelfth day of gestation was not carcinogenic to the offspring. Tumor development in the offspring increased significantly when administration of the carcinogen commenced on the thirteenth day of gestation. Maximum tumor yield was obtained when treatment was done on the eighteenth day of gestation; the tumor yield remained constant during the perinatal period.

The fetal age element in the postnatal develpment of a tumor suggests that a certain stage of development or differentiation is required in order for the neoplastic potential of susceptible cells to be expressed. Even dimethylnitrosamines and diethylnitrosamines, which are potent carcinogens to the adult rat, are not carcinogenic to the fetus if administered on the fifteenth day of gestation. These agents are carcinogenic to offspring if administered right before birth — the twenty-second day of gestation (Druckrey 1973b; Ivankovic 1972). It has been suggested that this fetal resistance toward these powerful carcinogens indicates the absence of activating enzymes, in this case, specific hydroxylases. These enzymes seem to develop during the latter part of gestation, since by then these carcinogens become active in the fetus. The results of Spatz and Lacquer (1967), showing the carcinogenicity of hydroxymethylazoxy methanol to the rat fetus, emphasize the importance of this hydroxylation process to the activity of the carcinogen in the rat fetus. It is carcinogenic even during the early stages of development and the inactivity of azoxymethane, an isomer of dimethylnitrosame (Druckrey 1973).

The sensitivity of the very young to carcinogens as observed in animals probably also applies to humans.

Fetal induction of cancer in humans is probably exemplified by recent observations of the development of a rare form of vaginal cancer in prepubertal girls. These girls were born of mothers treated with sufficient doses of the synthetic estrogen diethyl-stilbestrol, which was used to prevent (although not conclusively proved) threatened or habitual abortion (Herbst et al. 1971; Miller 1971, 1973).

Even though cancer is predominantly a disease of old age, there is at present an increasing frequency of cancer in childhood and youth. The average annual incidence per 100,000 for the years 1969 to 1971 was 20.43, 11.64, and 11.52 for the 0 to 4-, 5 to 9-, and 10 to 14-year-old children, respectively (Third National Cancer Survey 1974). One may conclude that exposure must have occurred during the prenatal or, at the most, neonatal stage of development (Peller 1960). This is proposed because of the essentially long latency of the carcinogenic process, especially in regard to weak carcinogens, or to the very low levels of exposure of these substances which must be assumed in these cases.

There are a number of possible explanations for the heightened susceptibility of the very young toward various carcinogens. In the first place, the developing young tissues have higher levels of cellular replication. This could, in part, increase the sensitivity of the very young to carcinogens, since, as can be shown in adults, increased susceptibility can be induced by increasing the rate of cell replication (Weisburger and Williams 1975). Second, enzymes involved in drug metabolism are usually at very low levels in the young (Brodie and Gillette 1971). Thus, detoxification of chemical carcinogens will be slow. For example, it has been shown that the rate of removal of 9,10-dimethyl-1,2-benzanthracene from the body of neonatal mice is lower than in adults (Domsky et al. 1963). Studies have shown the capability of fetuses to metabolize carcinogens to their active forms (Gillette et al. 1973; Pelkonen et al. 1973). For example, the fetus has been shown to possess nitroreductases and enzymes required for the epoxidation of polycyclic aromatic hydrocarbons, but to be deficient in glucuronic acid conjugase and epoxide hydrase; both of the latter enzymes are involved in the detoxification process (Brodie and Gillette 1971). Therefore, the increased sensitivity of the fetus and the neonate to carcinogens has firm molecular and cellular bases.

Prevalence of Cancer in Older Persons

The other age-related aspect of carcinogenesis is the observed high incidence of cancer with increasing age. This fact is illustrated in Figures 9 and 10. Note that in Figure 9, a log-log plot of the annual number of cases shows a linear relationship. A similar relationship exists for cancer of the large intestine (Fig. 10). The curves in Figure 9 depict the cancer incidence in both white males and females. The data were obtained from a survey from 1969 to 1971 in the United States (Third National Cancer Study 1974). There are three parts to the curve, represented by the three pairs of lines. The first slope, culminating at age 30 in males and age 25 in females, is called the juvenile cancer latency curve. If these curves are extrapolated to values approaching zero incidence, the age values for prenatal or neonatal exposure to unknown carcinogens can be proposed. Again, bearing in mind the prolonged latency of cancer induction, this hypothesis based on such projections becomes plausible. The latency of 25 to 30 years is within the known latency values deduced from human epidemiological studies.

The second set of curves in Figure 9 shows a steep rise in cancer incidence, culminating in a sharp peak or vertex. This point in the male curve corresponds to age 66 years, which is approximately the estimated average lifespan of white males in the United States during that period. The vertex in the female curve corresponds to age 62 years. This point may have a relationship with the average age of the end of the menopausal period. This point suggests that tissues under significant hormonal control such as the breasts, cervix, and ovaries account for the most frequent cancer sites in women (Third National Cancer Survey 1974). This part of the cancer incidence-age

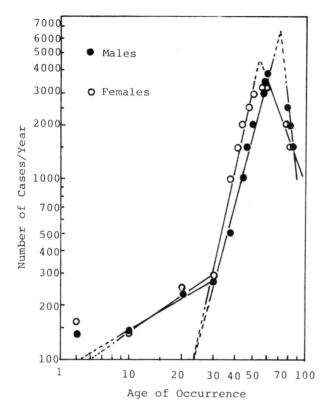

Figure 9. Log-log plot of the age specific cancer incidence rates for all sites (except skin and carcinoma in situ) by sex in the United States, all races combined for 1969 to 1971. Note the presence of three different slopes representing three age groups: below age 30, between age 30 and 65 or 75, and above 65 or 75. Extrapolation of these slopes to zero incidence would intersect a point in the abscissa representing the age of initiation of most cancers. The slope for the below 30 group would show a negative age value, suggesting a transplacental initiation. (From National Cancer Institute 1974, used with permission.)

curve is termed the adult cancer latency curve. By projecting the adult cancer latency curve downward to values approaching zero incidence, the age values suggest child-hood or pubertal exposure to carcinogens. A latency period of 20 to 50 years is also consistent with observed epidemiological data on certain human cancers with known causative agents.

The clustering of cancer with advancing age reflects an important aspect of car-cinogenesis. The events leading to cancer begin very much earlier in life, and have been postulated to be specific mutations (Cairns 1975). These mutational events may be initiated in the cell or its progeny at any time during the life of the individual. There-fore, the probability that a mutation will occur inducing neoplastic transformation in-creases with age.

The third set of cancer incidence-age curve shows a sharp drop in cancer inci-dence after age 66 to 70 years in men and 62 to 65 years in women. One may construe this drop as indicating that the probability of contracting cancer decreases significant-ly once past the critical ages corresponding to the vertices in the cancer incidence curves. In other words, persons who pass this critical age with no subclinical lesions of cancer have a greater probability of being cancer-free for the rest of their lifetime.

The logarithmic relationship between age and cancer incidence indicates an accelerated process similar to that exhibited by the dose-latency curves shown previously (Figs. 4 and 5). This means that the rate of cancer development increases quite rapidly with advancing age, especially between age 25 and 70 years.

The characteristic logarithmic plot of the relationship between age and cancer incidence appears to hold true for individuals with cancer of the large intestine, shown in Figure 10. Calculation of the slope of this curve gives a value of approximately 5. Cairns (1975) believes that this value reflects the number of mutations required for the development of tumors.

Extrapolation of the curve in Figure 10 to zero incidence again suggests that initiation of this cancer occurs at a very young age. Initiation at puberty is consistent with the physiological events occurring at this stage in life. The involvement of hormones in this case is unmistakable. As discussed later in this chapter (pp. 181—192), hormones play a significant role in cancer development.

The curve in Figure 10 differs from those in Figure 9 because it has no juvenile latency slope. This is consistent with the observed rarity of this form of cancer in very young people.

It has been established that the cancer observed later in life may have been initiated at a very early age. However, the specific sensitivity of the very young to a particular carcinogen will determine whether or not such an exposure will result in a neoplastic change. It is therefore important that exposure of children, especially of the newborn, to these substances be minimized. It has been argued that the very small quantities of carcinogens to which the newborns and children are exposed are inconsequential and harmless. However, one must bear in mind the specific sensitivity of the newborn, the multiple exposures of long duration, the multiplicity of carcinogenic compounds to which one may be exposed, and the presence of other factors which can enhance the carcinogenic process. Again, there is mounting evidence to indicate that a single neoplastic cell under the optimum conditions may be all that is necessary for the development of a clinical tumor (Nowell 1976).

Effect of Sex

There is a difference in the sensitivity of the males and females toward the development of neoplasia. This has been clearly shown in Figure 9, which is discussed in the previous section.

Because men and women, in general, have different personal habits, occupations, and other sex-related factors, their exposures to carcinogens and therefore their susceptibility to carcinogenesis is expected to differ if only because of these exogenous factors. Thus, when comparing differences between the male and female, it is probably more accurate to examine the cancer incidence among children, since in this population the carcinogenic effect will probably be less influenced by the factors affecting adults. Table 4 shows a comparison between the cancer incidence in 5 major sites among children below the age of 15 (Schottenfeld 1975). There is a highly statistically significant difference in susceptibility for some cancers in boys and girls. Girls are more highly susceptible to kidney cancers, ($p < 0.005$) while the opposite is seen with lymphoma ($p < 0.005$). Boys tend to show only a slightly greater tendency toward developing leukemia and other cancers. Both appear to have equal susceptibility to bone, brain, and other CNS cancers.

In overall cancer deaths during that survey period, boys accounted for more than 56% of all cancer deaths.

In older persons, it is difficult to compare the male-female susceptibility because, as already mentioned, personal habits and occupational hazards can influence the observed cancer incidence. For example, according to a 1970 survey, the lung cancer incidence in men is more than seven times that of women (Third National Cancer Survey 1974). This is because men smoke cigarettes more often and to a greater degree than women. Since tobacco smoking has also been correlated to other forms of cancer,

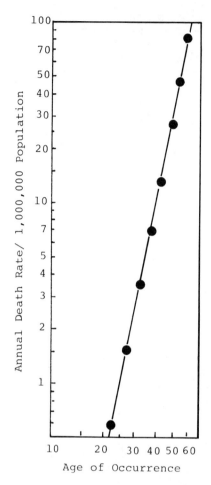

Figure 10. Log-log plot of the annual mortality rate of cancer of the large intestines in men. Extrapolation of the curve to the zero rate also bisects the abscissa at a point between age 10 and 20 (not shown in figure). This point is virtually the same as that in Figure 9. (From Cairns 1975, used with permission.)

cancer susceptibility in organs or tissues common to the male and female cannot be definitely related to specific gender susceptibility (Wynder et al. 1975). Nevertheless, even considering the influence of exogenous factors, a greater innate cancer susceptibility in the adult male may still be the underlying factor in the observed phenomenon, as shown in Table 5. A comparison in the age-adjusted incidence rate of cancer in various anatomical sites shows that except for cancer of the thyroid and the gall bladder males showed greater susceptibility to cancer than females. This fact holds true for both the white and black populations in the United States (Third National Cancer Survey 1974).

The differences between males and females have been demonstrated quite unequivocally in experimental animals. For example, liver cancer can be induced by N-2-fluorenylacetamide much more readily in male than in female rats, although some strains of female rats are not completely resistant (Gutmann et al. 1972; Miller and Miller 1971b). Male mice are less resistant than females to liver cancer induced by dimethylor diethylnitrosamines (Rao and Vesselinovitch 1973; Vesselinovitch 1969). Examples of

Table 4. Differences in Cancer Incidence in Five Major Sites Between Boys and Girls under 15 years of Age (U.S., 1966)

Cancer site	Percentage of total cancer deaths	
	Boys	Girls
Leukemia	47	44
Brain and CNS	22	23
Lymphomas	9	5
Bone	4	5
Kidney	3	6
Other sites	15	17
All sites	56.3	43.7

Source: Schottenfeld (1975), used with permission.

differences in male and female susceptibility to various carcinogens are given in Table 6. Clearly, in most instances, male rats or mice show greater sensitivity to cancer induction.

Aside from the obvious hormonal differences in males and females which can have an effect on cancer susceptibility, other sex-linked biochemical differences exist which may account for the greater cancer susceptibility in one sex compared to the other. For example, the higher susceptibility of male rats to liver cancer induced by N-2-fluorenylacetamide is due to the higher levels of the enzyme sulfotransferase (six to eight times) in the male rat than in the female. This enzyme is responsible for the activation of this procarcinogen to its sulfate ester, the active carcinogen (Weisburger et al. 1972). The increased susceptibility to carcinogens may reflect the greater activities of drug metabolizing enzymes as observed in the male (Conney 1967; Conney and Burns 1972).

The sex-linked differences in cancer susceptibility in children, as discussed earlier, has its counterpart in the newborn or sexually immature experimental animals (Toth 1968).

Hormonal Influences in Chemical Carcinogenesis

Hormones are regulatory substances which are produced by specialized groups of cells or glands and secreted directly into the bloodstream. These substances have a profound influence on the function, activity, and metabolic processes in target tissues or cells. Specialized hormone-producing glands include the hypothalamus, pituitary, thyroid, pineal, pancreas, adrenals, parathyroids, ovaries, and testes. Specialized hormone-producing cells are also located in the gastrointestinal mucosa and other tissues.

Hormones are secreted in response to external or internal stimuli or according to predetermined rhythms or cycles. They may be secreted according to certain time-dependent internal body indicators. For example, certain sexual hormones are not secreted or do not manifest their effects until a specific time in the life cycle. The diurnal rhythmic secretions of adrenal hormones and the cyclical monthly secretion of the gonadotropins in the pituitary glands are examples of the complex and still not well understood processes regulating hormonal secretions.

Some of these rhythmic secretions may be influenced to some extent by external factors such as light and temperature. The secretion of many hormones may also

Table 5. Differences in Cancer Incidence Rates Between Men and Women (U.S.)[a]

Cancer site	Whites		Blacks	
	Male	Female	Male	Female
All sites except cervix in situ	337.4	268.9	381.4	253.8
Lip, tongue, mouth	10.5	4.4	9.6	2.8
Esophagus	4.6	1.4	16.0	3.3
Stomach	15.2	6.8	21.0	8.2
Colon	34.5	29.5	29.6	26.0
Rectum	17.4	11.0	13.8	9.8
Liver	3.1	1.3	6.5	1.7
Gallbladder and ducts	2.5	3.1	1.6	3.0
Pancreas	11.9	7.3	14.9	8.5
Lung and bronchus	69.6	13.1	77.4	13.5
Bladder	22.6	6.0	12.4	3.9
Kidney	8.0	3.8	7.1	3.7
Bones and joints	1.2	0.8	1.3	0.3
Soft tissues	2.3	1.7	1.8	1.8
Melanomas — skin	3.3	3.3	0.5	0.6
Eye and nervous system	6.8	5.3	5.3	4.2
Thyroid	2.1	5.1	1.3	3.5
Lymphomas	15.6	9.8	16.6	8.2
Leukemias	12.4	7.4	10.6	5.7
Other sites	20.7	15.5	23.0	19.9

[a]Age-adjusted, 1970 standard population.
Source: The Third National Cancer Survey (1974).

depend on the level of specific exogenous or endogenous substances in the body fluids or tissues. For example, insulin and thyroxine secretions respond to the levels of glucose and iodine in body fluids and tissues.

Hormones regulate certain critical or rate-limiting reactions in metabolic and physiological processes. Thus, hormones have far reaching influences in metabolic activities of cells. Their influence in carcinogenesis is therefore to be expected. This is particularly true in tissues which are highly hormone dependent; e.g., the mammary gland. The hormonal interplay in the chemical induction of tumors in this tissue has been well documented (even though information in this respect is still incomplete), and is discussed in the following section.

Table 6. Differences in Susceptibility to Various Carcinogens Between Male and Female Rats or Mice

Carcinogens	Tumor type	Species	Male	Female	Ref.
4-Diemethylaminobenzeneazo-1-naphthalene	liver	rat	>[a]	<[b]	Mulay and O'Gara (1959)
4-Dimethylaminoazobenzene	liver	rat	>	<	Mulay and O'Gara (1959)
4-Dimethylaminobenzeneazo-2-naphthalene	liver	rat	=[c]	=[c]	Mulay and O'Gara (1959)
o-Aminotoluene	liver	mouse	<	>	Miller and Miller (1952)
1-Phenylazo-2-naphthol	liver	mouse	>	<	Kirby and Peacock (1949)
N-2-fluorenylacetamide	liver	rat	>	<	Gutman et al. (1972)
Dimethylnitrosamine	liver	mouse	>	<	Magee (1971)
	liver	rat	<	>	Magee et al. (1976)
Diethylnitrosamine	liver	mouse	>	<	Magee (1971)
	liver	rat	<	>	Magee et al. (1976)

[a]Greater susceptibility.
[b]Lesser susceptibility;
[c]Equal susceptibility but shorter latency in males than females.

Hormones and Chemical Mammary Carcinogenesis

Mammary cancer, as shown in Table 5 in the preceding section, is the leading cancer form in women of all races in the United States. It outranks all other types of cancer in women (American Cancer Society 1983; Third National Cancer Survey 1974). Thus, for this reason, this form of cancer has attracted intense interest.

As we shall see, mammary cancer has strong hormonal aspects. The metabolic pathways leading to the biosynthesis of hormones that have important bearing on the mammary gland are shown in Fig. 11. The mammary tissues are particularly sensitive to hormones. Foremost among these are the pituitary gonadotropic hormones (gonadotropins), prolactin, and the luteinizing hormones (LH). Note that these hormones stimulate the ovaries to synthesize progesterone, which is the precursor of various androgens and estrogens. The latter hormones also have effects on the tissues of the mammary gland. The pathways shown in Figure 11 are indicative of the complex interplay of hormones in processes in the mammary tissues, particularly in mammary carcinogenesis. However, the actual mechanisms by which these hormones regulate mammary carcinogenesis is largely unknown. Much progress in this direction has occurred in recent years.

Human Studies The induction of cancer in the mammary tissues is particularly influenced by those hormones that have specific effects on these tissues under normal conditions. Certain hormones, or their analogs, for example, estrogen and its

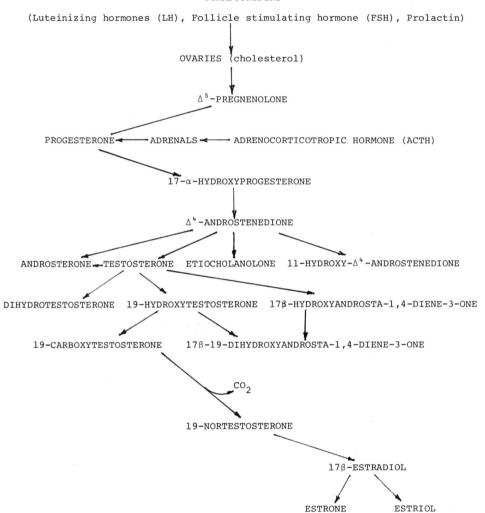

Figure 11. Schematic representation of the metabolic interrelationships between different sexual hormones.

synthetic analog, diethylstilbestrol, are carcinogens in their own right. While this fact is essential to the overall knowledge of carcinogenesis, a discussion of this subject is beyond the scope of this book.

Hormonal abnormalities have been observed to accompany carcinogenesis of the breast (Bodansky 1975). However, it is difficult to determine whether these abnormalities precede or result from cancer induction. Nevertheless, some studies have indicated that such abnormalities may predispose certain women to mammary cancer. Prospective studies undertaken in Guernsey, United Kingdom (Bulbrook 1970; Bulbrook and Hayward 1967) showed that a majority of women who were diagnosed subsequently with breast cancer excreted urinary 17-hydroxycorticosteroids, androsterone, and etiocholanolone in amounts that were significantly below the median value of the control group. The latter were matched for age, weight, menopausal status, and other parameters. This result may suggest an abnormal progesterone metabolism, since, as shown in Figure 11, these are metabolites of this hormone.

Progesterone is secreted by both the ovaries and the adrenal glands. The progesterone secretion in the ovaries is controlled by the gonadotropins, and that in the adrenals, by adrenocorticotropic hormone (ACTH). Progesterone levels in the blood vary with the menstrual cycle and are produced in a significant amount by the corpus luteum in preparation for pregnancy. In addition to other functions associated with ovulation and reproduction, progesterone also influences the growth of the mammary gland. The continuing production of progesterone in the corpus luteum is controlled by prolactin.

The excretion of 17-hydroxycorticosteroids also gives an indication of the status of progesterone metabolism in the adrenals. The degree of excretion of androsterone and etiocholanolone suggests the status of not only progesterone metabolism in the ovaries but also of that of the androgens and estrogens. The decreased excretion of etiocholanolone and androsterone that have been noted in certain women by Bulbrook and Hayward (1967) may suggest a diminished synthesis of progesterone, or an increased conversion of this hormone to testosterone, and consequently, to the estrogens.

It should be noted that the abnormality of sex hormone metabolism observed by Bulbrook et al. (1971), indicated by the decreased excretion of etiocholanolone, occurred long before breast cancer was detected in these women. The shortest time interval between urinary collection and analysis and breast cancer diagnosis was 5 months; the longest interval was 108 months; the mean interval was 44 months. Seven of the 21 women who developed breast cancer already gave low etiocholanolone excretion 5 to 9 months earlier.

It is noteworthy that in one study the excretion of estradiol and estriol in breast cancer patients was significantly lower than in the normal populations (Marmorston et al. 1965). If this were true in precancer patients, then by reference to Figure 11 these results may suggest that there is a hormonal defect predisposing women to mammary cancer. The hormonal abnormality indicated by the decreased excretion of etiocholanolone and androsterone (Bulbrook et al. 1971) may not be in the immediate steps leading to testosterone production, but rather in the steps preceding the synthesis of the above metabolites, probably in the production of progesterone.

The difference in cancer susceptibility between single, married, nulliparous, and multiparous women also suggests a significant hormonal influence. It is observed, for example, that single women between 30 and 68 years of age show a significantly higher breast cancer incidence than married women. This age bracket represents most of the active reproductive years in a woman's life. The significant increase in cancer incidence approaching middle age can be explained in terms of the unusually long cancer latency in humans. It also has been observed that the breast cancer incidence is significantly higher in those who were older at their first pregnancy, who were younger at menarche, and who had fewer pregnancies (Zippin and Petrakis 1971). Mazzoleni's study (1960), also supporting the hormonal influence in breast cancer, found that the number of children of breast cancer patients can be correlated with the cancer incidence. These observations are illustrated in Figure 12. Note that there is almost a linear inverse relationship between the number of children born to a woman and her susceptibility to breast cancer. Thus, the evidence shows that childbearing tends to protect a woman against breast cancer and that the greater the number of children, the less susceptible a woman becomes. The steepness of the curve in Figure 12 points to the strong influence that multiple pregnancies has in protecting women against mammary cancer. The hormonal mechanisms involved which increase a multiparous woman's resistance to breast cancer have not been determined. However, if results from animal studies are any indication, the increased resistance of women to breast cancer may be a result of lactation (Marchant 1958).

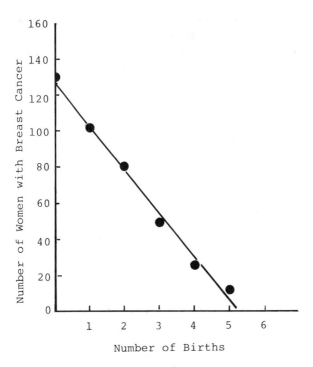

Figure 12. Inverse relationship between the number of births and breast cancer incidence among a group of women subjects (From Mazzoleni 1960, used with permission.)

Animal Studies   Likewise, animal studies have abundantly demonstrated the strong hormonal influences in the induction of mammary cancer by certain chemicals. However, in terms of latency and cancer incidence, earlier studies have demonstrated that the effect of breeding and pregnancy in animals on mammary chemical carcinogenesis is opposite to that of the general mammary cancer induction observed in women. This is also the case with spontaneous animal tumors. For example, early workers in the field of experimental carcinogenesis reported that breeding mice had shorter mammary cancer latency and greater cancer incidence than did virgin mice (Muhlbock and Van Rijssel 1954). The cancer incidence was even much lower in ovariectomized mice. Likewise, mice which were experimentally manipulated in order to have a rapid succession of pregnancies had a higher tumor incidence than normally breeding mice; virgin mice had zero incidence (Muhlbock and Van Rijssel 1954). It has been observed, however, that the increased susceptibility to cancer in mice during pregnancy is decreased or avoided if the mice are allowed to lactate normally (Marchant 1958). Thus, suppression of lactation in one side of the set of breasts of carcinogen-treated mice by excision of the nipples caused increased tumor incidence on this side as compared to the normal side (Biancifiori and Caschera 1972; Marchant 1958, 1959).

In mammary cancer induced by 20-methylcholanthrene (20-MC), for example, breeding or pregnancy resulted in a shorter latent period in dab mice (Kirschbaum et al. 1944) or in Sprague Dawley rats (Dao et al. 1959). In the case of the rats, as reported by the latter researchers, 50% of those treated with 20-MC for 60 days developed mammary cancer in 60 to 65 days. On the other hand, 95% of the rats treated with the same amount of chemical, 20 to 25 days prior to pregnancy, developed mammary cancer during the first 2 weeks of pregnancy. In fact, the tumors increased in size and number as the pregnancy progressed. However, the tumors in this case started to regress within 1 to 3 weeks after parturition. This regression is probably due to the increased lactation after parturition.

The opposite effects of pregnancy in mice and women on the induction of mammary cancer is to be expected considering the differences in hormonal characteristics betweeen these species. For example, Muhlbock (1958) points out that there is no luteal phase in the estrous cycle of the mice, and therefore, progesterone production is not increased during that cycle as observed in women. Mice also do not undergo menopause, so that the decreased mammary cancer incidence in women after the menopause is not seen in mice.

Notwithstanding these hormonal differences, the experimental demonstration of the hormonal influence in mammary cancer induction in these animals provides valuable information toward the understanding of the mechanism of mammary carcinogcnesis.

The following sections discuss several animal studies showing the roles of hormones in mammary chemical carcinogenesis. Considering the relationships among hormones, these studies have shown that hormones high in the hierarchy of endocrine control and metabolism, such as the gonadotropin-releasing factors, prolactin and progesterone, tend to increase the potency of certain polycyclic aromatic hydrocarbons with respect to the induction of mammary cancer. On the other hand, those in the lower level, i.e., estrogens and androgens, tend to depress mammary carcinogenesis, except when the latter hormones are administered in combination with progesterone.

Pituitary hormones: The hormonal dependency of mammary chemical carcinogenesis in rats and mice has been established by several workers using hypophysectomized (Noble and Walters 1954), bilaterally ovariectomized (Jull 1954) animals, or hormonal antagonists, such as Analog I (D-Leu^6-DesGlyNH$_2$^{10}-Pro-ethylamide^9) (GnRH), an antagonist of the gonadotropin-releasing factor (Johnson et al. 1976). The use of these procedures clearly inhibited the induction of mammary cancer with 9,10-dimethyl-1,2-benzanthracene (DMBA), and in the case of ovariectomized animals, with 20-MC as well (Jull 1954).

The rat mammary gland appears to be highly sensitive to DMBA carcinogenesis between the ages of 29 and 60 days (Huggins et al. 1961). This sensitivity coincides with the significant increase in the prolactin level in the blood. This hormone begins to appear in the serum about 15 days after birth and becomes distinctly detectable at 30 days of age (Furth 1973). Likewise, there is a rapid increase in serum estrogen level at age 19 days (Weisz and Gunzalus 1973). These increases in hormonal activity coincide with the unusual sensitivity of these animals to DMBA mammary carcinogenesis, and probably partly explains this phenomenon.

The very strong influence of prolactin on mammary carcinogenesis has been demonstrated by the effect of subcarcinogenic doses of 3-methylcholanthrene (same compound as 20-MC). No tumors developed in rats when a subcarcinogenic dose of 10 mg was applied. However, when this dose was combined with prolactin administration, an 85% mammary cancer incidence resulted (Kim and Furth 1960). Prolactin by itself is noncarcinogenic. These results have significant implications on human mammary carcinogenesis, since it is quite likely that most humans will be exposed frequently to very small doses of carcinogens in food, water, and the environment. The carcinogenic hazard is, of course, aggravated by the possibility of prolonged exposure to even very small doses of carcinogen.

Prolactin probably exerts its influence in conjunction with progesterone and estrogen, since normally the development of the mammary alveolar system is stimulated by the latter hormones, sensitizing these tissues to the action of prolactin (Cantarow and Schepartz 1967). Prolactin, in turn, stimulates RNA and protein synthesis in the mammary tissues (Orten and Neuhaus 1975). It is noted in the next section how a combination of progesterone and estrogen resulted in an increased incidence of mammary cancer induced by 20-MC (Jull 1954).

Ovarian hormones: In ovariectomized IF mice, the induction of mammary cancer by 20-MC requires the administration of both estrogen and progesterone (Jull 1954).

In this case, the increase in tumor incidence depended on the dose of the combined hormones. Thus, a weekly application increased tumor incidence from 6 to 10% without the hormones, and to 29% with the hormones; however, three applications of the hormones at biweekly intervals gave an 82% tumor incidence (Jull 1954). In intact female mice, the incidence following the application of 20-MC applied three times at biweekly intervals was 38%. In ovariectomized mice, under the same conditions, except that estrogen was also administered, the incidence was 10%. In the weekly application with 20-MC, the tumor incidence was 45%, if testosterone plus estrogen were used instead of progesterone plus estrogen (Jull 1954).

Progesterone injected three times per week in intact rats treated with 2-acetamido-fluorene (2-AF) produced a pronounced increase in tumor incidence, from 30 to 85% (Cantarow et al. 1948). This had little effect on rats receiving 2 mg of 20-MC daily (Shay et al. 1952). Progesterone, however, reduced the latency of mammary cancer induced by 20-MC from 50 to 41 days. This decrease may not seem significant, but when one considers the relatively short latency and the good reproducibility obtained by these researchers, a decrease of 7 days is significant.

The placental hormone lactogen has both prolactin and growth hormone activity, and like prolactin, it also promotes progesterone secretion in the ovaries (Nagasawa and Yanai 1973). Thus, it is not surprising that these workers reported that lactogen also promotes mammary carcinogenesis during pregnancy. It is possible that this hormone exerts its cocarcinogenic activity in conjunction with progesterone and other sex hormones.

An interesting observation is that the estrogen estradiol, by itself or in combination with progesterone, causes a significant delay in the latency of tumors induced by DMBA (McCormick and Moon 1973).

Similarly, the androgen dihydrotestosterone* also causes a delay in the latency of mammary tumors induced by DMBA (Huggins et al. 1959). This is in contrast to the effect of estrogen plus testosterone mentioned earlier in this section (Jull 1954). The fact that dihydrotestosterone (Fig. 11) does not serve as a precursor for the biosynthesis of the estrogens estrone and estradiol (Orten and Neuhaus 1975) may be relevant in these observations. However, testosterone is a precursor to the estrogens (Fig. 11), and its administration may increase the level of the later hormones. Consequently, a greater sensitivity to mammary cancer may be expected.

Mammary Chemical Carcinogenesis in the Male   Mammary cancer in the male is extremely rare. The Third National Cancer Survey (1974) has shown an age-adjusted incidence rate in men of all races in the United States as one-hundredth of the incidence in women. Nevertheless, hormonal influence of breast cancer in men is manifested by the effects of orchidotomy and adrenalectomy. Both these surgical procedures have resulted in substantial regression of mammary cancer in men.

Animal studies likewise have demonstrated the influence of hormones in mammary chemical carcinogenesis in males. For example, in male Wistar rats, a higher incidence of mammary tumors was observed when both estrogen and 20-MC were administered, than when either one was administered alone (Shay et al. 1952). With 2-AF and estrogen, the incidence was lower, but the observation is significant, since none has been observed with the carcinogen alone (Cantarow et al. 1948). Eleven of 16 IF mice administered estrogen and receiving repeated biweekly intranasal instillation of 20-MC developed mammary cancer. With a smaller dosage of the carcinogen, i.e., three biweekly paintings of 20-MC, two mammary cancers developed in 77 mice when estrogen was administered. With both progesterone and estrogen, four tumors developed in 14 animals (Jull 1954). Again, as in female animals, this latter result demonstrates the greater cocarcinogenic effect of progesterone combined with estrogen.

The importance of ovarian hormones in the induction of mammary tumors in the male rats treated with a carcinogen has been dramatically demonstrated in castrated

---

*This hormone is not produced in the ovaries.

animals. These castrates showed increased incidence of mammary tumors if the ovaries were also grafted at the same time (Dao et al. 1962). The induction of breast cancer in males who obviously have relatively "dormant" mammary tissues demonstrates the relative potency of hormones in augmenting the carcinogenicity of chemicals. Chemicals alone cannot induce mammary tumors in the male mice, but tumors will develop after chemical treatment if the animals also possess a transplanted ovary (Marchant 1958).

The mammary gland is a good example of a tissue where hormones have a very significant influence on carcinogenesis. No doubt, there are other hormone-dependent reproductive tissues, e.g., the ovaries, vagina, testes, prostate, penis, and others, in which the development of neoplasms also have strong hormonal influences. However, for the purposes of our discussion regarding the effects of hormones on chemical carcinogenesis in hormone-dependent tissues, the example of the mammary gland will suffice.

Hormonal Influences on Chemical Carcinogenesis in Nonreproductive Tissues

Even though mammary tumors are highly hormone dependent, these are not good examples of hormonal dependency of tumors in general. Hormonal dependency of the induction and growth of tumors arising from nonreproductive tissues has been reported, especially in experimental animals. These observations demonstrate the influence of hormones in chemical carcinogenesis without the added complication of the comparatively high hormonal dependency. Again, the mechanisms by which these hormones influence carcinogenesis in less hormone-dependent tissues is far from clear.

The term hormone-dependent used in this context means that a particular tissue is stimulated into mitotic and secretory activity over and beyond the normal metabolic requirements of that tissue. These tissues are stimulated into activity by specific hormones in response to special needs of the body. For example, the thyroid gland becomes hyperplastic in response to stimulation by the thyroid-stimulating hormone (TSH) following iodine deficiency.

Pituitary Hormones   Some of the influences of pituitary hormones on chemical carcinogenesis have been demonstrated in liver tumors. Clearly, the influence of these hormones becomes evident when the pituitary is removed and the carcinogen is applied. Thus, hepatocarcinogenesis, for example, from 3'-methyl-4-dimethylaminoazobenzene (3'-Me-DAB) was inhibited when the pituitary was excised (Griffin et al. 1955). The inhibition in this case is more significant, since food consumption of the experimental and control animals was equalized. Compared to hypophysectomized rats, the control animals rapidly developed liver cirrhosis, extensive bile duct proliferation, and increased protein-bound dye in the liver. Individually, both growth hormone and adrenocorticotropic hormone (ACTH) partially reversed the effect of hypophysectomy on hepatic tumor inhibition. Nonpituitary hormones such as cortisone, deoxycortisone, and testosterone had no effect. Thus, the pituitary hormone-dependence of liver tumor induction is demonstrable, but the occurrence of partial reversal only suggests the possible influence of other pituitary hormones.

Drugs such as 4-hydroxypropiophenone which suppress pituitary function also inhibit liver tumor induction by 4-dimethylaminoazobenzene (Baba 1957).

Since in studies on the influence of hormones in carcinogenesis some questions arise regarding the removal of the pituitary gland, "pituitary dwarf" mice would probably be more suitable experimental subjects. These animals do not show the general malaise following hypophysectomy and resultant decreased food intake. As discussed in Chapter 7, a decrease in food intake may affect tumor induction, beclouding the effect of hypophysectomy. Pituitary dwarf mice fail to secrete one or more tropic hormones (Smith and MacDowell 1930). Consequently, they remain infantile and sluggish and fail to develop normally. As would be expected, the induction of hepatoma in these animals with 2-acetamidofluorene (2-AF) is delayed (Bielschowsky 1961).

The effect of pituitary hormones is also seen in the induction of tumors of the skin by various chemicals. Removal of the pituitary gland results in a delay in the induction of local sarcomas in rats with 1,2,5,6-dibenzanthracene (Ball and Samuels 1936), 3,4-benzpyrene (Agate et al. 1955) and 20-MC (Moon and Simpson 1955).

An increased latency in 3,4-benzopyrene-induced papillomas has also been observed in hypophysectomized mice (Korteweg and Thomas 1939). An excess of growth hormone appears to cause increased latency in the induction of skin tumors in mice painted with DMBA (Engelbreth-Holm and Jensen 1953). The latter result suggest that a critical hormone concentration range or ratio may be required for tumor induction in the skin. An excess is tantamount to curtailing hormone biosynthesis by a feedback mechanism. However, the observation that growth hormone only partially reverses the inhibitory effects of hypophysectomy on hepatic tumor development (Griffin et al. 1955) suggests that growth hormone alone is not the principal hormone acting on the induction of tumors. It appears that other hormones whose biosynthesis may be affected by growth hormone concentrations in tissues and body fluids may be the controlling factors in tumorigenesis of the liver or skin.

In pituitary dwarf mice, there is also a delay in the latency of skin tumors induced by 20-MC (Bickis et al. 1956) or DMBA (Bielschowsky 1959).

With the exception of hepatoma induction, the fact that hypophysectomized animals show only a delay in tumor induction with different carcinogenic hydrocarbons suggests that pituitary hormones may only have a supporting role in tumorigenesis. These hormones most probably are involved in the accelerated rate of proliferation of established clones of tumorigenic cells. The size of the clones probably grow quite slowly in the absence of these hormones.

Adrenal Hormones   The influence of adrenal hormones is seen by the effect of adrenalectomy on hepatocarcinogenesis. In this case, liver tumors induced by 4-DAB are inhibited (Symeonidis et al. 1954). However, this effect is not seen with stronger carcinogens such as 3'-methyl-4-dimethylaminozaobenzene. Again, this result suggests a role for adrenal hormones in carcinogenesis similar to that of pituitary hormones; in this case, however, the cocarcinogenic potential of adrenal hormones is probably much weaker than that of the pituitary hormones. As recent developments show, there is mounting evidence suggesting that a critical clone size is required for incipient tumors in order to maintain an autonomous status and obtain a growth advantage over normal tissues (Nowell 1976). As with the pituitary hormones, one or more adrenal hormones may also be involved in accelerating the growth of such clones to a critical mass.

Insulin   Insulin is a hormone with far reaching effects on the general metabolism. Its effect in promoting tumorigenesis may be expected. However, the effects of insulin may be more limited than those of the pituitary hormones. For example, alloxan-induced diabetes in rats inhibits the formation of hepatomas induced by 3'-Me-4-DAB (Salzberg and Griffin 1952) or 2-AF (Bielschowsky and Bielschowsky 1959). The effect of the latter carcinogen has been observed in male Wistar rats. Likewise, alloxan-induced diabetes also inhibits 2-AF-induced mammary cancer in female Wistar rats (Bielschowsky and Bielschowsky 1959). However, in the induction of local sarcomas with 3,4-benzpyrene, both control and diabetic rats easily and equally develop the tumors (Dunning et al. 1949). In hooded female rats, diabetes appears to facilitate the induction of liver tumors with 2-AF, since no such tumors were shown to develop in the nondiabetic controls (Bielschowsky and Bielschowsky 1959).

The effect of insulin on carcinogenesis may be quite different in certain respects from that of the pituitary or adrenal hormones. This is to be expected, since there is generally an antagonism between insulin on one hand and growth hormone and the glucocorticoids on the other. The latter hormones promote hepatic glucogenesis, whereas insulin does the opposite. Whereas insulin causes increased utilization of glucose, growth hormone decreases it. There are also direct insulin antagonists present in the blood plasma whose synthesis or activity is promoted by growth hormone and the glucocorticoids (Cantarow and Schepartz 1967). In other words, growth hormone possesses an anti-insulin effect and its administration induces hyperglycemia. In certain species, growth hormone may result in hyperactivity and hyperplasia of the islets of Langerhans. The consequent destruction of islet beta cells results in permanent diabetes.

The promotion of carcinogenesis by insulin most probably is related to its role in glucose metabolism, and consequently, in energy metabolism, which certainly is of primary importance in the development and maintenance of tumor growth. Its absence will be akin to calorie deprivation which, as shown in Chapter 7, causes regression of tumors or failure in their induction. Tumor induction in diabetic animals with certain chemicals may be influenced by genetic factors or others affecting insulin function, which may account for the variability in the observed effects.

Thyroid Hormones Like insulin, the thyroid hormones also have broad effects on the general metabolism. One of their most important roles is in energy production which is obviously vital to tumorigenesis. Therefore, their influence on the induction and growth of tumors is also expected. Thus, hepatoma formation induced by 2-AF (Paschkis et al. 1948) or 4-DAB (Cantarow and Stasney 1948; Leathern and Barken 1950) can be prevented by administration of a goitrogen such as thiouracil or 3-amino-1,2,4-triazole (Hoshino 1960). The effect of the latter goitrogen has been demonstrated with 4-DAB, and was shown to be similar to thyroidectomy provided the carcinogen was applied after the operation (Bielschowsky and Hall 1953). The latter observation suggests that the hormone may initiate carcinogenesis. This effect of thyroidectomy can be reversed by growth hormone administration (Bielschowsky 1958). This may not be hard to explain considering the parallelisms in the metabolic effects of thyroid and growth hormones. However, it should be borne in mind that the fundamental effects of these hormones on the tumorigenic process may be distinct but related to their functions in the general metabolism.

Whereas the thyroid hormones influence the suppression of chemical carcinogenesis in extrathyroid tissues, the opposite effect is observed in the thyroid itself. For instance, either iodine deficiency or the administration of a goitrogen increases the rate of thyroid tumor formation following administration of a carcinogen (Bielschowsky 1955). This situation has been encountered in rats administered the carcinogen 2-AF and the goitrogen allylthiourea (Bielschowsky 1944). The effect of the goitrogen is similar, whether applied simultaneously with the carcinogen or several weeks later (Bielschowsky 1945; Hall 1948). Multiple adenomas form in a rat with both a goitrogen and carcinogen, whereas a single adenoma is produced with the goitrogen alone.

Pretreatment with 2-AF for 1 week followed by the goitrogen, 4-methyl-2-thiouracil, for up to 94 weeks resulted in more benign thyroid adenomas. This has been observed only in younger animals — those killed before 65 weeks (Hall and Bielschowsky 1949). The difference in the tumor incidence in rats treated with the goitrogen alone, or those pretreated with 2-AF followed by the goitrogen, has been demonstrated to slowly disappear as the animals age, and vanish after the animals are 1.5 years old. Essentially similar malignant tumor incidence was found in both groups. This result suggests that the brief carcinogenic treatment accelerated benign thyroid tumor formation only. However, malignant tumor induction and development in the thyroid following treatment with a carcinogen, as these workers concluded, is probably dependent on continued stimulation by the thyroid-stimulating hormone (TSH) (Hall and Bielschowsky 1949).

While thyroxine alleviates thiouracil-induced hyperplasia of the thyroid tissues, it has no effect on hyperplasia resulting from 2-AF administration. The carcinogen produces a decrease in latency and an increase in incidence in benign and malignant thyroid tumor formation.

Even though administration of thyroid hormones has no effect on thyroid hyperplasia when both a goitrogen and carcinogen are applied together, transplanted malignant thyroid tumors do not thrive in intact animals. These tumors grow only in animals with impaired thyroid function (Morris et al. 1951). One possible explanation for these tumors established in situ by a carcinogen is that the necessary tissue environment, e.g., adequate vascularity, needs to be established in order for tumors to thrive over normal tissues. Such an environment is obviously absent in intact animals.

Conclusions

It is evident from the preceding discussion that the interaction of hormones and carcinogens modifies the development of neoplasms. Our understanding of the role of hormones in carcinogenesis is unfortunately still very incomplete. There is a strong possibility that there are several hormones affecting carcinogenesis that still remain to be
identified; likewise, the exact role in carcinogenesis of known hormones needs further
clarification. The neoplastic cells themselves may elaborate hormones which may play a
role in counteracting or in outpacing the action of the restraining influences in the
body. For example, it has been shown that a clone of tumor cells produces a hormone,
the so-called tumor angiogenesis factor (TAF), which stimulates nearby blood vessels
to form large numbers of new capillaries which subsequently enmesh the tumor (Folkman 1976; Folkman et al. 1974). Thus, this neovascularization permits the tumor to
acquire nutrients and other developmental factors, and to remove metabolic wastes.
Consequently, the clone of tumor cells so vascularized is able to proliferate advantageously over normal cells.

Substances inhibiting mitosis have also been postulated to occur in normal cells.
These substances have been assumed to control unrestrained proliferation of cells.
They are called chalones (Bullough 1975), to indicate their inhibitory nature in con-
trast to the stimulatory effects of hormones.

Several lines of evidence support the contention that in most cases, each type of
tumor arises from a corresponding specific type of single mutant cell which has gained
a mitotic advantage over neighboring normal cells (Nowell 1976). If so, the proliferation of such a cell against the restraining influence of chalones in nearby normal cells
must depend on the ability of the mutant cell to overcome the inhibitory effects of
chalones. There is also experimental evidence which suggests that normal cells contain
diffusible chalones with the ability to inhibit the mitotic activity of malignant cell lines
(Houck and Irausquin 1973; Lipkin and Knecht 1974). Additionally, malignant cells
have been shown to be deficient in chalones. It is tempting to suggest from these observations that carcinogenic promoters, such as hormones, may inhibit or assist the
mutant cells in overcoming the chalones from neighboring cells, and thus gain a tremendous growth advantage over them.

Genetic Influences in Carcinogenesis

The term genetic, as applied to carcinogenesis, includes not only familial hereditary
factors, but also intraracial as well as interracial factors. (In animals, this would
translate into intra- and interspecies differences.) However, it should be pointed out
that international differences in cancer incidences may not be entirely due to racial or
hereditary susceptibility. Strong environmental and occupational as well as cultural
influences are likely to be involved. Similarly, within a country, the influence of heredity in the differences between racial and/or ethnic groups is obscured by, among
other factors, the regional differences in cancer incidence. Nevertheless, studies of
isolated cases or human pedigrees demonstrate a definite hereditary influence in cancer induction. Unfortunately, many factors associated with this pathological process
obscure, even under close scrutiny, the underlying hereditary influences as they
apply to cancer induction in the general population.

Animal studies are clearly a different matter. In these instances, conditions can
be controlled and short lifespans allow the observation of several generations of hybrids from parent strains with diverse susceptibilities. Species differences are also
observable. Thus, the heritability of the susceptibility to cancer induction is readily
demonstrable in animals.

The following discussion on genetic influences in chemical carcinogenesis does not
include the alteration of the DNA genome by exogenous factors in the postzygotic
state; ultimately such alterations result in the mutational transformation of the cell to
a malignant state (i.e., somatic mutation). Rather, this discussion is limited to

heritable changes in the DNA genome, so that cancer susceptibility is vertically transmitted to subsequent generations.

Whether all types of cancer or their susceptibilities are heritable is still being debated, as data do not yet lead to any definite conclusion. Nevertheless, as the following discussion shows, enough evidence from human and especially from animal studies has been obtained to indicate that at least in certain forms of cancer, heredity plays a significant role in cancer induction.

Most studies on the metabolism of carcinogens show that the metabolic activation of a procarcinogen is a prerequisite for carcinogenicity. This observation immediately points to a possible variation in this capacity among individuals, ethnic groups, or races. Biochemical individuality is an accepted phenomenon; both human (Brodie 1964) and animal studies (Hucker 1970) on drug metabolism demonstrate this fact definitively.

That susceptibility toward chemical carcinogenic induction has a genetic basis may be suspected by the gross observations of the effects seen in cigarette smoking: Not every heavy cigarette smoker develops cancer, and in those who do, the latency varies.

Cancer susceptibility presumes, in part, a heritable condition in which the individual responds to an exposure to a chemical carcinogen by developing a neoplastic growth. In contrast, those who do not possess the heritable susceptibility do not develop cancer, in spite of exposure to the carcinogen.

Several models of the mechanism of carcinogenesis assume two or more mutational steps or stages in the DNA genome leading to the development of neoplasms (Armitage and Doll 1957; Ashley 1969a). It has been speculated that one or more of these mutational steps may be inherited, so that postnatally, the number of steps toward neoplastic development is considerably reduced (Burch 1965). Thus, the fewer the number of steps, the more susceptible the individual to tumor induction. A shorter latency and lower dosages of carcinogens for cancer induction are indications of greater susceptibility. For example, from comparing the occurrence of colon cancer in the general population to those with polyposis of the colon, Ashley (1969b) concludes that the number of stages leading to colon cancer in the latter is reduced by one or two stages, depending on the growth rate of the resultant mutant cells.

The hereditary susceptibility or resistance to cancer may come in the form of immunological (Gatti and Good 1970, 1971), hormonal (pp. 181—192), and other biochemical characteristics (e.g., inducibility of metabolic enzymes (Kellerman et al. 1973). Evidence of the influence of heredity on the susceptibility to certain forms of cancer from both human and animal studies are given in the following section. That genetic factors increase or decrease the predisposition to chemical induction of cancer has been shown clearly from animal studies.

Human Studies

There are many hereditary human diseases which predispose one to specific types of cancer. Several of these diseases or syndromes are known. The specific types of cancer associated with the corresponding disease are also known. It should be pointed out that each type of cancer has an incidence in the specific population group significantly greater than comparable groups in the general population.

Several of the disorders have manifest chromosomal abnormality. However, these may comprise only a part of the syndrome. Thus, in mongolism, or Down's syndrome, the chromosomal abnormality consists of an extra chromosome 21, appearing oftentimes as trisomy 21. The disorder is associated with a group of specific symptoms including mental retardation, "mongoloid features," immunological defects, disturbance in nucleic acid metabolism (Mertz et al. 1963), and other biochemical disturbances. Above all, an increased predisposition to leukemia (Miller 1970c) as well as to other forms of cancer (Young 1971) has been observed. Thus, the mongoloid child is 10 to 20 times more susceptible to leukemia than normal children (Miller 1970c). Siblings of mongoloids have been reported also to have increased risk for leukemia (Miller 1963).

In other forms of trisomy, such as Klinefelter's syndrome and trisomy D, similar susceptibility to leukemia has been reported (Fraumeni 1969). However, in these conditions, as in Down's syndrome, the increased susceptibility to leukemia may not be directly attributable to the aneuploid state. Perhaps the trisomy may be the only visible sign of a chromosomal abnormality which includes, among other things, a greater chance of mitotic error in the hematopoietic system leading to leukemia. It should be pointed out that the abnormal purine metabolism in mongolism, as indicated by hyperuricemia (Mertz et al. 1963), is also observed and amply confirmed in leukemia (Krakoff and Meyer 1965; Weissberger and Perskey 1953).

In another type of chromosomal abnormality, called chromosome D deletion syndrome, a high predisposition to a rare form of cancer of the eye, retinoblastoma, has been observed (Wilson et al. 1973). In this syndrome, the chromosomal abnormality consists of a deletion of the long arm of chromosome 13, one of the D chromosomes. Again, in this condition, retinoblastoma is only a part of the syndrome which includes a number of congenital defects. As with the aneuploid states mentioned previously, the visible chromosomal abnormality may just be the result of a more general or specific chromosomal defect which, among other effects, produces increased susceptibility to retinoblastoma. Indeed, as will be discussed later, predisposition to retinoblastoma may be genetically transmitted unrelated to the D deletion syndrome (Knudson 1971).

In other genetic conditions with increased susceptibility to cancer, the only noticeable chromosomal abnormality is the increased fragility of the chromosomes with or without specific exogenous agents. For example, in Bloom's syndrome there is an increased rate of spontaneous chromosome breakage both in vivo and in vitro (German 1972). In Fanconi's syndrome, in addition to this type of chromosome breakage, cells from affected patients have abnormal responses to environmental carcinogens. In addition, there is observed chromosome breakage which is easily induced by x-rays (Higurashi and Conen 1971); cells in vitro manifest increased rate of endoreduplication and tetraploidy following treatment with 3,4-benz(a)pyrene (Hirschhorn and Bloch-Shtacher 1970). Leukemia has been observed in greater frequency in both syndromes compared to the general population; however, in Bloom's syndrome, other forms of cancer, for example, cancer of the GI tract occur in greater incidence (German 1972).

Increased spontaneous chromosome breakage in vitro is also an essential feature of ataxia-telangiectasia. This inherited disorder shows, among other abnormalities, an increased incidence of lymphoid cancer, including leukemia (Hecht et al. 1973). This syndrome is notable for immunodeficiencies in those afflicted (Waldmann et al. 1972). The studies of Hecht et al. (1973) appear to suggest that the chromosomal abnormality in this condition may result in a strong tendency for chromosomal translocation, particularly in the D group. A single lymphocyte from a patient with the disease contains a translocation in the D chromosomes. This lymphocyte, cultured for a period of 52 months, produced about 75% abnormal daughter lymphocytes with a translocation in the same site.

Abnormalities in the chromosomes may be translated ultimately into specific enzyme deficiencies. This is probably the case, for example, in xeroderma pigmentosum, a heritable condition with enhanced predisposition to skin cancer induced by ultraviolet radiation or chemicals. It has been shown that the basic defect in this condition is a deficiency in the enzyme endonuclease in the skin fibroblasts. This enzyme is required for the excision of the damaged portion of DNA. The damage may be caused by ultraviolet radiation (Cleaver 1968, 1969; Setlow et al. 1969) or a chemical carcinogen, such as N-acetoxy-2-acetylaminofluorene (Setlow and Regan 1972). The excision process is an essential step in the repair of DNA damage, with DNA polymerase I and DNA ligase (Orten and Neuhaus 1975).

Several genetically transmitted conditions have specific tumors in certain tissues as principal phenotypic manifestations. In a number of cases, there may be tumors at other sites also. For example, in the so-called cancer family syndrome, tumors may occur at several sites, particularly the colon and the endometrium (Anderson 1970; Lynch and Krush 1971). Warthin (1913) reported a large pedigree afflicted with this malady. This disease is similar to another heritable cancer-predisposing condition, called polyposis of the colon. The dominant feature in this condition is the presence of multiple benign polyps which invariably transform into adenocarcinomas (Neel 1971). Likewise, tumors may develop at other sites, particularly in the connective tissues. Thus, fibromas, osteomas, and fibrosarcomas may occur, and in some families, a very high incidence of these tumors has been observed (Gardner and Richards 1953).

A syndrome involving multiple tumors of the endocrine glands, such as the adrenal cortex, anterior pituitary, parathyroid, thyroid, and the islets of Langerhans, has also been reported; predisposition to these tumors also appears to be genetically transmitted (Anderson 1970). Clinically, the syndrome expectedly has a varied appearance depending on the type of tumor. In addition, the occurrence of the specific tumors may occur much earlier than in the general population. Penetrance of some aspects of the syndrome is quite high in young adults (Anderson 1970). The types of tumors that have been observed include pheochromocytoma of the adrenal medulla and medullary carcinoma of the thyroid. Both these tumors have high penetrance for expression, and even though subjects may have no familial history of the malady, their offspring generally have a 50% chance of developing the tumor. In this case, the number of tumors and the age of appearance are similar whether there is a family history or not (Knudson and Strong 1972a).

Retinoblastoma is a childhood tumor which is also dominantly inherited. As indicated earlier, it is a significant feature of the D deletion syndrome. However, in many cases, its dominant transmission may have nothing to do with this syndrome. Like the above tumors, it is an essential phenotypic expression of the genetically transmitted condition. It is a rare disease with an incidence of one or slightly more per 25,000 children (Croce and Koprowski 1978) or 23,000 live births according to other estimates (Altman and Schwartz 1978; Devesa 1975). However, because of the advances in cancer management more carriers have survived to reproduce. Indeed, this increased survival has permitted the observation of its genetic transmission (Knudson 1971, 1973). The data, however, indicate that only about 40% of cases may be hereditary. The data also seem to support the hypothesis that the genetic predisposition to cancer does not result in spontaneous cancer without additional stimuli. That is, the development of cancer from the inherited abnormality requires an actuating factor. Thus, about 5% of the defective gene carriers do not develop the disease, and most of those that do develop the cancer do not have affected parents or close relatives (Neel 1962). A small percentage of affected subjects have affected siblings as well. The penetrance for expression is very high, about 95% (Auerbach 1956; Neel 1962).

The greater cancer susceptibility of patients with familial retinoblastoma is indicated by their greater tendency than the general population to develop other types of cancer; e.g., leukemia and bone, kidney, and other tumors (Croce and Koprowski 1978).

Two other lethal childhood tumors with genetically transmitted predisposition are Wilms' tumor of the kidney and neuroblastoma (Knudson and Strong 1972a,b). Estimates of hereditary cases run as high as approximately 38% for Wilm's tumor and 22% for neuroblastoma. Like retinoblastoma, advances in cancer management have permitted survival of carriers, and in several cases have allowed the observation of the genetic transmissability and the predisposition to the disease.

Pheochromocytoma is a catecholamine-producing tumor arising from the chromaffin cells of the sympathoadrenal system. About 22% of all cases are estimated to be hereditary (Knudson and Strong 1972a). A number of pedigrees show dominant genetic transmission. In the familial form, 50% of cases have multiple tumors compared to 12% in all cases, and by age 50, approximately 90% of gene carriers would be expected to develop at least one tumor, with a mean of two or three tumors for each carrier. Pheochromocytoma is a rare type of tumor, accounting for only about 0.053% of all deaths in the United States related to hypertension (Roth and Kvale 1956). The latter is a common symptom associated with the tumor, often accompanied by severe head-aches, perspiration, palpitation, pallor, and other symptoms (Thomas et al. 1966). Most of the tumors originate in the adrenal glands, and in a smaller number of cases, in abdominal, pelvic, thoracic, and neck regions (Gjessing 1968; Strauss and Wurm 1960).

Thus far, examples of tumors or syndromes with an inherited predisposition to cancer have been cited. A question that comes to mind is whether all forms of cancer have genetic influences of the types just discussed. In particular, it would be of in-terest to know whether the most common forms of cancer have identifiable genetic carriers. The previous discussion cited cases whereby common cancers, such as leu-kemia and skin, colon, and endometrium cancers have familial cases associated with particular, genetically transmitted syndromes. To these might be added carcinoma of the breast. Several pedigrees showing genetic transmission of the susceptibility to the disease have been reported (Knudson et al. 1973). In addition, there is also a high concordance between identical and fraternal twins. Estimates run as high as 28 and 12%, respectively (Knudson et al. 1973). Similarly, dominant inheritance of cancer of the gastrointestinal and gastrourinary system has also been observed (Knudson et al. 1973).

The most common cancer, bronchogenic carcinoma, which accounts for most cases of cancer death, especially among males in the United States, may also have a genetic component (Tokuhata 1964). However, the environmental factors appear to have such profound effects that the hereditary component is obscured. Nevertheless, both her-editary and environmental effects have been shown by an analysis of the data to have synergistic effects (Tokuhata 1964). In this connection, the studies reported by Kel-lermann et al. (1973) identify those individuals with genetic cancer susceptibility, at least for tumor induction from carcinogenic hydrocarbons. It should be recalled that these groups of substances require a specific enzyme, arylhydrocarbon hydroxylase (AHH) for activation. This enzyme is highly inducible by a number of substances, and it is estimated that genetically, about 50% of the United States population have low in-ducibility for the enzyme; i.e., homozygous for the low inducibility allele. These groups are, therefore, less susceptible to arylhydrocarbon-induced tumors compared to those with high inducibility for the enzyme. Thus, individuals who are homozygous for the allele for low inducibility may be more resistant to lung cancer, even though they may be heavy smokers. In studies of patients with lung cancer, only two of 50 patients who were all heavy smokers were low inducers for the enzyme (Kellermann et al. 1973).

These findings may be extended to the induction of cancer by other procarcino-gens which also require metabolic activation. It will be shown in the next section that the resistance of certain species to chemical cancer induction is associated with the in-ability to transform the chemical to active forms.

Animal Studies

The observed effects on the chemical induction of cancer in animals clearly demon-strate that cancer susceptibility is an inherited characteristic. Thus, it has been es-tablished that the susceptibility of an animal to chemical carcinogenesis depends to a large extent on the animal's genetic make-up. The influence of genetics to susceptibil-ity to cancer induction is readily observed for low dosages of a carcinogen. Suscepti-bility is measured in terms of tumor incidence and latency. Thus, the variation in tumor incidence and latency may be a function of the genetic susceptibility.

It became clear to early investigators in cancer research that different species behave differently in their response to carcinogens. This is particularly true with low dosages of chemicals. For example, with coal tar as the carcinogen, the neoplastic re-sponse in the skin can be easily elicited in the mouse or rabbit, but not in the rat or guinea pig (Itchikawa and Baum 1924). Other species such as the chicken (Choldin 1927), dog (Passey 1938), and monkey (Bonne et al. 1930) are likewise resistant.

However, these animals ultimately will respond provided the dose or the carcinogen is potent enough, or the application continued long enough. Thus, the very resistant skin of the guinea pig yields to the carcinogenic action of such a powerful carcinogen as DMBA (Berenblum 1949).

The responses of these animals differ with the type of carcinogen. For example, both mouse and rabbit skin are highly responsive to coal tar, but the rabbit is only weakly responsive to 3,4-benz(a)pyrene, whereas the mouse remains strongly affected (Oberling and Guerin 1947). These two animals respond in reverse with certain coal tar fractions; i.e., the rabbit is in this case less resistant than the mouse (Berenblum and Schoental 1947b).

The animals also differ considerably with respect to the site of the carcinogenic response. For example, while the rat (Cook and Kennaway 1940), the chicken (Burrows 1933), and other birds (Duran-Reynals et al. 1945) are highly resistant to skin carcinogenesis, they will readily respond to subcutaneous sarcoma induction; the rat, in this case, even more readily than the mouse. The rabbit, however, which is very susceptible to skin carcinogenesis fails to respond to subcutaneous cancer induction (Berenblum 1949). The guinea pig, which is highly resistant to skin cancer induction, will respond to subcutaneous carcinogenesis with large enough doses of a specific carcinogen (Russell and Ortega 1952).

Species also differ considerably in the type of susceptible tissues remote from the point of application of the carcinogen. For example, estrone enhances mammary tumor response in the mouse (Lacassagne 1932) and the rat (McEuen 1939), whereas fibroid-like growths are produced in the uterus and abdominal viscera of the guinea pig (Lipschutz 1950), and kidney and liver tumors in hamsters (Kirkman 1952). No mammary tumors are induced by estrone in the rabbit, guinea pig, dog, or monkey (Gardner 1947). While the rat and mouse both easily produce liver tumors with o-aminoazotoulene (Shear 1937), they differ in their response to liver carcinogenesis with DAB — the rat being highly susceptible (Rusch et al. 1945a); the mouse is only weakly so (Andervont et al. 1944; Miller and Miller 1953). Likewise, the squirrel, chicken, cavy, hamster, chipmunk, and cotton rat are resistant to DAB hepatocarcinogenesis (Miller and Miller 1953). The dog develops invasive bladder tumors instead of liver tumors when fed DAB (20 mg/kg b.w., 3 to 4 years) (Nelson and Woodard 1953). β-Napthylamine is highly carcinogenic to the bladder of the dog and man (Hueper et al. 1938), but very weakly so in the rat and rabbit, tumors appearing only after very long, latent periods; i.e., about 100 weeks in the rat and 285 weeks in the rabbit (Bonser et al. 1951). The ferret, hamster, and guinea pig do not respond at all to this chemical (Bonser and Jull 1952) which induces liver tumors in the mouse (Bonser et al. 1956). Similarly, whereas diethylstilbestrol induces vaginal cancer in women (Herbst et al. 1972), it induces adenomammary carcinoma in the mouse (Huseby 1953).

Finally, while many animal species readily respond to the potent carcinogen 2-acetylaminofluorene (2-fluorenylacetamide), the guinea pig and steppe lemming are highly resistant (Miller et al. 1964; Weisburger and Weisburger 1966). Animals that are susceptible to this carcinogen also differ in the responding tissue. Thus, following oral administration of 2-acetylaminofluorene, the cat develops liver, kidney, and lung tumors, whereas the chicken responds with tumors of the kidney and ureter (Hartwell 1951); the syrian golden hamster with liver tumors (Della Porta et al. 1959); and the rabbit with bladder and ureter tumors (Shubik and Hartwell 1957).

Differences in genetic susceptibility to cancer is also clearly demonstrated in the response of the different strains of the same species. For example, in terms of latency in 3,4-benz(a)pyrene-induced skin tumors, these strains of mice exhibit the following responses (Berenblum 1954):

IF mice	18 weeks
C mice	30 weeks
dba mice	32 weeks
A and CBA mice	34 weeks

| C 3H mice | 42 weeks |
| C57 mice | resistant |

Similarly, with 3-MC skin carcinogenesis, the latent period for IF mice is 10.5 weeks compared to 20 weeks in CBA mice (Bonser 1938). While C57 mice are resistant to 3,4-benz(a)pyrene-induced skin cancer, they are less resistant than the C3H mice to dibenzanthracene (Lauridsin and Eggers 1943).

Regarding subcutaneous carcinogenesis, the species specificity appears to hold true in mice. Thus, IF mice, which are most sensitive to skin cancer, are less sensitive to subcutaneous carcinogenesis, whereas the opposite effect is seen in C3H mice (Burdette and Strong 1943).

There are also differences in the susceptibility of strains of mice to lung cancer induced by dibenzanthracene. The A strain is highly susceptible, whereas again the C57 black mice are particularly resistant (Andervont 1937a).

Of interest is the observation that the inherited susceptibility is not a general somatic phenomenon, but rather resides in specific tissues. Thus, when lung tissues are transplanted into hybrids of susceptible and resistant mice strains, the same response is observed. That is, after injection with dibenzanthracene (Heston and Dunn 1951) or urethane (Shapiro and Kirschbaum 1951), the transplanted lung of the susceptible species develops higher tumor incidence compared to the transplanted lung from the resistant species.

Genetic transmission has also been established from cross-breeding experiments. For example, when a resistant strain C57L mice are crossed with the susceptible strain A, the observed response in terms of pulmonary tumors following dibenz(a,h)anthracene treatment is characteristic of multiple-factor quantitative inheritance (Heston 1942a). F_1 and F_2 hybrids show an intermediate response between the parent strains, except that the F_2 indicate a segregation of genes by showing a greater spread than the F_1. It has been estimated that the parent strains differ by at least four pairs of genes controlling pulmonary tumor response.

Multiple gene inheritance with respect to chemically induced pulmonary tumor susceptibility has been similarly observed; in this case, using latency as the criterion (Heston 1942a). In these strains, similar multiple gene control has been observed with spontaneous pulmonary tumors.

Using tumor incidence and latency, linkage studies have demonstrated specific genes associated with either resistance or susceptibility to lung tumors. Thus, lethal yellow (A^{l}), on chromosome 1, has been associated with decreased tumor resistance. Vestigial tail (vt) and other genes in chromosome 11, obese (ob) in chromosome 6, flexed-tail (f) in chromosome 13, hairless (hr) in chromosome 14, and fused (fu) in chromosome 17 have been associated with increased resistance (Burdette 1952; Heston 1957). Another gene, dwarf (dw) has been associated with resistance to lung tumors. Each of these genes affects normal growth in the same manner as the number of induced tumors. The incidence of spontaneous tumors is also affected. Based on their results with crosses between susceptible strain A and resistant strain C57L mice, Bloom and Falconer (1964) propose the presence of ptr, a pulmonary tumor resistant gene. However, this gene has not been located in any linkage group.

Similar genetic transmissions of subcutaneous carcinogenesis have been demonstrated. F_1 hybrids of susceptible strain C3H mice crossed with resistant strains I and Y are intermediate between the parent mice in susceptibility to subcutaneous carcinogenesis (Andervont 1938). Similarly, the F_1 hybrids resulting from crosses between two susceptible strains, C3H and JK mice, demonstrate intermediate susceptibility to the parent strains to subcutaneous carcinogenesis induced by 3-methylcholanthrene (Burdette 1943). These workers concluded from these studies that there is more than one gene controlling susceptibility.

As already stated, genetic factors in cancer induction may be ultimately translated in terms of biosynthesis of the appropriate enzymes required in the metabolism of carcinogens. The metabolism of aflatoxins appears to be genetically determined and varies

greatly among species (Patterson 1973). As demonstrated in many cases, the variability in the metabolism of xenobiotic chemicals between and within species is genetically controlled (Weisburger and Rall 1972). Such differences may account for the
variability among individuals in susceptibility to cancer induction. Thus, because the
guinea pig cannot metabolize the insecticide 2-fluorenylacetamide (2-acetylaminofluor-
ene, 2-AAF) to its sulfate ester, the ultimate carcinogen, this species is resistant to
the hepatocarcinogenic effects of this chemical. In contrast, the rat is highly susceptible. The former lacks the ability to N-hydroxylate the procarcinogen. As shown in
the following scheme, N-hydroxylation is an essential step in the activation of the
insecticide (Miller 1970a; Miller et al. 1964; Weisburger and Weisburger 1973).

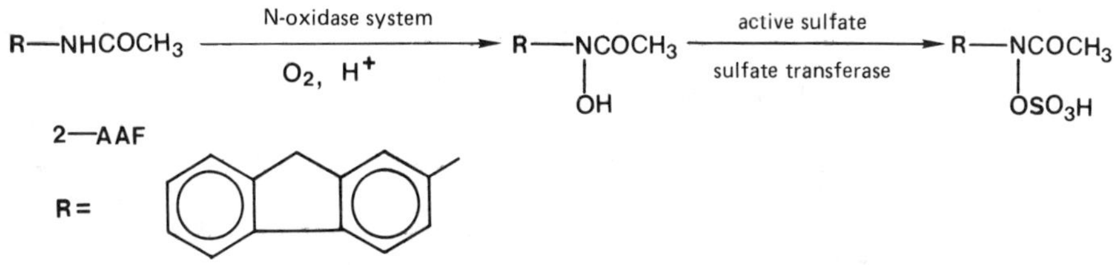

$$\text{R—NHCOCH}_3 \xrightarrow[\text{O}_2,\ \text{H}^+]{\text{N-oxidase system}} \underset{\overset{|}{\text{OH}}}{\text{R—NCOCH}_3} \xrightarrow[\text{sulfate transferase}]{\text{active sulfate}} \underset{\overset{|}{\text{OSO}_3\text{H}}}{\text{R—NCOCH}_3}$$

2—AAF

R =

Effect of Immunological Factors on Carcinogenesis

The immune mechanism appear to have a significant effect on carcinogenesis, judging
from the considerable data that have been accumulated in recent years (Bodansky
1975; Harris and Sinkovics 1970; Melief and Schwartz 1975; National Cancer Institute
1972). The initial postulate regarding the involvement of the immune response was
enunciated by Paul Ehrlich, the father of immunology, as early as 1908. In effect,
Ehrlich (1957) stated that aberrant, cancer-prone cells formed during fetal and post-
fetal development are held in check by the natural immunity of the body. When this
natural immunity fails, for one reason or another, neoplastic growth is manifested.
This immunosurveillance theory was ignored for several decades and was revived with
greater interest beginning in the early 1940s. There is now an increasing body of data
confirming Ehrlich's contention that immune competence significantly affects the development and promotion of neoplasia.

Recent concepts in immunology pertinent to neoplasia will be reviewed briefly in
order to put the role of immunological factors in carcinogenesis in a clearer perspective.

Cellular Basis of the Immune Function

It has been shown that the bone marrow contains stem cells which elaborate three kinds
of parent cells. The latter, in turn, give rise to specific cell types which are involved
in the immune response: the blood monocytes, or immature macrophages, and precursors for bursal (B), and thymus (T) lymphocytes (Cooper and Lawton 1974; Eisen
1973). However, the immune mechanism may be viewed to consist of two main branches:
the bursal system or its mammalian equivalent, and the central thymus system. The
bursal system is responsible for the production of humoral antibodies, whereas the
thymus system is involved with cell-mediated immunity. The latter manifests as delayed
hypersensitivity or delayed allergy, and homograft rejection. Whereas these two systems are distinct in both morphology and function, there is cooperation between them
when responding to antigens.

The thymus is derived from epithelial cells formerly lining the third and fourth
pharyngeal pouches in the region that becomes the throat during embryonic development. In the thymus, stem cells entering it become the so-called T lymphocytes, or T
cells. Maturation of the T cells is under the control of thymosin or thymus maturational
hormone. The T lymphocytes after leaving the thymus may take temporary residence in
the thymus-dependent zones of the lymph nodes and the spleen. The T cells then enter

the lymphatic circulation and reenter the bloodstream by way of the subclavian vein where the main lymphatic vessel, the thoracic duct, empties. The T lymphocytes encountering an antigen, such as a foreign protein or cell, or an autochthonous malignant cell, may repeatedly divide to form a clone of cells which is responsive to that particular antigen. During division, the T lymphocytes release protein molecules, the lymphokines, which participate in the elimination of the foreign materials.

A delayed hypersensitivity reaction has been usually evaluated by the presence of redness or induration at the site of the intracutaneous injection of an antigenic material. This reaction suggests a prior sensitivity to the antigen. A positive reaction develops generally within 5 to 24 hr (Uhr 1966) and reaches maximum reaction in 16 to 72 hr after injection. This delay in development represents the time required for the accumulation of the appropriate sensitized cells — lymphocytes and macrophages or monocytes — at the site of antigen exposure.

The bursal lymphocytes, or B cells, are derived, in the case of birds, from the bursa of Fabricus (Good 1971), a pouchlike organ attached to the intestine near the cloaca. In mammals, the origin of the B cells has not been definitely established. Some evidence indicates that the liver and the spleen may be the site of B cell formation (Cooper and Lawton 1974). Stem cells entering the bursa, or its mammalian equivalent, differentiate into B lymphocytes. The lymphocytes are stimulated by specific antigens to divide repeatedly into a clone of plasma cells. Each cell secretes about 2000 identical molecules per second (Cooper and Lawton 1974); the cell dies a few days after maturity. Exposure to an antigen also causes the production of a class of B lymphocytes, which has the ability to respond promptly and vigorously to a second encounter of the same antigen. These are called memory cells. The antibodies initiate the elimination of the foreign substance by activating a group of enzymes, collectively called the complement (Mayer 1973). The antibodies cause the complement to bind to the invading protein or cell, whereupon a complex series of reactions lead to the destruction of the invading material.

There seems to be cooperation between the two immune systems in their response to the presence of an antigen. It appears that this cooperation is brought about by the macrophages which arise from the third type of precursor cell of the bone marrow, the monocyte (Eisen 1973). In this case, the macrophages cooperate with the T cells in causing the B cells to respond to the antigens. The initial effect here is the transformation of the B cells into plasma cells, the latter being the source of antibody synthesis.

In a particular type of immune reaction, there appears to be an antagonism between these two immunological systems, particularly in relation to the neoplastic cells. This will be discussed later in this section.

Immunodeficiency and Malignancy

Numerous examples of increased incidence of malignancy in persons with immunodeficiency have been reported (Creysell et al. 1958; Gatti and Good 1971; Kersey et al. 1973a). Gatti and Good (1971) estimate that in persons with primary immunodeficiency diseases, the frequency of malignant neoplasms is 10,000 times that in the general age-matched population.

Immunosurveillance Theory

These observations in relation to the increased incidence of malignancy in immuno-incompetent persons have given support to the immunosurveillance theory, first proposed by Ehrlich in 1908 (1957), and propounded later by Thomas (1959) and Burnett (1964). The theory, in its present form, states that the immune mechanism is the primary means of natural defense against neoplastic growth. This theory implies that tumor cells possess specific antigens which are different from those of normal cells. These tumor antigens are, in fact, autoantigens in that they provoke the immune response of the host into activity, resulting in the destruction of the aberrant cells. The logical implication of this theory would be that immunoincompetence would lead to increased incidence of malignancy (Melief and Schwartz 1975).

Immunosuppression and Chemical Carcinogenesis

While the theory holds true for virus-induced tumors in experimental animals, other results, particularly in humans, seem to indicate that other factors must be incorporated into the theory in order to give it general validity (Melief and Schwartz 1975). In particular, in chemical oncogenesis, contradictory results have been recorded regarding the role of immunosuppression. For example, using antilymphocyte serum (ALS), which selectively depletes T cells in rodents (Lance et al. 1973), several investigators have reported enhanced chemically induced oncogenesis in terms of tumor incidence and/or decreased latency. Thus, ALS enhances the oncogenicity of 3-methylcholanthrene (Balner and Dersjant 1969; Rabbat and Jeejeebhoy 1970), diethylnitrosamine (Friedrich-Fresca and Hoffman 1969), and dimethylbenzanthracene (Woods 1969). On the other hand, Wagner and Haughton (1971) found no enhancing effect on the oncogenicity of 2-methylcholanthrene in ALS-treated animals, nor did Fisher et al. (1970) with other chemicals.

Still, others have found different results under varied conditions with the same carcinogen. For example, Grant and Roe (1969) found that germ-free mice treated with ALS do not develop tumors with dimethylbenzanthrazene, whereas about 50% of conventional mice did. Whereas no tumors of the nervous tissues have been shown to develop in ALS-treated rats with N-methyl-N-nitrosourea, which normally strongly induces tumors in these tissues, bladder tumors have been found in 25% of the rats so treated. None of the rats treated with either ALS or the carcinogen were shown to develop bladder tumors (Denlinger et al. 1973). Mice of the I strain, which normally are resistant to the carcinogenicity of methylcholanthrene, become more susceptible to the carcinogen after prolonged treatment with ALS (Stutman 1969).

Obviously, immunoincompetence alone cannot be responsible for increased carcinogenicity with chemicals. As shown in the previous sections, many other factors can modify the complex process and the immune mechanism is just one of these. The fact that a number of carcinogenic chemicals have been shown to suppress both humoral and cell-mediated immunities (Ball 1970; Stutman 1969; Szakall and Hanna 1972) further supports the theory that suppression of the immune function predisposes the cell to carcinogenic effects. The following observations appear to be pertinent: First, hydrocarbons which are carcinogenic have also been found to be immunosuppressive, whereas those that are noncarcinogenic are not (Stjernsward 1966). Second, mice which are resistant to the carcinogenic effects of 3-methylcholanthrene also resist immunosuppression by this carcinogen (Stutman 1969). Third, in general, the time required for antibody production to be halted after carcinogen administration corresponds to the latency of the tumor (Szakall and Hanna 1972), and the time of maximum suppression of antibody production also coincides with the time of appearance of the skin tumors induced by 7,12-dibenzanthracene. Cell-mediated immunity in this case appears to be depressed permanently.

While immunosuppression may enhance carcinogenesis, it does not follow that this will invariably be so. Immunoincompetence does not induce carcinogenesis or cause an increase of the number of preneoplastic cells. This condition may be viewed as facilitating the free expression of the carcinogenic potential already present in the cells, either during fetal development, or by prior exposure to a carcinogen. Susceptibility to a carcinogen appears to have a certain specificity in terms of the host animal or individual cells. Exposure to a carcinogen does not guarantee that all cells so exposed will become neoplastic. Likewise, depression of the immune function is not a primary requirement of carcinogenesis. For example, the carcinogen dimethylbenzanthrazene is immunosuppressive to antibody production caused by sheep red blood cells, whereas other carcinogens, such as 3.4-benz(a)pyrene and 3-methylcholanthrene, when injected to CFW/D mice (Ball 1970) are not. Note that in some other strains, 3-methylcholanthrene has been reported to be immunosuppressive (Stutman 1969). Further suppression of the immune function by thymectomy or ALS treatment neither increases the tumor incidence nor influences the development of tumors. Tumors can regress under these conditions (Andrews 1971).

Cytolytic T Lymphocytes and Blocking antibodies

It appears that the thymic branch of the immune system is responsible, to a large extent, for the elimination of aberrant cells. Almost all human cancers studied have demonstrated cell-mediated immunity against antigens of each type of tumor, whether derived from the patient or from histologically similar allogenic tumors; i.e., bladder tumor (Bubenik et al. 1970), Burkitt's lymphoma (Fass et al. 1970), melanoma (Hellstrom and Hellstrom 1973), neuroblastoma (Hellstrom et al. 1970a), colon carcinoma (Hellstrom et al. 1970b), and sarcoma (Cohen et al. 1973). However, the cytotoxic functions of the T lymphocytes are impaired or blocked by antibodies that bind to the surface of the tumor in response to its antigens. These antibodies protect the tumor from destruction (Hellstrom et al. 1969, 1971; Jose 1973; Jose et al. 1971). As shown in Chapter 7, the formation of "blocking antibodies" may be diminished or eliminated by moderate protein malnutrition (Cooper et al. 1970; Jose and Good 1971, 1973a) or moderate deficiency of specific amino acids (Jose 1973; Jose and Good 1973b).

It is obvious from the preceding discussion that the immune function is an essential factor in the regulation of carcinogenesis. The apparent successes that have been reported in the immunotherapy of cancer (Harris and Sinkovics 1970; National Cancer Institute 1972) suggest that the immune mechanism has more than a minor role in the development and control of neoplastic diseases. Admittedly, more information is needed in order to define this role more precisely.

Chemical Modifiers of Carcinogenesis

A number of exogenous chemicals can alter the course of the carcinogenic process. Some of these substances enhance the induction, promotion, and growth of tumors, whereas others either inhibit or retard the carcinogenic process, or reverse the growth of tumors. Three general types of substances which enhance the carcinogenic process are known: (a) promoters; (b) cocarcinogens; and (c) "syncarcinogens." Promoters and cocarcinogens have been discussed in a previous section. A chemical syncarcinogen acts additively or synergistically with another carcinogen in inducing a tumor in the same target organ(s). Cocarcinogens or tumor promoters are non-carcinogenic or at most, weakly so.

Two types of inhibitory substances are identified: (1) anticarcinogens, and (2) tumor inhibitors. These two terms, often used interchangeably by oncologists, refer to substances which reduce the incidence, increase the latency, or suppress the growth of tumors induced by chemical carcinogens (Homburger 1974). However, a distinction should be made. A chemical anticarcinogen interferes in the initiation or induction of neoplasm by a carconogen(s). In other words, it prevents the neoplastic transformation of a cell. Thus, an anticarcinogen may be expected to act at the enzyme or hormonal level during the initial inductive stages of carcinogenesis, or compete with the binding of carcinogens in specific cell receptors. In contrast to the anticarcinogen, a tumor inhibitor interferes in the growth of established tumors, or acts only after the cell's transformation to the neoplastic state has taken place. A special type of tumor inhibitor is the chemotherapeutic agent which acts on clinically established tumors. Indeed many of these agents are probably more effective during the early stages of tumor development. These substances may also interfere with the enzyme system(s) of the tumor, or with the hormones involved in its promotion. Additionally, tumor inhibitors may also enhance the immunological mechanisms. Thus, one may consider the anticarcinogens as preventive or prophylactic agents, whereas the tumor inhibitors as therapeutic agents.

This section will discuss syncarcinogens and inhibitory substances. These inhibitory or syncarcinogenic substances of nutritional nature will be discussed in Chapter 7.

In practice, the distinction between an anticarcinogen and a tumor inhibitor may be difficult because, in most cases, the manner in which these substances affect a cell undergoing neoplastic transformation is not known. Thus, it is possible that substances which are reported to inhibit the growth of established tumors may also act during the preneoplastic stages of tumor development. This section, therefore, discusses anticarcinogens and tumor inhibitors reported in the literature without differentiation. Nevertheless, known aspects of the mode of action of inhibitory substances will be discussed. This is particularly important since certain naturally occurring substances in food and many types of chemical contaminants show parallel responses in specific cells. Except for a few instances, it is not known whether or not they are inhibitors of tumorigenic processes.

Chemical Inhibitors of the Tumorigenic Process

Table 7 lists several examples of inhibitors of tumorigenesis. Note that a number of substances are carcinogens in their own right: 3-methylcholanthrene (3-MC), 1,2-benzanthracene (1,2-BA), 9,10-dimethyl-1,2-benzanthracene (DMBA), chrysene (Dipple 1976), urethane (Yamamoto et al. 1971); and trypan Blue (Gillman and Gillman 1952). Most striking is the fact that 3-MC, which can induce cancer in the mammary gland of female rats (Dunning et al. 1940), produces no additive or synergistic effects with other mammary carcinogens, such as DMBA (Wheatley 1968), 4-dimethylamino-stilbene (DAS) (Taufic 1965), and 2-acetylaminofluorene (2-AAF) (Miller et al. 1958). Rather, 3-MC inhibits carcinogenesis induced in this site by these carcinogens. There is no observed correlation between the potency of carcinogenicity at one site and inhibitory effects at other sites. For example, 3-MC is rarely a liver carcinogen, but is a potent one on the skin and other tissues. Many inhibitory substances are noncarcinogenic aromatic hydrocarbons; i.e., perylene and benzofluorene isomers (Dipple 1976). Many other inhibitory, noncarcinogenic organic compounds are not aromatic hydrocarbons; e.g., β-naphthoflavone, 7,8-benzoflavone, phenobarbital, phenobarbitone. Thus, unrelated substances appear to elicit similar inhibitory effects on cancerous tumors in the same site. For example, 3-MC acetanilide, or 8-hydroxyquinoline, produces similar inhibitory effects on hepatocarcinogenesis induced by 2-AAF. However, as will be seen later, these dissimilar substances appear to operate, understandably, by different mechanisms.

Results of several studies have shown that an exogenous compound may inhibit tumorigenesis by one or more of the following mechanisms: (1) promotion of increased rates of biosynthesis of microsomal enzymes, consequently, the detoxification of the carcinogen; (2) competition with specific procarcinogen-activating chemical groups or metabolites; (3) interference with hormones involved in the initiation of the tumor induced by the carcinogen; (4) enhancement of the rate of excretion of a specific metabolite; (5) interference with the binding of the carcinogen with a specific cell component, and thus with the reaction with critical cell receptors; and (6) inhibition of the enzymes involved in the metabolic activation of the carcinogen. Examples of each of these will be cited further.

Promotion of Increased Rates of Microsomal Enzyme ("Mixed Function Oxidase") Biosynthesis Such tumor inhibitors as those listed in Table 7 — 3-MC, phenobarbital, DMBA, 1,2-benzanthracene, β-naphthoflavone (5,6-benzoflavone), and 7,6-benzoflavone — have been shown to induce microsomal enzymes which are usually involved in the detoxification of xenobiotic compounds. The chemical natures of these compounds probably suggest that various types of microsomal enzymes, or at least different isozymes, may be induced. Among the different microsomal enzymes that can be induced by these compounds are the following.

Table 7. Chemical Carcinogens and Corresponding Chemical Inhibitors

Carcinogen	Inhibitor	Test animal	Tumor site inhibited[a]	Ref.
2-AAF, 7-F-2-AAF	3-MC	Rat	Liver Mammary gland Ear duct Small intestine	Miller et al. (1958)
2-AAF	Acetanilide	Rat	Liver	Yamamoto et al. (1968)
	8-HQ	Rat	Liver	Yamamoto et al. (1971)
Aflatoxin	Phenobarbitone	Rat	Liver	McLean and Marshall (1971)
3,4-BP	BHA	Mouse	Forestomach Lung	Wattenberg (1972)
	B(a)E, B(a)F, B(k)F, B(m,n,o)F chrysene, 2-naphthol, PNX and perylene	Rat	Subcutaneous	Falk et al. (1964)
	β-NpFv	Mouse	Lung, skin	Wattenberg and Leong (1970)
4-DAB	Copper salts	Rat	Liver	Howell (1958)
	4', 3-diMe-4-AB	Rat	Liver	Crabtree (1955)
	4-HPP	Rat	Liver	Baba (1957)
	Trypan blue	Rat	Liver	Fujita et al. (1952)
2', 4'-diF and 4-DAB	3-MC, 1,2-BA	Rat	Liver	Miller et al. (1958)
4'-F-4-DAB, 3'-Me-4-DAB	DMBA; 1,2,5,6-DBA			
	3-MC	Rat	Liver[a]	Meechan et al. (1953)
			Liver[a] Lymph nodes[b] Peritoneum[b] Adrenal[b] Heart[b] Spleen[b]	Richardson et al. (1952)
4-DAS	3-MC	Rat	Ear duct[a] Mammary gland	Taufic (1965)
DENA	Phenobarbital	Mouse	Liver	Kunz et al. (1969)

Table 7. (continued)

Carcinogen	Inhibitor	Test animal	Tumor site inhibited	Ref.
DMBA	7,8-BFv	Mouse	Skin	Gelboin et al. (1970)
	Chrysene 6-Aminochrysene 1-Me-7-IPrP, Sudan III	Rat	Mammary gland Liver Adrenal	Huggins et al. (1964)
	3-MC	Rat	Mammary gland	Wheatley (1968)
	β-NpFv	Mouse	Lung Mammary gland	Wattenberg and Leong (1968)
	Leupeptin	Mouse	Skin	Hozumi et al. (1972)
	TLCMK	Mouse	Skin	Troll et al. (1970)
DMNA	Acetonitrile	Rat	Liver	Hadjiolon (1971); Fiume (1964)
3-MC	Chrysene	Mouse	Skin	Lacassagne
	1,2,5,6-DBF	Mouse Rat	Skin Liver	et al (1934) Riegel et al. (1951)
	Urethane, uracil mustard	Mouse	Lung	Wattenberg (1972); Yamamoto et al. (1971)
	BHA	Mouse	Lung	Wattenberg (1972)
Urethane	Chlordane, β-NpFv and phenobarbital	Mouse	Lung	Yamamoto (1971)
	BHA	Mouse	Lung	Wattenberg (1972)

Abbreviations (in alphabetical order): Carcinogens: 2-AAF — 2-Acetylaminofluorene; 3,4-BP — 3,4-Benzo(a)pyrene; 1,2,5,6-DBA — 1,2,5,6-Dibenzanthracene; 4-DAB — 4-Dimethylaminoazobenzene; 4-DAS — 4-Dimethylaminostilbene; DENA — Diethyl-nitrosamine; 2',4'-diF-4-DAB — 2',4'-Difluoro-4-dimethylaminoazobenzene; DMBA — 9,10-Dimethyl-1,2-benzanthracene; 7-F-2-AAF — 7-Fluoro-2-acetylaminofluorene; 4'-F-4-DAB — 4'-Fluoro-4-dimethylaminoazobenzene; 3-MC — 3-Methylcholanthrene; 3'-Me-4-DAB — 3'-Methyl-4-dimethylaminoazobenzene. Anticarcinogens: 1,2-BA — 1,2-Benzanthracene; B(a)C — Benzo(a)carbazole; B(a)F — Benzo(a)fluorene; B(k)F — Benzo(k)fluorene; B(m,n,o)F — Benzo(m,n,o)fluorene; 7,8-BFv — 7,8-Benzo-flavone; BHA — Butylhydroxyanisole; 1,2,5,6-DBF — 1,2,5,6-Dibenzofluorene; 4',3-DiMe-4-AB — 4',3-Dimethyl-4-amino-azobenzene; DMBA — 9,10-Dimethyl-1,2-benzanthracene; 4-HPP — 4-Hydroxypropiophenone; 8-HQ — 8-Hydroxyquinoline; 3-MC — 3-Methylcholanthrene; 1-Me-7-IPrP — 1-Methyl-7-isopropylphenanthrene; β-NpFv — β-Naphthoflavone (5,6-Benzoflavone); PNX — Perinaphthoxanthine; TLCMK — Tosyllysinechloromethylketone
[a]Primary tumor site.
[b]Metastatic tumor site.

Hydroxylases: As stated in Chapter 4, hydroxylation is one way in which the body facilitates the elimination of toxic or foreign compounds; this process increases the polarity of these compounds and, therefore, their solubility in an aqueous medium. All the inhibitors listed previously (pp. 203−205) induce increased hydroxylation. In some cases, whether hydroxylation enhances or diminishes the carcinogenicity of a compound, depends on the position of hydroxylation in the molecule. For example, 2-acetylaminofluorene (2-AAF) may be hydroxylated at the nitrogen atom or at specific carbon atoms in the ring system by microsomal hydroxylases induced by 3-MC (Lotlikar et al. 1965). The C-hydroxylated metabolites (ring hydroxylated) are non-carcinogens, whereas the N-hydroxy products are carcinogens. Experiments by Lotlikar et al. (1965) using rat liver homogenates have shown that 3-MC increases ring hydroxylation 10-fold, twice that of N-hydroxylation. Thus, the production of both C- and N-hydroxy metabolites explains why carcinogenicity of 2-AAF is not completely abolished by 3-MC treatment.

Another example of mixed hydroxylation is that induced by β-naphthoflavone on DMBA. Hydroxylases are induced by this tumor inhibitor in the small intestines, lung, and liver (Wattenberg and Leong 1968). These workers reported at least two types of hydroxy metabolites produced by these hydroxylases:

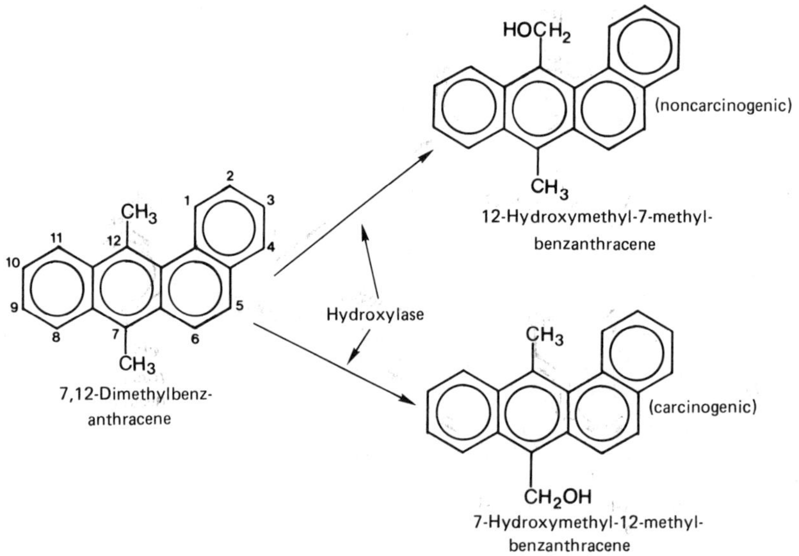

HOCH₂

(noncarcinogenic)

CH₃
12-Hydroxymethyl-7-methyl-
benzanthracene

CH₃

Hydroxylase

CH₃

(carcinogenic)

CH₂OH
7-Hydroxymethyl-12-methyl-
benzanthracene

7,12-Dimethylbenz-
anthracene

Thus, the production of carcinogenic and noncarcinogenic metabolites also explains the reduced, rather than complete, abolition of the carcinogenicity of DMBA administered with the flavone. Both lung and mammary tumor inductions are significantly inhibited.

Another flavone, 7,8-benzoflavone, also significantly reduces DMBA tumorigenesis in mouse skin; likewise, inhibition is incomplete (Kinoshita and Gelboin 1972). This flavone, however, is a good inhibitor for 3,4-benz(a)pyrene-induced skin tumors. Instead, when this compound was administered at a slightly higher dose — no more than two applications separated by a 3-day interval — 7,8-benzoflavone stimulated tumor formation by two fold.

Gelboin and Wiebel (1971) reported that β-naphthoflavone (5,6-benzoflavone) and 7,8-benzoflavone differ in their activity toward aryl hydrocarbon hydroxylase. The inhibition of DMBA-induced tumorigenesis by these compounds is the result of the inactivation of this enzyme. The effects of these flavones vary with the route of administration. When injected intraperitoneally, these compounds induce AHH activity in mouse skin. However, when applied topically, they elicit enzyme inhibition; 7,8-benzoflavone showed greater inhibition than 5,6-benzoflavone. The latter is one-third as active when applied topically than when injected intraperitoneally. Nevertheless, these flavones are potent inhibitors of AHH activity. At 10^{-17}M concentration, which is one-tenth of substrate concentration, 7,8-benzoflavone inhibits 60 to 70% of the enzyme activity. Increasing the flavone concentration 10-fold results in 77 to 91% inhibition.

The mechanism of tumor inhibition is different in tissues other than in the skin. Thus, 5,6-benzoflavone, which inhibits DMBA-induced tumor formation in lungs and mammary glands in rodents, induces rather than inhibits AHH activity in these tissues (Gelboin and Wiebel 1971).

There are at least two isozymes of microsomal AHH in tissues. One isozyme, the constitutive enzyme, is inherent in the tissues. The other is an induced isozyme, which is biosynthesized in response to the xenobiotic flavones and aromatic hydrocarbons. Flavones affect each of these isozymes differently. The constitutive isozyme is inhibited to a lesser extent than its induced counterpart (Wiebel et al. 1974). The isozymes in the liver also appear to be affected differently, depending on age and sex of the rodent. In 6-day-old rats, 7,8-benzoflavone increases the activity of the constitutive isoenzyme in both males and females, whereas the 3-MC-induced isozyme is inhibited. In adults, both isozymes are inhibited almost equally, by 75 to 86%, except in the male where the degree of inhibition is much less (19%). Thus, it appears that in the adult male rat, the constitutive isozyme is much more resistant to 7,8-benzoflavone and slightly stimulatory of the constitutive isozyme; the 3-MC-induced isozyme remains inhibited.

The importance of these flavones lies in the fact that a number of these substances occur naturally in food. They present significant biological activity, and have been observed by several investigators to have vitamin like properties (Baier et al. 1955; Scarborough and Bacharach 1949; Szent-Gyorgyi 1955). The flavones are often in the form of glycosides; e.g., as rhamnoglycosides. They are found in many fruits and vegetables and are most abundant in citrus fruits (Scarborough and Bacharach 1949). Several types of flavones and isoflavones found in natural products have been chemically identified and the structures of some of these are shown below.

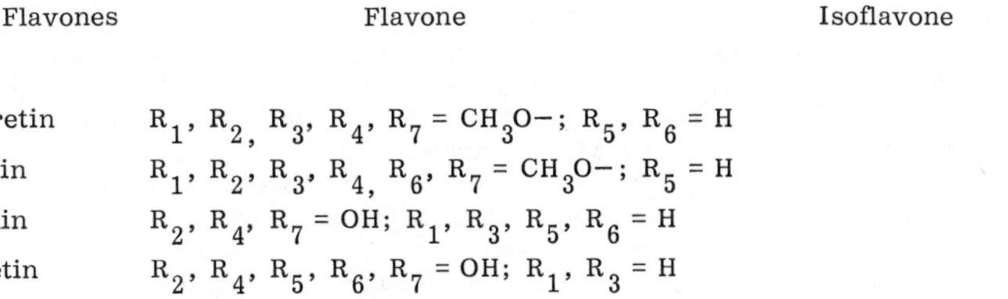

Flavones   Flavone   Isoflavone

Tangeretin	R_1, R_2, R_3, R_4, R_7 = CH$_3$O−; R_5, R_6 = H
Nobiletin	R_1, R_2, R_3, R_4, R_6, R_7 = CH$_3$O−; R_5 = H
Apigenin	R_2, R_4, R_7 = OH; R_1, R_3, R_5, R_6 = H
Quercetin	R_2, R_4, R_5, R_6, R_7 = OH; R_1, R_3 = H
Rutin	R_2, R_4, R_6, R_7 = OH; R_1, R_3 = H
	R_5 = rhamnoglucose

Hesperetin R_2, R_4, R_6 = OH; R_1, R_3, R_5 = H; R_7 = CH_3O-

Hesperidin R_1, R_3, R_5 = H; R_2, R_4, R_6 = OH; R_7 = CH O–

                  R_2 = rhamnoglucose

Catechin R_2, R_4, R_5, R_6, R_7 = OH; R_1, R_3 = H; H at C_4

Phloretol R_1, R_3, R_5 = OH; R , R , R = H; 2 and 3 positions in the ring are

                  saturated

Eriodictyol R_2, R_4, R_6, R_7 = OH: R_1, R_3, R_5 = H; 2 and 3 positions in the ring

                  are saturated

Naringin R_2, R_4, R_7 = OH; R_1, R_3, R_5, R_6 = H

Isoflavones

Formononetin R_2 = OH; R_6 = CH_3O-; R_1, R_3, R_4, R_5, R_7 = OH

Daidzein R_2, R_6 = OH; R_1, R_3, R_4, R_5, R_7 = H

Genistein R_2, R_4, R_6 = OH; R_1, R_3, R_5, R_7 = H

Biochanin A R_2, R_4 = OH; R_6 = CH_3O-; R_1, R_3, R_5, R_7 = H

The naturally occurring methoxyflavones, tangeretin and nobiletin, differ from the hydroxyflavones, apigenin and quercetin, in their activity toward AHH. The first two cause an enhanced activity of the constitutive isozyme, but a decreased activity of the 3-MC-induced AHH isozymes; the latter two result in an inhibition of both types of isozymes (Wiebel et al. 1974). Tangeretin is slightly more effective in enhancing constitutive AHH activity. Some isoflavones have estrogenic activity (Chap. 8).

Demethylases and Reductases: Table 7 demonstrates that the polycyclic aromatic hydrocarbons 3-MC, 1,2-BA, DMBA, and 1,2,5,6-DBA inhibit the hepatocarcinogenicity of 4-DAB and its respective derivatives (Miller et al. 1958). It has been observed that these hydrocarbons are able to maintain a high concentration of the hepatic enzymes, N-demethylase and azoreductase.

The detoxification of DAB or its derivatives such as 3-Me-4-DAB occurs in the presence of a series of enzymes, the major ones being N-demethylase and azoreductase (Chap. 4). The complete N-demethylation of DAB or its derivatives results in an almost complete loss of carcinogenicity, since the product of demethylation, 4-amino-azobenzene (4-AB) is essentially noncarcinogenic. Kirby (1947) reported that only hepatomas and cholangiomas developed in rats with diets containing 4-AB after a long latency. Derivatives of DAB require at least one N-methyl group in order to be an effective hepatocarcinogen (Clayson 1962).

Hydrocarbons such as 3-MC elicit rapidly increased tissue levels of N-demethylase (Conney et al. 1956). Within 24 hr, 0.1 mg of 3-MC increases the enzyme activity by a maximum of threefold. The activity increases in 6 hr and returns to normal in 7 days. The amount of enzyme induced increases with the dose of 3-MC. This increase occurs much earlier, and the enzyme persists at higher levels longer. Thus, 1 mg of 3-MC produces in 24 hr almost 1.5 times the activity produced with 0.1 mg; a slight increase to a maximum value (1.7 times) has been observed in 48 hr. This value persists for 5 days, and apparently, slowly drops off to control values.

N-Demethylases apparently can be induced only by specific compounds, such as those mentioned previously. Many polycyclic aromatic hydrocarbons, such as pyrene, fluorene, fluoranthrene, benzene, phenanthrene, and DMBA, are either inactive or very weak inducers (Conney et al. 1956). On the other hand, oxides of cholesterol, other steroids, such as dihydrocholesterol and ergosterol, and cyclic organic peroxides are effective N-demethylase inducers (Reif et al. 1954). Similarly, the quinones of 1,2,5,6-DBA are also active inducers (Conney et al. 1956). The activity of these oxides probably explains the increased azo dye N-demethylase activity in rats or mice fed commercial diets, or diets supplemented by animal products stored for long periods or crude tissue extracts. In contrast, purified semisynthetic diets or grain diets produce lower activity (Brown et al. 1954).

The induction of N-demethylases is by no means limited only to enzymes for azo dye demethylation. Many other kinds of N-demethylases for different types of compounds with susceptible N-methyl groups are also induced by such compounds as BP (Conney et al. 1959; von der Decken and Hultin 1960). In some cases, however, BP inhibits N-demethylation (Conney et al. 1959).

Other types of demethylases besides those specific for the N-methyl groups are also induced by hydrocarbons. Thus, there are O-methyl (Conney et al. 1959; Gillette 1963) and S-methyl (Henderson and Mazel 1964) demethylases.

The induction of N-demethylases by hydrocarbons such as 3-MC also occurs in other tissues besides the liver. The induction of demethylases in the lung and kidney has also been observed (Gilman and Conney 1963). However, certain demethylase inducers such as phenobarbital appear to be specific to the liver.

Azo reductases are also induced by polycyclic aromatic hydrocarbons, such as BP and 3-MC (Conney et al. 1956, 1959; Jervell et al. 1965). 3-MC can also produce a large increase in reductase activity (von der Decken and Hultin 1960). As with the N-demethylases, the level of enzyme activity also increases with the dose of the hydrocarbon. However, unlike the former, the attainment of a maximum level of activity is delayed for at least 24 hr. The observed differences in response of these two types of enzymes probably reflect the sequence of degradation of DAB, as shown in Chapter 4 on page 99.

Other types of reductases besides those degrading azo dyes are also induced by the hydrocarbons. The induction of these enzymes has been observed in the liver, lungs, adrenal and mammary glands, and even mammary tumors (Huggins and Fukunishi 1964).

Glucuronyltransferases: This enzyme, as discussed in Chapter 4, catalyzes glucuronide formation during the detoxification reaction of compounds. This enzyme can also be induced by certain compounds. Thus, 3,4-BP and 3-MC induce hepatic uridinediphosphate (UDP)-glucuronyl transferase in fetal and neonatal rats (Arias et al. 1963; Inscoe and Axelrod 1960). Induction of glucuronyl transferase by 3-MC reportedly occurs also in guinea pig liver (Inscoe and Axelrod 1960) and by 3,4-BP in mouse skin (Dutton and Stevenson 1962).

Phenobarbital also appears to be an effective inducer of glucuronyl transferase. Tracer studies suggest that phenobarbital enhances conjugation of BP metabolites with glucuronic acid (Schlede et al. 1970). This inducer also increases the excretion of 2-AAF glucuronide in rats (Matsushima et al. 1972; Wyatt and Cramer 1970). Whether or not phenobarbital treatment and glucuronyl transferase induction will promote or inhibit tumor formation depends on the time of phenobarbital administration relative to that of the carcinogen. If given prior to 2-AAF treatment, it reduces hepatoma formation; on the other hand, if the inducer is given after 2-AAF has been fed for 11 to 26 days, hepatic tumor formation is enhanced (Weisburger and Weisburger 1973). The reason for the latter observation is unknown.

The antioxidant butylhydroxytoluene also induces glucuronyl transferase activity, and like phenobarbital, also increases excretion of 2-AAF as the N-hydroxy glucuronide (Ulland et al. 1972).

Tumor Inhibition by Competition for Procarcinogen-Activating Chemical Groups or Metabolites There are not many examples in this mechanism of carcinogenic inhibition. For example, activation reactions involving groups which occur in relatively limited amounts in biological systems are easy targets for inhibition by competitive utilization of the required activating groups. For example, the activation of 2-AAF involves both hydroxylation and sulfation steps (Miller et al. 1961, 1964; p. 199). The biological system can provide more than enough oxygen and hydrogen atoms for the hydroxylation reaction, but not the sulfate ions for the sulfation reaction. The

latter is highly dependent on the dietary supply of sulfur amino acids, which in themselves are also limited in proteins. Therefore, compounds such as acetanilide (Miller
1970a; Weisburger et al. 1972) and possibly 8-hydroxyquinoline (Yamamoto et al. 1971)
may compete for sulfate groups. As expected, these compounds inhibit the carcinogenicity of 2-AAF, which apparently requires the final sulfate esterification for activation. Thus, addition of excess sulfate eliminates the inhibitory effects of acetanilide
(Weisburger et al. 1972) and increases the toxicity of 2-AAF (DeBaum et al. 1970).

Tumor Inhibition by Substances Interfering with Hormone Action Because hormones have a significant role in carcinogenesis, especially in highly hormone-
dependent tissues (pp. 181—189), substances which interfere with their activity may
be expected to inhibit tumorigenesis also. A few examples of these substances have
already been discussed; e.g., interference of Analog I with gonadotropin-releasing
factor (Johnson et al. 1976); 4-hydroxypropiophenone with pituitary hormones (Baba
1957); and goitrogens with thyroid hormones (Hoshino 1960; Leathern and Barken 1950;
Paschkis et al. 1948).

Tumor Inhibition by Substances Increasing Excretion of Carcinogen Biliary and
urinary excretion are the two major processes for eliminating foreign compounds. However, many substances eliminated by these routes require biotransformation to more
soluble as well as less toxic forms. Glucuronide formation is a common excretory biotransformation reaction allowing foreign compounds, such as carcinogens, to be excreted either in the bile or urine. Thus, conjugation of p-aminohippuric acid (PAH)
metabolites with glutathione (Boyland and Sims 1964a,b) and glucuronic and sulfuric
acids (Boyland and Sims 1962), leading to mercapturic acids, glucuronides and sulfates, respectively, have been observed with PAH. Glucuronides of nitrosoamines have
also been demonstrated (Okada and Suzuki 1972). Certain exogenous chemicals will induce specific enzymes to catalyze glucuronide formation of carcinogens, and thus promote rapid excretion. The route of excretion depends on the organism. For example,
phenobarbital enhances formation and biliary excretion of 2-AAF-glucuronide (Irving
et al. 1967; Matsushima et al. 1972; Wyatt and Cramer 1970) and BP-glucuronide
(Schlede et al. 1970) in the rat. However, in the rabbit, 2-AAF glucuronide is excreted mostly in the urine (Irving et al. 1967).
     The metabolic excretory products of several carcinogens are known, but whether
their formation is affected by other exogenous compounds has not been determined for
most of these compounds. It is conceivable that the induction of microsomal enzymes by
exogenous compounds, which result in hydroxylation and other reactions, will also
produce a "spin-off" in the induction of conjugative enzymes.

Inhibition of Tumorigenesis by Interference of the Binding or Reaction of
Carcinogens with Critical Cellular Molecules Carcinogens have been shown to bind to
both cellular proteins and nucleic acids. There appears to be a positive correlation between such types of binding and carcinogenic activity. A correlation has been reported, for example, between the carcinogenicity of several polycyclic aromatic hydrocarbons (PAH) (Heidelberger and Moldenhauer 1965) and their binding to soluble mouse
skin proteins, particularly with specific electrophoretic fractions (Abell and Heidelberger 1962). Binding also has been observed with nucleic acids (Brookes and Lawley
1964).
     Correlation between carcinogenicity and binding to cellular proteins also has been
noted with carcinogenic azo dyes, such as DAB and MAB (Bonser 1947; Miller and
Miller 1947) and their derivatives as well as others (Miller et al. 1949). Binding has
been observed not only to cellular proteins, but also to nucleic acids (Salzberg et al.
1951). Other carcinogenic aromatic amines also have been found to bind to cellular
proteins; thus, 2-AAF (2-fluorenylacetylamide) binds to the same mouse epithelial proteins as the PAH (Heidelberger and Weiss 1951). Like the PAH, the azo dyes appear to
bind to specific cellular proteins (Ketterer et al. 1967; Sorof et al. 1951).

The carcinogenic nitrosamines alkylate both proteins (Craddock 1965; Magee and Hultin 1962) and nucleic acids (Loveless 1969; Swann and Magee 1971; Wunderlich et al. 1970). While the binding of many carcinogens with cellular macromolecules correlates well with carcinogenicity, there are exceptions. Noncarcinogens in each class of compounds, i.e, PAH and aromatic amines, also bind strongly to these macromolecules. For example, the noncarcinogenic hydrocarbon dibenz(a,c)anthracene (Heidelberger and Moldenhauer 1956) and certain noncarcinogenic aniline and toluidine derivatives (Miller et al. 1949) bind extensively to proteins. However, in the case of the azo dyes, the carcinogenic compounds attained maximum binding more rapidly than the noncarcinogens (e.g., DAB in 3 to 4 weeks, compared to 12 weeks with the noncarcinogens) (Miller et al. 1949). Litwack et al. (1971) noted that carcinogens bind to proteins covalently, whereas noncarcinogens bind noncovalently.

It might be inferred from the data that for many carcinogens, the ability to bind or react with critical cellular macromolecules may be a requirement for carcinogenicity. Thus, if such binding can be inhibited, a corresponding decrease in carcinogenic potency or activity can be expected. There are, in fact, many exogenous compounds which inhibit such binding, and thus, tumor induction is inhibited as well. For example, 7,8-benzoflavone inhibits DNA, RNA, and protein binding of 7,12-dimethylbenz(a)anthracene (7,12-DMBA) by 50 to 70% (Kinoshita and Gelboin 1972), and the formation of skin tumors in mice by 55 to 80%. This compound which inhibits covalent binding of benz(a)pyrene to RNA and protein by as much as 50%, reportedly does not inhibit to a large extent skin tumorigenesis induced by benz(a)pyrene. Whatever its significance, the flavone inhibits binding to DNA by only 18% (Kinoshita and Gelboin 1972). The inhibition of tumorigenesis by the flavone is not associated with induction of specific microsomal enzymes which, as mentioned previously, are also involved in the inhibition of tumor induction and/or promotion (Gelboin et al. 1970).

However, the PAHs, which inhibit the aromatic amine-induced tumors, both induce microsomal enzymes as well as inhibit protein binding (Miller et al. 1958). This suggests that the binding species may be a metabolite of the carcinogen. Examples of compounds which reduce or inhibit protein binding by DAB, include 3-MC, benzo(a)-pyrene, dibenz(a,h)anthracene), and its 7,14- and 5,6-quinone derivatives.

Chloramphenicol and indole, which inhibit liver cancer induced by N-hydroxy-2AAF, also inhibit binding of the carcinogen to liver nuclear DNA (Weisburger et al. 1967). Whereas prefeeding chloramphenicol to experimental animals for 7 to 20 days inhibits liver tumors induced by 3'-methyl-DAB, protein binding by this carcinogen is not affected (Blunck 1971).

The binding of liver protein to N-nitrosodimethylamine is also significantly inhibited by acetonitrile as well as by dimethyl- and diethylformamide (Mirvish and Sidransky 1971). Protein binding with this carcinogen is only slightly inhibited by phenobarbitone and 3-methylcholanthrene. It should be recalled that phenobarbitone reduces liver and stomach tumors induced by diethylnitrosamine in NMRI mice (Kunz et al. 1969). 3-MC induces lung tumors in mice given dimethylnitrosamine (Hoch-Ligeti et al. 1968), even though this hydrocarbon reduces the acute toxicity of the nitrosamine (Venkatesan et al. 1970a,b).

The data appear to show that the binding of carcinogens to macromolecules in the cell may be related to the metabolic activation of some carcinogens, whereas in others, this is not necessarily so. This suggests that metabolic transformation is required in some cases prior to binding. Nevertheless, binding without activation does not imply that carcinogenic activity is not preceded by metabolic activation. In this case, binding simply allows longer residence of the compound in the cell, so that there are delayed excretion and longer contact with specific molecules necessary for carcinogenic induction.

Inhibition of Tumorigenesis by Interference with Specific Enzymes   Since most carcinogens require metabolic activation of their precursors, it is reasonable to expect that substances which can inhibit the enzymes involved would also inhibit tumorigenesis. Thus, actinomyocin D, at doses which do not cause skin damage, has been reported to inhibit the early stages of tumor formation induced by DMBA and β-propiolactone (Hemings et al. 1968) or urethane (Gelboin et al. 1965). It appears that this inhibitory activity is present even if the application of the inhibitor is delayed for as long as 30 to 40 days after tumor initiation. Such carcinogens as aflatoxin, diepoxy-butane, and acridine orange also exhibit tumor-inhibiting activity (Sporu et al. 1966). Apparently, these substances as well as actinomyin D are inhibitory because of their ability to bind or interact with DNA and RNA and/or inhibit their biosynthesis.

Mycophenolic acid, a product of the fungus *Penicillium stoniferum*, effectively inhibits certain types of tumors, such as Walker carcinoma 256 and other solid tumors. However, this compound is only moderately effective or completely ineffective with certain other types (Sweeney et al. 1972a). Its mode of action, as reported by Sweeney and coworkers (1972b), involves an interference in the interconversion of inosine, xanthosine, and guanosine monophosphates (IMP, XMP, and GMP, respectively) by inhibiting IMP dehydrogenase and GMP synthetase. Since these enzymes occur in normal cells, it is conceivable that mycophenolic acid may also be involved in specific processes during the initial cellular transformation. The activity of this inhibitor depends on the presence of β-glucuronidase in the tumor. Since mycophenolic acid is detoxified as the glucuronide, it cannot enter the cell in this form. Whether or not β-glucuronidase is produced by mycophenolic acid-sensitive cells in the preneoplastic state is not known. Normally, this enzyme occurs largely in the liver, spleen, and in certain reproductive and endocrine tissues (Fishman 1955). Sensitivity to mycophenolic acid also depends on whether the cell possesses a low activity of hypoxanthine-guanine phosphoribosyltransferase. This enzyme circumvents the interconversion of inosine, xanthosine, and guanosine monophosphates, the latter being required in RNA synthesis. Whether or not this enzyme is increased or decreased during preneoplastic transformation of a cell also is not known.

Certain structural analogs of carcinogens may exert a competitive inhibition for enzymes involved in the metabolism of a carcinogen. Thus, the inhibitory activity of butylcarbamates against skin cancer induced by ethylcarbamate (urethane) (Garcia 1963) may be explained on the basis of competitive inhibition between these two compounds. Similarly, other structural analogs of urethane show competitive inhibitory activity (Kaye 1960).

Other Inhibitory Mechanism   Certain substances exert their inhibitory action on the activity of cocarcinogens. For example, griseofulvin, a fungal antibiotic and a carcinogen (Epstein et al. 1967), inhibits the promotion of skin tumor induced by benz(a)-pyrene and promoted by croton oil (Vesselinovitch and Mihailovich 1968). Griseofulvin has not only carcinogenic activity, but also cocarcinogenic activity with 3-MC in inducing skin tumors (Barich et al. 1962). The inhibitory activity of griseofulvin arises from its interference in DNA replication, resulting in the arrest of cell division in the metaphase stage (Paget and Walpole 1960).

The detergent Tween 60 (polyoxyethylenesorbitan monostearate) promotes DMBA-induced skin tumors. Zephiran (benzalkonium chloride) inhibits this promoting activity (Dammert 1961). Cholesterol added to Tween 60 solution also inhibits the promoting activity of the latter (Setälä 1961). In the latter case, the added cholesterol prevents the leakage of membrane-bound sterol in the presence of Tween 60. This action explains the inhibitory activity of the added cholesterol.

A promising development in tumor inhibition is the discovery of the diffusible inhibitor, tumor angiogenesis factor (Brem and Folkman 1975; Brem et al. 1975). The diffusible factor was first demonstrated in neonatal rabbit cartilage. Its activity is destroyed by heating, and this fact suggests that the inhibitor is possibly a protein. It has been shown that rapid tumor growth understandably depends on the rapid vascularizaiton of the clone of tumor cells. To accomplish this, tumors produce a humoral substance which stimulates nearby blood vessels to develop vascular extensions toward the tumor. The latter grow rapidly when sufficient blood vessels have enmeshed it (Folkman 1975). Obviously, extensive vascularization is required for effective nutrification and removal of waste from the tumor.

There are also many other nonnutritive carcinogenesis inhibitors which have been reported (Homburger 1974; Wattenberg 1978). For example, butylhydroxyanisole (BHA), an antioxidant and a food additive, possesses marked inhibitory activity on tumors of the forestomach in mice induced by BP and DMBA (Wattenberg 1973); it also inhibits tumors remote from the site of application; e.g., pulmonary tumors, following application of BP, DMBA, urethane, or uracil mustard (Wattenberg 1973). Its mode of action in this case is not known, but like many other xenobiotic chemicals, it can also induce microsomal enzyme activity (Creaven et al. 1966); thus, deactivation of carcinogens may be enhanced. Perhaps relevant to the inhibitory activity of BHA is the effect of a similar antioxidant, butylhydroxytoluene (BHT). This antioxidant causes a decrease in the number of cultured monkey kidney cells by interfering with the incorporation of precursors into DNA, RNA, or proteins (Milner 1967). This effect is correlated to dosage. Additionally, BHT also causes shortening of the cell cycle and decreases survival of cultured human leukocytes stimulated by phytohemagglutinin. BHT also produces extensive cell membrane damage (Sciorra et al. 1974). This effect is dose related.

In relation to the role of antioxidants in carcinogenesis, an exciting development has been reported by Novi (1981). Advanced aflatoxin B_1-induced hepatocellular carcinomas were regressed in rats treated for 8 months with 100 mg/day of reduced glutathione (GHS). The GHS treatment, which commenced after 16 months following discontinuance of the aflatoxin treatment, resulted in 81% survival of the test animals 24 months after the last exposure to aflatoxin compared to 100% mortality after 20 months in those which received the carcinogen only. These results are consistent with the inhibitory effects of antioxidants (Shamberger et al. 1976; Wattenberg 1978) on tumor induction. As far as is known, this is the first time that a naturally occurring reducing agent has been reported to reverse the course of advanced tumors. These results provide valuable clues as to the role of oxidizing and reducing agents in carcinogenesis as well as the exciting possibility of finding a cure for cancer.

Syncarcinogenic Compounds

Understandably, more than one carcinogen may be ingested at any given time or for a prolonged period. We have noted in earlier sections that a carcinogen may inhibit or diminish the activity of another carcinogen. Thus, the question arises: Is there also syngerism or additive effects between carcinogens? The term syncarcinogenesis is meant to include both additive and synergistic effects. Syncarcinogenicity should be distinguished from cocarcinogenicity, since cocarcinogenic substances are noncarcinogens or, at worst, weak carcinogens. A number of studies have demonstrated syncarcinogenic effects, even though in some instances where a complex mixture is present, such as in tobacco smoke, tar, or similar mixtures, the distinction between these three effects is obscured. Nevertheless, tests using a mixture of pure carcinogens demonstrates the phenomenon of syncarcinogenesis. Some of the syncarcinogenic compounds that have been reported are shown in Table 8.

Syncarcinogenesis is of great significance when related to the human situation, since possible multiple exposures to several carcinogens may be the norm rather than the exception. Nevertheless, it is difficult to predict what direction such multiple exposures will take, since as seen in the preceding discussion, many factors come into play. The pluses and minuses together do not always follow a simple algebraic summation.

The Significance of Exogenous Chemical Modifiers of Carcinogenesis

The complex modern environment exposes humans to countless chemicals of varying biological activities. Nonnutritional exogenous compounds are metabolized for the purpose of facilitating excretion from the body, and in many cases, detoxification as well. Unfortunately, these metabolic processes also produce metabolites, which biologically, may be more harmful than their precursors. In many instances, the beneficial or

Table 8. Syncarcinogenic Compounds

Syncarcinogen	Test Animal	Tumor Site	Ref.
Tannic acid and 2-AAF		liver	Mosonyi and Korpassy (1953)
DMNA and CCl$_4$	rat	kidney	Pound et al. (1973)
DMNA and 3-MC	rat	lung	Hoch-Ligeti et al. (1968)
	mouse	kidney and lung	Cardesa et al. (1973)
DENA and 3,4-BP	hamster	lung	Montesano et al. (1970)
DENA and 3,4-BP plus ferric oxide	hamster	lung	Montesano et al. (1974)
DAB and DENA		liver	Epstein and Fugi (1970) Schmähl (1970)
Piperonylbutoxide and freon mice	mouse	liver	Epstein et al. (1967b)

Abbreviations: 2-AAF-2- — acetylaminofluorene; 3,4-BP — 3,4-benz(a)pyrene; DAB — dimethylazobenzene; DENA — diethylnitrosamine; DMNA — dimethylnitrosamine.

harmful effects resulting from the metabolism of these compounds cannot be predicted because other factors are involved. Thus, two or more carcinogens together may inhibit or reduce their carcinogenicity, or enhance markedly each separate effect. A noncarcinogen may also reduce the effect of a carcinogen or enhance it.

Of prime significance to the question of exogenous chemicals is the activity of microsomal enzymes which are responsible for the metabolism of these compounds. Two types of exogenous chemicals may be identified in terms of their effects on the activity of these enzymes: (1) Compounds which stimulate microsomal enzyme activity; and (2) compounds which inhibit these enzymes. In the first group are food additives — food dyes (Radonnski 1961), food preservatives (Botham et al. 1970; Gilbert and Goldberg 1965), chemical food contaminants in the form of insecticides such as DDT (Conney et al. 1967; Hart and Fouts 1965) and herbicides (Kinoshita et al. 1966); naturally occurring compounds, such as caffeine (Mitoma et al. 1969), flavones (Wattenberg et al. 1968), and essential oils, such as eucalyptol (Jori et al. 1970), and derived substances, such as the polycyclic aromatic hydrocarbons (Arcos et al. 1961; Welch et al. 1969). Compounds in the second group include certain organophosphate insecticides (Welch et al. 1967), insecticide synergists (Jaffe et al. 1968, 1969), aliphatic halogenated hydrocarbons, such as CCl$_4$ (Dingell and Heimberg 1968; Levin et al. 1970), CO (Conney et al. 1968; Cooper et al. 1965), and various drugs (Conney and Burns 1962). Because of their effects on microsomal enzymes, all of these compounds pose significant influence on the whole question of chemical carcinogenesis.

Results of studies on the influence of these compounds on microsomal enzyme induction in man have been reported. One of the most extensively studied insecticides is DDT. By comparing 6-β-hydroxycortisol urinary excretion and the serum half-life of phenylbutazone in DDT-exposed individuals and controls, one obtains an indication of liver microsomal enzyme activity. Studies by Poland et al. (1970) showed that 6-β-hydroxycortisol excretion of factory workers exposed to DDT was 291 ±36 mg/24 hr compared to 185 ±17 mg/24 hr in controls. The former showed a 65.5 ±3.5 hr half-life for phenylbutazone compared to 81.0 ±3.7 in the control. Both these values are statistically significant (p <0.01) even though there is great variability in the response of subjects. The total DDT level in serum of the factory workers was 1359 ±162 µg/ml (p <0.01) compared to 51 ±5 µg in controls. The observed variability may be ascribed to genetic and environmental factors.

The metabolism of other drugs can also be enhanced by DDT and other halogenated hydrocarbons. Thus, DDT enhances the metabolism of antipyrine (Kolmodin et al. 1969). DDT also produces increased hepatic glucuronyl transferase activity in rats (Thompson et al. 1969); this observation may explain the observed decreased bilirubin levels in humans with nonhemolytic jaundice (Thompson et al. 1969). This effect of DDT is similar to phenobarbital, which also increases glucuronyl transferase activity; the increased activity results in a decrease in bilirubin levels in newborns (Maurer et al. 1968). The occurrence of hyperbilirubinemia normally seen in newborns during the first few days of life is prevented when phenobarbital is administered daily for 2 weeks or more before delivery.

That polycyclic aromatic hydrocarbons also stimulate microsomal enzymes in human tissue has been demonstrated in studies with placentas from smokers and nonsmokers. In these studies (Nebert et al. 1969), Welch et al. 1969, 1968), there was a marked difference in the benz(a)pyrene (BP) hydroxylase activity. Those who smoked 10 to 40 cigarettes/day showed a 50-fold increase in BP activity compared to a control group, and a 70-fold increase in those who smoked 15 to 20 cigarettes. Similarly, placentas of smokers showed N-demethylase activity in contrast to nonsmokers who showed little or no activity (Welch et al. 1969). When several PAHs found in cigarette smoke were tested individually on rat placentas, all were able to induce marked BP hydroxylase activity. In this case, 1,2-benzanthracene was the most active (Welch et al. 1969). PAH also enhanced the metabolism of nicotine.

All exogenous chemicals, as would be expected, do not induce the activity of all microsomal enzymes. Thus, in humans, the insecticide piperonyl butoxide has no effect on the enzymes metabolizing antipyrene (Conney et al. 1971). Similarly, the induction of these enzymes also show species differences as well as genetic differences (Conney et al. 1971; Vessell and Page 1968a,b).

Thus, studies discussed in the preceding sections indicate that exogenous chemicals can stimulate or inhibit metabolism. The toxicological effects due to multiple exposures to all kinds of chemicals are hard to predict. Nevertheless, it is possible that substances which have little or no toxic effects at certain levels, but are markedly inhibitory to carcinogenesis, may provide another means of controlling this process.

REFERENCES

Abell, C. W. and Heidelberger, C. 1962. Interaction of carcinogenic hydrocarbons with tissues. VIII. Binding of tritium-labeled hydrocarbons to the soluble proteins of mouse skin. *Cancer Res.* 22: 931—946.

Agate, F. J. et al. 1955. The nonessentiality of the hypophysis for the induction of tumors with 3,4-benzpyrene. *Cancer Res.* 15: 6—8.

Altman, H. J. and Schwartz, A. D. 1978. Malignant diseases of infancy, childhood and adolescence. Saunders, Philadelphia.

American Cancer Society, 1983. Cancer Facts and Figures. American Cancer Society, New York.

Ames, B. N., Sims, P. and Grover, P. L. 1972. Epoxides of carcinogenic polycyclic hydrocarbons are frameshift mutagens. *Science* 176: 47—49.

Anderson, D. E. 1970. Genetic varieties of neoplasia. In: The University of Texas M.D. Anderson Hospital and Tumor Institute at Houston, 23rd Annual Symposium on Fundamental Cancer Research, 1969. *Genetic Concepts and Neoplasia*. Williams & Wilkins, Baltimore.

Anderson, D. E. 1971. Clinical characteristics of the genetic variety of cutaneous melanoma in man. *Cancer* 28: 728—725.

Andervont, H. B. 1937. Pulmonary tumors in mice — The susceptibility of the lungs of albino mice to carcinogenic action of 1,2,5,6-dibenzanthracene. *Public Health Rep.* 52: 212—221.

Andervont, H. B. 1938. The incidence of induced subcutaneous and pulmonary tumors and spontaneous mammary tumors in hybrid mice. *Public Health Rep.* 53: 1665—1671.

Andervont, H. B. 1950. Induction of hemangio-endotheliomas and sarcomas in mice with o-aminoazotoluene. *J. Natl. Cancer Inst.* 10: 927—941.

Andervont, H. B. and Dunn, T. B. 1950. Response of mammary-tumor-agent-free strain of DBA female mice to percutaneous application of methylcholanthrene. *J. Natl. Cancer Inst.* 10: 895—926.

Andervont, H. B., White, J. and Edwards, J. E. 1944. Effect of two azo compounds when added to the diet of mice. *J. Natl. Cancer Inst.* 4: 583—586.

Andrews, E. J. 1971. Evidence of the nonimmune regression of chemically induced papillomas in mouse skin. *J. Natl. Cancer Inst.* 47: 653—665.

Arcos, J. C., Conney, A. H. and Buu-Hoi, N. P. 1961. Induction of microsomal enzyme synthesis by polycyclic aromatic hydrocarbons of different molecular sizes. *J. Biol. Chem.* 236: 1291—1296.

Arcos, J. C., Argus, M. F. and Wolf, G. 1968. *Chemical Induction of Cancer, Structural Bases and Biological Mechanisms.* Academic Press, Inc., New York.

Arias, I. M., Gartner, I., Furman, M. and Wolfson, S. 1963. Studies on the effect of several drugs on hepatic glucuronide formation in newborn rats and humans. *Ann. N.Y. Acad. Sci.* 111: 274—280.

Armitage, P. and Doll, R. 1957. A two-stage theory of carcinogenesis in relation to the age distribution of human cancer. *Br. J. Cancer* 11: 161—169.

Ashley, D. J. B. 1969a. The two "hit" and multiple "hit" theories of carcinogenesis. *Br. J. Cancer* 23: 313—328.

Ashley, D. J. B. 1969b. Colonic cancer arising in polyposis coli. *J. Med. Genet.* 6: 376—378.

Atkin, N. B. 1970. Cytogenetic studies on human tumors and premalignant lesions. In: *Genetic Concepts and Neoplasia.* M.D. Anderson Hospital Symposium. Williams & Wilkins, Baltimore.

Auerbach, C. 1956. A possible case of delayed mutation in man. *Ann. Hum. Genet.* 20: 266—269.

Baba, T. 1957. Inhibitory effect of p-hydroxypropiophenone (PHP) upon experimental induction of hepatoma in rats fed butter-yellow (DAB). *Gann* 48: 145—158.

Badger, G. M. 1962. *The Chemical Basis of Carcinogenic Activity.* Charles Thomas, Springfield, Illinois.

Baier, W. E. et al. 1955. Bioflavonoids and the capillary. *Ann. N.Y. Acad. Sci.* 61: 637—736.

Ball, J. K. 1970. Immunosuppression and carcinogenesis. Contrasting effects with 7,12-dimethyl benz(a)anthracene, benz(a)pyrene, and 3-methylcholanthrene. *J. Natl. Cancer Inst.* 44: 1—10.

Ball, H. A. and Samuels, L. T. 1936. The relation of the hypophysis to the growth of malignant tumors. III. The effect of hypophesectomy on autogenous tumors. *Am. J. Cancer* 26: 547—551.

Balner, H. and Dersjant, H. 1969. Increased oncogenic effect of methyl cholanthrene after treatment with antilymphocyte serum. *Nature* 224: 376—378.

Barich, L. L., Schwartz, J. and Barich, D. J. 1962. Oral griseofulvin: A co-carcinogenic agent to MC-induced cutaneous tumors. *Cancer Res.* 22: 53—55.

Bartsch, H., Dworkin, C., Miller, E. C. and Miller, J. A. 1973. Formation of electrophilic N-acetoxyarylamines in cytosols from rat mammary gland and other tissues by transacetylation from the carcinogen N-hydroxy-4-acetylaminobiphenyl. *Biochim. Biophys. Acta* 304: 42—55.

Bates, R. R. et al. 1968. Inhibition by actinomycin D of DNA synthesis and skin tumorigenesis induced by 7,12-dimethylbenz(a)anthracene. *Cancer Res.* 28: 27–34.

Berenblum, I. 1949. The carcinogenic action of 9,10-dimethyl-1,2-benzanthracene on the skin and subcutaneous tissues of the mouse, rabbit, rat and guinea pig. *J. Natl. Cancer Inst.* 10: 167–174.

Berenblum, I. 1954. Carcinogenesis and tumor pathogenesis. *Adv. Cancer Res.* 2: 129–175.

Berenblum, I. and Schoental, R. 1947. Carcinogenic constituents of coal tar. *Br. J. Cancer* 1: 157–165.

Biancifiori, C. and Caschera, F. 1962. The relation between pseudo pregnancy and the chemical induction by four carcinogens of mammary and ovarian tumors in BALB/C Mice. *Br. J. Cancer* 16: 722–730.

Bickis, I., Estwick, R. R. and Campbell, J. S. 1956. Observations on initiation of skin carcinoma in pituitary dwarf mice. I. *Cancer* 9: 763–767.

Bielschowsky, F. 1944. Tumours of the thyroid produced by 2-acetylaminofluorene and allylthiourea. *Br. J. Exp. Pathol.* 25: 90–95.

Bielschowsky, F. 1945. Experimental nodular goiter. *Br. J. Exp. Pathol.* 26: 270–275.

Bielschowsky, F. 1955. Neoplasia and internal environment. *Br. J. Cancer* 9: 80–116.

Bielschowsky, F. 1958. Carcinogenesis in thyroidectomized rat. The effect of injected growth hormone. *Br. J. Cancer* 12: 231–233.

Bielschowsky, F. 1959. Carcinogenesis in dwarf mice. *Ann. Rep. Br. Emp. Cancer Camp.* 37: 482.

Bielschowsky, F. 1961. The role of hormonal factors in the development of tumors induced by 2-aminofluorene and related compounds. *Acta Un. Int. Canc.* 17: 121–130.

Bielschowsky, F. and Bielschowsky, M. 1959. Carcinogenesis in alloxan-diabetic rats. In: Ciba Foundation Symposium *Carcinogenesis: Mechanism of Action.* Wolstenholme and O'Connor (eds.). Churchill, London.

Bielschowsky, F. and Hall, W. H. 1953. Carcinogenesis in the thyroidectomized rat. *Br. J. Cancer* 7: 358–366.

Bischoff, F. 1972. Organic polymer biocompatibility and toxicology. *Clin. Chem.* 18: 869–894.

Bischoff, F. and Bryson, G. 1964. Carcinogenesis through solid state surfaces. *Prog. Exp. Tumor Res.* 5: 85–133.

Bloom, J. L. and Falconer, D. S. 1964. A gene with major effect on susceptibility to induced lung tumors in mice. *J. Natl. Cancer Inst.* 33: 607–618.

Blunck, J. M. 1971. Inhibition by chloramphenicol of aminoazo dye carcinogenesis in rat liver: Morphological studies. *Pathology* 3: 99–106.

Bodansky, O. 1975. *Biochemistry of Human Cancer.* Academic Press, New York.

Bonne, C., Lodder, J. and Streef, G. M. 1930. Skin cancers in monkeys (Macacus cynomolgus). *Z. Krebsforsch.* 32: 310–326 (German).

Bonser, G. M. 1938. The hereditary factor in induced skin tumours in mice: Establishment of a strain specially sensitive to carcinogenic agents applied to the skin. *J. Pathol. Bacteriol.* 46: 581–602.

Bonser, G. M. 1947. Experimental cancer of the bladder. *Br. Med. Bull.* 4: 379–382.

Bonser, G. M. and Jull, J. W. 1952. *Cited by* Berenblum, I. 1954. Carcinogenesis and tumor pathogenesis. *Adv. Cancer Res.* 2: 129–175.

Bonser, G. M., Clayson, D. B. and Jull, J. W. 1951. An experimental inquiry into the cause of industrial bladder cancer. *Lancet* 2: 286–288.

Bonser, G. M., Clayson, D. B. and Jull, J. W. 1956. The induction of tumours of the subcutaneous tissues, liver and intestine in the mouse by certain dyestuffs and their intermediates. *Br. J. Cancer* 10: 653–667.

Borchert, P., Miller, J. A., Miller, E. C. and Shires, T. K. 1973a. 1'-Hydroxy-safrole, a proximate carcinogenic metabolite of safrole in the rat and mouse. *Cancer Res.* 33: 590–600.

Borchert, P., Wislocki, P. G., Miller, J. A. and Miller, E. C. 1973b. The metabolism of the naturally occurring hepatocarcinogen safrole to 1'-hydroxysafrole and the electrophilic reactivity of 1'-acetoxysafrole. *Cancer Res.* 33: 575–589.

Botham, C. M. et al. 1970. Effects of butylated hydroxytoluene on the enzyme activity and ultrastructure of rat hepatocytes. *Food Cosmet. Toxicol.* 8: 1–8.

Boutwell, R. K. and Bosch, D. K. 1959. The tumor-promoting action of phenol and related compounds of mouse skin. *Cancer Res.* 19: 413–424.

Boutwell, R. K., Colburn, N. H. and Muckerman, C. C. 1969. In vivo reactions of β-propiolactone. *Ann. N.Y. Acad. Sci.* 163: 751–763.

Boyland, E. 1967. A chemist's view of cancer prevention. *Proc. R. Soc. Med.* 60: 93–89.

Boyland, E. and Sims, P. 1962. Metabolism of polycyclic compounds. 21. The metabolism of phenanthrene in rabbits and rats: Dihydro-dihydroxy compounds and related glucosiduronic acids. *Biochem. J.* 84: 571–582.

Boyland, E. and Sims, P. 1964a. Metabolism of polycyclic compounds. 23. The metabolism of pyrene in rats and rabbits. *Biochem. J.* 96: 391–398.

Boyland, E. and Sims, P. 1964b. Metabolism of polycyclic compounds. 24. The metabolism of benz(a)anthracene. *Biochem. J.* 91: 493–506.

Boyland, E. and Williams, K. 1965. An enzyme catalyzing the conjugation of epoxides with glutathione. *Biochem. J.* 94: 190–197.

Brem, H. and Folkman, J. 1975. Inhibition of tumor angiogenesis mediated by cartilage. *J. Exp. Med.* 141: 427–439.

Brem, H., Arensman, R. and Folkman, J. 1975. Inhibition of tumor angiogenesis by a diffusible factor from cartilage. In: *Extracellular Matrix Influences on Gene Expression.* H. Slavkin (ed.). Academic Press, New York.

Brodie, B. B. 1964. Distribution and fate of drugs: Therapeutic implications. In: *Absorption and Distribution of Drugs.* T. B. Burns (ed.). Livingston, London.

Brodie, B. B. and Gillette, J. R. 1971. *Concepts in Chemical Pharmacology.* Part II. Springer, New York.

Brookes, P. and Lawley, P. D. 1964a. Evidence for the binding of polynuclear aromatic hydrocarbons to the nucleic acids of mouse skin: Relation between carcinogenic power of hydrocarbons and their binding to deoxyribonucleic acid. *Nature* 202: 781–784.

Brookes, P. and Lawley, P. D. 1964b. Reaction of some mutagenic and carcinogenic compounds with nucleic acids. *J. Cell. Comp. Physiol.* (Suppl. 1) 64: 111–128.

Brown, R. R., Miller, J. A. and Miller, E. C. 1954. The metabolism of methylated aminoazo dyes. IV. Dietary factors enhancing demethylation in vitro. *J. Biol. Chem.* 209: 211–222.

Bubenik, J., Perlmann, P., Helmstein, K. and Moberger, G. 1970. Cellular and humoral immune responses to human urinary bladder carcinomas. *Int. J. Cancer* 5: 310–319.

Bulbrook, R. D. 1970. Prognostic value of steroid assays in human breast cancer. *Adv. Steroid Biochem. Pharmacol.* 1: 387–417.

Bulbrook, R. D. and Hayward, J. L. 1967. Abnormal urinary steroid excretion and subsequent breast cancer. *Lancet* 1: 519–522.

Bulbrook, R. D., Hayward, J. L. and Spicer, C. C. 1971. Relation between urinary androgen and corticoid excretion and subsequent breast cancer. *Lancet* 2: 395–398.

Bull, L. B., Culvenor, C. C. J. and Dick, A. T. 1968. *The Pyrrolizidine Alkaloids. Their Chemistry, Pathogenicity and Other Biological Properties.* Elsevier

North Holland, Amsterdam.

Bullough, W. S. 1975. Chalone control mechanisms. *Life Sci.* 16: 323–330.

Burch, P. R. J. 1965. Natural and radiation carcinogenesis in man. II. Natural leukemogenesis initiation. *Proc. R. Soc. Lond. (Biol.)* 162: 240.

Burdette, W. J. 1943. The inheritance of susceptibility to tumors induced in mice. II. Tumors induced by methylcholanthrene in the progeny of C3H and JK mice. *Cancer Res.* 3: 318–320.

Burdette, W. J. 1952. Induced pulmonary tumors. *J. Thoracic Surg.* 24: 427–433.

Burdette, W. J. and Strong, L. C. 1943. The inheritance of susceptibility to tumors induced in mice. I. Tumors induced by methylcholanthrene in five inbred strains of mice. *Cancer Res.* 3: 13–20.

Burnet, M. 1964. Immunological factors in the process of carcinogenesis. *Br. Med. Bull.* 20: 154–158.

Burrows, H. 1933. A spindle-celled tumor in a fowl following injection of 1:2:5:6-dibenzanthracene in a fatty medium. *Am. J. Cancer* 17: 1–6.

Butzow, J. J. and Eichhorn, G. L. 1965. Interactions of metal ions with polynucleotides and related compounds. IV. Degradation of polyribonucleotides by zinc and other divalent metal ions. *Biopolymers* 3: 95–107.

Cairns, J. 1975. The cancer problem. *Sci. Am.* 233(5): 64–79.

Cairns, J. and Logan, J. 1983. Step by step into carcinogenesis. *Nature* 304: 582–583.

Cantarow, A. and Schepartz, B. 1967. *Biochemistry*. 4th ed. Saunders, Philadelphia.

Cantarow, A., Stasney, J. and Paschkis, K. E. 1948. The influence of sex hormones on mammary tumors induced by 2-acetylaminofluorene. *Cancer Res.* 8: 412–417.

Cardesa, A. et al. 1973. The syncarcinogenic effect of methylcholanthrene and dimethylnitrosamine in Swiss mice. *Z. Krebsforsch.* 79: 98–107.

Chan, J. T. and Black, H. S. 1978. The mitigating effect of dietary antioxidants on chemically-induced carcinogenesis. *Experientia* 34: 110–111.

Chasseaud, L. F. 1979. The role of glutathione and glutathione s-transferases in the metabolism of chemical carcinogens and other electrophilic agents. *Adv. Cancer Res.* 29: 175–274.

Choldin, S. 1927. Tumors in chicken caused by coal tar. *Z. Krebsforsch.* 25: 235–246. (German)

Clayson, D. B. 1962. *Chemical Carcinogenesis*. Little Brown, Boston.

Clayson, D. B., Gardner, R. C. 1976. Carcinogenic aromatic amines and related compounds. In: *Chemical Carcinogens*. C. E. Searle (ed.). American Chemical Society, Washington, D. C.

Cleaver, J. E. 1968. Defective repair replication of DNA in xeroderma pigmentosum. *Nature* 218: 652–656.

Cleaver, J. E. 1969. Xeroderma pigmentosum: A human disease in which an initial stage of DNA repair is defective. *Proc. Natl. Acad. Sci.* 63: 428–435.

Cohen, A. M., Ketcham, A. S. and Morton, D. L. 1973. Tumor-specific cellular cytotoxicity to human sarcomas: Evidence for a cell-mediated host immune response to a common sarcoma cell-surface antigen. *J. Natl. Cancer Inst.* 50: 585–589.

Conney, A. H. 1967. Parmacological implications of microsomal enzyme induction. *Pharmacol. Rev.* 19: 317–366.

Conney, A. H. and Burns, J. J. 1962. Factors influencing drug metabolism. *Adv. Pharmacol.* 1: 31–58.

Conney, A. H. and Burns, J. J. 1972. Metabolic interactions among environmental chemicals and drugs. *Science* 178: 576–586.

Conney, A. H., Miller, E. C. and Miller, J. A. 1956. The metabolism of methylated aminoazo dyes. V. Evidence for induction of enzyme synthesis in the rat by 3-methylcholanthrene. *Cancer Res.* 16: 450–459.

Conney, A. H. et al. 1959. Induced synthesis of liver microsomal enzymes which metabolize foreign compounds. *Science* 130: 1478–1479.

Conney, A. H., Welch, R. M., Kuntzman, R. and Burns, J. J. 1967. Effects of pesticides on drug and steroid metabolism. *Clin. Pharmacol. Ther.* 8: 2–11.

Conney, A. H. et al. 1968. Inhibitory effect of carbon monoxide on the hydroxylation of testosterone by rat liver microsomes. *J. Biol. Chem.* 243: 3912–3915.

Conney, A. H. et al. 1971. Effects of environmental chemicals on the metabolism of drugs, carcinogens, and normal body constituents. *Ann. N.Y. Acad. Sci.* 179: 155–172.

Cook, J. W. and Kennaway, E. L. 1940. Chemical compounds as carcinogenic agents. *Am. J. Cancer* 39: 381–428.

Cookson, M. J., Sims, P. and Grover, P. L. 1971. Mutagenicity of epoxides of polycyclic hydrocarbons correlates with carcinogenicity of parent hydrocarbons. *Nature New Biol.* 234: 186–187.

Cooper, M. D. and Lawton, A. R. 1974. The development of the immune system. *Sci. Am.* 231(5): 59–72.

Cooper, D. Y. et al. 1965. Photochemical spectrum of the terminal oxidase of mixed function oxidase system. *Science* 147: 400–402.

Cooper, W. C., Mariani, T. and Good, R. A. 1970. Effects of chronic protein depletion on immune response. *Fed. Proc.* 29: 364.

Crabtree, H. G. 1955. Retardation of azo-carcinogenesis by non-carcinogenic azo-compounds. *Br. J. Cancer* 9: 310–319.

Craddock, V. M. 1965. Reaction of the carcinogen dimethylnitrosamine with proteins and with thiol compounds in the intact animal. *Biochem. J.* 94: 323–330.

Creaven, P. J., Davies, W. H. and Williams, R. T. 1966. The effect of butylated hydroxytoluene, butylated hydroxyanisole and octyl gallate upon liver weight and biphenyl-4-hydroxylase activity in the rat. *J. Pharm. Pharmacol.* 18: 485–489.

Creysell, R. et al. 1958. Deficiency in gamma-globulins and complications of infection in chronic lymphatic leukemia. Le Sang 29: 383–398. (French)

Croce, C. M. and Koprowski, H. 1978. The genetics of human cancer. *Sci. Am.* 238(2): 117–125.

Culvenor, C. C. J. et al. 1971. Optical rotary dispersion and circular dichroism. LXXVI. Circular dichroism of pyrrolizidine alkaloids and related compounds. *J. Chem. Soc.* (C): 3653–3664.

Dacre, J. C. 1970. Transport and fate of substances absorbed in the gastrointestinal tract with special reference to the significance of blood and tissue level. In: *Metabolic Aspects of Food Safety.* F. J. C. Roe (ed.). Academic Press, New York.

Daly, J. 1971. Enzymatic oxidation at carbon. In: *Concepts in Chemical Pharmacology.* Part II. B. B. Brodie and J. R. Gillette (eds.). Springer, New York.

Dammert, K. 1961. The effect of five ulcerating doses of alkyldimethylbenzylammonium chloride (Zephiran) on the tumor promoting action of polyoxyethylene sorbitan monostearate (Tween 60). *Acta Pathol. Microbiol. Scand.* 53: 22–32.

Dao, T. L. 1962. The role of ovarian hormones in initiating the induction of mammary cancer in rats by polynuclear hydrocarbons. *Cancer Res.* 22: 973–981.

Dao, T. L., Greiner, M. and Sunderland, H. 1959. The effect of pregnancy, parturition, and pseudopregnancy on the growth of mammary adenocarcinoma induced by intragastric instillation of 3-methylcholanthrene. *Proc. Am. Assoc. Cancer Res.* 3: 14–15.

DeBaum, J. R., Miller, E. C. and Miller, J. A. 1970. N-Hydroxy-2-acetylaminofluorene sulfotransferase: Its probable role in carcinogenesis and in protein-(Methion-S-yl) binding in rat liver. *Cancer Res.* 30: 577–595.

Della Porta, G. and Terracini, B. 1969. Chemical carcinogenesis in infant animals. *Prog. Exp. Tumor Res.* 11: 334–363.

Della Porta, G., Shubik, P. and Scortecci, V. 1959. The action of N-2-fluorenyl acetamide in the Syrian golden hamster. *J. Natl. Cancer Inst.* 22: 463–487.

Denlinger, R. H., Swenberg, J. A., Koestner, A. and Wechsler, W. 1973. Differential effect of immunosuppression on the induction of nervous system and bladder tumors by N-methylnitrosourea. *J. Natl. Cancer Inst.* 50: 87–93.

Devesa, S. S. 1975. The incidence of retinoblastoma. *Am. J. Opthalmol.* 80: 263–265.

Dingell, J. V. and Heimberg, M. 1968. The effects of aliphatic halogenated hydrocarbons on hepatic drug metabolism. *Biochem. Pharmacol.* 17: 1269–1278.

Dipple, A. 1976. Polynuclear aromatic carcinogens. In: *Chemical Carcinogens*. C. E. Searle (ed.). American Cancer Society, Washington, D.C.

Domsky, I. I., Linjinsky, W., Spencer, K. and Shubik, P. 1963. Rate of metabolism of 9,10-dimethyl-1,2-benzanthracene in newborn and adult mice. *Proc. Soc. Exp. Biol. Med.* 113: 110–112.

Druckrey, H. 1954. Studies on the mechanism of carcinogenesis. *Acta Un. Int. Cancr.* 10: 29–43.

Druckrey, H. 1959. Pharmacological approach to carcinogenesis. In: *Carcinogenesis Mechanism of Action*. Ciba Foundation Symposium. G. E. W. Wolstenholme and M. O'Connor (eds.). Little Brown, Boston.

Druckrey, H. 1973a. Specific carcinogenic and teratogenic effects of "indirect" alkylating methyl- and ethyl-compounds and their dependency on stages of ontogenic development. *Xenobiotica* 5: 271–303.

Druckrey, H. 1973b. Chemical structure and action in transplacental carcinogenesis and teratogenesis. In: *Transplacental Carcinogenesis*. IARC Publications No. 4. International Agency for Research on Cancer, Lyon.

Druckrey, H. 1975. Chemical carcinogenesis on N-nitroso derivatives. In: *Recent Topics in Chemical Carcinogenesis*. S. Odashima, S. Takayama, and H. Sato (eds). University Park Press, Baltimore.

Druckrey, H. and Kupfmuller, K. 1948. Quantitative analysis of the carcinogenic process. Z. Naturforschung 3b: 254–266. (German)

Druckrey, H. et al. 1963. Quantitative analysis of the carcinogenic effect of diethylnitrosamin. *Arzneimittelforschung.* 13: 841–851. (German)

Druckrey, H., Preussman, R., Ivankovic, S. and Schmahl, S. 1967. Organotropic carcinogenic effects of 65 different N-nitroso compounds on BD-rats. *Z. Krebsforsch* 69: 103–201. (German)

Druckrey, H., Landschutz, C. and Ivankovic, S. 1970a. Transplacental production of malignant tumor of the nervous system. I. Ethylnitrosourea applied to ten genetically defined rat strains. *Z. Krebsforsch.* 73: 371–386. (German)

Druckrey, H., Schagen, B. and Ivankovic, S. 1970b. Induction of neurogenic malignancies by one single dose of ethylnitrosourea (ENU) given to newborn and juvenile BD IX-strain rats. *Z. Krebsforsch* 74: 141–161. (German)

Dunning, W. F., Curtis, M. R. and Eisen, M. J. 1940. The carcinogenic activity of methylcholanthrene in rats. *Am. J. Cancer* 40: 85–127.

Dunning, W. F., Curtis, M. R. and Friedgood, C. 1949. The incidence of benzpyrene induced sarcomas in the diabetic and alloxan refractive rats of three strains. *Cancer Res.* 9: 546.

Duran-Reynals, F., Shrigley, E. W. and de Hostos, E. 1945. Carcinogenesis induced by methylcholanthrene in pigeons, guinea fowls, and ducks. *Cancer Res.* 5: 11–17.

Dutton, G. J. and Stevenson, I. H. 1962. Stimulation by 3,4-benzopyrene of glucuronide synthesis in skin. *Biochim. Biophys. Acta* 58: 633–634.

Ehrlich, P. 1957. On the present status of cancer research (German). In: *Collected Papers of Paul Ehrlich*. Vol. II. F. Himmelweit (ed). Pergamon Press, London.

Eichhorn, G. L., Clark, P. and Becker, E. D. 1966. Interactions of metal ions with polynucleotides and related compounds. VII. The binding of copper (II) to nucleosides, nucleotides and deoxyribonucleic acids. *Biochemistry* 5: 245–252.

Eisen, H. N. 1973. Antibody formation. In: *Microbiology*. 2nd ed. B. D. Davis et al. (eds.). Harper & Row, Hagerstown, Maryland.

Engelbreth-Holm, J. and Jensen, E. 1953. On the mechanism of experimental carcinogenesis. X. The influence of age and of growth hormone on skin carcinogenesis in mice. *Acta Path. Microbiol. Scand.* 33: 257–262.

Epstein, S. S. and Fuji, K. 1970. Synergism in carcinogenesis with particular reference to synergistic effect of piperonyl butoxide and related insecticidal synergist. In: *Chemical Tumor Problems*. W. Nakahara (ed.). Japanese Society for Promotion of Science, Tokyo.

Epstein, S. S., Andrea, J., Joshi, S. and Mantel, N. 1967a. Hepatocarcinogenicity of griseofulvin following parental administration to infant mice. *Cancer Res.* 27: 1900–1906.

Epstein, S. S. et al. 1967b. Synergistic toxicity and carcinogenicity of freons and piperonyl butoxide. *Nature* 214: 526–528.

Falk, H. L., Kotin, P. and Thompson, S. 1964. Inhibition of carcinogenesis — The effect of polycyclic hydrocarbons and related compounds. *Arch. Environ. Health* 9: 169–179.

Farber, E. and Cameron, R. 1980. The sequential analysis of cancer development. *Adv. Cancer Res.* 31: 125–226.

Fass, L., Herberman, R. B. and Ziegler, J. 1970. Delayed cutaneous hypersensitivity reactions to autologous extracts of Burkitt-lymphoma cells. *N. Engl. J. Med.* 282: 776–780.

Fialkow, P. J. 1970. Genetic marker studies in neoplasia. In: *Genetic Concepts and Neoplasia*. M. D. Anderson Hospital Symposium. Williams & Wilkins, Baltimore.

Fisher, J. C., Davis, R. C. and Mannick, J. A. 1970. The effects of immunosuppression on the induction and immunogenicity of chemically induced sarcomas. *Surgery* 68: 150–157.

Fishman, W. H. 1955. Beta-glucuronidase. *Adv. Enzymol.* 16: 361–409.

Fiume, L. 1964. Aminoacetonitrile action on the inhibition of protein synthesis produced in the rat by dimethylnitrosamine. *Nature* 201: 615.

Folkman, J. 1974. Tumor angiogenesis. *Adv. Cancer Res.* 19: 331–358.

Folkman, J. 1975. Tumor angiogenesis. In: *Cancer, A Comprehensive Treatise. Biology of Tumors*. Vol. 3. F. F. Becker (ed). Plenum Press, New York.

Folkman, J. 1976. The vascularization of tumors. *Sci. Am.* 234(5): 59–73.

Folkman, J., Hochberg, M. and Knighton, D. 1974. Self-regulation of growth in three dimensions. The role of surface area limitation. In: *Control of Proliferation in Animal Cells*. B. Clarkson and R. Baserga (ed.). Cold Spring Harbor Laboratory, New York.

Fong, Y. Y. and Walsh, E. O'F. 1971. Carcinogenic nitrosamines in Cantonese salt-dried fish. *Lancet* 2: 1032.

Fowler, J. S. L. 1969. Carbon tetrachloride metabolism in rabbit. *Br. J. Pharmacol.* 37: 733–737.

Fraumeni, J. F. 1969. Constitutional disorders of man predisposing to leukemia and lymphoma. *Natl. Cancer Inst. Monogr.* 32: 221–232.

Fridewald, W. F. and Rous, P. 1944. The initiating and promoting elements in tumor production: An analysis of the effects of tar, benzpyrene, and methylcholanthrene on rabbit skin. *J. Exp. Med.* 80: 101–126.

Fridewald, W. F. and Rous, P. 1950. The pathogenesis of deferred cancer. A study of the after-effects of methylcholanthrene upon rabbit skin. *J. Exp. Med.* 91: 459–484.

Friedman, M. a. 1979. Subchronic effects of piperonyl butoxide on carcinogen metabolism in hamster liver. *Bull. Environ. Contam. Toxicol.* 21: 815–821.

Friedrich-Fresca, H. and Hoffman, M. 1969. Immunological defense against preneo-
    plastic stages of diethylnitrosamine-induced carcinomas in rat liver. *Nature*
    223: 1162–1163.
Fujita, K. et al. 1956. Biochemical interaction of trypan blue and p-dimethylamino-
    azobenzene in the liver of rat. *Gann* 47: 181–206.
Furst, A. and Haro, R. T. 1969. A survey of metal carcinogenesis. In: *Prog. Exp.*
    Tumor Res. 12: 102–133.
Furth, J. 1973. Role of prolactin in mammary carcinogenesis. Human Prolactin,
    Proceedings International Symposium. J. L. Pasteels and C. Robyn (eds.).
    Excerpta Medica, Amsterdam.
Fuwa, K. et al. 1960. Nucleic acids and metals. II. Transition metals as determin-
    ants of the conformation of ribonucleic acids. *Proc. Natl. Acad. Sci.* 46:
    1298–1307.
Gandolfi, A. J. and Van Dyke, R. A. 1973. Dechlorination of chloroethane with re-
    constituted microsomal system. *Biochem. Biophys. Res. Commun.* 53: 687–692.
Garcia, H. 1963. Inhibition of tumorigenic action of urethane by butyl carbamate.
    Biologica 34: 11–13.
Gardner, W. U. 1947. Tumors in experimental animals receiving steroid hormones.
    In: *Endocrinology of Neoplastic Diseases.* G. H. Twombly and George T. Pack
    (eds.). Oxford University Press, London.
Gardner, E. J. and Richards, R. C. 1953. Multiple cutaneous and subcutaneous
    lesions occurring simultaneously with hereditary polyposis and osteomatosis.
    Am. J. Hum. Genet. 5: 139–147.
Gatti, R. A. and Good, R. A. 1970. The immunological deficiency diseases. *Med.*
    Clin. N. Am. 54: 281–307.
Gatti, R. A. and Good, R. A. 1971. Occurrence of malignancy in immuno-deficiency
    disease: A literature review. *Cancer* 28: 89–98.
Gelboin, H. V. 1969. A microsome-dependent binding of benzo(a)pyrene to DNA.
    Cancer Res. 29: 1272–1276.
Gelboin, H. V., Klein, M. and Bates, R. R. 1965. Inhibition of mouse skin tumori-
    genesis by actinomycin D. *Proc. Natl. Acad. Sci.* 53: 1353–1360.
Gelboin, H. V., Huberman, E. and Sachs, L. 1969. Enzymatic hydroxylation of
    benzopyrene and its relationship to autotoxicity. *Proc. Natl. Acad. Sci.* 64:
    1188–1194.
Gelboin, H. V., Wiebel, F. and Diamond, L. 1970. Dimethylbenzanthracene tumori-
    genesis and aryl hydrocarbon hydroxylase in mouse skin: Inhibition by 7,8-
    benzoflavone. *Science* 170: 169–171.
Gelboin, H. V. and Wiebel, F. J. 1971. Studies on the mechanism of arylhydro-
    carbon hydroxylase induction and its role in cytotoxicity and tumorigenicity.
    Ann. N.Y. Acad. Sci. 179: 529–547.
Gelboin, H. V., Wiebel, F. J. and Kinoshita, N. 1974. Aryl hydrocarbon hydroxy-
    lase: Regulation and role in polycyclic hydrocarbon action. In: *Chemical*
    Carcinogenesis. Part A. P. O. Ts'o and J. A. DiPaolo (eds.). Marcel Dekker,
    New York.
German, J. 1972. Genes which increase chromosomal instability in somatic cells and
    predispose to cancer. *Prog. Med. Genet.* 8: 61–101.
Gilbert, D. and Goldberg, L. 1965a. Liver response tests. III. Liver enlargement
    and stimulation of microsomal processing enzyme activity. *Food Cosmet. Toxicol.*
    3: 417–432.
Gilbert, D. and Goldberg, L. 1965b. Liver weight and microsomal processing (drug-
    metabolizing) enzymes in rats treated with butylated hydroxytoluene or butylated
    hydroxyanisole. *Biochem. J.* 97: 28.
Gillette, J. R. 1963. Factors that affect the stimulation of the microsomal drug en-
    zyme induced by foreign compounds. *Adv. Enzyme Regul.* 1: 215.
Gillette, J. R., Menard, R. H. and Stripp, B. 1973. Active products of fetal drug
    metabolism. *Clin. Pharmacol. Ther.* 14: 680–692.

Gillman, J. and Gillman, T. 1952. The pathogenesis of experimentally produced lymphoma in rats (including Hodgkin's-like sarcoma). *Cancer* 5: 792—846.

Gilman, A. G. and Conney, A. H. 1963. The induction of aminoazo dye N-demethylase in nonhepatic tissues by 3-mechylcholanthrene. *Biochem. Pharamacol.* 12: 591—593.

Gjessing, L. R. 1968. Biochemistry of functional neural crest tumors. *Adv. Clin. Chem.* 11: 81—131.

Goldblatt, M. W. 1947. Occupational cancer of the bladder. *Br. Med. Bull.* 4: 405—416.

Good, R. A. 1971. Disorders of the immune system. In: *Immunobiology.* R. A. Good and D. W. Fisher (eds.). Sinauer, Stamford, Connecticut.

Grant, G. A. and Roe, F. J. C. 1969. Effect of germ-free status and antilymphocyte serum on induction of various tumors in mice by a chemical carcinogen given at birth. *Nature* 223: 1060.

Griffin, A. C. et al. 1955. The role of hormones in liver carcinogenesis. *J. Natl. Cancer Inst.* 15: 1623—1628.

Grover, P. L. et al. 1971. In vitro transformation of rodent cells by K-region derivatives of polycyclic hydrocarbons. *Proc. Natl. Acad. Sci.* 68: 1098—1101.

Grover, P. L., Hewer, A. and Sims, P. 1972. Formation of K-region epoxides as microsomal metabolites of pyrene and benzo(a)pyrene. *Biochem. Pharmacol.* 21: 2713—2726.

Gutmann, H. R., Malejka-Giganti, D., Barry, E. J. and Rydell, R. E. 1972. On the correlation between the hepatocarcinogenicity of the carcinogen N-2-fluourenylacetamide, and its metabolic activation by the rat. *Cancer Res.* 32: 1554—1561.

Hadjiolov, D. 1971. The inhibition of dimethylnitrosamine carcinogenesis in rat liver by aminoacetonitrile. *Z. Krebsforsch.* 76: 91—92.

Haenszel, W. and Kurihara, M. 1968. Studies of Japanese migrants. I. Mortality from cancer and other diseases among Japanese in the United States. *J. Natl. Cancer Inst.* 40: 43—68.

Hall, W. H. 1948. The role of initating and promoting factors in the pathogenesis of tumours of the thyroid. *Br. J. Cancer* 2: 273—280.

Hall, W. H. and Bielschowsky, F. 1949. The development of malignancy in experimentally induced adenomata of the thyroid. *Br. J. Cancer* 3: 534—541.

Harris, P. N. 1947a. Production of sarcoma in rats with light green SF. *Cancer Res.* 7: 35—36.

Harris, P. N. 1947b. The effect of diet containing dried egg albumin upon p-dimethylaminoazobenzene carcinogenesis. *Cancer Res.* 7: 178—179.

Harris, J. E. and Sinkovics, J. G. 1970. The immunology of malignant diseases. Mosby, St. Louis.

Harris, P. N., Krahl, M. E., and Clowes, G. H. A. 1947a. p-Dimethylaminoazobenzene carcinogenesis with purified diets varying in content of cysteine, cystine, liver extract, protein, riboflavin, and other factors. *Cancer Res.* 7: 162—175.

Harris, P. N., Krahl, M. E. and Clowes, G. H. A. 1947b. The effect of biotin upon p-dimethylaminoazobenzene carcinogenesis. *Cancer Res.* 7: 176—177.

Hart, L. and Fouts, J. 1965. Further studies on the stimulation of hepatic microsomal drug-metabolizing enzymes by DDT and its analogs. *Naunyn Schmeidebergs Arch. Exp. Pathol.* 249: 486—500.

Hartwell, J. L. 1951. Survey of compounds which have been tested for carcinogenic activity. Publ. Health Service Publ. No. 149, 2nd ed. U.S. Government Printing Office, Washington, D.C.

Hecht, F., McCaw, B. K. and Koler, R. D. 1973. Ataxia-telangiectasia — Clonal growth of translocation lymphocytes. *N. Engl. J. Med.* 289: 286—291.

Hecker, E. 1968. Cocarcinogenic principles from the seed oil of Croton tiglium and from other Euphorbiaceae. *Cancer Res.* 28: 2338—2349.

Hecker, E. 1971. Isolation and characterization of cocarcinogenic principles from croton oil. In: *Methods in Cancer Research.* H. Busch (ed.). Academic Press, New York.

Heidelberger, C. and Moldenhauer, M. G. 1956. The interaction of carcinogenic hydrocarbons with tissue constituents. IV. A quantitative study of the binding to skin proteins of several C^{14} labeled hydrocarbons. *Cancer Res.* 16: 442–449.

Heidelberger, C. and Weiss, S. M. 1951. The distribution of radioactivity in mice following administration of 3,4-benzpyrene-5-C^{14} and 1,2,5,6-dibenzanthracene-9, 10-C^{14}. *Cancer Res.* 11: 885–891.

Hellström, I and Hellström, K. E. 1973. Some recent studies on cellular immunity to human melanomas. *Fed. Proc.* 32: 156–159.

Hellström, I. et al. 1969. Serum-mediated protection of neoplastic cells from inhibition by lymphocytes immune to their tumor-specific antigen. *Proc. Natl. Acad. Sci.* 62: 362–368.

Hellström, I. et al. 1970a. Studies on cellular immunity to human neuroblastoma cells. *Int. J. Cancer* 6: 172–188.

Hellström, I., Hellström, K. E. and Shepard, T. H. 1970b. Cell-mediated immunity against antigens common to human colonic carcinomas and fetal gut epithelium. *Int. J. Cancer* 6: 346–351.

Hellström, I., Hellström, K. E., Sjogren, H. O. and Warner, G. A. 1971. Serum factors in tumor-free patients cancelling the blocking of cell-mediated tumor immunity. *Int. J. Cancer* 8: 185–191.

Hemings, H., Smith, H. C., Colburn, N. H. and Boutwell, R. K. 1968. Inhibition by actinomycin D of DNA and RNA synthesis and of skin carcinogenesis initiated by 7-12-dimethylbenz(a)anthracene or β-propiolactone. *Cancer Res.* 28: 543–552.

Henderson, J. F. and Mazel, P. 1964. Demethylation of purine analogs by microsomal enzymes from mouse liver. *Biochem. Pharmacol.* 13: 207–210.

Hendry, N. W. 1965. The geology, occurrences, and major uses of asbestos. *Ann. N.Y. Acad. Sci.* 132: 12–22.

Henry, S. A. 1947. Occupational cutaneous cancer attributable to certain chemicals in industry. *Br. Med. Bull.* 4: 389–401.

Herbst, A. L., Ulfelder, H. and Poskanzer, D. C. 1971. Adenocarcinoma of the vagina. *N. Engl. J. Med.* 284: 878–881.

Herbst, A. L., Kurman, R. J., Scully, R. E. and Poskanzer, D. C. 1972. Clear-cell adenocarcinoma of the genital tract in young females. *N. Engl. J. Med.* 287: 1259–1263.

Heston, E. W. 1942a. Genetic analysis of susceptibility to induced pulmonary tumors in mice. *J. Natl. Cancer Inst.* 3: 69–78.

Heston, E. W. 1942b. Inheritance of susceptibility to spontaneous pulmonary tumors in mice. *J. Natl. Cancer Inst.* 3: 79–82.

Heston, E. W. 1957. Effects of genes located on chromosomes III, V, VII, IX, and XIV on the occurrence of pulmonary tumors in the mouse. In: *Proceedings of International Genetics Symposia, 1956. Cytologia* (Suppl.) Vol. 219.

Heston, E. W. and Dunn, T. B. 1951. Tumor development in susceptible strain A and resistant strain L lung transplants in LA F_1 hosts. *J. Natl. Cancer Inst.* 11: 1057–1071.

Higginson, J. 1969. Present trends in cancer epidemiology. *Can. Cancer Conf.* 8: 40–75.

Higginson, J. 1976. Chronic toxicology — An epidemiologist's approach to the problem of carcinogenesis. In: *Essays in Toxicology.* Vol. 7. W. J. Hayes, Jr. (ed.). Academic Press, New York.

Higurashi, M. and Conen, P. E. 1971. In vitro chromosomal radiosensitivity in Fanconi's anemia. *Blood* 38: 336–342.

Hirschhorn, K. and Bloch-Shtacher, N. 1970. Transformation of genetically abnormal cells. In: *Genetic Concepts and Neoplasia.* M.D. Anderson Hospital Symposium. Williams & Wilkins, Baltimore.

Hoch-Ligeti, C., Argus, M. F. and Arcos, J. C. 1968. Combined carcinogenic effects of dimethylnitrosamine and 3-methylcholanthrene in the rat. *J. Natl. Cancer Inst.* 40: 535–549.

Homburger, F. 1972. Chemical carcinogenesis in Syrian hamsters. *Prog. Exp. Tumor Res.* 16: 152–175.

Homburger, F. 1974. Modifiers of carcinogenesis. In: *The Physiopathology of Cancer: Biology and Biochemistry* 1. Karger, Basel.

Homburger, F. and Boger, E. 1968. The carcinogenicity of essential oils, flavors, and spices. A review. *Cancer Res.* 28: 2372–2374.

Hoshino, M. 1960. Effect of 3-amino-1,2,4-triazole on the experimental production of liver cancer. *Nature* 186: 174–175.

Houck, J. C. and Irausquin, H. 1973. Some properties of the lymphocyte chalone. In: *Chalones: Concepts and Current Researches.* National Cancer Insitute Monograph 38. B. K. Forscher and J. C. Houck (eds.). National Institutes of Health, Bethesda, Maryland.

Howard, J. W., Fazio, T. 1969. Review of polycyclic aromatic hydrocarbons in foods. *J. Agric. Food Chem.* 17: 527–531.

Howell, J. S. 1958. The effect of copper acetate on p-dimethylaminoazobenzene carcinogenesis in the rat. *Brit. J. Cancer* 12: 594–608.

Hozumi, M. et al. 1972. Inhibition of tumorigenesis in mouse skin by leupeptin, a protease inhibitor from Actinomycetes. *Cancer Res.* 32: 1725–1728.

Hsu, I. C., Shumaker, R. C., Allen, J. R. 1973. Tissue distribution of tritium-labeled dehydroretronecine. *Chem. Biol. Interact.* 8: 163–170.

Huberman, E. et al. 1971. Mutagenicity to mammalian cells of epoxides and other derivatives of polycyclic hydrocarbons. *Proc. Nat. Acad. Sci.* 68: 3195–3199.

Huberman, E. et al. 1972. Transformation of hamster embryo cells by epoxides and other derivatives of polycyclic hydrocarbons. *Cancer Res.* 32: 1391–1396.

Hucker, H. B. 1970. Species differences in drug metabolism. *Ann. Rev. Biochem.* 10: 99–118.

Hueper, W. C., Conway, W. D. 1964. Chemical Carcinogenesis and Cancers. C. C. Thomas Publishers, Springfield, Ill.

Hueper, W. C., Wiley, F. H., Wolfe, H. D. 1938. Experimental production of bladder tumors in dogs by administration of beta-naphthylamine. *J. Indust. Hyg. & Toxicol.* 20: 46–84.

Huggins, C., Fukunishi, R. 1964. Induced protection of adrenal cortex against 7,12-dimethylbenz(a)anthracene. *J. Exp. Med.* 119: 923–942.

Huggins, C., Briziarelli, G., Sutton, H. 1959. Rapid induction of mammary carcinoma in the rat and the influence of hormones on the tumors. *J. Exp. Med.* 109: 25–42.

Huggins, C., Grand, L. C., Brillantes, F. P. 1961. Mammary cancer induced by single feeding of polynuclear hydrocarbon and its suppression. *Nature* 189: 204–207.

Huggins, C., Grand, L., Fukunishi, R. 1964. Aromatic influences on the yields of mammary cancers following administration of 7,12-dimethylbenz(a)anthracene. *Proc. Nat. Acad. Sci.* 51: 737–742.

Huseby, R. A. 1953. The effect of testicular function upon stilbestrol-induced mammary and pituitary tumors in mice. *Proc. Am. Ass. Cancer Res.* 1: 25.

Innes, J. R. M. et al. 1969. Bioassays of pesticides and industrial chemicals for tumorigenicity in mice. A preliminary note. *J. Natl. Cancer Inst.* 42: 1101–1114.

Inscoe, J. K., Axelrod, J. 1960. Some factors affecting glucuronide formation in vitro. *J. Pharmacol. Exptl. Therap.* 129: 128–131.

Irving, C. C., Wiseman, R., Hill, J. T. 1967. Biliary excretion of the O-glucuronide of N-hydroxy-2-acetylaminofluorene by the rat and rabbit. *Cancer Res.* 27: 2309–2317.

Itchikawa, K., Baum, S. M. 1924. Local reaction of animals resistant to cancer production following application of coal tar (rat and guinea-pig). *Bull. Assoc.
Franc. Etude Cancer* 13: 386–395.

Ivankovic, S. 1972. Prenatal carcinogenesis. In: *Topics in Chemical Carcinogenesis.*
W. Nakahara, S. Takayama, T. Sugimura and S. Odashima (eds.). University
of Tokyo Press, Tokyo.

Ivankovic, W., Druckrey, H. 1968. Transplacental induction of malignant tumors of
the nervous system. I. Ethylnitrosourea in BDIX rats. *2. Krebsforsch.* 71:
320–360.

Jaffe, H. et al. 1968. In vivo inhibition of mouse liver microsomal hydroxylating
systems by methylenedioxyphenyl insecticidal synergists and related compounds.
Life Science 7: 1051–1062.

Jaffe, H. et al. 1969. Bimodal effect of piperonyl butoxide on the O- and p-
hydroxylation of biphenyl by mouse liver microsomes. *Biochem. Pharmacol.*
18: 1045–1051.

Jervell, D. F., Christoffersen, T., Morland, J. 1965. Studies on the 3-methyl-
cholanthrene induction and carbohydrate repression of rat liver dimethylaminoazobenzene reductase. *Arch. Biochem. Biophys.* 111: 15–22.

Johnson, E. S., Seely, J. H., White, W. F., DeSombre, E. R. 1976. Endocrine-
dependent rat mammary tumor regression: use of a gonadotropin releasing hormone analog. *Science* 194: 329–330.

Jori, A., Bianchetti, A., Prestini, P. E. and Garattini, S. 1970. Effect of eucalyptol (1,8-cineole) on the metabolism of other drugs in rats and in man. *Europ. J.
Pharmacol.* 9: 362–366.

Jose, D. G. 1973. The cancer connection with immunity and nutrition. *Nutrition
Today* 8(2): 4–9.

Jose, D. G. and Good, R. A. 1971. Absence of enhancing antibody in cell-mediated
immunity to tumor heterografts in protein deficient rats. *Nature* 231: 323–325.

Jose, D. G. and Good, R. A. 1973a. Quantitative effects of nutritional protein and
calorie deficiency upon immune responses to tumors in mice. *Cancer Res.* 33:
807–812.

Jose, D. G. and Good, R. A. 1973b. Quantitative effects of nutritional essential
amino acid deficiency upon immune responses to tumors in mice. *J. Exp. Med.*
137: 1–9.

Jose, D. G., Cooper, W. C. and Good, R. A. 1971. How protein deficiency enhances cellular immunity (editorial). *J. Am. Med. Ass.* 218: 1428–1429.

Jull, J. W. 1954. The effects of oestrogen and progesterone on the chemical induction of mammary cancer in mice of the IF strain. *J. Path. Bact.* 68: 547–559.

Jull, J. W. 1956. Hormones as promoting agents in mammary carcinogenesis. *Acta
Un. Int. Contra Cancr.* 12: 653–660.

Kato, R., Shoji, H. and Takanaka, A. 1967. Metabolism of carcinogenic compounds.
1. Effect of phenobarbital and methylcholanthrene on the activities of N-
demethylation of carcinogenic compounds by liver microsomes of male and female
rats. *Gann* 58: 467–469.

Kaye, A. M. 1960. A study of the relationship between the rate of ethyl carbamate
(urethan) catabolism and urethan carcinogenesis. *Cancer Res.* 20: 237–241.

Kellermann, G., Shaw, C. R. and Luyten-Kellerman, M. 1973. Aryl hydrocarbon
hydroxylase inducibility and brochogenic carcinoma. *New Engl. J. Med.* 289:
934–937.

Kersey, J. H., Spector, B. D. and Good, R. A. 1973a. Immunodeficiency and cancer. *Advan. Cancer Res.* 18: 211–230.

Kersey, J. H., Spector, B. D. and Good, R. A. 1973b. Primary immunodeficiency
diseases and cancer: the immunodeficiency-cancer registry. *Int. J. Cancer*
12: 333–347.

Ketterer, B., Ross-Mansell, P. and Whitehead, J. K. 1967. The isolation of
carcinogen-binding protein from livers of rat given 4-dimethylaminobenzene.
Biochem. J. 103: 316–324.

Kim, U. and Furth, J. 1960. Relation of mammary tumors to mammotropes. I. Induction of mammary tumors in rats. *Proc. Soc. Exp. Biol. Med.* 103: 640–645.

Kinoshita, N. and Gelboin, H. V. 1972. Aryl hydrocarbon hydroxylase and polycyclic hydrocarbon tumorigenesis: Effect of the enzyme inhibitor 7,8-benzoflavone on tumorigenesis and macromolecule binding. *Proc. Natl. Acad. Sci.* 69: 824–828.

Kinoshita, F. K., Frawley, J. P. and duBois, K. P. 1966. Effects of subacute administration of some pesticides on microsomal enzyme systems. *Toxicol. Appl. Pharmacol.* 8: 345–346.

Kirby, A. H. M. 1947. Studies in the carcinogenesis of azo compounds. III. The action of (A) four azo compounds in Wistar rats fed restricted diets; (B) N,N-diethyl-p-aminoazobenzene in mice. *Cancer Res.* 7: 333–341.

Kirby, A. H. M. and Peacock, P. R. 1949. Liver tumors in mice injected with commercial food dyes. *Glasg. Med. J.* 30: 364.

Kirkman, H. 1952. The effect of different estrogens on the induction of renal tumors and hepatomas in male golden hamsters. *Cancer Res.* 12: 274–275.

Kirschbaum, A., Lawrason, F. D., Kaplan, H. S. and Bittner, J. J. 1944. Influence of breeding on induction of mammary cancer with methylcholanthrene in strain dba female mice. *Proc. Soc. Exp. Biol.* 55: 141–142.

Klarner, P. 1962. Formation of sarcoma from foreign body implant of polymethacrylate (German). *2. Krebsforsch.* 65: 99–100.

Kmet, J., Mahboubi, E. 1972. Esophageal cancer in the Caspian littoral of Iran: Initial studies. *Science* 175: 846–853.

Knudson, A. G. 1971. Mutation and cancer: Statistical study of retinoblastoma. *Proc. Natl. Acad. Sci.* 68: 820–823.

Knudson, A. G. 1973. Mutation and human cancer. *Adv. Cancer Res.* 17: 317–352.

Knudson, A. G. and Strong, L. C. 1972a. Mutation and cancer: Neuroblastoma and pheochromocytoma. *Am. J. Hum. Genet.* 24: 514–532.

Knudson, A. G. and Strong, L. C. 1972b. Mutation and cancer: A model for Wilms' tumor of the kidney. *J. Natl. Cancer Inst.* 48: 313–324.

Knudson, A. G., Strong, L. C. and Anderson, D. E. 1973. Heredity and cancer in man. *Prog. Med. Genet.* 9: 113–158.

Kolmodin, B., Azarnoff, D. and Sjoqvist, F. 1969. Effect of environmental factors on drug metabolism: Decreased plasma half-life of antipyrine in workers exposed to chlorinated hydrocarbon insecticides. *Clin. Pharmacol. Ther.* 10: 638–642.

Korteweg, R. and Thomas, F. 1939. Tumor induction and tumor growth in hypophysectomised mice. *Amer. J. Cancer* 37: 36–44.

Krakoff, I. H., Meyer, R. L. 1965. Prevention of hyperuricemia in leukemia and lymphoma. *J. Amer. Med. Ass.* 193: 1–6.

Kriek, E. 1969/1970. On the mechanism of action of carcinogenic aromatic amines. I. Binding of 2-acetylaminofluorene and N-hydroxy-2-acetylaminofluorene to rat-liver nucleic acids in vivo. *Chem.-Biol. Interactions* 1: 3–17.

Kruger, F. W. 1972. New aspects in metabolism of carcinogenic nitrosamines. In: *Topics in Chemical Carcinogenesis.* W. Nakahara, S. Takayama, T. Sugimura, and S. Odashima (eds.). University of Tokyo Press, Tokyo.

Kruger, F. W. 1973. Metabolism of nitrosamines in vivo. II. On the methylation of nucleic acids by aliphatic di-n-alkyl-nitrosamines in vivo, caused by β-oxidation. The increased formation of 7-methylguanine after application of β-hydroxypropyl-propyl-nitrosamine compared to that after application of di-n-propyl-nitrosamines. *Z. Krebsforsch* 79: 90–97.

Kruger, F. W. and Bertram, B. 1973. Metabolism of nitrosamines in vivo. III. On the methylation of nucleic acids by aliphatic di-n-alkyl-nitrosamines in vivo resulting from β-oxidation: the formation of 7-methylguanine after application of 2-oxo-propyl-propyl-nitrosamine and methyl-propylnitrosamine. *Z. Krebsforsch* 80: 189–196.

Kunz, W., Schande, G. and Thomas, C. 1969. The effect of phenobarbital and halogenated hydrocarbons on nitrosamine carcinogenesis. *Z. Krebsforsch.* 72: 291—304.

Lacassagne, A. 1932. Carcinogenesis and tumor pathogenesis. *Cited by* I. Berenblum, 1954. *Adv. Cancer Res.* 2: 129—175.

Lacassagne, A., Buu-Hoi, N. P., Dandel, R. and Rudali, G. 1934. *Cited by* H. V. Gelboin, 1967. Carcinogens, enzyme induction and gene action. *Adv. Cancer Res.* 10: 1—81.

Lacquer, G. L., Spatz, M. 1968. Toxicology of cycasin. *Cancer Res.* 28: 2262—2267.

Lance, E. M., Medawar, P. B. and Taut, R. N. 1973. Antilymphocyte serum. *Advan. Immunol.* 17: 1—92.

Land, H., Parada, C. F. and Weinberg, R. A. 1983. Tumorigenic conversion of primary embryo fibroblasts requires at least two cooperating oncogenes. *Nature* 304: 596—602.

Lauridsen, J. and Eggers, H. E. 1943. Carcinogenesis after multiple irritation. *Cancer Res.* 3: 43—46.

Lawley, P. D. et al. 1968. Methylated bases in liver nucleic acids from rats treated with dimethylnitrosamine. *Biochim. Biophys. Acta* 157: 646—648.

Lawley, P. D. et al. 1973. Reaction products from N-methyl-N-nitrosourea and deoxyribonucleic acid containing thymidine residues: Synthesis and identification of a new methylation product O^4 methylthymidine. *Biochem. J.* 135: 193—201.

Leathern, J. H. and Barken, H. B. 1950. Relationship between thyroid activity and liver tumor induction with 2-acetylaminofluorene. *Cancer Res.* 10: 231.

Lee, K. Y. and Lijinsky, W. 1966. Alkylation of rat liver RNA by cyclic N-nitrosamines in vivo. *J. Natl. Cancer Inst.* 37: 401—407.

Lee, D. J., Wales, J. H., Ayres, J. L. and Sinnhuber, R. O. 1968. Synergism between cyclopropenoid fatty acids and chemical carcinogens in rainbow trout (Salmo gairdneri). *Cancer Res.* 28: 2312—2316.

Leiter, J. and Shear, M. J. 1942-1943. Quantitative experiments on the production of subcutaneous tumors in strain A mice with marginal doses of 3,4-benzpyrene. *J. Natl. Cancer Inst.* 3: 455—477.

Levin, W., Welch, R. M. and Conney, A. H. 1970. Effect of carbon tetrachloride and other inhibitors of drug metabolism on the metabolism and action of estradiol-17 and estrone in the rat. *J. Pharmacol. Exp. Ther.* 173: 247—255.

Lijinsky, W., Loo, J. and Ross, A. E. 1968. Mechanism of alkylation of nucleic acids by nitrosodimethylamine. *Nature* (Lond.) 218: 1174—1175.

Lipkin, G., Knecht, M. E. 1974. A diffusible factor restoring contact inhibition of growth to malignant melanocytes. *Proc. Natl. Acad. Sci.* 71: 849—853.

Lipschutz, A. 1950. *Steroid Hormones and Tumors.* Williams & Wilkins, Baltimore.

Litwack, G., Ketterer, B. and Arias, I. M. 1971. Ligandin: a hepatic protein which binds steroids, bilirubin, carcinogens and a number of exogenous organic anions. *Nature* 234: 466—467.

Lotlikar, P. D., Miller, E. C., Miller, J. A. and Margreth, A. 1965. The enzymatic reduction of the N-hydroxy derivatives of 2-acetylaminofluorene and related carcinogens by tissue preparations. *Cancer Res.* 25: 1743—1752.

Loveless, A. 1969. A possible relevance of O-6 alkylation of deoxyguanosine to the mutagenicity and carcinogenicity of nitrosamines and nitrosamides. *Nature* 223: 206—207.

Lu, A. Y. H. et al. 1972. Reconstituted liver microsomal enzyme system that hydroxylates drugs, other foreign compounds, and endogenous substrates. II. Role of cytochrome P-450 and P-448 fractions in drug and steroid hydroxylations. *J. Biol. Chem.* 247: 1727—1734.

Lynch, H. T. and Krush, A. J. 1971. Cancer family "G" revisited: 1895-1970. *Cancer* 27: 1505—1511.

Maenza, R. M., Pradhan, A. M. and Sunderman, F. 1971. Rapid induction of sar-
    comas in rats by combination of nickel sulfide and 3,4-benzpyrene. *Cancer Res.*
    31: 2067−2071.
Magee, P. N. 1971. Toxicity of nitrosamines: their possible human health hazards.
    Food Cosmet. Toxicol. 9: 207−218.
Magee, P. N. and Hultin, T. 1962. Toxic liver injury and carcinogenesis. Methyla-
    tion of proteins of rat liver slices by dimethylnitrosamine in vitro. *Biochem. J.*
    83: 106−114.
Magee, P. N. and Schoental, R. 1964. Carcinogenesis by nitroso compounds. *Brit.*
    Med. Bull. 20: 102−106.
Magee, P. N., Montesano, R. and Preussmann, R. 1976. Nitroso compounds and
    related carcinogens. In: *Chemical Carcinogens*. C. E. Searle (ed.). American
    Chemical Society, Washington, D.C.
Malanoski, A. J. et al. 1968. Survey of polycyclic aromatic hydrocarbons in smoked
    foods. *J. Ass. Offic. Anal. Chem.* 51: 114−121.
Marchant, J. 1958. The induction of breast tumours by methylcholanthrene in
    castrated male and female mice of the IF strain bearing ovarian grafts. *Br. J.*
    Cancer 12: 62−64.
Marchant, J. 1959. Local inhibition by lactation of chemically induced breast tumours
    in mice of the IF strain. *Nature* 183: 629.
Marmorston, J. et al. 1965. II. Urinary excretion of estrone, estradiol and estriol
    by patients with breast cancer and benign breast disease. *Amer. J. Obstet.*
    Gynecol. 92: 460−467.
Martin, A. E. 1970. *Cited by* W.H.O. 1972. Health hazards of the human environ-
    ment. World Health Organization, Geneva.
Matsushima, T., Grantham, P. H., Weisburger, E. K. and Weisburger, J. H. 1972.
    Phenobarbital-mediated increase in ring- and N-hydroxylation of the carcinogen
    N-2-fluorenylacetamide, and decrease in amounts bound to liver deoxyribonucleic
    acid. *Biochem. Pharmacol.* 21: 2043−2051.
Mattocks, A. R. 1968. Toxicity of pyrrolizidine alkaloids. *Nature* 217: 723−728.
Mattocks, A. R. 1969. Dihydropyrrolizine derivatives from unsaturated pyrrolizidine
    alkaloids. *J. Chem. Soc.* Sect. C, 1155−1162.
Mattocks, A. R. and White, I. N. H. 1973. Toxic effects and pyrrolic metabolites in
    the liver of young rats given the pyrrolizidine alkaloid retrorsine. *Chem. Biol.*
    Interact. 6: 297−306.
Maurer, H. M. et al. 1968. Reduction in concentration of total serum-bilirubin in
    offspring of women treated with phenobarbitone during pregnancy. *Lancet* 2:
    122−124.
Mayer, M. M. 1973. The complement system. *Scientific American* 229(5): 54−66.
Mazzoleni, G. F. 1960. Correlation between the incidence of mammary cancer and
    number of births. *Riv. Anat. Path. Oncol.* 17: 243.
McCormick, G. M. and Moon, R. C. 1973. Effect of increasing doses of estrogen and
    progesterone on mammary carcinoma in the rat. *Europ. J. Cancer* 9: 483−486.
McEuen, C. S. 1939. Observations on rats treated with the sex hormones estrin and
    testosterone. *Am. J. Cancer* 36: 551−566.
McLean, A. E. M. and Marshall, A. 1971. Reduced carcinogenic effects of aflatoxin
    in rats given phenobarbitone. *Br. J. Exp. Oath.* 52: 322−329.
Meechan, R. A., McCafferty, D. C. and Jones, R. S. 1953. 3-Methylcholanthrene
    as an inhibitor of hepatic cancer induced by 3'-methyl-4-dimethylaminoazo-
    benzene in the diet of the rat. A determination of the time relationship. *Cancer*
    Res. 13: 802−806.
Melick, W. F. et al. 1955. The first reported cases of human bladder tumors due to
    a new carcinogen — xenylamine. *J. Urol.* 74: 760−766.
Melief, C. J. M. and Schwartz, R. 1975. Immunocompetence and malignancy. In:
    Cancer — a Comprehensive Treatise. Etiology: Chemical and Physical Carcino-
    genesis. V. 1. F. F. Becker (ed.). Plenum Press, New York.

Mertz, E. T., Fuller, R. W. and Concon, J. M. 1963. Serum uric acid in young mongoloids. *Science* 141: 535.

Mickelson, O. 1972. Introductory remarks, Symposium on Cycads. *Fed. Proc.* 31: 1465—1546.

Miller, R. W. 1963. Down's syndrome (mongolism), other congenital malformations and cancer among the sibs of leukemic children. *New Engl. J. Med.* 268: 393—401.

Miller, E. C. 1970a. Reactive forms of chemical carcinogens: Interactions with tissue components, historical review and perspectives. In: *Oncology.* R. C. Clark, R. W. Cumley, J. E. McCay and M. M. Copeland (eds.). Yearbook Medical Publishers, Inc., Chicago, Vol. 1.

Miller, J. A. 1970b. Carcinogenesis by chemicals: An overview. G. H. A. Clowes Memorial Lecture. *Cancer Res.* 30: 559—576.

Miller, R. W. 1970c. Neoplasia and Down's syndrome. *Ann. N.Y. Acad. Sci.* 171: 637—640.

Miller, R. W. 1971. Transplacental chemical carcinogenesis in man. *J. Natl. Cancer Inst.* 47: 1169—1191.

Miller, R. W. 1973. New hypotheses on the etiology of cancer. Proceedings of the Seventh National Cancer Conference (1972). J.B. Lippincott Co., Philadelphia.

Miller, E. C. and Miller J. A. 1947. The presence and significance of bound aminoazo dyes in the livers of rats fed p-dimethylazobenzene. *Cancer Res.* 7: 468—480.

Miller, E. C. and Miller, J. A. 1952. In vivo combinations between carcinogens and tissue constituents and their possible role in carcinogenesis. *Cancer Res.* 12: 547—556.

Miller, J. A. and Miller, E. C. 1953. The carcinogenic aminoazo dyes. *Adv. Cancer Res.* 1: 339—369.

Miller, E. C. and Miller, J. A. 1971a. The mutagenicity of chemical carcinogens: Correlations, problems, and interpretations. In: *Chemical Mutagens.* A. Hollander (ed.). Plenum Press, New York.

Miller, J. A. and Miller, E. C. 1971b. Chemical carcinogenesis: Mechanism and approaches to its control. *J. Natl. Cancer Inst.* 47: V—XIII.

Miller, J. A. and Miller, E. C. 1974. Some current thresholds of research in chemical carcinogenesis. In: *Chemical Carcinogenesis.* Part A. P. O. P. Ts'o and J. A. DiPaolo (eds.). Marcel Dekker, Inc., New York.

Miller, E. C., Miller, J. A., Sapp, R. W. and Weber, G. M. 1949. Studies on the protein-bound aminoazo dyes formed in vivo from 4-dimethylaminoazobenzene and its C-monomethyl derivatives. *Cancer Res.* 9: 336—343.

Miller, E. C., Plescia, A. M., Miller, J. A. and Heidelberger, C. 1952. The metabolism of methylated aminoazo dyes. I. The demethylation of 3'-methyl-4-dimethyl-C^{14}-aminoazobenzene in vivo. *J. Biol. Chem.* 196: 863—874.

Miller, E. C., Miller, J. A., Brown, R. R. and MacDonald, J. M. 1958. On the protective action of certain polycyclic aromatic hydrocarbons against carcinogenesis by aminoazo dyes and 2-acetylaminofluorene. *Cancer Res.* 18: 469—477.

Miller, E. C., Miller, J. A. and Hartman, H. A. 1961. N-Hydroxy-2-acetylaminofluorene: A metabolite of 2-acetylaminofluorene with increased carcinogenic activity in the rat. *Cancer Res.* 21: 815—824.

Miller, E. C., Miller, J. A. and Enomoto, M. 1964. The comparative carcinogenicities of 2-acetylaminofluorene and its N-hydroxy metabolite in mice, hamsters, and guinea pigs. *Cancer Res.* 24: 2018—2031.

Milner, S. M. 1967. Effects of the food additive butylated hydroxytoluene on monolayer cultures of primate cells. *Nature* 216: 557—560.

Mirvish, S. S. and Sidransky, H. 1971. Labeling in vivo of rat liver proteins by tritium-labeled dimethylnitrosamine. Effect of prior treatment with 3-methylcholanthrene, phenobarbitone, dimethylformamide, diethylformamide, aminoacetonitrile, ethionine, and carbon tetrachloride. *Biochem. Pharmacol.* 20: 3493—3499.

Mitoma, C., Lombrozo, L., LeValley, S. and Dehn, F. 1969. Nature of the effect of caffeine on the drug-metabolizing enzymes. *Arch. Biochem.* 134: 434—441.

Montesano, R., Saffiotti, U. and Shubik, P. 1970. The role of topical and systemic factors in experimental respiratory carcinogenesis. In: *Inhalation Carcinogenesis*. M. G. Hanna, P. Nettesheim, and J. R. Gilbert (eds.). AEC Symposium.

Montesano, R., Saffiotti, U., Ferrero, A. and Kaufman, D. G. 1974. Synergistic effects of benzo(a)pyrene and diethylnitrosamine on respiratory carcinogenesis in hamsters. *J. Natl. Cancer Inst.* 53: 1395—1397.

Moon, H. D. and Simpson, M. E. 1955. Effect of hypophysectomy on carcinogenesis: Inhibition of methylcholanthrene carcinogenesis. *Cancer Res.* 15: 403—406.

Morris, H. P., Dalton, A. J. and Green, C. D. 1951. Malignant thyroid tumors occurring in the mouse after prolonged hormonal imbalance during the ingestion of thiouracil. *J. Clin. Endocr.* 11: 1281—1295.

Mosonyi, M. and Korpassy, B. 1953. Rapid production of malignant hepatomas by simultaneous administration of tannic acid and 2-acetylaminofluorene. *Nature* 171: 791.

Mühlbock, O. 1958. Mammary cancer in human beings and in animals. A comparison. In: *International Symposium on Mammary Cancer*. L. Severi (ed.). Division of Cancer Research, University of Perugia.

Mühlbock, O. and Van Rijssel, T. G. 1954. Studies on mammary tumors in the O20 Amsterdam strain of mice. *J. Natl. Cancer Inst.* 15: 73—97.

Mulay, A. S. and O'Gara, R. W. 1959. Incidence of liver tumors in male and female rats fed carcinogenic azo dyes. *Proc. Soc. Exp. Biol.* 100: 320—322.

Muth, O. H. (ed.). 1967. *Selenium in Biomedicine*. AVI Publishing, Westport, Connecticut.

Nagasawa, H. and Yanai, R. 1973. Effect of human placental lactogen on growth of carcinogen-induced mammary tumors in rats. *Int. J. Cancer* 11: 131—137.

National Cancer Institute. 1972. Monograph 35. Conference on Immunology of Carcinogenesis. U.S. Department of Health, Education, and Welfare Public Health Service. National Institutes of Health. National Cancer Institute.

National Cancer Institute. 1974. Third National Cancer Survey. Monograph 41. U.S. Government Printing Office, Washington, D.C.

Nebert, D. W. and Gelboin, H. V. 1968. Substrate-inducible microsomal aryl hydroxylase in mammalian cell cultures. *J. Biol. Chem.* 243: 6250—6261.

Nebert, D. W. and Gelboin, H. V. 1969. In vivo and in vitro induction of aryl hydrocarbon hydroxylase in mammalian cells of different species, tissues, strains, and developmental and hormonal states. *Arch. Biochem. Biophys.* 134: 76—89.

Nebert, D. W., Winker, J. and Gelboin, H. V. 1969. Aryl hydrocarbon hydroxylase in human placenta from cigarette smoking and nonsmoking women. *Cancer Res.* 29: 1763—1769.

Neel, J. V. 1962. Mutations in the human population. In: *Methodology in Human Genetics*. W. J. Burdette (ed.). Holden-Day, San Francisco.

Neel, J. V. 1971. Familial factors in adenocarcinoma of the colon. *Cancer* 28: 46—50.

Nelson, A. A. and Woodard, G. 1953. Tumors of the urinary bladder, gall bladder, and liver in dogs fed O-aminoazotoluene or p-dimethylaminoazobenzene. *J. Natl. Cancer Inst.* 13: 1497—1509.

Newbold, R. F. and Overell, R. W. 1983. Fibroblast immortality is a prerequisite for transformation by E J C-Ha-ras oncogene. *Nature* 304: 648—651.

Noble, R. L. and Walters, J. H. 1954. The effect of hypophysectomy on 9,10-dimethyl-1,2-benzanthracene-induced carcinogenesis. *Proc. Am. Ass. Cancer Res.* 1: 35—36.

Nothdurft, H. 1955. The experimental formation of sarcomas in rats and mice by implantation of round disc made of gold, platinum, silver or ivory. *Naturwissenschaften*. 42: 75—76. (German)

Novi, A. N. 1981. Regression of aflatoxin B_1-induced hepatocellular carcinomas by reduced glutathione. *Science* 212: 541–542.

Nowell, P. D. 1976. The clonal evolution of tumor cell populations. *Science* 194: 23–28.

Oberling, Ch. and Guerin, M. 1947. Epitheliomatous reaction of rat skin after painting with benzpyrene. *Bull. Assoc. franc. etude Cancer* 34: 30–42. (French)

O'Connor, P. J., Capps, M. J. and Craig, A. W. 1973. Comparative studies of the hepatocarcinogen N,N-dimethylnitrosamine in vivo: Reaction sites in rat liver DNA and the significance of their relative stabilities. *Br. J. Cancer* 27: 153–166.

Oesch, F. et al. 1972. A reconstituted microsomal enzyme system that converts naphthalene to trans-1,2-dihydroxy-1,2-dihydronaphthalene via naphthalene-1,2-oxide: Presence of epoxide hydrase in cytochrome P-450 and P-448 fractions. *Arch. Biochem. Biophys.* 153: 62–67.

Okada, M. and Suzuki, E. 1972. Metabolism of butyl-(4-hydroxybutyl)nitrosamine in rats. *Gann* 63: 391.

Orten, J. M. and Neuhaus, O. W. 1975. *Human Biochemistry*. Mosby, St. Louis.

Ottoboni, A., Gee, R., Stanley, R. L. and Goetz, M. E. 1968. Evidence from conversion of DDT to TDE in rat liver. II. Conversion of p,p'-DDT to p,p'-DTE in axenic rats. *Bull. Environ. Contam. Toxicol.* 3: 302–308.

Paget, G. E. and Walpole, A. L. 1960. The experimental toxicity of griseofulvin. *Arch. Dermatol.* 81: 750–757.

Pantuck, E. J., Kuntzman, R. and Conney, A. H. 1972. Decreased concentration of phenacetin in plasma of cigarette smokers. *Science* 175: 1248–1250.

Paschkis, K. E., Cantarow, A. and Stasney, J. 1948. Influence of thiouracil on carcinoma induced by 2-acetaminofluorene. *Cancer Res.* 8: 257–263.

Passey, R. D. 1938. Experimental tar tumours in dogs. *J. Pathol. Bacteriol.* 47: 349–351.

Patterson, D. S. P. 1973. Metabolism as a factor in determining the toxic action of the aflatoxins in different animal species. *Food Cosmet. Toxicol.* 11: 287–294.

Payne, W. W. and Hueper, W. C. 1960. Carcinogenic effects of single and repeated doses of 3,4-benzpyrene. *Am. Ind. Hyg. Ass. J.* 21: 350–355.

Pelkonen, O., Kaltiala, E. O., Larmi, T. K. I. and Kärki, N. T. 1973. Comparison of activities of drug metabolism of enzymes in human fetal and adult livers. *Clin. Pharmacol. Ther.* 14: 840–846.

Peller, S. 1960. *Cancer in Childhood and Youth*. Wright, Bristol, England.

Peterson, J. E. and Robison, W. H. 1964. Metabolic products of p,p'-DDT in rat. *Toxicol. Appl. Pharmacol.* 6: 321–327.

Poland, A. et al. 1970. Effect of intensive occupational exposure to DDT on phenylbutazone ans cortisol metabolism in humans. *Clin. Pharmacol. Ther.* 11: 724–732.

Pollack, E. S. and Horn, J. W. 1980. Trends in cancer incidence and mortality in the United States, 1969-1976. *J. Natl. Cancer Inst.* 64: 1091–1103.

Pound, A. W., Lawson, T. A. and Horn, L. 1973. Increased carcinogenic action of dimethylnitrosamine after prior administration of carbon tetrachloride. *Br. J. Cancer* 27: 451–459.

Rabbat, A. G. and Jeejeebhoy, H. F. 1970. Heterologous antilymphocyte serum (ALS) hastens the appearance of methyl-cholanthrene-induced tumors in mice. *Transplantation* 9: 164–166.

Radonnski, J. L. 1961. The absorption, fate, and excretion of citrus red No. 2 (2,5-dimethoxyphenyl-azo-2-naphthol) and external D and C No. 14 (1-xylyl-azo-2-naphthol). *J. Pharmacol. Exp. Ther.* 134: 100–109.

Rajewsky, M. F., Dauber, W. and Frankenberg, H. 1966. Liver carcinogenesis by diethylnitrosamine in the rat. *Science* 152: 83.

Rao, K. V. N. and Vesselinovitch, S. D. 1973. Age and sex-associated diethyl-nitrosamine dealkylation activity of the mouse liver and hepatocarcinogenesis. *Cancer Res.* 33: 1625–1627.

Reif, A. E. et al. 1954. Effect of diet on the antimycin titer of mouse. *J. Biol. Chem.* 209: 223—226.

Reuber, M. D. and Lee, C. W. 1968. Effect of age and sex on hepatic lesions in buffalo strain rats ingesting diethylnitrosamine. *J. Natl. Cancer Inst.* 41: 1133—1140.

Richardson, H. L., Stier, A. R. and Borsos-Nachtnebel, E. 1952. Liver tumor inhibition and adrenal histologic responses to rats to which 3'-methyl-4-dimethylaminoazobenzene and 20-methylcholanthrene were simultaneously administered. *Cancer Res.* 12: 356—361.

Riegel, B. et al. 1951. Delay of methylcholanthrene skin carcinogenesis in mice by 1,2,5,6-dibenzofluorene. *Cancer Res.* 11: 301—303.

Roe, F. J. C. and Pierce, W. E. H. 1960. Tumor promotion by citrus oils. Tumors of the skin and urethral orifice in mice. *J. Natl. Cancer Inst.* 24: 1389—1403.

Roth, G. M. and Kvale, W. F. 1956. Pheochromocytoma, factors in accurate pharmacologic diagnosis. *Dis. Chest* 29: 366—375.

Rous, P. and Kidd, J. G. 1941. Conditional neoplasms and subthreshold neoplastic states. A study of the tar tumors of rabbits. *J. Exp. Med.* 73: 365—390.

Ruley, H. E. 1983. Adenovirus early region 1A enables viral and cellular transforming genes to transform primary cells in culture. *Nature* 304: 602—606.

Rusch, H. P., Baumann, C. A., Miller, J. A. and Kline, B. E. 1945. Experimental liver tumors. Research Conf. on Cancer (1944). *Publ. Am. Assoc. Adv. Sci.*

Rusch, H. P., Bosch, D. and Boutwell, R. K. 1955. The influence of irritants on mitotic activity and tumor formation in mouse epidermis. *Acta Unio. Int. Contra Cancrum* 11: 699—703.

Russell, W. O. and Ortega, L. R. 1952. Methylcholanthrene-induced tumors in guinea pigs. *Arch. Pathol.* 53: 301—314.

Saffioti, U. and Shubik, P. 1956. The effects of low concentration in epidermal carcinogenesis: A comparison with promoting agents. *J. Natl. Cancer Inst.* 16: 961—969.

Saffioti, U. et al. 1972. Respiratory tract carcinogenesis in hamsters induced by different numbers of administrations of benzo(a)pyrene and ferric oxide. *Cancer Res.* 32: 1073—1081.

Salaman, M. H. and Roe, F. J. C. 1964. Cocarcinogenesis. *Br. Med. Bull.* 20: 139—144.

Salzberg, D. A. and Griffin, A. C. 1952. Inhibition of azo dye carcinogenesis in alloxan-diabetic rat. *Cancer Res.* 12: 294.

Salzberg, D. A., Hane, S. and Griffin, A. C. 1951. The distribution of 3'-methyl-(C^{14})-4-dimethylaminoazobenzene in the rat. *Cancer Res.* 11: 276.

Scarborough, H. and Bacharach, A. L. 1949. Vitamin P. *Vitam. Horm.* 7: 1—55.

Schlede, E., Kuntzman, R. and Conney, A. H. 1970. Stimulatory effect of benzo(a)pyrene and phenobarbital pretreatment on the biliary excretion of benzo(a)pyrene metabolites in the rat. *Cancer Res.* 30: 2898—2904.

Schmähl, D. 1970. Syncarcinogenesis: Experimental investigations. In: *Chemical Tumor Problems*. W. Nakahara (ed.). Japanese Society for Promotion of Science, Tokyo.

Schneiderman, M. 1980. *Cited by* Toxic Substances Strategy Committee. 1980. Chemicals and public protection, A report to the president. Government Printing Office, Washington, D. C.

Schottenfeld, D. 1975. Introduction: The magnitude of cancer. In: *Cancer Epidemiology and Prevention*. D. Schottenfeld (ed.). Charles Thomas, Springfield, Illinois.

Sciorra, L. J., Kaufmann, B. and Maier, R. 1974. Effect of butylated hydroxytoluene on cell cycle and chromosome morphology of phytohemagglutinin-stimulated leucocyte cultures. *Food Cosmet. Toxicol.* 12: 33—44.

Segal, A. et al. 1972. Tumor inhibition, persistence and binding of actinomycin D in mouse skin. *Cancer Res.* 32: 1384—1390.

Segi, M., Kurihara, M. and Matsuyame, T. 1969. *Cancer Mortality for Selected Sites in 24 Countries (1964-1965)*, No. 5. Sanko, Sendai, Japan.

Selikoff, I. J., Hammond, E. C. and Heimann, H. 1971. *Cited by* World Health Association 1972. *Health Hazards of the Human Environment.* W.H.O., Geneva.

Selkirk, J. K., Huberman, E. and Heidelberger, C. 1972. An epoxide is an intermediate in the microsomal metabolism of the chemical carcinogen dibenz(a,h)-anthracene. *Biochem. Biophys. Res. Commun.* 43: 1010—1016.

Setälä, K. 1961. Nature and mechanism of tumour promotion in skin carcinogenesis in mice. *Acta Un. Int. Cancer* 17: 31—44.

Setälä, K., Setälä, H. and Holsti, P. 1954. A new and physicochemically well-defined group of tumor-promoting (cocarcinogenic) agents for mouse skin. *Science* 120: 1075—1076.

Setälä, K., Setälä, H., Merenmies, L. and Holsti, P. 1957. Investigations on the tumor promoting effect of non-ionic surface active substances on mouse and rats. *Z. Krebsforsch.* 61: 534—547. (German)

Setlow, R. B. and Regan, J. D. 1972. Defective repair of N-acetoxy-2-acetylamino-fluorene-induced lesions in the DNA of xeroderma pigmentosum cells. *Biochem. Biophys. Res. Commun.* 46: 1019—1024.

Setlow, R. B., Regan, J. D., German, J. and Carrier, W. L. 1969. Evidence that xeroderma pigmentosum cells do not perform the first step in the repair of ultraviolet damage to their DNA. *Proc. Natl. Acad. Sci.* 64: 1035—1041.

Shamberger, R. J., Tytko, S. A. and Willis, C. E. 1976. Antioxidants and cancer. Part VI. Selenium and age-adjusted human cancer mortality. *Arch. Environ. Health.* 31: 231—235.

Shapiro, R. 1968. Chemistry of guanine and its biologically significant derivatives. *Prog. Nucleic Acid Res. Mol. Biol.* 8: 73—112.

Shapiro, J. R. and Kirschbaum, A. 1951. Intrinsic tissue response to induction of pulmonary tumors. *Cancer Res.* 11: 644—647.

Shay, H., Harris, C. and Gruenstein, M. 1952. Influence of sex hormones on the incidence and form of tumors produced in male or female rats by gastric instillation of methylcholanthrene. *J. Natl. Cancer Inst.* 13: 307—331.

Shear, M. J. 1937. Studies in carcinogenesis. IV. Development of liver tumors in pure strain mice following the injection of 2-amino-5-azotoluene. *Am. J. Cancer* 29: 269—284.

Shubik, P. and Hartwell, J. L. 1957. Survey of compounds which have been tested for carcinogenic activity. Public Health Service Publ. No. 149, Suppl. 1. U.S. Govt. Printing Office, Washington, D.C.

Shubik, P., Saffiotti, U., Feldman, R. and Ritchie, A. C. 1956. Studies on promoting action in skin carcinogenesis. *Proc. Am. Assoc. Cancer Res.* 2: 146—147.

Sice, J. 1966. Tumor-promoting activity of n-alkanes and 1-alkanols. *Toxicol. Appl. Pharmacol.* 9: 70—74.

Smith, P. E. and MacDowell, E. c. 1930. An hereditary anterior-pituitary deficiency in mouse. *Anat. Rec.* 46: 249—257.

Sorof, S., Cohen, P. P., Miller, E. C. and Miller, J. A. 1951. Electrophoretic studies on the soluble proteins from livers of rats fed amino azo dyes. *Cancer Res.* 11: 383—387.

Spatz, M. and Lacquer, G. L. 1967. Transplacental induction of tumors in Sprague-Dawley rats with crude cycad material. *J. Natl. Cancer Inst.* 38: 233—245.

Sporu, M. B., Dingman, C. W. and Phelps, H. L. 1966. Aflatoxin B_1 binding to DNA in vitro and alteration of RNA metabolism in vivo. *Science* 151: 1539—1541.

Stewart, B. W. and Magee, P. H. 1972. Metabolism and some biochemical effects of N-nitrosomorpholine. *Biochem. J.* 126: 21.

Stjernsward, J. 1966. Effect of non-carcinogenic and carcinogenic hydrocarbons on antibody forming cells measured at cellular level in vitro. *J. Natl. Cancer Inst.* 36: 1189—1195.

Strauss, R. and Wurm, M. 1960. Catecholamines and the diagnosis of pheochromo-cytoma. *Am. J. Clin. Pathol.* 34: 403—425.

Stutman, O. 1969. Carcinogen-induced immune depression: Absence in mice resist-ant to chemical oncogenesis. *Science* 166: 620—621.

Sunderman, F. W. Jr. 1971. Metal carcinogenesis in experimental animals. *Food Cosmet. Toxicol.* 9: 105—120.

Swan, P. F. and Magee, P. N. 1968. Nitrosamine-induced carcinogenesis. The alky-lation of nucleic acids of the rat by N-methyl-N-nitrosourea, dimethylnitros-amine, dimethylsulfate and methylmethane sulphonate. *Biochem. J.* 110: 39—47.

Swan, P. F. and Magee, P. N. 1971. Nitrosamine induced carcinogenesis. The alky-lation of N-7 guanine of nucleic acids of the rat by diethylnitrosamine, ethyl-nitrosourea, and ethyl-methane sulfonate. *Biochem. J.* 125: 841—847.

Sweeney, M. J. et al. 1972a. Experimental antitumor activity and preclinical toxi-cology of mycophenolic acid. *Cancer Res.* 32: 1795—1802.

Sweeney, M. J., Hoffman, D. H. and Esterman, M. A. 1972b. Metabolism and bio-chemistry of mycophenolic acid. *Cancer Res.* 32: 1803—1809.

Swenson, D. H., Miller, J. A. and Miller, E. C. 1973. 2,3-Dihydro-2,3-dihydroxy-aflatoxin B_1: An acid hydrolysis product of an RNA-aflatoxin B_1 adduct formed by hamsters and rat liver microsomes in vitrol. *Biochem. Biophys. Res. Commun.* 53: 1260—1267.

Swenson, D. H., Miller, J. A. and Miller, E. C. 1974. Aflatoxin B_1-2,3-dichloride: A toxic and reactive derivative of aflatoxin B_1. *Proc. Am. Assoc. Cancer Res.* 15: 43.

Symeonidis, A., Mulay, A. S. and Burgoyne, F. H. 1954. Effect of adrenalectomy and of desoxycorticosterone acetate on the formation of liver lesions in rats fed p-dimethylaminoazobenzene. *J. Natl. Cancer Inst.* 14: 805—818.

Szakall, A. K. and Hanna, M. G. 1972. Immune suppression and carcinogenesis in hamsters during topical application of 7,12-dimethylbenz(a)anthracene. In: Con-ference on Immunology of Carcinogenesis. National Cancer Institute Mongraph 35. National Institutes of Health. Bethesda, Maryland.

Szent-Györgyi, A. 1955. Perspectives for bioflavinoids. *Ann. N.Y. Acad. Sci.* 61: 732—735.

Taufic, H. N. 1965. Studies on ear duct tumors in rats. Ii. Inhibitory effect of methylcholanthrene and 1,2-benzanthracene on tumor formation by 4-dimethyl-aminostilbene. *Acta. Pathol. Jpn.* 15: 255—260.

Thomas, L. 1959. Discussion in cellular and humoral aspects of the hypersensitive states. H. S. Laurence (ed.). Hoeber-Harper, New York.

Thomas, J. E., Rooke, E. D. and Kvale, W. I. 1966. the neurologist's experience with pheochromocytoma. *J.A.M.A.* 197: 754—758.

Thompson, R. P. H. et al. 1969. Treatment of unconjugated jaundice with dicophane. *Lancet* 2: 4—6.

Tokuhata, G. K. 1964. Familial factors in human lung cancer and smoking. *Am. J. Public Health* 54: 24—32.

Toth, B. 1968. A critical review of experiments in chemical carcinogenesis using newborn animals. *Cancer Res.* 28: 727—738.

Toxic Substances Strategy Committee. 1980. *Chemicals and Public Protection, a Report to the President.* Government Printing Office, Washington, D.C.

Troll, W., Klassen, A. and Janoff, A. 1970. Tumorigenesis in mouse skin: Inhibi-tion by synthetic inhibitors of proteases. *Science* 169: 1211—1213.

Truhaut, R. and Dechambre, R. P. 1972. Modality of induction of mouse pulmonary tumor by benz(a)pyrene. Influence of the dose of aromatic hydrocarbon and of environmental factors. *C.R. Acad. Sci.* 274: 2263—2267. (French)

Turusov, V., Day, N., Andrianov, L. and Jain, D. 1971. Influence of dose on skin tumors induced in mice by single application of 7,12-dimethylbenz(a)anthracene. *J. Natl. Cancer Inst.* 47: 105—111.

Uehleke, H., Hellmer, K. H. and Tabarelli, S. 1973. Binding of ^{14}C-carbon tetra-chloride to microsomal proteins in vitro and formation of $CHCl_3$ by reduced liver microsomes. *Xenobiotica* 3: 1—11.

Uhr, J. W. 1966. Delayed hypersensitivity. *Physiol. Rev.* 46: 359—419.

Ulland, B. M., Weisburger, J. H., Yamamoto, R. S. and Weisburger, E. K. 1972. Antioxidants and carcinogenesis: Butylated hydroxytoluene, but not diphenyl-p-phenylenediamine, inhibits cancer induction by N-2-fluorenylacetamide and by N-hydroxy-N-2-fluorenylacetamide in rats. *Toxicol. Appl. Pharmacol.* 22: 281.

U.S. Environmental Protection Agency. 1971. *Background Information: Proposed National Emission Standards for Hazardous Air Pollutants: Asbestos, Beryllium, Mercury.* Research Triangle Park, N.C.

U.S. Public Health Service 1964. *Smoking and Health.* U.S. Department of Health, Education, and Welfare. Public Health Service. Publication No. 1103, Washington, D.C.

U.S. Public Health Service. 1971. *The Health Consequences of Smoking. A report to the Surgeon General.* U.S. Department of Health, Education, and Welfare. DHEW Publication No. (HSM) 72-6516, 1972. Washington, D.C.

U.S. Public Health Service. 1972. *The Health Consequences of Smoking. A Report to the Surgeon General.* U.S. Department of Health, Education, and Welfare. DHEW Publication No. (HSM) 71-7513, 1971, Washington, D.C.

U.S. Public Health Service. 1973. *The Health Consequences of Smoking.* U.S. Department of Health, Education, and Welfare. DHEW Publication No. (HSM) 73-8704, Washington, D.C.

Van Duuren, B. L. 1976. Tumor-promoting and co-carcinogenic agents in chemical carcinogenesis. In: *Chemical Carcinogens.* C. E. Searle (ed.). American Chemical Society, Washington, D.C.

Venkatesan, N., Arcos, J. C. and Argus, M. F. 1970a. Amino acid induction and carbohydrate repression of dimethylnitrosamine demethylase in rat liver. *Cancer Res.* 30: 2563—2567.

Venkatesan, N., Argus, M. F. and Arcos, J. C. 1970b. Mechanism of 3-methyl-cholanthrene-induced inhibition of dimethylnitrosamine demethylase in rat liver. *Cancer Res.* 30: 2556—2562.

Vesselinovitch, S. D. 1969. The sex-dependent difference in the development of liver tumors in mice administered dimethylnitrosamine. *Cancer Res.* 29: 1024—1027.

Vesselinovitch, S. D., Mihailovich, N. 1968. The inhibitory effect of griseofulvin on the promotion of skin carcinogenesis. *Cancer Res.* 28: 2463—2465.

Vesselinovitch, S. D. et al. 1972. Aflatoxin B_1, a hepatocarcinogen in the infant mouse. *Cancer Res.* 32: 2289—2291.

Vesell, E. S., Page, J. G. 1968a. Genetic control of drug levels in man: Antipyrene. *Science* 161: 72—73.

Vesell, E. S., Page, J. G. 1968b. Genetic control of drug levels in man: Phenyl-butazone. *Science* 159: 1479—1480.

Vesell, E. S. and Page, J. G. 1969. Genetic control of the phenobarbital-induced shortening of plasma antipyrine half lives in man. *J. Clin Invest.* 48: 2202—2209.

Von Der Decken, A. and Hultin, T. 1960. Inductive effects of 3-methylcholanthrene on enzyme activities and amino acid incorporation capacity of rat liver micro-somes. *Arch. Biochem. Biophys.* 90: 201—207.

Wagner, J. L. and Haughton, G. 1971. Immunosuppression by antilymphocyte serum and its effects on tumors induced by 2-methylcholanthrene in mice. *J. Natl. Cancer Inst.* 46: 1—10.

Wagner, J. C., Gibson, J. C., Berry, G. and Timbrell, V. 1971. Epidemiology of asbestos cancers. *Br. Med. Bull.* 27: 71—76.

Waldmann, T. A., Strober, W. and Blaese, R. M. 1972. Immunodeficiency disease and malignancy. Various immunologic deficiencies of man and the role of immune processes in the control of malignant disease. *Ann. Int. Med.* 77: 605—628.

Warthin, A. S. 1913. Heredity with reference to carcinoma: As shown by the study of the cases examined in the pathological laboratory of the University of Michigan, 1985-1913. *Arch. Int. Med.* 12: 546—555.

Wattenberg, L. W. 1972. Inhibition of carcinogenic and toxic effects of polycyclic hydrocarbons by phenolic antioxidants and ethoxyquin. *J. Natl. Cancer Inst.* 48: 1425—1430.

Wattenberg, L. W. 1973. Inhibition of chemical carcinogen-induced pulmonary neoplasia by butylated hydroxyanisole. *J. Natl. Cancer Inst.* 40: 1541—1544.

Wattenberg, L. W. 1978. Inhibition of chemical carcinogenesis. *J. Natl. Cancer Inst.* 60: 11—18.

Wattenberg, L. W. and Leong, J. L. 1952. Histochemical demonstration of reduced pyridine nucleotide dependent polycyclic hydrocarbon metabolizing systems. *J. Histochem. Cytochem.* 10: 412—420.

Wattenberg, L. W. and Leong, J. L. 1968. Inhibition of the carcinogenic action of 7,12-dimethylbenz(α)anthracene by beta-naphthoflavone. *Proc. Soc. Exp. Biol. Med.* 128: 940—943.

Wattenberg, L. W. and Leong, J. L. 1970. *Inhibition of the Carcinogenic Action of Benzo(a)pyrene by Flavones.* Abstr. Tenth International Cancer Congress, Houston, Texas.

Wattenberg, L. W., Page, M. A. and Leong, J. L. 1968. Induction of increased benzopyrene hydroxylase activity by flavones and related compounds. *Cancer Res.* 28: 934—937.

Weil, C. S. 1972. Statistic vs safety factors and scientific judgment in the evaluation of safety for man. *Toxicol. Appl. Pharmacol.* 21: 454—463.

Weisburger, J. H. 1973. Chemical carcinogensis. In: *Cancer Medicine.* J. F. Holland and E. Frei (eds.). Lea & Febiger, Philadelphia.

Weisburger, J. H. 1975. Chemical carcinogenesis. In: *Toxicology — The Basic Science of Poisons.* L. J. Casarett and J. Doull (eds.). Macmillan, New York.

Weisburger, J. H. et al. 1970. A comparison of the effect of the carcinogen N-hydroxy-N-2-fluorenylacetamide in infant and weanling rats. *J. Natl. Cancer Inst.* 45: 29—35.

Weissberger, A. S. and Perskey, L. 1953. Renal calculi and uremia as complications of lymphoma. *Am. J. Med. Sci.* 225: 669—673.

Weisburger, J. H. and Rall, E. P. 1972. Do animal models predict carcinogenic hazards for man? In: Environment and Cancer. M. D. Anderson Symposium. Williams & Wilkins, Baltimore.

Weisburger, E. V. and Weisburger, J. H. 1958. Chemistry carcinogenicity, and metabolism of 2-fluorenamine and related compounds. *Adv. Cancer Res.* 5: 333—432.

Weisburger, J. H. and Weisburger, E. K. 1966. Chemicals as causes of cancer. *Chem. Eng. News* 43: 112—142.

Weisburger, J. H. and Weisburger, E. K. 1973. Biochemical formation and pharmacological, toxicological, and pathological properties of hydroxylamines and hydroxamic acids. *Pharmacol. Rev.* 25: 1—66.

Weisburger, J. H. and Williams, G. M. 1975. Metabolism of chemical carcinogens. In: *Cancer.* Vol. 1. F. Becker (ed.). Plenum Press, New York.

Weisburger, J. H., Shirasu, Y., Grantham, P. H. and Weisburger, E. K. 1967. Chloramphenicol, protein synthesis, and the metabolism of the carcinogen N-2-fluorenyldiacetamide in rats. *J. Biol. Chem.* 242: 372—378.

Weisburger, J. H. et al. 1972. On the sulfate ester of N-hydroxy-N-2-fluorenylacetamide as a key ultimate hepatocarcinogen in the rat. *Cancer Res.* 32: 491—500.

Weisz, J. and Gunzalus, P. 1973. Estrogen levels in immature female rats: True or spurious; ovarian or adrenal. *Endocrinology* 93: 1057—1065.

Welch, R. M., Levin, W. and Conney, A. H. 1967. Insecticide inhibition and stimulation of steroid hydroxylase in rat liver. *J. Pharmacol. Exp. Ther.* 155: 167—173.

Welch, R. W. et al. 1968. Cigarette smoking: Stimulatory effect on metabolism of 3,4-benzpyrene by enzymes in human placenta. *Science* 160: 541—542.

Welch, R. M. et al. 1969. Stimulatory effect of cigarette smoking on the hydroxylation of 3,4-benzpyrene and the N-demethylation of 3-methyl-4-monomethylaminoazobenzene by enzymes in human placenta. *Clin. Pharmacol. Ther.* 10: 100—109.

Wheatley, D. N. 1968. Enhancement and inhibition of the induction by 7,12-dimethylbenz(a)anthracene of mammary tumors in female, Sprague-Dawley rats. *Br. J. Cancer* 22: 787—797.

White, I. N. H. and Mattocks, A. R. 1972. Reaction of dihydropyrrolozines with deoxyribonucleic acid in vitro. *Biochem. J.* 128: 291—297.

Whitlock, N. P., Cooper, H. L. and Gelboin, H. V. 1972. Aryl hydrocarbon (benzopyrene) hydroxylase is stimulated in human lymphocytes by mitogens and benz-(a)anthracene. *Science* 177: 618—619.

Wiebel, F. J. et al. 1974. Flavones and polycyclic hydrocarbons as modulators of aryl hydrocarbon (benzo(a)pyrene) hydroxylase. In: *Chemical Carcinogenesis*. Part A. P. O. P. Ts'o and J. A. DiPaolo (eds.). Marcel Dekker, New York.

Wilson, M. G., Towner, J. W. and Fujimoto, A. 1973. Retinoblastoma and D-chromosome deletions. *Am. J. Hum. Genet.* 25: 57—61.

Wogan, G. N. 1974. Naturally occurring carcinogens. In: *The Physiopathology of Cancer*. F. Homburger (ed.). S. Karger, Basel.

Woods, D. A. 1969. Influence of antilymphocyte serum on DMBA induction of oral carcinomas. *Nature* 224: 276—277.

World Health Organization. 1972. Health hazards of the human environment. W.H.O. Geneva.

Wright, W. G. 1969. Asbestos and health in 1969. *Am. Rev. Respir. Dis.* 100: 467—479.

Wunderlich, V., Schütt, M., Böttger, M. and Graffi, A. 1970. Preferential alkylation of mitrochondrial deoxyribonucleic acid by N-methyl-N-nitrosourea. *Biochem. J.* 118: 99—109.

Wyatt, P. L. and Cramer, J. W. 1970. Urinary excretion of N-hydroxy-2-acetylaminofluorene (N-HO-AAF) by rats given phenobarbital (PB). *Proc. Am. Assoc. Cancer Res.* 11: 83.

Wynder, E. L. and Mabuchi, K. 1972. Etiological and preventive aspects of human cancer. *Prev. Med.* 1: 300—334.

Wynder, E. L., Mabuchi, K. and Hoffmann, D. 1975. Tobacco. In: *Cancer Epidemiology and Prevention*. D. Schottenfeld (ed.). Charles C Thomas, Springfield, Illinois.

Yamamoto, R. S. et al. 1968. Inhibition of the toxicity and carcinogenicity of N-2-fluorenylacetamide by acetanilide. *Toxicol. Appl. Pharmacol.* 13: 108—117.

Yamamoto, R. S., Williams, G. M., Frankel, H. H. and Weisburger, J. H. 1971. 8-hydroxyquinoline: Chronic toxicity and inhibitory effect on the carcinogenicity of N-2-fluorenylacetamide. *Toxicol. Appl. Pharmacol.* 19: 687—698.

Young, D. 1971. The susceptibility to SV40 fibroblasts obtained from patients with Down's syndrome. *Europ. J. Cancer* 7: 337—339.

Zippin, C. and Petrakis, N. L. 1971. Identification of high risk groups in breast cancer. *Cancer* 28: 1381—1387.

7

Nutritional Factors and Carcinogenesis

Nutritional factors can be expected to affect tumor initiation and promotion in several ways: (1) Adequate supply of nutrients is needed for the energy and metabolic requirements of the rapidly proliferating tumor mass, particularly for the biosynthesis of tissue components such as proteins. (2) Certain vitamins and trace metals which are components of coenzymes and cofactors, respectively, are required by the enzymes which either activate or inactivate carcinogens and toxicants. (3) Also, the presence of certain nutrients may inhibit the formation of carcinogens in vivo from innocuous precursors. Other nutrients may enhance the induction or facilitate the promotion of tumors. (5) Nutrients, by themselves, may be precursors of carcinogens formed in vivo. (6) Fats may act as solvents of carcinogens, facilitating their absorption, transport, and storage in tissues. (7) It appears that nutritional status may affect immunological competence, and thus tumor development. (8) The nature of the diet may also influence the type and quantity of intestinal bacteria, which may produce carcinogens from bile acids and sterols.

EFFECT OF CALORIC INTAKE

With very rare exception, obesity involving endocrine dysfunction is related to excess caloric intake over caloric expenditure. Actuarial data show that mortality from all forms of cancer in adults of both sexes appears to increase with the degree of obesity (Dublin 1930; Society of Actuaries 1959). Epidemiological studies on specific cancer types show a significant relationship between obesity or overweight and cancer of the breast, endometrium, and gallbladder (deWaard 1975; Wynder and Mabuchi 1972). In a study of Wynder et al. (1966), 48% of patients with endometrial cancer were obese compared to 18% of the control; among 59 breast cancer patients, 78% were obese compared to 54% of the control (deWaard et al. 1960). A similar statistical association between obesity and cancer of the large bowel in men, unexpectedly, not in women, and cancer of the uterus has been reported (Shils 1973).

The validity of the conclusions from the epidemiological data regarding the role of obesity in carcinogenesis appears to be strengthened by results obtained with experimental animals. These results indicate that caloric restriction has a marked influence in the development of neoplasms (Tannenbaum 1959). Many types of tumors are inhibited by chronic caloric restriction (Comings 1973). The degree of inhibition of tumor formation varies with the type of tumor, including the so-called spontaneous tumors, and the type of carcinogens (Ross and Bras 1971; Shils 1973; Tannenbaum 1959). For example, caloric restriction most easily inhibits spontaneous breast and lung tumors in mice, and

Table 7.1 Inhibition of Spontaneous Mammary Cancer in Two Strains of Mice by Caloric Restriction or Underfeeding

Strain	Dietary regimen	Amount of Restriction (Fraction of control)	Age Restriction ended (months)	Period of Restriction (months)	Breeding	% tumor incidence Control	% tumor incidence Experiment
dba	CR	1/2	20	17.5	NP	38	0
C3H	CR	1/3	18	17.0	NP	67	0
C3H	CR	1/2	22	21.0	NP	100	12.5
C3H	CR	1/2	22	18.0	P	100	18.5
dba	UF	1/3–1/2	18	12.5	NP	40	2
dba	UF	1/3–1/2	24	15.0	27% NP 73% NP	30	7

Abbreviations: NP, nulliparous; P, parous; CR, caloric restriction; UF, underfeeding.
Source: Morris (1945).

to a lesser degree, carcinogen-induced tumors of the skin (Tannenbaum 1944) and sarcomas (i.e., malignant tumors of the mesenchymal tissues, e.g., connective tissues, muscles, bone).

Data presented by Morris (1945) show the effect of caloric restriction or underfeeding on spontaneous mammary cancer development in two strains of parous and nulliparous mice.

In Table 7.1, note that in a strain showing 100% tumor incidence without caloric restriction, this regimen produced 12.5% incidence only in the nulliparous, and somewhat higher in the parous animals. In those mice which normally produced 30 to 67% spontaneous tumor incidence, caloric restriction reduced tumor incidence from 0 to 7%. Similar studies in mice support these findings (King et al. 1951; Tannenbaum 1944).

An excellent work by Ross and Bras (1971) on the effect of caloric restriction throughout the lifespan in rats as well as for 7 weeks after weaning underscores the marked inhibitory effect of these dietary regimens on spontaneous tumor development. The animals were started with 2 g of diet containing 22% casein, 58.5% sucrose, 13.5% corn oil, and adequate vitamins and minerals. The amount of diet given was gradually increased to 6.0 g in 0.1 g increments, up to age 273 days; the total amount of diet given at this age was maintained thereafter (in the case of the restricted group [R]). The amount of feed given to the rats on 7-week restriction was increased from 2.0 g to 4.3 g, then switched to ad libitum feeding (RAL). Control animals were fed the same diet ad libitum (AL).

Table 7.2 shows a comparison of tumor risk between all three dietary regimen; ad libitum feeding is taken as standard and is assumed to produce a tumor incidence ratio (TIR) of 100 for purposes of comparison. A lifetime restriction in caloric intake reduces the tumor risk to around 6% for both benign and malignant tumors. Even if the caloric restriction is maintained after weaning for only 7 weeks, significant reduction in tumor risk is obtained, even though the risk involving malignant tumors is not decreased as much as benign tumors.

The tumor risk varies with the tissue of origin; it seems highest for the lymphoreticular, hematopoietic, and soft tissues in animals on RAL regimen, and for

Table 7.2 Long Term Effects of Caloric Restriction on Tumor Risk

Tumor	Tumor incidence ratio (%) Dietary Regimen		
	AL	RAL	R
All tumor-bearing animals	100	62.8	10.0
Benign tumors	100	50.9	6.0
Malignant tumors	100	84.1	6.5
Tissue of origin			
Epithelial tissues	100	52.4	6.0
Lymphoreticular and hematopoietic tissues	100	86.1	3.4
Soft tissues	100	84.7	15.3
Connective tissues	100	19.6	18.3

Abbreviations: AL, ad libitum; RAL, 7-week restriction, and then switched to ad libitum feeding thereafter; R, restrictive.
Source: Ross and Bras (1971).

connective tissues in rats on R regimen. The study of Ross and Bras (1971) has shown many interesting features of the effects of caloric restriction on tumor incidence. (The experiment used equal numbers of animals, in the groups fed ad libitum and lifetime restricted diets. However, 40% fewer animals were in the group fed restricted diet for 7 weeks post-weaning. The results were mathematically adjusted in order to make all values comparable.) Fewer animals developed tumors in the group on lifetime caloric restriction than in the group on ad libitum feeding. Furthermore, with calorie restriction, the development of tumors was markedly delayed. Thus, only six cases were noted in the calorie-restricted group in the 700-day period, in contrast to 30 in the ad libitum group. In the ad libitum feeding regimen, there was a rapid increase in tumor incidence after 500 days, whereas in the restricted group, tumors developed slowly and gradually. Even though more animals lived longer in the restricted group, the combined tumor incidence was still lower than in the ad libitum animals. More animals on the RAL diet developed tumors than the R group, but their combined totals were still less than the AL group.

The rate of tumor development in the RAL group was similar to that of the AL group. However, the appearance of tumors in the former seemed to be delayed by 70 to 100 days. Thus, it seems that processes leading to tumor development may be present early in the life of these animals, and that caloric restriction during this period has a significant effect on these processes.

One other interesting observation in this study was the effects of body weight. Within each dietary group, the percentage of animals developing tumors was greater in heavier rats. For this purpose, animals weighing less than the average weight of the dietary group were considered in the lightweight group, and those equal to, or above the average was considered in the heavy group.

The results indicate that benign tumor incidence in the all-tumor group of the heavier rats in the RAL regimen are slightly greater than in the AL group. However, this trend is reversed when a number of factors are taken into account, such as the age when a specified mature body weight is attained and when the tumors appears, and the rates of attrition among the subpopulation.

In the RAL and AL dietary groups, it has been shown that the tumor incidence increases with increasing body weight; tumor incidence does not appear to have a significant correlation with age, especially in the AL group.

Analysis of the data, however, suggests that for the RAL group, when the incidence for each tumor type is considered, the reduction in risk for RAL rats is largely attributable to the long-term effects of the dietary restriction early in life.

All in all, the authors conclude that (1) the initiating factors which determine tumor formation later in life are already present early in the development of the animals, and the age and rate of appearance of tumors in a specific organ depends on the diet-dependent rate of development of the animals; (2) the sequential carcinogenic changes occurring under conditions conducive to rapid growth are inhibited or arrested by dietary restrictions; (3) the growth of both normal and preneoplastic cell variants may be partially inhibited by food restriction during the hyperplastic phase of oncogenesis of an organ.

A number of concepts have been proposed to explain the effect of caloric restriction on tumor development. Among these is the inhibition of mitotic activity resulting from a deficiency of glucose and its metabolites needed for energy production (Kraybill 1963; Tannenbaum 1959). In the rat, undernutrition early in life alters the total cell population of an organ even with subsequent adequate feeding (Winick and Noble 1966); the reverse is observed with overnutrition (Winick and Noble 1967). It seems that the maximum cell number for all organs in these rats, except the spleen and thymus, is attained after age 65 days (Winick and Noble 1966). There appears to be a direct and exponential correlation between the instantaneous increase of parenchymal cells of the liver during the early postweaning period and the relative risk of tumor development with aging (Ross and Bras 1965).

Caloric restriction can also alter the hormonal status of the host. For example, reduction in the estrogen level as a result of caloric restriction may reduce the formation of mammary cancer in mice (Huseby et al. 1945; Loeb 1940; Tannenbaum 1959). Reduction in the incidence of tumors of the endocrine organs as a result of early dietary restriction also has been reported (Huseby et al. 1945; Loeb 1940).

Caloric restriction may also produce immunological changes which may have a beneficial effect on carcinogenesis (Good and Finstad 1968).

Whether there is a critical caloric intake influencing carcinogenic development is not known; it is likely that this can be defined only by considering other factors, such as the tumor site, characteristics of the carcinogen, the age of duration of exposure, other components of the diet, and genetic predisposition.

EFFECTS OF DIETARY EXCESSES OR DEFICIENCY OF PROTEINS

There are epidemiological data showing a significant correlation between meat consumption and intestinal cancer incidence and mortality. Berg et al. (1973) demonstrated with national statistical data that the rapid rise in intestinal cancer mortality in 23 countries can be associated with the rapid increase in intake of animal protein over a period of 8 to 12 years. Figure 7.1 shows a positive correlation between daily per capita meat consumption and the annual intestinal cancer incidence in women in 23 countries (Cairns 1975). No doubt other factors influence intestinal cancer incidence in these countries. Whether one can definitely separate meat consumption from other factors, such as fat and cereal consumption in a correlation of this sort, cannot easily be ascertained. However, other epidemiological studies also show a positive correlation between increased beef consumption and increased intestinal cancer incidence. For example, studies by Haenszel et al. (1973) on Japanese migrants in Hawaii, and studies reported by Howell (1975) on international and United States food-consumption patterns, tend to support the correlation between higher animal protein consumption in Hawaii and the increased intestinal cancer incidence.

Animal experiments designed to study the effect of high or low protein diets on tumor development show variable results depending on the type of tumor. Several examples can be cited. In a study by Ross and Bras (1965) with rats, the incidence of spontaneous malignant lymphoma correlated with high protein intake. However, the incidence of fibromas and fibrosarcomas were highest in the group with low intakes of protein, carbohydrates, and total calories. In a later study by the same authors (Ross and Bras 1971), restriction of these nutrients resulted in the lowest spontaneous tumor incidence, the longest latency of tumors, absence of malignant epithelial tumors, and of course, highest life expectancy.

When food intake was restricted, spontaneous tumor incidence has been directly related to the protein level in the diet (Ross et al. 1970), and the greatest depression in tumor incidence has been shown to occur when both protein and calories are restricted.

Dimethylnitrosamine-induced liver cancer is suppressed in rats on protein deficient diets, but the same diet enhances the formation of kidney cancer which appears later in life (McLean and Magee 1970). The decreased hepatocarcinogenicity of nitrosamines in the rat correlates with the decrease in N-demethylase activity; this enzyme is essential for the metabolic activation of nitrosamines (Swann and McLean 1971). However, the fact that the activity of the carcinogen is enhanced in the kidney suggests a probably different metabolic regulation in this organ.

The carcinogenicity of tannic acid is doubled in rats fed a diet containing 3% casein and 20% fat compared to one with 25% casein and 5% fat (Korpassy 1959). The carcinogenicity of safrole is enhanced by a high protein diet (Warwick 1971). In contrast, the carcinogenicity of 2-acetylaminofluorene appears to be depressed with high casein diets, and enhanced by a low protein diet (Engel and Copeland 1952). Protein intake also influences the rate of metastasis of injected Walker carcinosarcoma 256 cells. With

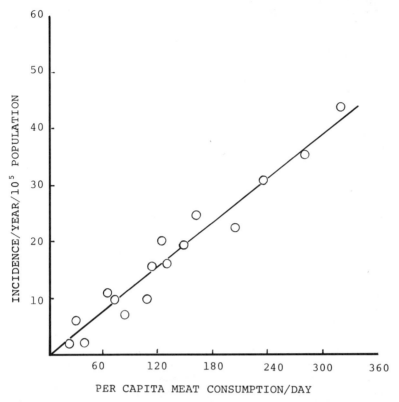

Fig. 7.1 Correlation between per capita meat consumption per day and the annual incidence of the cancer of the large intestines in women in various countries. Each point represents a country. The highest point is that of New Zealand, followed by the United States (upper right hand corner). The lowest point is that of Nigeria (lower left hand corner). Most developed countries are found in between. (From Cairns 1975, used with permission.)

higher protein intakes, more animals show hepatic metastasis and at the same time, larger tumors. Protein intake influences the level of hepatic proteins which in turn affect the growth of metastatic tumors rather than the "take" of the tumor cells (Fisher and Fisher 1961).

As shown by the effect on N-demethylase activity, the level of proteins in the diet certainly affects the activity of many liver enzymes (Rumack et al. 1973), and possibly, other organs. Indeed, with protein deficient diets, aryl hydrocarbon hydroxylase activity, which is essential for the activation of benzo(a)pyrene and similar hydrocarbons, is reduced in the liver, kidneys, and lungs in rats (Paine and McLean 1973).

EFFECTS OF AMINO ACIDS

The effect of the protein level in the diet certainly reflects the influence of individual amino acids, particularly the essential ones. For example, nulliparous C3H mice fed a lysine-deficient diet 1 month after birth, for 27 months, showed a marked inhibition of spontaneous mammary tumor development; these animals produced a 25% tumor incidence compared to the 97.6% in the controls (Morris 1945). Cystine deficiency in the diet for 21 months has been shown to be more effective in inhibiting spontaneous mammary tumor formation — resulting in zero incidence compared to 97.4% of the control. There was either atrophy or a marked decrease in mammary gland development and an occasional estrus with lysine deficiency, and an apparent complete absence of estrus with cystine deficiency. Expectedly, both diets inhibit growth; only a 20% increase in body weight was seen with lysine deficient diets, and zero growth with diets deficient in cystine.

The administration of diethylstilbestrol stimulates mammary gland development and the occurrence of estrus in rats with cystine-deficient diets. It also increases tumor incidence, but only approximately half that of the controls. Apparently, mammary tumor formation is contingent upon full development of the mammary gland following hormonal stimulation. However, the development of mammary tumors, like every other tissue, is highly dependent on cystine.

Hui et al. (1971) determined the transformation (Table 7.3) of transplanted hyperplastic alveolar nodules to typical adenocarcinomas for different levels of phenylalanine in the diet. They found that the extent of tumor transformation from transplanted hyperplastic alveolar nodules in Crgl female mice appeared to decrease, in some complex relationship, with the decrease in phenylalanine in the diet. With this diet, growth rate diminished with the decrease in phenylalanine level. At the 0.09 and 0.12% phenylalanine levels, the tumor incidence was roughly 42 and 51% of controls, respectively. The mammary glands of the mice on the phenylalanine diet were immature and poorly developed, and at the same time, there was atrophy of the ovaries and fewer corpora lutea and interstitial tissues. The observed results with the pair-weight control indicates that about a third of the inhibition of tumor formation is due to a depression of food intake. A possible explanation of the results, as suggested by these researchers, is that the deficiency in phenylalanine affects the development of the ovary, so that a deficiency in key ovarian hormones is produced; in turn, the hormonal deficiencies lead to an inhibition of mammary gland development, and consequently, tumorigenesis in that gland.

Other tumor forms in experimental animals are also inhibited by phenylalanine-deficient diets. Similar results have also been observed with tyrosine-restricted diets.

Table 7.3 Effect of Different Levels of Phenylalanine on the Extent of Malignant Transformations of Transplanted Hyperplastic Alveolar Nodules

% Phenylalanine in Lofnalec	No. tumors/ no. transplants/100	TE_{50} (days)	Mean latent period (days)
0.090	42.4	300	149
0.120	51.4	280	152
0.135	62.5	264	188
0.150	71.1	160	130
0.300	89.7	112	129
SD	90.00	132	131
PWC	75.00	170	142

Abbreviations: TE_{50}, number of days required for 50% of transplants to develop tumors; SD, stock diet; PWC, pair-weight control.
Source: Hui et al. (1971).

For example, S91 melanoma (malignant brown pigmented skin tumor) in mice has been shown to be inhibited by limitation of these two amino acids (Demopoulos 1966). BW7756 hepatoma in mice and three types of adenocarcinoma were inhibited when phenylalanine in the diet has been shown to be restricted to 0.17% (Lorincz et al. 1969, 1968). In contrast, Ryan and Elliott (1968) have reported that fluorphenylalanine has little effect on this hepatoma, or on C3HBA mammary adenocarcinoma in certain strains of mice on a phenylalanine deficient diet.

Theuer (1971) systematically studied the effect of the restriction of each essential amino acid on the growth of implanted BW10232 adenocarcinomas in female C57BL/J6 mice. He found that restriction of isoleucine, phenylalanine, and valine inhibits tumor growth without causing weight loss in the mice. Restriction of leucine, methionine, threonine, and tryptophan significantly inhibits tumor growth as well as loss in body weight.

Increased amounts of certain amino acids in the diet, such as tryptophan, may actually enhance tumor formation. Thus, increased amounts of this amino acid and other indoles markedly enhance bladder tumor formation induced by 2-acetylaminofluorene (Dunning et al. 1950). On the other hand, when a diet contains a very large amount of a particular amino acid, an imbalance may be produced that has a significant harmful effect on the metabolic processes of tumors. A preliminary report suggested that large quantities of phenylalanine and tyrosine in the diet of leukemic children may provide a partial remission of symptoms (Allan et al. 1965).

Certain types of tumors may have a greater need for particular amino acids than normal tissues. For example, asparagine appears to be required by neoplasms in several animals: mice, rats, dogs, and man (Cooney and Handschumacher 1970). Therefore, the enzyme asparaginase, which deaminates asparagine to aspartic acid, inhibits certain tumor growth in these species, especially lymphocytic anemia in man. Unfortunately, the leukemic cells probably develop the capability to cope with the lack of asparagine, since the remission of symptoms of leukemia cannot be sustained (Capizzi et al. 1970; Cooney and Handschumacher 1970).

Effect of Protein and Amino Acid Deficiency on the Immune System

There is ample evidence from animal experiments to suggest that the effect of protein and amino acid deficiency on tumor inhibition can involve the immune system (Jose and Good 1973). The role of the immune system in carcinogenesis is discussed in Chapter 6. The role of amino acids in modifying the immune response to tumor growth should be mentioned. Jose and Good (1973) have shown that deficiency of phenylalanine, tyrosine, valine, threonine, methionine, cystine, isoleucine, or tryptophan separately increases the immune resistance of mice to tumor growth. Deficiency of each of these amino acids depresses or removes blocking antibody (B cell) response without affecting the lymphocytes (T cells); the latter are cytotoxic toward tumor cells. As will be shown in the next section, the B cells protect tumor cells from the "killing" action of T cells. The deficiency of the basic amino acids, lysine, arginine, and histidine, has little effect on inhibiting tumor growth or in depressing blocking antibodies. Leucine deficiency depresses the cytotoxic lymphocytes with little effect on the serum-blocking antibody secretion. Thus, deficiency of this amino acid has been shown to enhance the growth rate of certain malignant tumors (Jose 1973).

EFFECTS OF DIETARY LIPIDS

Epidemiological studies show a direct correlation between fat intake and mortality from breast cancer (in several countries) (Carroll et al. 1968; Lea 1966). Other studies note an association between Western diets which are generally high in fat and colon cancer (Howell 1975; Wynder et al. 1969).

Polyunsaturated Fatty Acids

There are conflicting studies regarding the carcinogenic effects of excessive consumption of unsaturated fatty acids. Pearce and Dayton (1971) report a higher incidence of fatality from cancer in Los Angeles men consuming diets calculated to contain four times as much polyunsaturated fatty acids and half as much cholesterol than those eating normal diets. Other clinical studies in different locations (Faribault, Minnesota; Helsinki, Finland; London, England) have failed to verify these results. Observations made in Oslo, however, supported Pearce and Dayton's results (Ederer et al. 1971). The statistical analysis of the data, both including and excluding the results of the Los Angeles findings, does not support the theory that diets high in polyunsaturated fatty acids increase cancer risk. However, the validity of the statistical analysis should not be held at its face value, considering the number of factors affecting carcinogenesis. Suffice it to say that the possibility exists, that under certain conditions, diets high in polyunsaturated fatty acids (PUFA) may enhance carcinogenesis. This hypothesis has been supported by further experiments. For example, Rose et al. (1974) reported that high PUFA intake may cause more bile salts to be secreted, and that intestinal bacteria may degrade these compounds to carcinogens. Therefore, the risk of cancer of the colon may be increased. Furthermore, heating oils high in PUFA may produce potentially carcinogenic substances such as polycyclic aromatic hydrocarbons (Michael et al. 1966). Not only carcinogens, but also cocarcinogens can be produced by heating such oils; this has been demonstrated by Sugai et al. (1962), who found that heated vegetable oils may function as cocarcinogen to 2-acetylaminofluorene.

Several other examples may be cited: 4-Dimethylaminoazobenzene is more hepatocarcinogenic in rats fed diets with corn oil than hydrogenated coconut oil (Miller et al. 1944); the fatty acids derived from coconut oil and corn oil show results similar to results with the intact oils (Kline et al. 1946). Miller and Miller (1953) gave evidence that hydrogenated coconut oil enables the rat to maintain higher levels of riboflavin in the liver than corn oil. Riboflavin, as will be shown later, has a protective effect on liver carcinogenesis with this dye (see next section). A diet high in corn oil enhances the development of mammary cancer in intact female rats treated with 7,12-dimethylbenzo(a)anthracene (DMBA) (Gammal et al. 1968, 1967) compared to diets high in coconut oil or low in fat. Highly unsaturated oils, compared to saturated fats, promote tumor induction with DMBA (Hopkins et al. 1976). These investigators have found that unsaturated oils, fed to female rats at 18.6% of the diet will affect tumor induction only when the fat diet is consumed after DMBA treatment. Even at lower levels of fat intake, colon tumors develop more readily in rats fed corn oil instead of lard; at higher levels, no difference in the carcinogenic response can be observed (Weisburger 1975).

The amount, source, and saturation level of fat appears to make a difference. Adding soybean oil or chicken fat to the diet of experimental animals produces the highest cancer incidence; whereas cottonseed oil and butter produce the lowest (Kaunitz and Johnson 1973). Cottonseed and soybean oils may differ in composition. In C3H female rats, increasing the degree of unsaturation of fats and/or the fat intake with isocaloric diets results in increased tumor incidence (Wynder et al. 1969). Mice fed higher levels of corn and safflower oil reportedly die earlier from gross mammary tumors than those consuming lower amounts of these oils (Harman 1971).

High Fat Diets

High fat diets per se may enhance carcinogenesis in experimental animals. The work of Tannenbaum (1942b, 1944), Silverstone and Tannenbaum (1951a,b) and Tannenbaum and Silverstone (1950) clearly have shown that with isocaloric diets, increased levels of fat from less than 5 to more than 20% gave greater skin tumor yields in three strains of mice treated with benzo(a)pyrene. Similarly, the incidence of spontaneous hepatomas in one strain increased. With respect to spontaneous mammary tumors, high fat diets either increased the tumor yield or reduced the latency of the tumor. In like manner, Boutwell et al. (1949a) confirmed the observations of Tannenbaum (1942b) that increased dietary fat can enhance skin carcinogenesis. However, a further increase to as much as 6% did not produce a proportional tumor yield. It also has been observed that increasing the level of dietary fat fourfold enhances the induction of colon cancer in the rat (Rogers and Newberne 1975; Weisburger 1973, 1975).

It has been demonstrated that the incidence of other types of tumors is not affected by increased levels of dietary fat; for example, induced sarcoma, spontaneous and induced leukemia, primary lung adenoma in mice (Tannenbaum 1959) and fibroadenomas and adenomas in general (Carroll and Khor 1971).

Restriction of fat intake can decrease mammary tumor induction with 7,12-dimethylbenz(a)anthracene (Carroll and Khor 1970; Chan and Cohen 1974; Dao 1971).

Thus, even though there are conflicting epidemiological data on the effect of dietary fat levels and the type of fat in the diet, the experimental results in animals warrant careful evaluation of fat intake in relation to carcinogenesis. It should be pointed out that many carcinogens are fat soluble, and therefore, as suggested by Tannenbaum and Silverstone (1957), a high fat intake will facilitate absorption of carcinogens from the intestines and transport to tissues and also modify lipid distribution. The latter situation may alter the availability of the carcinogen in the tissues. It is also possible that the fat-soluble carcinogens, i.e., polycyclic aromatic hydrocarbons, such as benzo(a)pyrene, may be persistent contaminants of fats and oils (Jung and Morand 1962). If so, the presence of these contaminants may enhance markedly the carcinogenic process.

EFFECTS OF VITAMINS

In addition to their role as coenzymes in many metabolic reactions, vitamins are also involved in other cellular processes, some mechanisms of which are still unknown. Among these is carcinogenesis. In addition to the regular metabolic reactions involved in the biosynthesis of tissue components (energy production, utilization, and storage) vitamins may also influence cellular differentiation, hormonal metabolism and regulation, immunological control, and metabolic activation or inactivation of carcinogens. All of these processes have a strong influence on the tumorigenic process. Thus, a deficiency or excess of a vitamin may enhance or diminish the tumorigenic process. These effects are evident in the discussion that follows.

Effects of Retinol and Derivatives

Bjelke (1975) has reported from Norway that a survey among more than 8000 Norwegian men showed an inverse relationship between intake of retinol or its derivatives and lung cancer incidence. When this 5-year lung cancer incidence was compared among various groups, this study indicated a significant and protective effect of this vitamin even among those who smoked heavily. This report is encouraging, since it is consistent with the results of many studies in animals showing a similar significant effect of this vitamin in decreasing tumor incidence.

The above observation of Bjelke (1975) regarding retinol has been supported by several other epidemiological studies, which include cancer of other sites. Thus, Hirayama (1979) reported a statistically significant correlation between per capita vitamin A intake among Japanese women and the age-adjusted uterine cancer mortality. The magnitude of the correlation coefficient ($r = 0.855$) indicates a rather close association. Retrospective data obtained with 569 bladder cancer patients and 1025 controls showed a high bladder cancer risk among those with low intakes of vitamin A (relative risk = 3.1) and carrots (relative risk = 3.0) (Mettlin and Graham 1979; Mettlin et al. 1979a). Compounding variables such as cigarette smoking, coffee drinking, and high cancer risk occupations had no influence on the results. Other epidemiological studies

also support the finding that low vitamin A or provitamin A intakes significantly increase the risk for cancer, especially lung cancer (Mettlin et al. 1979b; Smith and Jick
1978).

A prospective study reported by Wald et al. (1980) has shown that low serum
retinol has a predictive value with respect to the future development of cancer, especially cancer of the lung and gastrointestinal tract. The study involving 16,000 men,
age 35 to 64 years, demonstrates that there is a significant correlation (p <0.025) between the level of serum retinol determined 1 to 4 years earilier and risk of developing
cancer. A statistically significant correlation (p <0.025) has been observed between decreasing levels of serum retinol concentration and an increasing risk for cancer. Thus,
those with the lowest level (20 I.U./dl) are 2.2 times more likely to develop cancer
than those at the highest level (267 to 346 I.U./dl).

Less direct but with more practical implication is the report of Hirayama (1979) on
the protective effects against several forms of cancer of the daily consumption of
green-yellow vegetables (GYVs). Based on a 10-year prospective study of 265,118
Japanese adults, daily consumption of GYVs resulted in a significant decrease in cancer of the lungs, prostate, and to some extent colon and stomach. In terms of lung
cancer, the effect was particularly dramatic when smokers were compared with nonsmokers, ex-smokers, and those who smoke later in life. These comparisons are shown
in Table 7.4. However, daily GYV consumption seems to offer no protection among
those who started to smoke as teen-agers.

The significant decrease in mortality among daily GYV consumers who also quit
smoking suggests an important role of GYVs on the repair mechanisms in the pulmonary
or bronchial epithelia. Thus, because GYVs contain high levels of provitamin A (in
this study, providing a daily intake of 640 I.U. as vitamin A), it can be assumed that
the principal component responsible for the protective effect is vitamin A in the form
of its provitamin, the carotenes. Of course, other factors may be involved such as
ascorbic acid. However, based on the accumulated epidemiological and experimental
evidence, vitamin A is definitely involved in the results reported by Hirayama (1979).

Table 7.4 Standard Mortality Rates per 100,000 Population for Lung Cancer Showing the Effects of Smoking, Cessation of Smoking, and the Daily Consumption of
Green-Yellow Vegetables (GYV)

| Subject | Standard mortality rate | |
	Daily GYV consumer	Occasional or nonconsumers of GYV
Smokers starting at age		
15-19	90.4	91.7
20-29	70.6	80.6
30 or over	17.5	80.6
Current smokers[a] (all subjects)	66.3	79.5
Ex-smokers for 4 years[b]	36.2	96.9
Ex-smokers for 5 years[b]	18.2	65.4
Nonsmokers	14.5	32.4

[a]Smokers at the end of survey.
[b]Represents years prior to end of survey when cessation of smoking occurred.
Source: Hirayama (1979).

Retinol controls the state of cellular differentiation in many epithelial tissues by an obscure mechanism (DeLuca et al. 1972; Wolbach and Howe 1925). When there is a retinol deficiency, as observed in the rat or guinea pig, normally nonkeratinizing epithelia such as the paraocular glands, salivary glands, larynx, trachea, bronchi, urogenital tract (Mori 1922; Wolbach and Howe 1925), and the intestinal mucosa (DeLuca et al. 1970) became keratinized. The antikeratinizing effects of retinol have been confirmed by in vitro studies (Kahn 1954; Lasnitzki 1961).

Since many forms of neoplasms arise from epithelial tissues, particularly those that are directly exposed to the environment (Cairns 1975), many studies have been conducted to assess the impact of a deficiency, adequacy, or excess of vitamin A on the carcinogenic process in epithelial tissues. Thus, the induction of tracheobronchial squamous metaplasia and squamous cell tumors have been shown to be inhibited by vitamin A (Saffioti et al. 1967). In mice, retinoic acid (200 mg/kg) also has been shown to retard the appearance of papillomas (Bollag 1972) induced by topical application of dimethylbenzanthracene and promoted by croton oil. The vitamin also reduces the number of papillomas in these animals, and retards tumor growth. Some papillomas also regressed. The vitamin in this case was applied during the promotion phase of carcinogenesis.

The induction of tumors of the forestomach and cervix of Syrian hamsters following benzo(a)pyrene administration also has been inhibited by vitamin A in the form of retinyl palmitate (Chu and Malmgren 1965). Cone and Nettesheim (1973) noted that intragastric administration of retinyl acetate prior to intratracheal injection of 3-methylcholanthrene and then maintained thereafter, twice a week, at 20 times the maintenance requirement of rats, significantly reduces the development of squamous metaplasias and squamous cell tumors. However, these researchers pointed out that very high doses of a carcinogen may minimize the actual protective potential of retinol. In other words, the protective effect of the vitamin in reducing tumor development may be more apparent at lower doses of the carcinogen.

A similar work by Smith et al. (1975) on benzo(a)pyrene carcinogenesis in hamsters instilled intratracheally with Fe_2O_3, did not show any significant suppression of respiratory tract tumors with vitamin A. This result was observed in spite of high doses of retinyl acetate (1600 to 2400 µg). However, these doses of the vitamin were shown to significantly reduce the total incidence of papillomas of the forestomach, compared to a much lower dose of 100 µg. As stated by the authors, the lack of significant inhibition of the respiratory tract tumors may have resulted from the high dose of the carcinogen (12 doses of 3 mg/week), which might have overcome the protective effect of the vitamin. In addition, Fe_2O_3 used as a vehicle for benzo(a)pyrene instillation may be a carcinogen, if not a cocarcinogen, in its own right. The latter may initiate a different carcinogenic mechanism for benzo(a)pyrene.

Hypervitaminosis A also has been demonstrated to inhibit Shope rabbit papillomas (McMichael 1965) and papillomas induced by 7,12-dimethylbenzo(a)anthracene on rhinomouse skin (Davies 1967).

Retinol or its derivatives are lysosome membrane labilizers (Weissman 1964); thus, the lysosomal enzyme activity of tissues may be enhanced by retinol treatment (Lucey and Dingle 1964). The lysosomes contain proteases, nucleases, and other enzymes which may cause lysis of tumor cells. Shamberger (1969), for example, reported that increased lysosomal enzyme activity is associated with regression of mammary tumors. In a subsequent study, Shamberger (1971) observed that retinyl acetate labilizes the lysosomes of mouse skin, as shown by the increased acid phosphatase and arylsulfatase activities. Another lysosome labilizer is the polyene antibiotic, filipin (Weissman et al. 1967). In one experiment, both retinyl acetate and filipin treatment have been shown to result in fewer animals with tumors; 46 to 26%, respectively, compared to 86.6% of the control. In both cases, low levels (0.015%) of retinyl acetate and filipin were applied 3 weeks after a 0.125-mg dose of 7,12-dimethylbenzo(a)anthracene (DMBA) for 16 or 18 weeks. In contrast, 90% of animals treated with lysosomal stabilizers, chloroquine, and hydrocortisone (Weissman 1964) developed tumors. In all cases, tumors were induced by application of DMBA concomitant with croton oil as the promoter.

Quite surprisingly, β-carotene, a retinol precursor, has been observed to produce more tumor-bearing animals than retinol. With corton resin as a promoter, 94% of DMBA-treated mice were shown to develop tumors in the presence of β-carotene as compared to 90 and 60% in the control and retinyl groups, respectively. The action of β-carotene in promoting tumorigenesis may be related to its property as a terpene. Terpenes are believed to be the tumor-promoting components of several essential oils (Roe and Field 1967). Phorbol esters, the active tumor-promoting component in croton oil, are diterpenes (Hecker et al. 1965).

A report by Prutkin (1975) confirms the tumor-inhibiting effect of retinyl palmitate on DMBA-treated rabbit ear. The inhibitory effect appears to be enhanced when fluorouracil is used with the vitamin. In this experiment, a low dose (0.1%) of retinyl palmitate was applied.

Retinol may also function as an immune adjuvant (Cohen and Cohen 1973; Dresser 1968; Spitznagel and Allison 1970). This vitamin, for example, may stimulate the production of humoral antibodies toward an otherwise nonantigenic protein (Dresser 1968). It has also been shown that retinol increases the serum or cell-mediated immunity in mice (Cohen and Cohen 1973, Taub et al. 1970), increases the resistance of mice to bacterial and fungal infections (Cohen and Elin 1974), and reduces the severity of viral infections in animals (Bang et al. 1972). Thus, retinol-deficient chickens are more susceptible to Newcastle disease virus (Bang et al. 1973).

The immune mechanism may be involved in the control of tumorigenesis (see next section). Thus, the reported antitumor effect of retinol may also result from a stimulation of the immune response. For instance, Seifter et al. (1973) found that mice fed large amounts of retinyl palmitate (15,000 u/kg diet) have a decreased probability of developing tumors when challenged by a large dose of murine sarcoma virus. In this case, only 65% of mice fed a high level of retinyl palmitate developed tumors compared to 100% of the control. Retinol enhanced the antitumor effect of bacille Calmette-Guérin (BCG) vaccine on transplanted mouse tumors (Meltzer and Cohen 1974); the vitamin by itself has no effect on this tumor.

Felix et al. (1975) reported a dramatic inhibition by retinyl palmitate on the growth and development of a transplanted, highly immunogenic, murine melanoma. That the antitumor activity of retinol may somehow involve the immune mechanism is indicated by the abrogation of this activity by mouse antilymphocyte serum (ALS). This antiserum itself will enhance tumor growth. These results are strikingly significant in view of the failure of previous attempts to prevent transplanted tumor growth with retinol pretreatment (Bollag 1971c).

Some investigators have been shown to obtain only partial success. For example, Rettura et al. (1975) found that in their system, retinyl palmitate does not affect tumor incidence in mice innoculated with 1×10^3 C3HBA tumor cells. However, the vitamin retards tumor growth for the first 19 days, after which, growth rate of the tumor is independent of retinyl palmitate treatment. The less successful results of Rettura et al. (1975), in contrast to those of Felix et al. (1975), may be ascribed to a possible lower vitamin consumption in the former system; i.e., 750 u, compared with 3100 u in the latter.

The antitumor activity of retinol may also result from its ability to counteract the possible effect of stress on tumorigenesis. The role of stress on the body's resistance to carcinogenesis has not been systematically evaluated. Some possible indication of the effect of stress on carcinogenesis has been shown by the higher cancer mortality or incidence among the divorced and widowed compared to married persons (Lilienfeld 1956). Riley (1975) demonstrated an increase in tumor incidence in mice innoculated with mammary tumor virus and chronically exposed to environmental stresses. Similarly, physical stress make mice more susceptible to oncogenic viruses and increase the severity and incidence of tumor development (Seifter et al. 1973).

Physical stress may cause involution of the thymus (Selye 1936). A similar change can be observed after treatment with glucocorticoids (Antopol 1950). Glucocorticoids can suppress immune competence, and this suppression can be reversed by thymic extracts (Zisblatt and Lilly 1972). These observations suggest that interference by glucocorticoids in the immune functions may result from its effects on the thymus. Indeed, earlier studies have shown that there is a relationship between stress, thymic function, and adrenocorticoid secretion, and that an elevation of plasma corticoids produces an involution of the thymus (Dougherty and White 1945; Santisteban and Dougherty 1954). Thus, another possible mechanism by which retinol can suppress tumorigenesis is its protective effect against thymus involution caused by stress and corticoids (Seifter et al. 1973; Zisblatt et al. 1973). Stress may increase production of adrenocorticoids (Selye 1936). Thus, 30% of retinol-treated mice subjected to the stress of casts on their bodies developed tumors after treatment with a low dose of murine sarcoma virus; in contrast, 90% of the controls developed tumors. At high virus dose, the corresponding values were 65 and 100%, respectively (Seifter et al. 1973). However, under severe stress, caused by burning, retinol appears to have no influence. Negative results also have been observed in the case of the glucocorticoid-augmented tumorigenesis. The amount of vitamin that was given in this case (150 u/ml or 510 u total, assuming a water and feed consumption of 5 ml and 5 g, respectively) might have been insufficient to overcome the effect of very severe stress or of high doses of the glucocorticoids.

Because retinol has an ameliorative or inhibitive effect on tumorigenesis, it follows that a deficiency of this vitamin will stimulate tumor initiation, or enhance growth. For example, retinol deficiency has been shown to promote the growth of rat odontomas (Orten et al. 1937) and salivary tumors (Rowe et al. 1970). Retinol deficiency also has been noted to result in the development of precancerous lesions of the stomach mucosa in experimental animals (Kraybill 1963). The hepatocarcinogenic aflatoxin B_1 can initiate colon cancer only in the presence of a retinol deficiency (Newberne and Rogers 1973, Rogers and Newberne 1975). Similarly, in retinol deficiency, an increased incidence and early appearance of respiratory tract tumors induced by 3-methylcholanthrene has been observed in experimental animals (Genta et al. 1974). A possible mechanism by which retinol deficiency enhances tumorigenesis is suggested by the increased binding of benzo(a)pyrene to tracheal epithelial DNA in retinol-deficient animals (Genta et al. 1974). This increased binding may result from the increased activity of aryl hydrocarbon hydroxylase (AHH) in the presence of retinol deficiency. This enzyme is involved in the oxidative hydroxylation of polycyclic aromatic hydrocarbons (Chap. 6). That AHH activity may be responsible for the increased binding of benzo-(a)pyrene to DNA is suggested from the results showing a reduction in the DNA binding in the presence of 7,8-benzoflavone, an AAH inhibitor (Diamond and Gelboin 1969). Deoxyribonucleic acid (DNA) binding of a carcinogen has been postulated to be an essential step in the carcinogenic process (Brookes 1966; Sporn and Dingman 1966).

The epidemiological findings discussed previously showing increased cancer risk when intakes of vitamin A are low are highly consistent with the aforementioned results.

Therapeutic Effects of Retinol

The observed tumor-inhibiting property of retinol and its derivatives immediately suggests a potential chemotherapeutic agent against neoplastic growth. Thus, Bollag (1971a,b) reported that retinyl palmitate and retinoic acid are effective chemotherapeutic agents against chemically induced and transplanted tumors. In one experiment, oral or intraperitoneal administration of retinoic acid has been shown to cause immediate shrinkage of tumors induced by 7,12-dimethylbenzo(a)anthracene and promoted by croton oil (Bollag 1971a). Bollag and Ott (1971) also reported the significant therapeutic value of retinoic acid applied locally on actinic keratoses and basal cell carcinomas. The observations are remarkable, since retinoic acid is found effective in those cancers in which other powerful cancer chemotherapeutic agents have been shown to have almost no effect; i.e., cyclophosphamide, fluorouracil, and procarbazine (Bollag 1971a). Retinol also enhances the effect of certain antileukemogenic alkylating agents, such as 1,3-bis(2-chloroethyl)-1-nitrosourea (BCNU) (Cohen and Carbone 1972). As tested in mice, timing in the administration of retinol appears to be essential for its effectiveness.

It also has been observed in this work (Cohen and Carbone 1972) that retinol enhances an irreversible and lethal membrane alteration of leukemic cells by BCNU. This combined effect of retinol and BCNU on leukemic cells is enhanced by caffeine (Cohen 1972) by an as yet unknown mechanism.

Promoting or Negative Effects of Retinol on Tumorigenesis

A few reports have shown that under certain conditions, retinol promotes carcino-genesis. Thus, Levij and Polliack (1968) and Polliack and Levij (1969) observed an enhancing effect of retinol on carcinogenesis induced by 9,10-dimethyl-1,2-benzanthra-cene on hamster cheek pouch. Smith et al. (1972) also noted a similar potentiation of pulmonary epithelia tumors in mice. Prutkin (1968) observed a marked increase in the yield of tumor in rabbit skin treated simultaneously with the carcinogen and high doses of retinoic acid. Finally, Rogers et al. (1973) noted that a deficiency or excess of retinol had no effect on cancer induced by 1,2-dimethylhydrazine.

In view of the many factors affecting carcinogenesis, it is not surprising that negative effects of retinol on tumorigenesis can occur. In many cases, the negative effects may be a matter of the dosage of both retinol and the carcinogen. The form of the vitamin, i.e., ester derivatives, alcohol, and acid, may have an important influence on its effectiveness. For example, Dingle and Lucy (1962) found that several derivatives of retinol hemolyze red blood cells in the following decending order: retinol > retinoic acid > retinyl acetate. Cohen and Carbone (1972) also found that retinol effectively enhances the antitumor effect of BCNU, whereas retinyl acetate has essentially no effect.

Effects of Riboflavin

Several studies have demonstrated three functions of riboflavin and their relation to tumorigenesis: (1) The essential coenzymes flavin adenine dinucleotide (FAD) and flavin mononucleotide (FMN) are required for many types of metabolic reactions in both normal and tumor cells, especially in energy metabolism. (2) These coenzymes are also required in the metabolic deactivation and, possibly, activation of carcinogens. (3) Maintenance of the integrity and repair of epithelial cells or tissues appears to be an essential function of riboflavin (Horwitt et al. 1949). Other functions of riboflavin are even less well understood, so that their significance with respect to tumorigenesis is not readily apparent.

The role of riboflavin as an essential coenzyme in metabolic reactions in tumor cells can be demonstrated by the effect of its deficiency in the development or induction of tumors. For example, the growth of spontaneous mammary cancers in mice, with respect to size and number, is markedly inhibited by riboflavin-deficient diets (Morris and Robertson 1943). There is a gradual decrease in the growth rate of the tumors, and this is most noticeable during later stages of the deficient diet. Normal growth rate of these tumors resumes upon riboflavin supplementation. Other studies (Morris 1947) have shown a similar reduction in tumor size in riboflavin deficiency. In addition, a direct relationship has been observed between dietary riboflavin concentration and the number of spontaneous mammary tumors formed. Similarly, transplanted lymphosarcoma cells in riboflavin-deficient mice are characterized by slow growth (Stoerk and Emerson 1949) which did not increase after riboflavin supplementation.

Diet-induced riboflavin deficiency occurs very slowly because of the relatively large volume of tissue stores and the slow turnover rates (Rivlin 1970). However, riboflavin antagonists can deplete riboflavin concentrations even more rapidly. Thus, 6,7-dichloro-9-(1'-D-sorbityl)-isoalloxazine depletes riboflavin and consequently causes a regression of a form of lymphosarcoma in experimental animals (Holly et al. 1950). Likewise, diethylriboflavin diminishes the growth rate of Walker carcinomas to two-thirds that of control tumor-bearing animals. In some cancer patients, the size and growth rate of tumors have been reduced after treatment with galactoflavin (Lane et al. 1964). Similar remission of tumors has been observed in some patients with Hodgkin's disease, lymphosarcoma, and polycythemia vera when dietary riboflavin deficiency is imposed by the riboflavin antagonist galactoflavin (Lane 1971).

Results of several studies suggest that tumors have a relatively greater need for riboflavin than normal tissues. Accordingly, the data presented by Morris and Robert-son (1943) has shown that the concentration of flavin in tumors decreases much more slowly than in normal liver or muscle tissues. Studies by Rivlin et al. (1973) with transplanted Novikoff hepatoma in rats have shown that the FAD levels in the tumor are not affected significantly by riboflavin deficiency, even though the levels of FMN and FAD in nontumor tissues are markedly reduced.

In the livers of tumor-bearing animals, the activity of FAD pyrophosphorylase, an enzyme required in the conversion of FMN to FAD, is elevated significantly. However, in terms of specific activity, the level of the enzyme in the hepatoma is higher. This suggests that there is a more active conversion of FMN to FAD in hepatomas than in normal liver tissues.

After riboflavin loading, patients with larynx cancer excrete less riboflavin in the urine and have a lower plasma concentration than those with benign diseases (Kits-manyuk 1967). In this case, the level of plasma riboflavin can be correlated with the stage of the malignancy. Thus, in these cancer patients, riboflavin concentration in the plasma has been shown to return to normal after successful treatment, but remains low when treatment is unsuccessful.

Although the protective role of riboflavin against hepatic chemical carcinogenesis has been demonstrated spectacularly by Yoshida and Kinosita in relation to the carcinogenicity of butter yellow or 4-dimethylaminoazobenzene (Haddow 1975), attempts to repeat their work in the United States have failed. Earlier, Miller and Miller (1953) demonstrated that the diets fed experimental animals in the United States had higher levels of riboflavin than the less nutritive polished rice-based diet given to the rats in Japan. Thus, riboflavin has been shown to protect the experimental rats in the United States from the carcinogenic effects of butter yellow. Several studies have confirmed the protective action of riboflavin on azo dye carcinogenesis (Bebawi et al. 1970; Griffin and Bauman 1946, 1948; Kensler 1947; Kensler et al. 1940; Lambooy 1970; Mulay and O'Gara 1968).

Riboflavin deficiency is extremely effective regarding the induction of hepatic tumors in rats. This has been demonstrated in animals made deficient by a riboflavin antagonist and administered a dose of azo dye too small to induce tumors under other experimental conditions (Mulay and O'Gara 1968). The essential requirement for the in-duction of tumors with an azo dye is the flavin concentration in the liver. In this case, the tumor incidence was observed to be inversely proportional to the flavin concentra-tion (Griffin and Bauman 1948).

It seems that carcinogenic azo dyes may lay their own groundwork for the induc-tion of tumors. This conclusion is based on the fact that treatment of animals with azo dyes decreases the concentration of flavin in the liver (Griffin and Bauman 1946, 1948; Kensler 1947; Kensler et al. 1940). This decrease is shown by the increased urinary excretion of riboflavin following treatment with azo dyes (Okuda and Haruna 1959). Thus, it has been reported that the carcinogenicity of several types of azo dyes may be correlated with their capacity to lower liver flavin concentration (Griffin and Bau-man 1946). The decrease in flavin concentration in the liver may be brought about possibly by the formation of azo dye riboflavin complexes, and by the increased water solubility of 4-dimethylaminoazobenzene (DAB) in the presence of riboflavin (Tung and Lin 1964). Possible complex formation is indicated by the quenching of riboflavin fluorescence in the presence of DAB.

The lowering of flavin concentration in the liver seems to be a specific property of the carcinogenic azo dyes. Accordingly, compounds which are structurally related to DAB, but do not lower the liver flavin concentration, are noncarcinogenic (Griffin and Bauman 1948).

The protective effect of riboflavin on azo dye carcinogenesis is dependent on two sets of enzyme systems which apparently require FAD or $FADH_2$ as coenzymes. One system, the demethylase system, requires both $NADPH + H^+$ and FAD, and possibly, also cytochrome P-450 as cofactors (Holtzman et al. 1968; Miller and Miller 1953, 1969); the other, the azoreductase system, probably requires $FADH_2$ (Conney et al. 1956). Based on the types of urinary metabolites recovered from animals fed 4-dimethylamino-azobenzene, the following deactivation scheme has been proposed (Conney et al. 1957; Kensler et al. 1940; Miller and Baumann 1945; Mueller and Miller 1953; Miller et al. 1945; Stevenson et al. 1942).

The activities of enzymes required in the deactivation of azo dyes also are reduced in riboflavin deficiency. In one case, it has been shown that FAD in riboflavin-deficient animals was reduced by one-third that of normal (Rivlin 1970). Williams et al. (1970) have confirmed previous observations of Conney et al. (1956) regarding the decreased azo dye reductase activity in the livers of riboflavin-deficient rats. In addition, these researchers also have found bacterial azo dye reductase activity in the cecal contents of the riboflavin-deficient rats to be decreased. This activity is normally six times that of the liver.

In addition to the increased urinary excretion of riboflavin after DAB treatment, one other possible mechanism which may account for the decreased FAD is the observed increased nucleotide pyrophosphatase activity in liver tumors induced by DAB. This enzyme catalyzes the degradation of FAD to FMN, and it is three times as active in the tumor as in the liver (Yang and Sung 1966).

The protective effect of riboflavin also has been seen in rats treated intragastrically with aflatoxin B_1 (7 mg/kg). In the absence of riboflavin, nine of 19 animals treated with aflatoxin B_1 developed hepatomas, whereas only five of 18 in the riboflavin-aflatoxin group developed the tumors (Lemonnier et al. 1975). Even though the number of animals used in this experiment was small, the proportion that developed tumors was significant enough to suggest an inhibition of the metabolic activation of aflatoxin (Patterson 1973). Riboflavin also might promote the transformation of aflatoxin B_1 to the less active forms, aflatoxin M_1 and P_1 (Bassir and Osiyemi 1967; Patterson 1971).

A similar experiment with aflatoxin and aflatoxin-CCl_4 and aflatoxin B_1-riboflavin combinations also have demonstrated the apparent protective effects of riboflavin against aflatoxin-induced hepatoma (Scotto et al. 1975). In this study, the tumor incidence with the CCl_4-aflatoxin combination was essentially the same as with aflatoxin alone.

It seems that the effect of riboflavin deficiency on hepatic enzyme activity is more general than previously realized, since under these conditions the metabolism of many other foreign compounds is also affected. For example, in addition to aflatoxin, the metabolism of 3,4-benzo(a)pyrene (Catz et al. 1970) and various drugs (Rivlin et al. 1968) is also reduced. In particular, the metabolism of drugs requiring the NADPH-cytochrome reductase system, which also requires FAD as coenzyme, is also reduced in riboflavin deficiency (Rivlin et al. 1968).

The function of riboflavin in maintaining integrity of the epithelial cells is clearly evident from the observed skin lesions in riboflavin deficiency, especially the mucous membranes (Wagner and Folkers 1964). Wynder and Klein (1965) noted the successive changes of the esophageal and stomach epithelia in riboflavin-deficient mice. Atrophy of these tissues, which progressed to hyperplasia and hyperkeratosis, was also observed. The riboflavin-deficient epithelia of the skin became more easily susceptible to the carcinogenic effects of 7,12-dimethylbenzanthracene (DMBA) promoted with croton oil. In this case, the tumors in riboflavin-deficient animals were more numerous, and appeared 2 weeks earlier than in the normal animals (Wynder and Chan 1970). It was also found that aryl hydrocarbon hydroxylase activity can be induced in deficient animals topically applied with DMBA following the feeding of diets with normal amounts of riboflavin.

Effects of Ascorbic Acid

Present studies regarding the role of ascorbic acid in carcinogenesis are confined mainly to its ability to prevent the in vivo nitrosation of secondary and tertiary amines and amides in the presence of nitrite. The nitrosamines produced by this reaction are usually carcinogenic (Chap. 12).

Ascorbic acid, being a reducing agent, competes for the nitrosating species, nitrous anhydride, N_2O_3, during the nitrosation reaction. At pH 3.5 to 5.0, ascorbic acid, as the monoanion, reacts rapidly with N_2O_3 to form dehydroascorbic acid and nitric oxide:

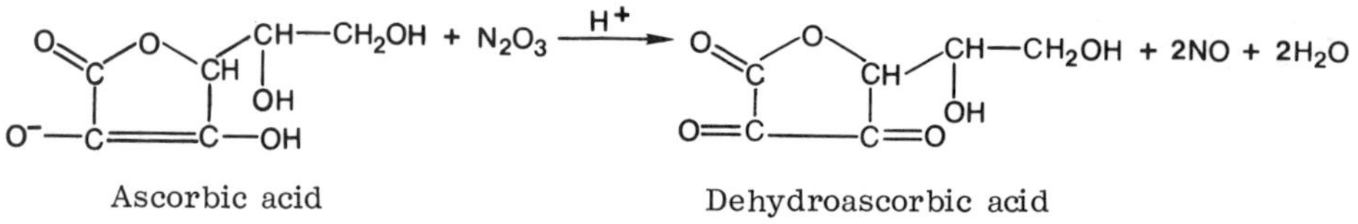

Ascorbic acid   Dehydroascorbic acid

The rate of the above reaction is much more rapid than the amine nitrosation reaction. Thus, in the presence of excess ascorbic acid, no N_2O_3 will be available to react with amines (Archer et al. 1975).

The extent of inhibition of the nitrosation reaction depends on the concentration of ascorbic acid, amines, nitrite, and other factors, such as oxygen. The latter can prevent the effective inhibition of nitrosation by reacting with ascorbic acid. For example, with morpholine, under anaerobic conditions, an ascorbic acid/morpholine ratio of 0.5 completely inhibits the nitrosation at pH 4. Whereas, in the presence of air, an equimolar concentration of ascorbic acid is needed to prevent nitrosation. In pure oxygen, not even an equimolar concentration of ascorbic acid can prevent the nitrosation reaction (Archer et al. 1975). Fan and Tannenbaum (1973) have found that an ascorbic acid/morpholine ratio of 2:1 is necessary for the complete blockage of the formation of nitrosomorpholine, and that only partial blocking is accomplished if the ratio is less than this.

Oxygen prevents the inhibition of the nitrosation reaction either by oxidizing ascorbic acid or at least by rendering it less effective. Indeed, the stability of ascorbic acid in packaged food, such as bacon, has been found to depend on the oxygen content of the package (Newark et al. 1974).

A curious observation is the formation of a more strongly carcinogenic dinitrosopiperazine from piperazine adipate in the presence of ascorbic acid (Mirvish 1975). However, the mononitrosopiperazine formation is completely inhibited by ascorbic acid. The presence of adipate probably promotes the formation of the dinitroso derivative, since the free base does not produce the compound (Mirvish 1975). The inhibition of the dinitroso derivative appears to be accomplished more effectively by glutathione than by ascorbic acid.

Compared to other inhibitors of the nitrosation reaction involving piperazine, ascorbic acid seems to be more effective than gallic acid, tannin, sulfite, and cysteine. Piperazine is more easily nitrosated than morpholine, and as such, presents a more critical test for the inhibitory action of ascorbic acid in the nitrosation reaction.

Table 7.5 shows the inhibitory effect of ascorbic acid on dimethylnitrosamine formation in model low moisture and aqueous systems (Gray and Dugan 1975). The low moisture system consisted of a freeze-dried mixture of carboxymethylcellulose (CMC), dimethylamine (1 mM) or proline, sodium nitrite (5 mM), and the appropriate buffer and inhibitor. The mixture contained 3.5% moisture and was heated to 69°C, the temperature used in the pasteurization of ham. With ascorbic acid, the results show a greater rate of nitrosation of the amine in the low moisture system than in the aqueous system. Thus, at pH 3.5 and 5.5 there is a 44.6 and 17.7% conversion in the low moisture system compared to the 40.3 and 6.2% conversion in the aqueous system. With ascorbic acid, the inhibition is essentially complete when the ratio of the vitamin to nitrite (mole/mole) is 2:1 or greater. The moderately greater inhibition at pH 5.5 may be explained by the smaller amount of nitrosamine formed at this pH. These results agree with the findings of Fan and Tannenbaum (1973).

Ascorbic acid inhibits the conversion of proline to N-nitrosopyrrolidine, when this amino acid is heated to 185°C with sodium nitrite in a freeze-dried mixture with CMC and appropriate buffer. A mixture of 2.5 mM proline and 12.5 mM $NaNO_2$ produces a 1.74% conversion of proline to the nitrosamine under these conditions.

The inhibitory effects of ascorbic acid on nitrosamine formation, as shown in in vitro model systems, has an actual counterpart in food systems. This has been demonstrated

Table 7.5 Inhibition of Dimethylnitrosamine Formation from Dimethylamine and Sodium Nitrite by Ascorbic acid in Both Low Moisture and Aqueous Systems

	PERCENT INHIBITION			
Ascorbic acid concentration (mM)[a]	pH 3.5		pH 5.5	
	Low moisture system[b]	Aqueous	Low moisture system[b]	Aqueous
2.5	60.8	67.4	71.9	71.6
5.0	91.3	96.7	92.0	97.9
10.0	99.0	98.5	95.0	99.1
20.0	99.4	99.5	99.5	99.8

[a]Concentrations of dimethylamine and sodium nitrite were 1 mM and 5 mM, respectively.
[b]Carboxymethylcellulose.
Source: Gray and Dugan (1975).

by Fiddler et al. (1973) with frankfurters. Frankfurters prepared with either 550 or 5500 ppm ascorbate and 1500 ppm nitrite do not produce any nitrosamines after 2 hr of processing. In contrast, frankfurters containing no ascorbic acid produce 10 ppb of nitrosamines.

Similarly, sodium ascorbate added to bacon at 500 to 2000 ppm effectively inhibits the formation of nitrosopyrrolidine (Herring 1973). The results of the work of Sen et al. (1976) regarding the inhibitory effect of ascorbyl palmitate and sodium ascorbate on the formation of nitrosopyrrolidine is shown in Table 7.6. Seven brands of bacon containing different levels of nitrite were tested. As the data show, there is no correlation between the initial amount of nitrite and the amount of nitrosamine that is formed. Ascorbyl palmitate appears to be more effective in inhibiting nitrosamine formation than sodium ascorbate. This may be due to differences in solubility. However, sodium ascorbate in the presence of propyl gallate appears to be quite effective.

The cooking condition may also affect the degree of inhibition. Inhibition has been shown to be more effective when starting with a cold pan and heating at 340 to 350°C for 13 min than when starting with a preheated pan at 400°C and maintaining the heat for 6 min. At any rate, ascorbyl palmitate causes from 73 to 97% inhibition of nitrosamine formation. It is obvious from the data that several factors may affect both the level of nitrosamine and the extent that this is inhibited by ascorbic acid.

Other inhibitors can, of course, influence nitrosamine formation, as discussed in Chapter 12.

The formation of nitrite from nitrate and the degradation of the latter by either ascorbic acid, its D isomer, erythorbic acid, or other endogenous reducing agents in food products are essential to the whole question of nitrosamine formation. This is partly because of the prevalence of nitrates over nitrites in food products.

Erythorbic Acid (Isoascorbic acid)

The increased levels of nitrites arising from nitrates in food products can also be prevented by ascorbic acid or erythorbic acid (Eakes and Blumer 1975). For example, in the presence of erythorbic acid, nitrites and nitrates in ham or ground pork are more rapidly depleted at 29°C (Eakes and Blumer 1975). Other researchers have also reported the rapid depletion of nitrite in ham in the presence of ascorbic or erythorbic acids (Brown et al. 1974; White 1975). Ascorbate added to ground potato containing nitrite and incubated at pH 1.5 and 37°C, to simulate conditions in the human stomach, diminish the nitrite content significantly when the ascorbate-nitrite ratio is greater than 2:1 (Raineri and Weisburger 1975). The formation of nitrates will be discussed in Chapter 18.

A number of studies show that ascorbic acid inhibits tumor formation produced by nitrite in the presence of the appropriate amines. It has been shown, for example, that a simultaneous administration of ascorbic acid will prevent the induction of neurogenic tumors in the offspring following gavage of ethyl urea plus $NaNO_2$ in pregnant rats. It does not, however, protect the mothers. Mirvish et al. (1973) found that the addition of 23 g ascorbic acid/kg food reduces the incidence of lung adenoma by 97% in mice induced by piperazine and $NaNO_2$ under the experimental conditions used. The tumor incidence is reduced by only 37% when the ascorbic acid/kg of food is reduced to 5.75g. Morpholine-$NaNO_2$-induced lung adenoma is inhibited by 89% at the higher ascorbic acid level compared to 72% at the lower level. Thus, the effective tumor inhibition at

Table 7.6 Inhibition of Nitrosopyrrolidine Formation in Bacon with Ascorbyl Palmitate and Sodium Ascorbate

Brand (ppm nitrite)	Cooking condition[a]	Nitrosopyrrolidine in control (ppb)	Additive[b] (1000 ppm)	% Inhibition
A (64)	1	22	Na ascorbate + propyl gallate	86
A (69)	2	20	Ascorbyl palmitate	80
A (30)	1	12	Ascorbyl palmitate	75
B (101)	1	30	Na ascorbate	40
			Ascorbyl palmitate	86
B (25)	1	25	Na ascorbate	40
			Ascorbyl palmitate	80
C (30)	1	15	Na ascorbate	40
C (59)	1	11	Na ascorbate	54
			Ascorbyl palmitate	73
D (90)	1	20	Na ascorbate + propyl gallate	80
D (10)	2	22	Ascorbyl palmitate	59
E (32)	1	30	Na ascorbate + propyl gallate	83
F (35)	1	40	Na ascorbate	77
			Ascorbyl palmitate	97
G (76)	2	10	Ascorbyl palmitate	0
			Ascorbyl palmitate, (sprinkled)	70

[a]Cooking condition: (1) 13 min, 340–350°C, starting with cold pan; (2) 6 min at 400°C, preheated pan.
[b]Additive was sprayed on bacon samples which were allowed to stand at room temperature for 30–60 min before cooking.
Source: Sen et al (1976).

lower levels of ascorbic acid depends on the type of amine. Ascorbic acid, at 12.6 g/kg of food, administered with methyl urea and $NaNO_2$ produces 98% tumor inhibition (Mirvish 1975).

In other experiments, however, ascorbic acid appears to enhance tumor formation by preformed nitrosamine. Thus, with nitrosopiperazine (34.5 mg/l drinking water), 23g ascorbic acid/kg of food increases the lung adenoma induction by 59%. Similar types of increased lung adenoma incidence also have been observed with nitrosomorpholine (Mirvish 1975). This effect, as pointed out by the investigator, might have been due to the increased consumption of nitrosamine-contaminated drinking water. The results may also be due to specific metabolic action of ascorbic acid. It has been shown in guinea pigs that the microsomal metabolism of drugs can be increased with high doses of the vitamin (Zannoni and Sato 1975). Such increased microsomal activity may enhance the activation of the nitrosamines. It would be interesting to see the results of this experiment under controlled amine consumption.

In this connection, it is notable that ascorbic acid together with butylhydroxytoluene inhibits skin tumor induction in hamsters subjected to ultraviolet light (Black 1974). Furthermore, hepatotoxicity induced by gavage of rats and mice with nitrite and dimethylamine is completely prevented by ascorbic acid. However, as in tumor induction, ascorbic acid appears to have no protective effect on the hepatotoxicity of preformed dimethylnitrosamine (Cardesa et al. 1974).

The induction of neurogenic tumors of the peripheral nervous system in the progeny of pregnant hamsters administered with ethylurea and $NaNO_2$ intragastrically and intraintestinally, has been shown to be completely prevented by the concurrent administration of sodium ascorbate (Rustia 1975).

Ascorbic acid at high doses also has been shown to inhibit the formation of bladder tumors induced by 3-hydroxyanthranilic acid pellets implanted in the mice bladders (Pipkin et al. 1969; Schlegel et al. 1969). In this case, ascorbic acid is believed to prevent the oxidation of 3-hydroxyanthranilic acid, an easily oxidizable tryptophan metabolite (Pipkin et al. 1967). As with 3-hydroxyanthranilic acid, other primary bladder carcinogens are believed to be oxidation products of corresponding compounds which are easily oxidizable; e.g., hydroxy-β-naphthylamine and a number of tryptophan metabolites. The oxidation of the latter, which are powerful bladder carcinogens, can be prevented by ascorbic acid, provided its concentration during the time urine is normally stored (i.e., 2 hr) is greater than 2 mg% (Schlegel 1975).

Effects of Pyridoxine

Bischoff et al. (1943) first reported the regression of murine sarcoma 180 in mice on pyridoxine-deficient diets. Similar observations were reported in that same year on three other transplantable tumors (Kline et al. 1943). Following this report, regression of transplanted lymphosarcoma in pyridoxine-deficient mice was also observed by Stoerk (1947). The deficiency in Stoerk's study was induced by the use of a pyridoxine-deficient diet simultaneouly with a pyridoxine antagonist such as 4-deoxypyridoxine. A pyridoxine antagonist alone was shown to be ineffective in inducing tumor regression (Brockman et al. 1956), especially when the experimental animals were fed regular diets.

Mihich and Nichol (1959) found that for optimum regression of mouse sarcoma 180 tumor, animals must be on the pyridoxine-deficient diet for at least 2 weeks prior to implantation. Longer periods of prior deficiency have no further influence on the extent of tumor regression. Placing animals on the pyridoxine-deficient diet at the time of tumor implantation has less effect in inducing tumor regression. For example, of 148 transplanted tumors about 15% regressed in mice fed the deficient diet on the day of transplantation, whereas less than 5% regressed completely. In contrast, feeding the deficient diet 2 weeks prior to transplantation produced a 58% regression of the total number of tumors transplanted; in this case, more than 36% regressed completely.

Pyridoxine and its derivatives, when supplied at the start of transplantation, prevents both inhibition and regression of tumor growth. Control experiments indicate that the effects of pyridoxine deficiency on tumor regression is not due to decreased dietary intake; as shown previously, decreased food intake has a significant effect on inhibition of tumor growth (pp. 241–245). Pyridoxine deficiency also causes regression of adenocarcinoma 755, and at least growth inhibition in six other types of tumors (Mihich et al. 1959). In the same study, pyridoxine deficiency was shown not to affect the growth of three other types of tumors.

Treatment with cortisone significantly reduces the number of tumors that regress, even though it has no effect on tumor growth. Additionally, those mice in which tumors have previously regressed and are subsequently put on a pyridoxine-deficient diet followed by 4 to 12 weeks on a regular diet show a remarkable resistance to retransplanted tumors. Even though a significant number of tumors grow very slowly in these mice, all tumors are eventually rejected. The results shown with cortisone treatment as well as the resistance of mice in which tumors have previously regressed to another transplanted tumor, indicate a possible stimulation of immune mechanisms against tumor growth. Similar resistance to retransplantation of tumors had been observed in other experimental conditions (Andervont 1932; Bradner et al. 1958).

The observed effects of pyridoxine deficiency on the immune response to tumor growth is similar to the effects noted in riboflavin deficiency (Stoerk and Emerson 1949) on the resistance of mice to reimplantation of lymphosarcoma 6C3H-CD.

Attempts to induce tumor regression with pyridoxine-deficient diets in patients with advanced cancers were unsuccessful (Gailani et al. 1968). This lack of effect is consistent with the observation of Mihich and Nichol (1959) that pyridoxine deficiency at the time of tumor transplantation in animals produces minimal tumor regression.

Effects of Folic Acid

The folic acid antagonist methotrexate, or 4-amino-N^{10}-methylpteroylglutamic acid, is a well-known antitumor agent; it is used as a chemotherapeutic agent, particularly in leukemia. Thus, as with the other vitamin deficiencies described previously, such antifolic acid compounds also produce a vitamin deficiency. In this case, the antifolic agent interferes in the activity of reductases which are required in the formation of tetrahydrofolic acid, the active form of folic acid. It appears that the requirement of tumor cells for these enzymes may be greater than in normal cells. For example, Bertino et al. (1963) found greater activities of tetrahydrofolate-dependent enzymes in leukemic cells compared to normal leukocytes. These enzymes are, therefore, likely targets by antifolic acid agents. However, in some cases, antifolic agents, such as methotrexate, have no effect on growth of certain tumors, such as Walker carcinoma in rats (Rosen and Nichol 1962), but this tumor can be significantly inhibited by dietary folic acid deficiency.

It has been shown in another earlier study (Walpole 1951) that dietary folic acid deficiency started 2 weeks prior to transplantation of tumor results in 95% inhibition of tumor growth 28 days after transplantation. Tumor growth is also inhibited by as much as 53%, expressed as tumor weight, even if the folic acid-deficient diet is given 14 days posttransplantation. Significant suppression of tumor growth is noted when animals are given diets supplying only 0.25 g folic acid/kg body weight, and almost complete inhibition when the diet contains as little as 50 µg/kg body weight. Tumors resume normal rapid growth when animals are given adequate diets again. Curiously, the tumors can not compete with the normal liver cells for the available folic acid. Even on an adequate ration, the folic acid contents of tumor cells is almost twice that in folic acid-deficient animals. Livers of animals on adequate diets contain 12 times as much folic acid as those on the deficient diet.

Again, in this experiment (Walpole 1951), it has been shown that treatment with 0.5 or 1.0 mg methotrexate does not affect tumor growth unless there is dietary folic acid deficiency. It is possible that the amount of antifolic acid agent used is insufficient to overcome the supply of folic acid in the liver when animals are fed a normal diet. Similarly, tumor-bearing animals on an adequate diet also may be able to detoxify the antifolic acid agents adequately.

Effects of Other Vitamins

Earlier work on pantothenic acid-deficient diets also have shown that this vitamin has an inhibitory effect on the growth of spontaneous mammary tumors in mice (Morris and Lippincott 1941). However, the diets used were extremely deficient in the vitamin. Like dietary folic acid deficiency, tumor growth resumes on supplementation with the vitamin.

Thiamin deficiency seems to enhance slightly the growth of spontaneous mammary tumor in mice, whereas increased intake of the vitamin results in a slight decrease in tumor growth (Morris 1947). Daily subcutaneous injection of 40 to 60 μg of thiamin also has been reported to retard the growth of spontaneous mammary tumors in mice (Dobrovolskaia-Zavadskaia 1945).

Studies on the anticarcinogenic effects of α-tocopherol and its natural analogues have not been as extensive as those of retinol. Nevertheless, some studies indicate significant anticarcinogenic effects of α-tocopherol with certain carcinogens. For example, the incidence of tumors induced by 3-methylcholanthrene (100 μg/ml in mineral oil, subcutaneously) has been shown to be reduced by 50% in C57 leaden female mice fed diets containing 30 to 100 times the normal intake of α-tocopherol (Haber and Wissler 1962). The same authors also found a 50% reduction in tumor incidence induced with the same carcinogen in C57 black male mice fed diets supplemented with α-tocopherol (7 mg/g feed).

The anticarcinogenic effects of wheat germ oil against methylcholanthrene have been reported (Jaffe 1946); a 50% reduction in sarcoma incidence was noted in this study. Wheat germ oil contains relatively high levels of α-tocopherol, approximately 0.5% (Eckey and Miller 1954). However, in view of the presence of other components in wheat germ oil, the anticarcinogenic effects in this case may not be ascribed entirely to the tocopherols.

Tocopherols may exercise their anticarcinogenic effects in three ways. First, as an antioxidant, it may enhance the antitumorigenic effects of retinol (pp. 250—255) by protecting the retinol from oxidation. Second, as an antioxidant, the carcinogenicity of peroxides, free radicals, and other oxidation products with carcinogenic potentials may be diminished by this vitamin. It should be recalled that many procarcinogens are converted to primary carcinogens by oxidation, and that the reactive species of carcinogenic alkylating agents may be free radicals (Chap. 6). Third, α-tocopherol may be a cofactor in detoxification mechanisms of a number of carcinogens. For example, liver ribosomes may be protected from the effects of large doses of the carcinogens, 2-aminofluorene, and 2-naphthylamine (Hultin and Arrhenius 1965). Furthermore, α-tocopherol may enhance N-demethylation and reduce N-hydroxylation processes. This has been demonstrated in the case of N-dimethylaniline (Arrhenius 1968). It should be recalled that the deactivation of 4-dimethylaminoazobenzene requires the process of N-demethylation (p. 257), and that N-hydroxylation is involved in the conversion of dimethylnitrosamine to reactive species (Chap. 12).

Biotin seems to counter the protective effects of riboflavin against azo dye carcinogenesis. Thus, it has been observed that when a highly protective, riboflavin-containing diet is supplemented with 2 to 4 μg of biotin, increased tumor formation occurs (du Vigneaud et al. 1942). This stimulation of azo dye carcinogenesis by biotin also has been observed by other researchers (Harris et al. 1947). However, with a nonprotective diet containing low levels of riboflavin, biotin does not cause further stimulation of the carcinogenicity of the azo dye (Harris et al. 1947; Miller and Miller 1952). Substitution of casein in the diet with egg albumin, presumably to bind biotin with avidin, causes a marked inhibition of tumor induction with 4-dimethylazobenzene (Harris et al. 1947; Kline et al. 1945). However, heating the egg albumin, presumably to destroy avidin, unexpectedly, does not alter the inhibitory effects of albumin. Thus, the inhibitory effects of albumin probably are due to other factors.

Cobalamin, the antipernicious anemia vitamin, has stimulatory effects on 4-dimethylazobenzene-induced liver tumors. In one experiment, it was shown that liver tumors in rats weaning on soy protein diets grow more rapidly when the diet contains cobalamin (Day et al. 1950; Miller and Miller 1952). It is possible that, since cobalamin is involved in methylation reactions, detoxification of the azo dye by demethylation may be countered by this vitamin (Day et al. 1950). It should be recalled that demethylation of this carcinogen is enhanced or promoted by riboflavin (p. 257).

It is an interesting observation that cobalamin as well as folic acid increases the inhibitory effects of 8-azaguanine on mammary adenocarcinoma 755 in C57 black mice (Shapiro and Gellhorn 1951).

Severe choline deficiency appears to have a unique effect in that this condition has been reported to induce spontaneous liver tumors (Copeland and Salmon 1946; Salmon et al. 1955) in rats and chickens. Riboflavin has been reported to counteract this effect (Schaefer et al. 1950). However, recent knowledge of the pathogenesis of liver tumors involving aflatoxins has led some investigators to suggest that the earlier observations on choline deficiency and liver tumor induction may have also involved aflatoxins (Butler and Newberne 1969; Salmon and Newberne 1963). It should be recalled that liver carcinogenesis caused by aflatoxins is also counteracted by riboflavin (Lemonnier et al. 1975).

General Remarks

The foregoing discussion on the effect of vitamins on carcinogenesis underscores the complex involvement of these micronutrients in this intriguing pathological process. It appears that no general principle can be stated for the role of vitamins in the inhibition or promotion of tumor induction and growth. In one situation, an inhibitory effect is observed; in another, there may be promoting effects. This has been illustrated in the case of retinol and ascorbic acid. While under certain conditions, some vitamin deficiencies promote tumor growth (i.e., retinol, riboflavin, ascorbic acid, tocopherols, choline); under other conditions, vitamin deficiencies have inhibitory effects (i.e., thiamin, pyridoxine, cobalamin, biotin, riboflavin, folic acid). Deficiencies of certain vitamins inhibit tumor growth; these same vitamins will enhance tumorigenesis when present in adequate amounts in the diet.

One serious defect in many studies involving the role of vitamins in cancer is the emphasis on one vitamin with little or no consideration of other vitamins as well as other nutrients. Metabolism of the vitamins are directly or indirectly interrelated in such a way that alteration in one or more vitamins may affect the functions of the others. Therefore, it is reasonable to propose that vitaminology in cancer should consider all vitamins taken as a group. Thus, the effect of the quantitative and qualitative balance of vitamins on tumor induction and progression may be more effectively assessed if these are studied as a group. Each type of tissue may require a different quantitative and qualitative vitamin involvement with respect to cancer induction or inhibition.

Other physiological factors which enter into the carcinogenic process, such as the immune response, undoubtedly would have vitamin involvement. To be able to ascertain the definite role of vitamins in these instances would have a profound impact on understanding the control of cancer. One significant observation that emerged from studies in oncology is the delicate balance among the factors in metabolism which lead to the induction and promotion of neoplasms.

EFFECTS OF INORGANIC NUTRIENTS

The metallic nutrients and other inorganic elements are closely related in function to the vitamins. This follows from the known role of inorganic elements in enzyme action which also involves many of the vitamins. Admittedly, the precise involvement and assignation of each vitamin or group of vitamins as well as the inorganic nutrients to enzymes are far from understood. Additionally, our understanding of many enzyme systems in terms of identity, tissue distribution and concentration, induction by exogenous and indogenous factors, and so on, is vague, if not unknown. Nowhere are these limitations in our understanding of the role of vitamins and inorganic nutrients more glaringly underscored than in oncology. Nevertheless, a few inroads have been made.

Some studies of the role of inorganic nutrients in tumorigenesis, particularly in induction and progression of tumors, are discussed in the following section. This discussion will not deal with the carcinogenicity of inorganic nutrients per se (see Chap. 18).

As with the vitamins, the deficiency or presence of metals which act as cofactors in enzyme action has also been found to modify tumorigenesis. Among these metals are magnesium, manganese, cobalt, copper, zinc, selenium, and vanadium.

Magnesium is an essential cofactor in many enzymes in intermediary metabolism, particularly in the glycolytic pathway, glycogen metabolism, oxidative phosphorylation, protein biosynthesis, and neuromuscular processes, to name a few. The widespread functions of magnesium immediately suggests serious metabolic repercussions in case of deficiency. One of these effects, as observed in the rat, is leukocytosis which appears to be irreversible even after magnesium supplementation (Battifora et al. 1968). A number of rats fed a synthetic diet containing between 4 and 6 mg magnesium/100 g of diet suffered a more severe leukocytosis with pathological alterations which are characteristic of myelogenous leukemia. The symptoms of leukocytosis and leukemia in these cases could not be reversed by magnesium supplementation. These studies revealed a 10% incidence of leukemia, which is significant since spontaneous myelogenous leukemia is rare among rats (Wilens and Sproul 1936). In the experiment of Battifora et al. (1968), the incidence of leukemia decreased with progressive reduction of magnesium in the diet. The latter results are consistent with observations which show that malnutrition following underfeeding has a protective effect in mice against the development of spontaneous leukemia (Saxton et al. 1944).

In related studies, magnesium deficiency has been shown to induce thymic lymphosarcoma in rats (Bois 1964; Bois and Beaulnes 1966; Bois et al. 1969). In the work of Bois et al. (1969), nine groups of rats developed tumor incidence ranging from 7 to 50% per group, with an average group incidence of 20.6%. Most tumors were usually invasive, and the larger tumors were accompanied by extensive metastases to the heart, esophagus, kidney, and bone marrow. In some cases, the tumor eventually produced leukemia (Bois 1968).

The effect of magnesium deficiency in inducing leukemia and thymic tumors may be related to its function in DNA replication and formation of the mitotic spindle (Battifora et al. 1968). In this case, magnesium deficiency may lead to abnormal changes in cell division, resulting in defective cell cones with hyperplastic or neoplastic capabilities. Magnesium deficiency also has been found to produce abnormal immune responses at cellular and serological levels (Battifora et al. 1968; McCreary et al. 1966). Such abnormality may hinder the immune response from inhibiting the proliferation of neoplastic cells, such as in leukemia.

Related to magnesium is manganese, which can function interchangeably with magnesium in a variety of enzyme systems. However, the use of manganous chloride rather than magnesium chloride causes a more rapid appearance of lymphosarcoma in mice (di Paolo 1964). Neither elemental magnesium nor manganese has been reported to be potentially carcinogenic (Furst and Haro 1969).

Cobalt is a transition element like magnesium and manganese; it functions in the body as part of the cobalamin molecule. It is potentially carcinogenic (Gilman and Ruckenbauer 1962; Heath 1956; Thomas and Thiery 1953). On the other hand, cobalt salts have been observed to reduce the incidence of skin tumors induced by 3-methylcholanthrene (Kasirsky et al. 1965; Orzechowski et al. 1965). As much as a 50% reduction in skin tumor incidence has been noted with sodium cobaltinitrite (Orzechowski et al. 1965).

Copper is another transition element with varied functions, notably, in electron transport; in iron, purine, and connective tissue metabolism and in phospholipid formation and nervous tissue development (O'Dell et al. 1961; Seelig 1972; Graham 1971).

There is some doubt about the potential carcinogenicity of copper compounds, although teratomas are reportedly produced in the testes of roosters injected with copper sulfate during periods of high gonadal activity (Falin and Anissimore 1940). Nevertheless, copper may accentuate the carcinogenicity of known carcinogens. For example, the induction of skin tumors in mice with 9,10-dimethyl-1,2-benzanthracene is accelerated by application with copper acetate (Fare 1965). Similarly, the carcinogenicity of

N-hydroxy-2-acetylaminofluorene is enhanced if the carcinogen is in the form of a copper chelate (Stanton 1967).

However, the opposite effect has been reported in the case of azo dye carcinogenesis. Cupric oxyacetate prevents liver cancer induced by 3-methoxy-4-aminoazobenzene, even though skin and ear duct tumors are not prevented (Fare and Howell 1964). Cupric oxyacetate also protects the liver from the harmful effects of not only 4-dimethylaminoazobenzene, but also other carcinogens; i.e., thioacetamide, acetaminofluorene, β-naphthylisothiocyanate, and dimethylnitrosamine (Fare and Woodhouse 1963). Essentially, complete protection from liver tumor induced by 4-dimethylaminoazobenzene is accomplished when rats are fed a mixture of yeast, beef extract, and cupric oxyacetate (Fare 1964).

The protective effects of copper salts toward azo dye carcinogenesis may be due to the destruction of the dye in the diet by copper-catalyzed oxidation. Perhaps more definitive results could have been obtained if the copper salt were administered separately from the diet. Nevertheless, the inhibitory effect of copper on azo dye carcinogenesis may follow from other mechanisms besides the in vitro oxidation of the dye, since the metal also protects the liver from thioacetamide, 2-acetylaminofluorene, and β-naphthylisothiocyanate (Fare and Woodhouse 1963). These specific carcinogens may not be oxidized as readily by copper as the azo dyes. In addition, the greater affinity for copper by tumors induced by aromatic hydrocarbons (Arnold and Sasse 1961) than by normal tissues suggests a possible involvement of this metal in cellular processes related to the carcinogenic induction.

Zinc is another nutrient metal of the transition series which appears to be a potential carcinogen. Injection of a zinc compound into the testes of rats has been shown to result in teratomas (Riviere et al. 1960) and fowl (Guthrie 1964, 1967). Zinc is involved in a wide variety of cellular processes, and is a component of metalloenzymes. In particular, it is involved in DNA, ribonucleic acid (RNA), and protein synthesis, especially skin keratin and collagen, and in the production and activities of several hormones (Food and Nutrition Board NAS-NRC 1970; Prasad 1966; Prasad et al. 1963; Vallee 1959). Like copper, zinc can also accelerate the growth of experimental tumors. For example, the rate of growth of sarcomas is increased following administration of zinc sulfate (Chahovitch 1955). Like copper, zinc also accumulates in tumor tissues, for example, in mammary tumors, more than in the surrounding normal mammary tissues (Tupper et al. 1955). Zinc exhibits an antagonism against cadmium-induced tumors of the interstitial cells in the testes of rats and mice (Gunn et al. 1963). With zinc, mice are afforded 100% protection, whereas rats develop only a few tumors.

Selenium is closely liked with the tocopherols as an antioxidant. Specifically, selenium protects cell membranes against oxidation and function in red blood cell formation (Sucommittee on Selenium 1971). This higher analog of sulfur may replace the sulfur atom in sulfur amino acids, such as methionine, to form selenomethionine. Its potential carcinogenicity has been reported from the production of low grade tumors at doses approaching chronic poisoning (Nelson et al. 1943; Tscherkes et al. 1963). Some researchers have been unable to confirm this potential carcinogenicity (Harr et al. 1967), possibly because of variables such as the strain of animal, the composition of the diet, or the type of selenium compound; e.g., selenates or selenites versus selenide or organoselenium.

The possibility that this element has protective effects against human stomach cancer has been suggested (Subcommittee on Selenium 1971). Likewise, Shamberger and Frost (1969) noted the inverse relationships between the occurrence of selenium in soil and forage crops and the human cancer death rate in the United States and Canada in 1965. They also cited an inverse relationship between selenium blood levels in humans and the cancer death rates in several cities.

Animal studies have demonstrated the anticarcinogenic effects of selenium. For example, a lower incidence of liver tumors induced by dimethylaminoazobenzene has been observed in rats fed diets with added sodium selenite (Clayton and Bauman 1949). The inhibitory effects of selenium salts on tumor induction with three types of carcinogenic hydrocarbons also has been demonstrated by Shamberger (1970). Although total protection from the carcinogenic effects was not achieved at the concentration of selenium compounds used by Shamberger (1970), a significant difference between the experimental and control mice was demonstrated. For example, 17% of the mice developed skin tumors compared to 43% of the control when 0.0005% sodium selenide was applied for 20 days, following the topical application of 0.125 mg of dimethylbenzanthracene with croton oil as the promoter. Under the same experimental conditions — except that *Torula* yeast containing 1 ppm sodium selenate was fed 2 weeks prior to the application of the carcinogen — 45 and 89% of experimental and control mice, respectively, developed tumors. Sodium selenide gave no protective effects if applied 3 weeks after the administration of the carcinogen. α-Tocopherol at a level of 0.13% gave less protection than selenium. In both of the preceding experiments 24 and 64% of the mice, respectively, bore tumors.

In the case of 3-methylcholanthrene, sodium selenide was shown not to be as protective, with 60% of the mice bearing tumors compared with 83% of the controls. α-Tocopherol gave no protection at all with this carcinogen. With benzo(a)pyrene, 1 ppm sodium selenate added to a *Torula* yeast diet produced tumors in 44% of the mice compared to 86% of the control. At this level of selenate, 24% of the mice had cancer compared to 40% of the control. Strangely enough, feeding a commercial diet instead of the *Torula* yeast diet produced tumors in 94.4% of the mice. Obviously, the commercial diet contained unknown potentiating factors.

Other antioxidants, such as ascorbic acid and lysosomal stabilizers, fail to reduce tumor incidence. This suggests that the protective action of selenium and α-tocopherol is highly specific, and may not be related to mechanisms which entail antioxidant effects or lysosomal stabilization.

REFERENCES

Allan, J. D., Ireland, J. T., Milner, J. and Moss, A. D. 1965. Treatment of leukemia by amino acid imbalance. *Lancet* 1: 302–303.

Andervont, H. B. 1932. Studies on immunity induced by mouse sarcoma 180. *Public Health Rep.* 47: 1859–1877.

Antopol, W. 1950. Anatomic changes produced in mice treated with excessive doses of cortisone. *Proc. Soc. Exp. Biol. Med.* 73: 262–265.

Archer, M. C., Tannenbaum, S. R., Fan, T.-Y. and Weisman, M. 1975. Reaction of nitrite with ascorbate and its relation to nitrosamine formation. *J. Natl. Cancer Inst.* 54: 1203–1205.

Arnold, M. and Sasse, D. 1961. Quantitative and histochemical analysis of Cu, Zn, and Fe in spontaneous and induced primary tumors of rats. *Cancer Res.* 21: 761–766.

Arrhenius, E. 1968. Effects on hepatic microsomal N- and C-oxygenation of aromatic amines by in vivo corticosteroid or aminofluorene treatment, diet, or stress. *Cancer Res.* 28: 264–273.

Bang, B. G., Bang, F. B. and Foard, M. A. 1972. Lymphocyte depression induced in chickens on diets deficient in vitamin A and other components. *Am. J. Pathol.* 68: 147–162.

Bang, B. G., Foard, M. A. and Bang, F. B. 1973. The effect of vitamin A deficiency and Newcastle disease on lymphoid cell systems in chicken. *Proc. Soc. Exp. Biol. Med.* 143: 1140–1146.

Bassir, O. and Osiyemi, F. 1967. Biliary excretion of aflatoxin in the rat after a single dose. *Nature* 215: 882.

Battifora, H. A. et al. 1968. Chronic magnesium deficiency in the rat: Studies of chronic myelogenous leukemia. *Arch. Pathol.* 86: 610–620.

Bebawi, G. M., Kim, Y. S. and Lambooy, J. P. 1970. Study of the carcinogenicity of a series of structurally related 4-dimethylaminoazobenzenes. *Cancer Res.* 30: 1520–1524.

Berg, J. W., Howell, M. A. and Silverman, S. J. 1973. Dietary hypotheses and diet-related research in the etiology of colon cancer. *Health Serv. Rep.* 88: 915–924.

Bertino, J. R. et al. 1963. Studies on normal and leukemic leukocytes. IV. Tetrahydrofolate-dependent enzyme systems and dehydrofolic reductase. *J. Clin. Invest.* 42: 1899–1907.

Bischoff, F., Ingraham, L. P. and Rupp, J. J. 1943. Influence of vitamin B_6 and pantothenic acid on growth of sarcoma 180. *Arch. Pathol.* 35: 713–716.

Bjelke, E. 1975. Dietary vitamin A and human lung cancer. *Int. J. Cancer* 15: 561–565.

Black, H. S. 1974. Effects of dietary antioxidants on actinic tumor induction. *Res. Commun. Chem. Pathol. Pharmacol.* 7: 783–786.

Bois, P. 1964. Tumour of the thymus in magnesium-deficient rats. *Nature* 204: 1316.

Bois, P. 1968. Peripheral vasodilation and thymic tumors in magnesium deficient rats. In: *Endocrine Aspects of Disease Processes.* G. Jasmin (ed.). Warren H. Green, St. Louis.

Bois, P. and Beaulnes, A. 1966. Histamine, magnesium deficiency and thymic tumors in rats. *Can. J. Physiol. Pharmacol.* 44: 373–377.

Bois, P., Sandborn, B. and Messier, P. E. 1969. A study of thymic lymphosarcoma developing in magnesium-deficient rats. *Cancer Res.* 29: 763–775.

Bollag, W. 1971a. Therapy of chemically induced skin tumors of mice with vitamin A palmitate and vitamin A acid. *Experientia* 27: 90–92.

Bollag, W. 1971b. Vitamin A in tumor therapy. Schweiz. Med. *Wochenschr.* 101: 11–17. (German)

Bollag, W. 1971c. Effects of vitamin A acid (NSC-122758) on transplantable and chemically induced tumors. *Cancer Chemother. Rep.* 55: 53–58.

Bollag, W. 1972. Prophylaxis of chemically induced benign and malignant epithelial tumors by vitamin A acid (retinoic acid). *Eur. J. Cancer* 8: 689–693.

Bollag, W. and Ott, F. 1971. Local treatment of premalignant lesions and basal cell carcinoma with vitamin A acid. Schweiz. Med. *Wochenschr.* 101: 17–19. (German).

Boutwell, R. K., Brush, M. K. and Rusch, H. P. 1949a. The stimulating effect of dietary fat on carcinogenesis. *Cancer Res.* 9: 741–746.

Bradner, W. T., Clarke, D. A. and Stock, C. C. 1958. Stimulation of host defense against experimental cancer. I. Zymosan and sarcoma 180 in mice. *Cancer Res.* 18: 347–351.

Brockman, R. W., Thomson, J. R., Schabel, F. M., Jr. and Skipper, H. E. 1956. The inhibition of growth of sarcoma 180 by combinations of B_6-antagonists and acid hydrazides. *Cancer Res.* 16: 788–795.

Brookes, P. 1966. Quantitative aspects of the reaction of some carcinogens with nucleic acids and the possible significance of such reactions in the process of carcinogenesis. *Cancer Res.* 26: 1994–2003.

Brown, C. L., Hedrick, H. B. and Bailey, M. E. 1974. Characteristics of cured ham as influenced by levels of sodium nitrite and sodium ascorbate. *J. Food Sci.* 39: 977–979.

Butler, W. H. and Newberne, P. M. 1969. Acute and chronic effects of aflatoxin on the liver of domestic and laboratory animals: A review. *Cancer Res.* 29: 236–250.

Cairns, J. 1975. The cancer problem. *Sci. Am.* 233: 64–79.

Capizzi, R. L., Bertino, J. R. and Handschumacher, R. E. 1970. L-asparaginase. *Ann. Rev. Med.* 21: 433–444.

Cardesa, A., Mirvish, S. S., Haven, G. T. and Shubik, P. 1974. Inhibitory effect of ascorbic acid on the acute toxicity of dimethylamine plus nitrite in the rat. *Proc. Soc. Exp. Biol. Med.* 145: 124–128.

Carroll, K. K. and Khor, H. T. 1970. Effects of dietary fat and dose level of 7,12-dimethylbenz(a)anthracene on mammary tumor incidence in rats. *Cancer Res.* 30: 2260-2264.

Carroll, K. K. and Khor, H. T. 1971. Effects of level and type of dietary fat on incidence of mammary tumors induced in female Sprague-Dawley rats by 7,12-dimethylbenzanthracene. *Lipids* 6: 415—420.

Carroll, K. K., Gammal, E. B. and Plunkett, E. R. 1968. Dietary fat and mammary cancer. *Can. Med. Assoc. J.* 98: 590—594.

Catz, C. S., Jachan, M. R. and Yaffe, S. J. 1970. Effects of iron, riboflavin, and iodine deficiencies on hepatic, drug-metabolizing enzyme systems. *J. Pharmacol. Exp. Ther.* 174: 197—205.

Chahovitch, X. 1955. The action of zinc on the growth of experimental tumours incited by carcinogens. G1. *Srpske. Akad. Nauka, Od. Med Nauka* 215: 143—146 (1955). Cited by Excerpta Med. (Amsterdam), Section XVI, 4: 459 (1956).

Chan, P. C. and Cohen, L. A. 1974. Effect of dietary fat, anti-estrogen and anti-prolactin on the development of mammary tumors in rats. *J. Natl. Cancer Inst.* 52: 25—30.

Chu, E. W. and Malmgren, R. A. 1965. An inhibitory effect of vitamin A on the induction of tumors of forestomach and cervix in the Syrian hamster by carcinogenic polycyclic hydrocarbons. *Cancer Res.* 25: 884—895.

Clayton, C. C., Bauman, C. A. 1949. Diet and azo dye tumors: Effect of diet during a period when the dye is not fed. *Cancer Res.* 9: 575—582.

Cohen, M. H. 1972. Enhancement of the antitumor effect of 1,3-bis(2-chloroethyl)-1-nitrosourea by vitamin A and caffeine. *J. Natl. Cancer Inst.* 48: 927—932.

Cohen, M. H. and Carbone, P. P. 1972. Enhancement of the antitumor effects of BCNU and cyclophosphamide by vitamin A. *J. Natl. Cancer Inst.* 48: 921—926.

Cohen, B. E., Cohen, I. K. 1973. Vitamin A adjuvant and steroid antagonist in the immune response. *J. Immunol.* 111: 1376—1380.

Cohen, B. E. and Elin, R. J. 1974. Enhanced resistance to certain infections in vitamin A-treated mice. *Plast. Reconstr. Surg.* 54: 192—194.

Comings, D. E. 1973. A general theory of carcinogenesis. *Proc. Natl. Acad. Sci.* 70: 3324—3328.

Cone, M. V. and Nettesheim, P. 1973. Effects of vitamin A on 3-methylcholanthrene-induced squamous metaplasias and early tumors in the respiratory tract of rats. *J. Natl. Cancer Inst.* 50: 1599—1606.

Conney, A. H., Miller, E. C. and Miller, J. A. 1956. The metabolism of methylated aminoazo dyes. V. Evidence for induction of enzyme synthesis in the rat by 3-methylcholanthrene. *Cancer Res.* 16: 450—459.

Conney, A. H., Brown, R. R., Miller, J. A. and Miller, E. C. 1957. The metabolism of methylated aminoazo dyes. VI. Intracellular distribution and properties of the demethylase system. *Cancer Res.* 17: 628—633.

Cooney, D. A. and Handschumacher, R. E. 1970. L-asparaginase and L-asparagine metabolism. *Ann. Rev. Pharmacol.* 10: 421—440.

Copeland, D. H. and Salmon, W. D. 1946. The occurrence of neoplasms in the liver, lungs and other tissues of rats as a result of prolonged choline deficiency. *Am. J. Pathol.* 22: 1059—1079.

Dao, T. L. 1971. Inhibition of tumor induction in chemical carcinogenesis in the mammary gland. *Prog. Exp. Tumor Res.* 14: 60—88.

Davies, R. E. 1967. Effect of vitamin A on 7,12-dimethylbenz(a)anthracene-induced papillomas in rhino mouse skin. *Cancer Res.* 27: 237—241.

Day, P. L., Payne, L. D. and Dinning, J. S. 1950. Procarcinogenic effect of vitamin B_{12} on p-dimethylaminoazobenzene-fed rats. *Proc. Soc. Exp. Biol. Med.* 74: 854—855.

DeLuca, L., Schumacher, M. and Wolf, G. 1970. Biosynthesis of a fucose-containing glycopeptide from rat small intestine in normal and vitamin-A-deficient conditions. *J. Biol. Chem.* 245: 4551-4556.

DeLuca, L., Maestri, N., Bonanni, F. and Nelson, D. 1972. Maintenance of epithelian cell differentiation: The mode of action of vitamin A. *Cancer* 30: 1326—1331.

Demopoulos, H. B. 1966. Effects of low phenylalanine-tyrosine diets on S91 mouse melanomas. *J. Natl. Cancer Inst.* 37: 185–190.

DeWaard, F. 1975. Breast cancer incidence and nutritional status with particular reference to body weight and height. Paper presented at the Conference on "Nutrition in the Causation of Cancer." Key Biscayne, Florida, May 1975.

DeWaard, F., DeLaive, J. W. J. and Baandersvan Halewijn, E. A. 1960. On the bimodal age distribution of mammary carcinoma. *Br. J. Cancer* 14: 437–448.

Diamond, L. and Gelboin, H. V. 1969. Alphanaphthoflavone: An inhibitor of hydrocarbon cytotoxicity and microsomal hydroxylase. *Science* 166: 1023–1025.

Dingle, J. T. and Lucy, J. A. 1962. Studies on the mode of action of vitamin A on the stability of the erythrocyte membrane. *Biochem. J.* 84: 611–621.

DiPaolo, J. A. 1964. Potentiation of lymphosarcomas in the mouse by manganous chloride. *Fed. Proc.* 23: 393.

Dobrovolskaïa-Zavadskaïa, N. 1945. The effect of aneurine (vitamin B1) on the growth of spontaneous tumors in mice. *C. R. Soc. Biol.* 139: 494–495. (French)

Dougherty, T. F. and White, A. 1945. Functional alteration in lymphoid tissue induced by adrenal cortical secretion. *Am. J. Anat.* 77: 81–116.

Dresser, D. W. 1968. Adjuvanticity of vitamin A. *Nature* 217: 527–529.

Dublin, L. I. 1930. The influence of weight on certain causes of death. *Human Biol.* 2: 159–184.

Dunning, W. F., Curtis, M. R. and Maun, M. E. 1950. The effect of added dietary tryptophane on the occurrence of 2-acetylaminofluorene-induced liver and bladder cancer in rats. *Cancer Res.* 10: 454–459.

DuVigneaud, V. et al. 1942. Procarcinogenic effect of biotin in butter yellow tumor formation. *Science* 95: 174–176.

Eakes, B. D. and Blumer, T. N. 1975. Effect of various levels of potassium nitrate and sodium nitrite on color and flavor of cured loins and country-style hams. *J. Food Sci.* 40: 977–980.

Eckey, E. W. and Miller, L. P. 1954. *Vegetable Fats and Oils.* American Chemical Society Monograph No. 123. Reinhold, New York.

Ederer, F., Leren, P., Turpeinen, O. and Frantz, I. D. 1971. Cancer among men on cholesterol-lowering diets. *Lancet* 2: 203–206.

Engel, R. W. and Copeland, D. H. 1952. The influence of dietary casein level on tumor induction with 2-acetylaminofluorene. *Cancer Res.* 12: 905–908.

Falin, L. I. and Anissimore, V. 1940. The pathogenesis of experimental tumor of the genital glands: Tumors in cocks caused by the injection of a solution of copper sulfate. *Bull. Biol. Med. Exp.* 9: 519–520. (French)

Fan, T. Y. and Tannenbaum, S. R. 1973. Natural inhibitors of nitrosation reactions: The concept of available nitrite. *J. Food Sci.* 38: 1067–1069.

Fare, G. 1964. The protective effects of beef and yeast extracts and copper acetate in the diet against rat liver carcinogenesis by 4-dimethylaminoazobenzene. *Br. J. Cancer* 18: 782–791.

Fare, G. 1965. Copper acetate as an accelerator in mouse skin carcinogenesis by 9,10-dimethyl-1,2-benzanthracene. *Experientia* 21: 415–416.

Fare, G. and Howell, J. S. 1964. The effect of dietary copper on rat carcinogenesis by 3-methoxy dyes. I. Tumors induced at various sites by feeding 3-methoxy-4-aminoazobenzene and its N-methyl derivative. *Cancer Res.* 24: 1279–1283.

Fare, G. and Woodhouse, D. L. 1963. The effect of copper acetate on biochemical changes induced in the rat liver by p-dimethylaminoazobenzene. *Br. J. Cancer* 27: 512–523.

Felix, E. L., Loyd, B. and Cohen, M. H. 1975. Inhibition of the growth and development of a transplantable murine melanoma by vitamin A. *Science* 189: 886–888.

Fiddler, W., Pensabene, J. W. and Piotrowski, E. G. 1973. Use of sodium ascorbate or erythorbate to inhibit formation of N-nitrosodimethylamine in frankfurters. *J. Food Sci.* 38: 1084–1085.

Fisher, B. and Fisher, E. R. 1961. Experimental studies of factors influencing hepatic metastases. VI. Effects of nutrition. *Cancer* 14: 547–554.

Food and Nutrition Board NAS-NRC. 1970. Zinc in human nutrition. Food and Nutrition Board, National Academy of Sciences-National Research Council, Washington, D.C.

Furst, A. and Haro, R. T. 1969. A survey of metal carcinogenesis. *Prog. Exp. Tumor Res.* 12: 102–133.

Gailani, S. D., Holland, J. F., Nussbaum, A. and Olson, K. B. 1968. Clinical and biochemical studies of pyridoxine deficiency in patients with neoplastic diseases. *Cancer* 21: 975–988.

Gammal, E. B., Carroll, K. K. and Plunkett, E. R. 1967. Effects of dietary fat on mammary carcinogenesis by 7,12-dimethylbenz(a)anthracene in rats. *Cancer Res.* 27: 1737–1742.

Gammal, E. B., Carroll, K. K. and Plunkett, E. R. 1968. Effects of dietary fat on the uptake and clearance of 7,12-dimethylbenz(alpha)anthracene by rat mammary tissue. *Cancer Res.* 28: 384–385.

Genta, V. M. et al. 1974. Vitamin A deficiency enhances binding of benzo(a)pyrene to tracheal epithelial DNA. *Nature* 247: 48–49.

Gilman, J. P. W. and Ruckenbauer, G. M. 1962. Metal carcinogenesis. I. Observations on the carcinogenicity of a refinery dust, cobalt oxide, and colloidal thorium dioxide. *Cancer Res.* 22: 152–157.

Good, R. A. and Finstad, J. 1968. Essential relationship between the lymphoid system, immunity and malignancy. *Natl. Cancer Inst. Monogr.* 31: 41–58.

Graham, G. G. 1971. Human copper deficiency. *N. Engl. J. Med.* 285: 857–858.

Gray, J. I. and Dugan, L. R., Jr. 1975. Inhibition of N-nitrosamine formation in model food systems. *J. Food Sci.* 40: 981–984.

Griffin, A. C. and Bauman, C. A. 1946. Effect of certain azo dyes upon storage of riboflavin in the liver. *Arch. Biochem.* 11: 467–476.

Griffin, A. C. and Bauman, C. A. 1948. Hepatic riboflavin and tumor formation in rats fed azo dyes in various diets. *Cancer Res.* 8: 279–284.

Gunn, A., Gould, T. C. and Anderson, W. A. D. 1963. Cadmium-induced interstitial cell tumors in rats and mice and their prevention by zinc. *J. Natl. Cancer Inst.* 31: 745–759.

Guthrie, J. 1964. Observations on the zinc-induced testicular teratomas of fowl. *Br. J. Cancer* 18: 130–142.

Guthrie, J. 1967. Specificity of the metallic ion in the experimental induction of tertomas in the fowl. *Br. J. Cancer* 21: 619–622.

Haber, L. and Wissler, R. W. 1962. Effect of vitamin E on carcinogenicity of methylcholanthrene. *Proc. Soc. Exp. Biol.* 111: 774–775.

Haddow, A. 1975. Professor Tomizo Yoshida. In: *Recent Topics in Chemical Carcinogenesis.* S. Odashima, S. Takayama and H. Sato (eds.). Gann Monograph on Cancer Research No. 17. University Park Press, Baltimore.

Haenszel, W. et al. 1973. Large bowel cancer in Hawaiian Japanese. *J. Natl. Cancer Inst.* 51: 1765–1779.

Harman, D. 1971. Free radical theory of aging: Effect of the amount and degree of unsaturation of dietary fat on mortality rate. *J. Gerontol.* 26: 451–457.

Harr, J. R. et al. 1967. Selenium toxicity in rats. II. Histopathology. In: *Selenium in Biomedicine.* O. H. Muth (ed.). AVI, Westport, Connecticut.

Harris, P. N., Krahl, M. E. and Clowes, G. H. A. 1947. Effect of biotin upon p-dimethylaminoazobenzene carcinogenesis. *Cancer Res.* 7: 176–177.

Heath, J. C. 1956. The production of malignant tumours by cobalt in the rat. *Br. J. Cancer* 10: 668–673.

Hecker, E., Jarczyk, H. and Meyer, H. 1965. On the effect of Croton oils. II. A systematic fractionation of Croton oil. *Z. Krebsforsch.* 66: 478–490.

Herring, H. K. 1973. Effect of nitrite and other factors on the physico-chemical characteristics of nitrosamine formation in bacon. In: Proceedings of Meat Industry Research Conference, Chicago, March 1973, American Meat Institute, Washington, D.C.

Hirayama, T. 1979. Diet and cancer. *Nutr. Cancer* 1: 67−81.

Holly, F. W., Peel, E. W., Mozingo, R. and Folkers, K. 1950. Studies on carcinolytic compounds. 1. 6,7-Dichloro-9-(1'-D-sorbityl) isoalloxazine. *J. Am. Chem. Soc.* 72: 5416−5418.

Holtzman, J. L., Gram, T. E., Gigon, P. L. and Gillette, J. R. 1968. The distribution of the components of mixed-function oxidase between the rough and the smooth endoplasmic reticulum of liver cells. *Biochem. J.* 110: 407−412.

Hopkins, G. W., West, C. E. and Hard, G. C. 1976. Effect of dietary fats on the incidence of 7,12-dimethylbenz(a)anthracene-induced tumors in rats. *Lipids* 11: 328−333.

Horwitt, M. K. et al. 1949. Effect of dietary depletion of riboflavin. *J. Nutr.* 39: 357−373.

Howell, M. A. 1975. Diet as an etiological factor in the development of cancers of the colon and rectum. *J. Chron. Dis.* 28: 67−80.

Hui, Y. H., DeOme, K. B. and Briggs, G. M. 1971. Inhibition of transformation of mammary preneoplastic nodules to tumors in C3H mice fed phenylalanine-deficient diet. *J. Natl. Cancer Inst.* 47: 245−251.

Hultin, T. and Arrhenius, E. 1965. Effect of carcinogenic amines on amino acid incorporation by liver systems. III. Inhibition by aminofluorene treatment and its dependence on vitamin E. *Cancer Res.* 25: 124−131.

Huseby, R. A., Ball, Z. B. and Visscher, M. B. 1945. Further observations on the influence of single caloric restriction on mammary cancer incidence and related phenomenon in C3H mice. *Cancer Res.* 5: 40−46.

Jaffe, W. 1946. Influence of wheat germ oil on production of tumors in rats by methylcholanthrene. *Exp. Med. Surg.* 4: 278−282.

Jose, D. G. 1973. The cancer connection with immunity and nutrition. *Nutr. Today* 8(2): 4−9.

Jose, D. G. and Good, R. A. 1973. Quantitative effects of nutritional essential amino acid deficiency upon immune responses to tumors in mice. *J. Exp. Med.* 137: 1−9.

Jung, L. and Morand, P. 1962. Presence of pyrene, 1,2-benzopyrene and 3,4-benzopyrene in different vegetable oils. *Compt. Rend.* 254(8): 1489−1491.

Kahn, R. H. 1954. Effect of oestrogen and of vitamin A on vaginal cornification in tissue culture. *Nature* 174: 317.

Kasirsky, G., Gautieri, R. F. and Mann, D. E., Jr. 1965. Effect of cobaltous chloride on the minimal carcinogenic dose of methylcholanthrene in albino mice. *J. Pharm. Sci.* 54: 491−493.

Kaunitz, H. and Johnson, R. E. 1973. Exacerbation of heart and liver lesions in rats by feeding of various mildly oxidized fats. *Lipids* 8: 329−336.

Kensler, C. J. 1947. Effect of diet on the production of liver tumors in the rat by N,N-dimethyl-p-aminoazobenzene. *Ann. N.Y. Acad. Sci.* 49: 29−40.

Kensler, C. J., Suguria, K. and Rhoads, C. P. 1940. Coenzyme 1 and riboflavin content of livers of rats fed butter yellow. *Science* 91: 623.

King, J. T., Casas, C. B. and Visscher, M. B. 1951. The estrous behavior and mammary cancer incidence in ovariectomized C3H mice in relation to caloric intake. *Cancer Res.* 11: 712−715.

Kitsmanyuk, Z. D. 1967. Riboflavin content in the blood and urine in patients with cancer of the larynx in dynamics. *Zn. Ushnykh, Nosovykh Gorlovykh, boleznei* 28: 80−83. (Russian)

Kline, B. E., Rusch, H. P., Baumann, C. A. and Lavik, P. S. 1943. The effect of pyridoxine on tumor growth. *Cancer Res.* 3: 825−829.

Kline, B. E., Miller, J. A. and Rusch, H. P. 1945. Certain effects of egg white and biotin on carcinogenicity of p-dimethylaminoazobenzene in rats fed sub-protective level of riboflavin. *Cancer Res.* 5: 641–643.

Kline, B. E., Miller, J. A., Rusch, H. P. and Baumann, C. A. 1946. Carcino-genicity of p-dimethylaminoazobenzene in diets containing the fatty acids of hydrogenated coconut oil or of corn oil. *Cancer Res.* 6: 1–4.

Korpassy, B. 1959. The hepatocarcinogenicity of tannic acid. *Cancer Res.* 19: 501–504.

Kraybill, H. F. 1963. Symposium on chemical carcinogenesis. II. Carcinogenesis associated with foods, food additives, food degradation products, and related dietary factors. *Clin. Pharmacol. Ther.* 4: 73–87.

Lambooy, J. P. 1970. Riboflavin and azo dye induced hepatomas in rat. *Fed. Proc.* 29: 296.

Lane, M. 1971. Induced riboflavin deficiency in treatment of patients with lymphomas and polycythemia vera. *Proc. Am. Assoc. Cancer Res.* 12: 85.

Lane, M. et al. 1964. The rapid induction of human riboflavin deficiency with gal-actoflavin. *J. Clin. Invest.* 43: 357–373.

Lasnitzki, I. 1961. Effect of excess vitamin A on the normal and oestrone-treated mouse vagina grown in chemically defined medium. *Exp. Cell Res.* 24: 37–45.

Lea, A. J. 1966. Dietary factors associated with death rates from certain neoplasms in man. *Lancet* 2: 332–333.

Lemonnier, F. J., Scotto, J. M. and Thuong-Trieu, C. 1975. Influence of riboflavin on distribution in tryptophan metabolism and hepatoma production after a single dose of aflatoxin B_1. *J. Natl. Cancer Inst.* 55: 1085–1087.

Levij, I. S. and Polliack, M. B. 1968. Potentiating effect of vitamin A on 9,10-dimethyl-1,2-benzanthracene carcinogenesis in the hamster cheek pouch. *Cancer* 22: 300–306.

Lilienfeld, A. M. 1956. Relationship of cancer of female breast to artificial meno-pause and marital status. *Cancer* 9: 927–934.

Loeb, L. 1940. The significance of hormones in the origin of cancer. *J. Natl. Cancer Inst.* 1: 169–195.

Lorincz, A. B., Kuttner, R. E. and Ryan, W. L. 1968. Essential amino acid re-stricted diets and tumor inhibition. *J. Reprod. Med.* 1: 461–475.

Lorincz, A. B., Kuttner, R. E. and Brandt, M. B. 1969. Tumor response to phenylalanine-tyrosine-limited diets. *J. Am. Diet. Assoc.* 54: 198–205.

Lucey, J. A. and Dingle, J. T. 1964. Fat soluble vitamins and biological membranes. *Nature* 204: 156–160.

McCreary, P. A., Battifora, H. A. and Laing, G. H. 1966. Protective effect of mag-nesium deficiency on experimental allergic encephalomyelitis in the rat. *Proc. Soc. Exp. Biol. Med.* 121: 1130–1133.

McLean, A. E. and Magee, P. N. 1970. Increased renal carcinogenesis by dimethyl nitrosamine in protein deficient rats. *Br. J. Exp. Pathol.* 51: 589–590.

McMichael, H. 1965. Inhibition of growth of Shope rabbit papilloma by hypervita-minosis A. *Cancer Res.* 25: 947–955.

Meltzer, M. S., Cohen, B. E. 1974. Tumor suppression by mycobacterium bovis (strain BCG) enhanced by vitamin A. *J. Natl. Cancer Inst.* 53: 585–587.

Mettlin, C. and Graham, S. 1979. Dietary risk factors in human bladder cancer. *Am. J. Epidemiol.* 110: 255–263.

Mettlin, C., Graham, S., Rzepka, T. and Swanson, M. 1979a. Vitamin A in human bladder cancer. *Am. J. Epidemiol.* 110: 353.

Mettlin, C., Graham, S. and Swanson, M. 1979b. Vitamin A and lung cancer. *J. Natl. Cancer Inst.* 62: 1435–1438.

Michael, W. R., Alexander, J. C. and Artman, N. R. 1966. Thermal reactions of methyl linoleate. I. Heating conditions, isolation techniques, biological studies and chemical changes. *Lipids* 1: 353–358.

Mihich, E. and Nichol, C. A. 1959. The effect of pyridoxine deficiency on mouse sarcoma 180. *Cancer Res.* 19: 279–284.

Mihich, E., Rosen, F. and Nichol, C. A. 1959. The effect of pyridoxine deficiency on a spectrum of mouse and rat tumors. *Cancer Res.* 19: 1244–1248.

Miller, J. A. and Baumann, C. A. 1945. The determination of p-dimethylaminoazobenzene, p-monomethylaminoazobenzene, and p-aminoazobenzene in tissue. *Cancer Res.* 5: 157–161.

Miller, E. C. and Miller, J. A. 1952. Symposium on immunogenetics and carcinogenesis; in vivo combinations between carcinogens and tissue constituents and their possible role in carcinogenesis. *Cancer Res.* 12: 547–556.

Miller, J. A. and Miller, E. C. 1953. The carcinogenic aminoazo dyes. *Adv. Cancer Res.* 1: 339–396.

Miller, J. A. and Miller, E. C. 1969. Metabolic activation of carcinogenic aromatic amines and amides via N-hydroxylation and N-hydroxyesterification and its relationship to ultimate carcinogen as electrophilic reactants. In: *The Jerusalem Symposia on Quantum Chemistry and Biochemistry, Physico-chemical Mechanisms of Carcinogenesis.* Vol. I. E. D. Bergmann and B. Pullman (eds.). Israel Academy of Sciences and Humanities, Jerusalem, Israel.

Miller, J. A., Kline, B. E., Rusch, H. P. and Baumann, C. A. 1944. Carcinogenicity of p-dimethylaminoazobenzene in diets containing hydrogenated coconut oil. *Cancer Res.* 4: 153–158.

Miller, J. A., Miller, E. C. and Baumann, C. A. 1945. On methylation and demethylation of certain carcinogenic azo dyes in rat. *Cancer Res.* 5: 162–168.

Mirvish, S. S. 1975. Blocking the formation of N-nitroso compounds with ascorbic acid in vitro and in vivo. *Ann. N.Y. Acad. Sci.* 258: 175–180.

Mirvish, S. S. and Shubik, P. 1974. Ascorbic acid and nitrosamines. *Nature* 250: 684.

Mirvish, S. S., Cardesa, A., Wallcave, L. and Shubik, P. 1973. Effect of sodium ascorbate on lung adenoma induction by amines plus nitrite. *Proc. Am. Assoc. Cancer Res.* 14: 102.

Mori, S. 1922. Changes in the para-ocular glands which follow the administration of diets low in fat-soluble A; with notes of the effect of the same diets on the salivary glands and the mucosa of the larynx and trachea. *Bull. Hopkins Hosp.* 33: 357–359.

Morris, H. P. 1945. Ample exercise and a minimum of food as measures for cancer prevention? *Science* 101: 457–459.

Morris, H. P. 1947. Effects on the genesis and growth of tumors associated with vitamin intake. *Ann. N.Y. Acad. Sci.* 49: 119–140.

Morris, H. P. and Lippincott, S. W. 1941. The effect on growth of the spontaneous mammary carcinoma in female C3H mice. *J. Natl. Cancer Inst.* 2: 47–54.

Morris, H. P. and Robertson, W. V. B. 1943. Growth rate and number of spontaneous mammary carcinomas and riboflavin concentration of liver, muscle, and tumor of C3H mice as influenced by dietary riboflavin. *J. Natl. Cancer Inst.* 3: 479–489.

Mueller, G. C. and Miller, J. A. 1953. The metabolism of methylated aminoazo dyes. II. Oxidative demethylation by rat liver homogenates. *J. Biol. Chem.* 202: 579–587.

Mulay, A. S. and O'Gara, R. W. 1968. Enhancing effect of a riboflavin analog on azo-dye carcinogenesis in rats. *J. Natl. Cancer Inst.* 40: 731–735.

Nelson, A. A., Fitzhugh, O. G. and Calvery, H. O. 1943. Liver tumors following cirrhosis caused by selenium in rats. *Cancer Res.* 3: 230–236.

Newark, H. L., Osadca, M. and Aranjo, M. 1974. Stability of ascorbate in bacon. *Food Technol.* 28: 28–31.

Newberne, P. M. and Rogers, A. E. 1973. Rat colon carcinomas associated with aflatoxin and marginal vitamin A. *J. Natl. Cancer Inst.* 50: 439–448.

O'Dell, B. L., Hardwick, B. C., Reynolds, G. and Savage, J. E. 1961. Connective tissue defect in the chick resulting from copper deficiency. *Proc. Soc. Exp. Biol. Med.* 108: 402–405.

Okuda, K. and Haruna, K. 1959. Changes of some flavin enzyme in the liver of rat during DAB carcinogenesis. *Gann* 51: 153−158.

Orten, A. U., Burn, C. G. and Smith, A. H. 1937. Effects of prolonged chronic vitamin A deficiency in rat, with special reference to ondontomas. *Proc. Soc. Exp. Biol. Med.* 36: 82−84.

Orzechowski, R. F., Gautieri, R. F. and Mann, D. E., Jr. 1965. Effect of sodium nitrite and p-aminopropiophenone on the minimal carcinogenic dose$_{50}$ of methylcholanthrene on mouse epidermis. *J. Pharm. Sci.* 54: 64−66.

Paine, A. J. and McLean, A. E. M. 1973. The effect of dietary protein and fat on the activity of aryl hydrocarbon hydroxylase in rat liver, kidney and lung. *Biochem. Pharmacol.* 22: 2875−2880.

Patterson, D. S. 1971. Hydroxylation and toxicity of aflatoxins. *Biochem. J.* 125: 19−20.

Patterson, D. S. 1973. Metabolism as a factor in determining the toxic action of the aflatoxins in different animal species. *Food Cosmet. Toxicol.* 11: 287−294.

Pearce, M. L. and Dayton, S. 1971. Incidence of cancer in men on a diet high in polyunsaturated fat. *Lancet* 1: 464−467.

Pipkin, G. E., Nishimura, R., Banowsky, L. and Schlegel, J. U. 1967. Stabilization of urinary 3-hydroxyanthranilic acid by oral administration of L-ascorbic acid. *Proc. Soc. Exp. Biol. Med.* 162: 702−704.

Pipkin, G. E., Schlegel, J. U., Nishimura, R. and Schultz, G. N. 1969. Inhibitory effect of ascorbate on tumor formation in urinary bladders implanted with 3-hydroxyanthranilic acid. *Proc. Soc. Exp. Biol. Med.* 131: 522−524.

Polliack, A. and Levij, I. S. 1969. The effect of topical vitamin A on papillomas and intraepithelial carcinomas induced in hamster cheek pouches with 9,10-dimethyl-1,2-benzanthracene. *Cancer Res.* 29: 327-332.

Prasad, A. S. 1966. *Zinc Metabolism*. Thomas, Springfield, Illinois.

Prasad, A. S. et al. 1963. Zinc metabolism in patients with the syndrome of iron deficiency anemia, hepatosplenomegaly, dwarfism, and hypogonadism. *J. Lab. Clin. Med.* 61: 537−549.

Prutkin, L. 1968. The effect of vitamin A acid on tumorigenesis and protein production. *Cancer Res.* 28: 1021−1030.

Prutkin, L. 1975. Inhibition of tumorigenesis by topical application of low doses of vitamin A acid and fluorouracil. *Experientia* 31: 494.

Raineri, R. and Weisburger, J. H. 1975. Reduction of gastric carcinogens with ascorbic acid. *Ann. N.Y. Acad. Sci.* 258: 181−189.

Rettura, G. et al. 1975. Antitumor action of vitamin A in mice inoculated with adenocarcinoma cells. *J. Natl. Cancer Inst.* 54: 1489−1491.

Riley, V. 1975. Mouse mammary tumors: alteration of incidence as apparent function of stress. *Science* 189: 465−467.

Riviere, M. R., Chouroulenkov, I. and Guerin, M. 1960. The production of tumours by means of intra-testicular injections of zinc chloride in the rat. *Bull. Assoc. franc. Cancer* 47: 55−87.

Rivlin, R. S. 1970. Medical progress: Riboflavin metabolism. *N. Engl. J. Med.* 283: 463−472.

Rivlin, R. S., Menendez, C. E. and Langdon, R. G. 1968. Biochemical similarities between hypothyroidism and riboflavin deficiency. *Endocrinology* 83: 461−469.

Rivlin, R. S., Hornibrook, R. and Osnos, M. 1973. Effects of riboflavin deficiency upon concentrations of riboflavin, flavin mononucleotide and flavin adenine dinucleotide in Novikoff hepatoma in rats. *Cancer Res.* 33: 3019−3023.

Roe, R. J. and Field, W. E. 1967. Chronic toxicity of essential oils and certain other products of natural origin. *Food Cosmet. Toxicol.* 3: 311−324.

Rogers, A. E. and Newberne, P. M. 1975. Dietary effects in chemical carcinogenesis in animal models for colon and liver tumors. Paper presented at the Conference on "Nutrition in the Causation of Cancer." Key Biscayne, Florida, May 1975.

Rogers, A. E., Herndon, B. J. and Newberne, P. M. 1973. Induction by dimethyl-hydrazine of intestinal carcinoma in normal rats and rats fed high or low levels of vitamin A. *Cancer Res.* 33: 1003—1009.

Rose, G. et al. 1974. Colon cancer and blood cholesterol. *Lancet* 1: 181—183.

Rosen, F. and Nichol, C. A. 1962. Inhibition of the growth of an amethpterin-refractory tumor by dietary restriction of folic acid. *Cancer Res.* 22: 495—500.

Ross, M. H. and Bras, G. 1965. Tumor incidence patterns and nutrition in the rat. *J. Nutr.* 87: 245—260.

Ross, M. H. and Bras, G. 1971. Lasting influence of early caloric restriction on prevalence of neoplasms in rats. *J. Natl. Cancer Inst.* 47: 1095—1113.

Ross, M. H., Bras, G. and Ragbeer, M. S. 1970. Influence of protein and caloric intake upon spontaneous tumor incidence of the anterior pituitary gland of the rat. *J. Nutr.* 100: 177—189.

Rowe, N. H., Grammer, F. C., Watson, F. R. and Nickerson, N. H. 1970. A study of environmental influence upon salivary gland neoplasia in rats. *Cancer* 26: 436—444.

Rumack, B. H., Holtzman, J. and Chase, H. P. 1973. Hepatic drug metabolism and protein malnutrition. *J. Pharmacol. Exp. Ther.* 186: 441—446.

Rustia, M. 1975. Inhibitory effect of sodium ascorbate on ethylurea and sodium nitrite carcinogenesis and negative findings in progeny after intestinal inoculation of precursors into pregnant hamsters. *J. Natl. Cancer Inst.* 55: 1389—1394.

Ryan, W. L., Elliot, J. A. 1968. Fluorophenylalanine inhibition of tumors in mice on a phenylalanine-deficient diet. *Arch. Biochem. Biophys.* 125: 797—802.

Saffioti, U., Montesano, R., Sellakumar, A. R. and Borg, S. A. 1967. Experimental cancer of the lung. Inhibition by vitamin A of the induction of tracheobronchial squamous metaplasia and squamous cell tumors. *Cancer* 20: 857—864.

Salmon, W. D. and Newberne, P. M. 1963. Occurrence of hepatomas in rats fed diets containing peanut meal as a major source of protein. *Cancer Res.* 23: 571—575.

Salmon, W. D., Copeland, D. H. and Burns, M. J. 1955. Hepatomas in choline deficiency. *J. Natl. Cancer Inst.* 15: 1549—1568.

Santisteban, G. A. and Dougherty, T. F. 1954. Comparison of the influences of adrenocortical hormones on growth and involution of lymphatic organs. *Endocrinology* 54: 130—146.

Saxton, J. A., Jr., Boon, M. C. and Furth, J. 1944. Spontaneous leukemia in mice by underfeeding. *Cancer Res.* 4: 401—409.

Schaefer, A. E., Copeland, D. H., Salmon, W. D. and Hale, O. M. 1950. The influence of riboflavin, pyridoxine, inositol, and protein depletion-repletion upon the induction of neoplasms by choline deficiency. *Cancer Res.* 10: 786—792.

Schlegel, J. U. 1975. Proposed uses of ascorbic acid in prevention of bladder carcinoma. *Ann. N.Y. Acad. Sci.* 258: 432—437.

Schlegel, J. U., Pipkin, G. E. and Shultz, G. N. 1969. The aetiology of bladder tumors. *Br. J. Urol.* 41: 718—723.

Schlegel, J. U., Pipkin, G. E. and Nishimura, R. 1970. The role of ascorbic acid in the prevention of bladder tumor formation. *J. Urol.* 103: 155—159.

Scotto, J. M., Stralin, H. G., Lageron, A. and Lemonnier, F. J. 1975. Influence of carbon tetrachloride or riboflavin on liver carcinogenesis with a single dose of aflatoxin B_1. *Br. J. Exp. Pathol.* 56: 133—138.

Seelig, M. S. 1972. Review: Relationships of copper and molybdenum to iron metabolism. *Am. J. Clin Nutr.* 25: 1022—1037.

Seifter, E., Zisblatt, M., Levine, N. and Rettura, G. 1973. Inhibitory action of vitamin A on a murine sarcoma. *Life Sci.* 13: 945—952.

Selye, H. 1936. Thymus and adrenals in response to injuries and intoxications. *Br. J. Exp. Pathol.* 17: 234—248.

Sen, N. P. et al. 1976. Inhibition of nitrosamine formation in fried bacon by propyl gallate and L-ascorbylpalmitate. *J. Agric. Food Chem.* 24: 397—401.

Shamberger, R. J. 1969. Lysosomal enzyme changes in growing and regressing
    mammary tumours. *Biochem. J.* 111: 375—383.
Shamberger, R. J. 1970. Relation of selenium to cancer. I. Inhibitory effect of
    selenium on carcinogenesis. *J. Natl. Cancer Inst.* 44: 931—936.
Shamberger, R. J. 1971. Inhibitory effect of vitamin A on carcinogenesis. *J. Natl.
    Cancer Inst.* 47: 667—673.
Shamberger, R. J. and Frost, D. V. 1969. Possible protective effect of selenium
    against human cancer. *Can. Med. Assoc. J.* 100: 682.
Shapiro, D. M. and Gellhorn, A. 1951. Combinations of chemical compounds in
    experimental cancer therapy. *Cancer Res.* 11: 35—41.
Shils, M. E. 1973. Nutrition and neoplasia. In: *Modern Nutrition in Health and
    Disease.* R. S. Goodhart and M. R. Shils (eds.). Lea & Febiger, Philadelphia.
Silverstone, H. and Tannenbaum, A. 1951a. Influence of dietary fat and riboflavin
    on formation of spontaneous hepatomas in mouse. *Cancer Res.* 11: 200—203.
Silverstone, H. and Tannenbaum, A. 1951b. Proportion of dietary protein and form-
    ation of spontaneous hepatomas in mouse. *Cancer Res.* 11: 442—446.
Smith, P. G. and Jick, A. 1978. Cancers among users of preparations containing
    vitamin A: A case control investigation. *Cancer* 42: 808—811.
Smith, W. E., Yazdi, E., Miller, L. 1972. Carcinogenesis in pulmonary epithelia in
    mice on different levels of vitamin A. *Environ. Res.* 5: 152—163.
Smith, D. M., Rogers, A. E., Herndorn, B. J. and Newbern, P. M. 1975. Vitamin
    A (retinyl acetate) and benzo(a)pyrene-induced respiratory tract carcinogenesis
    in hamsters fed a commercial diet. *Cancer Res.* 35: 11—16.
Society of Actuaries. 1959. *Build and Blood Press Study.* Vol. 1. Society of
    Actuaries, Chicago.
Spitznagel, J. K. and Allison, A. C. 1970. Mode of action of adjuvants. Retinol and
    other lysosome-labilizing agents as adjuvants. *J. Immunol.* 104: 119—127.
Sporn, M. B. and Dingman, C. W. 1966. 2-Acetaminofluorene and 3-methylcholan-
    threne: differences in binding to rat liver deoxyribonucleic acid in vivo.
    Nature 210: 531—532.
Stanton, M. F. 1967. Primary tumors of bone and lungs in rats following local de-
    position of cupria-chelated N-hydroxy-2-acetylaminofluorene. *Cancer Res.* 27:
    1000—1006.
Stevenson, E. S., Dobriner, K. and Rhoads, C. P. 1942. The metabolism of di-
    methylaminoazobenzene (butter yellow) in rats. *Cancer Res.* 2: 160—167.
Stoerk, H. C. 1947. The regression of lymphosarcoma in plants in pyridoxine-
    deficient mice. *J. Biol. Chem.* 171: 437—438.
Stoerk, H. C. and Emerson, G. A. 1949. Complete regression of lymphosarcoma
    implants following temporary induction of riboflavin deficiency in mice. *Proc.
    Soc. Exp. Biol. Med.* 70: 703—704.
Subcommittee on Selenium. 1971. *Selenium in Nutrition.* Committee on animal nutri-
    tion, Agricultural Board and National Research Council, National Academy of
    Sciences, Washington, D.C.
Sugai, M., Witting, L. A., Tsuchiyama, H. and Kummerow, F. A. 1962. The ef-
    fect of heated fat on the carcinogenic activity of 2-acetylaminofluorene. *Cancer
    Res.* 22: 510—519.
Swann, P. F. and McLean, A. E. M. 1971. The effect of a protein-free high-
    carbohydrate diet on the metabolism of dimethylnitrosamine in the rat. *Biochem.
    J.* 124: 283—288.
Tannenbaum, A. 1942. The genesis and growth of tumors. III. Effects of a high fat
    diet. *Cancer Res.* 2: 468—475.
Tannenbaum, A. 1944. The dependence of the genesis of induced skin tumors on the
    caloric intake during different stages of carcinogenesis. *Cancer Res.* 4: 683—
    687.
Tannenbaum, A. 1959. Nutrition and cancer. in: *Physiopathology of Cancer.*
    2nd ed. F. Homburger (ed.). Hoeber-Harper, New York.

Tannenbaum, A. and Silverstone, H. 1950. Failure to inhibit the formation of mammary carcinoma in mice by intermittent fasting. *Cancer Res.* 10: 577–579.

Tannenbaum, A. and Silverstone, H. 1957. Nutrition and the genesis of tumours. In: *Cancer.* Vol. 1. R. W. Raven (ed.). Butterworth, London.

Taub, R. N., Krantz, A. R. and Dresser, D. W. 1970. The effect of localized injection of adjuvant material on the draining lymph node. *Immunology.* 18: 171–186.

Theuer, R. C. 1971. Effect of essential amino acid restriction on the growth of female $C_{57}B1$ mice and their implanted BW10232 adenocarcinomas. *J. Nutr.* 101: 223–232.

Thomas, J. A. and Thiery, J. P. 1953. Induced production of liposarcoma in rabbits with the trace elements zinc and cobalt. *C. R. Acad. Sci.* 236: 1387–1389.

Tscherkes, L. A., Volgarev, M. N. and Aptekar, S. G. 1963. Selenium-caused tumors. *Acta Un. Int. Cancer* 19: 632–633.

Tung, T. C. and Lin, J. K. 1964. The interaction of riboflavin with 4-dimethylaminoazobenzene and 4-aminoazobenzene. *J. Formosa Med. Assoc.* 63: 225–233.

Tupper, R., Watts, R. W. E. and Normall, A. 1955. The incorporation of ^{65}Zn in mammary tumours and some other tissues of mice after injection of the isotope. *Biochem. J.* 59: 264–268.

Vallee, B. L. 1959. Biochemistry, physiology and pathology of zinc. *Physiol. Rev.* 39: 443–490.

Wagner, A. F. and Folkers, K. 1964. Vitamins and coenzymes. Interscience, New York.

Wald, N., Idle, M., Boreham, J. J. and Bailey, A. 1980. Low serum-vitamin A and subsequent risk of cancer. *Lancet* 2: 813–815.

Walpole, A. L. 1951. Walker carcinoma 256 in screening of tumour inhibitors. *Br. J. Pharmacol.* 6: 135–143.

Warwick, G. P. 1971. Metabolism of liver carcinogens and other factors influencing liver cancer induction. In: *Liver Cancer.* International Agency of Research on Cancer, World Health Organization, Lyon.

Weisburger, J. H. 1973. Chemical carcinogens and their mode of action in colonic neoplasia. *Dis. Colon Rectum* 16: 431–437.

Weisburger, J. H. 1975. Dietary factors and cancer of the large bowel. Paper presented at the Conference on "Nutrition in the Causation of Cancer." Key Biscayne, Florida, May 1975.

Weissman, G. 1964. Labilization and stabilization of lysosomes. *Fed. Proc.* 23: 1038–1044.

Weissman, G., Hirschhorn, R. and Pras, M. 1967. Studies of lysosomes. 8. The effect of polyene antibiotics on lysosomes. *Biochem. Pharmacol.* 16: 1057–1069.

White, J. W., Jr. 1975. Relative significance of dietary sources of nitrate and nitrite. *J. Agric. Food Chem.* 23: 886–891.

Wilens, S. L. and Sproul, E. E. 1936. Spontaneous leukemia in the rat. *Am. J. Pathol.* 12: 249–275.

Williams, J. R., Jr., Grantham, P. H., Yamamoto, R. S. and Weisburger, J. H. 1970. Effect of dietary riboflavin on azo dye reductase in liver and bacterial contents in rats. *Biochem. Pharmacol.* 19: 2523–2525.

Winick, M. and Noble, A. 1966. Cellular response in rats during malnutrition at various ages. *J. Nutr.* 89: 300–306.

Winick, M. and Noble, A. 1967. Cellular response with increased feeding in neonatal rats. *J. Nutr.* 91: 179–182.

Wolbach, S. B. and Howe, P. R. 1925. Tissue changes following deprivation of fat soluble A vitamin. *J. Exp. Med.* 47: 753–777.

Wynder, E. L. and Chan, P. C. 1970. The possible role of riboflavin deficiency in epithelial neoplasia. II. Effect of skin tumor development. *Cancer* 26: 1221–1224.

Wynder, E. L. and Klein, U. E. 1965. The possible role of riboflavin deficiency in epithelial neoplasia. I. Epithelial changes in mice in simple deficiency. *Cancer* 18: 167–180.

Wynder, E. L., Mabuchi, L. 1972. Etiological and preventive aspects of human cancer. *Prevent. Med.* 1: 300–334.

Wynder, E. L., Escher, G. and Mantal, N. 1966. An epidemiological investigation of cancer of the endometrium. *Cancer* 19: 487–520.

Wynder, E. L. et al. 1969. Environmental factors of cancer of the colon and rectum. II. Japanese epidemiological data. *Cancer* 23: 1210–1220.

Yang, W. K. and Sung, J. L. 1966. Riboflavin metabolism in liver diseases. IV. Enzymatic splitting and synthesis of flavin adenine dinucleotide in the p-dimethylaminoazobenzene induced rat liver carcinoma tissue. *J. Formosan Med. Assoc.* 65: 299–305.

Zannoni, V. G. and Sato, P. H. 1975. Interaction with drugs and environmental chemicals. Effects of ascorbic acid on microsomal drug metabolism. *Ann. N.Y. Acad. Sci.* 258: 119–131.

Zisblatt, M. and Lilly, F. 1972. The effect of immunosuppression on oncogenesis by murine sarcoma virus. *Proc. Soc. Exp. Biol. Med.* 141: 1036–1040.

Zisblatt, M., Hardy, G., Rettura, G. and Seifter, E. 1973. Partial inhibition of a murine sarcoma by vitamin A. *J. Nutr.* 103: Abst. No. 30, XXIV.

8

Endogenous Toxicants in Foods Derived from Higher Plants

Because products derived from higher plants comprise the bulk of the food for humanity, the existence of endogenous toxicants in these foodstuffs is a fundamental concern. Various types of toxic plant metabolites have been found and chemically characterized. There are also many other types of compounds present in plant foodstuffs that still need to be precisely identified. The presence of these toxicants in foods is suspected from the biological effects seen in animals or humans. Both acute and chronic toxicities following consumption of certain food products have been observed. In fact, many cases of poisonings from endogenous toxicants have been fatal or have led to prolonged and serious disabilities.

Certain toxicants are present in plant-derived foods at levels which pose no serious or immediate threat of acute toxicity. These substances may present toxic hazards, since it is possible, as shown by examples in this chapter, that chronic toxicity may occur from chronic consumption. It is, therefore, essential that these compounds be identified and quantified so that their significance to human health can be evaluated, and possibly, preventive or corrective measures can be instituted to minimize any toxic hazards.

CLASSIFICATION OF TOXIC PLANT METABOLITES IN FOOD

There appears to be no simple way of classifying toxic plant metabolites in food because of the many different types of compounds that this group comprises. Nevertheless, attempts have been made and these substances have been advantageously classified by: (1) common functional groups, e.g., plant phenols; (2) physiological actions, e.g., acetylcholinesterase inhibitors, stimulants, and so on; (3) type of toxin produced, e.g., cyanogenic glycosides; (4) type of disease produced, e.g., carcinogens, lathyrogens, and so on; and (5) effect on nutrients, e.g., antinutritives. The latter is a special group — their primary effect being to deprive the organism of the value of certain nutrients, and thus elicit nutritional deficiency symptoms depending on the conditions. This group of substances is discussed in Chapter 9.

Cyanogenic Glycosides

At least 1000 plant species from 90 families and 250 genera are reported to be cyanophoric (Dilleman 1958; Hegnauer 1963). The cyanide in plants exists in the bound form as a glycoside. At least 20 of such glycosides are known and have been positively identified in less than 50 species (Conn 1973). Most of these compounds are found in nonfood plants.

The cyanogenic glycoside molecule consists of a monosaccharide (glucose) or disaccharide (Gentiobiose or vicianose) and an β-hydroxynitrile. The glycoside breaks down to the sugar and the nitrile in the presence of β-glucosidase; the nitrile is similarly decomposed by a lyase to generate hydrogen cyanide, an aldehyde, ketone, or in rare instances, an acid.

$$\text{Sugar}-O(1)-\underset{R_2}{\overset{\overset{\displaystyle CN}{|}}{\underset{}{C}}}\overset{R_1}{\diagup} \quad \xrightarrow[\text{β-glucosidase}]{H_2O} \quad \text{Sugar} \; + \; \underset{R_2}{\overset{\overset{\displaystyle OH}{\diagdown}}{R_1}}-C-CN$$

$$\underset{R_2}{\overset{\overset{\displaystyle OH}{|}}{R_1}}-C-CN \quad \xrightarrow[]{\text{hydroxynitrile lyase}} \quad HCN + \underset{R_2}{\overset{}{R_1}}\diagup C{=}O$$

When R_1 and R_2 are different groups, the sugar moiety becomes attached to an asymmetric carbon and two diastereomers are produced.

β-Glucosidase and hydroxynitrile lyase are present in plant cells, possibly in specific organelles, and are released to act on the glycosides when the plant tissue is damaged. Damage to such tissues is inevitable when foodstuffs are prepared for consumption. The rate of HCN production following contact between the glycoside and enzymes depends on the particular product and the conditions. Maximal amounts of cyanide may be produced within 45 min at 37°C or 2 hr at 23°C (Viehoever 1940). In the cold, expectedly, greater yields may be obtained only after 24 hr (Winkler 1951).

Mammals appear to be unable to produce such enzymes endogenously, but intestinal bacteria may possess the necessary enzymes that hydrolyze the glycosides (Winkler 1958). There is evidence to indicate that intestinal bacteria in mammals can, in fact, hydrolyze these glycosides. For example, amygdalin is practically harmless to mice when injected, but highly toxic when given orally. This is evident from the intraperitoneal LD_{50} of >5000 mg/kg, compared to the oral LD_{50} of 300 mg/kg (Williams 1970). Furthermore, seven of 10 rats given 50 mg linamarine by stomach tube died. The rats completely absorbed the glycoside, of which 18.8% was excreted in the urine unchanged, and about 58% was metabolized to thiocyanate in 72 hr (Barrett et al. 1977). It also has been reported that lima beans high in cyanogens, which were boiled for 2.5 hr to destroy the glucosidase, still cause serious poisoning in human subjects, with symptoms of vomiting (Gabel and Kruger 1920). These subjects excreted cyanide in the urine. Other cases of human poisoning due to cooked lima beans have also been reported (Viehoever 1940). More convincingly, human fecal extracts and a strain of *Escherichia coli* that usually inhabits the human gastrointestinal tract were found to release significant amounts of HCN from cooked lima beans (Winkler 1951). Thus, the toxicity of orally administered cyanogenic glycosides appears to depend on hydrolytic activity of intestinal bacteria (Chap. 3).

Hydrochloride in the stomach cannot hydrolyze the glycoside to any significant degree (Montgomery 1964). In fact, in vitro tests show that even after 7 to 9 hr, hydrolysis at 100°C is incomplete, and at 60°C, acid hydrolysis of these compounds appears not to occur at all (Montgomery 1964; Viehoever 1940).

Table 8.1 lists seven cyanogenic glycosides in plant foodstuffs. There are three major types based on the sugar moiety: glucosides, vicianosides, and gentiobiosides. Most are glucosides which are found in sorghum, kaffir corn, cassava, and certain legumes. The cyanogen in the common vetch (*Vicia sativa*) and similar legumes is a vicianoside, whereas those of the rose family are gentiobiosides (Conn 1973, 1969; Dilleman 1958; Eyjolfsson 1970). Many edible legumes release cyanide, obviously from cyanogenic glycosides which have not been as yet characterized; e.g., Bengal gram

Table 8.1 Cyanogenic Glycosides in Foodstuffs (Conn 1973, 1979)

Glycosides	Aglycone	Sugar	Food found
Amygdalin	D-mandelonitrile	Gentiobiose	Rosaceae Prunus spp.: almonds, apple, apricot, cherry, peach, pear, plum, quince.
Dhurrin	L-p-hydroxymandelonitrile	D-Glucose	Sorghums, kaffir corns
Isolinamarin		D-Glucose	Cassava (Clapp et al. 1966)
Linamarin	α-hydroxyisobutyronitrile	D-Glucose	Lima beans (Phaseolus lunatus varieties); flax seed (Linum usitatissimum); cassava or manioc (Manihot spp.)
Lotoaustralin	α-Hydroxy-α-methylbutyronitrile	D-Glucose	Same as linamarin cassava (Bissett 1969)
Prunasin	D-Mandelonitrile	D-Glucose	Prunus spp. and other Rosaceae
Sambunigrin	L-Mandelonitrile	D-Glucose	Legumes; elderberry (Sambucus nigra)
Vicianin	D-Mandelonitrile	Vicianose	Common vetch (Vicia angustifolia), and other vicias

(*Cicer arietinum*) (Food Agricultural Organization 1959), fava beans (*Vicia fava*) (Cugudda et al. 1953), and others (Jaffe 1950). Many other cyanogenic glycosides have been identified in nonfood plant species.

Cyanogen Content (as HCN) in Foodstuffs Implicated in Human Poisonings

A dose of cyanide lethal to humans can easily be produced and exceeded by many cyanogenic foodstuffs. The reported lethal doses in humans are from 0.5 to 3.5 mg/kg body weight (Montgomery 1969), and the amounts of HCN produced by the Burmese (white variety), Puerto Rican (black variety), and Javanese (colored variety) lima beans are 210 mg (Kohn-Abrest 1906), 300 mg (Viehoever 1940) and 312 mg/100 g (Guignard 1907). Human and animal fatalities from consumption of these beans have been reported (Anonymous 1912; Auld 1912-1913; Viehoever 1940); in addition, there also have been numerous nonfatal poisonings from these foodstuffs (Montgomery 1969); this is particularly true with cassava and lima beans, as mentioned earlier. In this connection, American varieties of lima beans, even the colored Arizona variety, produce less than 20 mg HCN/100 g (Montgomery 1964; Viehoever 1940). Importation of lima beans into the United States is limited to products producing less than 20 mg HCN/100 g (Conn 1973).

Fresh cassava (Manihot spp.) cortex produces HCN anywhere from 1.0 to 60.0 mg or more per 100 g depending on the variety, source, period of harvest, field conditions, and so forth (Muthuswamy et al. 1976; Obigbesan and Fayemi 1976; Oke 1968). The amount of cyanide produced by cassava varies considerably with the variety. For example, 101 varieties of cassava examined by Raymond et al. (1941) gave cyanide values ranging from 16 to 434 mg/kg, with an average of 158 mg/kg for the whole tuber. While the bitter variety *(M. utilissima)* may be more cyanophoric than the sweet variety *(M. palmata,* or *M. aipi),* this is only a matter of morphological distribution. Boulos (1975) reported that both sweet and bitter cassava may contain relatively large amounts of glycoside, except that in the bitter variety the toxicant is more evenly distributed in the whole root, whereas in the sweet variety it is concentrated in the rind and outer cortical layers. For example, a Singapore sweet variety contains 20 mg/100 g in the cortex and 90 mg/100 g in the rind (Joachim and Pandittesekere 1944). In some other varieties, the rind may contain four to 10 times as much cyanide or more compared to the cortex (Muthuswamy et al. 1976; Wood 1965). Thus, the peeling of sweet cassava may render the product quite harmless. However, there may be sweet varieties in which the cyanogen may be found at relatively high levels throughout the root (Ketiku et al. 1978; Wood 1965).

The manner of preparation of cassava may also modify the cyanide content. For example, drying the root cortex may increase the cyanide content to as much as 245 mg/100 g (Collens 1915). A preparation called "purupuru" may contain some 32 to 48 mg HCN/100 g (Osuntokun 1968). However, local practices in cassava preparation may reduce the cyanide content even more, down to safe levels (Charavanapavan 1944; Descartes de Garcia; Paula and Rangel 1939; Ketiku et al. 1978).

Attention should be also directed to the leaves of cassava which are also eaten in some cultures. These leaves are also highly cyanogenic, containing as much as 78.6 mg HCN/100 g (Charavanapavan 1944).

Certain legume seeds, such as those of *Vicia sativa,* may also contain as much as 52 mg HCN/100 g (Montgomery 1964).

The young growth of sorghum *(Sorghum vulgare)* may also contain toxic levels of the cyanogen dhurrin. Values of as much as 0.2% have been reported. On germination, the seeds may contain from 3 to 5% dhurrin on a dry weight basis (Akazawa et al. 1960; Pinckney 1924).

Thus, while the cyanide contents of these foodstuffs vary depending on many endogenous and exogenous factors, in many instances these values may be within the range of lethal doses in humans. Furthermore, individual susceptibility may also vary, so that low doses which are innocuous to certain individuals may be deleterious to others (Clark 1936).

Symptoms of Cyanide Poisoning

Cyanide poisoning from cyanogenic glycoside may manifest in one of three forms: (1) acute poisoning, indicative of cytotoxic anoxia; (2) chronic poisoning, indicative of degenerative neuropathy; and (3) chronic poisoning, manifested by goitrogeny.

Acute Poisoning   As mentioned earlier in this section, deaths due to acute cyanide poisoning from consumption of lima beans (Anonymous 1912; Gabel and Kruger 1920; Viehoever 1940); manioc (Clark 1936; Oke 1968), and unripe sorghum (Clark 1936) have been reported. In addition, there have been reported fatalities, particularly among children, from eating bitter almonds (Cleland 1931; Pack et al. 1972); apricot kernels (Cleland 1931; Morbidity and Mortality Weekly Reports 1975); and apple seeds (Kingsbury 1964).

Acute cyanide poisoning is characterized by symptoms suggestive of cellular oxygen deprivation. Signs of poisoning begin initially with hyperventilation, headache, nausea, vomiting, general weakness, abdominal distention, and pain (Byam and Archibald 1921-1923; Worden 1940). Fatal doses produce, in addition, not only tachypnea and dyspnea, but also paralysis, convulsions, unconsciousness, respiratory arrest, and collapse (Stecher et al. 1960; Worden 1940). The sequence of symptoms may occur rapidly, terminating in death within 20 min or even much less (Worden 1940).

Unlike pure cyanide, the acute symptoms from ingesting cyanogenic foods may be delayed because of slower absorption for one reason or another (Montgomery 1965).

Free cyanide is absorbed rapidly in the gastrointestinal tract. Once in the cell, it binds reversibly to cytochrome a_3 in the cytochrome c oxidase complex. Therefore, the enzyme is unable to function in the electron transport chain. The tissues are thus unable to accept oxygen from the blood. Neuronal depression in the medullary centers leads to respiratory arrest and death (Scheffer et al 1970; Worden 1940). This binding can be reversed by hydroxycobalamin, since CN^- has a stronger affinity for cobalt in cyanocobalamin than the iron in cytochrome c oxidase (Vieira Lopes and Campello 1975).

Cyanide damages the brain consistent with the effect of cytotoxic anoxia, in common with similar agents (Reiders 1971). Under this condition, many areas of the brain are damaged, such as the corpora stricta, hippocampus, cortical gray matter, and the substantia nigra. Cyanide is especially damaging to the white matter, particularly the corpus callosum (Bass 1968; Hicks 1950; Levine et al. 1967). Oxygen deprivation by cyanide results in substantial metabolic changes in the brain cells (Estler 1965). Changes in the metachromatic material of the central nervous system (CNS) also has been observed (Ibrahim and Levine 1967).

Chronic Cyanide Poisoning Manifested by Degenerative Neuropathy Two types of neurological degenerative diseases have been described and linked to chronic cyanide poisoning from high consumption of cassava. One disease, tropical ataxic neuropathy, is endemic in some parts of Nigeria and Senegal (Monekosso and Wilson 1966; Osuntokun 1968, 1973, 1981; Osuntokun et al. 1969, 1970a,b; Williams and Osuntokun 1969). The disease is believed to be caused in part by the failure of the body to dispose of cyanide owing to cobalamin deficiency. Examination of the peripheral nerves of ataxic patients has revealed demyelination. Under the electron microscope two types of demyelinating processes are recognized: (1) disintegration and lysis of the myelin lamellae, and (2) presence of ovoid or myelin bodies inside macrophages, indicating digestion of myelin. The segmental demyelination of peripheral nerves is consistent with the fact that the axons of nerve fibers are unaffected. Even though these changes may not be considered as specific to cyanide-induced damage, chronic cyanide ingestion may indeed be a main cause of the disease. This contention is supported by the observed demyelination of rat sciatic nerve injected weeks earlier with cyanide. The damage is strikingly similar to that observed in ataxic patients.

Further evidence implicating chronic cyanide consumption as a cause of this neurological disorder is shown by the elevated thiocynate levels in the blood plasma and urine of patients with the disease. It is also noted that the levels of both free and bound cyanide are also markedly increased in these patients (Osuntokun et al. 1970b).

The other disease believed to be caused by chronic cyanide intoxication is called tropical amblyopia, a form of blindness which is common in countries in Western Africa (Clark 1936). It appears that this malady and related diseases may result from secondary cobalamin deficiency. Cobalamin has a high affinity for cyanide (Vieira Lopes and Campello 1975), and may be inactivated by the vitamin. Thus, hydroxycobalamin treatment of cases of tropical amblyopia may bring about improvement (Degazon 1956; Mclaren 1960). (A related disease, tobacco amblyopia, also thought to be due to poisoning from HCN in tobacco smoke, also has been treated effectively with hydroxycobalamin [Anonymous 1969; Heaton et al. 1958; Wilson et al. 1971].)

Chronic Poisoning Manifested by Goitrogeny As stated earlier, cyanide is also a goitrogen, since it is metabolized in the presence of the enzyme rhodanase to thiocyanate, a known goitrogen (Barrett et al. 1978; Greer et al. 1966; Vanderlaan and Vanderlaan 1947). Thus, the high consumption of dry unfermented cassava, which contains high levels of cyanogen, has been implicated in the widespread incidence of goiter in eastern Nigeria (Ekpechi et al. 1966) and other parts of Africa (Ermans et al. 1980).

The mechanism by which thiocyanate causes goiter has been clarified by Ermans and his colleagues (Delange and Ermans 1979; Ermans 1979). In their studies with both human subjects in Zaire and iodine-deficient rats, they found that prolonged consumption of cassava definitely causes changes in the adaptation mechanism of the thyroid gland in iodine deficiency. In this deficient condition, the adaptation mechanism ensures that the iodine uptake to the gland remains unchanged by increasing the unidirectional iodine clearance into the gland. Thus, even with high CNS level in the blood due to cassava consumption, the iodine uptake is unchanged. However, the abnormal CNS level causes a depression of iodine clearance by increasing the rate iodine leaves the gland, so that the CNS overload produces even more severe iodine deficiency, resulting in enhanced goiter formation. The adaptation mechanism explains the failure in past attempts to find evidence of the role of goitrogenic substances in food in goiter.

Detoxification of Cyanide

The enzyme rhodanase is widely distributed in tissues, with the highest activity being found in the liver (Himwich and Saunders 1948; Lang 1933a,b). This enzyme catalyzes the conversion of cyanide to thiocyanate ($-SCN$), contingent on the presence of sulfur, which is the limiting factor. For rapid detoxification of large amounts of cyanide, preformed thiosulfate is necessary (Chen et al. 1934; Gillman et al. 1946). Cysteine provides the necessary sulfur for detoxification of normal levels of cyanide. The amino acid is converted by transamination to 3-mercaptopyruvic acid, which donates its sulfur to cyanide in the presence of sulfur transferase (Fiedler and Wood 1956; Wood and Fiedler 1953) (Chap. 4).

Other pathways for cyanide detoxification involve the previously mentioned reaction with hydroxycobalamin (Smith 1961; Wokes 1952; Wokes and Pikard 1955), and the reaction with cystine to form cysteine and β-thiocyanoalanine (I) (Schobert and Hamm 1948; Voegtlin et al. 1926; Wood and Cooley 1956). The latter tantomerizes to 2-amino-thiazoline-4-carboxylic acid (II) or 2-imino-4-thiazolidine carboxylic acid (III).

These alternate pathways are probably of minor importance compared to the rhodanase or sulfur transferase mechanisms.

Vasoactive (Pressor) Amines

One of the main physiological actions of naturally occurring amines is vascular contraction or dilation; thus, these substances have marked effects on blood pressure.

Some of the known vasoactive or pressor amines found in plants are given in Table 8.2.

The banana fruit appears equipped for the enzymatic transformation of these amines. Thus, Deacon and Marsh (1971) found an enzyme capable of hydroxylating monophenols to diphenols and tyramine to dopamine. Nagatsu et al. (1972) found similar enzymes which hydroxylate tyrosine. The presence of such metabolites in banana pulp as metanephrine, normetanephrine, and methoxytryptamine (Kenyhercz and Kissinger 1978) suggest the presence of enzymes which reduce the toxicity of parent amines. In banana, dopamine is converted to salsolinol (1-methyl-6,7-dihyroxy-1,2,3,4-tetrahydroquinoline) by reaction with acetaldehyde (Riggin et al. 1976). The toxicological significance of this alkaloid, which increases in quantity during ripening (40 μg/g), is unknown.

Table 8.2   Vasoactive (Pressor) Amines in Fruits and Vegetables (mg/100 g fresh weight)

Amines	Avocado	Banana pulp	Eggplant	Orange	Red plum	Tomato (ripe)
Dopamine	0.4-0.5	66-70		0.1		
Epinephrine		<.25				
Norepinephrine		10.8				
Octopanine		0.37				
Serotonine	1.0	2.5-8.0	0.2		1.0	1.2
Tryptamine		0.12			0.2	0.4
Tryamine	2.3	6.5-9.4	0.3	1.0	0.6	0.4

				Pineapple			Plantain		
	Dates	Figs	Pawpaw	Grn	Ripe	Jce	Grn	Ripe	Ckd
Dopamine	<0.08	<0.02	0.1-0.2						
Epinephrine	<0.08	<0.02							
Norepinephrine	<0.08	<0.02					0.2	0.25	
Serotonine	0.9	1.3	0.1-0.2	5.0-6.0	2.0	2.5-3.5	2.0-6.0	4.0-10.0	4.7

	Blue plum	Potato
Norepinephrine		0.01-0.02
Tryptamine	0.5	
Tyramine		0.1

Abbreviations: Grn, Green; Jce, Juice; Ckd, Cooked
Source: Data compiled from Bruce 1961; Foy and Parratt 1960; Kenyhercz and Kissinger 1978; Marshall 1959; Stachelberger et al. 1977; and West 1959.

The amounts of amines listed in Table 8.2 may appear minimal. However, these compounds are highly active, so that if the amounts present in the quantity of foods normally eaten at one time were injected intravenously, disastrous consequences might be expected. The body is equipped with efficient detoxification mechanisms which render these substances innocuous. The amines are rapidly inactivated in the body by the mitochrondrial enzymes, the monoamine oxidases; these are present in many tissues. However, extreme cases of intoxications have been reported concerning persons taking monoamine oxidase inhibitors with amine-containing foods (Blackwell et al. 1967). This poisoning phenomenon is discussed in more detail in Chapter 21 on derived toxicants. In this connection, the effects of these amines can also be potentiated by hyperthyroidism because of the effects of thyroxine (Halpern et al. 1964).

The possible chronic effects of pressor amines have been discussed by several authors (Arnott 1959; Crawford 1962; Foy and Parratt 1962, 1961). A case frequently cited is the prevalence of endomyocardial fibrosis among West Africans. Plantain, which is quite rich in 5-hydroxytryptamine (5-HT), constitutes the staple food in these populations. From the amount normally eaten, a West African may have a daily dose of about 200 mg of 5-HT. Since there is a similarity between the lesions in carcinoid heart disease — a condition which is accompanied by an increased production of endogenous 5-HT — and those of endomyocaridal fibrosis, the suspicion that 5-HT has some role in the etiology of the latter is greatly reinforced (Arnott 1959).

Tyramine not only causes hypertension but also intense throbbing headache among those taking monoamine oxidase inhibitory drugs (Blackwell et al. 1967; Hanington and Harper 1968). The individuals taking these drugs often suffer from the headache following consumption of foods high in tyramine. A group of investigators have identified a subpopulation of individuals suffering from migraine headaches who are sensitive to tyramine (Bonnet and Lepreux 1971; Ghose et al. 1977; Hanington et al. 1970; Smith et al. 1970). It has been shown that a migraine attack among sensitive persons can be provoked within a few hours following ingestion of 125 mg of tyramine (Hanington et al. 1970; Smith et al. 1970). This level is, of course, much higher than the amount that can be reasonably ingested in high-amine natural food, such as a banana, which contains about 10 mg tyramine/100 g of pulp (Kenyhercz and Kissinger 1978). However, if it is assumed that other vasoactive amines are similarly headache producing, then it might be possible to provoke such a headache with one to five bananas. As shown in Table 8.2, some varieties of bananas contain high levels of amines.

Another vasoactive amine causing headaches is phenylethylamine (Sandler et al. 1974), which is present in chocolates, cheeses, and red wines (Chaytor et al. 1975; Schweitzer et al. 1975). As little as 3 mg of phenylethylamine has been shown to provoke migraine headache in 50% of subjects compared to 15% after placebo challenge (Sandler et al. 1974).

The mechanism by which these amines cause headache is unknown. Both amines are present in the human brain (Sabelli et al. 1978; Spector et al. 1963) and may function as modulators of catecholamine function. For example, the tyramine causes a release of norepinephrine from its binding sites and its hypertensive effects may be related to this process (Burn and Rand 1958). Phenylethylamine causes dramatic changes in blood flow through the brain (McCulloch and Harper 1979).

Two other amines not listed in Table 8.2 are synephrine and octopamine, which are found in lemons (Stewart and Wheaton 1964). Octopamine is also present in bananas at about 4 mg/g of wet pulp (Kenyhercz and Kissinger 1978).

Synephrine   Octopamine

It should be recalled that octopamine is found in the octopus and the squid. Synephrine is used widely as dilator and decongestant (Crosby 1969).

Many other types of endogenous amines have been identified. Thus, citrus fruits contain not only tyramine, but also methylated tyramine derivatives such as octopamine, synephrine, feruloylputrescine, hordenine (N,N-dimethyltyramine), and N-methyltyramine (Wheaton and Stewart 1969). The tyramine derivatives are also found in the sawa millet seeds (Sato et al. 1970). Hordenine is found in barley, and markedly increases in concentration upon germination.

Hordenine

It is also an hypertensive agent and a psychostimulant, and in large doses causes convulsions and respiratory failure (Concon 1979).

Vasoactive amines may be formed by metabolic transformation of precursors which are endogenously present in plant foodstuffs. Thus, dihydroxyphenylalanine (DOPA) is present in broad beans (*Vicia fava*) (Hodge et al. 1964). This compound has been implicated in hypertensive episodes following the consumption of broad beans by patients on monoamine oxidase inhibitors (pargyline). DOPA appears to have been found only in the pods and seeds of certain legumes (Sealock 1949). It is decarboxylated to dopamine, which is responsible for the pressor activity.

Undoubtedly many other kinds of plant foodstuffs contain vasoactive amines. A systematic study needs to be undertaken.

Stimulants and Other Psychoactive Compounds

The best examples of stimulants are caffeine in coffee, tea, cocoa, and kola nuts; theophyllin in tea; and theobromine in cocoa. Perhaps these substances are of no significance because of the universal consumption of beverages which contain them. Nevertheless, these are toxicants and their effects are not generally appreciated. Sensitivity to these substances varies with the individual.

Coffee is probably the most popular beverage all over the world. In the United States alone, it is estimated that more than a billion kilograms are consumed annually. This beverage undoubtedly owes its immense popularity to its aroma, flavor, and caffeine content. More than 200 compounds that are volatile under reduced pressure have been identified in the aqueous extract of roasted coffee (Goldman et al. 1967; Stoll et al. 1967). The compounds include hydrocarbons, acids, acid anhydrides, alcohols, aldehydes, esters, ethers, furans, ketones, lactones, mercaptans, phenols, pyrroles, picolines, pyrazines, pyridines, sulfides, thiazoles, and thiophenes. Obviously, these do not constitute all the compounds in coffee. Whether all these compounds contribute to the aroma and flavor of coffee is not known. The toxicological properties of these compounds have not been determined, except for a few which have been studied independent of their presence in coffee.

Toxicological Studies on Coffee, Caffeine, and Related Xanthines

Toxicological studies on whole or brewed coffee and caffeine have been undertaken to determine their deleterious effects, in view of the widespread consumption of coffee. The results with whole or brewed coffee have revealed some interesting observations. Bauer et al. (1977) gave a pure-bred strain of mice brewed coffee as the sole source of fluid throughout their adult lifespan. Standard commercial regular grind coffee was brewed in the proportion of 5.2 g/100 ml of water. Food and coffee were allowed ad libitum. The mice on coffee drank and ate as much as, or more, fluid and food than the control mice, which were given boiled water, but the longevity of the former was significantly reduced. The experimental animals seemed to age faster, showed markedly deteriorated physical conditions, and had lower body weights. Whereas all the control mice were still alive by the seventy-fifth or eightieth week, more than 50% of the coffee drinkers were dead by the same period. No gross pathological lesions were observed among the coffee drinkers at autopsy, although pneumonia seemed to be a terminal event common to both experimental and control animals. Thus, death appeared to be precipitated by premature aging.

In experiments with rats fed commercial diets containing 6% instant coffee, Wurzner et al. (1977) found no difference in longevity between experimental and control groups, but the coffee animals had significantly lower growth rates or body weights even though the food consumption was similar or higher than in the controls. The plasma cholesterol and phospholipid levels were also significantly elevated in the experimental animals; the cholesterol level showed consistent positive correlation with the caffeine content of the diets. A similar observation of cholesterol levels has been noted by other investigators with similar doses of caffeine (Naismith et al. 1969). Bellet et al. (1965) found that ingestion of 5 g instant coffee containing 218 mg caffeine markedly raise the serum free fatty acids of human subjects, and that these results are similar to pure caffeine administered as the sodium benzoate derivative. Although these changes are not considered toxic effects by the investigators, these abnormalities indicate that coffee can induce biochemical changes which may have harmful effects in the long run. These changes may be considered significant when compared with the results obtained by other workers with respect to caffeine.

Caffeine is the principal pharmacologically active component of coffee and similar beverages. The structures of caffeine and related xanthines are shown below:

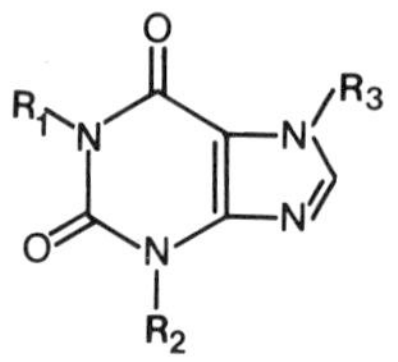

	R_1	R_2	R_3
Caffeine:	CH_3	CH_3	CH_3
Theobromine:	H	CH_3	CH_3
Theophylline:	CH_3	CH_3	H

<u>Biochemical and Physiological Effects of Caffeine and related Xanthines</u>   These pharmacologically active compounds elicit varied physiological effects which may have toxicological significance.

Effect on catecholamine activity: The biochemical activity of caffeine may be related to its action on the release or synthesis of catecholamines. In rats and guinea pigs, caffeine reportedly stimulates the synthesis of norepinephrine and causes it to be released to the brain tissues. In addition, caffeine also induces the release of epinephrine from the adrenal medulla (Berkowitz et al. 1970). A test conducted on non-coffee drinkers has shown that a single oral dose of 250 mg caffeine increases the level of plasma epinephrine and norepinephrine by 75 and 207%, respectively (Robertson et al. 1978). The relationship of catecholamine activity to the action of caffeine also can be demonstrated when the increased oxygen consumption in rats following intraperitoneal injection of 6.6 mg caffeine/kg is abolished by pretreatment with reserpine (Strubelt and Siegers 1969).

The increase in catecholamines has repercussions in glucose or glycogen and lipid metabolism. These amines stimulate the synthesis of 3', 5'-cyclic AMP which, in turn, promotes glycogenolysis and lipolysis as well as inhibits glycogenesis and lipogenesis. Caffeine or theophylline can also maintain the concentration of 3', 5'-cyclic AMP by inhibiting phosphodiesterase; this enzyme causes the hydrolysis of the cyclic nucleotide to inactive 5'-AMP. Thus, in this manner, these xanthines also enhance the action of the catecholamines (Kruse and Scholz 1978; Orten and Neuhaus 1975; Weinstein et al. 1975).

However, the evidence indicates that inhibition of phosphodiesterase may not be the principal mechanism by which caffeine exerts its pharmacological effects. The reason is that the amount required to inhibit the enzyme is too large (of the order of 0.5 to 1.0 mM) to be compatible with life (von Borstel 1983). Developments indicate that caffeine exerts its effects by competing with the receptors for adenosine on cellular membranes (Bruns et al. 1980). Adenosine, which structurally resembles caffeine, exerts a sedative and other effects opposite to those of caffeine, and thus the latter, by competing with these receptors produces its well-known effects (Daly et al. 1981, 1983; Snyder et al. 1981). Caffeine has been shown to compete with these receptors at levels that are normally detected in human plasma (Bruns et al. 1980). Other lines of evidence which support this theory are: (1) the increased sensitivity of rats to the hypotensive effects of adenosine (von Borstel et al. 1983), and (2) the compensatory increase in adenosine receptors in the brain (Boulenger et al. 1983) following several weeks of exposure to caffeine in either drinking water or food.

Caffeine may also produce some of its observed effects (e.g., diuresis) by promoting enhanced production of prostaglandins (Takeuchi et al. 1980).

The hyperglucosemic and hyperlipemic effects of caffeine have been demonstrated in both human and animal studies. For example, in normal and diabetic mice, the blood glucose level increases and the liver glycogen level decreases after 2 hr following subcutaneous injection of 25 mg caffeine/kg. It also has been demonstrated that the serum free fatty acids and total liver fatty acids also increase 2 hr after subcutaneous injection of 50 mg caffeine/kg (Ammon and Estler 1969). The effect is much greater in diabetic mice, since in these animals, lipolysis occurs already at a greater rate than lipogenesis; caffeine further aggravates this imbalance, so that ketonemia is greatly exaggerated in diabetic mice.

Similar findings have been reported for rats fed coffee or pure caffeine equivalent to 12 cups of the beverage, equivalent to what a 70-kg man would consume (Naismith et al. 1969). Plasma cholesterol and phospholipids have been found to be elevated in rats given coffee or pure caffeine compared to control animals or those given decaffeinated coffee. The rise in plasma lipids is roughly proportional to the amount of caffeine in the diet. However, the plasma triglycerides are depressed. This latter result is understandable, since lipogenesis is depressed by the xanthines. There is a significant rise in the plasma triglyceride level when starch in the basal diet is replaced by sucrose.

Observations in human subjects given caffeine or coffee have been similar to those seen in animals. For example, pregnant nondiabetic women given 2 cups of coffee containing a total of 250 to 300 mg caffeine show a decrease in intravenous glucose tolerance (Goldman and Ovadia 1969); the magnitude of the decrease, however, does not constitute a danger to the mother or to the unborn child. In healthy male and female volunteers who habitually ingested an average of 560 mg caffeine/day in the form of coffee or tea, the blood glucose falls when these subjects are placed on decaffeinated coffee for 14 days. Their plasma cholesterol and phospholipids rise slightly, but the triglycerides drop markedly. The levels of the lipids rise again when 875 mg caffeine/day is administered during a 20-day period, but there is no effect on the blood glucose. These results, which are different from the rat studies, may have been due to species differences, as has been demonstrated in animals regarding caffeine toxicity (Boyd et al. 1965; Salant and Rieger 1912; Vacca 1926). On the other hand, caffeine withdrawal, which produces marked clinical symptoms, might produce different transient metabolic effects, so that interpretation of the above results becomes difficult. Resistance to the toxic effect of caffeine (Peters 1967) is also another phenomenon which may cause a difference in response between habitual and nonhabitual drinkers when caffeine is withdrawn and then readministered.

As mentioned before, a marked rise (four times over control) in serum free fatty acids also has been observed in volunteers ingesting 218 mg caffeine in the form of 5 g instant coffee or injected with 0.5 g caffeine as sodium benzoate derivative intramuscularly (Bellet et al. 1965).

Potential Mutagenicity of Caffeine and Related Xanthines Many studies have demonstrated that caffeine and related xanthines may be potential mutagens. First of all, it has been shown that caffeine can bind not only to fully denatured DNA (Ts'o and Lu 1961), but also especially with the partially denatured nucleic acid (Domon et al. 1970). In the latter case, with calf thymus DNA, maximum binding occurs when only 50% of DNA is denatured by ultraviolet (UV) light. This binding can explain the observed interference in the de novo synthesis of DNA in Chinese hamster cells irradiated by UV light (Cleaver and Thomas 1969). In fact, caffeine has been found to be a potent inhibitor of postreplication repair of Chinese hamster DNA damaged by UV irradiation (Nilsson and Lehmann 1975) and by the carcinogen N-acetoxy-2-acetylaminofluorene (Trosko et al. 1973). Theobromine, theophylline, and other xanthines were moderate inhibitors of postreplication DNA repair (Nilsson and Lehmann 1975). This inhibitory effect of caffeine apparently occurs only with postreplication DNA repair and not on normal DNA synthesis (Fujiwara and Kondo 1972; Lehmann 1972; Lehmann and Kirk-Bell 1974; Trosko and Chu 1973). No such inhibition has been observed in normal human cells (Buhl and Regan 1974; Lehmann et al. 1975).

It also has been established in the latter work that caffeine potentiates UV-induced chromosome damage. The observed damage consists of abnormal metaphases, chromosome breakage, and chromatid exchanges (Nilsson and Lehmann 1975).

Caffeine also potentiates chromosome-breaking activity of several alkylating agents (Kihlman et al. 1974; Roberts et al. 1974; Sturelid and Kihlman 1975). In addition, this alkaloid can also enhance the lethal effects of alkylating agents on cultured mouse and hamster cells (Rauth et al. 1970; Walker and Reid 1971).

Caffeine, theophylline, and theobromine also have been found to be clastogenic on human lymphocytes in cultures (Ostertag 1966; Weinstein et al. 1973, 1975). The damage results in the suppression of mitosis in these cell cultures (Timson 1972; Weinstein et al 1975).

However, by means of the dominant lethal test, caffeine has been found to have no mutagenic effects (Adler 1969; Adler and Röhrborn 1969; Epstein et al. 1970). In this test, male mice to be mated to untreated females are injected with a relatively large dose of caffeine or given a caffeine solution of specified concentration for drinking water. Chromosomal aberrations are indicated by zygote lethality, F_1-progeny sterility, and postimplantation deaths or resorption of embryos. But none of these effects is seen with caffeine. Obviously, in vivo metabolic transformation dilution, and other factors may dissipate whatever mutagenic property caffeine may possess.

In a review of the experimental evidence, Thayer and Palm (1975) concluded that caffeine as a mutagen to humans, as yet, has not been established to be "of great concern or being dismissible." At most, it can be considered as a weak mutagen in some nonmammalion systems. Questions remain concerning caffeine and DNA repair mechanisms, for it appears possible that caffeine, on the contrary, may possess anticarcinogenic and/or antimutagenic properties.

Teratogenicity of Caffeine   Even though in the dominant lethal test no abnormality has been observed, the situation may be quite different when caffeine is administered directly to pregnant animals. Thus, Fujii and co-workers (1969) injected 200 mg caffeine/kg subcutaneously and intraperitoneally separately to two groups of 20 pregnant 1CR-JCL mice. Both groups showed a significant range of fetal abnormalities, the highest incidence being in mice injected with the alkaloid subcutaneously. Two separate doses of 100 mg/kg injected at intervals of 2 or 4 hr had lesser effects, and there was little difference when the doses were separated by 2 or 4 hr. Thus, the degree of caffeine toxicity to unborn mice varies with the route of administration, and the dose reaching the embryo at any given time influences the effect. It appears that the subcutaneous route affords a greater caffeine concentration to the embryo than the intraperitoneal route. Similar fatal effects of caffeine on the embryo have been described in rabbits (Stieve 1938). Fetal abnormalities have also been described earlier in mice given the maximum tolerated dose of caffeine (Nishimura and Nakai 1960), with abortions being described as the early sign of caffeine toxicity. However, some early reports showed that abortions in humans even with very high doses of caffeine are quite rare (Lewin 1904).

Many investigators also have demonstrated that repeated oral doses of 125 mg caffeine/kg or greater produces teratogenic effects in the rat (Bertrand et al. 1970; Fujii and Nishimura 1972; Leuschner and Czok 1973). Some skull malformations (5.8%) in rat fetuses develop when pregnant rats are given rapid oral intubation of 30 mg caffeine/kg daily from day 0 to 19 of pregnancy. None has been observed when the same total dose is consumed in drinking water (Palm et al. 1978, quoted by Thayer and Palm 1975). Similar works with low oral doses of 22.5 mg/kg or less given on days 6 to 15 of pregnancy in Wistar rats, 30 mg/kg or less given to hamsters on days 6 to 10 of pregnancy, or 32.5 mg/kg or less in rabbits on days 6 to 18 of pregnancy have shown no increased malformations (Food and Drug Research Labs, Inc. 1973a,b). Teratogenic effects appear to vary with the strain of animal, stage of embryonic development, rate of caffeine administration, the size of the dose, and other factors (Thayer and Palm 1975).

Thus, caffeine may possess greater teratogenic than mutagenic effects in mammalian systems, but a demonstration of its teratogenic effects in humans has not been made. However, Jacobson et al. (1981) reported three cases of birth defects which may have some relationships to coffee drinking. One case involved a woman who gave birth to an infant with severe ectodactyly. She took neither drugs nor alcohol nor smoked cigarettes, but drank large quantities of coffee during pregnancy. The two other cases were infants with missing metacarpals and phalanges whose mothers ingested as much as 25 cups of coffee per day during pregnancy. In the latter cases, however, the relationship of the birth defects to coffee drinking was obscured because these women also took alcohol and drugs as well as smoked cigarettes. These birth defects are consistent with teratogenic effects in rats reported by Collins et al. (1981), which were primarily ectodactyly. In this study, the mothers were gavage fed with 80 mg caffeine/kg body weight. The no-effect dose was 40 mg/kg.

The exposure of the fetus to caffeine is certainly prolonged because in pregnancy its rate of metabolism is altered, so that its half-life in the tissues is increased from 5 to 6 hr in the nonpregnant state to 18 hr in pregnancy (von Borstel 1983). The fetal and neonatal liver metabolizes caffeine very slowly, so that its half-life in the tissues during this stage is 3 to 4 days. In the newborn, at least 80% of administered caffeine is eliminated unchanged (Aldridge et al. 1979).

It must be stated that in rats, caffeine tends to accumulate in the fetal brain and diminishes more slowly in this tissue other than in the mother (Galli et al. 1975). Thus, these results suggest that prolonged pharmacological effects of caffeine during the early development of the central nervous system is possible. How this translates in terms of the teratogenicity of caffeine remains to be determined.

Absorption and Excretion of Caffeine   Caffeine is absorbed rapidly in the human gastrointestinal tract so that maximum plasma level is attained in 0.25 to 1.0 hr (Axelrod and Reichenthal 1953; Bonati et al. 1982; Dobmeyer et al. 1983; Sant'Ambrogio et al. 1964). In six healthy volunteers given a test meal with 500 mg caffeine in a 350 ml solution, the absorption of caffeine depended on the residence time in the stomach (Chvasta and Cooke 1971). In 20 min, 86% of the test meal had emptied from the stomach and 16% of the caffeine was absorbed. With buffered meals (pH 1 to 9) given with 100 g glucose/L, the peak absorption in 20 min of 21% was observed at pH 7; negligible absorption was noted at pH 1. Caffeine increased gastric acidity more so than water.

Diffusion of caffeine in human tissues also occurs rapidly. Thus, in humans the onset of the pharmacological effects of caffeine is noted from as early as 10 min (Blum et al. 1964) to as long as 50 min (Weiss and Laties 1962), with peak activity reported at 2 hr (Cheney 1935). The half-life of caffeine in humans has been reported to be 3 to 3.5 hr (Axelrod and Reichenthal 1953; Sant'Ambrogio et al. 1964).

A man who swallowed a fatal dose of caffeine (5 to 10 g) afforded investigators an opportunity to determine the distribution of caffeine in the body. In this case, Parish et al. (1965) reported that excluding the stomach, the highest concentration was found in the liver, which was two to three times as high as in the kidneys and more than four times as high as in the brain. A similar tissue distribution has been found in rats given a fatal oral dose of 1 g/kg.

In mice, an oral dose of 25 mg caffeine/kg has been found in most tissues in 5 min, being generally distributed in 1 hr; the half-life of caffeine in these tissues is 3 hr (Burg and Werner 1972).

The maximum caffeine concentration in the urine of rats was measured 5 hr after administration (Czok et al. 1969). It seems, however, that there may be factors in tea which tend to diminish absorption of caffeine. Chlorogenic acid tends to delay excretion caffeine in rats. The mechanism for this delaying action is not known.

Caffeine is efficiently reabsorbed in the kidneys (98%) (von Borstel 1983). Thus, conversion to a more readily excretable form is necessary for its rapid excretion. That this biotransformation must occur in the liver explains why in liver disease the elimination of caffeine can take several days (Statland and Demas 1980).

Other factors can modify the excretion of caffeine. Oral contraceptives can increase its half-life in the tissues to about 11 hr (Patwardhan et al. 1980). Cigarette smoking (Parsons and Neims 1978) as well as exposure to certain exogenous compounds (Aldridge et al. 1977) can also markedly enhance elimination of caffeine.

Acute Toxicity of Caffeine   Reported fatal oral doses of caffeine for man range from 150 to 200 mg/kg (Khodasevich 1965; McGee 1980). This is similar to the values that have been reported for the oral minimal lethal doses for cats, 100 to 150 mg/kg; and for dogs, 140 to 150 mg/kg (Spector 1956). The oral LD_{50} for the rat is around 200 mg/kg (Boyd 1959; Spector 1956); the oral LD_{50} in humans is estimated to be over 140 mg/kg (Gemmill 1958). Concerning the nonlethal toxicity of caffeine, humans are reported to be more sensitive than animals. It is estimated that the minimum toxic dose for humans is 2 to 5 mg caffeine/kg; the corresponding values for rats or mice are between 25 and 50 mg/kg (Ulrich 1958).

The symptoms elicited by large doses or overdoses of caffeine in humans include insomnia, nausea, nervousness, diuresis, tinnitus, scintillating scotomas, restlessness, vomiting, and tachycardia; moderate doses may produce only the first four symptoms (Stecher et al. 1960).

In rats given a lethal oral dose of caffeine, some of the symptoms observed by Boyd (1959) during the first or second hour include weakness, tenseness, ataxia, withdrawn behavior, catalepsy, and phonation when the rats were moved. After 6 to 24 hr, the animals developed mild diarrhea, eye infections, excitement, pallor, and tremors. In addition, CNS depression, blepharitis, hypothermia, anorexia, and loss of weight were also recorded. Death from respiratory failure following tetanic convulsions or cardiac collapse occurred after 20 to 40 hr. Similar signs had been observed by earlier investigators (Holck 1949; Maloney 1935). Other species had been reported to show similar toxic signs (Salant and Rieger 1909; Sollmann and Pilcher 1911).

A lethal dose of caffeine produces severe damage to the internal organs, e.g., gastroenteritis, congestion of the liver, kidneys, heart, and lungs; degenerative changes in the pancreas, spleen, and thymus; and dehydration of most tissues was also recorded (Boyd 1973).

The average caffeine contents, respectively, per 5-oz cup of ground-roasted, instant and decaffeinated coffee are 85, 60, and 3 mg; 40 and 30 mg for leaf or bag and instant teas; 4 mg for cocoa in hot chocolate. A 6-oz glass of cola drinks and an 8-oz glass of chocolate milk contain 18 mg and 5 mg caffeine, respectively (Roberts and Barone 1983).

For a 70-kg person, two and one-half to four 5-oz cups of coffee from ground-roasted beans consumed within a short period (30 min or less) will bring the plasma concentration to 15 to 30 µM. This will cause mild anxiety, respiratory stimulation, diuresis, and increased gastric secretion, especially among those who are not regular coffee drinkers (Robertson et al. 1981). Individual tolerance can, of course, occur, so that higher doses may be necessary for these effects to happen in regular drinkers. Even considering the caffeine content of other beverages, it appears difficult to attain such levels of plasma caffeine, since it will be almost impossible to consume the required amount of beverage within a short period of time.

Serious poisoning indicated by severe restlessness, tachycardia, delirium, muscular tension, and twitching will require 10 to 20 times the amount of coffee shown above. The caffeine concentration in the plasma in these cases will be 150 to 200 µM (von Borstel 1983).

Other Effects   Caffeine can produce transient hypertension in humans (Robertson et al. 1978). Regular coffee given to two groups of men produced a transient but significant elevation of blood pressure of 5 to 10 mm Hg. The effect was more distinct in

(53- to 70-year-old) men than in younger ones (22 to 44 years old) (Horst and Jenkins 1935). These effects were compared in the same subjects consuming decaffeinated coffee; measurements were obtained 1 to 2 hr after consumption. Robertson et al. (1978) found a blood pressure increase of 14/10 mm Hg (systolic/diastolic) in their non-coffee drinking subjects given a single oral dose of 250 mg caffeine. This increase in blood pressure appears to be mediated through the enhanced renin and catecholamine activity.

Ammon and Estler (1970) demonstrated the hypertensive effects of caffeine in rats. Its effects were also more pronounced in older animals. As in the human studies (Horst and Jenkins 1935), the heart rate in rats also increased with caffeine (Ammon and Estler 1970).

Caffeine, and especially theophylline, at 100 mg/kg produce necrosis of the myocardium in rats. Theophylline produces more severe necrosis in all rats after 16 hr. Caffeine is less cardiotoxic, producing moderate necrosis of the myocardium in only 20% of the rats.

Heart attacks: The reported effect of caffeine on cardiac function as well as on the myocardium may be significant, since some studies (Boston Collaborative Drug Surveillance Program 1972; Jick et al. 1973) appear to suggest a high statistical correlation between daily coffee consumption and the incidence of acute myocardial infarction. However, this observation has been disputed (Hennekens et al. 1976; Jick et al. 1974; Kannell and Dawber 1973; Klatsky et al. 1973, 1974; Nichols 1973). Among other things, drinking tea, which also contains similar concentration of caffeine, has been found to have no correlation with the disease. In addition, studies with rats have indicated that caffeine, which until recently has been presumed to be the only biologically active ingredient in coffee, may have no atherogenic activity. This conclusion has been deduced from the fact that rats given tea infusions, which contain similar amounts of caffeine as in coffee, have shown significant lowering of cholesterol and triglyceride levels in the blood (Akinyanju and Yudkin 1967). Thus, other pharamacologically active compounds responsible for these observed effects must be present in coffee, but not in tea, in order to explain the differences in activity between these beverages. It is conceivable that these noncaffeine fractions in coffee may act synergistically with caffeine. In addition, even though atherogenesis is a predisposing factor in coronary heart disease, it should be emphasized that heart failure does not always involve apparent disease of the coronary arteries.

The presence of other active factors in coffee is suggested in the work of Würzner et al. (1977). These researchers found that regular and decaffeinated coffee produce similar significant elevations in the plasma levels of phospholipids and other plasma constituents in male rats. More importantly, Kalsner (1977) found that coffee contains an unknown vasoactive material with potent constrictor action on the coronary arteries; in contrast, pure caffeine and tea produce only vascular relaxation. These actions were tested on beef coronary artery strips. Since regular and decaffeinated coffees produced vasoconstrictor responses of similar magnitude, the presence of vasoactive materials in coffee is indicated. From the response, the material(s) may be highly potent or present in a sufficiently high concentration, or both, to overcome the vasodilatory effects of caffeine. The unknown vasoactive material in coffee appears to be a cholinomimetic substance, since its effect is blocked or neutralized by atropine, a known cholinergic receptor antagonist.

Kalsner (1977) points out that this observation may be pertinent to the greater incidence of acute myocardial infarction among coffee drinkers, as suggested by the results of studies undertaken in the Boston Collaborative Drug Surveillance Program (1972) and by Jick et al. (1973). The possibility that constrictions or spasms of coronary arteries are factors in the etiology of myocardial infarction has been proposed by a number of investigators (Chahine et al. 1975; Cheng et al. 1972; Lange et al. 1972). Indeed, some cases of angina pectoris and sudden death from heart failure appear to involve coronary artery constriction or spasm (Kalsner 1976; MacAlpin 1973; Oliva et al. 1973; Prchkov et al. 1974).

It is interesting to note that an earlier epidemiological survey reported by Paul et al. (1963) also showed a positive correlation between coffee intake and coronary heart disease.

In this connection, the effect of caffeine on the heart is underscored by the positive correlation between tea and coffee drinking and ventricular ectopic activity, as reported by Prineas et al. (1980). These workers found that consumption of more than nine cups of coffee or tea daily induces or increases the prevalence of ventricular premature beats. Similarly, Dobmeyer et al. (1983) found arrhythmias in their series of subjects who drank three to five cups of coffee per day containing 200 mg of caffeine, or who were injected intravenously with the same amount of caffeine. Even though these effects may be provoked by other factors (Graboys and Lown 1983), this does not obscure the fact that caffeine is an arrhythmogenic compound which may have serious effects on those with underlying heart disease.

Gastric ulcers: The cholinomimetic action of the vasoconstrictive component of coffee may be related to the reported association between coffee drinking and gastric ulcers and other deleterious effects (Harvey 1975; Hayreh 1973). It is known that gastric acid secretion involves a cholinergic mechanism (Ritchie 1975), and it appears that both regular and decaffeinated coffee produce similar responses in terms of acid production in the stomach (Cohen and Booth 1975; Roth and Ivy 1944; Roth et al. 1944). In healthy adult male and female volunteers, doses of caffeine and both decaffeinated and regular instant coffees exhibited greater rates of gastric acid secretion than caffeine. This suggests that other pharmacologically active compounds are present in coffee (Cohen and Booth 1975). Further evidence of the presence of other active compounds in coffee is that regular or decaffeinated coffee at high doses produces a significant increase in sphincter pressure in the lower esophagus of the same volunteers; caffeine produces only a modest but significant rise in pressure (Cohen and Booth 1975). The compound(s) producing these effects remains to be identified.

Cancer: Another possible deleterious effect of coffee is the reported association between coffee drinking and cancer of the lower urinary tract (Cole 1971). It has been observed that among coffee drinkers, the relative risk of the disease is 1.24 among males and 2.58 among females, compared to 1.0 among non coffee drinkers in both sexes.

Simon et al. (1975) found a similar association between coffee drinking and cancer of the lower urinary tract. But Armstrong et al. (1976) did not find any association in their retrospective study involving renal cancer.

MacMahon et al. (1981) found that for both sexes coffee consumption is significantly associated with pancreatic cancer. When adjustment for other risk factors is made, the relative risk for drinking two cups/day was 1.8, and for 3 or more cups, 2.7. Lin and Kessler (1981) found that drinking decaffeinated coffee is one of the three risk factors for men and women for pancreatic cancer. (The two other risk factors are different for either sex.) An interesting case study reported from Australia by Ferguson and Watts (1980) involved a husband and wife with pancreatic cancer. This couple had the dietary idiosyncrasies of adding a liquid coffee concentrate to their ground coffee before percolation and consuming copious amounts of margarine. The authors placed a greater weight as possible causative factor on the use of the coffee concentrate.

Even though these observations do not show an association between urinary tract and pancreatic cancers, the possibility of this association is enhanced by the observed effect of coffee on the carcinogenic potency of cycasin in rats (Mori and Hirono 1977). Rats given coffee in their drinking water throught their lifespans and administered a single dose of 150 mg cycasin/kg, developed a high incidence of tumors, especially colorectal adenoma. Control animals given coffee or cycasin alone developed significantly fewer tumors. Thus, coffee contains a substance(s) which promotes the carcinogenic activity of cycasin. The proximate carcinogenic metabolite of cycasin is similar to nitrosamine (Laqueur et al. 1963), and Challis and Bartlett (1975) found that the nitrosation reaction can be catalyzed by easily oxidizable compounds similar in structure to chlorogenic acid, which is 13% (W/W) of standard coffees. Thus, one or more

of the myriad coffee substances can act as tumor promoters, not only for those of carcinogens in coffee (endogenous, contaminants, or derived).

It should be mentioned here that roasted coffee contains polycyclic aromatic hydrocarbons (Kuratsune and Hueper 1960) (Chap. 12).

Psychoactive Compounds

There are psychoactive compounds which are of lesser importance. These compounds
are found in food products that normally have limited consumption. Nevertheless,
these compounds are potent enough that isolated cases of intentional or accidental
excessive consumption have resulted in severe poisonings. Some of these are discussed in the following sections.

Myristicin   Myristicin is present in nutmeg and mace to the extent of 4% of the
volatile oils (Shulgin et al. 1967). It is also present in lesser quantities in black pepper (Richard and Jennings 1971), parsley (Small 1949), celery (Karmazine 1955), dill
(Karow 1969), and carrots (Buttery et al. 1968). There is some structural relationship
between myristicin and mescaline. This fact may explain the psychoactivity of myristicin (Truit 1967; Truit et al. 1961). Myristicin may also act as a weak monoamine

Myristicin   Mescaline

oxidase inhibitor (Truit and Ebersberger 1962; Truit et al. 1961). However, nutmeg
and mace (*Myristica fragrans*) produce greater narcotic and psychomimetic activity
than an equivalent amount of myristicin or elemicin, also a component of nutmet (Truit
et al. 1961).

Nutmeg produces effects similar to alcoholic intoxication. Reportedly these spices
have been frequently used as narcotics by prison inmates (Jacobziner and Rayibin
1965; Weiss 1960). Nutmeg poisoning (Green 1959; Weil 1965) results in part from the
mistaken notion that it is an abortifacient and emmenagogue (Weil 1965). Around 5 to
15 g of nutmeg powder can produce euphoria, hallucinations, and narcosis. However,
it has very unpleasant and severe side effects — headache, nausea, abdominal pain,
delerium, hypotension, depression, acidosis, stupor, shock (Green 1959; Weiss 1960)
— and in large doses, liver damage and death (Truit et al. 1961). Nutmeg poisoning
may induce prolonged sleep, followed by euphoria lasting from 24 hr (Truit et al.
1961; Weiss 1960) to 10 days, in some cases (Akesson and Walinder 1965). Expectedly,
whole nutmeg oil has been shown to enhance ethanol-induced sleep in subjects (Sherry
and Burnett 1978).

Dioscorine   Of the more than 600 species of yams of the genus *Dioscorea,* a few
species which are found in West Africa, Nigeria, Indonesia, the Philippines, and possibly many other places, are poisonous. These species include *D. dumetorum, D.
hirsuta* (Bevan and Hirst 1958), and *D. hispida* (Leyva and Gutierrez 1937; Pinder
1953). These poisonous species may be mistaken for the edible ones, and have been
reported to have caused fatal poisonings (Corkill 1948; Leyva and Gutierrez 1937; Oke
1972). These yams contain the tropane alkaloids dioscorine (in *D. dumetorum* and *D.
hispida)* and dihydrodioscorine (in *D. hirsuta*). These alkaloids are central nervous
system depressants and convulsants (Bevan and Hirst 1958; Gorter 1911). Injected
into mice, the alkaloids produce clonic and tonic convulsions which, in several cases,
precede death. The highly poisonous nature of dioscorine is shown by its ability to

Dioscorine

induce general paralysis (Gorter 1911). Its intraperitoneal LD_{50} in mice is about 65 mg/kg; at 20 mg/kg, it enhances the pressor effect of epinephrine, but in cats, it depresses the effect of acetylcholine on blood pressure (Bevan and Hirst 1958).

In humans, dioscorine produces a burning sensation in the mouth and throat, abdominal pain, vomiting, diarrhea, and speech disturbances; these symptoms are followed by vertigo, salivation, lachrymation, sensation of heat, exosphthalmos, deafness, and delirium. In severe cases, death may occur between 3 and 168 hr (Corkill 1948). *D. dumetorum* and *D. hispida* have been implicated in many cases of poisonings.

Dihydrodioscorine has pharmacological activity similar to dioscorine, only weaker (Bevan and Hirst 1958).

Carotatoxin Carrots and celery contain this acetylenic alcohol. Carrots yield about 2 mg/kg. This compound resembles the powerful CNS stimulant cicutoxin, a very poisonous substance from the water hemlock (*Cicuta masculata*) (Anet et al. 1953; Haggerty and Conway 1936). Carotatoxin has been shown to be highly neurotoxic to mice (Crosby and Aharonson 1967), but is much less toxic than cicutoxin.

$$(C_9H_{17})C \equiv C - C \equiv C - CH_2 - CH - CH = CH_2$$
$$OH$$

Carotatoxin

Psychoactive Compounds of Lesser Toxicological Importance Such psychoactive compounds as psilocybin, psilocin from the mushroom *Psilocybe mexicana*, and muscarine and bufotenine from *Amanita muscaria* and other mushrooms are discussed in Chapter 10.

Several other psychoactive compounds are known but are of little food toxicological importance. In many cases, interest in these compounds arises as a result of mistaken identity, contamination of foodstuffs, and accidental or innocent ingestion by children. To cite a few examples: the berries of the deadly nightshade have caused fatal poisoning in children (Innes and Nickerson 1970). It was also reported that an adult was poisoned from eating liver from cattle that grazed on deadly nightshade (Clarke 1970). This plant contains another tropane alkaloid, L-hyoscyamine, a potent CNS depressant as well as a hallucinogen. The plant's leaves and berries also contain scopolamine, which has an action similar to atropine.

A strong depressant alkaloid appears to be present in the death camas (*Zigadenus venenosus*), which can be mistaken for the edible camas lily (Cameron 1952).

Cholinesterase Inhibitors

Cholinesterase inhibitors have been detected in several edible fruits and vegetables by Orgell (1963) and other investigators (Menn et al. 1964; Orgell et al. 1959). These foodstuffs include broccoli, Valencia oranges, sugar beets, rutabagas, cabbage, peppers (*Capsicum frutescence*), pumpkins, squash, carrots, strawberries, tomatoes, Jonathan and Stayman apples, lima beans, eggplant, asparagus, turnips, radishes, and several species of potatoes. The inhibitors are found in the edible portions of the plant. The most active inhibitor is found in potatoes.

The nature of the acetylcholinesterase inhibitors in these foodstuffs has not been chemically characterized, with the exception of the principal alkaloids in potatoes, tomatoes, and eggplant; all these plants are members of the family Solanaceae. The principal acetylcholinesterase inhibitor in potatoes is solanine, a glycoalkaloid. The action and toxicity of this alkaloid have been extensively studied, although there is

Solanine

more than one alkaloid in potatoes. Solanine is also found in other poisonous Solan-aceae, such as the common nightshade (*Solanum nigrum* and *S. americanum*). Solanine is also found in eggplant (*S. melongena*) and in green and red peppers (*Capsicum anum*) at 7.6 to 8.2, 6.1 to 11.33 and 7.7 to 9.2 mg/100 g, respectively (Jones and Fenwick 1981). The solanine content of commercial potatoes ranges from 2 to 15 mg/100 g fresh weight (Cronk et al. 1974; Jones and Fenwick 1981; Wolf and Duggar 1946). Most commercial varieties contain less than 12 mg/100 g, normally between 2 and 13 mg/ 100 g (Wolf and Duggar 1946). However, a new variety, lenape (USDA B 5141-6), with good chipping properties — high solids and low sugar content (Akeley et al. 1968) — has been shown to contain over 20 mg/kg (Zitnak and Johnson 1970). This cultivar was withdrawn by USDA for commercial production because of its possible harmful effects (Anonymous 1970). Tubers containing 20 mg or more solanine/100 g have an acrid taste, and it is generally held that potatoes containing solanine above 20 mg/100 g may be unsafe (Bömer and Mattis 1924; Oslage 1956; Sapeika 1969; Willimott 1933). Solanine is heat stable and insoluble in water, and hence, toxic potatoes cannot be made harm-less in the cooking process.

The solanine content of tubers may vary with the degree of maturity at harvest, rate of nitrogen fertilization, storage conditions (Cronk et al. 1974), biological stress, such as blight infection (*Phytophthora infestans*) (Gull and Isenburg 1960; Schreiber 1968; Locci and Kue 1967), and greening by exposure to light (Wolf and Duggar 1946).

The variation in solanine content, with conditions, may depend on the variety: A variety may increase or decrease in solanine content with maturation, and increase, decrease, or remain unaffected by fertilization (Cronk et al. 1974). Storage conditions may increase the solanine content, but again, this may depend on the variety (Cronk et al. 1974; Wang 1970). Several varieties have shown increased solanine upon storage. The potato lenape, high in solanine content, may show a significant increase in alka-loid content upon storage, and tends to have a greater concentration in smaller tubers weighing around 100 g (Cronk et al. 1974).

Greening in potatoes may increase the solanine content to as high as 80 to 100 mg/ 100 g; most of the alkaloid is concentrated in the skin (Wolf and Duggar 1946). The sprouts may contain lethal amounts of solanine (Willimott 1933).

Several cases of potato poisoning have been reported, some of which were fatal (Bömer and Mattis 1924; Hansen 1925; Terbrüggen 1936; Willimott 1933). Since potatoes contain not just solanine, but also other glycoalkaloids, e.g., chaconine and tomatine (Nishie et al. 1975), it is possible that symptoms seen in potato poisoning are due to the combined effects of the alkaloids. Thus, it has been shown that the solanine content of potatoes did not correlate very well with its anticholinesterase activity (Abbot et al. 1960). Furthermore, when injected into rabbits, little cholinergic effects have been noted in spite of the anticholinesterase activity observed in vitro (Nishie et al. 1975).

Solanine has relatively high oral LD_{50}s in animals, which is also described as a low oral toxicity. There are three reasons why this is so: (1) It is poorly absorbed in the gastrointestinal tract, as shown by the low blood levels following ingestion. (2) It is also excreted rapidly, usually within 12 hr, through the feces and urine, so it does not accumulate in the tissues for any significant period of time. (3) Hydrolysis of the glycoside by intestinal bacteria releases the aglycone solanidine, which is poorly absorbed and much less toxic than solanine; 500 mg solanidine/kg, i/p. was nontoxic to mice, whereas the intraperitoneal (i.p.) LD_{50} of solanine is from 1/12 to 1/16 of this value (Nishie et al. 1971; Patil et al. 1972).

Nevertheless, in spite of its general low oral toxicity, serious or severe toxic effects and even fatal poisonings in humans and animals have been documented. In humans, an oral dose of about 2.8 mg/kg body weight has been shown to cause both neurological symptoms in the form of hyperesthesia, dyspnea, itchiness in the neck, and drowsiness, and gastrointestinal effects such as vomiting and diarrhea (Rühl 1951). Symptoms of solanine poisoning may begin about 8 hr after ingestion; tachycardia, pupil dilation, and cardiovascular and respiratory depression may follow. Confusion and a semicomatose state may precede death (Sapeika 1960; Willimot 1933). In a fatal solanine poisoning of a child, headache and increased cerebrospinal fluid pressure were reported by Terbrüggen (1936). The increased intracranial pressure caused by solanine is indicated by the appearance of delta waves, as seen in rabbits administered a lethal i.p dose of 20 to 30 mg/kg. Such waves are also observed in humans with increased intracranial pressure (Hughes 1961).

Solanine also has saponinelike properties; it can cause hemolytic and hemorrhagic damage to the gastrointestinal tract (König and Stafze 1953) and the retina (Rühl 1951; von Oettingen 1952).

There are apparent interspecific differences in the oral lethal dose of this alkaloid. In rats, the LD_{50} is 590 mg/kg (Gull 1961). Mice are highly resistant; 1000 mg/kg given orally had no effect (Nishie et al. 1971). Sheep are likewise resistant; 225 mg/kg did not kill these animals, but produced undefined blood abnormalities; e.g., increased concentration of leukocytes and erythrocytes of unequal, irregular or abnormal shapes.

However, solanine is more toxic when administered parenterally. The i.p. LD_{50} values in rats (Gull 1961), and mice (Nishie et al. 1971) are 75 mg and 42 mg/kg, respectively. The i.p. LD_{50} for mice (Patil et al. 1972), is 32.3 mg/kg. In rabbits, 20 mg/kg is lethal in approximately 6 hr; 30 mg/kg kills rabbits overnight. An intravenous dose of 10 mg/kg kills rabbits in 2 min. The LD_{50} for chick embryos is 18.8 mg/kg; 19 to 25 mg/kg produces high mortality within 1 day after injection. Death in rabbits appears to be caused by central nervous system depression, as shown by the initial loss of electroencephalographic (EEG) signals, followed by respiratory cessation and terminal loss of EEG signals (Nishie et al. 1971).

Higher concentrations of solanine affect animal nervous systems compared to other cholinesterase inhibitors. For example, 50 to 100 µg/ml of solanine, compared to 0.005 to 0.01 µg/ml of acetylcholine, causes guinea-pig ileum strips to contract.

Solanine as well as solanidine has cardiac effects which are similar to those induced by cardiac glycosides, such as K-strophanthoside. Solanine is equal in potency to K-strophanthoside on a molar basis in producing positive inotropic effects on electrically driven frog ventricle. Solanidine has one-fifth the activity of solanine or K-strophanthoside. At high concentrations, solanine causes terminal contraction of the heart (Nishie et al. 1971).

The alkaloids chaconine and tomatine, also found in potatoes and similar solanaceous foodstuffs, possess pharmacological properties similar to solanine; chaconine and solanine have similar toxicities, as tested in mice, rabbits, and chick embryos (Nishie et al. 1975).

An interesting hypothesis was presented by Renwick (1972) regarding the relationship between the incidence of anencephaly and spina bifida among white infants, and the consumption of potatoes high in solanine. The phenomenon which led to Renwick's hypothesis was the correlation between the geographical pattern of average severity of late blight (*Phytophthora infestans*) fungal infection in potatoes and the aforementioned birth abnormality. In this case, Renwick stated that the glycoalkaloid concentration in potatoes may have been increased following stress produced by the fungal infection. Locci and Kuc (1967) suggested that such an increase was possible. Other researchers (Gull and Isenburg 1960; Schreiber 1968) similarly demonstrated the increased concentration of solanine in potatoes following infection by the fungus. Mun and co-workers (1975) found that solanine or a preparation of mixed glycoalkaloids from potatoes naturally infected with the fungus significantly produces abnormalities in chick embryos when injected after 0 and 26 hr of incubation. However, this observation could not be verified by Nishie et al. (1971, 1975), who failed to observe a statistically significant incidence of abnormalities in chicks treated with the alkaloid. Notwithstanding, these researchers did find abnormal embryos in eggs injected with solanine. The contradictory observations may have been due to differences in experimental conditions (e.g., solvents, time of injection, and nutritional status of embryos). Ruddick et al. (1974) also failed to see any teratogenic effects of blighted potatoes in rat embryos; similar negative findings involving rat, rabbit, and chick embryos also have been reported by Swinyard and Chaube (1973).

However, the observation of Mun et al. (1975) has been confirmed by Jelinek et al. (1976), who produced deformities in chick embryos treated with ethanol extracts of boiled potatoes previously infected with *P. infestans*. The deformities consisted of caudal regression, myeloschisis at the somite stage, cranioschisis, celeosoma, and cardiac septal defects. The safe effects have been observed with extracts of healthy potatoes or solanine at the same concentration as those in extracts. Keeler et al. (1976a, 1978) produced teratogenic deformities which included spina bifida and exencephaly in hamsters gavaged with extracts of high alkaloid sprouts of various potato cultivars. Keeler et al. (1976a,b) also showed that solasodine, which is found in eggplants (and perhaps also in potatoes), produces teratomas in fetus of hamsters gavaged with 1.2 to 1.6 g/kg. The defects included spina bifida, exencephaly, and cranial bleb.

It is clear, as discussed in Chapter 5, that teratogenesis is dependent on many external and internal factors. One of these external factors is molecular structure, as demonstrated by Brown and Keeler (1978) in the case of the solanidan epimers.

These steroids are pharmacologically potent compounds and many compounds in this class are teratogenic in experimental animals (Kalter 1968; Keeler 1979). One possible mechanism might be in the direction of producing secondary nutritional deficiencies, as certain steroids are known to cause changes in tissue levels of retinol, ascorbic acid, and other water-soluble vitamins (Millen and Woollam 1957; Warkany 1971).

Lathyrogens

Human lathyrism is a neurological disease associated with the consumption of legumes of the genus Lathyrus, particularly chickling vetch (*L. sativus*), Spanish vetch (*L. clymenum*), and flat-podded vetch (*L. cicera*). The disease is quite insidious; it may be precipitated by fatigue and exposure to cold and wetness. The symptoms begin with back pain, and weakness and stiffness of the legs. Muscular weakness, and in severe cases, paralysis of the legs follow, limiting the victim's mobility to crawling. Males between 20 and 29 years old appear to be most sensitive to lathyrogenic agents, and are the ones usually affected (McPhee 1956; Selye 1957; Stockman 1929). Presently, lathyrism is confined mostly to the Indian subcontinent.

Toxic Factors in Lathyrus Seeds

Four types of toxic substances have been identified in the seeds of Lathyrus plants. The species containing these compounds are listed in Table 8.3 with their

Table 8.3 Lathyrogens in Seeds of Various *Lathrus* spp.

Species	Lathyrogen[a,f]	Species	Lathyrogen[a,f]
alatus	ODPA**	*leteus*	DBA**
articulatus	ODPA**	*megallanicus*	ODPA**
arvense	ODPA**	*multiflora*	DBA**, ODBA*
aurantius	DBA**		ODPA[d]
cicera	ODPA[d]		
cirrhosus	ODPA**	*ochrus*	ODPA**
clymenum	ODPA**	*odoratus*	GAPN*
gorgoni	DBA**, ODBA*,	*pannonicus*	ODPA*
	ODPA*	*pseudocicera*	ODPA[d]
		pusillus	GAPN*
grandiflora	DBA**, ODBA*, ODPA*	*quadrimarginatus*	ODPA[d]
		roseus	GAPN[d]
		rotundifolius	DBA**, ODBA*
heterophyllus	DBA**, ODBA*		ODPA*
	ODPA*	*sativus*[b,e]	ODPA**
		setitolius	ODPA***
hirsutus	GAPN[c]	*sylvestris*	DBA**
laevigatus var		*tremolsianus*	ODPA[d]
aureus	DBA**	*tuberosus*	DBA**, ODBA*
latifolius	DBA**, ODBA*		ODPA*
	ODPA*	*undulatus*	DBA**, ODBA*
			ODPA[d]

Abbreviations: DBA, diaminobutyric acid; ODBA, N-γ-oxalyl-α-γ-diaminobutyric acid; ODPA, N-β-oxalyl-α-β-diaminopropionic acid; GAPA, γ-glutamyl-β-aminopropionitrile.
[a]All toxicants are neurolathyrogens except GAPN, which is an osteolathyrogen.
[b]Associated with human lathyrism.
[c]Osteolathyrogen.
[d]Trace.
[e]Contains also N-β-D-glucopyranosyl-N-L-arabinosyl-α-β-diaminopropionitrile.
[f]Asterisk(s) on each toxicant represent a range of approximate values on a dry basis: *0.5-1.0%; **1-2%; ***2.%.
Source: Bell (1973).

corresponding toxic compounds. As demonstrated in animals, three of these compounds are neurolathyrogens; e.g., α-γ-diaminobutyric acid (DBA), N-γ-oxalyl-α-γ-diamino-butyric acid (ODBA), N-β-oxalyl-α-β-diaminopropionic acid (ODPA); one compound, γ-glutamyl-β-aminopropionitrile (GAPN), is an osteolathyrogen. Structures of these compounds are shown below.

$$H_2NCH_2CH_2CH-COOH$$

DBA NH_2

$$HOOC-\overset{O}{\overset{\|}{C}}-NHCH_2\overset{NH_2}{\overset{|}{C}H}-COOH$$

ODPA

$$HOOC-\overset{O}{\overset{\|}{C}}-NHCH_2CH_2\overset{NH_2}{\overset{|}{C}H}-COOH$$

ODBA

$$\overset{CN}{\overset{|}{C}H_2}CH_2NH\overset{O}{\overset{\|}{C}}CH_2\overset{NH_2}{\overset{|}{C}HCOOH}$$

GAPN

An osteolathyrogen is distinguished from a neurolathyrogen in that the former produces its characteristic toxicity by interfering in the cross-linking of component chains of collagen (Levene 1962) and elastin (O'Dell et al. 1966). Severe skeletal deformities result from the weakened bones, and aortic aneurysms are possible from the abnormal walls of blood vessels. Severe skeletal deformities in young rats (McKay et al. 1954) and aortic aneurysms in both rats and chicks (Bachhuber et al. 1955) have been observed when these animals have been fed β-aminopropionitrile, the active moiety of GAPN (Dasler 1954; Dupuy and Lee 1954).

Among the neurolathyrogens, only ODPA may be associated with human lathyrism, since it is found to be the only lathyrogen in Lathyrus species implicated in this crippling disease. This compound has been found to produce neurological effects in young dogs, rats, and guinea pigs (Rao and Sarma 1967) and birds (Adiga et al. 1963). Intraperitoneal injections of 10 to 20 mg and 100 mg, have proved to be toxic to day-old chicks and 12-day-old dogs, respectively. It has been shown to be a powerful excitant of the spinal interneurons in cats (Watkins et al. 1966) and the brain cells of young rats (Cheema et al. 1970). Most importantly, the evidence regarding ODPA's possible involvement in human lathyrism has been greatly strengthened by the observation that when adult monkeys are injected intrathecally with the lathyrogen typical hind leg paralysis develops (Rao et al. 1967). However, the toxin has no effect when injected intraperitoneally in adult animals except in those made acidotic with calcium chloride (Cheema et al. 1969). It has been suggested that this lack of toxicity by intraperitoneal injection in adults, in contrast to young animals, may be due to the exclusion of the compound by the blood-brain barrier, which is still imperfect in the young (Curtis and Watson 1965). Acidosis, elicited by calcium chloride, and other factors may allow compounds to permeate this barrier. Even though this explanation is plausible, the actual toxic factor in human lathyrism is still not conclusively known.

N-β-D-glucopyranosyl-N-α-L-arabinosyl-α,β-diaminopropionitrile, a neurotoxin, also has been isolated from L. sativus (Rukmini 1969, 1968). It is present in low concentrations in the seed (0.003%), and is toxic to day-old chicks at 50 mg/100 g body weight. Its role in human lathyrism is also unclear, partly because of its low concentration.

L. sativus also contains the α-oxalyl isomer of ODPA; but its toxicity is not known (Bell and O'Donovan 1966).

L-α-γ-diaminobutyric acid (DBA), another neurotoxin, is present in high concentrations in certain Lathyrus species. As shown in Table 8.3, it is found in at least 13 species. For example, L. sylvestris seeds contain 2.7% DBA (as the monohydrochloride) by weight (VanEtten and Miller 1963). Other researchers have reported a lower value of 1.4% (Ressler et al. 1961). At least six other species from five related genera contain DBA. These species and corresponding DBA values, expressed as the percentage of total nitrogen, are: *Abrus precatorius* (0.04%), *Cicer arietinum* (0.03%), *Lens culimaris* (0.14%), *Pisum sativum* (0.12%), *Vicia cracca* (0.14%), and *Vicia fava* (0.05%). DBA is not limited exclusively to Lathyrus and related genera; it is also found in at least 80 other species, particularly in the Cruciferae and Leguminosae families (VanEtten and Miller 1963). In these species, the amount of DBA range from 0.01 to 0.07% of the total nitrogen. These values are low enough to be of little toxicological significance.

The γ-, α, N-γ; and N-α-oxalyl derivatives of L-α,γ-diaminobutyric acid (DBA) are also found in at least 10 species of Lathyrus (Bell and O'Donovan 1966). These compounds coexist in these seeds with ODPA, ODBA, and DBA. The γ-oxalyl derivative have been shown to be neurotoxic to young chicks at doses of 30 to 35 mg/chick (Rao and Sarma 1966). Thus, the toxicity of Lathyrus seeds, most probably, is the result of the combined effects of these compounds.

In addition to the aforementioned compounds, many unusual amino acids have been found in Lathyrus species. These amino acids include L-homoarginine, isolated from *L. cicera* (Bell 1964), *L. sativus* (Rao et al. 1963), and 39 other Lathyrus species (Bell 1964); lathyrine, a major constituent of at least 12 of 16 species of Lathyrus containing lathyrine (Bell 1962), with *L. tingitanus* and *L. variegatus* containing the highest concentration; γ-hydroxyhomoarginine, in four Lathyrus species (Bell 1964); γ-methylglutamic acid, from *L. maritimus* (Przybylska and Strong 1968); and γ-hydroxynorvaline, from *L. odoratus* (Fowden 1966). Except for L-homoarginine, which was found to be nontoxic to the rat (Rao et al. 1963; Stevens and Bush 1950), the toxic properties of the other unusual amino acids have not been determined. However, because of the similarity of γ-hydroxynorvaline to threonine, the former might be toxic to animals because of a possible antagonism with protein amino acid.

It has been reported that *L. sativus* harvested in localities with endemic lathyrism is frequently contaminated with the common vetch *Vicia sativa* (Anderson et al. 1924). It also has been found to be a contaminant of wheat eaten during several outbreaks of lathyrism in India (Shah 1939). This observation is significant, since *V. sativa* produces neurological symptoms in ducks and adult monkeys in contrast to *L. sativus* which does not. The toxic factors in *V. sativa* have been identified by Ressler et al. (Ressler 1962; Ressler et al. 1964, 1967) as β-cyanoalanine and its γ-glutamyl derivative. β-cyanoalanine is present to the extent of 0.1% of the seed. The subcutaneous LD_{50} of β-cyanoalanine in young or adult rats is 13.5 mg/100 g; when injected or fed to young or adult rats and chickens at specific levels, this compound causes convulsions, rigidity, prostration, and death (Ressler et al. 1964, 1967). This amino acid interferes with the rat liver enzyme cystathionase, the pyridoxal phosphate-requiring enzyme which is needed to convert cystathionine to cystine. Thus, expectedly, β-cyanoalanine added to the diets of rats causes large excretion of cystathionine (Pfeffer and Ressler 1967).

Even though the role of *V. sativa* in human lathyrism is not known, its occurrence as a contaminant in human foodstuffs, and its demonstrated neurotoxicity in adult animals has led to the suggestion that perhaps β-cyanoalanine or its bound form, γ-L-glutamyl-β-cyano-L-alanine, may be a factor in human lathyrism (Resser 1962).

β-cyano-L-alanine is also found in the narrow-leaf vetch *V. angustifolia* (Ressler 1962).

A possible practical procedure for detoxification of Lathyrus seeds has been suggested by Mohan et al. (1966). These researchers maintain that most of the toxin in the seed can be leached out by soaking the seeds in hot water for several minutes. Of course, a more effective means of controlling human lathyrism is total avoidance of the lathyrogenic legumes, and replacement of these species by nontoxic varieties.

Favic Agents

Consumption of faba beans (*Vicia faba*) or inhalation of its pollen has been associated with the disease known as favism. The infirmity is characterized by hemolytic anemia, hemoglobinuria, and shock (Luisada 1941; McPhee 1956; Stockman 1929). The favic attack may occur rapidly with hemolysis starting within a few minutes. In most cases, however, the attack is delayed from 5 to 24 hr (Luisada 1941). Mortality of less than 8% of those exposed has been reported (Crosby 1956). In mild cases, malaise, dizziness, gastrointestinal upset, pallor, jaundice, vomiting, and lumbar pain are often observed. The disease is usually self-limiting in adults, with the acute stage lasting 24 to 48 hr. Recovery is spontaneous and complete. However, repeated attacks will occur with each new exposure.

Cooked or raw fresh beans, even without skins, are most often associated with favism. Dried beans seem to have less favic activity (Luisada 1941). Thus, the incidence of favism rises during periods when freshly harvested beans are available, generally during spring and early summer. However, it is claimed that the practice of storing dried beans underground under anaerobic conditions in certain parts of Egypt is associated with the rise in incidence of favism in that country in the fall (Patwardhan and White 1973). Thus, it appears that drying or possibly exposure to oxygen and light may decrease favic activity in these seeds.

Favism is present in the Mediterranean area in such countries as Sardinia, Sicily, Southern Italy, Greece, Turkey, Cyprus, Israel, Egypt, and Spain (Belsey 1970; Luisada 1941). Sardinia has recorded the highest number of cases, five per 1000 population annually (Crosby 1956). In 1965, Iran had a high incidence of favism, from two to nine per 10,000 population (Donoso et al. 1969). Favism also has been recorded in China (Du 1952) and sporadically in the United States (McPhee 1956).

Male children appear to be most susceptible to favism. Susceptibility to favism is an inherited deficiency, characterized by very low concentrations of reduced glutathione (GSH) and glucose-6-phosphate dehydrogenase (G-6-PD) in erythrocytes (Luisada 1941; Sansone et al. 1958; Szeinberg and Chari-Bitron 1957; Zinkham et al. 1958). The latter deficiency seems to be compensated by an increase in transketolase and transaldolase activities (Bonsignori et al. 1961), possibly as an attempt by the body to by-pass the pathway utilizing glucose-6-phosphate dehydrogenase.

The hemolysis caused by faba beans is similar to one caused by premaquine, a hemolytic drug, in individuals with the inborn defects in erythrocytes mentioned above (Crosby 1956; Carson et al. 1956). Thus, the total quality of glutathione is reduced, but the proportion of oxidized glutathione (GSSG) is higher than in normal erythrocytes (Srivastava and Beutler 1968).

Glucose-6-phosphate dehydrogenase deficiency is a sex-linked trait transmitted by an incompletely dominant gene located on the X chromosome. Among Sardinian males, up to 48% are G-6-PD deficient (Siniscalco et al. 1961); the corresponding figure among male Kurdish Jews is 53% (Szeinberg et al. 1958a,b,c). Similarly, black Africans, as well as Asian and Egyptian males, appear to have a high incidence of G-6-PD deficiency; as much as 24 to 26% of these population groups may have this deficiency (Mager et al. 1969).

There are variants or isozymes of G-6-PD, and a deficiency of any of these can result in drug sensitivity. However, not all cases of favism are seen in G-6-PD-deficient persons, even though most of them may be susceptible to hemolysis induced by certain drugs (World Health Organization 1967). The Mediterranean variants have very low enzyme activity (less than 5% of normal) in the erythrocytes and low Michaelis constants for the substrate glucose-6-phosphate (Kirkman 1968). While these factors may partly explain the sensitivity of the Mediterranean variants to favism, it is not always true that a G-6-PD deficiency in the Mediterranean area is positively correlated with the incidence of favism. This situation is underscored by the observation that favism is rare in certain parts of Greece, even though about 20% of the population may be G-6-PD deficient (Stamatoyannopolos et al. 1966). Thus, susceptibility to favism appears not to rest solely on G-6-PD deficiency. Other factor(s) which remain to be demonstrated must act in conjunction with G-6-PD deficiency in order to elicit the disease.

Toxic Compounds in the Faba Bean

In the presence of raw faba bean extracts, G-6-PD-deficient erythrocytes show a significant decrease in GSH concentration compared to normal erythrocytes (Bowman and Walker 1961). There is some analogy in the activity of faba bean extract and primaquine, an hemolytic drug (Panizon and Zacchello 1965), except that the latter causes loss of potassium ions from the G-6-PD-deficient erythrocytes, whereas the faba bean extract does not. The structures of toxicants in the faba bean are shown below.

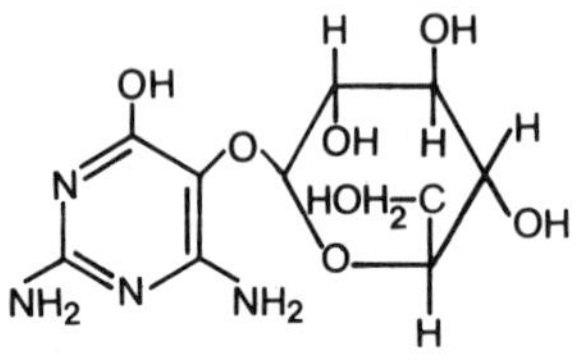

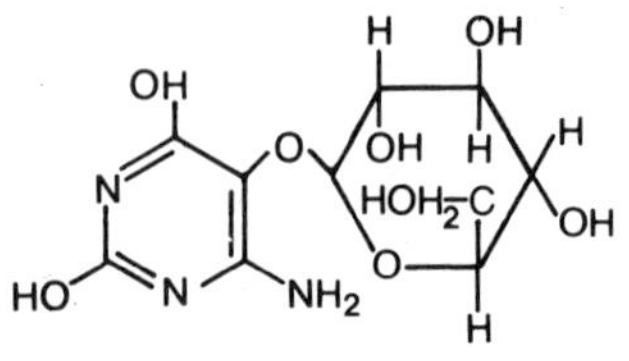

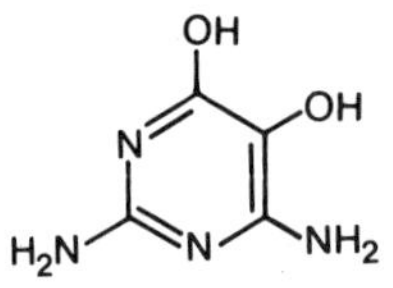

Divicine 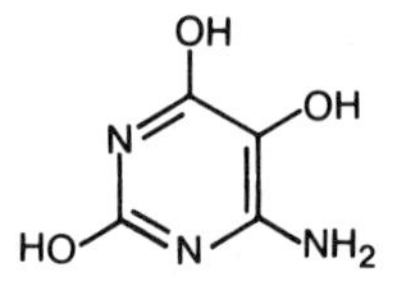   Isouramil

Favic Glycosides and corresponding aglycones

Vicine, a nucleoside, has been reported to inhibit G-6-PD activity in vitro. It also has been found to produce mild hemoglobinuria when given to dogs by stomach tube at 0.2 g/kg, and to retard growth in rats. On the basis of these activities, Lin and Ling (1962a,b) have posulated that this compound may be the hemolytic agent in the faba bean. Another nucleoside, convicine, is also present in faba beans (Bien et al. 1968).

Vicine and convicine (note structures) can be hydrolyzed by emulsin, a β-glucosidase, in a mild acid solution to yield the aglycones divicine and isouramil, respectively (Bendich and Clements 1952; Bien et al. 1968). Both aglycones can decrease the GSH content of human erythrocytes suspended in phosphate buffer-saline at pH 7.4 (Mager et al. 1965). Apparently, the decrease in GSH follows from the inability of the erythrocytes to reduce oxidized glutathione (GSSG). This is because the hemolytic aglycones interfered in the activity of G-6-PD, which was already deficient (Mager et al. 1969). This interference results in a lack of NADPH which is necessary for the reduction of GSSG.

In normal erythrocytes, glucose abolishes the effect of these compounds; this is not the case with G-6-PD-deficient cells. Thus, the active components are the aglycones, since the presence of glycosidic bond at position 5 in the pyrimidine ring makes the parent glucosides completely inactive. Hydrolysis, for example, by intestinal bacteria may be necessary for the activity of vicine and convicine (Mager et al. 1969).

Faba bean also contains 3,4-dihydroxy-L-phenylalanine (L-DOPA) (Kosower and Kosower 1967). DOPA may be transformed to dopaquinone by action of tyrosinase. The quinone is active in causing a decrease in GSH in erythrocytes in G-6-PD-deficient subjects, whereas L-DOPA is not (Buetler 1970). Indeed, L-DOPA is present in garden peas (*Pisum sativum*), which rarely causes, if at all, acute hemolysis as seen in favism.

It is possible that L-DOPA and divicine or isouramil may act synergistically in causing a lowering of erythrocyte GSH in these subjects (Razin et al. 1968). For that matter, ascorbic acid will also enhance the hemolytic property of divicine and isouramil (Razin et al. 1968).

Photodynamic Substances

In Chapter 1, the theoretical aspects of the photosensitization reaction are discussed. It is shown that photodynamic substances, in response to the action of light, are transformed into highly reactive compounds. These photoactivated compounds in turn react with susceptible receptors in the cell, producing characteristic lesions. The skin, under the influence of the photodynamic substance, becomes hypersensitive to light. It becomes inflamed, blisters, and eventually becomes phlegmonous and gangrenous. Inflammation of the conjuctiva, pharynx, larynx, and bronchus may accompany the skin condition which resembles erysipelas. Animals so affected may show convulsion and delerium (Blum 1938, 1941; Clare 1955).

The photodynamic substances accumulate in the skin of animals owing to inefficient excretion. Photodynamism, also known as fagopyrism (from the buckwheat genus, Fagopyrum), has so far been observed only in white-skinned animals. No human cases have been reported, although it may easily be mistaken for sunburn or tanning. In this case, fagopyrism may be distinguished by exposing the suspected skin to light filtered through plate glass which does not allow ultravoilet light to pass through (Clare 1955).

The above symptoms are characteristics of primary fagopyrism, which is generally observed in animals ingesting buckwheat (*F. esculentum*) (Clare 1955). The photodynamic substance is identified as fagopyrin; the chemical structure of this compound is similar to hypericin, a napthodianthrone derivative which also has potent photodynamic activity (see structures below). The latter is obtained from the klamath weed, or St. Johnswort (*Hypericium perforatum*). Fagopyrin is found in all parts of the buckwheat plant, including the seed (Brockmann 1957). Another pigment identified in buckwheat is photofagopyrin, whose structure is similar to fagopyrin, except that in the former, there are only seven fused rings as compared to eight in the latter. Buckwheat, however, seems to be devoid of fagopyritic effects in man, most probably because of the efficient excretory mechanism.

Hypericin is fatal to rats and mice, when the animals are exposed to sunlight following treatment. Thus, 1 to 2 mg hypericin has been shown to kill rats in 1 to 2 hr after administration of the photosensitive compound followed by exposure to sunlight; 0.25 to 0.5 mg of hypericin has been shown to kill mice within 24 hr following exposure of animals to a 2000-W lamp for 30 min (Brockman and Kluge 1951; Brockman et al. 1942, 1957).

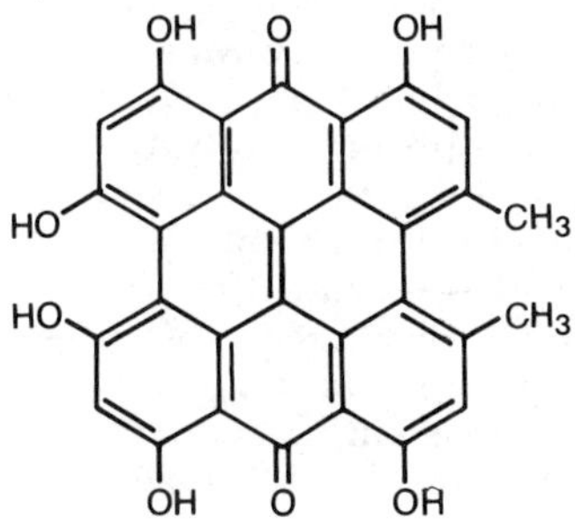

Hypercin

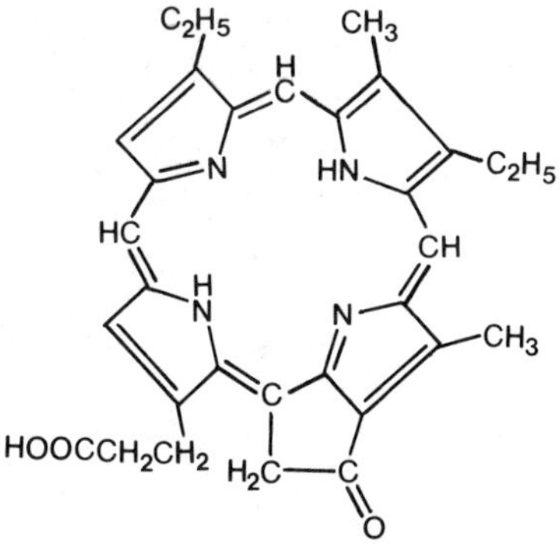

Phylloermythrin

The furocoumarins, such as isopimpinellin, are also photodynamic. These pigments are found in the juice and oils of citrus fruits, celery, parsley, and other plants (Bernhard 1958; Fitzpatrick et al. 1955).

Isopimpinellin

There are also chemically uncharacterized, as yet, photodynamic substances in oats, sorghum, and various species of Vicia (Arscott and Harper 1963).

Phylloerythrin, a photodynamic derivative of chlorophyll, may be deposited in the skin in the presence of liver dysfunction and biliary obstruction. The resulting fagopyrism is characterized by general icterus, which results from liver damage. This type of photodynamism, known as ictrogenic fagopyrism, has been observed only in animals (Torlone and Rampichini 1959).

Phylloerythrin has been identified as the photodynamic substance that causes the disease in South African sheep known as "geeldikkop." These animals develop the disease after eating species of Tribulus and Lippia plants. These plants contain ictrogenic compounds which interfere with bile excretion. Thus, bile accumulates in the blood, and phylloerythrin, which is normally excreted through the bile, is deposited in the skin instead.

The ictrogenic compounds in *Lippia rehmanni* have been identified as icterogenin and rehmannic acid. These compounds are steroidal in nature (Heikel and Rimington 1968; Rimington and Quin 1934, 1937). Intraperitoneal injection of icterogenin in rabbits causes a marked decrease in bile flow, and consequently, a severe reduction in the excretion of bile pigments and porphyrin.

Phylloerythrin is produced normally during digestion in animals by action of intestinal bacteria on chlorophyll (Quin et al. 1935).

Certain flavones, such as quercetin, can enhance the effect of photodynamic substances (Horsley 1934).

Toxic Plant Phenolic Substances and Alcohols

Probably more than 800 phenolic compounds are recognized in plants, not including sugars and closely related compounds (Geissman and Hinreiner 1952; Karrer 1958). These compounds may be divided into two major groups based on frequency of occurrence, similarity in structure, and relative toxicity: (1) phenolic compounds having widespread and common occurrence in plant-derived foods and beverages; approximately 25 compounds are identified (Bate-Smith 1965, 1968; Swain 1965); and (2) more heterogeneous groups of compounds, including a few dozen phenolic derivatives which are highly toxic or have potent pharmacological activities (Singleton and Kratzer 1969).

In the first group, some of the compounds occur in relatively high concentrations in some plant foodstuffs; a majority of these compounds are present in trace quantities. Because of widespread consumption, it can be presumed that these substances normally are devoid of acute toxicity at the levels they are usually found in food. Evolutionary adaptation probably gave animals, including man, the capability to detoxify these compounds very easily (Singleton and Kratzer 1973). This first group includes phenolic acids such as caffeic, ferulic, sinapic, and gallic acids, their derivatives, flavonoids, lignin, hydrolizable and condensed tannins, ellagic acids, and derivatives of these compounds. As seen in Chapter 9, some of these compounds have antinutritive properties. The tannins are carcinogens and will be discussed in another section.

Examples of the second group include gossypol, phlorizin, coumarins, myristicin, urushiols, and phenolic amines or cathecholamines. Some of these compounds are discussed elsewhere in this chapter in connection with compounds having specific pharmacological effects. Some toxic phenolic compounds found contaminating foodstuffs are discussed in Chapter 17.

Gossypol

Gossypol, or 1,1', 6,6', 7,7'-hexahydroxy-5,5'-diisopropyl-3,3'-dimethyl-(2,2'-binaphthalene)-8,8'-dicarboxaldehyde, is a yellow pigment present in the pigment glands of the leaf, stem, laproot bark, roots, and especially the seed of the cotton plant (Gossypium spp.) (Royce et al. 1941; Smith 1962). This pigment was thought to be confined to this genus, but another source of gossypol, the tropical tree *Thepesia populnea*, has been identified (Datta et al. 1968; King and DeSilva 1968). Gossypol occurs in three tautomeric forms, the phenolic quinoid tautomer (I), aldehyde (II), and the hemiacetal (III). This is illustrated below:

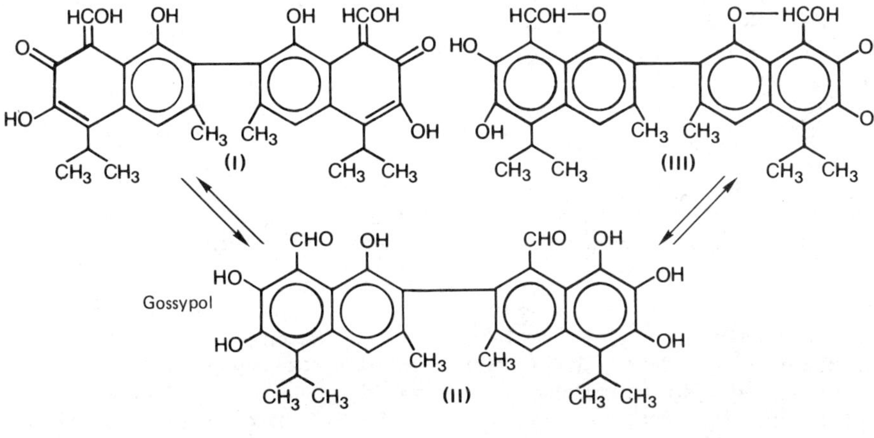

As a potential toxicant, this pigment would have remained a mere scientific curiosity were it not for the fact that cottonseed protein has gained in importance as a supplement to both animal and human diets. Cottonseed protein is now widely available for supplementation of nutritionally poor diets in many developing nations (Decossass et al. 1968; Harper and Smith 1968).

Large amounts of cottonseed are processed in the production of cotton fiber. For each metric ton of cotton fiber, 1.68 metric ton of cottonseed can be produced (Altschul et al. 1958). From 1 metric ton of cottonseed, 470 kg of feed-grade meal can be obtained (Altschul et al. 1958); from 150 to 200 kg of food-grade flour can be processed from a ton of meal. The refined cottonseed flour may contain up to 60% protein. It is obvious that cottonseed is a valuable and abundant source of supplementary protein for human consumption. Thus, the presence of gossypol in the meal is of toxicological importance.

The pigment gland represents about 2 to 5% of the kernel of cotton plants raised in the United States, and 20 to 39% of the weight of the gland is gossypol; the gland also contains about 2% other related pigments (Berardi and Goldblatt 1969). Processing removes 80 to 99% of the gossypol. The pigment is extracted with the oil and is removed by alkaline treatment. About 0.5 to 1.2% of the total gossypol generally remains in the processed meal. Less than 0.06% is free gossypol. In the United States, maximum allowable gossypol content of cottonseed preparations for human food has been set at 0.045% (Berardi and Goldblatt 1969).

Toxicity of Gossypol   The toxicity of gossypol is influenced by many factors, and is attributed mainly to the unbound pigment. However, it has been suggested that the several forms of both free and bound gossypol have different activities (Berardi and Martinez 1966). In addition, other toxicants in the seed may also contribute to its over-all toxicity (Eagle 1960).

Gossypol affects mainly nonruminants; ruminants are generally resistant (Reiser and Fu 1962), except the young animals whose rumens are not yet fully functional (Adams et al. 1960).

The LD_{50} of gossypol is quite high, indicating a low acute oral toxicity: The value for rats is about 2.6 g/kg when administered in water; it is 10% more toxic when given in oil. Similarly, the oral LD_{50} values of gossypol administered in water for mice, rabbits, and guinea pigs have been reported to be 500 to 950, 350 to 600, and 280 to 300 mg/kg, respectively (Eagle et al. 1948). The toxicity also increases by 10% when the pigment is administered in oil. The oral LD_{50} for pigs, as determined by Lyman et al. 1963), is 550 mg/kg; over 0.02% gossypol in diet was established as toxic to pigs (Clawson et al. 1961). A level of 0.01% or less is considered safe (Hale et al. 1958). This safe level is equivalent, usually, to about 9% cottonseed meal.

Dogs are very sensitive to gossypol; 10 to 200 mg/kg/day reportedly would kill dogs in less than a month (Eagle 1960). Chickens are slightly more sensitive than rats. Thus, as with many other poisonous substances, there are interspecific differences regarding gossypol toxicity.

the oral LD_{50} in rats for the intact pigment glands suspended in water is from 0.925 to 2.17 g/kg; in oil, it is slightly less toxic (Eagle 1960). The higher toxicity of the gland compared to the isolated pigment may be due to three factors: (1) potentiation by unidentified toxicants in the seed; (2) increased absorption due to the presence of oil; and (3) decreased rate of inactivation in the gut, or a combination of all these factors. However, the presence of other toxicants in cottonseed has not yet been established.

Symptoms of Gossypol Poisoning in Animals   The symptoms of gossypol poisoning have been observed in rats (Gallup 1931; Tone and Jensen 1970); rabbits (Menaul 1923; Schwartze and Alsberg 1924); cats (Schwartze and Alsberg 1924); pigs (Smith 1957); dogs (Eagle 1960); and chicks (Hill and Totsuka 1964). In most of these animals, feeding or treatment with gossypol results in weight reduction, loss of appetite, and consequently, growth retardation. In addition, rabbits, dogs, and pigs also develop diarrhea. Spastic paralysis has been observed in rabbits and cats. The poisoning can be quite severe and fatal.

A significant manifestation of gossypol poisoning is seen in the effect on blood or hematopoiesis. Thus, after 14 days on a diet containing gossypol, rats develop anemia characterized by a decreased concentration of erythrocytes and their hemoglobin content (Tone and Jensen 1970) — signs which are typical of iron deficiency anemia. These signs, and the fact that treatment with iron-dextran complex partially prevents growth retardation, suggest that gossypol interferes with normal iron utilization in hemoglobin synthesis. A decrease in hemoglobin content in the blood and hematocrit level also has been observed in pits fed a ration containing 240 ppm gossypol for 15 weeks (Braham et al. 1967). Hemoglobin and hematocrit levels have been shown to decrease even before the pigs show signs of poisoning. Serum proteins and their iron-binding capacity are also reduced. The investigators (Skutches et al. 1974) attribute this to the inhibitory effect of gossypol on protein synthesis. Chicks fed the pigment have shown decreased blood hemoglobin (Chang 1955), hemolytic anemia (Rigdon et al. 1958), and lowering of total serum proteins (Narain et al. 1961, 1958).

Rabbits and pigs (Harms and Holley 1951) fed gossypol develop hypoprothrombin-emia and also hemorrhaging in the pigs' livers, stomachs, and small intestines. It has been suggested that the effects of gossypol in swine may result from the chelation of iron, interfering in the synthesis of hemoglobin and iron-containing enzymes, such as respiratory enzymes. The symptoms usually seen with gossypol poisoning also suggest iron deficiency: palpitation, weakness, and shallow breathing (Skutches et al. 1973).

Gossypol poisoning also causes severe damage to internal organs. For example, rats develop in addition to hemorrhage, gastritis and enteritis in the distal part of the duodenum, liver damage, and congestion in the kidneys, which sometimes affect most parts of the intestines (El-Nockrashy et al. 1963). Edema, an excessive accumulation of fluids in the peritoneal, pleural, and/or pericardial cavities, has been shown to occur in gossypol-poisoned cats (Schwartze and Alsberg 1924), digs (Eagle 1960), and pigs (Smith 1957). Cats develop dyspnea with rapid pulse. Gossypol poisoning in these animals is also characterized by emaciation, progressive weakness, and thumping. Pigs also show degeneration of the spleen, cardiac muscle, and liver, the latter with intralobular necrosis; dilatation and hypertrophy of the heart; deficiency of lymphoid cells; edema of the heart and lymph nodes; and dyspnea. Hydropericardium and congestion of the splanchnic organs has been shown to develop in gossypol-poisoned dogs.

In chicks, gossypol causes hypertrophy of the gall bladder (Lillie and Bird 1950) and pancreas (Hill and Totsuka 1964).

Mechanism of Gossypol Toxicity   Gossypol is, in fact, an antinutritive substance. It forms an insoluble chelate with many essential metals (Ramaswamy and O'Connor 1969, 1970), such as iron (Braham et al. 1967), and binds with amino acids in proteins, especially lysine (Conkerton and Frampton 1959). Thus, this amino acid becomes unavailable, and secondary lysine deficiency occurs (Kuiken et al. 1948). Gossypol also forms complexes with other amino acids (Cater and Lyman 1969).

More importantly, the binding of gossypol to proteins indicates that it can inactivate important enzymes. Indeed, studies have shown that gossypol can inhibit the activity of enzymes. This pigment can combine with pepsinogen in vitro inhibiting its conversion to pepsin (Finlay et al. 1973; Tanksley et al. 1970; Wong et al. 1972). Pyridoxal phosphate, which forms a Schiff base with amino groups, can protect the proenzyme (Finlay et al. 1973). Gossypol also inhibits in vivo the livery cytochrome oxidase and succinic dehydrogenase in chicks, but not in the livers of hens. These enzymes from normal hens are inhibited in vitro (Ferguson et al. 1959). This difference between young and adult chickens suggests that the detoxification mechanism in the young bird is still not fully functional. This fact may also explain the failure of gossypol to inactivate these enzymes in the liver of adult pigs, rabbits, and rats (Meksongsee et al. 1970).

Ingested gossypol concentrates in the microsomal fraction and mitochondria of the rat (Abou-Donia and Dieckert 1971; Dieckert and Abou-Donia 1972). In the case of the microsomes, the pigment stimulates the synthesis of oxidative dealkylases, so that in the rat, the dealkylation of many carbamate pesticides is enhanced when the pigment is fed. Its presence in high concentrations in the mitochondria suggests that many oxidative enzymes in this organelle can be affected. In fact, gossypol uncouples the respiratory chain phosphorylation in rat liver mitochondria (Abou-Donia and Dieckert 1974). This uncoupling could explain certain relevant observations, such as the significant reduction of metabolizable energy in hens fed high levels of the pigment (Hill and Totsuka 1964).

To a significant degree, then, gossypol toxicity may be explained on the bases of the aforementioned effects.

The binding of iron to gossypol occurs on a one-to-one molar ratio (Ramaswamy and O'Connor 1969, 1970). As already mentioned, iron deficiency anemia is one manifestation of gossypol toxicity. Therefore, toxicity is decreased if additional iron is given to animals (Braham et al. 1967). Toxicity is abolished only if calcium hydroxide is also administered (Braham et al. 1967). This effect may be explained in part by the fact that the ferrous-gossypol complex is less soluble in the presence of calcium (Shieh et al. 1968).

   The binding of amino acid residues to gossypol lowers the digestibility of proteins (Lyman et al. 1959; Smith and Clawson 1970), and, in fact, makes other amino acids even less available than lysine (Cater and Lyman 1970). In addition, gossypol is bound at high levels to tissue proteins in the stomach, liver, muscles, kidney, spleen, and blood (Abou-Donia et al. 1970; Buitrago et al. 1970; Lyman et al. 1969; Smith and Clawson 1970). The bound gossypol may remain in the tissues over an extended period. The half-life of the pigment in the body tissues of the rat, including the gastrointestinal (GI) tract, is about 48 hr (Abou-Donia et al. 1970); in pig liver, the bound gossypol may decrease to about one-fifth of the original value in 34 days (Buitrago et al. 1970). The half-life in the pig, based on the radioactivity count of administered ^{14}C-gossypol, is 78 hr (Abou-Donia and Dieckert 1975). In trout fed gossypol over an extended period, gossypol accumulation in the tissues increases slowly, and when subsequently fed a gossypol-free diet, the bound pigment is eliminated very slowly. In some tissues, the pigment even increased over a 10-week period (Roehm et al. 1967).

   Gossypol toxicity is therefore decreased by high intakes of protein containing excess lysine (Clawson et al. 1961; Tone and Jensen 1970). The excess protein in the diet serves to bind gossypol. Since the gossypol-protein complex is not easily digestible, less gossypol is absorbed (Lyman et al. 1969, 1959; Smith and Clawson 1970).

   The addition of excess iron also diminishes toxicity for similar reasons: The iron-gossypol complex, especially with ferric metal, is less water soluble and is eliminated in the feces (Abou-Donia et al. 1970; Braham et al. 1967). Excess iron also hastens the removal of bound or accumulated pigment in the tissues (Buitrago et al. 1970). For example, in the presence of added iron, the half-life of gossypol bound in the body tissues of the rat is 23 hr, compared to 48 hr without iron (Abou-Donia et al. 1970).

   Effect of Gossypol in Humans   While there are a limited number of studies regarding the effect of gossypol in humans, the few observations that have been made indicate that consumption of diets containing moderate amounts of cottonseed meal may be safe even for children. Thus, bread containing small amounts of cottonseed meal has been shown to produce no ill effects in humans after 1 year (Bydagyan et al. 1947). Similarly, no harmful effects have been noted when 60 g cottonseed cake originally containing 0.11 to 0.20% free gossypol has been fed daily to humans for 4.5 months (Harper and Smith 1968). A cottonseed-containing product known as Incaparina has been commercially produced in some countries, notably, Guatemala for several years without any signs of harmful effects (Berardi and Goldblatt 1969; Gillham 1969; Harper and Smith 1968). This product, when given to children under close supervision for over 2 years, improved their nutritional status and showed no signs of toxicity.

   Nevertheless, the toxic potential of gossypol is evident from animal studies, so that limits of gossypol content in foodstuffs have been set: 0.45% in the United States and 0.06 and 1.2% free and total gossypol, respectively, by internal organizations (Berardi and Goldblatt 1969).

   Reduction of Free Gossypol in Cottonseed Meal   The formation of an insoluble iron-gossypol complex, especially in the presence of $Ca(OH)_3$, has been the basis for reducing the free gossypol content of cottonseed meal preparations to very low levels (Mayorga et al. 1975). The use of such additives as $FeSO_4$ and $Ca(OH)_3$ also protects lysine from reacting with gossypol even in the presence of heat (Bressani et al. 1964).

   A glandless cotton plant, *Gossypium hirsutum*, is available (McMichael 1960). Another glandless variety, *G. barbadense*, has been developed by seed irradiation (Afifi et al. 1965); this character is dominantly genetically transmissible (Nassar 1969). The meals from glandless varieties are equal, if not superior, to ether-extracted, commercial cottonseed meals (Smith et al. 1961).

Alkylated Catechols and Related Phenolic Compounds

The mango (*Mangifera indica*) (see Fig. 1), cashew (*Anacardium occidentale*), and pistachio (*Pistacia vera*) are tropical plants of the family Anacardiaceae. These plants

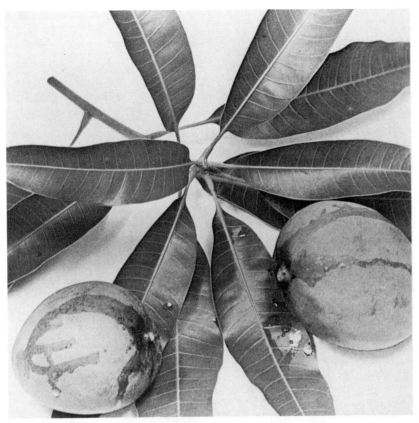

Fig. 8.1 Mango *(Mangifera indica)*. (Courtesy of Julia F. Morton, Director, Morton Collectanea, University of Miami, Coral Gables, Florida.)

yield edible fruits, nuts, and seeds — indeed, the extremely delicious mango is considered the queen of tropical fruits. However, this family is notorious for its many poisonous members, notably the poison ivy *(Toxicodendron radicans)*, and its variants *(Rhus toxicodendron)*, and other members of the genus Rhus such as poison sumac *(Rhus toxicodendron vernix)*, poison oak *(R. toxicodendron diversilobum)*, and the lac tree *(R. verniciflua)*. All these species exude an oily sap when their leaves, or bark, or peel is injured. The sap polymerizes upon exposure to air, to form a hard, dark resin. The sap of incompletely polymerized resin contains a vesicant which upon contact with the skin produces the typical poison ivy dermatitis (Dawson 1954).

The active principle in poison ivy is a mixture of alkylated catechols which differs in the degree of unsaturation of the hydrocarbon substituent (Dawson 1954, 1956; Markiewitz and Dawson 1965). There are four alkylated catechols in this mixture, consisting of approximately 2% β-n-pentadecylcatechol (I), 10% $\Delta^{8'}$-3-n-pentadecenyl-catechol (II), 23% $\Delta^{8'}$, 11', 14-3-n-pentadecatrienylcatechol (III), and 64% $\Delta^{8'}$, 11'-3-n-pentadecadienylcatechol (IV).

Urushiols
(3-n-Alkylcatechol)

(I):   R =   β-n-Pentadecyl (3-n-pentadecyl)

(II):   R = $\Delta 8'$- 3-n-Pentadecenyl

(III): R = $\Delta 8',11'$- 3-n-pentadecatrienyl

(IV):   R = $\Delta 8', 11'$ 3-n-Pentadecadienyl

Mango dermatitis is very similar to poison ivy; in fact, considerable allergic cross reactions between these two poisonous principles have been known to occur. In other words, persons sensitive to poison ivy may also be sensitive to mango (Keil et al. 1946). The active principle of mango is located principally in the bark, stem, leaves, and peel of the fruit. The pulp of the fruit is safe. This poisonous compound(s) in mango has not been formally identified. But some preliminary findings suggest that the active compound(s) may be catechol derivative(s) (Vasistha and Siddiquiy 1938). Furthermore, the demonstrated cross-reactivity of mango with poison ivy saps and especially 3-n-pentadecylcatechol, a component of poison ivy sap, strongly suggests that the mango irritant is chemically very similar to that of poison ivy.

Mango dermatitis is similar to other forms of what Merrill (1944) has called ana-cardiaceous dermatitis. For those who peel the fruit before eating it, mango dermatitis is manifested by acute erythematovesicular eruptions with some swelling in the lips, cheeks, chin, and sometimes the hands. The dermatitis is largely indistinguishable from poison ivy dermatitis except that the linear arrangement of vesicles characteristic of the latter is absent in the former (Keil et al. 1946). Sometimes stomatitis and acute gastrointestinal disturbance may also occur. The reaction generally appears within 6 to 24 hr after exposure, beginning with smarting and erythema followed by an intense burning sensation and itching accompanied by vesiculation and sometimes edema. Depending on susceptibility, one may experience from only slight erythema to mild dermatitis with little pain to intense itchiness with vesicular eruptions, disfiguring edema, and lesions, which can last from 5 to 15 days (Kirby-Smith 1938).

It has also been reported that excessive eating of mangoes may cause renal inflammation. Bloat, atony, and ruminal impaction reportedly have been seen in cattle eating excessive quantities of the unripe, or even the ripe fruit (Watt and Breyer-Brandwijk 1962).

It should be emphasized that adverse reaction to the toxic principle in mangoes is dependent on individual susceptibility. The available evidence indicates that immunity to mango dermatitis may develop, so that individuals who are constantly exposed to mangoes may soon become resistant to mango dermatitis (Kirby-Smith 1938).

It is appropriate to mention at this point that mangoes contain several other phenolic compounds. These phenolics include the xanthones, mangiferin (1,3,6,7,-tetra-hydroxy-2-C-β-D-glucopyranosyl xanthone), and to some extent isomangiferin (1,3,6, 7-tetrahydroxy-4-C-β-D-glucopyranosylxanthone), the flavonoid, quercetin, and hydrolyzable tannins (Saleh and El-Ansari 1975). The subject of tannins will be discussed in another section (pp. 319—323). The toxic property of the xanthones has not been determined. From studies with specific mango varieties, it appears that the phenolics are concentrated in the peel (Lakshminarayana et al. 1970), and tend to decline with age or period of storage.

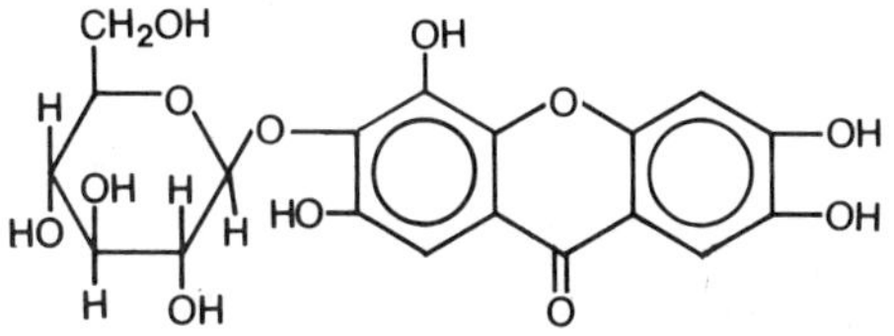

Mangiferin

(Structure of
quercitin in
Chapter 6, p. 207)

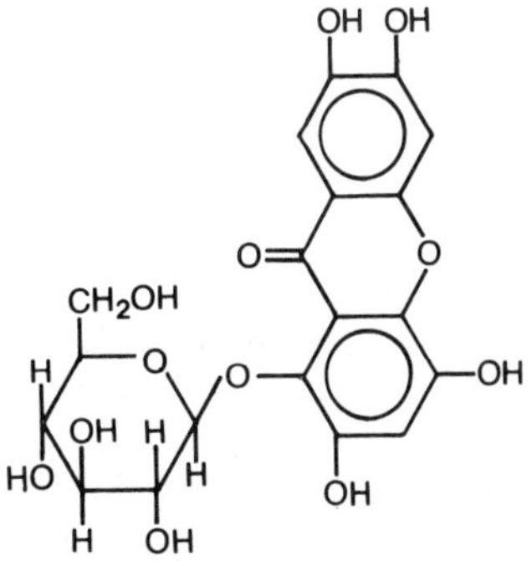

Isomangiferin

Among species of *Mangifera*, *M. caesia* and *M. lagenifera*, known as binjai and lanjut, respectively, in the Malay Peninsula are the most poisonous; even vapor of freshly cut tissues or raindrops in contact with the leaves of these species may cause dermatitis. Other species, *M. foetida* and *M. adorata*, are also contact poisons. All these bear edible fruits and are cultivated as such (Merrill 1944).

Related to the urushiols are the salicylic acid derivatives in cashew nut oil and the ginkgo nut *(Ginkgo biloba)*. These derivatives are the anacardic acids. There are at least 11 types of anacardic acids, which differ in the length and the degree of unsaturation of the alkyl side chains; the chain may be 13, 15, or 17 carbons long. These structures are shown below (Gellerman and Schlenk 1968).

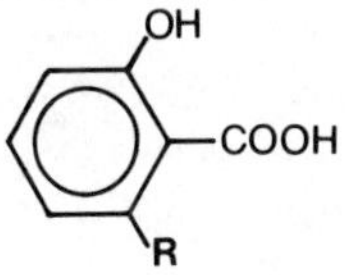

Anacardic Acids

R = n-tridecyl; Δ^6, Δ^8, Δ^{10}-*n*-pentadecenyl; $\Delta^{8,11}$, $\Delta^{6,9}$ *n*-pentadecadienyl; *n*-pentadecyl; *n*-heptadecyl; Δ^8-n-heptadecenyl; $\Delta^{8,11}$, $\Delta^{5,8}$-*n*-heptadecadienyl; $\Delta^{8,11,14}$, $\Delta^{10,13,16}$-n-heptadecatrienyl.

The anacardic acids can decarboxylate on heating at high temperatures to form the anacardols or cardanols (Dawson 1956).

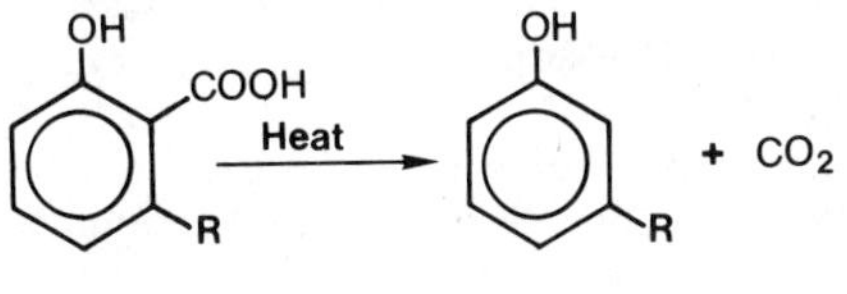

Anacardic
acids

Cardanols

R = hydrocarbon chains as in the previous structure.

A resorcinol derivative, cardol, is also present in the cashew nut shell oil (Dawson 1956).

OH

HO $C_{15}H_{27}$

Cardol

All these compounds can cause dermatitis. The most active among these is cardol, producing the most intense group reaction among the components of cashew nut oil (Keil et al. 1945a). Again, as with mango dermatitis, sensitivity to poison ivy also predetermines one's sensitivity to these toxic substances in cashew oil.

In the spring of 1982, a large outbreak of anacardiaceous dermatitis occurred in Pennsylvania involving 24% of persons who ate cashew nuts. The pruritic rash developed 1 to 8 days (median 2 days) following cashew nut consumption, and lasted 5 to 21 days (median 7 days). The rash developed principally on the extremities, and in a large proportion of patients, on the trunk, groin, axilla, and buttocks. A few had perianal itching and blistering of the mouth. It appeared that the nuts were contaminated by the cashew shell oil, as indicated by the presence of cashew shells in some of the bags (Morbidity and Mortality Reports 1983). Another outbreak reported in 1974 resulted from consumption of raw cashew nuts. Five individuals who were highly sensitive to the anacardiaceous antigen developed generalized eczematous dermatitis (Ratner et al. 1974). Other reports of anacardiaceous dermatitis involved persons who handled cashew nuts (Downing and Gurney 1940; Orris 1958).

The oil of cashew shells is extremely potent in those sensitive to poison ivy. But tests with purified poison ivy urushiols have indicated that sensitivity to these substances is time conditioned; i.e., the closer to the previous reactive exposure, the faster the appearance of symptoms (Johnson et al. 1972).

The urushiols of poison ivy and related plants and the toxic principles in cashew oil share a common structure, the long, unsaturated side chain meta to a phenolic hydroxy group. The 3-position, as shown in the structures, is important to reactivity; the location of the alkyl group para or ortho to the phenolic hydroxyl abolishes the reactivity. The presence of unsaturation and the length of the side chain also determine the incidence and intensity of group reactivity. Thus, hydrogenation and shortening of the side chain diminish the reactivity (Keil et al. 1945b). The compounds with free phenolic groups, and 1,2- and 1,3-dihydric phenols are more reactive than 1,4-dihydric and monohydric phenols (Dawson 1956).

Toxic Flavones and Chalcones

The flavones are methylated phenolics. Examples of flavones or flavonoids are nobiletin, tangeretin, and 3,3',4',5,6,7,8-heptamethoxyflavone. These are commonly found in citrus fruits, tangerines, mandarines, and oranges; the latter is found in grapefruit (Kefford and Chandler 1970). They are generally located in the oil vesicles of the fruit peel. However, they may be found in the juice following the pressing process. Thus, the oily material pressed from orange peel may contain about 2 mg nobiletin/100 ml and 0.3 mg tangeretin/100 ml.

These flavones appear to be devoid of acute toxicity. In mice, intraperitoneal administration of tangeretin and other flavones and flavonones at 500 mg/kg, and oral administration in dogs of the same substances at 1 g/kg had no acute toxic effects, except slight diarrhea in the dogs (Stout et al. 1963, 1964). While these flavones are nontoxic to adults, they are quite deadly to certain animal embryos that have been tested. For example, when administered subcutaneously to rats during gestation at 10/mg/kg/day, 83% of the offspring were stillborn or dead within 3 days, even though they

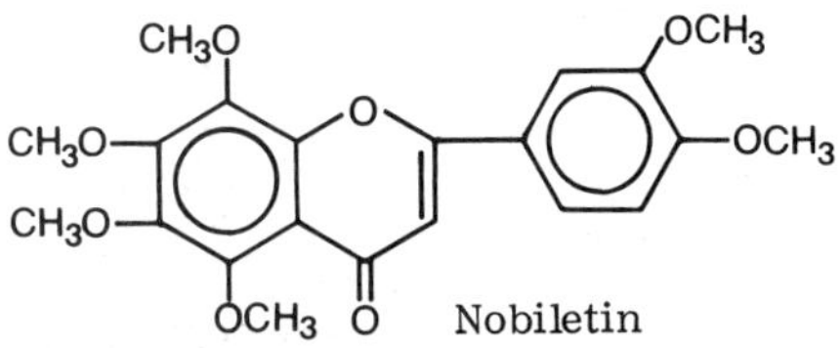

Nobiletin

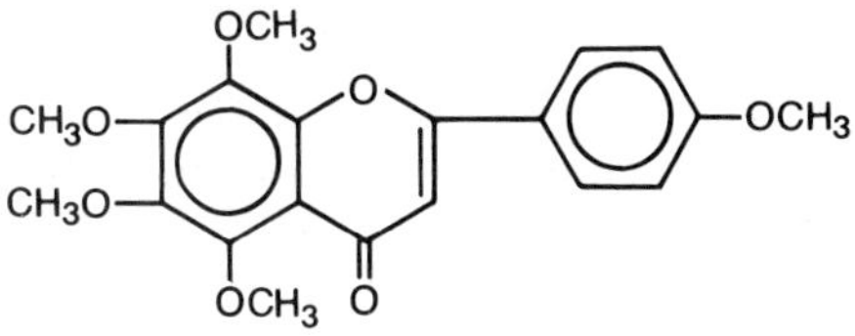

Tangeretin

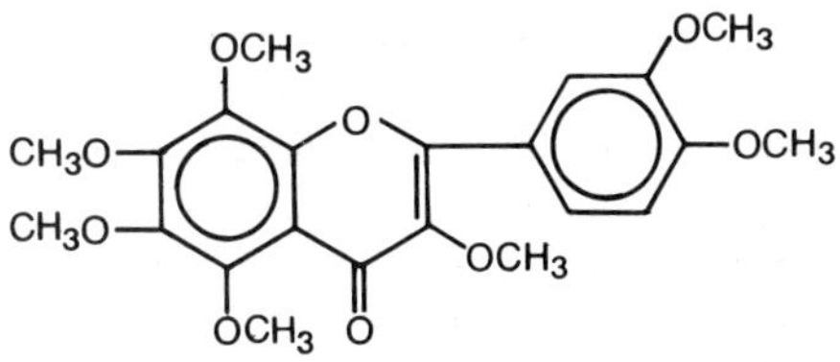

3,3',4',5,6,7,8-Heptamethoxyflavone

appeared normal (Stout et al. 1964). When zebra fish embryos were exposed to tangeretin at 0.2 to 0.4 mg/L, it proved to be cytotoxic in 24 hr to 50% of the embryos. Its analog, nobiletin, was less active, even up to 1 mg/L (Jones et al. 1964); no data are available beyond 1 mg/L. The bioflavonoids at 5% in the diet depress the growth of chickens but 2.5% does not (Deyoe et al. 1962). While there appears to be no hazard to humans at their exogenous levels in fruit, regular excessive consumption of the fruit peel, even though remote, should be discouraged, pending further results.

The toxicity of tangeretin may be due to several factors; e.g., high lipid solubility, nonglycoside structure, and the difficulty of completely metabolizing the compound to CO_2, particularly the phloroglucinol A ring, which is completely substituted (De Eds 1968).

The chalcones are similar to the flavones except that the middle flavone ring is open and they may not be methylated; thus, chalcones may be present in plants as glycosides. The chalcones apparently have a limited distribution in plants. Only one chalcone, phlorizin, as far as this author is aware, has been studied somewhat extensively in relation to its effects in animals, including man. Phlorizin is the 2'-glucoside of phloretin (2',4',6'-trihydroxy-3-(p-hydroxyphenyl)propiophenone. It is present in apples to the extent of 300 to 400 mg/kg in the fruit core and seeds.

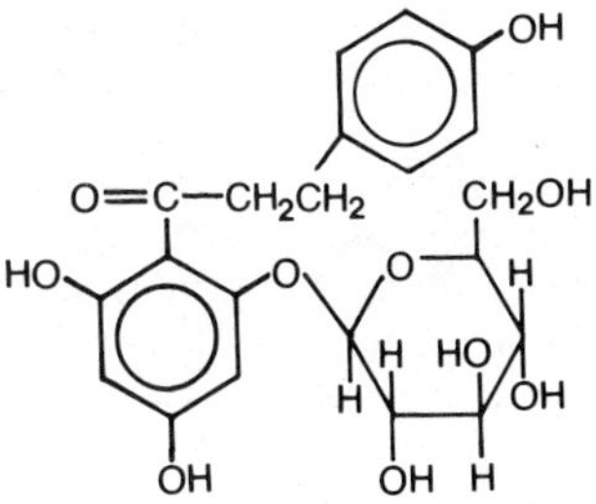

Phlorizin

The concentration of phlorizen is much higher in the fresh leaves (up to 1%) and in the root bark (over 12%) (Durkee and Poapst 1965; Williams 1966).

Phlorizin causes abnormally pronounced urinary glucose excretion when fed to humans and animals at doses of 200 to 400 mg/kg. It appears that this glucoside specifically blocks the reabsorption by active transport of glucose in the kidney tubules to the peritubular blood. Its principal targets are the epithelial cells lining the convoluted kidney tubules. As expected, phlorizin interferes in the absorption of glucose in the small intestines. Similarly, it antagonizes glucose absorption in the muscles following insulin administration. Phlorizin is a highly potent promoter of glucosuria; only a small amount is needed to bind to the active site in the kidney to be effective (Lotspeich 1960-1961; McKee and Hawkins 1945). It is absorbed rapidly and firmly by receptors in hamster kidney and intestinal epithelium (Diedrich 1968).

Rats injected subcutaneously with phlorizin at 500 mg/kg for 6 days develop drowsiness, slight weight loss, and accumulation of glycogen in the kidney in spite of the glucosuria (Babu et al. 1967).

The actual toxicant in phlorizin is the aglycone phloretin, which is released from the glucoside by hydrolases in the cell membranes (Diedrich 1968). Phloretin inhibits mitochondrial adenosine triphosphatase (ATPase) noncompetitively (Tellez de Inon 1968). Thus, the efficiency of mitochondrial phosphorylation is decreased, so that these organelles swell; the addition of ATP prevents swelling.

In plant cells, phloretin has been found to inhibit photophosphorylation by chloroplasts, by inhibiting both electron transport and transphosphorylation (Uribe 1970). Both phlorizin and phloretin have a distinct uncoupling effect on oxidative phosphorylation (Stenlid 1968).

Oral administration of phloretin, however, appears to have no activity in the kidney as well as the small intestine. Methylated phloretin is inactive. This apparent discrepancy between the activity of phloretin and phlorizin may be resolved if one considers that the glycoside form is necessary to facilitate transport and penetration of the aglycone into the cell. In other words, the glycoside acts as a carrier.

Other Toxic Phenolic Compounds

There are several other phenolic compounds endogenous in plant foodstuffs that show varying degrees of toxicity in animals. Some of these, such as the tannins, safrole, and related compounds are carcinogens, and are discussed in the following section. Another group of phenolics is the estrogenic compounds, which are discussed later in this chapter.

Finally, a toxic lignan podophyllotoxin from the Mayapple (Podophyllum peltatum) should be mentioned. Whereas the ripe fruit contains little of the toxin, the green fruit contains relatively large quantities and may be dangerous (Chatterjee 1952). The plant exudes a resin, podophyllin, which when collected from the dry roots is about 20% podophyllotoxin. About 130 mg of this resin reportedly has caused death in humans (Spector 1956). The oral LD_{50} of the lignan in mice is 90 mg/kg (Stecher et al. 1960). The resin is an irritant and produces cytotoxic as well as cathartic effects (Kelly and Hartwell 1954; Spector 1956). Even podophyllotoxin is under suspicion of being a carcinogen. It is able to induce hyperplastic changes and tumors when administered orally, or especially when applied to the uterine cervix of the mouse (Kaminetzky and McGrew 1962; O'Gara 1968). It is also suspected as one of the possible carcinogens in red cedar (Juniperus virginiana) wood chips. This is an attempt to explain the increased incidence of "spontaneous" liver and mammary tumors in C_3HA^{vy} mice when their bedding was switched from Douglas fir (Pseudotsuga spp.) to red cedar shavings (Sabine et al. 1973).

Carcinogens

It was once thought that chemical carcinogens were mostly man-made products. However, in 1950, Cook et al. (1950) reported that alkaloids of certain Senecio plants induced liver tumors in rats. Also in that year, the hepatocarcinogenicity of tannic acid was reported (Korpassy 1950; Korpassy and Mosonyi 1950, 1951). In succeeding years, a number of carcinogens were discovered in various higher plants, particularly in foodstuffs derived from them. Thus, it is now evident that carcinogens are present endogenously throughout the hierarchy of the plant kingdom.

This section will focus on the carcinogens in foodstuffs derived from higher plants. Other carcinogens like the Senecio alkaloids which are contaminants are discussed in Chapter 17.

Tannins

The tannins are a group of poorly characterized heterogenous substances in plants (Humphries 1967; White et al. 1952); and most authorities consider tannins to include all plant polyphenolic substances having a molecular weight greater than 500. Swain and Bate-Smith (1962) define tannins as water-soluble phenolic compounds, having molecular weights between 500 and 3000, and besides giving the usual phenolic reactions, having the ability to precipitate alkaloids, gelatin, and other proteins. This definition obviously will include substances which have no commercial value in the tanning of leather. However, two types of tannins can be distinguished based on certain properties, breakdown products, and botanical distribution. These are the hydrolyzable and condensed tannins (Haslam 1966; Ribereau-Gayon 1972).

The hydrolyzable tannins are gallic, digallic, and ellagic acid esters of glucose or quinic acid. One type of hydrolyzable tannin is tannic acid (or gallotannic acid, gallotannin, or simply tannin), and as shown by its structure, all the hydroxyl groups of glucose are esterified with gallic or digallic acid. Tannic acid in the form of flakes, spongy masses, or a bulky powder, is light yellow or brown and amorphous, with a characteristic faint odor and astringent taste. It will gradually darken on exposure to light and air, and produces insoluble precipitates with albumin, starch, gelatin, alkaloidal, and metallic salts. Tannic acid is very soluble in water (2.9 g/ml), warm glycerol (1 g/ml), alcohol, and acetone, but insoluble in less polar organic solvents; e.g., benzene, ethylether, and chloroform (Stecher 1960).

Gallotannic acid

The condensed tannins, also called flavolans, are polymers of flavonoids which, in most cases, are leukoanthocyanidins. The monomers are linked through carbon-carbon bonds at position 4 in one unit to position 6 or 8 in another (Haslam 1966). The monomers may also be catechins or anthocyanidins. Condensed tannins are not degraded enzymatically in the body, and their monomeric units are released only under drastic conditions. A proposed structure of condensed leukoanthocyanidin units is shown below. Further C_4 to C_8 condensation of the flavan-3,4-diol units produces specific tannin molecules.

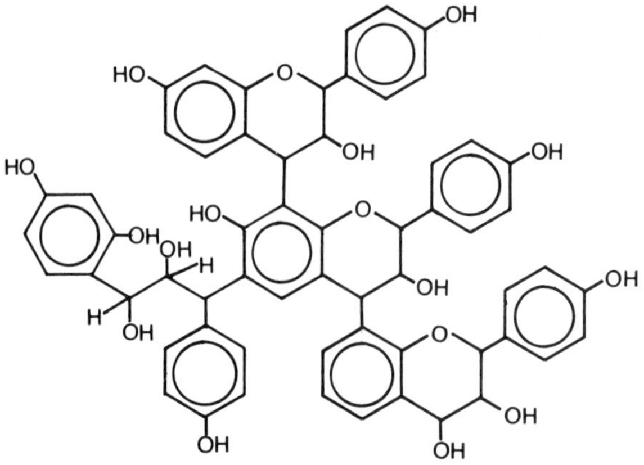

Segment of a condensed tannin molecule (proposed structure [Freudenberg and Weinges 1961])

Tannins are widely distributed in plants; many edible fruits contain significant quantities of tannins. Mango fruit contains gallotannins (El Ansari et al. 1971; El Sissi et al. 1971; Saeed et al. 1976). This substance is particularly abundant in the unripe fruit — about 8 to 10% of the seed pulp.

Many other tropical fruits are rich in tannins. These include dates (Maier and Metzler 1965a,b,c), persimmons (Ito 1980; Ito and Oshima 1962), and the sopota fruit (Achraszapota) (Lakshminarayana and Moreno-Rivera 1979; Lakshminarayana and Subramanyam 1966). The tannins, of course, diminish in amounts as the fruits ripen. In the case of persimmons, the tannin contents and, therefore, the astringency may be reduced by treatment with CO_2 or alcohol (Ito 1980; Matsuo et al. 1976).

Tannins in beverages Of particular significance to the total tannin load of humans are the tannins of tea, coffee, and cocoa. These beverages contain variable quantities of tannins (Martinek and Wolman 1955).

Martinek and Wolman (1955) obtained some interesting results: random samples of four brands of regular coffee gave an average of about 1.1% tannins; three brands of instant coffee gave about 4.3%; two brands of decaffeinated ground coffee, 1.2%; and two brands of instant decaffeinated coffee, 5.2%. Thus, as expected, instant coffees will yield more tannins than regular coffee, since instant coffee is prepared by extracting ground-roasted coffee beans with water and then evaporating the water. A cup of regular ground coffee from the brands investigated yielded from 72 to 104 mg of tannins; the instant type, from 111 to 128 mg. Decaffeinated instant coffee gave the highest, 134 to 187 mg. A brand of unsweetened cocoa had 2.5% tannin, yielding 215 mg/cup. A brand of cocoa made by the Dutch process (treatment with alkali) had 4% tannin and yielded 371 mg tannins per cup. It was estimated by Mueller (1942) that a child whose total milk intake is consumed as chocolate milk and who eats some additional chocolate candies may consume a total tannin load of 160 mg/kg/day. Panda et al. (1979) found values as high as 7.0 to 18.8% soluble tannins in coffee, so that each cup of strong coffee could contain as much as 109 to 159 mg of tannic acid.

Among the beverages, tea has the highest tannin yield on a percentage or per cup basis. The average amount of tannins in two brands of bulk black tea and one brand of green tea ranged from 10.5 to 11.8%; in tea bags (four brands of black and one of green) the tannins constituted 9.1 to 13.1% of the tea. One brand of black instant tea had 14.7% tannins. It was shown that on a per cup basis, when the tea was prepared with longer steeping to obtain maximum extraction, the black, bulk tea brands produced from 431 to 450 mg tannins; the green tea, 475 mg. The tannin yields of the tea bags were from 212 to 284 mg/ the instant black tea, 94 mg. The lower yields of tea bags on a per cup basis were due to the smaller amounts of tea used in the infusion. Certain Japanese green tea may contain 4% tannins; Formosan Oolong tea, as much as 23% (Jacobs 1951).

Green tea, however, may yield more soluble tannins, as shown, for example, by the data on one brand of bulk tea, since during fermentation in the production of black tea, oxidation of phenolic precursors by polyphenol oxidases increases the molecular weight of the tannins; these high molecular weight tannins have a greater tendency to form insoluble complexes with tea leaf proteins (Bokuchava 1962).

Thus, it can be estimated that from the above sources, a person may very easily ingest an amount of tannins on the order of 1 g or more per day.

Other important sources of tannins are grapes and the juice and wines derived from them (Singleton and Esau 1969); the tannins in grapes are mostly the condensed type and may average to about 500 mg/kg of grapes. Large quantities of tannins in grapes are found in the skins and are reflected in the high levels of tannins in wines, particularly red wines. For example, in one study, the average tannin content of several red wines of each of 27 varieties of grapes from the same cellar ranged from 1152 to 1318 mg/L (Amerine and Winkler 1963). Light clarets may contain 0.1 to 0.15% tannic acid; the heavy clarets, 0.2 to 0.3%. The tannic acid content of certain French red wines of vintages prior to 1948 ranged from 2.7 to 4.4 g/L; the range of vintages from 1952 to 1962 was 1.5 to 2.5 g/L (Ribereau-Gayon and Stonestreet 1966).

Tannins are also quite high in many varieties of sorghum grains (Chavan et al. 1979; Fuller et al. 1966; Price et al. 1978), and in bracket ferns. In the latter, a yield of 2.45 g/kg has been reported (Wang et al. 1976).

Tannins as Carcinogens Tannins were probably the first products derived from higher plants found to be carcinogenic (Korpassy 1950; Korpassy and Mosonyi 1950, 1951). Purified tannin in the form of gallotannic acid is probably a weaker carcinogen than a mixture of tannins in the form of tannin extracts. Thus, a subcutaneous dose of 9 g/kg body weight was needed in the case of gallotannic acid to induce hepatomas in the rat (Korpassy and Mosonyi 1950, 1951). Kirby (1960) produced hepatomas by subcutaneous injection of only 350 mg tannin extract/kg body weight in rats, and 750 mg/kg in mice. These results with low dosages of tannin extracts may not be comparable to those of Korpassy and Mosonyi (1950, 1951), who used purified gallotannic acid, since the same strain of animals was not used.

The demonstration that these groups of substances may be responsible for bracken carcinogenicity is most significant to tannic carcinogenicity (Wang et al. 1976). Bracken fern (Pteridium aquilimum) is widely distributed from the Arctic Circle in Norway to the tropics (Evans 1976). The plant is eaten as a delicacy in the United States, New Zealand, and particularly in Japan (Hirono et al. 1972; Pamukcu et al. 1970). This plant has been shown to induce urinary bladder tumors in cows eating 0.5 to 1.0 kg bracken daily (Price and Pamukcu 1968; Pamukcu et al. 1967), and in rats on diets of 30 to 50% bracken (Evans and Mason 1965; Pamukcu and Price 1969). It has been shown that when both rats and mice were fed a basal diet containing 33% bracken, rats develop adenomas, adenocarcinomas, and sarcomas, C57BL/6 mice develop jejunal tumors, and dd mice develop lung adenomas (Hirono et al. 1975). Bracken fern also has induced adenocarcinomas, predominantly in the two ceca and in the colon and distal ileum in 80% of 34 Japanese quails (Evans et al. 1967). Leukemias, gastric cancers, and pulmonary adenomas also have been induced in mice (Evans 1972, 1968; Evans et al. 1967, 1969; Pamukcu et al. 1972).

Bracken, of course, has other toxicants, one of which is a thiaminase (Chap. 9). Bracken is extremely toxic to cattle when sufficient quantities are eaten; animals dying from "cattle bracken poisoning" show anorexia, extensive intestinal ulceration and damage, general hemorrhage with massive blood loss, intense fever (41.7° to 42.8°C), and death within a few weeks or months (Boddie 1947). The toxin destroys the bone marrow, leading to acute leukopenia and thrombocytopenia in addition to the afore-mentioned severe damage to the intestinal mucosa (Evans et al. 1951, 1954a,b,c). Note that both bone marrow and intestinal mucosa consist of cells which have a rapid turn-over and rate of cell division, so that interference in this activity can be expected to result in severe and usually irreversible damage. Even though sheep are more resist-ant to the hemorrhagic effects of bracken fern, symptoms of bracken poisoning have also been observed in the field (Parker and MaCrea 1965), and can be induced experi-mentally in these animals (Evans 1968; Moon and McKeand 1953; Moon and Raafat 1951). In addition, the so-called "bright blindness" in sheep, characterized by stenosis of the blood vessels and progressive retinal atrophy, has been blamed on the eating of brack-en fern. This also has been experimentally induced (Barnett and Watson 1968; Watson et al. 1972a,b; 1965).

As already stated, the tannins in bracken have been shown to be the carcinogens (Wang et al. 1976), and have a mean lethal dose of 0.16 mg/g, i.p., in female Swiss albino mice (average weight 10 g). Shikimic acid (3,4,5-trihydroxy-1-cyclohexene-1-carboxylic acid) has been isolated by Evans and Osman (1974) from bracken fern and a

HO
HO—$\bigcirc$—COOH
HO

Shikimic acid

single injection of the commercially purified product produces precancerous and cancer-ous lesions in the gastric mucosa and malignant leukemias in mice. However, this com-pound is probably not the principal carcinogen of bracken (Evans and Osman 1974; Wang et al. 1976).

Hirono et al. (1975) have shown that the bracken carcinogen increases in concen-tration from the stalks to the young fronds and rhizomes. Immature bracken fronds are more carcinogenic than mature ones. The carcinogen can be removed or partially de-toxified by boiling water, but treatment with potassium carbonate (wood ash), $NaHCO_3$, or NaCl reduces the carcinogenicity considerably. It should be noted that tannins are alkali labile. This may explain the effect of K_2CO_3 or $NaHCO_3$ and the findings (Evans 1976) that an alkaline condition greatly reduces or destroys the carcinogenicity of bracken fern. However, the effect of NaCl probably is due to the greater rate of ex-traction of the tannins.

Morton (1970) suggests that catachin tannins are strongly suspected as being etio-logical agents of esophageal cancer, which occurs at high incidence in many parts of the world where the local population consumes high tannin food, teas, wine, and medic-inal plants. The carcinogenicity of these plants has been borne out by a series of studies on extracts of these plants. Thus, the tannin fraction of *Quercus falcata pagodaefolia, Diospyros virginiana,* and *Camellia sinensis* (common tea) and three other plants has been shown to be tumorigenic at the site of subcutaneous (s.c.) injection. The total aqueous extracts of five of six plants also have been demonstrated to be tumorigenic in NIH Black rats (Kapadia et al. 1976). Extracts of the root of *Acacia villosa* and *Melochia tomentosa, Heliotropium angiospermum,* and *Krameria ixina* have been shown to be highly sarcomagenic to female NIH Black rats following s.c. injection on the lower back. The first two plants in this series are highly carcinogenic; these plants produce not only 100% tumor incidence but also short latent periods. Other plants administered similarly do not produce tumors. (The alcohol extract is more tumorigenic than the residue of the aqueous extract following alcohol extraction [O'Gara et al. 1964].)

In a continuing study on these types of plants, Kapadia et al. (1978) have found further evidence by subcutaneous injection of the carcinogenicity of high tannin plants such as *Areca catechu* and *Rhus copalina*. Extracts of these plants produce mesenchymal tumors after 78 weeks. These workers also have found that some plants not rich in tannins also induce a high incidence of tumors in rats. These plants included *Sassafras albidum, Diospyros virginiana,* and *Chenopodium ambrosioides.*

Tea or oak extracts containing 1% tannins also have been shown to shorten the latency of tumors induced by 3,4-benzpyrene on mouse skin (Bogovski and Day 1977). Extracts of roasted coffee beans, instant coffee, caffeine-free instant coffee, black tea, green tea, and roasted tea are mutagenic to *Salmonella typhimurium* TA 100 without activation (i.e., without treatment with activated liver microsomal enzyme preparation) (Nagao et al. 1979).

While the case for tannins as causative agents of esophageal cancer is circumstantial epidemiologically, their experimentally proven carcinogenicity and toxicity in animals are cause for further investigation. These substances must be considered as potential carcinogens in humans. It must be reiterated that in most cases the cause of esophageal cancer may be highly multifactorial (Burrell 1962), as may be the case in most types of cancer, and that carcinogens may act synergistically in eliciting tumors.

Cycasin and Related Azoxyglycosides

The species of the ancient plant family Cycadaceae thrive in the tropical and subtropical regions of the Pacific and Caribbean Islands, Mexico, Florida, Japan, and Southeast Asia (Whiting 1963). They are extremely hardy and are able to withstand adverse climatic conditions. When most other food crops are destroyed, for example, during the typhoon season, they become the principal source of subsistence (Hirono et al. 1970). There are nine genera in Cycadaceae, and at least four species from three genera, *Cycas circinalis* (Nishida et al. 1955), *C. revoluta* (Nagahama 1964; Nishida 1959; Nishida et al. 1955; Riggs 1956), *Encephalartos barkeri* (Riggs 1954), and *Macrozamia spiralis* (Cooper 1941) have been found to contain toxic compounds which have been chemically identified.

The discovery that cycads contain potent carcinogens came about during investigations in search of a neurotoxin. On the island of Guam where cycads grow abundantly, there is a high incidence of amyotrophic lateral sclerosis, and cycad nuts, which are consumed by the islanders, are a prime suspect as the causative agent. In addition, the presence of cycads on grazing lands in many parts of the world has been linked to the occurrence of irreversible hindleg paralysis in cattle (Lacquer and Spatz 1968; Whiting 1963). Unexpectedly, however, when untreated cycad flour prepared from cycad nuts from Guam was fed to rats, benign and malignant tumors developed, mainly in the liver and kidney, and in a few animals, in the lung and intestines (Lacquer et al. 1963). The tumors in the lungs and kidneys resembled those produced in the rat by dimethylnitrosamine (DMN) (Chap. 12). The liver tumors were described as hepatocellular carcinomas and reticuloendothelial neoplasms. The tumors in the lungs resembled those in the liver; there was a massive hemorrhage into the tumor and adjacent lung tissue. The renal tumors were both epithelial and mesenchymal types. Chronic feeding (6 to 9 months) resulted mostly in liver tumors; short-term feeding (13 to 21 days) resulted preferentially in renal tumors. It appears that the preferential induction of hepatic tumors, depending on the length of exposure to the carcinogen, was also observed with dimethylnitrosamine (Magee and Barnes 1959). The formation of tumors in the colon was not affected by the duration of exposure, but the male rat appeared to be more prone to this type of tumor (Lacquer 1965).

The toxic principles from cycads have been identified, isolated, and crystallized. These differed only in the sugar moieties, having the same aglycone. Cycasin has been isolated from *C. circinalis* from Guam (Riggs 1956) and *C. revoluta* from Japan (Nishida et al. 1955). *C. revoluta* yields several other azoxyglycosides, called neocycasins, which also have the identical aglycone as cycasin (Nagahama 1964; Nishida 1959).

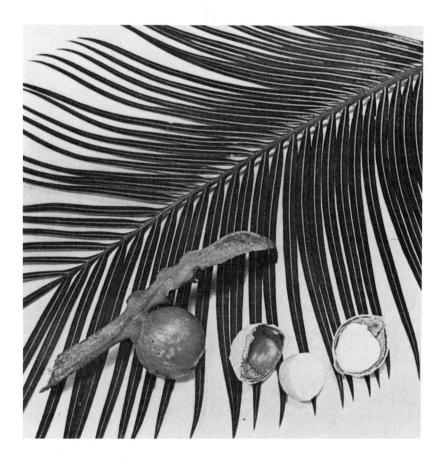

Fig. 8.2 *Cycas circinalis*. (Courtesy of Julia F. Morton, Director, Morton Collectanea, University of Miami, Coral Gables, Florida.)

Macrozamin has been crystallized from *Macrozamia spiralis* by Cooper (1941), and also has been identified in the African cycad, *Encephalartos barkeri* (Riggs 1954). As shown in the structures below, cycasin and macrozamin differ only in that the former contains glucose and macrozamin has primeverose (6-[β-D-xylosido]-D-glucose).

Cycasin

Macrozamin

The azoxyglycosides of cycads are harmless when administered parenterally, and only when taken orally are their toxic effects evident (Cooper 1941; Nishida et al. 1956). The aglycone methylazoxymethanol has been shown to be toxic parenterally (Matsumoto and Strong 1963). The toxicity is independent of the route of administration (Kobayashi and Matsumoto 1965). Methylazoxymethanol or the synthetic methyl-azoxymethyl acetate also is oncogenic independent of the route of administration in both conventional and germ-free animals, and under various experimental conditions (Kobayashi and Matsumoto 1965; Lacquer and Matsumoto 1966; Lacquer et al. 1967; Narisawa and Nakano 1973). As with cycad meal, both malignant and benign tumors of the liver, duodenum, colon, rectum, and kidneys have been induced by methylazoxy-methanol or its acetate form. These results suggest that the toxicity of the glycosides is dependent on their hydrolysis in the gastrointestinal tract to the aglycone form. Studies with germ-free rats versus conventional animals have demonstrated the importance of intestinal bacteria to effect this hydrolysis. In this case, 200 mg% cycasin — a relatively large dose — in the diet was shown to produce death in almost all animals by the twentieth day, whereas all germ-free animals were shown to remain healthy (Lacquer et al. 1967). Furthermore, it has been shown that germ-free rats identically treated do not develop tumors even after 2 yr of treatment. It was shown that the germ-free animals excreted 97% of intact cycasin in the feces and only 27% in the conventional animals (Spatz et al. 1966). In addition, it was noted that when the germ-free animals are contaminated with selected, individual β-glucosidase-producing bacteria, survival time, degree of severity of hepatic injury, and extent of cycasin hydrolysis are correlated with the enzymic activity of the bacteria (Spatz et al. 1967).

However, the tissues of rats less than 1 month old were noted to exhibit the ability to hydrolyze cycasin; these neonatal animals, whether conventional or germ-free, develop tumors following parenteral administration (Hirono et al. 1968). The skin and subcutaneous tissues of perinatal Sprague-Dawley and Fisher rats (Spatz 1968) as well as the liver, kidney, small intestine, and skin of Wistar albino rats (Matsumoto et al. 1972) are able to hydrolyze cycasin. In both instances, there was a marked increase in enzymatic activity after the first postnatal month. The enzyme activity has been noted even before birth in the skin of Sprague-Dawley rats and it starts to drop after the fourth or sixth day postpartum. In the Wistar rats, the highest activity has been noted on the sixteenth postnatal day. The highest tumor yield of the treated rats later in life has been seen in those rats treated with cycasin during the peak of enzyme activity, and no tumors have been observed when the animals are injected on the twenty-fifth postnatal day. The β-glucosidase activity, however, has been shown to remain active at low levels in the intestines and kidneys even as late as 90 days after birth (Matsumoto et al. 1972). The enzyme has not been induced by cycasin.

The carcinogenicity of cycasin or cycad meal also has been demonstrated in mice (Hirono et al. 1969; O'Gara et al. 1964), hamsters (Hirono et al. 1971; Spatz 1970), and guinea pigs (Spatz 1964, 1970). The sensitivity of neonatal animals to the carcinogenicity of cycasin also has been observed in mice and hamsters (Hirono 1972). Transplacental carcinogenesis also has been observed in hamsters (Spatz and Lacquer 1968).

Methylazoxymethanol also has been found to pass into the milk of dams (Spatz and Lacquer 1968; Yang et al. 1969) and across the placenta (Nagata and Matsumoto 1969; Spatz and Lacquer 1968). In one experiment, 18.5% of the 81 offsprings of rats fed cycad meal during pregnancy developed tumors at several sites (Spatz and Lacquer 1967). In experiments with Fisher rats, mostly receiving 20 mg methylazoxymethanol/kg body weight, 12.3% of 340 offspring developed tumors, and 45% of those having tumors were progeny of mothers treated on the twenty-first day of pregnancy (Lacquer and Spatz 1973). In addition, most of the latter offspring developed pulmonary and brain tumors. This also has been observed in neonatal Fischer rats receiving a single subcutaneous dose of cycasin (0.5 mg/g body weight) (Hirono et al. 1968). The reason for the preponderance of tumor development in animals treated with carcinogen during the perinatal period has been already explained by the presence of high β-glucosidase activity in their tissues. However, the reason for the preferential development of pulmonary and cerebral tumors is not clear. This sensitivity of perinatal rats to the cycad toxin and the preferential development of pulmonary and cerebral tumors is not unique to this carcinogen, since similar behavior also has been observed with urethane (Klein 1952; Larsen 1947).

The probability that cycasin is a human carcinogen is enhanced by the observation that one of eight monkeys developed hepatocellular carcinoma after ingestion over a period of 69 months, a total of 31.69 g of cycasin and 18.13 of methylazoxymethanol acetate (MAMA). In other monkeys, all but one had hepatic lesions such as toxic hepatitis with centrilobular necrosis. These animals received an average of 27 to 38 g of cycasin and/or 0.13-56.08 g of MAMA for 2 to 133 months. Six of 10 monkeys receiving an average of 6.14 g MAMA for 10 to 89 months developed tumors in various internal organs (Adamson et al. 1979).

Other Toxic Effects of Cycasin and Methylazoxymethanol The transplacental passage of cycasin or its aglycone immediately suggests a possible teratogenic effect. Indeed, this has been confirmed in hamsters (Spatz et al. 1967). When the aglycone (20 mg/kg body weight) is injected intravenously in hamsters on the eighth day of pregnancy, many types of malformations are seen in the offspring, including hydrocephalus, microcephalus, exencephaly, anophthalmia, microophthalmia, oligodactyly, spina bifida, cranioschisis, and rachischisis. Doses larger than 20 mg/kg result in many fetal deaths as well as many sites of fetal resorption. Smaller doses do not produce malformations in a majority of living fetuses. Microencephaly has been also observed in the offspring of rats injected with the aglycone intraperitoneally on the fourteenth or fifteenth day of pregnancy (Hirono et al. 1970). Defective mentation has been observed in the offspring of dams similarly treated (Haddad et al. 1972).

The demonstrated mutagenicity of methylazoxymethanol in histidine-dependent mutants of *Salmonella typhimurium* (Smith 1966) and in Drosophila (Teas and Dyson 1967) is to be expected from its carcinogenicity. Cycasin has been shown to be inactive in both systems because of the lack of β-glucosidase in both the Salmonella mutants and Drosophi. However, this mutagenicity has been demonstrated by means of a host-mediated assay in mice, in which the Salmonella mutants and cycasin, respectively, were injected intraperitoneally and orally (Gabridge et al. 1969). The result of the latter again attests to the importance of intestinal bacteria in the toxicity of cycasin.

The effect of the aglycone on the liver is similar to that seen with dimethylnitrosamine (Lacquer et al. 1963). The pathological changes in rats occur within 24 hr after feeding the carcinogen. Loss of glycogen and cytoplasmic basophilia occur in isolated liver cells around central veins; cytoplasmic eosinophilia and focal cellular necrosis follow after 48 hr. These changes involved all liver lobules uniformly and there are hemorrhages into the necrotic areas. Continued feeding of methylazoxymethanol acetate result in megalocytosis (Zedeck and Sternberg 1975).

The acute toxicity of cycad nuts in humans and animals has been described by Whiting (1963). Eaten raw or improperly prepared, cycad nuts or flour can be dangerously toxic. The signs of poisoning may range from minor or vague feelings of illness to severe and often fatal illness. This, of course, depends on the dose and the degree of toxicity of the nuts. Cycad nuts do differ in the degree of toxicity (Haring 1952). The symptoms in humans include headache, vertigo, stupor, euphoria, depression, violent retching, swelling of the abdomen and legs, abdominal cramps, tenesmus, diarrhea, rheumatism, and muscle paralysis. Some of these are acute symptoms, appearing almost immediately after ingestion. In some places, cycad nuts are sometimes used for criminal poisonings. There are numerous accounts of human poisonings from eating cycad nuts (Whiting 1963).

Poisoning of livestock following ingestion of various parts of the cycad plant has resulted in innumerable losses. Most prominent symptoms are irreversible hindleg paralysis, with slight staggering and weaving gait, and gastrointestinal disturbance. In acute poisoning, the common symptoms, in the order of appearance, include anorexia, hyperthermia, bloody diarrhea, fecal impaction, and respiratory distress; icterus develops after a few days if the animal survives the acute condition the first few days. Other signs are rapid twitching of eyelids, nostrils, lips, jaw muscles, and muscular tremor, impaired vision, and photophobia. Death is due to respiratory paralysis (Whiting 1963).

The amounts causing death in animals have been variously reported. A dose of 13.3 g/kg body weight in the form of fresh kernels of *Macrozamia spiralis* has been shown to produce death in a sheep within 2 days; the boiled nuts to produce death in 4 days; 5.6 g or more/kg in the form of fresh kernels of *Encephalartos horridus* fed to rabbits to result in death in a few hours; and 3 mg/g of cycasin or macrozamin given orally to mice as a single dose to result in death within a few hours. The lethal dose in guinea pigs has been shown to be 1 g/kg (Whiting 1963).

Pathological findings have been extensive internal organ damage; e.g., liver, lungs, heart, intestines, spleen, kidneys, and adrenals.

<u>Biochemical Effects of Cycasin and Its Aglycone</u> The toxicity of methylazoxymethanol or cycasin is reflected by its inhibitory effect on ribonucleic acid (RNA) (Williams and Lacquer 1965) and protein synthesis (Shank and Magee 1967) in the liver, and in the case of the latter, also in the small intestines and kidneys. The decrease in RNA, and consequently, protein synthesis is indicated by loss of ribosomes from the endoplasmic reticulum (Williams and Lacquer 1965), and inhibition of thymidine incorporation in the liver, small intestines, and kidneys in rats (Zedeck et al. 1970). More directly, the aglycone inhibits cytidine uptake into nucleolar RNA, and uridine triphosphate (UTP) incorporation into RNA of hepatic nuclei. The latter suggests an effect on RNA polymerase acitvity or deoxyribonucleic acid (DNA) template (Zedeck et al. 1972). The inhibition of RNA synthesis probably results from an interference with the enzyme system involved (Grab et al. 1973) by changing the protein conformation of the enzyme "aggregate" (as shown by circular dichroism analysis). Methylazoxymethanol can also react with histidine to form N-1- and N-3-methylhistidine in vitro (Morita et al. 1971); it also can methylate nucleic acids in vivo in rat livers (Shank and Magee 1967), and in fetal rat livers (Nagata and Matsumoto 1969). Like other methylating agents, methylazoxymethanol acetate produces breaks in single strands of rat liver DNA, and the repair process for the DNA damage occurs more slowly than for certain noncarcinogenic methylating agents. In general, cycasin and its aglycone resemble the nitrosoamines in their biochemical action, which is also reflected by the similarity in oncogenic, mutagenic, and other toxic properties of these two groups of powerful toxicants.

<u>Detoxification of Cycad Nuts</u> Fortunately, the toxic compound in cycads is highly water soluble, and the powdered or grated endosperm is rendered nontoxic by washing and thorough soaking (Whiting 1963).

Methylenedioxy- and Methoxyalkyl- and Methoxyalkenylbenzenes

<u>Safrole and Derivatives</u> A number of alkenyl- and alkylbenzenes with a methylenedioxy substituent in the 3,4 position have been already proven to be carcinogenic. These include safrole, its isomer isosafrole, and their derivatives. Safrole and isosafrole are 3,4-methylenedioxy-1-allylbenzene and 3,4-methylenedioxy-1-propenylbenzene, respectively. The structures of other carcinogenic derivatives are shown below. Safrole is a hepatocarcinogen in rats (Homburger et al. 1962, 1961; Lehman 1961; Long et al. 1963) and mice (Epstein et al. 1969; Lipsky et al. 1980). It is also a pulmonary carcinogen in mice (Epstein et al. 1969). Dihydrosafrole has been shown to be weakly esophagotumorigenic in rats (Long and Jenner 1963), but is not a liver tumorigen in at least the strain of rats studied. Isosafrole also has been shown to be weakly hepatocarcinogenic in mice (Innes et al. 1969). Both the methylenedioxybenzene group and the allylic side chain appear to be necessary for the carcinogenic activity of safrole (Hagan et al. 1965).

Safrole: R = $-CH_2CH=CH_2$

Isosafrole: R = $-CH=CHCH_3$

Dihydrosafrole: R = $-CH_2CH_2CH_3$

1'-Hydroxysafrole: R = $-CHCH=CH_2$

$\qquad\qquad\qquad\qquad$ OH

1'-Acetoxysafrole: R = $-CHCH=CH_2$

$\qquad\qquad\qquad\qquad\qquad$ OCOCH$_3$

3'-Hydroxysafrole: R =

$-CH=CHCH_2OH$

In a series of structure-activity carcinogenicity studies, Miller et al. (1983) once more confirmed the hepatocarcinogenicity of safrole to male CD-1 mice administered by stomach tube or by i.p. injection during the first 4 or 5 weeks after birth. The animals received a total of 125 µmol safrole/g body weight for the per os treatment and 9.45 µmol for the i.p. treatment. Among mice treated per os, 61% developed hepatomas after 11 to 14 months; among those treated i.p., 67% developed the tumors, compared to 24 to 26% of those treated the vehicle only. Safrole was not active in female mice in these series of treatments.

On the other hand, diets containing 0.25 and 0.50% safrole fed to CD-1 female mice for 12 months, starting at 8 weeks of age, produced hepatomas in 72 and 80% of the mice after 10 mo.

Transplacental as well as lactational carcinogenesis also has been demonstrated with safrole (Vesselinovitch et al. 1979a,b), Thus, renal tumors developed in 7% of female mice (none among males) exposed to safrole in utero; the tumors were observed 94 weeks after birth. On the other hand, 34% of the male offspring and none among the females nursed by mothers fed safrole developed hepatocellular tumors after 94 weeks. The pregnant mice received 120 µg safrole/g body weight for four times on days 12, 14, 16, and 18 of gestation. The lactating mice received the same dose every second day following parturition. Greater incidence of hepatocellular tumors (48%) was obtained among female mice exposed to 120 µg safrole/g body weight for two times per week for 90 weeks, but only 8% in males.

Safrole has an oral MLD in rabbits of 1 g/kg body weight (Stecher et al. 1960). In rats, at 1% of the diet, safrole produced weight loss, atrophy of the testes, and depletion of the bone marrow (Homburger and Boger 1968). At 0.1% in the diet safrole seems to be devoid of toxicity.

Several factors modify the carcinogenicity of safrole. In Carworth Farms CFN rats, riboflavin, α-tocopherol, and protein-deficient diets produce smaller hepatic adenomas, whereas casein supplementation increases the size of tumors during the same period of time. Biotin supplementation inhibits the carcinogenicity of safrole; pyridoxine deficiency, which reduces the carcinogenicity of butter yellow, has no effect on safrole (Homburger et al. 1961, 1962). Genetics also influences safrole carcinogenicity in that Osborne-Mendel rats are more sensitive than Carworth Farms CFN rats (Homburger et al. 1965).

Safrole is present endogenously in sassafras tea (Sassafras albidum), particularly in the root bark of this plant, from which oil of sassafras is obtained; it constitutes 85% of the oil (Dodsworth 1945). It is also present to the extent of 95% in the oil of Cinnamomum micranthum (Guenther 1950), in the volatile oil of the leaf of Cinnamomum camphora var. glaucescence (Naito 1943), and in small quantities in Cinnamomum cassia, C. zeylanicum, and C. lourerii, from which the flavoring agent oil of cinnamon is obtained. Safrole is a trace constituent in cocoa (Van der Wal et al. 1968), nutmeg, and mace (Myristica fragrans) (Power and Salway 1907), California bay laurel (Umbellularia californica), black pepper (Piper nigrum) (Richard and Jennings 1971), anise (Pimpiorella anisum) (Klein 1965), Japanese star anise (Illicium anisatum) (Concha and

Wungwira 1964; Stecher et al. 1960) and the Japanese wild ginger (Harada and Saika 1956). This carcinogen also has been detected in tamarind (*Tamarindus indica*) (Lee et al. 1975), and in the oil fraction of banana (Tressl et al. 1970, 1969). Thus, safrole has widespread occurrence as a component in many naturally occurring essential oils.

Isosafrole and dihydrosafrole are synthetic products. Safrole and its synthetic derivatives were once used as flavoring ingredients; safrole was used in root beer at approximately 20 ppm. However, to comply with the Delaney clause in the Food Additives Amendment of 1958, these flavoring ingredients have been dropped from commercial use.

Safrole is metabolized to 1'-hydroxysafrole and excreted as the glucuronide in rats, mice, hamsters, and guinea pigs (Borchert et al. 1973a). This metabolite accounts for 1 to 3% of the administered dose in rats, hamsters, and guinea pigs, and about 30% in mice (Borchert et al. 1973). It is considered to be the proximate carcinogenic metabolite of safrole (Borchert et al. 1973), but a major portion of the administered dose is still unaccounted for. 1'-Hydroxysafrole, unlike safrole, induces not only liver tumors in rats and mice but also a few stomach tumors in rats and sarcomas in the interscapular tissues in mice when fed for prolonged periods at the same level in the diet as safrole — about 0.5% (Borchert et al. 1973b). Oral application of a synthetic acetate ester of 1-hydroxysafrole produces stomach tumors, whereas subcutaneous applications create sarcomas at the site of injection. Thus, it has been postulated that a putative ester of safrole may be the ultimate carcinogenic metabolite of safrole; it is possible that there may be other carcinogenic metabolites because, as stated previously, a major portion of the metabolites of safrole remain to be identified. A putative epoxide of safrole 1'-hydroxysafrole-2',3'-epoxide has been shown to be a carcinogenic metabolite (Wislocki et al. 1977). In addition, the metabolic formation of 1'-ketosafrole has been suggested by the isolation of 1'-keto-3'-dimethylamino-2'-3'-dihydrosafrole as well as the corresponding N-piperidyl and N-pyrrolidinyl derivatives from rat and guinea pig urine (Oswald et al. 1971). The double bond in safrole also readily migrates from the 2',3' to 1',2' position and, thus, 3'-hydroxysafrole forms easily from 1'-hydroxysafrole.

Miller et al. (1983) have confirmed the tumorigenicity of 1'-hydroxysafrole and 1'-hydroxysafrole-2',3'-oxide in mice by i.p. administration and by topical application with croton oil as promoter. Whereas safrole-2',3'-oxide is not significantly tumorigenic by i.p. administration, it is so by topical application.

These studies confirm the importance of metabolic 1'-hydroxylation in the hepato-carcinogenicity of safrole. However, there is strong evidence that the more proximate carcinogenic metabolite of safrole is the sulfuric acid ester conjugate of 1'-hydroxysafrole (Dallacker 1969), and this conjugation is mediated by hepatic sulfotransferases (Wislocki et al. 1976).

Other Methylenedioxybenzenes   Scattered throughout many species which are food sources are other methylenedioxybenzenes. Some of the most common are myristicin and related compounds, which are found in nutmeg and other spices (p. 297); apiol, which is found in the oleo resin of parsley (*Petroselinum crispum* and *p. sativum*) and celery (*Apium graveoleus*) (Watt and Breyer-Brandwijk 1962); sesamol, sesamolin, and sesamin, which are from the oil of sesame (*Sesamum indicum*); and the alkaloids of black pepper (*Piper nigrum*), piperine, chavicine, and piperettine. Piperine is also found in other species in the family Piperaceae (Stecher et al. 1960). The structures of these compounds are shown in Figure 8.3. Note that all have very similar structures to safrole (p. 328). However, Miller et al. (1983) have shown that in male B6C3F1 mice, myristicin, dill apiol, and parsley apiol did not significantly produce tumors after 13 months. The compounds were administered i.p. during the more sensitive preweaning period at a total dose of 4.75 μmol. Nevertheless, these results are by no means conclusive, for their activity may be weakened by the methoxy substituents *meta* and/or *ortho* to the allyl group. Thus, tests using higher doses on the same or different strains may reveal their carcinogenic potential.

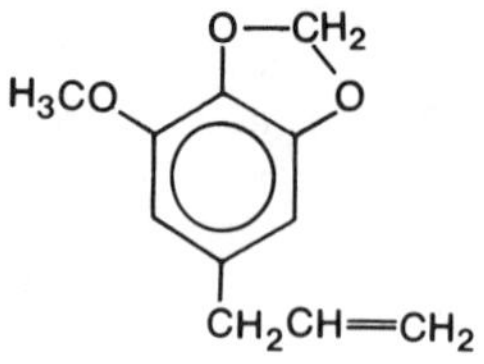

Myristicin

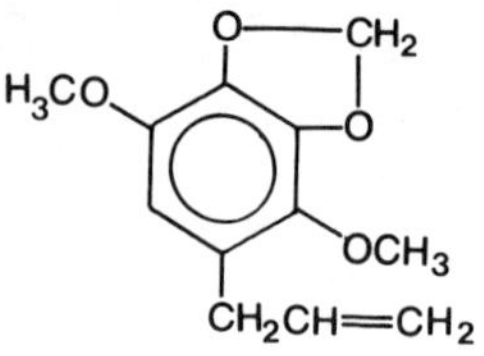

Apiol

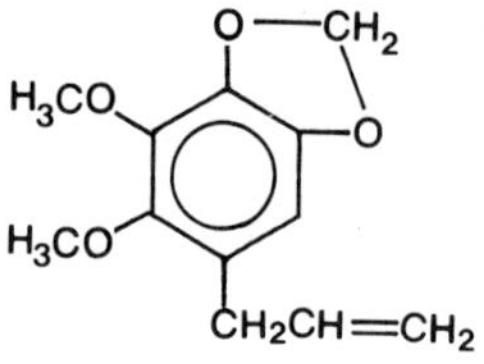

Dillapiol

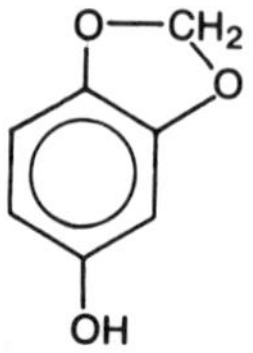

Sesamol

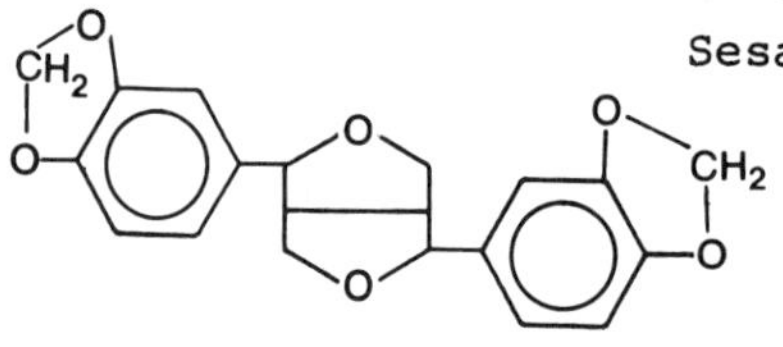

Sesamin

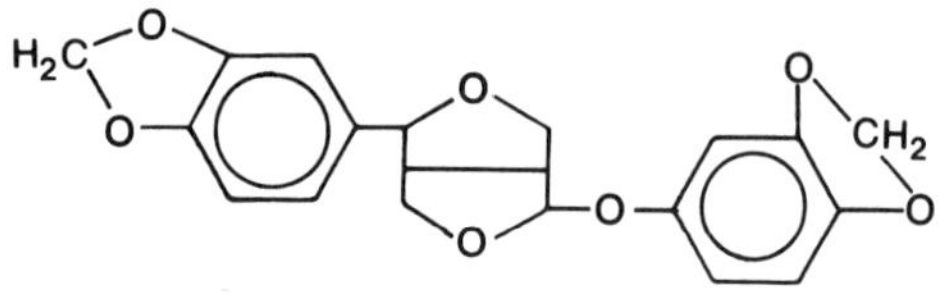

Sesamolin

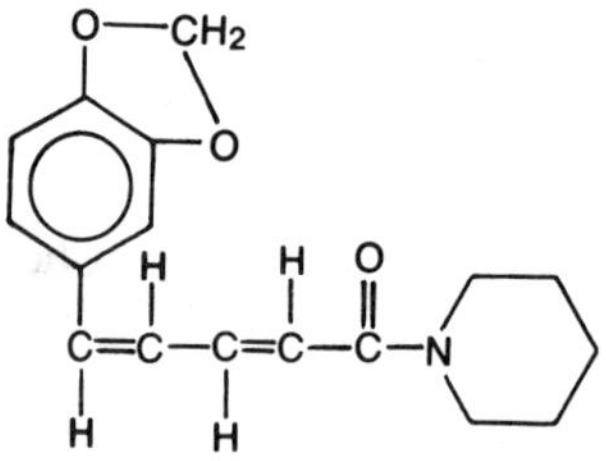

Piperine

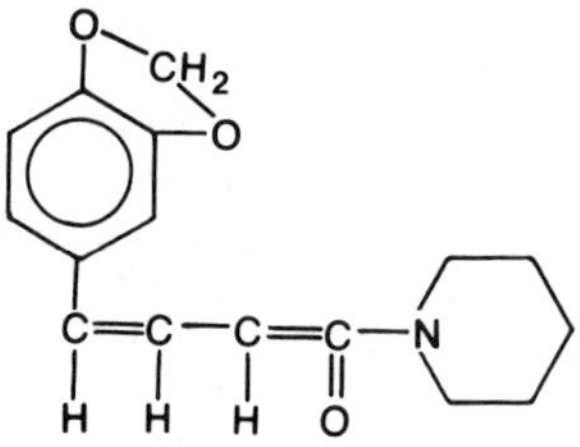

Chavicine

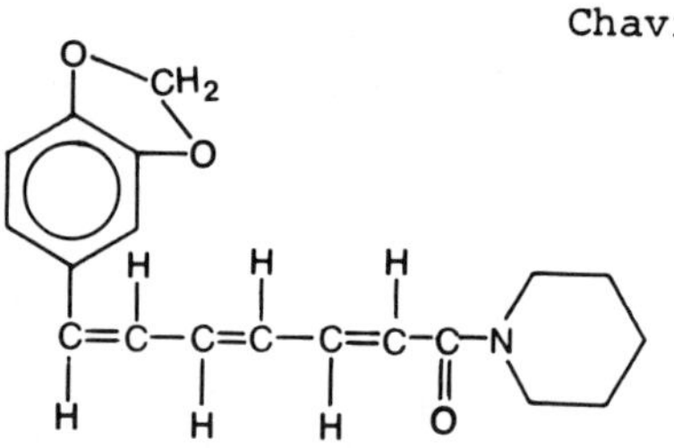

Piperettine

Fig. 8.3 Carcinogenic methylenedioxybenzenes from various foodstuffs.

The potential carcinogenicity of black pepper has been reported by Concon et al. (1979, 1981). Some preliminary results indicating that black pepper is a potential carcinogen are discussed in the next section. In addition, the tumorigenicity of sesamol also has been evaluated by Ambrose et al. (1958), who reported that an increased incidence of benign proliferative lesions is observed in rats fed for several months a diet containing sesamol.

Sanguinarine, a benzphenanthridine alkaloid from the poppy-fumaria species *Argemone mexicana*, contains two methylenedioxy groups. This carcinogen is discussed under plant-derived biological contaminants (Chap. 17).

<u>Methoxyalkyl- and Methoxyalkenylbenzenes</u>   These compounds and safrole have common structural features (Table 8.4). Among the few methoxybenzenes to be evaluated for tumorigenicity is 3,4,5-trimethoxycinnamaldehyde, which induces tumors, including nasal squamous carcinomas, when administered to young rats by subcutaneous and intraperitoneal injections (Schoental and Gibbard 1972). While there have been no reports that this compound is found in food, the demonstration of its carcinogenicity is significant because there are many methoxy-substituted aromatic compounds in food products, and it appears that the methoxy substituent may enhance or promote carcinogenic potentials. This fact has been demonstrated with unsubstituted cinnamaldehyde compared with the aforementioned trimethoxy derivative (Schoental and Gibbard 1976). Indeed, a number of methoxybenzenes have already been shown to possess some carcinogenic activity: Podophyllotoxin, which is present in the May apple, has already been mentioned (p. 318). Another carcinogen is β-asarone (1-propenyl-2, 4,5-trimethoxybenzene), which is the principal component of oil of calamus (*Acorus calamus*). A few rats fed diets containing up to 0.5% oil of calamus for 2 years have shown dose-related mesenchymal tumors of the small intestines (Gross et al. 1967; Hagan et al. 1967; Taylor et al. 1967), and the same type of tumor has been seen in rats fed β-asarone (Taylor 1973). Oil of calamus was not only carcinogenic, but at levels of 0.05 to 1.0%, the Jammu variety of the oil, also have been shown to inhibit growth in rats, increased fluid accumulation in the abdominal cavity, cause pathological changes in the liver and heart, and increase mortality (Hagan et al. 1967). This oil is a flavoring agent, and has been withdrawn from commercial use in the United States and other countries.

Estragole has been shown to be a strong hepatocarcinogen in mice (Drinkwater et al. 1976). Mice injected s.c. with 4.4 and 5.2 μM of estragole, starting at age 1 day and weekly thereafter, up to age 22 days, have been shown to develop 23 to 39% incidence of hepatocellular carcinoma after 12 to 15 months. A metabolite of estragole, 1'-hydroxyestragole, also has been proven to be a more potent carcinogen than the parent compound; in this case a 59 to 70% incidence of hepatocellular carcinoma has been observed.

Miller et al. (1983) have confirmed the hepatocarcinogenicity of estragole in male CD-1 mice. This carcinogen was administered by stomach tube, i.p. injection, and in the diet with identical protocol as that described for safrole. A metabolite of estragole, 1'-hydroxy-estragole A, was even more stronly tumorigenic by i.p. administration in 136C3F$_1$ mice; but its 2',3'-oxide derivative was not. However, the latter derivative and 1'-hydroxy-estragole-2',3'-oxide was tumorigenic by topical application with croton oil as promoter.

In this series of tests using the same level of test substances and protocol as with estragole, several methoxyallylbenzenes, such as elemicin, eugenol, and anethole, have been shown to be inactive. However, methyleugenol and its 1'-hydroxy derivative are strongly tumorigenic in male B6C3F$_1$ mice.

These results present some interesting structural relationships with respect to tumorigenic activity. Thus, the simultaneous presence of a methoxy and 2'-alkenyl group, *para* to each other appears essential to tumorigenicity. But a third methoxy group *meta* to the allyl group nullifies or perhaps weakens this effect. These relationships can be seen by comparison of the structures of these compounds shown in Fig-

Table 8.4 Methoxybenzenes of Essential Oils and Spices

Methoxybenzene	Structure	Source
Acetyl eugene	$CH_2{=}CHCH_2$—〈ring〉—$OCOCH_3$	Cloves
Anethole	CH_3O—〈ring with OCH_3〉—$CH{=}CHCH_3$	Anise oil (80-90%), fennel (50-60%)
Anisole	CH_3O—〈ring〉	Anise oil
Anisaldehyde	CH_3O—〈ring〉—CHO	Anise oil
Asarone[a]	$CH_3CH{=}CH$—〈ring with OCH_3, OCH_3〉, CH_3O	Calamus oil
Elemicin	CH_3O—〈ring with CH_3O, CH_3O〉—$CH_2CH{=}CH_2$	Nutmeg
Eugenol[b]	HO—〈ring with CH_3O〉—$CH_2CH{=}CH_2$	Anise oil; bay leaf (myrcia) (40-50%); Calamus; Chinese cinnamon; Ceylon cinnamon (64-68%); cloves (82-87%); pimento; sweet bay; sassafras
Estragole[a]	CH_3O—〈ring〉—$CH_2CH{=}CH$	Basil oil; tarragon (60-75%)
Lemettin[b]	CH_3O〈bicyclic lactone with OCH_3, O, =O〉	Lime oil

Table 8.4 (continued)

Methoxybenzene	Structure	Source
Methylchavicol	CH_3O—⬡—$CH_2CH{=}CH_2$	Anise oil; basil; bay leaf; sweet bay
Methyleugenol[b]	CH_3O, CH_3O—⬡—$CH_2CH{=}CH_2$	Asarum oil; bay leaf
Vanillin	CH_3O, HO—⬡—CHO	Cloves; vanilla (2.75%)
Vanillic acid	HO—⬡—$COOH$, CH_3O	Vanilla
Capsaicin[a]	HO—⬡—$CH_2NHC(CH_2)_4CH{=}CHCH(CH_3)_2$, CH_3O	Capsicum peppers
Bergapten[b]	furanocoumarin structure with OCH_3	Lime oil

[a]Asarone, methyleugenol and estragole already shown to be carcinogenic in animals; capsaicin is presumed to be the carcinogenic factor in *Capsicum* peppers.
[b]Eugenol possesses some cocarcinogenic activity. Limettin and bergapten may contribute to the cocarcinogenic activity in lime oil; the latter is photodynamic.

ure 8.1 and Table 8.4. For example, carcinogenic estragole is structurally similar to the inactive or perhaps weakly active anethole except for the 1'-alkenyl substituent in the latter. Likewise, inactive eugenol and active methyleugenol are similar except for the absence of the *para* methoxy group in eugenol, which has an hydroxy group. Other examples need to be tested in order to verify this hypothesis.

Another methoxybenzene found to be tumorigenic is the amide capsaicin, the "hot" or pungent substance in red peppers (Capsicum spp.). This potent irritant and vesicant produces liver tumors when fed at levels of 10% in the diet (Hoch-Ligeti 1952). This compound may cause injury to the gastrointestinal mucosa. For example, when injected or administered by stomach tube into a ligated duodenum of Sprague-Dawley rats, morphological changes in the duodenal cells occur within 2 min of exposure, and injury increases with time of exposure — swelling of mitochondria with rarefication of the matrix and disorganization of the cristae; dilation of the endoplasmic reticulum and Golgi complexes; shrinking of the nuclei and clumping of chromatin, which were marginated near the nuclear envelope; and increased concentration of free ribosomes and lysosomes (Nopanitaya and Nye 1974). These morphological changes occur even if the concentration of administered capsaicin is as low as 0.014% in physiological saline (0.85%).

Another study has shown that capsaicin inhibits respiratory response of isolated liver mitochondria in the presence of adenosine diphosphate (ADP), and inorganic phosphate; 2,4 dinitrophenol; or $CaCl_2$ plus inorganic phosphate. Similar inhibition of oxidative phosphorylation also has been observed with other NAD^- link substrates such as β-hydroxybutyrate and malatepyruvate. At much higher doses, capsaicin uncouples oxidative phosphorylation. It also depresses adenosine triphosphatase activity activated by dinitrophenol in rat liver mitochondria (Chudapongse and Janthasoot 1976).

Several other methoxybenzenes which have not been tested for carcinogenicity also are listed with their structures in Table 8.4. There is a compelling reason to determine the carcinogenicity of compounds like elemicin, which is found in nutmeg; it shares similar substituents with trimethyoxycinnamaldehyde and safrole; i.e., the trimethoxy groups and the allyl side chain, respectively. Note, for example, that a similar trimethoxybenzene asarone which has a propenyl side chain as in isosafrole and methoxy substituents in the 2,4,5 positions already has been shown to be carcinogenic (p. 331).

Some of these methoxybenzenes may show cocarcinogenic activity. For example, eugenol, which is present in large quantities in the essential oils of bay leaf (*Myrcia* or *Pimenta acris*), cloves (*Eugenia caryophyllata*), and tarragon (*Artemesia dracunculus*), is probably a weak cocarcinogen with benzo(a)pyrene (Van Duuren 1976); the former applied at a dose of 10 mg simultaneously with the latter, three times weekly. The weak response may be due to the dose. Lime oil also has cocarcinogenic activity, and it contains the coumarins, limettin, or 5,7-dimethoxycoumarin, and bergapten, or 5-methoxypsoralen. The coumarin structure together with the methoxy substituent probably enhances their activity. Lime oil increases markedly the incidence of epithelial tumors in the forestomach of mice administered via stomach tube a single 50-mg dose of dimethylbenzanthracene, or 3,4-benzo(a)pyrene in polyethyleneglycol (Field and Roe 1965). The action of 8-methoxypsoralen (xanthotoxin) confirms the photodynamic and tumorigenic qualities of the psoralens. This compound produced ear tumors in mice which were irradiated after treatment with the compound. This psoralen is used in suntan preparations (Hakim et al. 1960).

There is compelling evidence that bergapten, or 5-methoxypsoralen, is a carcinogenic hazard (Ashwood-Smith and Poulton 1981; Ashwood-Smith et al. 1980; Forlot 1980). Furocoumarins such as bergaptene can have a devastating effect on the DNA in the presence of ultraviolet (u.v.) light. This damage appears to be a function of both concentration of the furocoumarin and the intensity of u.v. radiation. This relationship was discovered by Burger and Simons (1979), who showed that the degree of chromosome damage - K (C × II), where C is the concentration of furocoumarin (ug/ml); I is the intensity of u.v. radiation (in joules/m^2), and K is a constant. This equation shows that the degree of DNA damage will be the same for a small or large amount of furocoumarins depending on the level of u.v. radiation. Thus, a small exposure to a furocoumarin will be just as hazardous as a large one, depending on the intensity of u.v. exposure (Ashwood-Smith and Poulton 1981). Stern et al. (1979) have shown that a related furocoumarin, 8-methoxypsoralen used in the treatment of a skin disorder, is not only an animal but also a probable human photocarcinogen.

Psoralens are also found in celery and parsnip (Ashwood-Smith and Poulton 1981; Ivie et al. 1981; Levin et al. 1982).

Many methoxy compounds have significant biological activity if only because of their phenolic character. For example, myristicin and elemicin from nutmeg have hallucinogenic properties. The flavones tangeretin (5,6,7,8,4'-pentamethoxyflavone), and and nobiletin (5,6,7,8,3',4'-hexamethoxyflavone) in certain citrus oils are inducers of microsomal hydroxylating enzymes (Wattenberg et al. 1968), as with safrole (Parke and Rahman 1970). Bergapten, a methoxypsoralen, is also a photodynamic substance.

Many flavones which are polyhydroxy compounds have been shown to be mutagenic to certain strains of *Salmonella*. These include quercetin, morin, kaempferol, fisetin, myricetin (Hardigree and Epler 1978; Nago et al. 1981), wogonin, galaugin, rhamnetin, and isorhamnetin (Nago et al. 1981). Quercetin has been shown to be mutagenic to *Salmonella* strains TA98 and TA1538 without metabolic activation. But its activity has been enhanced by metabolic activation by liver enzyme preparation (Bjeldanes and Chang 1977; MacGregor and Jurd 1978). The flavones are of special food toxicological interest because they are widely distributed in the plant kingdom. Quercetin occurs widely in fruits, vegetables, and tea as the glycoside quercitrin and rutin. Feeding tests in ddY mice with quercetin at 2% in the diet did not unequivocally show carcinogenicity, although the test showed that quercetin produced more tumors than the control (Saito et al. 1979, 1980). Feeding tests in inbred ACI rats have been shown to produce no significant indication of carcinogenicity (Hirono et al. 1981). However, Meltz and MacGregor (1981) have found that quercetin is able to cause genetic damage to a mouse leukemia cell line without rat liver microsomal enzymes treatment. But with microsomal enzyme treatment, higher concentrations are required to cause significant damage. This suggests that the microsomal enzymes detoxify the flavone. Additionally, Pamukcu et al. (1980) have found quercetin to be a relatively strong intestinal and bladder carcinogen when fed at 0.1% in the diet to noninbred, weanling albino rats. The ileal tumors include adenoma, fibroadenoma, and adenocarcinoma with mesenteric metastasis.

Terpenes and Other Isoprenoid Compounds

Because the composition of a food product is extremely complex, it is not at all surprising that other potentially carcinogenic compounds are being discovered in these products. Investigators are just beginning to identify other potential carcinogens, cocarcinogens, and tumor-promoting agents in spices and flavoring agents. Among these substances are a class of compounds known as the terpenes, or more accurately isoprenoid compounds. These are cyclic or acyclic hydrocarbons whose derivatives are exact multiples of C_5H_8, the isoprene unit

$$\overset{\displaystyle CH_3}{(CH_2{=}\underset{|}{C}{-}CH{=}CH_2).}$$

The simplest isoprenoids are the C_{10} compounds, the monoterpenes, or simply terpenes. The C_{15} compounds are called sesquiterpenes; C_{20}, diterpenes, and C_{30}, triterpenes.

These compounds may be bicyclic or polycyclic, and may have oxygen substituents. The isolates of mixtures of these products by ether extraction or steam distillation are known as essential oils.

Examples of essential oils or terpenes that have been shown to be carcinogenic, cocarcinogenic, or tumor promoting are those found in oranges, lemons, limes, and grapefruits. These oils have been shown to promote the development of a large number of malignant and benign tumors on the skin of mice pretreated with subcarcinogenic doses of 3,4-penzpyrene, 7,12-dimethylbenzo(a)anthracene (DMBA), or urethan (Roe and Pierce 1960). Orange oil has no carcinogenic effects (Roe 1959), but the terpene fraction containing mostly D-limonene (Table 8.5) gives rise to epidermic hyperplasia, and eventually tumors (Roe 1960). It has been postulated that the active species is not D-limonene as such, but possibly its auto-oxidized form D-limonene-4-hydroperoxide (see below). This has been deduced from two lines of evidence. First, a related compound 1-vinylcyclohexyl-3-ene, which differs from D-limonene, by the absence of the methyl groups is carcinogenic only in the crude form, but noncarcinogenic when purified and protected from oxygen. The primary carcinogen in this case has been shown to be 1-vinylcyclohex-3-ene-1-hydroperoxide. Another related compound without the vinyl group, cyclohex-3-ene-1-hydroperoxide also is carcinogenic (Van Duuren 1965;

D-Limonene hydroperoxide

Table 5. Terpenes in Essential Oils of Spices and Other Flavoring Products

Terpenes	Structure	Plant Sources
α-*cis* Bergamotene		Black pepper (Muller and Jennings 1967) bergamot fruit rind (Balavoine 1952)
α-*trans*-Bergamotene		Black pepper (Muller and Jennings 1967)
β-Bisabolene		Black pepper (Muller and Jennings 1967; Richard et al. 1971)
Borneol		Asarum, cardamon, coriander, ginger, nutmeg, thyme (acetate form) Stecher et al. (1960)
Cadinene		Juniper, peppermint (Russell and Jennings 1967) black pepper (Tikhonova and Goryaen 1957)
Calamenene		Cubeb oil; black pepper (Muller and Jennings 1967)
Camphene		Ginger, juniper (Stecher et al. 1960) black pepper (Ikeda et al. 1962; Richard et al. 1971)
Δ 3- Carene		Black pepper (Richard et al. 1971; Wrolstad and Jennings 1965)
cis-Carveol		Black pepper (Russell and Jennings 1969)
trans-Carveol		Black pepper (Russell and Jennings 1969)
Carvacrol		Origanum, thyme (Stecher et al. 1960)
Carvone		Caraway (53-63%), dill, spearmint (Stecher et al. 1960); black pepper (Richard et al. 1971; Russell and Jennings 1969)

Table 5. (continued)

Terpenes	Structure	Plant Sources
Caryophyllene		Black pepper (Hasselstrom et al 1957; Muller and Jennings 1967; Richard et al. 1971); clove (Stecher et al. 1960)
Caryophyllenone		Black pepper (Richard et al. 1971)
Citronellal	$CH_2=C(CH_2)_3CHCH_2CHO$ CH_3 CH_3	Lemon; lemon grass (Stecher et al. 1960)
Citral	$CH_3C=CHCH_2CH_2C=CHCHO$ CH_3 CH_3	Balm, bay, bitter orange, ginger, lemon, lemon grass, orange (Stecher et al. 1960)
Copaen		Black pepper (Hasselstrom et al. 1957; Muller and Jennings 1967)
Cryptone		Black pepper oil (Hasselstrom et al. 1957; Russell and Jennings 1969)
Cubebene		Black pepper (Richard and Jennings 1971)
Cuminal		
ar-Curcumene		Black pepper (Russell and Jennings 1969)
p-Cymene		Coriander, cumin, origanum, thyme (Stecher et al. 1960); black pepper (Richard et al. 1971; Wrolstad and Jennings 1965)
p-Cymene-8-ol		Black pepper (Russell and Jennings 1969)
Eucalyptol (cineol)		Artimisia, basil, cardamon, ginger, lavender, niaouli, sweet bay (Stecher et al. 1960)

Table 8.5 (continued)

Terpenes	Structure	Plant Sources
cis-p-2- Menthane-1-ol	H₃C—⬡—CHCH₃ / HO / CH₃	Black pepper (Richard and Jennings 1971)
cis-p-2-8- Menthadien-1-ol	H₃C—⬡—C=CH₂ / HO / CH₃	Black pepper (Richard and Jennings 1971)
Menthol	H₃C—⬡—CHCH₃ / OH CH₃	Peppermint (also esters of menthol (Stecher et al. 1960)
Menthone	H₃C—⬡—CHCH₃ / O CH₃	Peppermint (Stecher et al. 1960)
Menthyl acetate	H₃C—⬡—CHCH₃ / CH₃ / OCOCH₃	Peppermint (Stecher et al. 1960)
Myrcene	$(CH_3)_2-C=CH(CH_2)-C-CH=CH_2$ $\qquad\qquad\qquad\quad \overset{\|}{C}H_2$	Bay (Stecher et al. 1960); black pepper (Richard et al. 1971; Wrolstad and Jennings 1965)
Nerol	$(CH_3)_2-C=CH(CH_2)\ _2C=CHCH_2OH$ $\qquad\qquad\qquad\qquad\quad \underset{CH_3}{\|}$	Orange flowers (Stecher et al. 1960)
Neral	$(CH_3)_2-C=CH(CH_2)_2-C=CHCHO$ $\qquad\qquad\qquad\qquad\quad \underset{CH_3}{\|}$	Orange flowers (Stecher et al. 1960)
Ocimene	$CH_2=C-(CH_2)_2CH=CCH=CH_2$ $\quad\ \underset{CH_3}{\|}\qquad\qquad\ \underset{CH_3}{\|}$	Black pepper (Ikeda et al. 1962)
Nerolidol	$(CH_3)_2-C=CH(CH_2)_2-C=CH(CH_2)_2-\overset{OH}{\underset{CH_3}{\|}}CH=CH_2$ $\qquad\qquad\qquad\qquad \underset{CH_3}{\|}$	Black pepper (Russell and Jennings 1969)
α-d-Pinene	H₃C—|—C—|—CH₃ / CH₃	Coriander, fennel, juniper lavender, lemon, niaouli, nutmeg, peppermint, sassafras, spearmint, sweet bay, thyme (Russell and Jennings 1969); black pepper (Hasselstrom et al. 1957; Richard et al. 1971; Wrolstad and Jennings 1965)

Table 8.5 (continued)

Terpenes	Structure	Plant Sources
β-Elemene		Black pepper (Muller and Jennings 1967; Richard et al. 1971)
∂-Elemene		Black pepper (Muller and Jennings 1967)
β-Farnesene	$(CH_3)_2-C=CH(CH_2)_2-\underset{CH_3}{C}=CHCH_2CH=\underset{CH_3}{C}-CH=CH_2$	Black pepper (Richard et al. 1971)
Farnesol	$(CH_3)_2-C=CH(CH_2)_2\underset{CH_3}{C}=CH(CH_2)_2-\underset{CH_3}{C}=CHCH_2OH$	Citronella, neroli, lemon grass (Stecher et al. 1960)
d-Fenchone		Fennel (Stecher et al. 1960)
Geraniol	$(CH_3)_2-C=CHCH_2CH_2-\underset{CH_3}{C}=CHCH_2OH$	Asarum, coriander, lavender, lemon (acetate form), lemon grass, nutmeg, orange flowers (Stecher et al. 1960)
Humulene		Black pepper (Ikeda et al. 1962; Richard and Jennings 1971)
d-Limonene		Bitter orange, caraway, (Stecher et al. 1960); celery, dill, fennel, lavander, lemon (90%), lemon grass, Naouli, orange (90%), peppermint, spearmint (Russell and Jennings 1969); black pepper (Hasselstrom et al. 1971; Wrolstad and Jennings 1965)
l-Linalool	$(CH_3)_2-C=CH_2-CH_2\underset{OH}{\overset{CH_3}{C}}CH=CH_2$	Asarum, basil, bitter orange, thyme (Stecher et al 1960); black pepper (Richard et al. 1971; Russell and Jennings 1969); lavander, orange, orange flowers (acetate form) Stecher et al. 1960)

Table 8.5 (continued)

Terpenes	Structure	Plant Sources
β-D-Pinene		Asarum, cumin (Stecher et al. 1960); black pepper (Hasselstrom et al. 1957; Richard et al. 1971; Wrolstad and Jennings 1965)
trans-Pinocarveol		Black pepper (Richard and Jennings 1965)
Peperitone		Japanese peppermint (Stecher et al. 1960)
α-Phellandrene		D isomer: Ceylon cinnamon, dill, ginger, ginger grass, star anise seed cinnamon, angelica, lemon peppermint, sassafras (Stecher et al. 1960); black pepper (Hasselstrom et al. 1957; Richard et al. 1971; Wrolstad and Jennings 1965)
β-Phellandrene		L isomer: Eucalyptus, bay (Stecher et al. 1960)
		D isomer: Lemon oil, fennel oil
		L isomer: Peppermint oil (Japanese) (Russell and Jennings 1969); black pepper (Richard et al. 1971; Wrolstad and Jennings 1965)
Sabinene		Black pepper (Richard et al. 1971; Wrolstad and Jennings 1965); cardamon (Russell and Jennings 1969)
D-Santalene		Black pepper (Muller and Jennings 1967)
α-Selinene		Black pepper (Muller and Jennings 1967; Richard et al. 1971); celery (Stecher et al. 1960)

Table 8.5 (continued)

Terpenes	Structure	Plant Sources
β-Selinene		Black pepper (Muller and Jennings 1967; Richard et al. 1971)
α-Terpinene		Lemon, cardamon (Stecher et al. 1960); black pepper (Wrolstad and Jennings 1965)
β-Terpinene		Lemon, marjoram (Stecher et al. 1960)
γ-Terpinene		Lemon (Stecher et al. 1960); black pepper (Richard et al. 1971; Wrolstad and Jennings 1965)
α-Terpineol		Black pepper (Richard et al. 1971; Russell and Jennings 1969); bitter orange, cardamon, juniper, marjoram, Niaouli, nutmeg, orange (Stecher et al. 1960)
L-Terpinen-4-ol		Cardamon (Stecher et al. 1960); black pepper (Richard et al. 1971; Russell and Jennings 1969)
Thymol		Thyme (20-40%) (Stecher et al. 1960)
α-Thujene		Black pepper (Richard et al. 1971; Wrolstad and Jennings 1965)
Thujone		Wormwood oil (Balavoine 1952); artimisia (Tikhonova and Goryaev 1957); sage (Brieskorn and Wenger 1960; Vernazza 1957)
Umbellulone		California bay laurel (Drake and Stuhr 1935; Guenther 1950)

Scientific names of plant sources of products: Angelica — *Angelica archangelica* (Umbelliferae); artimisia — *Artimisia cina* (Compositae); asarum — *Asarum canadense* (Canadian snakeroot) (Aristolochiaceae); balm — *Melissa officinalis* (Labiatae); basil — *Ocimum basilicum* (Labiatae); bay (myrcia) — *Pimenta (Myrcia) acris* (Myrtaceae); California bay laurel — *Umbellularia californica* (Umbelliferae); bitter orange — *Citrus aurantium* (Rutaceae); calamus — *Acornus calamus* (Araceae); caraway — *Carum carvi* (Umbelliferae); cardamon — *Eletaria cardamomum* (Zingiberaceae); celery — *Apium graveolens* (Umbelliferae); Ceylon cinnamon — *Cinnamomum zeylanicum* (Lauraceae); clove — *Eugenia caryophyllata* (Myrtaceae); coriander — *Coriander sativum* (Umbelliferae); cumin — *Cuminum cyminum* (Umbelliferae); dill — *Anethum graveoleus*

Table 8.5 (continued)

(Umbelliferae); fennel — *Foeniculum vulgare* (Umbelliferae); ginger — *Zingiber officinale* (Zingiberaceae); juniper — *Juniperus communis* (Pinaceae) lavender — *Lavandula officinalis* (Labiatae); lemon — *Citrus limonum* (Rutaceae); lemon grass — *Cymbopogon (Andropogon); citratus (Verbena melissa* (Gramineae); marjoram — *Origanum marjorana* (Labiatae); niaouli — *Melaleuca viridiflora* (Myrtaceae); nutmeg — *Myristica fragrans* (Myristicaceae); orange — *Citrus aurantium* var. *sinensis* (Rutaceae); origanum — *Origanum vulgare* (wild marjoram) (Labiatae); origanum cretan — *Origanum creticum* (Labiatae); parsley — *Petroselinum hortense* or *P. sativum* (Umbelliferae); pepper (black and white) — *Piper nigrum* (Piperaceae); peppermint — *Mentha piperita, Mentha arvensis* var. *piperacens* (Japanese peppermint) (Labiatae); sassafras — *Sassafras albidum* (Lauraceae); spearmint — *Mentha spicata* (Labiatae); sweet bay laurel — *Laurus nobilis* (Lauraceae); thyme — *Thymus vulgaris* (Labiatae)

Van Duuren et al. 1963). Second, D-limonene exposed to air shows inhibitory activity on various microorganisms and none when purified. The inhibitory activity increases with increasing exposure to oxygen and decreases in the presence of ascorbic acid (Zukerman 1951). It is evident that the concentration of the hydroperoxide of D-limonene determines the degree of carcinogenic activity. One may assume that other factors in orange oil may modify the rate and extent of auto-oxidation of D-limonene, and therefore its carcinogenic activity. Thus, the observations that orange oil alone has no carcinogenic effects on mouse skin (Roe 1959) and that it has relatively low tumorigenic activity on the urethral orifice of female mice, with or without DMBA (Roe and Pierce 1960), are consistent with the assumption.

D-Limonene is a component of many spices and flavoring agents, e.g., oils of caraway, cardamon, celery, dill, fennel, lavender, lemon grass, niaouli, peppermint, and spearmint. Orange and lemon oil contain about 90% D-limonene (Stecher et al. 1960).

Other terpenes reported to have tumor-promoting activity are L-pinene (MacKenzie and Rous 1941), phellandrene, and linalool (Roe and Field 1965). L-Pinene is found in the essential oil fraction of many spices, such as lemon, nutmeg, and peppermint (Table 8.5); it has been shown to promote tumor development in rabbits (MacKenzie and Rous 1941), but not in mice (Shubik 1950). Similarly, phellandrene, which is also widely distributed among spices and flavoring products, is more effective as a tumor-promoting agent than linalool (Roe and Field 1965). Linalyl acetate, found in bergamot (*Citrus aurantium* var. *bergamia*), lavender (*Lavandula officinalis*), and orange flowers (Stecher et al. 1960), and linalyl oleate are cocarcinogens with benzo(a)pyrene (Van Duuren et al. 1971).

A majority of the terpenes listed in Table 8.5 have not been tested for crucial oncological activity. As discussed later in this chapter, a number of these compounds have other significant biological activities. Because certain terpenes already have been shown to possess carcinogenic, cocarcinogenic, or tumor-promoting activity, e.g., D-limonene and L-pinene, many other terpenes in Table 8.5 with similar structures should be prime candidates for carcinogenicity testing.

Miscellaneous Endogenous Oncological Substances in Plant Foodstuffs

The previous sections have shown that there are many types of endogenous oncological substances (carcinogens, cocarcinogens, and tumor promoters) in plants which belong to a few general classes of compounds. The grouping of oncological compounds into special classes based on certain chemical characteristics has repeatedly been shown to have significant predictive value, even though correlations between structure and oncological activity may not always be true (Chap. 6 and 21), as in the case of nitrosamines and polycyclic aromatic compounds.

Black Pepper Carcinogens The presence of alkaloids in black pepper which are structurally similar to safrole, i.e., methylenedioxybenzene structures and terpenes (Table 8.5), make one suspect this product as a potential carcinogenic agent. The structures of the alkaloids piperine, chavicine, and piperettine are shown in Figure 8.1. The first two are stereoisomers. Chavicine is soluble in organic solvents, such as alcohol, ethyl ether, and petroleum ether. It is an oily substance with a sharp peppery taste, and is one of the most active constituents of black pepper. Piperine is sparingly soluble in water (4 mg/100 ml), but more soluble in ethanol, chloroform, and ethyl ether. It is almost insoluble in petroleum ether. This compound is tasteless initially but gives a burning aftertaste (Stecher et al. 1960). Piperine also has a strong insecticidal property against the housefly (Harvill et al. 1943).

Another alkaloid in black pepper is α-methylpyrroline (Pictet and Pictet 1927). Piperidine has also been detected in black pepper, constituting about 0.1% of the volatile oil (Hasselstrom et al. 1957).

Piperidine   α-Methylpyrroline

These compounds are secondary amines and have the potential of being nitrosated in vivo as well as in vitro (Chapter 21). N-Nitrosopiperidine is a strong carcinogen; animals treated with this compound developed tumors in various sites (Garcia and Lijinsky 1972). Among 30 male and 30 female Swiss mice treated with 0.01% of the carcinogen in drinking water five times a week for 26 weeks, the investigators counted 57 lung adenomas and tumors developing in 17 mice (Greenblatt and Lijinsky 1972). Piperidine itself has been reported to produce tumors in a significant number of rats treated with the compound (Garcia and Lijinsky 1973); this result suggests that nitrosation of piperidine may have occurred in vivo.

Piperine has been reported to be directly nitrosable, producing N-nitrosopiperidine (Lijinsky et al. 1972). Therefore, piperine and similar alkaloids in black pepper are potentially carcinogenic in two ways. Gershbein (1977) reported that piperine stimulates liver regeneration in rats, as do the known oncogens, safrole, isosafrole, dihydrosafrole, and estragole. Noncarcinogens with similar structures do not. Osawa et al. (1981) showed that piperine treated with nitrite is highly mutagenic in bacterial test systems.

Black pepper contains 1 to 2.6% (Furia and Bellance 1971) essential oils and 6 to 12% piperine and chavicine combined (Marion 1950). To date, more than 43 terpenes have been identified in black pepper oil (Table 8.5), consisting mostly of monoterpenes, sesquiterpenes, and oxygen-containing terpenes. The predominant terpenes are α- and β-pinenes, D-limonene, β-caryophyllene as well as savinene and 3-carene, and moderate amounts of α-phellandrene (Hasselstrom et al. 1957; Wrolstad and Jennings 1965). In addition, the volatile fraction of black pepper also contains safrole, myristicin, methyleugenol (Russell and Jennings 1969), piperidine, piperonal, and various alcohols (Hasselstrom et al. 1957). Note that the predominant terpenes already have been shown to possess carcinogenic or cocarcinogenic activity — α- and β-pinene and phellandrene are cocarcinogenic, D-limonene is carcinogenic in its peroxide form (pp. 335—342).

It is against this background that Concon et al. (1979, 1981) tested the carcinogenic activity of black pepper. Preliminary experiments with Swiss albino mice have shown that this spice may be potentially a strong carcinogen. Weanling mice were treated on the skin with 1 mg pepper extract in 0.1 ml acetone solution for 3 months (three times weekly the first month, twice a week the second, and once a week, the third). Animals surviving after 19 to 22 months developed lung tumors with nearly 85%

tumor incidence compared to 31% in the control. In addition, a significant incidence of liver tumors (4/13) and skin tumors (4/13), and somewhat lower incidence of pancreatic (3/13) and other tumors (total, 4/13) developed. The controls showed none of these other tumors.

Fractionation of the pepper extract produced a fraction which had significant mutational activity on histidine-dependent strain of *Salmonella typhimurium* (Concon et al. 1981). Such mutational activity on bacterial systems has been highly correlated with carcinogenic activity (Ames et al. 1973; Legator and Malling 1971).

The development of liver and pulmonary tumors in mice also has been observed with safrole. However, in this case, there was a lower incidence of pulmonary tumors and a much higher incidence (50% to 58%) of liver tumors (Epstein et al. 1970); the control animals showed 5 to 6% incidence of liver tumors but no pulmonary tumors.

In view of the widespread use of black pepper and products derived from it (world consumption estimated at several thousand tons per year [Furia and Bellanca 1971]), these preliminary findings deserve serious attention.

Polycyclic Aromatic Hydrocarbons (PAH)   These have been found in several raw green vegetables, in cabbage, leeks, lettuce, tomatoes, and spinach. Cabbage and spinach contains particularly high levels of the carcinogens benzo(a)pyrene and dibenzo(a,h)anthracene (Graf and Diehl 1966; Grimmer and Hildebrandt 1965). The levels of benzo(a)pyrene and benzo(a)anthracene detected in fresh vegetables were 2.85 to 24.5 ppb and 0.3 to 43.6 ppb, respectively. PAHs also have been detected in unrefined vegetable oils, such as sunflower seed and palm kernel oils, which also contain relatively high levels of benzo(a)pyrene (Grimmer and Hildebrandt 1967, 1968). The sample of crude coconut oil was found to contain 44 ppb benzo(a)pyrene, 1 ppm phenanthrene, and from 129 to 402 ppb of other noncarcinogenic PAHs. Sunflower seed and palm oil have a higher benzo(a)pyrene content. The presence of PAHs in crude oil rather than in the refined products is emphasized in order to distinguish those PAHs which may have been transferred to the oil during refining, as was suggested (Howard et al. 1966). Evidence is accumulating which suggests that PAH may be endogenously synthesized by plants. For example, it has been observed that there is an increase in the PAH content of leaves during yellowing and germination and in starchy bulbs (Graf and Diehl 1966).

It also has been observed that plants grown on artificial media and those grown in locations distant from sources of pollution have similar levels of PAHs (Graf and Diehl 1966). The PAH content of vegetables depends on the surface area and time of exposure. However, thorough washing of the vegetable reduces the PAH content by only one-tenth (Grimmer and Hildebrandt 1965). This observation suggested to these investigators that most of the PAH is in the interior of the tissues and that these may have been of endogenous origin. Further evidence has been reported by Borneff et al. (1968), who demonstrated by use of a ^{14}C-acetate medium that algae biosynthesized PAHs. No doubt a significant portion of the PAH content of plants may come from the soil and atmospheric pollution. This aspect of the PAH occurrence in foodstuffs is discussed in Chapter 19; further discussion on this subject is found in Chapter 6.

Nitrosamines   These compounds are among the most potent and versatile of carcinogens, producing tumors in several sites in experimental animals (Chap. 12). Of interest here is the possible endogenous synthesis of nitrosamines in plants processed for food, particularly because of the reported isolation of dimethylnitrosamines in samples of wheat flours, grains, and certain plants (Hedler and Marquardt 1968). The precursors, secondary amines, and nitrates (which can be easily reduced to nitrites) have been found in many plants (Miller 1973). Nitrosamines are easily formed from these amines and nitrites even at low concentrations (Mirvish 1970). There is some evidence that certain plants may synthesize nitrosamines under conditions of molybdenum deficiency. Du Plessis et al. (1969) isolated dimethylnitrosamine from an ethanolic extract of the fruit of *Solanum incantum* growing in a molybdenum-deficient medium. The juice of this fruit is used by Bantus in certain parts of Africa to curdle milk. The high incidence of esophageal cancer in these areas coincides with the occurrence of molybdenum deficiency in corn, beans, and pumpkins (Burrell et al. 1966; Du Plessis et al. 1969). Schoental (1969) has suggested that these plants are possible etiological agents in liver cancer in Central and East Africa because of their wide use as herbal remedies.

Carcinogenic Goitrogens Thiourea is a goitrogen, and thus a carcinogen. Rats fed diets containing 0.1 to 1.0% thiourea have been shown to develop not only thyroid tumors (adenomas and carcinomas) (Purves and Griesbach 1947), but also liver tumors (Fitzhugh and Nelson 1948), and malignant tumors of the eyelid and ear duct glands (Rosin and Ungar 1957). Thiourea is produced endogenously in the seeds of Laburnum species of the Leguminosae family (Klein and Farkass 1930). Fortunately, these plants do not constitute a source of human foodstuffs. The carcinogenic activity of thiourea makes one suspect other sulfur-containing goitrogens; e.g., those containing the 5-vinyl-oxazolidine-2-thione moiety. As discussed in Chapter 9, these glucosinolates are present in many food-bearing crucifers, particularly cabbages, kales, turnips, and rapes of the genus *Brassica*. Indeed, thyroid have been shown to develop adenomata in rats fed a diet containing 45% rapeseed (Griesbach et al. 1945). Other glucosinolates deserve similar tests.

Coumarinic Lactones Many types of coumarinic lactones have been reported to have significant toxicological activity. Most prominent in this group are the aflatoxins and related mycotoxins (Chap. 13). Also, mention has been made of limettin and bergapten, which appear to be the principal cocarcinogenic and photodynamic substances in limes, respectively (p. 334). Another structurally simple coumarinic lactone, parasorbic acid, or 5-methyl-2-hexenoic acid lactone, has been shown to produce local sarcomas in Wistar rats when 0.2- or 2-mg doses in peanut oil were injected twice a week for a total of 64 injections (Dickens and Jones 1963). Parasorbic acid is the major constituent of the oil obtained by steam distillation from acidified ripe berries of the mountain ash *Sorbus ancuparia* (family Rosaceae) (Kuhn and Jerchel 1943).

Yet, the simplest lactone in this group, coumarin, has been shown to be inactive in the rat by subcutaneous injection (Dickens and Jones 1965). Subsequently, it has

Coumarin

been reported by other researchers (Bär and Griepentrog 1967; Griepentrog 1973) that bile duct adenomas and carcinomas are induced in rats when fed diets containing 5000 ppm coumarin for prolonged periods. These results are to be expected, since earlier researchers (Hazelton et al. 1956; Sporn 1960) reported that coumarin fed at 2500 ppm in the diet produces extensive liver damage. Subsequently, Hagan et al. (1967) confirmed the hepatotoxicity of coumarin in rats fed diets containing 5000 and 2500 ppm coumarin, and in dogs with diets containing 25, 50, and 100 ppm. These workers observed liver enlargement, fatty changes, and bile duct proliferation and fibrosis. In addition, the animals showed growth retardation and testicular atrophy. The interpretation of the bile duct changes caused by coumarin seems in conflict with the earlier reports.

Humans differ from rats with regard to the metabolism of coumarin. Man converts it almost completely to 7-hydroxycoumarin with only traces of o-hydroxyphenylacetic acid (Shilling et al. 1969). Rats, on the other hand, metabolize this lactone chiefly to o-hydroxyphenylacetic acid, in addition to several other metabolites: o-hydroxyphenylacetic acid and 7-hydroxycoumarin (Feuer et al. 1966; Kaighen and Williams

1961). These acids are potent inhibitors of glucose-6-phosphatase in the hepatic microsomes, whereas 7-hydroxycoumarin is inactive. Whether these findings have any significance to the hepatotoxicity of coumarin in rats or humans is not known. Glucose-6-phosphatase facilitates the conversion of glucose-6-phosphate to free glucose, thus facilitating the conversion of other monosaccharides to glucose. o-Hydroxyphenyl-acetic acid is a normal but minor product of phenylalanine metabolism.

Coumarin has moderate acute toxicity in animals including man. About 5 g is fatal to sheep, and about 4 g produces mild toxic effects in humans; about 40 g is lethal to horses (Dean 1950). Rats are killed in 8 weeks when fed diets containing 1% coumarin (Hagan et al. 1967). Coumarin also possesses narcotic, hypnotic, and sedative effects in many animal species (Dean 1950).

Coumarin once was used as a flavoring agent in food products, particularly in imitation vanilla, but it has been banned since 1954 (Food and Drug Administration 1977).

There are many other simple coumarinic lactones, which also show varied physio-logical and pharmacological effects in animals. There are at least 115 such naturally occurring lactones (Soine 1964). An estrogenic coumarinic lactone, coumestrol, is dis-cussed in the next section.

Coumarin is a minor constituent of certain edible fruits, e.g., strawberries, cher-ries, apricots, and a major constituent of tongka beans (*Dipteryx odorata*), its prin-cipal source. Coumarin is present in many flavoring agents — for example, cassie (*Acacia farnesiana*) (LaFace 1950), woodruff (*Asperula odorada*) (Stecher et al. 1960), lavender (*Lavandula officinalis*) (Seidel et al. 1944), and lovage (*Levisticum officinale*) (Naves 1943). These flavoring agents are used extensively in candies, liqueurs, and certain wines. Trace quantities of coumarin are also found in citrus oils (DiGiacomo 1966) and carrotseed oil (Seifert et al. 1968).

Petasites as a Carcinogen   *Petasites japonicus*, which resembles the weed coltsfoot (*Tussilago farfara*), is cultivated and used in Japan as a food and herbal remedy. Rats given a diet containing 4% Petasites for 480 days developed a 42% incidence of liver tumors characterized as hemangioendothelial sarcoma. Significantly lower inci-dences (9 to 10%) have been observed when the Petasites diet was alternated with nor-mal diet at weekly intervals. No tumors were observed when these animals were given diets containing 16.6% Petasites for 134 days followed by 8.3% diet for 86 days; mega-locytosis, proliferation of the bile duct, nodular hyperplasia, and finally, cirrhosis developed instead. The carcinogen appeared to occur predominantly in the flower stalks than in the vegetative parts. However, the flower stalks of cultivated plants are significantly less carcinogenic than the wild variety (Hirono et al. 1975).

Hirono et al. (1977) has identified a carcinogen in *Petasites japonicus*, petasiten-ine, a pyrrolizidine alkaloid. Administered at 0.01% in drinking water, this alkaloid has been shown to produce liver tumors in 8/10 animals within 160 days. When given at 0.05% in the drinking water, all rats died in 72 days with liver necrosis, hemor-rhage, and bile duct proliferation. The structure of petasitenine is shown below:

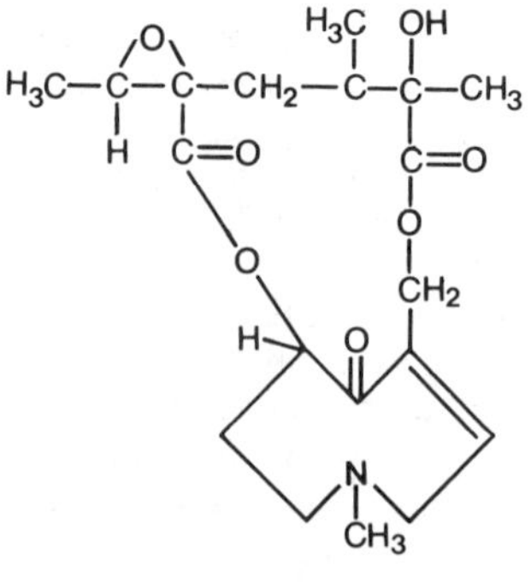

Petasitenine

Carrageenans These hydrophillic colloidal substances are obtained from red algae or seaweeds (*Chondrus crispus* and other species). Carrageenans are probably examples of "solid-state" carcinogens. These are nonspecific solids which when entrapped in tissues for long periods induce tumors at the site of contact under certain conditions (Chap. 6). Thus, after 2 years following a single subcutaneous injection of 50 mg carrageenans in 5 ml saline, a significant incidence of sarcomas (11/39) at the injection site has been observed in rats (Cater 1961). It has been shown that the latency of tumor development following multiple subcutaneous injections of carrageenans is accelerated when another carcinogen, 2-acetylaminofluorene, is fed simultaneously (Walpole 1962). Feeding carrageenans for 2 years does not produce tumors in rats or mice. However, the survival rates of these animals are lower (Nilson and Wagner 1959).

These high molecular weight sulfated polysaccharides of galactose and anhydrogalactose are used as food additives as stabilizers and bulking agents. As discussed in Chapter 9, animal experiments indicate that excessive consumption of these polysaccharides decreases mineral and nitrogen absorption.

Remarks No doubt this list of endogenous carcinogens in foodstuff-producing plants will be extended as more substances from these plants are tested. A notable example is black pepper, which may yield other types of carcinogens besides those already identified. Plants have consistently yielded many pharmacologically active compounds.

Phytoestrogens

The subject on phytoestrogens probably belongs in the previous section, since the primary significance of estrogens lies in their oncological activity. However, there has as yet been no reported direct evidence that phytoestrogens possess such activity, although this potential may indeed be present. The subject of the carcinogenicity of estrogens is discussed in Chapters 6 and 19.

Estrogen is a generic term applied to substances which induce estrus. In rats and mice, the occurrrence of estrus is accompanied by characteristic proliferative changes in the vaginal epithelium. Microscopical examination of vaginal smears will indicate whether estrus is indeed occurring. This is the basis of the Allen-Doisy test, which has been described in detail by Emmens (1950).

Since the development of this test, it has been possible to demonstrate the estrogenic activity of many substances, particularly those from plants. There is no doubt that phytoestrogens possess specific physiological activity, the degree of which depends on the dose. Table 8.6 lists several foodstuffs which contain estrogenic activity. Unfortunately not all observed estrogenic activities are quantified. Estrogenic activity is usually expressed in mouse or rat units. One mouse unit (MU) of activity is equivalent to 0.1 µg of estrone. Note that certain products have high estrogenic activity, especially garlic, sage, and palm kernel. The reported estrogenic activity in certain foodstuffs may be an artifact because other researchers have been unable to confirm such findings. For example, the estrogenic activity could not be confirmed in coffee oil (Hauptmann et al. 1943) and potatoes (Walker and Janney 1930).

The nature of chemicals responsible for the estrogenic activity of most of the products listed in Table 8.6 have not been determined. However, the few phytoestrogens for which the chemical structures (Fig. 8.4) have been established show that the estrogenicity is not uniquely correlated with a special structural type or class of compounds. Thus, there are phytoestrogens among triterpenes, stilbenes, phenanthrenes, steroids, bitter acids, isoflavones, and coumestans. Zearalenone, a mycoestrogen produced by several Fusarium molds, is a resorcylic acid lactone (Chap. 13). However, as will be discussed later, there is a certain feature in these structures which seems to be shared by all known estrogens.

Phytoestrogens with triterpene and phenanthrene structures have not been reported to be present in plant foodstuffs. The stilbenes are represented by that

Table 8.6 Estrogenic Activity in Foodstuffs

Foodstuff	Part tested	Activity[a] MU or RU/kg
Alfalfa (Medicago sativa)	Hay	1.9-3.5 µg DES[b]/kg hay[c]; contains coumestrol
Anise (Pimpinella anisum)	Oil	+
Apple (Malus sylvestris)	Fruit flesh	+
Barley (Hordeum vulgare)	Germ	+
Beet (Beta vulgaris)	Seeds	500 MU
Cherry (Prunus avium)	Fruit flesh	+
Cinnamon (Cinnamomum zeylanicum)	Bark (oil)	+
Coffee (Coffea arabica)	Seed (oil)	+
Fennel (Foeniculum vulgare)	Oil	+
Garlic (Allium sativum)	Bulb	4000 MU
Licorice (Glycyrrhiza glabra)	Root	++
Oats (Avena sativa)	Seeds Sprouted seeds	6.6 RU, 50 RU 50 RU-16,000 RU
Palm (Elaeis guineensis)	Kernel (residues)	20,000 MU
Parsley (Petroselinum crispum)	Root	+
Plum (Prunus avium)	Fruit flesh	+
Potato (Solanum tuberosum)	Tubers	+
Rape (Brassica campestris)	Seeds	+
Rhubarb (Rheum rhaponticum)	Leaves	5 MU
Rice (Oryza sativa)	Germ	+
Rye (Secale cereale)		+
Sage (Salvia officinalis)	Leaves	6000 MU
Soybean Soya hispida)	Oil	$\simeq$ 0.1% genistin[d]; also contains coumestrol[e]

[a]1 MU = 0.1 µg estrone; IRU = 0.5 µg estrone.
[b]Diethylstilbestrol.
[c]Contains coumestrol: 1 µg coumestrol = 3.5×10^{-4} µg DES, = 5.1×10^{-3} estrone (Bickoff et al. 1962).
[d]1 µg genistin = $1-2 \times 10^{-5}$ µg DES (Bickoff et al. 1962; Cheng et al. 1955).
[e]Present in both soybean seed and sprouts (Wada and Yuhara 1964).
Source: From Bradbury and White (1954), except data on alfalfa and soybeans which were taken from Cheng et al. (1955).

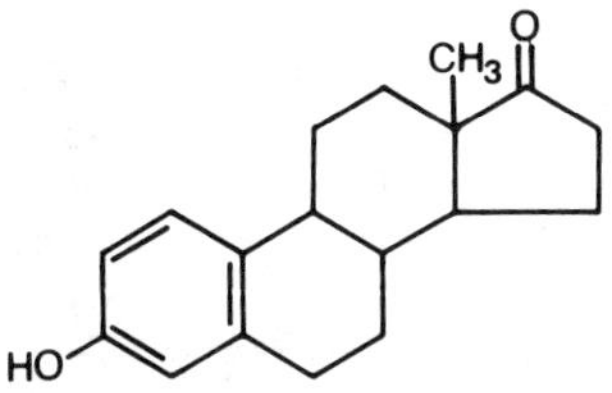

ESTRONE

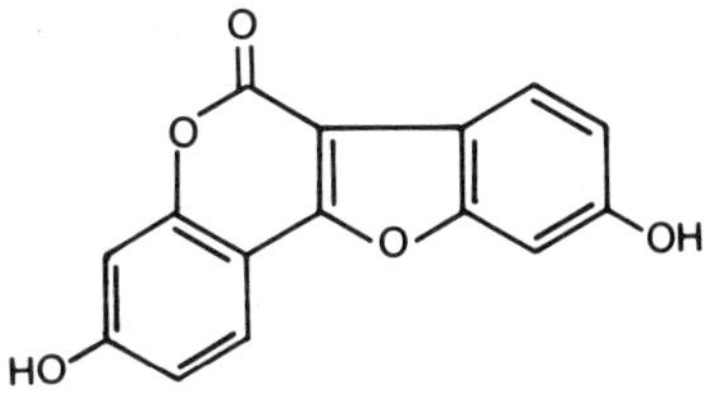

COUMESTROL

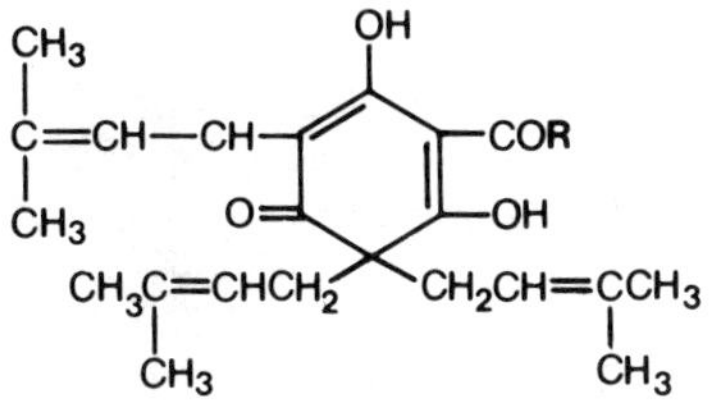

BITTER ACID

	R
COLUPULON	-CHCH3 CH3
LUPULON	-CH2CHCH3 CH3
ADLUPULON	-CHCH3 CH2CH3

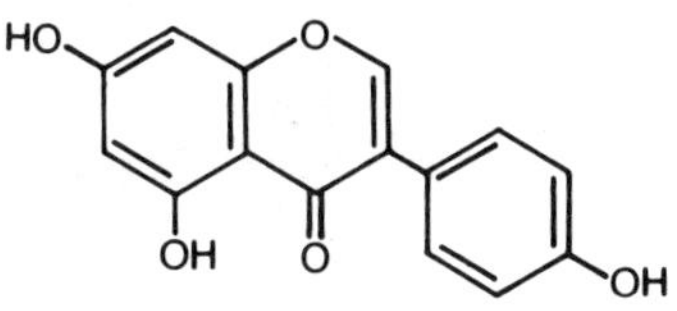

GENISTEIN
(AN ISOFLAVONE)

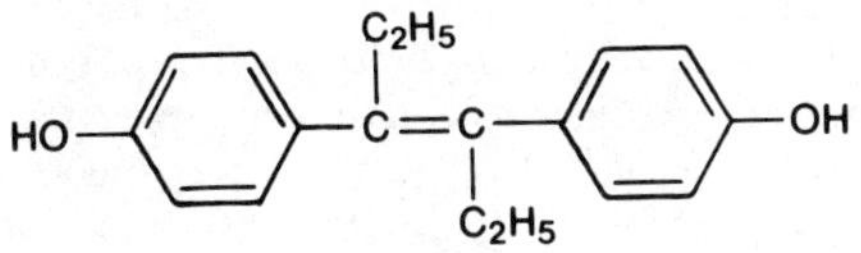

Figure 8.4 Phytoestrogens. Estrone is found in palm kernels (*Elaeis guineesis*); coumestrol in alfalfa (*Mendicago sativa*); the bitter acids in hops (*Humulus lupulus*) used to impart bitter flavor in beer; isoflavones in soybeans and other sources.

powerful estrogen, the synthetic diethylstilbestrol (DES). Apparently there have been no reports of endogenous stilbenes in plant foodstuffs, except perhaps a possible transformation product of anethole. The latter is present in several spices and flavoring products such as anise and fennel oils (Table 8.6). Estrogenic stilbenes have been reported to be present endogenously in the heartwoods of certain trees (Lindstedt 1951).

Estrogenic bitter acids are represented by lupulon and related compounds (Zenisek and Bednar 1960), which are found in hops. The hops or dried strobiles of *Humulus lupulus* of the Moraceae family are used in the brewing of beer. The estrogenic activity of hops has been reported to be 12,500 IU/g (1 IU = 0.1 μg estradiol). However, there is as yet no reported evidence that beer is estrogenic.

A steroidal estrogen has been isolated from the oil of palm kernel (*Elaeis guineesis*) residues left after pressing (Butenandt and Jacobi 1933). After careful chemical work, the phytoestrogen from these kernels has been identified as estrone. The oil from the press-cake has been determined to contain an estrogenic activity of about 417,000 MU/ kg. This is the only clear cut case of an ovarian hormone which is endogenous in a plant foodstuff. However, another phytoestrogen resembling the animal estrogen, estriol, also has been reported. This was isolated from willow flowers (Skarzynski 1933a,b). It resembles estriol chemically but has only one-fourth of its activity. Its true identity is not known.

Estrogenic isoflavones have been more thoroughly evaluated and studied. A number of these isoflavones have been isolated and their structures established. These include genistein, biochanin A, prunetin, daidzein, and formononetin. Biochanin A and prunetin are the 4'-methylether and 7-methylether of genistein, respectively.

Genistein occurs freely and as the 7-glucoside, genistin, in soybeans (Cheng et al. 1953); the aglycone is also present in subterranean clover (*Trifolium subterraneum*) and other species of clover (Biggers and Curnow 1954; Bradbury and White 1951). A sample of hexane-extracted soybeans was shown to contain 0.1% genistin (Walter 1941); the estrogenic activity of a kilogram of unextracted soybeans may be equivalent to 6 μg DES (Wada and Fukushima 1963). On a molar basis, genistein and genistin have equal activity based on the mouse uterine weight assay[*] (Cheng et al. 1955). Biochanin A is similarly found in red clover (Pope et al. 1953).

Genistein occurs also in the form of 4'-glucoside, sophoricoside, and 4'-glucosidorhamnoside; sophorabioside in the fruit of the Japanese pagoda tree *Sophora japonica*. The fruit of this tree is sometimes processed into flour and used for food during difficult times. Presumably, when properly prepared, the flour is safe, but otherwise it may be dangerous and even lethal (King-Li-Pin 1931). The toxicity is not due to these glycosides but probably mostly owing to other toxicants present in fruit (Watt and Breyer-Brandwijk 1962).

Prunetin is present in certain species of Prunus (Finnemore 1910; King and Jurd 1952).

Daidzein is a dihydroxyisoflavone differing from genistein by the absence of an hydroxyl group in the 5 position. Its 4'-methylether is formononetin. Daidzein has been identified in soybeans in the form of the glycoside daidzin (Walz 1931). Formononetin has been isolated from subterranean clover (Bradbury and White 1951). The estrogenic activity of 1 μg of daidzein, formononetin, genistein, and biochanin A are equivalent to 1.7×10^{-5}, 3.6×10^{-6}, 1.32×10^{-5}, 1.32×10^{-5} μg DES, respectively, based on the uterine weight assay. Thus, daidzein has slightly higher activity than genistein and biochanin A, both of the latter being equal (Cheng et al. 1955). Formononetin has the least activity in the group.

Two coumestans are known: coumestrol, which is obtained from alfalfa (Bickoff et al. 1957), soybeans, and soybean sprouts (Wada and Yuhara 1964), and its 4'-O-methylether, which is also found in alfalfa (Bickoff et al. 1962). Coumestrol is heat stable, and the estrogenic activity of 1 μg of coumestrol is equivalent to 3.5×10^{-4} μg of DES or 1×10^{-2} μg estrone. It is, however, more estrogenic than genistin, 1 μg coumestrol being equivalent to 35 μg genistein (Bickoff et al. 1962).

Possible Relationships Between Estrogenicity and Structure

Figure 8.4 shows the structures of most of the phytoestrogens that have been identified. For purposes of comparison, the structure of DES is also given. Note that four classes of compounds are represented: a stilbene (DES), steroid (estrone), isoflavone

---

[*]Uterine weight assay measures the increase in uterine weight in immature mice following four daily doses of estrogenic compound.

(e.g., genistein), and coumestan or coumarinic lactone (coumestrol and its 4'-methyl derivative). However, one is impressed by a certain feature of the configuration of each estrogen. Note that all structures in Fig. 8.4 may be drawn to assume the "rolling pin" form of DES.

One can assume that this similarity in form may explain why such diverse structures are associated with a specific physiological effect. However, the manner in which these compounds stimulate estrus is unknown.

Toxicological Effects of Estrogens

The physiological action of estrogen is discussed in standard textbooks of endocrinology or biochemistry, and therefore need not be reviewed here. Suffice it to say that the plant estrogens are able to produce similar, if not identical, effects as the animal estrogens: They have been shown to stimulate uterine hypertrophy in intact immature rodents, such as the mouse (Bickoff et al. 1962), and to stimulate protein synthesis in the uterus of ovariectomized rats (Noteboom and Gorski 1963). But unlike the animal hormone, they cannot induce ovum implantation in ovariectomized rodents maintained on gestagen (Perel and Lindner 1970). Genistein reportedly can displace estradiol from receptor sites in the uterus (Shutt 1967), and coumesterol has been shown to inhibit gonadotropin function (Leavitt and Wright 1965).

A dramatic demonstration that phytoestrogens can produce serious reproductive damage has been reported by Australian researchers. Ewes grazing on pastures laden with subterranean clover (*Trifolium subterraneum*) were afflicted with the so-called "clover disease." The disease syndrome is described as consisting of dystokia, uterine prolapse (Bennetts and Underwood 1951), and progressive, severe, and irreversible infertility (Schinkel 1948). The affected ewes develop cystic endometria (Bennetts and Underwood 1951). There were also neuronal damage and neuronophagia in the hypothalamus, atrophy in the adrenal cortex (Gardiner and Nairn 1969), and cystic changes and squamous metaplasia in the cervix (Adams 1976; Hearnshaw et al. 1972). The affected animals had abnormal mucin secretion (Adams 1976; Smith 1971) with low viscosity (Smith 1971). It is believed that this abnormal mucin prevents the proper orientation of the sperm during migration through the cervix (Smith 1971).

It also has been shown that ewes grazing on estrogenic clover develop morphological changes not only in the reproductive tissues, but also in other organs, particularly in the pituitary, hypothalamus, and thyroid glands (Adams 1977). These changes have been observed to occur in ewes as early as within 3 weeks after feeding.

Heifers grazing on grass stands with at least 42% clover have shown metabolic changes; e.g., increased urea production, decreased phenol sulfate secretion, and slightly decreased productivity than those grazing on stands containing about 13% clover (Palfii et al. 1975). It also has been shown that a high level of subterranean clover in the feed causes increased glucose-6-phosphate and malate dehydrogenases in the teats of sheep and cattle. Similar observations have been made with DES (Smithard et al. 1975). These results again verify the estrogenicity of subterranean clover.

The aforementioned results affirm the hidden hazard of estrogenic foodstuffs, eaten in excess, on the reproductive system. In view of the rigid interrelationships of the hormonal systems, related endocrine functions may also be endangered.

One hazard that deserves serious attention is the possible oncological activity of phytoestrogens. There have been already numerous reports confirming the oncological activity of animal and synthetic estrogens such as DES (Schoental 1976). Phytoestrogens may be expected to have similar activity, but perhaps to a lesser degree. There are some indications that phytoestrogens in the diet may in fact enhance oncogenesis. For example, it has been reported that C3HAvy mice exported to Australia developed markedly fewer spontaneous mammary tumors compared to those raised in the United States, but the incidence of mammary tumors significantly increased when the mice were fed American mice chow (Sabine et al. 1973); the incidence was restored to the original American level when the mice were also bedded on red cedar instead of

Douglas fir shavings. The estrogenic activity of batches of laboratory rat chow has been in fact reported by Drane et al. (1975).

Toxic Fatty Acids

The fatty acids in foodstuffs that are of nutritional value are without exception saturated or unsaturated straight chains, and rarely exceed 20 carbon atoms in length.

The double bonds in unsaturated fatty acids follow a specific pattern: The double bond(s) is in the 9 position in the monoenes, palmitoleic and oleic acids; the bonds are in positions 9 and 12 in the diene, linoleic acid; 9,12, and 15 in the triene, linolenic acid; and 5, 8, 11, and 14 in the tetraene, arachidonic acid. The 24-carbon nervonic acid with the double bond on carbon-15 has no dietary significance, and in the animal body is usually associated with nervous tissues. It cannot accumulate in certain tissues without specific damage. For example, hemolytic anemia in hamsters is believed to be partly due to the accumulation of nervonic acid in the erythrocyte membrane (Vles and Abdellatif 1970).

The specific structures of nutritional fatty acids suggest that any deviation from the norm may result in adverse effects, unless the animal system can successfully degrade the acid to nontoxic metabolites. Thus, several unusual fatty acids have been shown to be toxic. These fatty acids include erucic acid, sterculic and malvalic acids (cyclopropene fatty acids), cetoleic acid, and in the presence of Refsum's syndrome, phytanic acid. Cetoleic acid is of animal origin, being found in herring oil (Beare-Rogers et al. 1971), and having toxic effect similar to erucic acid. Phytanic acid does not occur endogenously in plant foodstuffs, so far as is known, even though its precursor, phytol, is a component of chlorophyll. Phytanic acid is a contaminant in ruminant fats and possibly dairy products (Hansen 1965a,b; Patton and Benson 1966).

Erucic acid and the cyclopropene fatty acids are the only ones in this group that are endogenous in plant foodstuffs.

Erucic acid

Erucic acid is found largely in the plant family Cruciferae, notably in Brassica. The oils from rapeseeds (*B. rapus* and *B. campestris*) and mustardseeds (*B. hirta* and *B. juncea*) are particularly high in erucic acid. These oils may contain from 20 to 55% erucic acid (Eckey 1954; Markley 1960; Miller et al. 1965).

Selective breeding in Canada (Stefansson et al. 1961; Krzymanski and Downey 1969) has resulted in a new variety of rape with seed oil low in erucic acid. Rapeseed and mustardseed oils have commercial value in many parts of the world, and thus, their potential toxicity is a fundamental concern.

The toxic effects of rapeseed oil were first reported by Roine et al. (1960). They fed rats high levels of

$$CH_3(CH_2)_7CH=CH(CH_2)_{11}COOH$$

Erucic acid

rapeseed oils — 50 to 70% of the caloric content — and these animals developed myocarditis. This observation was soon confirmed by later researchers (Abdellatif and Vles 1970a; Beare-Rogers et al. 1971; Rocquelin et al. 1968). Weanling rats fed high levels of rapeseed oil accumulate fat in the heart muscles even after the first day of feeding; the fat droplets are scattered throughout the myocardium. The level of fat in the heart muscle sometimes exceeds four times normal values. Similar changes occur in the skeletal muscles (Abdellatif and Vles 1970a). The fat droplets are mainly triglycerides containing a large proportion of erucic acid (Beare-Rogers et al. 1971; Houtsmuller et al. 1970). The fatty accumulation decreases and finally disappears with time even with continued feeding of rapeseed oil. This disappearance is soon followed by mononuclear cell infiltration, and eventually myocardial fibrosis (Abdellatif and Vles 1970a,b). However, the accumulation of fats in the myocardium was (Engfeldt 1975) persistent throughout a 160-day experiment even when the diet contained small amounts of erucic acid.

Experiments confirming that erucic acid is the toxic principle in rapeseed oil have shown that trierucin produces similar lesions in the rat (Abdellatif and Vles 1970a), and that feeding rapeseed oil low in erucic acid does not produce these characteristic lesions (Beare-Rogers et al. 1971; Vles et al. 1976).

Rapeseed oil fed at high levels also has been shown to retard growth in the rat (Beare et al. 1957, 1959; Boer et al. 1947; Rocquelin et al. 1968), and when fed throughout the lifespan at such levels, it causes a high incidence of degenerative changes in the liver, nephrosis (Abdellatif and Vles 1970a; Thomasson 1955), and smaller size and weight of litter in these animals (Beare et al. 1961). The lifespan, however, is not affected in spite of these degenerative changes. Rapeseed oil containing 0.6 to 85% erucic acid also produces dermal lesions and alopecia in male rats (Hulan et al. 1976b). The feet and tails of these rats become scaly, hemorrhagic, and necrotic after 4 to 5 weeks on the diet; the lesions increase in severity after 5 to 8 weeks and disappeared after 14 weeks. These lesions develop no matter whether the rapeseed oil contains higher (23.6%) or lower (0.6%) erucic acid levels. The lesions have been attributed to inhibition of prostaglandin synthesis.

Rapeseed oil also interferes with the ability of the mitochondria in heart muscle to oxidize substrates such as glutamate, and thus impairs the rate of ATP synthesis (Houtsmuller et al. 1970). This does not occur with liver mitochondria; thus the fatty accumulation in the heart muscle is due to the failure of the myocardium to oxidize erucic acid and/or convert it to oleic acid.

Fatty accumulation following feeding with rapeseed oil also has been observed in hamsters (Thomasson et al. 1970), minipigs, squirrel monkeys (Beare-Rogers 1970), and ducklings (Abdellatif and Vles 1970c; Thomasson et al. 1970). The latter also develop hydropericardium and cirrhosis of the liver. Guinea pigs fed large amounts of rapeseed oil develop not only enlargement of the spleen, but also hemolytic anemia (Thomasson et al. 1970; Vles and Abdellatif 1970). The hemolytic anemia has been attributed to the accumulation of erucic acid in addition to nervonic acid, in erythrocyte membrane, so that the permeability of the cell is increased.

High levels of erucic acid in the diet also impair the growth of chickens (Salmon 1969a), ducklings, guinea pigs, hamsters, mice (Thomasson et al. 1970), pigs (Thoron 1969), and turkeys (Salmon 1969b). The retardation of growth in rats also can be accomplished by feeding other fats mixed with erucic acid (Beare et al. 1959; Thomasson and Boldingh 1955).

Growth retardation in rats caused by rapeseed oil has been prevented by partial hydrogenation of the oil and/or addition of saturated fats to the oil (Beare et al. 1963; Craig et al. 1963). This not only improves the consistency of the diet, but also increases the levels of palmitic and myristic acids; both the improvement in consistency (Alexander and Mattson 1966) and the increased level of these acids (Beare et al. 1963; Thomasson et al. 1970) improve growth performance in the rat in the presence of erucic acid. Palmitic acid not only has been shown to prevent growth retardation, but also decreases the severity and incidence of hydropericardium in ducklings, and prevents hemolytic anemia in hamsters (Vles and Abdellatiff 1970). The pathological effects take place only in the presence of erucic acid in diet; thus, these effects cannot be attributed to the unfavorable ratio of saturated and unsaturated fatty acids (Rocquelin et al. 1970; Vles and Abdellatif 1970).

Rapeseed oil becomes damaging only at high doses; i.e., 10 to 20% of calories fed to the weanling rat (Abdellatif and Vles 1970a; Beare-Rogers et al. 1971; Hulan et al. 1976a,b), 30% in duckling (Abdellatif and Vles 1970b) and 25% in guinea pigs (Vles and Abdellatif 1970).

Refining procedures which lower the erucic acid contents to as low as 1.4% render rapeseed oil relatively safe, as has been shown in the weanling Wistar rat (Vles et al.

1976). However, some workers have reported that the low erucic acid Canbra oil still can produce cardiac lesions, even though it has a lower incidence and is less severe than the regular variety (Roine et al. 1960).

Toxic response to erucic acid seems to be dependent on age — weanling rats suffer more massive damage to the heart muscles than those 2 to 3 months past the weanling stage (Beare-Rogers 1970); however, even in these older animals, mononuclear cell infiltration of the myocardium still occurs when fed a diet containing significant levels of erucic acid (Abdellatif and Vles 1970a).

Erucic acid also may be ingested indirectly from body fats of animals fed rapeseed oil. For example, the fatty acid has been found in the fat of chicken (Salmon 1969a; Sell and Hodgson 1962), lambs (Stokes and Walker 1970), and turkeys (Salmon 1969b); it also has been detected in rat milk (Beare et al. 1961). However, erucic acid has not been reported as being present also in cow's milk.

Because a large intake of erucic acid is necessary to induce myocardial damage in animals, the hazard of erucic acid toxicity in humans is probably minimal. Nevertheless, Canadian authorities prudently are replacing the normal rapeseed variety with the low-erucic acid varieties. It is also possible that any low toxic effects in humans would be unsuspected and their significance to the total health of an individual would not be recognized. That such possible toxic effects may go unrecognized is shown by the fact that the lifespan of rats is not shortened even in the presence of erucic acid-induced degenerative changes in the liver and nephrosis in the kidneys (Thomasson 1955; Vles and Abdellatif 1970). And neither is there an inhibition of the reproductive performance of these animals; only the sizes of their litter are reduced (Beare et al. 1961).

Cyclopropene Fatty Acids

The oils or fat of every plant of the order Malvales that have been examined so far, with one exception, contain cyclopropene fatty acids (Eckey 1954; Phelps et al. 1965). The exception is cocoa butter from *Theobroma cocoa* (Hilditch and Williams 1964). Two important acids in this group are sterculic (19 carbons) and malvalic (18 carbons) acids. Their structures are as follows:

$$CH_3(CH_2)_7 \overset{\overset{\displaystyle CH_2}{\displaystyle \diagup \diagdown}}{C=C} - (CH_2)_n COOH$$

Malvalic acid: n = 6; Sterculic acid: n = 7

From the food toxicological standpoint, only the cyclopropene fatty acids in the oil of cottonseeds (*Gossypium hirsutum*) are of significance. Crude cottonseed oil may contain from 0.6 to 1.2% cyclopropene fatty acids in the form of sterculic and malvalic acids (Bailey et al. 1966). Processing may reduce these levels from 0.1 to 0.5% (Hammonds and Shone 1966; Harris et al. 1964). The cottonseed meal may contain about 0.01% depending on the quantity of residual oil (Levi et al. 1967). Hydrogenation probably destroys some of the biological effects of these acids (Masson et al. 1957).

Another source of high levels of cyclopropene fatty acids is kapok seed oil from *Ciba peutandra* and *Bombax malavaricum*. The oil from these species contain from 10 to 14% of these acids. However, another species of kapok, *Sterculia foetida*, may contain more than 70% sterculic acid (Hilditch and Williams 1964). The oil from *S. foetida* is bland or slightly sweet, and is used for cooking (Hilditch and Williams 1964).

The interest in the cyclopropene fatty acids developed when it was determined that these were responsible for the pinkish or reddish discoloration of egg whites (Masson et al. 1957; Phelps et al. 1965; Shenstone and Vickery 1959). It also has been observed that hens stopped laying eggs when fed 250 mg of these fatty acids daily (Shenstone and Vickery 1959). Sexual maturity in chickens fed kapok oil also is delayed with slow or inhibited comb development, and with liver and gallbladder enlargement (Schneider et al. 1962. The reproductive capability of female rats fed diets containing 3% *S. foetida* oil also is suppressed, with inhibition or retardation in the development of the follicles and uteri. Male rats are otherwise unaffected (Rascop et al. 1966). Rats fed kapok seed oil containing 10 to 14% cyclopropene fatty acids at a level of 10% of the calories in the diet fail to grow normally; at 40% of the total calories, the diet is lethal to the animals in a few weeks (Thomasson 1955). Expectedly, *S. foetida* oil, with its very high level of cyclopropene fatty acids, causes death at only 10% of the total caloric intake (Schneider et al. 1968). Mice appear to be insensitive to the effect of sterculic acids at levels of up to 200 mg/kg body weight per day, at least in terms of reproductive performance (Phelps et al. 1965).

More important perhaps in terms of human health is the carcinogenic activity of these acids. This has been demonstrated in rainbow trout. In the presence of the cyclopropene fatty acids, the carcinogenic activity of aflatoxin B_1 has been shown to be considerably enhanced (Lee et al. 1967; Sinnhuber et al. 1966).

An important biochemical effect of sterculic acid is the observed inhibition of the conversion of exogenous stearic acid to oleic acid. In hens, this inhibition results in the increased levels of saturated fatty acids in body fat at the expense of mono-unsaturated fatty acids (Allen et al. 1967; Evans et al. 1962; Johnson et al. 1967). This shift to high melting point body fats also has been observed in pigs fed a high ration of cottonseed meal (Deuel 1955). This increase in saturated fatty acids in body fat cannot be overcome by addition of oleic or linoleic acids in the diet (Evans et al. 1963).

The cyclopropene group in these fatty acids reacts with the SH groups of cysteine and glutathione (Raju and Reiser 1969); thus it is believed that one possible mechanism for the observed interference in the conversion of stearic acid to oleic acid is the inhibition of stearate desaturase (Johnson et al. 1967; Raju and Reiser 1969). In the alga Chlorella, sterculic acid blocks the conversion of oleic acid to linoleic acid when both acids are combined in the algal culture, but not when oleic acid is added first, sufficiently long enough for it to be incorporated into the tissue triglycerides (James et al. 1968). This effect on Chlorella is similar to that observed in hens.

Presently, the importance of cyclopropene fatty acids to human health is unknown. Cottonseed oil has been used for several years in food preparation, with apparently no ill effects. This statement must be qualified, since experimental or epidemiological evidence to this effect is lacking. The carcinogenicity of these fatty acids together with their biological and biochemical effects gives them greater toxicological significance than hitherto realized.

Miscellaneous Endogenous Toxicants

A number of toxicants which do not fall under any of the categories in the preceding sections will be discussed in this section. To a large extent, the toxicants included here have not been structurally identified or characterized.

Many foodstuffs may contain more than one toxic substance; e.g., the legumes, spices and many fruits. Thus, it would be convenient and advantageous to discuss the toxicants in this section under each type of food.

Avocado Persea americana

Avocados are consumed in great numbers, particularly in the tropics, with no ill effects, but apparently certain varieties contain toxic principles of as yet an undetermined nature. There are at least 500 varieties of avocado pear (Watt and Breyerbrandwijk 1962). The fruit has been used for therapeutic purposes. The Fuerte and Naval varieties are toxic, since rabbits fed the leaves have been shown to die within 24 hr. There have been reported poisonings of animals — canaries, cattle, fish, goats, and rabbits — consuming not only leaves, bark, and seeds, but also the fruit pulp (Kingsbury 1964). Toxicity of some varieties of avocado also have been confirmed experimentally (Appleman 1944; Valeri and Gimeno 1954). The primary symptom of avocado poisoning in cattle, goats, and horses is severe, noninfectious, sensitive mastitis with reduced milk flow. The milk-producing capacity of these animals remains subnormal even after the mastitis is under control.

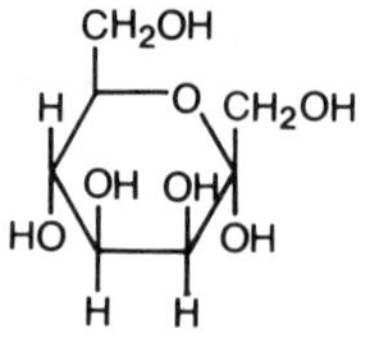

Mannoheptulose

The avocado is the only known source for the isolation of D-mannoheptulose (structure above) in relatively large amounts (Simon and Kraicer 1966). Thus, for this reason, the avocado appears unique among the more common edible tropical fruit (Ogata et al. 1972). In four avocado varieties, the amount of mannoheptulose ranges from 0.64 to 2.5% of the unripe pulp. The amounts tend to drop drastically on ripening; values of 0.03 to 0.5% have been obtained. Other tropical fruit contains 0.0 to <0.01% of the sugar (Ogata et al. 1972). The amounts vary considerably among varieties. Simon and Kraicer (1966) found values as high as 3.9% in the tree-ripened Lula variety. Similar wide variation has been reported by Nagy et al. (1979), who also found that Florida avocados contain more mannoheptulose than the California varieties.

In both human and animal subjects, consumption of avocados has been shown to result in hyperglycemia or a depression in plasma insulin and the insulogenic index, which is the ratio of the plasma insulin concentration ($\mu U/ml$) to the glucose concentration (mg%) (Viktora et al. 1969). In humans, as little as about 3 g avocado/kg body weight, or an intake of 22.5 mg mannoheptulose/g avocado pulp has been shown to be sufficient to cause a drop in plasma insulin (Viktora et al. 1969).

In studies with isolated rabbit pancreas, Coore et al. (1963) have concluded that mannoheptulose completely but reversibly suppresses the stimulating effect of D-glucose on insulin secretion. This sugar is potent enough to inhibit the rat pancreas from secreting insulin at doses which do not induce hyperglycemia. At larger doses, the level of hyperglycemia is in direct proportion to the amount of mannoheptulose administered (Simon and Kraicer 1966). It also has been shown that the diabetogenic effect is due to both a blockage of insulin secretion and an acceleration of gluconeogenesis from amino acids (Simon and Kraicer 1966). Malaisse et al. (1968) have shown that this sugar inhibits the phosphorylation of glucose, and that this process appears to be essential in the stimulation of insulin.

For normal individuals, this temporary drop in insulin levels from occasional consumption of avocados may be harmless. However, the effect of persistent consumption is unknown, especially in tropical regions where there is an abundance of fruit. Furthermore, for marginal or incipient diabetics, will a summer of daily consumption of a variety of tropical fruits induce the appearance of frank diabetes?

The pericarp of the avocado contains a resinous substance; when injected intraperitoneally in guinea pigs, at a dose of about 0.9 g/kg body weight, it produces excitement, semiparalysis, brain and myocardial hemorrhage, and death within 8 hours. Subcutaneous doses in the same amounts also produce similar effects, in addition to swelling of the legs and abdomen (Watt and Breyer-Brandwijk 1962).

California Bay Laurel (Umbellularia californica)

Contrary to some claims, California bay laurel is still sold as a condiment or seasoning agent in the United States. An irritating oil constitutes about 0.5 to 4% of this spice.

The oil contains from 40 to 60% umbellulone, a ketonic monoterpene. According to Drake and Stuhr (1935), contact with the oil, or even exposure to the vapors, can cause skin irritation, headache, and in some cases, the effect can be serious enough to cause unconsciousness. When 2 ml of a 0.1% solution of the terpene in olive oil was injected into guinea pigs, three times a week for 6 weeks, the terpene produced marked hemolysis. Umbellulone possesses an atropinelike effect on the nerves and muscle fibers of frog heart. It has been concluded that umbellulone blocks the pulmonary circulation (Drake and Stuhr 1935). California bay laurel should not be mistaken

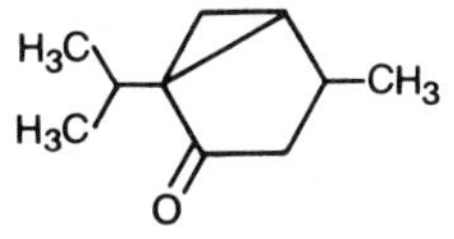

Umbellulone

for the conventional bay leaves, or laurel (*Laurus nobilis*), which is devoid of this toxic effect.

Figs (Ficus carica)

Like prunes, figs contain a laxative principle which has not been identified (Watt and Breyer-Brandwijk 1962). If unripe, figs are emetic (Ulmann et al. 1945). The latex of this plant contains a proteolytic enzyme ficin. High doses of ficin can be extremely toxic; the LD_{50} in rats and mice is 10 g/kg, being lower in rabbits and guinea pigs, approximately 5 g/kg (Stecher et al. 1960). At sublethal oral doses, severe irritation of the gastrointestinal mucosa, at times with erosion, is accompanied by vomiting, bloody diarrhea, and general prostration (Molitor et al. 1941).

Licorice (Glycyrrhiza glabra)

The extract of the root of the licorice plant has been used for medicinal purposes for many years. It has a pleasant flavor, and is used to mask the taste of unpleasant medicines. Licorice is also widely used in candies and other confections. However, this flavoring agent contains a glycoside which constitutes about 5 to 10% of the root (Osol and Farrar 1955). The glycoside consists of two glucuronic acid moieties and a steroidal aglycone glycyrrhetinic acid. The calcium or potassium salt of the glycoside is called glycyrrhizin. Glycyrrhizin is approximately 50 times as sweet as sucrose so that its sweetness is detectable at a dilution of 1:15,000 (Osol and Farrar 1955).

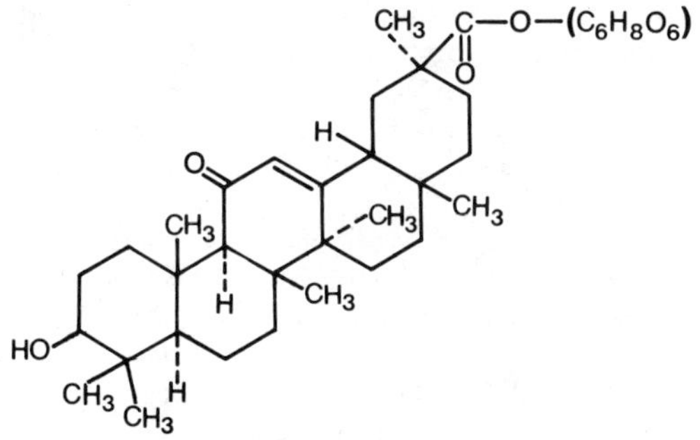

Glycyrrhizin

Because of the steroidal character, the aglycone licorice extracts, expectedly, possess marked physiological activity. Indeed, licorice has been reported to have a deoxycorticosterone activity, as shown by the usual water and sodium retention and potassium loss following consumption (Conn et al. 1968; Menkyna 1954). Consequently, excessive consumption of licorice candy can cause not only sodium and water retention, but also severe hypertension, hypokalemia, aldosteronopenia, suppressed plasma renin activity, and cardiac enlargement (Conn et al. 1968; Koster and David 1968). A case of licorice poisoning is on record in which consumption of candy containing approximately 0.5 g ammonium glycyrrhizate for a prolonged period at a rate approaching 100 g/day resulted in pseudoaldosteronism and fulminant congestive heart failure (Chamberlain 1970). Excessive licorice ingestion by a patient also has been shown to produce hypokalemic myopathy with myoglobinuria (Gross et al. 1966). The aldosterone effect of licorice produces other complications as a result of electrolyte imbalance. Therefore, licorice may pose a considerable hazard in those with heart or kidney disease. Occasional consumption of licorice probably has little adverse effect, if any: it has been shown that a dose of 0.5 g/70 kg apparently causes no harmful effect in a human being (Berger and Höller 1957).

Oil of Wormwood (Artemisia absinthium)

The oil of the wormwood plant contains the ketoterpene thujone as a major component.

Thujone

The oil was once used as the main flavoring agent of liqueur absinthe. Because of the serious toxicological effects, its use was abolished in France in the early part of this century (Balavoine 1952). It is still used as a flavoring agent in wines such as vermouth, but only in trace quantities (i.e., less than 10 ppm). Thujone is a convulsant; about 30 mg/kg body weight will produce convulsions in experimental animals, with lesions of the cerebral cortex (Keith and Stavraky 1935; Opper 1939). Thujone is also a component of sage (Salvia officinalis) (Brieskorn and Wenger 1960; Vernazza 1957).

Onions, Garlic, and Related Species (Allium spp.)

A number of species of Allium Liliaceae family, have been used by diverse populations not only as spices or condiments, but also for medicinal purposes. The most common members of this group are the onion (Allium cepa), garlic (A. sativum), leek (A. porrum), shallot or scallion (A. ascalonicum), and chives (A. schoenaprasum). The species that have been used more commonly for medicinal purposes are onions and garlic.

The most distinctive characteristic of these species is the odor which emanates from any tissue when these plants are bruised or crushed. This distinctive odor or flavor is due to a number of sulfur compounds, including alliin (allylthiosulfinate) (Cavallito and Bailey 1944). The latter is derived from alliine, or (+)-S-allyl-L-cysteine sulfoxide (Stoll and Seebeck 1949). Garlic contains about 2.4 mg allicin/g (Stoll and Seebeck 1948). The odor of garlic develops upon enzymatic cleavage of allicine. In onions, compounds similar to allicin have been isolated; these compounds have methyl, propyl, or trans1-propenyl groups instead of the allyl group in alliin (Carson and Wong 1961; Carson et al. 1966; Virtanen and Matikkala 1959). These cysteine sulfoxides are decomposed by alliinase, an enzyme produced by the plant, to the

corresponding thiosulfinates. These labile thiosulfinates slowly decompose to thiosul-
fonates and disulfides (Mazelis 1963; Moisio et al. 1962). These reactions are shown
schematically as follows:

$$\overset{O}{\underset{\uparrow}{R-S}}-CH_2-CH(NH_2)COOH \xrightarrow{\text{Alliinase}} \overset{O}{\underset{\uparrow}{R-S}}-S-R + 2CH_3COCOOH + 2NH_3$$

(I)   (II)

$$\overset{O}{\underset{\uparrow}{R-S}}-S-R \xrightarrow{\text{Disproportionation}} RSSR + R-\overset{O}{\underset{\underset{O}{\uparrow}}{\underset{\downarrow}{S}}}-S-R$$

(III)   (IV)

I: Alliin; R = allyl = CH_2=CH-CH_2-, in garlic; R = methyl, propyl, or *trans*-
      1-propenyl, in onions
II: Allicine or 2-propenyl-2-propenethiosulfinate
III: Allyldisulfide
IV: Allylthiosulfonate

The volatile disulfides are also partly responsible for the characteristic odor and
flavor of these products (Small et al. 1947). Many types of sulfides and thiosulfate
have been isolated from fresh onions, dehydrated onions (Bernhard 1968; Boelens et
al. 1971), distilled onion oil (Brodnitz and Pollock 1970; Brodnitz et al. 1969), and
garlic (Jacobsen et al. 1964).
      Onions contain about 2 mg *trans*-(+)-S-(propen-1-yl)-L-cystein sulfoxide per
gram (Matikkala and Virtanen 1967). This is converted, by the action of alliinase, to
propenylsulfenic acid (Moisio et al. 1962). Propenylsulfenic acid converts to thiopropanal-S-oxide, which has been shown to be the lacrimatory factor from onions (Brodnitz and Pascale 1971).

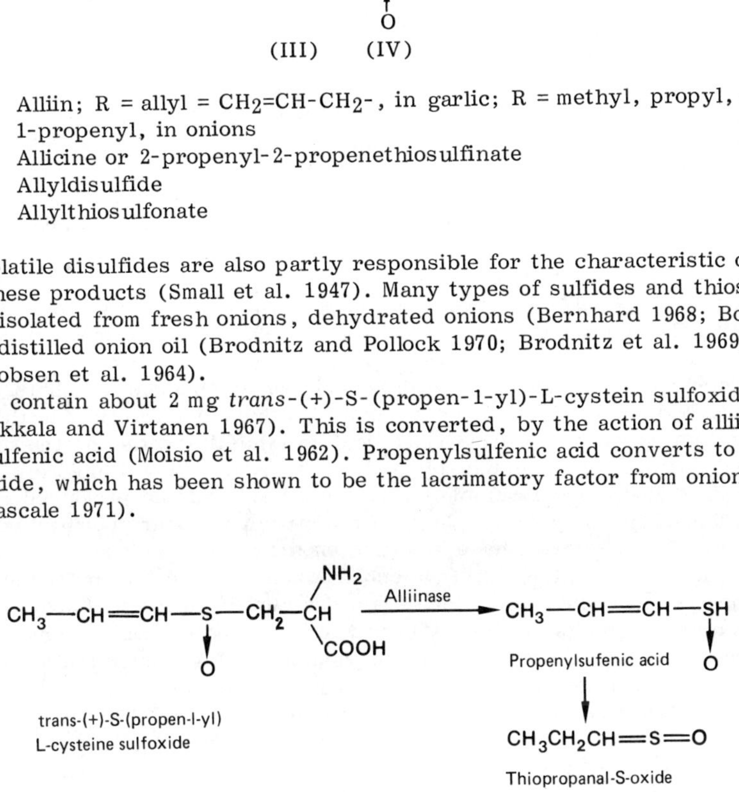

$$CH_3-CH=CH-\overset{O}{\underset{\downarrow}{S}}-CH_2-\overset{NH_2}{\underset{COOH}{CH}} \xrightarrow{\text{Alliinase}} CH_3-CH=CH-\overset{O}{\underset{\downarrow}{SH}}$$

trans-(+)-S-(propen-l-yl)   Propenylsufenic acid
L-cysteine sulfoxide

$$CH_3CH_2CH=S=O$$

Thiopropanal-S-oxide

      As most users know, the alliums, especially onions and garlic, are strong irritants
not only to the eye — hence, the lacrimatory effect — but also to the hands and nose.
The pattern of distribution of the topical dermatitis on the fingers reveals the manner
of contact — the thumb on both hands, and the index and middle fingers on the left
hand (Burks 1954). Excessive ingestion can also irritate the gastrointestinal tract, resulting in vomiting and diarrhea; irritation to the kidneys can also occur. Excessive
comsumption of onions has been shown to fatally poison cattle (Goldsmith 1909; Koger
1956) and horses (Thorp and Harshfield 1939). The symptoms in cattle have been
shown to include gastroenteritis, vomiting, constipation or sometimes diarrhea, and
dark-colored urine (hemoglobinuria) with a strong onion odor. Horses have been observed to devlop anemia, icterus, and also dark-colored urine. Seven of nine horses
in the study of Thorp and Harshfield (1939) died. The symptoms appear after 6 or

more days following consumption, and death is precipitated by sudden forced activity. The younger horses tend to be more susceptible than the older animals. Sebrell (1930) reported that severe anemia also develops in dogs fed raw or cooked onions in amounts of 0.5% of body weight, or 15 g or more per day; in this case, both erythrocyte concentration and hemoglobin content of these cells were shown to decrease and the red blood cell concentration was sometimes observed to drop to less than 2 million/mm^3.

The anemia-producing compound has not been identified; it is not extractable by water or ether but by ethanol (Maiori and Squeri 1955-56).

Onions also possess hypoglycemic action. This has been demonstrated by oral administration of onion extracts to rabbits and pancreatomized dogs (Laland and Havrevold 1933). The maximum effect has been noted from 1 to 5 hr following treatment, and the activity is lost when the extracts are allowed to stand for 1 to 10 days even under refrigeration and in the presence of a preservative. The hypoglycemic fraction has been found in the nondialyzable fraction of the extract and not in the lipid fraction (Laurin 1931). It has been shown to be present in fresh onion juice (Janot et al. 1930; Kreitmair 1936), and in extracts of the green tops of sprouts, in the roots, and bulbs (Collip 1923a,b,c). Laland and Havrevold (1933) reported that the hypoglycemic principle is alkaloidal in nature and is active only in the presence of the sulfides. A similar hypoglycemic principle also has been demonstrated in garlic (Laland and Havrevold 1933). The hypoglycemic activity explains the use of garlic in India as an antidiabetogenic agent (Mukerji 1957). However, this action reportedly is not analogous to that of insulin.

The gonadotropic activity of garlic has been mentioned in connection with phytoestrogens (pp. 347-350). Androgenic activity also is present in garlic in equipotent amounts with the estrogens (Glaser and Drobnik 1939). Gonadotropic activity also has been reported in onion extracts (Klosa 1951).

A hypotensive factor also may be present in garlic (Lio and Agnoli 1927). A chloroform-soluble fraction from garlic has a weak hypotensive effect in the cat, a slight stimulant action on the frog heart, and an inhibiting action on the movement of the isolated intestine of the guinea pig, even with very highly diluted extracts (0.0025%). The chloroform-insoluble fraction has a marked and prolonged hypotensive effect in the cat, but only slight effect on the other parameters (Umberto de Torrescasana 1946). These extracts have no effect on the isolated guinea-pig uterus, but the alcohol extracts increase the amplitude and frequency of uterine contractions and slightly increase the tone of the uterine muscles (Mateo Tinao and Calvo Terren 1955).

Garlic oil also inhibits pepsin action and forms methaemoglobin (Lehmann 1929-1930). The oil is absorbed in the intestines and some of it is excreted via the lungs.

Garlic has been regarded in India as a nerve stimulant, especially in children. Oral administration is said to be dangerous or even fatal to children. Even the fumes may have such an effect (Watt and Breyer-Brandwijk 1962).

The oral toxicity of garlic also has been shown in the mouse, rat, and guinea pig (Maxwell et al. 1939). All animals tested with garlic oil have shown stimulant-narcotic effects, and 0.775 ml/kg has proved toxic to rabbits (Perrin et al. 1924).

The goitrogenicity of onions is discussed in Chapter 9.

Similarly, chives contain an irritant oil, and like onions, have been shown to poison horses (Kobayashi 1950).

Peppermint Oil (Mentha piperita)

Peppermint oil contains approximately 40% menthol (Smith and Levi 1961; Stecher et al. 1960). This terpene is also found in other foodstuffs such as cocoa (Van der Wal et al. 1971). As a flavoring agent, menthol is used in candies, chewing gum, liqueurs, and other products. Aside from sensitization reactions in the form of urticaria (Papa and Shelley 1964), some adverse reaction can result from excessive consumption of menthol-containing products. Two patients were shown to develop heart fibrillation after prolonged addictive consumption of up to 225 g peppermint candy per day (Thomas 1962).

Toxic psychosis also has been reported to develop in a woman who was habituated to mentholated cigarettes (Luke 1962). The symptoms in these cases disappeared when the incriminating products were avoided.

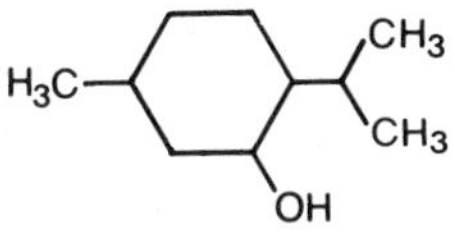

Menthol

Prunes (Prunus domestica)

Prunes are a type of plum which can dry partially without spoiling. They are sold commercially as the dried product, and eaten either cooked or uncooked. The plant is cultivated in many countries. As discussed previously (p. 282), one of its many toxicants is the cyanogenic glycoside amygdalin, which occurs commonly in other members of the family Rosaceae, which comprises many common edible fruit.

However, prunes, particularly the French or Santa Clara varieties, are also noted for their cathartic effects. Both the dried and fresh prunes possess this purgative action. While it has been claimed that this effect is due to the indigestible pectins and other emollient materials, Emerson (1933) showed that the cathartic action is not entirely due to these emollient materials; to a large extent, catharsis is due to a specific chemical substance(s). Although the compounds has not been chemically identified, a comparison of the physiological action of known laxatives with that of prune extracts on isolated rabbit jejunum or duodenum strongly indicates that the cathartic compound is dihydroxyphenylisatin, or 3,3-bis(p-hydroxyphenyl)-oxindole. Similar to a prune extract, this compound produces the same immediate increase in tonus and amplitude of contraction of the intestinal segments and chlorogenic and caffeic acids also may contribute to the laxative action of prunes.

Turmeric (Curcuma longa)

The powdered rhizome of *Curcuma longa* of the ginger family is turmeric or curcuma. This yellow powder is used as a condiment — mixed with curry powders and other spices. It also has been used for medicinal purposes (Watt and Breyer-Brandwijk 1962). The pigment in turmeric is curcumin, which has been shown to be a cholagogue; that is, it increases bile flow and stimulates contraction of the gallbladder (Ramprasad and Sirsi 1956, 1957a,b).

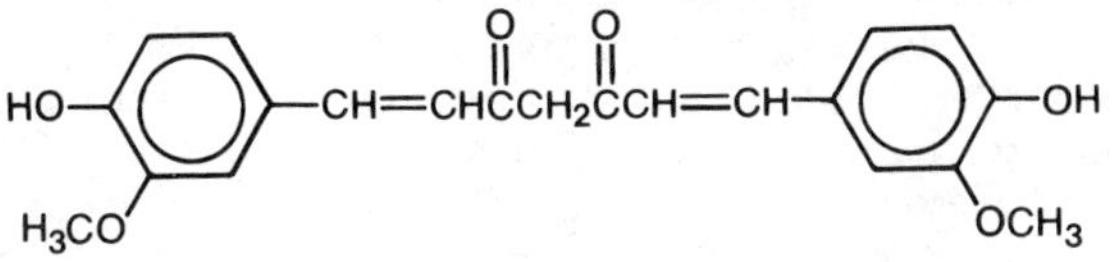

Curcumin

It has been shown that when a curcumin extract of turmeric is added to cultures of cells from Chinese hamsters, cactus mouse, Indian muntijac, and human lymphocytes, it arrests mitosis, affects chromosome morphology, and inhibits nucleic acid synthesis. Thus, the rate of incorporation of tritium-labeled thymidine and uridine into Chinese hamster cells is reduced to 25% of control values within 30 min after adding 10 μg turmeric per ml; a slight rate reduction has been noted with 1 μg/ml. Turmeric interferes with cell cycle progression. The effect on chromosome morphology is reflected by the progression of changes of the metaphase forms; i.e., uncoiling, chromatid separation, fragmentation, and disintegration (Goodpasture and Arrighi 1976).

Miscellaneous Foodstuffs

There are many types of foodstuffs which are consumed only by a limited number of people, usually within a certain geographical area. Such uncommon foods often contain toxic substances, and in many cases, the population at large in the area has learned procedures to eliminate or minimize them, undoubtedly by experience.

In certain areas in Southeast Asia, India, and Africa, the fruit, root, and young shoots of the palmyrah tree (*Borassus flabellifer*) of the palm family are used for food (Watt and Breyer-Brandwikj 1962). It has been shown that the flour from the young palmyrah shoots when fed to Wistar rats for up to 12 months produces chronic hepatic veno-occlusive lesions, which include intraluminal fibrosis of the centrilobular and portal veins, bile duct proliferation, increased reticulin formation, and fibrosis (Panabokke and Arseculeratne 1976). The flour also has been shown to produce malignant lymphomas in rats after prolonged feeding (Panabokke and Arseculeratne 1977). Aqueous extracts of this flour are clastogenic to human lymphocytes (Kangwanpong et al. 1981). The investigators believe that the unknown toxin may be different from the pyrrolizidine alkaloids and dimethylnitrosamine in spite of the similarity of the lesions. This is reminiscent of another toxic starch, the cycad flour (pp. 323–327).

Finally, many highly edible plant products when eaten in excess may produce toxic effects. Thus, an overconsumption of tomato juice may result in lycopenia, a condition characterized by deep orange discoloration of the skin owing to accumulation of lycopene; this pigment can also accumulate in the liver, causing illness (Arena 1963; Reich et al. 1960). Tomato also contains the alkaloid tomatine, which has a similar action to solanine, except that it is milder in its effect (pp. 298–301).

The very delicious papaya (*Carica papaya*) not only contains the powerful protease papain, but also an alkaloid, carpain. This alkaloid is present at around 0.02% in

O=C———(CH$_2$)$_7$

NH

O—

CH$_3$

Carpaine

the peeled fruit (Noble 1946-47; Webb 1948). Nevertheless, it has a powerful cardiac and diuretic action (Henry 1949; Stecher et al. 1960; Tuffey and Williams 1951; Watt and Breyer-Brandwijk 1962). It also has an effect similar to emetine (Tuffley and Williams 1951). This alkaloid is probably responsible for the slightly bitter taste of papaya. Carpain depresses atrial, followed by ventricular contractions of the heart without interference to the conduction system. The depression of cardiac action causes hypotension. At higher concentrations, carpain causes vasoconstriction which is not reversed by epinephrine. The irritability of the smooth muscles of the cat and guinea pig intestines, and the guinea pig uterus and bronchiole is depressed by this alkaloid. Its cardiac effect is also similar to digitalis action at certain dose levels; e.g., 20 mg/day (Noble 1946–1947).

Conclusions

As discussed in this chapter, a whole range of toxic substances are endogenous in plant foodstuffs. Many of these substances occur in trace amounts; nevertheless, their toxic potentialities must be recognized, since it must be realized that certain toxic effects do not require more than trace amounts; e.g., carcinogens and urushiols. Furthermore, excessive quantities of these foodstuffs may be consumed, sometimes with disastrous effects.

Hereditary traits are another aspect that must be considered in terms of the endogenous toxicants in plant foodstuffs — "Quod ali cibus est, aliis, fiat acre venenum" — What is food to one may be fierce poison to others (Lucretius, 95-55 B.C. *De Rerum Natura:* IV, 637).

Thus, poisonings can occur in abnormal situations; e.g., excessive consumption of foods containing cyanogens (e.g., goitrogens, acetylcholinesterase inhibitors), and unusual individual susceptibility to foodstuffs containing such substances as urushiols and favic agents.

Some toxicants occur in amounts sufficiently high that toxicity is manifested even at normal levels of consumptions of the corresponding foodstuffs; e.g., discorine in yams, carcinogens, and lathyrogens.

Present fadism involving the so-called superior qualities of natural foods undoubtedly arises from ignorance of the potential toxicity of the unadulterated products of nature. The facts, to the contrary, speak for themselves.

REFERENCES

Abbott, D. C., Field, K. and Johnson, E. I. 1960. Observations on the correlation of anticholinesterase effect with solanine content of potatoes. *Analyst* 85: 375—376.

Abdellatif, A. M. M. and Vles, R. O. 1970a. Pathological effects of dietary rapeseed oil in rats. *Nutr. Metab.* 12: 285—295.

Abdellatif, A. M. M. and Vles, R. O. 1970b. Physiopathological effects of rapeseed oil and canbra oil in rats. Proceedings of the International Conference on the Science, Technology and Marketing of Rapeseed and Rapeseed Products. Rapeseed Association of Canada, Winnipeg, Manitoba.

Abdellatif, A. M. M. and Vles, R. O. 1970c. Pathological effects of dietary rapeseed oil in ducklings. *Nutr. Metab.* 12: 296—305.

Abou-Donia, M. B. and Dieckert, J. W. 1971. Gossypol: Subcellular localization and stimulation of rat liver microsomal oxidases. *Toxicol. Applied Pharmacol.* 18: 507—516.

Abou-Donia, M. B. and Dieckert, J. W. 1974. Gossypol: Uncoupling of respiratory chain and oxidative phosphorylation. *Life Sci.* 14: 1955-1963.

Abou-Donia, M. B. and Dieckert, J. W. 1975. Metabolic fate of gossypol: The metabolism of [14C] gossypol in swine. *Toxicol. Applied Pharmacol.* 31: 32—46.

Abou-Donia, M. B., Lyman, C. M., and Dieckert, J. W. 1970. Metabolic fate of gossypol: The metabolism of 14C-gossypol in rats. *Lipids* 5: 938—946.

Adams, N. R. 1976. Pathological changes in the tissue of infertile ewes with clover disease. *J. Comp. Pathol.* 86: 29—35.

Adams, N. R. 1977. Morphological changes in the organs of ewes grazing oestrogenic subterranean clover. *Res. Vet. Sci.* 22: 216—221.

Adams, R., Geissman, T. A., and Edwards, J. D. 1960. Gossypol, a pigment of cottonseed. *Chem. Rev.* 60: 555—574.

Adamson, R. H., Sieber, S. M. and Gargus, J. L. 1979. Carcinogenic effects of cycasin and methylazoxymethanol (MAM)-acetate in non-human primates (meeting abstract). *Proc. Am. Assoc. Cancer Res.* 20: 218.

Adiga, P. R., Rao, S. L. N., and Sarma, P. S. 1963. Some structural features and neurotoxic action of a compound from *Lathyrus sativus* seeds. *Curr. Sci.* 32: 153—155.

Adler, I.-D. 1969. Does caffeine induce dominant lethal mutations in mice? *Humangenetik* 7: 137—148.

Adler, I.-D., and Röhrborn, G. 1969. Cytogenic investigation of meiotic chromosomes of male mice after chronic caffeine treatment. *Humangenetik* 8: 81—85.

Afifi, A., Abdel-Bari, A., Kamel, S. A., and Heickal, I. 1965. Bahtim-110. A new Egyptian cotton free of gossypol induced by radiation. *Bahtim Exp. Sta. Tech. Bull.* 80: 1—35.

Akazawa, T., Miljanich, P., and Conn, E. E. 1960. Cyanogenic glycoside of *Sorghum vulgare*. *Plant Physiol.* 35: 535—538.

Akeley, R. V., Mills, W. R., Cunningham, C. E. and Watts, J. 1968. Lenape: A new potato variety high in solids and chipping quality. *Am. Potato. J.* 45: 142—145.

Akesson, H. O., and Walinder, J. 1965. Nutmeg intoxication. *Lancet* 1: 1271—1272.

Akinyanju, P., and Yudkin, J. 1967. Effect of coffee and tea on serum lipids in the rat. *Nature* 214: 426—427.

Aldridge, A., Parsons, W. D. and Neims, A. H. 1977. Stimulation of caffeine metabolism in the rat by 3-methylcholanthrene. *Life Sci.* 21: 967—974.

Aldridge, A., Aranda, J. V. and Neims, A. H. 1979. Caffeine metabolism in the newborn. *Clin. Pharmacol. Ther.* 25: 447.

Alexander, J. C. and Mattson, F. H. 1966. A nutritional comparison of rapeseed oil and soybean oil. *Can. J. Biochem.* 44: 34—43.

Allen, E. et al. 1967. Inhibition by cyclopropene fatty acids of the desaturation of stearic acid in hen liver. *Lipids* 2: 419—423.

Altschul, A. M., Lyman, C. M. and Thurber, F. H. 1958. Cottonseed meal. In: *Processed Plant Protein Foodstuffs*. A. M. Altschul (ed.). Academic Press, New York.

Ambrose, A. M., Cox, A. J., Jr. and DeEds, F. 1958. Antioxidant toxicity: Toxicological studies on sesamol. *J. Agric. Food Chem.* 6: 600—604.

Amerine, M. A. and Winkler, A. J. 1963. California wine grapes: Composition and quality of their musts and wines. *Calif. Univ. Agric. Exp. Sta. Bull.* 794: 1—83.

Ames, B. N., Lee, F. D. and Durstan, W. E. 1973. An improved bacterial test system for the detection and classification of mutagens and carcinogens. *Proc. Natl. Acad. Sci. U.S.A.* 70: 782—786.

Ammon, H. P. T. and Estler, C.-J. 1969. The influence of caffeine on carbohydrate and lipid metabolism in alloxan-diabetic mice. *Med. Exp.* 19: 161—169.

Ammon, H. P. T. and Estler, C.-J. 1970. Role of age in the caffeine effect on the function and metabolism of the heart. *Arzneimmittelforsch.* 20: 471—473. (German)

Anderson, L. A. P., Howard, A. and Simonsen, J. L. 1924. Studies on lathyrism. *Indian J. Med. Res.* 12: 613—643.

Anet, E. F. L. J., Lythgoe, B., Silk, M. H. and Trippett, S. 1953. Enanthotoxin and cicutoxin. Isolation and structures. *J. Chem. Soc. 1953:* 309—322.

Anonymous. 1912. *Phaseolus lunatus* beans. *Bull. Imp. Inst.* 10: 653—655.

Anonymous. 1969. Chronic cyanide neurotoxicity. *Lancet* 2: 942—943.

Anonymous. 1970. Name of potato variety Lenape withdrawn. *Am. Potato J.* 47: 103.

Appleman, D. 1944. *Preliminary Report on Toxicity of Avocado Leaves*. California Avocado Society Yearbook. Santa Ana, California.

Arena, J. M. 1963. *Poisoning*. Thomas, Springfield, Illinois.

Armstrong, B., Garrod, A., and Doll, R. 1976. A retrospective study of renal cancer with special reference to coffee and animal protein consumption. *Br. J. Cancer* 33: 127—136.

Arnott, W. M. 1959. A problem in tropical cardiology. *Br. Med. J.* 2: 1273—1285.

Arscott, T. H. and Harper, J. A. 1963. Relationship of 2,5-diamino-4,6-diketopyrimidine, 2,4-diaminobutyric acid and a crude preparation of β-cyano-L-alanine to the toxicity of the common and hairy vetch seed fed to chicks. *J. Nutr.* 80: 251—254.

Asatoor, A. M. and Simenhoff, M. L. 1965. The origin of urinary dimethylamine. *Biochem. Biophys. Acta* 111: 384—392.

Askar, A., Rubach, K. and Schormüller, J. 1972. Thin layer chromatographic separation of the amine fraction in banana. *Chem. Microbiol. Technol. Lebensm.* I: 187–190. (German)

Ashwood-Smith, M. J. and Poulton, G. A. 1981. Inappropriate regulations governing the use of oil of bergamot in suntan preparations. *Mutat. Res.* 85: 389–390.

Ashwood-Smith, M. J., Poulton, G. A., Barker, M. and Mildenberger, M. 1980. 5-Methoxypsoralen, an ingredient in several suntan preparations, has lethal, mutagenic and clastogenic properties. *Nature* 285: 407–409.

Auld, S. J. M. 1912–1913. Cyanogenesis under digestive conditions. *J. Agric. Sci.* 5: 409–417.

Axelrod, J. and Reichenthal, J. 1953. The fate of caffeine in man and a method for its estimation in biological material. *J. Pharmacol. Exp. Ther.* 107: 519–523.

Babu, S., Madhavan, T. V. and Rao, K. R. 1967. Effect of phlorhizin and related compounds on glucose excretion, kidney glycogen content and alkaline phosphatase activity of treated rats. *Indian J. Med. Res.* 55: 1226–1230.

Bachhuber, T. E., Lalich, J. J., Schilling, E. D. And Strong, F. M. 1965. Lathyrus factor activity of beta-aminopropionitrile. *Fed. Proc.* 14: 175.

Baer, H. 1979. The poisonous anacardiaceae. In: *Toxic Plants*. A. D. Kinghorn (ed.). Columbia University Press, New York.

Bailey, A. V., Harris, J. A., Skau, E. L. and Kerr, T. 1966. Cyclopropenoid fatty acid content and fatty acid composition of crude oils from twenty-five varieties of cottonseed. *J. Am. Oil Chem. Soc.* 43: 107–110.

Balavoine, P. 1952. Thujone in absinthe and its imitations. *Mitt. Lebensm. Hyg.* 43: 195–196. (French)

Baldry, J., Dougan, J. and Howard, C. E. 1972. Volatile flavoring constituents of durian. *Phytochemistry* 11: 2081–2084.

Bär, F. and Griepentrog, F. 1967. Health considerations of aromatic substances in foods. *Med. Ernaehr.* 8: 244. (German)

Barnett, K. C. and Watson, W. A. 1968. Bright blindness in sheep — The results of further investigations. *Veterinarian* 5: 17–27.

Barrett, M. D., Hill, D. C., Alexander, J. C. and Zitnak, A. 1977. Fate of orally dosed linamarin in the rat. *Can. J. Physiol. Pharmacol.* 55: 134–136.

Barrett, M. D. P., Alexander, J. C. and Hill, D. C. 1978. Effects of dietary cyanide on growth, and thiocyanate levels in blood and urine in rats. *Nutr. Rep. Int.* 18: 413–419.

Bass, N. H. 1968. Pathogenesis of myelin lesions in experimental cyanide encephalopathy. *Neurology* 18: 167–177.

Bate-Smith, E. C. 1965. Recent progress in the chemical taxonomy of some phenolic constituents of plants. Mem. Soc. Bot. France 1965: 16–27, Appendix 27–28.

Bate-Smith, E. C. 1968. Phenolic constituents of plants and their taxonomic significance. II. Monocotyledons. *J. Linnean Soc. Lond. Botany* 60: 325–326.

Bauer, A. R., Jr. et al. 1977. The effects of prolonged coffee intake on genetically identical mice. *Life Sci.* 21: 63–70.

Beare, J. L., Murray, T. K. and Campbell, J. A. 1957. Effects of varying proportions of dietary rapeseed oil on the rat. *Can. J. Biochem. Physiol.* 35: 1225–1231.

Beare, J. L., Murray, T. K., Grice, H. C. and Campbell, J. A. 1959. A comparison of the utilization of rapeseed oil and corn oil by the rat. *Can. J. Biochem. Physiol.* 37: 613–621.

Beare, J. L., Gregory, E. R. W., Smith, D. M. and Campbell, J. A. 1961. The effect of rapeseed oil on reproduction and on the composition of rat milk fat. *Can. J. Biochem. Physiol.* 39: 195–201.

Beare, J. J., Campbell, J. A., Youngs, C. G. and Craig, B. M. 1963. Effects of saturated fat in rats fed rapeseed oil. *Can. J. Biochem. Biophysiol.* 41: 605–612.

Beare-Rogers, J. L. 1970. Nutritional aspect of long-chain fatty acids. Proceedings of the International Conference on the Science, Technology and Marketing of Rapeseed and Rapeseed Products. Rapeseed Association of Canada, Winnipeg, Manitoba.

Beare-Rogers, J. L., Nera, E. A. and Heggtviet, H. A. 1971. Cardiac lipid changes in rats fed oils containing long-chain fatty acids. *Can Inst. Food Technol. J.* 4: 120—124.

Beier, R. C., Ivie, G. W., Oertli, E. H. and Holt, D. L. 1983. HPLC analysis of linear furocoumarins (psoralens) in healthy celery *(Apium graveolens). Food Chem. Toxicol.* 21: 163—165.

Bell, E. A. 1962. Associations of ninhydrin-reacting compounds in seeds of 49 species of *Lathyrus. Biochem. J.* 83: 225—229.

Bell, E. A. 1964. Relevance of biochemical taxonomy to the problem of lathyrism. *Nature* 203: 378—380.

Bell, E. A. 1973. Aminonitriles and amino acids not derived from proteins. In: *Toxicants Occurring Naturally in Foods.* 2nd ed. National Research Council. Committee on Food Protection, Washington, D.C.

Bell, E. A. and O'Donovan, J. P. 1966. The usolation of α- and γ-oxalyl derivatives of α,γ-diaminobutyric acid from seeds of *Lathyrus latifolius* and the detection of the α-oxalyl isomer of the neurotoxin α-amino-β-oxalylaminopropionic acid which occurs together with the neurotoxin in this and other species. *Phytochemistry* 5: 1211—1219.

Bellet, S., Kershbaum, A. and Aspe, J. 1965. The effect of caffeine on free fatty acids. A preliminary report. *Arch. Intern. Med.* 116: 750—752.

Belsey, M. A. 1970. *Favism in the Middle East. An Epidemiological Appraisal of the Problem in Relationship to Infant Nutrition and Public Health.* Final Report to the World Health Organization, Geneva.

Bendich, A. and Clements, G. C. 1952. A revision of the structural formulation of vicine and its pyrimidine aglucone, divicine. *Biochim Biophys. Acta* 12: 462—477.

Bennetts, H. W. and Underwood, E. J. 1951. The estrogenic effects of subterranean clover *(Trifolium subterraneum).* Uterine maintenance in the ovariectomized ewe on clover grazing. *Australian J. Exp. Biol. Med. Sci.* 29: 249—253.

Berardi, L. C. and Goldblatt, L. A. 1969. Gossypol. In: *Toxic Constituents of Plant Foodstuffs.* I. E. Liener (ed). Academic Press, New York.

Berardi, L. C. and Martinez, W. H. 1966. Gossypol source versus biological activity. Proceedings of the Conference on Inactivation of Gossypol with Mineral Salts. National Cottonseed Products Association, Memphis.

Berger, H. and Höller, H. 1957. Flavonoids. I. Spasmolytic material in *Glycyrrhiza glabra. Sci. Pharm.* 25: 172—175.

Berkowitz, B. A., Tarver, J. H. and Spector, S. 1970. Release of norepinephrine in the central nervous system by theophylline and caffeine. *Eur. J. Pharmacol.* 10: 64—71.

Bernhard, R. A. 1958. Occurrence of coumarin analogues in lemon juice. *Nature* 182: 1171.

Bernhard, R. A. 1968. Comparative distribution of volatile aliphatic disulfides derived from fresh and dehydrated onions. *J. Food Sci.* 33: 298—304.

Bertrand, M., Girod, J. and Rigaud, M. F. 1970. Electrodactyl induced by caffeine in rongeurs. The role of specific genetic factors. *C. R. Soc. Biol.* 164: 1488—1489. (French)

Beutler, E. 1970. L-Dopa and favism. *Blood* 36: 523—525.

Bevan, C. W. L. and Hirst, J. 1958. A convulsant alkaloid of *Dioscorea dumentorum. Chem. Ind.* 4: 103.

Bevenue, A., White, L. M., Secor, G. E. and Williams, K. T. 1961. The occurrence of two heptuloses in the fig plant. *J. Assoc. Off. Anal. Chem.* 44: 265—266.

Bickoff, E. M. et al. 1957. Coumestrol, a new estrogen isolated from forage crops. *Science* 126: 969–970.

Bickoff, E. M., Livingston, A. L., Hendrickson, A. P. and Booth, A. N. 1962. Relative potencies of several estrogen-like compounds found in forages. *J. Agric. Food Chem.* 10: 410–412.

Bien, S., Salemnik, G., Zamir, L. and Rosenblum, M. 1968. Structure of convicine. *J. Chem. Soc. C*: 496–499.

Biggers, J. D. And Curnow, D. H. 1954. Oestrogenic activity of subterranean clover. 1. The oestrogenic activity of genistein. *Biochem. J.* 58: 278–282.

Bissett, R. H. et al. 1969. Cyanogenesis in manioc. Concerning Lotaustralin. *Phytochemistry* 8: 2235–2247.

Bjeldanes, L. F. and Chang, G. W. 1977. Mutagenic activity of quercetin and related compounds. *Science* 197: 577–578.

Blackwell, B., Marley, E., Price, J. and Taylor, D. 1967. Hypertensive interactions between monoamine oxidase inhibitors and foodstuffs. *Br. J. Psychiatry* 113: 349–365.

Blauch, J. L. and Tarka, S. M., Jr. 1983. HPLC determination of caffeine and theobromine in coffee, tea and instant hot cocoa mixes. *J. Food Sci.* 48: 745–747.

Blum, H. F. 1938. Domestic animal diseases produced by light. *J. Am. Vet. Med. Assoc.* 93: 185–191.

Blum, H. F. 1941. *Photodynamic Action and Diseases Caused by Light*. American Chemical Society Monograph Series. Reinhold, New York.

Blum, B., Stern, M. H. and Melville, K. I. 1964. A comparative evaluation of the action of depressant and stimulant drugs on human performance. *Psychopharmacologia* 6: 173–177.

Boddie, G. F. 1947. Toxicological problems in veterinary practice. *Vet Rec.* 59: 471–478.

Boelens, M., deValois, P. J., Wobben, H. J. and van der Gen, A. 1971. Volatile flavor compounds from onion. *J. Agric. Food Chem.* 19: 984–991.

Boer, J., Jansen, B. C. P. and Kentie, A. 1947. On the growth-promoting factor for rats present in summer butter. *J. Nutr.* 33: 339–360.

Bogovski, P. and Day, N. 1977. Accelerating action of tea on mouse skin carcinogenesis. *Cancer Lett.* 3: 9–13.

Bokuchava, M. A. 1962. Chemical and physical properties and biological action of tea tannin. In: *Seminar on Vegetable Tannins*. S. Rajadurai and K. U. Bhanu (eds.). Central Leather Research Institute, Madras, India.

Bömer, A. and Mattis, H. 1924. The solanine content of potatoes. *Z. Nahr. Genussm.* 47: 97–127.

Bonati, M. et al. 1982. Caffeine disposition after oral doses. *Clin. Pharmacol. Ther.* 32: 98.

Bonnet, G. F. and Lepreux, P. 1971. The tyramine migraine headache. *Semin. Hosp. Paris* 47: 2441–2445. (French)

Bonsignori, A., Fornaini, G., Segni, G. and Seitun, A. 1961. Transketolase and transaldolase reactions in the erythrocytes of human subjects with favism history. *Biochem. Biophys. Res. Commun.* 4: 147–150.

Borchert, P., Miller, J. A., Miller, E. C. and Shires, T. K. 1973. 1'-Hydroxysafrole, a proximate carcinogenic metabolite of safrole in the rat and mouse. *Cancer Res.* 33: 590–600.

Borneff, J., Selenka, F., Kunte, H. and Maximas, A. 1968. Experimental studies on the formation of polycyclic aromatic hydrocarbons in plants. *Environ. Res.* 2: 22–29.

Boston Collaborative Drug Surveillance Program. 1972. Report. Coffee drinking and acute myocardial infarction. *Lancet* 2: 1278–1281.

Boulenger, J.-P. et al. 1983. Chronic caffeine consumption increases the number of brain adenosine receptors. *Life Sci.* 32: 1135.

Boulos, N. N. 1975. Hydrogen cyanide content of cassava root. *Sudan. J. Food Sci. Technol.* 7: 94–96. (English summary)

Bowman, J. E. and Walker, D. G. 1961. Action of *Vicia faba* on erythrocytes: Possible relationship to favism. *Nature* 189: 555–556.

Boyd, E. M. 1959. The acute oral toxicity of caffeine. *Toxicol. Appl. Pharmacol.* 1: 250–257.

Boyd, E. M. 1973. The toxicity of food adjuvants. In: *Toxicity of Pure Foods.* C. E. Boyd (ed.). CRC Press, Cleveland, Ohio.

Boyd, E. M., Dolman, M., Knight, L. M. and Shepard, E. P. 1965. The chronic oral toxicity of caffein. *Can. J. Physiol. Pharmacol.* 43: 995–1007.

Bradbury, R. B. and White, D. E. 1951. Chemistry of subterranean clover. I. Isolation of formononetin and genistein. *J. Chem. Soc.* 1951: 3447–3449.

Bradbury, R. B. and White, D. E. 1954. Estrogens and related substances in plants. In: *Vitamins and Hormones.* Vol. XII. R. S. Harris, G. F. Marrian and K. V. Thimann (eds.). Academic Press, New York.

Braham, J. E., et al. 1967. Effect of gossypol on the iron-binding capacity of serum in swine. *J. Nutr.* 93: 241–248.

Bressani, R., Elias, L. G., Jarquin, R. and Braham, J. E. 1964. All-vegetable protein mixtures for human feeding. XIII. Effect of cooking mixtures containing cottonseed flour on free gossypol content. *Food Technol.* 18: 1599–1603.

Brieskorn, C. H. and Wenger, E. 1960. Constituents of *Salvia officinalis.* XI. The analysis of ethereal sage oil by means of gas and thin-bedded chromatography. *Arch. Pharm.* 293: 21–26.

Brockmann, H. 1957. Centenary lecture — Photodynamically active plant pigments. *Proc. Chem. Soc.* p. 304–312.

Brockmann, H. and Kluge, F. 1951. The synthesis of hypericin. *Naturwissenschaften* 38: 141.

Brockmann, H., Pohl, F., Maier, K. and Haschad, M. N. 1942. On hypericin, the photodynamic substances of St. John's bread *(Hypericum perforatum).* *Ann. Chem.* 553: 1–52.

Brockmann, H., Kluge, F. and Muxfeldt, H. 1957. Total synthesis of hypericin. *Chem. Ber.* 90: 2302–2318.

Brodnitz, M. H. and Pascale, J. V. 1971. Thiopropanol S-oxide: A lachrymatory factor in onions. *J. Agric. Food Chem.* 19: 269–272.

Brodnitz, M. H. and Pollock, C. L. 1970. Gas chromatographic analysis of distilled onion oil. *Food Technol.* 24: 78–80.

Brodnitz, M. H., Pollock, C. L. and Vallon, P. P. 1969. Flavor components of onion oil. *J. Agric. Food Chem.* 17: 760–763.

Brown, D. and Keeler, R. 1978. Structure-activity relation of steroid teratogens. 3. Solanidan epimers. *J. Agric. Food Chem.* 26: 566–569.

Bruce, D. W. 1961. Carcinoid tumours and pineapples. *J. Pharm. Pharmacol.* 3: 256.

Bruns, R. F., Daly, J. W. and Snyder, S. H. 1980. Adenosine receptors in brain membranes: Binding of N[6]cyclohexyl (^{3}H) adenosine and 1,3-diethyl-8-(^{3}H) phenylxanthine. *Proc. Nat. Acad. Sci.* 77: 5547.

Buhl, S. N. and Regan, J. D. 1974. Effect of caffeine on postreplication repair in human cells. *Biophys. J.* 14: 519–527.

Buitrago, J. A., Clawson, A. J. and Smith, F. H. 1970. Effects of dietary iron on gossypol accumulation in and elimination from porcine liver. *J. Anim. Sci.* 31: 554–558.

Bunker, M. L. and McWilliams, M. 1979. Caffein content of common beverages. *J. Am. Diet. Assoc.* 74(1): 28–32.

Burg, A. W. and Werner, E. 1972. Tissue distribution of caffeine and its metabolites in the mouse. *Biochem. Pharmacol.* 21: 923–936.

Burger, P. M. and Simons, J. W. I. M. 1979. Mutagenicity of 8-methoxypsoralen and long-wave ultraviolet irradiation in diploid human skin fibroblast. An improved risk estimate in photochemotherapy. *Mutat. Res.* 63: 371–380.

Burks, J. W., Jr. 1954. Classic aspects of onion and garlic dermatitis in housewives. *Ann. Allergy* 12: 592–596.

Burn, J. H. and Rand, M. J. 1958. The action of sympathomimetic amines in animals treated with reserpine. *J. Physiol.* 144: 314–316.

Burrell, R. J. W. 1962. Esophageal cancer among Bantu in the Transkei. *J. Natl. Cancer Inst.* 28: 495–514.

Burrell, R. J. W., Roach, W. A. and Shadwell, A. 1966. Esophagael cancer in the Bantu of the Transkei associated with mineral deficiency in garden plants. *J. Natl. Cancer Inst.* 36: 201–209.

Butenandt, A. and Jacobi, H. 1933. The female sexual hormone. X. The preparation of a crystalline plant tokokinin (thelykinin) and its identification with the α-follicular hormone. *Z. Physiol. Chem.* 218: 104–112.

Buttery, R. G. et al. 1968. Characterization of some volatile constituents of carrots. *J. Agric. Food Chem.* 16: 1009–1015.

Byam, W. and Archibald, R. G. 1921–1923. *The Practice of Medicine in the Tropics.* Oxford Medical Publications, Henry Frowde and Hodder & Stroughton, London.

Bydagyan, F. E., Vladimirov, B. D., Levitskii, L. M. and Shchurov, K. A. 1947. Influences of prolonged consumption of small amounts of cottonseed meal on the human organism. *Gig. Sanit.* 7: 28–33.

Cameron, K. 1952. Death camas poisoning. *N.W. Med.* 51: 682–683.

Campbell, L. D. and Marquardt, R. R. 1977. Performance of broiler chicks fed diets of varying energy density and containing varied levels of raw or heat-treated faba beans. *Poultry Sci.* 56: 442–448.

Carson, J. F. and Wong, F. F. 1961. Isolation of (+)S-methyl-L-cysteine sulfoxide derivatives. *J. Org. Chem.* 26: 4997–5000.

Carson, P. E., Flanagan, C. L., Ickes, C. E. and Alving, A. S. 1956. Enzymatic deficiency in primaquine-sensitive erythrocytes. *Science* 124: 484–485.

Carson, J. F., Lundin, R. E. and Lukes, T. M. 1966. The configuration of (+)-S-(1-propenyl)-L-cysteine S-oxide from *Allium cepa. J. Org. Chem.* 31: 1634–1635.

Cater, D. B. 1961. The carcinogenic action of carrageenin in rats. *Br. J. Cancer* 15: 607–614.

Cater, C. M. and Lyman, C. M. 1969. Reaction of gossypol with amino acids and other amino compounds. *J. Am. Oil Chem. Soc.* 46: 649–653.

Cater, C. M. and Lyman, C. M. 1970. Effect of bound gossypol in cottonseed meal on enzymic degradation. *Lipids* 5: 765–769.

Cavallito, C. J. and Bailey, J. H. 1944. Allicin, the antibacterial principal of *Allium sativum.* I. Isolation, physical properties and antibacterial action. *J. Am. Chem. Soc.* 66: 1950–1951.

Chahine, R. A. et al. 1975. The incidence and clinical implications of coronary artery spasm. *Circulation* 52: 972–978.

Challis, B. C. and Bartlett, C. D. 1975. Possible cocarcinogenic effects of coffee constituents. *Nature* 254: 532–533.

Chamberlain, T. J. 1970. Licorice poisoning, pseudoaldosteronism, and heart failure. *J.A.M.A.* 213: 1343.

Chang, W. Y. 1955. "The Chemical Characteristics of Cottonseed Meal as Related to the Biological Utilization." M.S. Thesis, Texas A & M University, College Station, Texas.

Charavanapavan, C. 1944. Studies in casava and lima beans with special reference to their utilization as harmless food. *Trop. Agric.* 100: 164–168.

Chatterjee, R. 1952. Indian podophyllum. *Econ. Bot.* 6: 342–354.

Chavan, J. K., Kadam, S. S., Ghonsikari, C. P. and Salunkhe, D. K. 1979. Removal of tannins and improvement of in vitro protein digestibility of sorghum seeds by soaking in alkali. *J. Food Sci.* 44: 1319–1321.

Chaytor, J. P., Crathorne, B. and Saxby, M. J. 1975. The identification and significance of 2-phenylethylamine in foods. *J. Sci. Food Agric.* 26: 539–598.

Cheema, P. S., Padmanaban, G. and Sarma, P. S. 1969. Neurotoxic action of β-N-oxalyl-L- α, β-diaminopropionic acid in acidotic adult rats. *Indian J. Biochem.* 6: 146–147.

Cheema, P. S., Padmanaban, G. and Sarma, P. S. 1970. Biochemical characterization of β-N-oxalyl-L- α,β-diaminoproprionic acid, the *Lathyrus sativus* neurotoxin as an excitant amino acid. *J. Neurochem.* 17: 1293–1298.

Chen, K. K., Rose, C. L. and Clowes, G. H. A. 1934. Comparative values of several antidotes in cyanide poisoning. *Am. J. Med. Sci.* 188: 767–781.

Cheney, R. H. 1935. Comparative effect of caffeine per se and a caffeine beverage (coffee) upon the reaction time in normal young adults. *J. Pharmacol. Exp. Ther.* 53: 304–313.

Cheng, E. et al. 1953. Estrogenic activity of isoflavone derivatives extracted and prepared from soybean oil meal. *Science* 118: 164–165.

Cheng, E. W., Yoder, L., Story, C. D. and Burroughs, W. 1955. Estrogenic activity of some naturally occurring isoflavones. *Ann. N.Y. Acad Sci.* 61: 652–659.

Cheng, T. O., Bashour, T., Singh, B. K. and Kelser, G. A. 1972. Myocardial infarction in the absence of coronary arteriosclerosis. Result of coronary spasm(?) *Am. J. Cardiol.* 30: 680–682.

Chudapongse, P. and Janthasoot, W. 1976. Studies on the effect of capsaicin on metabolic reactions of isolated rat liver mitochondria. *Toxicol. Appl. Pharmacol.* 37: 263–270.

Chvasta, T. E. and Cooke, A. R. 1971. Emptying and absorption of caffeine from the human stomach. *Gastroenterology* 61: 838–843.

Clapp, R. C., Bissett, F. H., Coburn, R. A. and Long, L., Jr. 1966. Cyanogenesis in manioc: Linamarin and isolinamarin. *Phytochemistry* 5: 1323–1326.

Clare, N. T. 1955. Photosensitization in animals. *Adv. Vet. Sci.* 2: 182–211.

Clark, A. 1936. Report on effects of certain poisons contained in food plants of West Africa upon health of native races. *J. Trop. Med. Hyg.* 39: 269–276.

Clarke, G. C. 1970. The forensic chemistry of alkaloids. In: *The Alkaloids.* Vol. XIII. R. H. F. Manske (ed.). Academic Press, New York.

Clawson, A. J., Smith, F. H., Osborne, L. C. and Barrick, E. R. 1961. Effect of protein source, autoclaving, and lysine supplementation on gossypol toxicity. *J. Anim. Sci.* 20: 547–552.

Cleaver, J. E. and Thomas, G. H. 1969. single strand interruptions in DNA and the effect of caffeine in Chinese hamster cells irradiated with ultraviolet light. *Biochem. Biophys. Res. Commun.* 36: 203–208.

Cleland, J. B. 1931. Plants, including fungi, poisonous or otherwise injurious to man in Australia. *Med. J. Aust.* 2: 775–778.

Cohen, S. and Booth, G. H., Jr. 1975. Gastric acid secretion and lower esophageal-sphincter pressure in response to coffee and caffeine. *N. Engl. J. Med.* 293: 897–899.

Cole, P. 1971. Coffee-drinking and cancer of the lower urinary tract. *Lancet* 1: 1335–1337.

Collens, A. E. 1915. Bitter and sweet casava — Hydrocyanic acid contents. *Bull. Dept. Agric. Trinidad Tobago* 14: 54.

Collins, T. F. X., Welsh, J. J., Black, T. N. and Collins, E. V. 1981. Caffeine teratogenic potential in rats. *Reg. Toxicol. Pharmacol.* 1: 355.

Collip, J. B. 1923a. Glucokinin. *J. Biol. Chem.* 57: 65–78.

Collip, J. B. 1923c. Glucokinin. A new hormone present in plant tissue. Preliminary paper. *J. Biol. Chem.* 56: 513–531.

Collip, J. B. 1923-1924b. Glucokinin. An apparent synthesis in the normal animal of a hypoglycemia-producing principle. Animal passage of the principle. *J. Biol. Chem.* 58: 163—208.

Concha, J. A. and Wungwira, L. 1964. Essential oil of *Illicium anisatum. J. Philippine Pharm. Assoc.* 50: 361—363.

Concon, J. M. 1979. Alkaloids. In: *Encyclopedia of Food Science.* Martin S. Peterson and Arnold H. Johnson (eds.). AVI, Westport, Connecticut.

Concon, J. M., Swerczek, T. W. and Newburg, D. S. 1979. Black pepper *(Piper nigrum)*: Evidence of carcinogenicity. *Nutr. Cancer* 1: 22—26.

Concon, J. M., Swerczek, T. W. and Newburg, D. S. 1981. Potential carcinogenicity of black pepper *(Piper nigrum).* In: *Antinutrients and Natural Toxicants in Foods.* R. L. Ory (ed.). Food & Nutrition Press, Westport, Connecticut.

Conkerton, E. J. and Frampton, V. L. 1959. Reactions of gossypol with free *epsilon*-amino groups of lysine of protein. *Arch. Biochem. Biophys.* 81: 130—134.

Conn. E. E. 1969. Cyanogenic glycosides. *J. Agric. Food Chem.* 17: 519—526.

Conn, E. E. 1973. Cyanogenetic glycosides. In: *Toxicants Occurring Naturally in Foods.* 2nd ed. National Academy of Sciences, Washington, D.C.

Conn, E. E. 1977. Biosynthesis of cyanogenic glycosides. *Naturwissenschaften* 66: 28—34.

Conn, J. W., Rovner, D. R. and Cohen, E. L. 1968. Licorice-induced pseudoaldosteronism. Hypertension, hypokalemia, aldosteronopenia, and suppressed plasma renin activity. *J.A.M.A.* 205: 492—496.

Cook, J. W., Duffy, E. and Schoental, R. 1950. Primary liver tumours in rats following feeding with alkaloids of *Senecio jacobaea. Br. J. Cancer* 4: 405—410.

Cooper, J. M. 1941. Isolation of a toxic principle from the seeds of *Macrozamia spiralis. Proc. R. Soc. New South Wales* 74: 450—454.

Coore, H. G. et al. 1963. Block of insulin secretion from the pancreas by D-mannoheptulose. *Nature* 197: 1264—1266.

Corkill, N. L. 1948. The poisonous wild cluster yam, *Dioscorea dumetorum* Pax. as a famine food in Anglo-Egyptian Sudan. *Ann. Trop. Med. Parasitol.* 42: 278—287.

Craig, B. M., Youngs, C. G., Beare, J. L. and Campbell, J. A. 1963. Influence of selective and non-selective hydrogenation of rapeseed oil on carcass fat of rats. *Can. J. Biochem. Physiol.* 41: 51—56.

Crawford, M. A. 1962. Excretion of 5-hydroxyindolyacetic acid in East Africans. *Lancet* 1: 352—353.

Cronk, T. C., Kuhn, G. D. and McArdle, F. J. 1974. The influence of stage of maturity, level of nitrogen fertilization and storage on the concentration of solanine in tubers of three potato cultivars. *Bull. Environ. Contam. Toxicol.* 11: 163—168.

Crosby, W. H. 1956. Favism in Sardinia. *Blood* 11: 91—92.

Crosby, D. G. 1969. Natural toxic background in the food of man and his animals. *J. Agric. Food Chem.* 17: 532—538.

Crosby, D. G. and Aharonson, N. 1967. Structure of carotatoxin, a natural toxicant from carrot. *Tetrahedron* 25: 465—472.

Cugudda, E., Gigli, C. and Massenti, S. 1953. Pathogenesis of favus. Hemoagglutination and hemolytic activity of some chemical constituents. *Minerva Med.* 44: I, 140—147.

Curtis, D. R. and Watson, J. C. 1965. The pharmacology of amino acids related to γ-aminobutyric acid. *Pharmacol. Rev.* 17: 347—391.

Cutillo, S., Costa, S., Vintuleddu, M. C. and Meloni, T. 1976. Salicylamide-glucuronide formation in children with favism and in their parents. *Acta Haematol. (Basel)* 55: 296—299. (Italian)

Czok, G. 1976. Metabolic effects of coffee and caffeine. *Z. Ernahrungswiss.* 15: 109—121. (German)

Czok, G., Schmidt, B. and Lang, K. 1969. Comparative experimental animal research with coffee and tea. *Z. Ernahrungswiss.* 9: 103–108. (German)

Dallacker, F. 1969. Derivatives of methylendioxybenzenes. 27. Synthesis of dimethoxymethylen-dioxy-allylbenzene. *Chem. Ber.* 102: 2663–2676. (German)

Daly, J. W., Bruns, R. F. and Snyder, S. H. 1981. Adenosine receptors in the central nervous system: Relationship to the central actions of methylxanthines. *Life Sci.* 28: 2083.

Daly, J. W., Butts-Lamb, P. and Padgett, W. 1983. Subclasses of adenosine receptors in the central nervous: Interaction with caffeine and related methylxanthines. *Cell. Mol. Neurobiol.* 3(1): 69–80.

Dasler, W. 1954. Isolation of toxic crystals from sweet peas *(Lathyrus odoratus).* *Science* 120: 307–308.

Datta, S. C., Murti, V. V. S. and Seshadri, T. R. 1968. A new component of the flowers of *Thespesia populnea*: (+)-Gossypol. *Curr. Sci.* 37: 135.

Dawson, C. R. 1954. The toxic principle of poison ivy and related plants. *Rec. Chem. Prog.* 15: 39–53.

Dawson, C. R. 1956. The chemistry of poison ivy. *Trans. N.Y. Acad. Sci.* (Ser. II) 89: 427–450.

Deacon, W. and Marsh, H. V., Jr. 1971. Properties of an enzyme from bananas *(Musa sapientum)* which hydroxylates tyramine to dopamine. *Phytochemistry* 10: 2915–2924.

Dean, F. M. 1950. Naturally occurring coumarines. *Fortschr. Chem. Org. Naturst.* 9: 225–291.

Decossas, K. M., Molaison, L. J., Kleppinger, A. de B. and Laporte, V. L. 1968. Cottonseed oil and meal utilization. *J. Am. Oil. Chem. Soc.* 45: 52A–85A.

De Eds, F. 1968. Flavonoid metabolism. In: *Comprehensive Biochemistry.* M. Florkin and E. H. Stotz (eds.). Elsevier, Amsterdam.

Degazon, D. W. 1956. Tropical amblyopia in Jamaica. *West Indian Med. J.* 5: 223–230.

Delange, F. M. and Ermans, A. M. 1979. Endemic goiter and cretinism. Naturally occurring goitrogens. In: *International Encyclopedia of Pharmacology and Therapeutics.* J. M. Hershman and G. A. Bray (eds.). Pergamon Press, Oxford, England.

Der Marderosian, A. and Roia, F. C., Jr. 1979. Literature review and clinical management of household ornamental plants potentially toxic to humans. In: *Toxic Plants.* A. D. Kinghorn (ed). Columbia University Press, New York.

Descartes de Garcia Paula, R. and Rangel, J. L. 1939. HCN or the poison of bitter or sweet manioc *(Manihot* spp). *Rev. Alimentar. (Rio de Janeiro)* 3(29): 215–217.

Deuel, H. J., Jr. 1955. The digestion and absorption of fats in the gastrointestinal tract. In: *Lipids.* Vol. II. Interscience, New York.

Deyoe, C. W., Deacon, L. E. and Couch, J. R. 1962. Citrus bioflavonoids in broiler diets. *Poult. Sci.* 41: 1088–1090.

Dickens, F. and Jones, H. E. H. 1963. The carcinogenic action of aflatoxin after its subcutaneous injection in the rat. *Br. J. Cancer* 17: 691–698.

Dickens, F. and Jones, H. E. H. 1965. Further studies on the carcinogenic action of certain lactones and related substances in the rat and mouse. *Br. J. Cancer* 19: 392–403.

Dieckert, J. W. and Abou-Donia, M. B. 1972. Metabolism of gossypol in mammals. In: *Swine Research.* Texas A & M University, College Station, Texas.

Diedrich, D. F. 1968. Is phloretin the sugar transport inhibitor in intestine? *Arch. Biochem. Biophys.* 127: 803–812.

DiGiacomo, A. 1966. Citrus essential oils. *Riechst. Aromen Koerperpflegem.* 16: 348–366. (German)

Dilleman, G. 1958. Cyanogenic compounds. In: *Handbook of Plant Physiology.* Vol. VIII. W. Ruhland (ed.). Springer, Eerlin. (French)

Dobmeyer, D. J. et al. 1983. The arrhythmogenic effects of caffeine in human beings. *N. Engl. J. Med.* 308: 814–815.

Dodsworth, M. R. 1945. Some considerations on sassafras oil. *Biol. Divulgacão Inst. Oleos* 3: 21–30.

Domon, M., Barton, B., Porte, A. and Rauth, A. M. 1970. The interaction of caffeine with ultraviolet-light-irradiated DNA. *Int. J. Radiat. Biol.* 17: 395–399.

Donoso, G., Hedayat, H. and Khayatian, H. 1969. Favism, with special reference to Iran. *Bull. W.H.O.* 40: 513–519.

Dorrell, D. G. 1976. Chlorogenic acid content of meal from cultivated and wild sunflowers. *Crop. Sci.* 16: 422–424.

Downing, J. G. and Gurney, S. W. 1940. Dermatitis from cashew nut shell oil. *J. Indust. Hyg. Toxicol.* 22: 169–174.

Drake, M. E. and Stuhr, E. T. 1935. Some pharmacological and bactericidal properties of umbellulone. *J. Am. Pharm. Assoc. Sci. Ed.* 24: 196–207.

Drane, H., Patterson, D. S. P., Roberts, B. A. and Saba, N. 1975. The chance discovery of oestrogenic activity in laboratory rat cake. *Food Cosmet. Toxicol.* 13: 491–492.

Drinkwater, N. R., Miller, E. C., Miller, J. A. and Pitot, H. C. 1976. Hepatocarcinogenicity of estragole (1-allyl-4-methoxybenzene) and 1'-hydroxyestragole in the mouse and mutagenicity of 1'-acetoxyestragole in bacteria. *J. Natl. Cancer Inst.* 57: 1323–1331.

Du, S. D. 1952. Favism in West China. *Chinese Med. J.* 70: 17–26.

Du Plessis, L. S., Nunn, J. R. and Roach, W. A. 1969. Carcinogen in a Transkeian Bantu food additive. *Nature* 222: 1198–1199.

DuPuy, H. P. and Lee, J. G. 1954. The isolation of a material capable of producing experimental lathyrism. *J. Am. Pharm. Assoc. Sci. Ed.* 43: 61–62.

Durkee, A. B. and Poapst, P. A. 1965. Phenolic constituents in core tissues and ripe seed of McIntosh apples. *J. Agric. Food Chem.* 13: 137–139.

Eagle, E. 1960. A review of some physiological effects of gossypol and cottonseed pigment glands. *J. Am. Oil Chem. Soc.* 37: 40–43.

Eagle, E., Castillon, L. E., Hall, C. M. and Boatner, C. H. 1948. Acute oral toxicity of gossypol and cottonseed pigment glands for rats, mice, rabbits, and guinea pigs. *Arch. Biochem. Biophys.* 18: 271–277.

Eckey, E. W. 1954. Rhoeadales. In: *Vegetable Fats and Oils.* Reinhold, New York.

Ekpechi, O. L., Dimitriadou, A. and Fraser, R. 1966. Goitrogenic activity of cassava (a staple Nigerian food). *Nature* 210: 1137–1138.

El Ansari, M. A., Reddy, K. K., Sastry, K. N. S. and Nayudamma, Y. 1971. Polyphenols of *Mangifera indica*. *Phytochemistry* 10: 2239–2241.

El-Nockrashy, A. S., Lyman, C. M. and Dollahite, J. W. 1963. The acute oral toxicity of cottonseed pigment glands and intraglandular pigments. *J. Am. Oil chem. Soc.* 40: 14–17.

El Sissi, H. I., Ishak, M. S., Abd El Wahid, M. S. and El Ansari, M. A. 1971. Gallotannins of *Rhus coriaria* and *Mangifera indica*. *Planta Med.* 19: 342–351.

Emerson, G. A. 1933. The laxative principle in prunes. *Proc. Soc. Exp. Biol. Med.* 31: 278–281.

Emmens, C. W. 1950. *Hormone Assay.* Academic Press, New York.

Engfeldt, B. (ed.). 1975. *Morphological and Biochemical Effects of Orally Administered Rapeseed Oil on Rat Myocardium.* Acta Medica Scandinavica, Suppl. 585, Stockholm, Sweden.

Epstein, S. M., Bartus, B. and Farber, E. 1969. Renal epithelial neoplasms induced in male Wistar rats by oral aflatoxin B_1. *Cancer Res.* 29: 1045–1050.

Epstein, S. S., Bass, W., Arnold, E. and Bishop, Y. 1970. The failure of caffeine to induce mutagenic effects or to synergize the effects of known mutagens in mice. *Food Cosmet. Toxicol.* 8: 381–401.

Ermans, A. M. 1979. New data on the pathogeny of endemic goiter: Role of certain goitrogenic foodstuffs. *Bull. Mem. Acad. R. Med. Belg.* 134: 137–153. (French)

Ermans, A. M. et al. (ed.). 1980. *Role of Cassava in the Etiology of Endemic Goiter and Cretinism.* International Development Research Center, Ottawa, Canada.

Estler, C. J. 1965. Metabolic changes of the brain in nonfatal KCN poisoning and its modification by cyanide antagonists. *Arch. Exp. Pathol.* 25: 413–432. (German)

Evans, I. A. 1968. The radio-mimetic nature of bracken toxin. *Cancer Res.* 28: 2252–2261.

Evans, I. A. 1972. Bracken fern toxin. Onocology 1970. Proc. 10th Int. Cancer Congress V: 178–195.

Evans, I. A. 1976. The bracken carcinogen. In: *Chemical Carcinogens.* C. E. Searle (ed.). American Chemical Society, Washington, D.C.

Evans, I. A. and Mason, J. 1965. Carcinogenic activity of bracken. *Nature* 208: 913–914.

Evans, I. A. and Osman, M. A. 1974. Carcinogenicity of bracken and shikimic acid. *Nature* 250: 348–349.

Evans, I. A. and Widdop, B. 1966. *Carcinogenic Activity of Bracken.* British Empire Cancer Campaign for Research Annual Report, London.

Evans, E. T. R., Evans, W. C. and Roberts, H. E. 1951. Studies on bracken *(Pteris aquilina)* poisoning in the horse. *Br. Vet J.* 107: 364–371; 399–411.

Evans, W. C., Evans, E. T. R. and Hughes, L. E. 1954a. Studies on bracken poisoning in cattle, Part 1. *Br. Vet J.* 110: 295–306.

Evans, W. C., Evans, E. T. R. and Hughes, L. E. 1954b. Studies on bracken poisoning in cattle, Part II. 1950 bracken poisoning experiments. *Br. Vet. J.* 110: 365–380.

Evans, W. C., Evans, E. T. R. and Hughes, L. E. 1954c. Studies on bracken poisoning in cattle, Part III. Field outbreaks of bovine bracken poisoning. *Br. Vet. J.* 110: 426–442.

Evans, R. J., Bandemer, S. L., Anderson, M. and Davidson, J. A. 1962. Fatty acid distribution in tissues from hens fed cottonseed oil or *Sterculia foetida* seeds. *J. Nutr.* 76: 314–319.

Evans, R. J., Davidson, J. A., LaRue, J. N. and Bandemer, S. L. 1963. Interference in fatty acid metabolism of laying hens caused by cottonseed oil feeding. *Poult. Sci.* 42: 875–881.

Evans, I. A., Widdop, B. and Barber, G. D. 1967. *Carcinogenic Activity of Bracken.* British Empire Cancer Campaign for Research Annual Report, London.

Evans, I. A., Barber, G. D., Jones, R. S. and Leach, H. 1969. *Carcinogenic Activity of Bracken.* British Empire Cancer Campaign for Research Annual Report, London.

Eyjolfsson, R. 1970. Recent advances in the chemistry of cyanogenic glycosides. *Fortsch. Chem. Org. Naturst.* 28: 74–108.

Ferguson, L. J. and Watts, J. McK. 1980. Simultaneous cancer of the pancreas occurring in husband and wife. *Gut* 21: 537–540.

Ferguson, T. M., Couch, J. R. and Rigdon, R. H. 1959. Histopathology of animal reactions to pigment compounds — chickens. In: *Proceedings of the Conference on Chemical Structure and Reactions of Gossypol and Nongossypol Pigments of Cottonseed.* National Cottonseed Products Association, Memphis, Tennessee.

Feuer, G., Golberg, L. and Gibson, K. I. 1966. Liver response tests. VII. Coumarin metabolism in relation to the inhibition of rat-liver glucose-6-phosphatase. *Food Cosmet. Toxicol.* 4: 157–167.

Fiedler, H. and Wood, J. L. 1956. Specificity studies on the β-mercaptopyruvate-cyanide transsulfuration system. *J. Biol. Chem.* 222: 387–397.

Field, W. E. H. and Roe, F. J. C. 1965. Tumor promotion in the forestomach epithelium of mice by oral administration of citrus oils. *J. Natl. Cancer Inst.* 35: 771—787.

Finlay, T. H., Dharmgrongartama, E. D. and Perlmann, G. E. 1973. Mechanism of the gossypol inactivation of pepsinogen. *J. Biol. Chem.* 248: 4827—4833.

Finnemore, H. 1910. Examination of a species of *Prunus*. *Pharm. J.* 85: 604—607.

Fitzhugh, O. G. and Nelson, A. A. 1948. Liver tumors in rats fed thiourea or thioacetamide. *Science* 108: 626—628.

Fitzpatrick, T. B., Hopkins, C. E., Blickenstaff, D. D. and Swift, S. 1955. Augmented pigmentation and other responses of normal human skin to solar radiation following oral adminstration of 8-methoxypsoralen. *J. Invest. Dermatol.* 25: 187—190.

Food Agricultural Organization. 1959. Report: *Legumes in Agriculture and Human Nutrition in Africa*. FAO Technical Meeting, Rome, Italy.

Food and Drug Administration. 1977. Substances prohibited from use in human food. S 189.130. Coumarin. In: *Food Drug Cosmetic Law Reports. Food for Human Use. Reorganization and Recodification*. 21 CFR Parts 100-197. Commerce Clearing House, Chicago.

Food and Drug Research Labs, Inc. 1973a. *Teratologic Evaluation of FDA 71-44 (Caffeine)*. National Technical Information Service Report, No. PB-221., January, 1973.

Food and Drug Research Labs, Inc., 1973b. *Teratologic Evaluation of FDA 71-44 (Caffeine)*. National Technical Information Service Report, No. PB-223, July 1973.

Forlot, P. 1980. Possible cancer hazard associated with 5-methoxypsoralen in suntan preparation. *Br. Med. J.* 280: 648.

Fowden, L. 1966. Isolation of γ-hydroxynorvaline from *Lathyrus odoratus* seed. *Nature* 209: 807—808.

Foy, J. M. and Parratt, J. R. 1960. A note on the presence of noradrenaline and 5-hydroxytryptamine in plantain *(Musa sapientum*, var. *paradisiaca)*. *J. Pharm. Pharmacol.* 12: 360—364.

Foy, J. M. and Parratt, J. R. 1961. 5-Hydroxytryptamine in pineapples. *J. Pharm. Pharmacol.* 13: 382—383.

Foy, J. M. and Parratt, J. R. 1962. Urinary excretion of 5-hydroxyindoleacetic acid in West Africans. *Lancet* 1: 942—943.

Freudenberg, K. and Weinges, K. 1961. Catechins and flavonoid compounds. In: *The Chemistry of Flavonoid Compounds*. T. A. Geissman (ed.). Macmillan, New York.

Fujii, T. and Nishimura, H. 1972. Adverse effects of prolonged administration of caffeine on rat fetus. *Toxicol. Appl. Pharmacol.* 22: 449—457.

Fujii, T., Sasaki, H. and Nishimura, H. 1969. Teratogenicity of caffeine in mice related to its mode of administration. *Jpn. J. Pharmacol.* 19: 134—138.

Fujiwara, Y. and Kondo, T. 1972. Caffeine-sensitive repair of ultraviolet light-damaged DNA of mouse L cells. *Biochem. Biophys. Res. Commun.* 47: 557-564.

Fuller, H. L., Potter, D. K. and Brown, A. R. 1966. The feeding value of grain sorghums in relation to their tannin content. *Ga. Agric. Exp. Sta. Bull.* No. 176.

Furia, T. E. and Bellanca, N. 1971. *Fenarolli's Handbook of Flavor Ingredients*. Chemical Rubber Company, Bleveland.

Gabel, W. and Kruger, W. 1920. The toxic action of Rangoon beans. *Muensch. Med. Wochschr.* 67: 214—215.

Gabridge, M. G., Denunzio, A. and Legator, M. S. 1969. Cycasin: Detection of associated mutagenic activity in vivo. *Science* 163: 689—691.

Galli, C., Spano, P. F. and Szyszka, K. 1975. Accumulation of caffeine and its
metabolites in rat fetal brain and liver. *Pharmacol. Res. Commun.* 7:
217–221.

Gallup, W. D. 1931. Concerning the use of cottonseed meal in the diet of the rat.
J. Biol. Chem. 91: 387–394.

Garcia, H. and Lijinsky, W. 1972. Tumorigenicity of five cyclic nitrosamines in MRC
rats. *Z. Krebsforsch.* 77: 257–261.

Garcia, H. and Lijinsky, W. 1973. Studies of the tumorigenic effect in feeding of
nitrosamino acids and of low doses of amines and nitrite to rats. *Z. Krebsforsch.*
79: 141–144.

Gardiner, M. R. and Nairn, M. E. 1969. Studies on the effect of cobalt and selenium in clover disease of ewes. *Aust. Vet. J.* 45: 215–222.

Geissman, T. H. and Hinreiner, E. 1952. Theories of the biogenesis of flavonoid
compounds. Part I and Part II. *Botan. Rev.* 18: 77–244.

Gellerman, J. L. and Schlenk, H. 1968. Methods for isolation and determination of
anacardic acids. *Anal. Chem.* 20: 739–743.

Gemmill, C. L. 1958. The xanthines. In: *Pharmacology in Medicine.* 2nd Ed. V. A.
Drill (ed). McGraw-Hill, New York.

Gershbein, L. L. 1977. Regeneration of rat liver in the presence of essential oils
and their metabolites. *Food Cosmet. Toxicol.* 15: 173–181.

Ghose, K., Coppen, A. and Carroll, D. 1977. Intravenous tyramine response in migraine before and during treatment with indoramin. *Br. Med. J.* L: 1191–1193.

Gillham, F. E. M. 1969. Cotton in a hungry world. *S. Afr. J. Sci.* 65: 173–179.

Gillman, A., Phillips, F. S. and Koelle, E. S. 1946. The renal clearance of thiosulfate with observations on its volume distribution. *Am. J. Physiol.* 146: 348–357.

Glaser, E. and Drobnik, R. 1939. Review of knowledge on the components of garlic.
Arch. Exp. Pathol. Pharmakol. 193: 1–9. (German)

Goldman, J. A. and Ovadia, J. 1969. The effect of coffee on glucose tolerance in
normal and prediabetic pregnant women. *Obstet. Gynecol.* 33: 214–218.

Goldman, I. M. et al. 1967. Research on aromas. XIV. Coffee aroma. 2. Pyrazines
and pyridine. *Helv. Chim. Acta* 50: 694–705. (French)

Goldsmith, W. W. 1909. Onion poisoning in cattle. *J. Comp. Pathol. Ther.* 22: 151.

Goldstein, N. 1968. The ubiquitous urushiols — contact dermatitis from mango,
poison ivy, and other "poison" plants. *Cutis* 4: 679–685.

Goodpasture, C. E. and Arrighi, F. E. 1976. Effects of food seasonings on the cell
cycle and chromosome morphology of mammalian cells in vitro with special reference to tumeric. *Food Cosmet. Toxicol.* 14: 9–14.

Gorter, S. 1911. Dioscorine. *Rec. Trav. Chim.* 30: 161–166.

Grab, D. J., Zedeck, M. S., Swislocki, N. I. and Sonenberg, M. 1973. In vitro
synthesis of RNA with aggregate enzyme, chromatin, and DNA from liver of
methylazoxymethanol acetate-treated rats. *Chem. Biol. Interact.* 6: 259–267.

Graboys, T. B. and Lown, B. 1983. Coffee, arrhythmias, and common sense.
N. Engl. J. Med. 308: 835-837.

Graf, W. and Diehl, H. 1966. Carcinogenic polycyclic aromatic hydrocarbons found
in natural amounts in vegetable materials. *Arch. Hyg. Bakteriol.* 150: 49–59.
(German)

Green, R. C. 1959. Nutmeg poisoning. *Va. Med. Monthly* 86: 586–590.

Greenblatt, M. and Lijinsky, W. 1972. Failure to induce tumors in Swiss mice after
concurrent administration of amino acids and sodium nitrite. *J. Natl. Cancer
Inst.* 48: 1389–1392.

Greer, M. A., Stott, A. K. and Milne, K. A. 1966. Effect of thiocyanate, perchlorate, and other anions on thyroidal iodine metabolism. *Endocrinology* 79:
237–247.

Griepentrog, F. 1973. Pathological-anatomical results on the effect of coumarin in
animal experiments. *Toxicology* 1: 93–102.

Griesbach, W. E., Kennedy, T. H. and Purves, H. D. 1945. Studies on experimental goitre. VI. Thyroid adenomata in rats on Brassica seed diet. *Br. J. Exp.*
Pathol. 26: 18–24.

Grimmer, G. and Hildebrandt, A. 1965. Content of polycyclic hydrocarbons in different vegetables. III. Hydrocarbons in the human surroundings. *Dtsch.*
Lebensm. Rundschau 61: 237–239. (German)

Grimmer, G. and Hildebrandt, A. 1967. Content of polycyclic hydrocarbons in crude
vegetable oils. *Chem. Ind.* 47: 2000–2002.

Grimmer, G. and Hildebrandt, A. 1968. Hydrocarbons in the human environment.
VI. Levels of polycyclic hydrocarbons in crude vegetable oils. *Arch. Hyg.*
Bakteriol. 152: 255–259. (German)

Gross, E. G. and Dexter, J. D., Roth, R. G. 1966. Hypokalemic myopathy with
myoglobinuria associated with licorice ingestion. *N. Engl. J. Med.* 274: 602–606.

Gross, M. A., Jones, W. I., Cook, E. L. and Boone, C. C. 1967. Carcinogenicity
of oil of calamus. *Proc. Am. Assoc. Cancer Res.* 8: 24.

Guenther, E. 1950. *The Essential Oils.* Vol. 4. Van Nostrand, New York.

Guignard, L. 1907. On the amount of hydrogen cyanide obtained from *Phaseolus*
lunatus cultivated under the Paris climate. *Bull. Sci. Pharmacol.* 14: 556–557.
(French)

Gull, D. D. 1961. "Chlorophyll and Solanine Changes in Tubers of *Solannum tuber-*
osum Induced by Fluorescent Light, and a Study of Solanine Toxicology by Bioassay Technique." Dissertation Abstr. 21: 2242–2243. Ph.D. Thesis, Cornell
University, Ithaca, New York.

Gull, D. D. and Isenburg, F. M. 1960. Chlorophyll and solanine content and distribution in four varieties of potato tubers. *Proc. Am. Soc. Hort. Sci.* 75:
545–556.

Haddad, R. K., Rabe, A. and Dumas, R. 1972. Comparison of effects of methyl-
azosymethanol acetate on brain development in different species. *Fed. Proc.,*
Fed Am. Soc. Exp. Biol. 31: 1520–1523.

Hagan, E. C. et al. 1965. Toxic properties of compounds related to safrols. *Toxicol.*
Appl. Pharmacol. 7: 18–24.

Hagan, E. C. et al. 1967. Food flavourings and compounds of related structure. II.
Subacute and chronic toxicity. *Food Cosmet. Toxicol.* 5: 141–157.

Haggerty, D. R. and Conway, J. A. 1936. Report of poisoning by *Cicuta maculata*
(water hemlock). *N. Y. State J. Med.* 36: 1511–1514.

Hakim, R. E., Griffin, A. C. and Knox, J. M. 1960. Erythema and tumor formation
in methoxysalen-treated mice exposed to fluorescent light. *Arch. Dermatol.* 82:
572–577.

Hale, F., Lyman, C. M. and Smith, N. A. 1958. Use of cottonseed meal in swine
rations. Bull. 898 Tex. Agric. Exp. Sta.

Halpern, B. N., Drudi-Barracco, C., and Bessirard, D. 1964. Exaltation of toxicity
of sympathomimetic amines by thyroxine. *Nature* 204: 387–388.

Hammonds, T. W. and Shone, G. G. 1966. The analysis of fats containing cyclopropenoid fatty acids. *Analyst* 91: 455–458.

Hanington, E. and Harper, A. M. 1968. The role of tyramine in the aetiology of migraine, and related studies on the cerebral and extracerebral circulations.
Headache 8: 87–97.

Hanington, E., Horn, M. and Wilkinson, M. 1970. Further observations on the effect
of tyramine. In: *Background to Migraine, 3rd Migraine Symposium.* J. N. Cum-
ings (ed). Springer, New York.

Hansen, A. A. 1925. Two fatal cases of potato poisoning. *Science* 61: 340–341.

Hansen, R. P. 1965a. 3, 7, 11, 15-Tetramethylhexadecanoic acid: Its occurrence in
sheep fat. *N. Z. J. Sci.* 8: 158–160.

Hansen, R. P. 1965b. Occurrence of 3, 7, 11, 15-tetramethylhexadecanoic acid in ox
perinephric fat. *Chem. Ind.* 7: 303–304.

Harada, T. and Saika, Y. 1956. Pharmaceutical studies of Japanese wild ginger. II. Paper chromatography of essential oils. *Pharm. Bull. (Japan)* 4: 223—224.

Harborne, J. B., Williams, C. G. and Greenham, J. 1974. Distribution of charged flavones and caffeylshikimic acid in Palmac. *Phytochemistry* 13: 1557—1559.

Hardigree, A. A. and Epler, J. L. 1978. Comparative mutagenesis of plant flavonoids in microbial systems. *Mutat. Res.* 58: 231—239.

Haring, D. G. 1952. The island of Amami Oshima in the northern Ryukyus. National Research Council, Pacific Sci. Bd., SIRI, Rept. 2, Mimeo.

Harms, W. S. and Holley, K. T. 1951. Hypoprothrombinemia induced by gossypol. *Proc. Soc. Exp. Biol. Med.* 77: 297—299.

Harper, G. A. and Smith, K. J. 1968. Status of cottonseed protein. *Econ. Bot.* 22: 63—72.

Harris, J. A., Magne, F. C. and Skau, E. L. 1964. Methods for the determination of cyclopropenoid fatty acids. IV. Application of the step-wise HBr titration method to the analysis of refined and crude cottonseed oils. *J. Am. Oil Chem. Soc.* 41: 309—311.

Harvey, S. C. 1975. Gastric antacids and digestants. In: *The Pharmacological Basis of Therapeutics*. 5th ed. L. S. Goodman and A. Gilman (eds). Macmillan, New York.

Harvill, E. K., Hartzell, A. and Arthur, J. M. 1943. Toxicity of piperine solutions to houseflies (*Musca domestica L.*). *Contrib. Boyce Thompson Inst.* 13: 87—91.

Haslam, E. 1966. *Chemistry of Vegetable Tannins*. Academic Press, London.

Hasselstrom, T. E., Hewitt, E. J., Konigebacher, K. S. and Ritter, J. J. 1957. Composition of volatile oil of black pepper. Piper nigrum. *J. Agric. Food. Chem.* 5: 53—55.

Hauptmann, H., Franca, J. and Bruck-Lacerda, L. 1943. Cafesterol. III. The supposed estrogenic activity of cafesterol. *J. Am. Chem. Soc.* 65: 993—994.

Hayreh, S. S. 1973. Coffee drinking and acute myocardial infarction. *Lancet* 1: 45.

Hazelton, L. W. et al. 1956. Toxicity of coumarin. *J. Pharmacol. Exp. Ther.* 118: 348—358.

Hearnshaw, H. et al. 1972. Endocrinological and histopathological aspects of the infertility in the ewe caused by oestrogenic clover. *J. Reprod. Fertil.* 28: 160—161.

Heaton, J. M., McCormick, A. J. A. and Freeman, A. G. 1958. Tobacco amblyopia: a clinical manifestation of vitamin B_{12} deficiency. *Lancet* 2: 286—290.

Hedler, L. and Marquardt, P. 1968. Occurrence of diethylnitrosamine in some samples of food. *Food Cosmet. Toxicol.* 6: 341—348.

Hegnauer, R. 1963. *Chemotaxonomy of Plants*. Vol. 1. Birkhausen, Basel.

Heikel, T. A. J. and Rimington, C. 1968. Inhibition of biliary secretion by icterogenin and related triperpenes. II. Effect of icterogenin, crude rehmannic acid, oleanolic acetate, and "mixed lippia acids" on mitochondria isolated from biliary fistula rabbits receiving the triterpenes. *Biochem. Pharmacol.* 17: 1091—1097.

Hennekens, C. H. et al. 1976. Coffee drinking and death due to coronary heart disease. *N. Engl. J. Med.* 294: 633—636.

Henry, T. A. 1949. *The Plant Alkaloids*. Blakiston, Philadelphia.

Hicks, S. P. 1950. Brain metabolism in vivo. I. The distribution of lesions caused by cyanide poisoning, insulin hypoglycemia, asphyxia in nitrogen and fluoroacetate poisoning in rats. *Arch. Pathol.* 49: 111—137.

Hilditch, T. P. and Williams, P. N. 1964. *The Chemical Constitution of Natural Fats*. 4th ed. Spottiswoode, Ballantyne, London.

Hill, F. W. and Totsuka, K. 1964. Studies on the metabolizable energy of cottonseed meals for chicks, with particular reference to the effect of gossypol. *Poult. Sci.* 43: 362—370.

Himwich, W. A. and Saunders, J. P. 1948. Enzymatic conversion of cyanide to thiocyanate. *Am. J. Physiol.* 153: 348—354.

Hirono, I. 1972. Carcinogenicity and neurotoxicity of cycasin with special reference to species difference. *Fed. Proc.* 31: 1493–1497.

Hirono, I., Lacquer, G. L. and Spatz, M. 1968. Tumor induction in Fischer and Osborne-Mendel rats by a single administration of cycasin. *J. Natl. Cancer Inst.* 40: 1003–1010.

Hirono, I., Shibuya, C. and Fushimi, K. 1969. Tumor induction in C57BL/6 mice by a single administration of cycasin. *Cancer Res.* 29: 1658–1662.

Hirono, I., Shibuya, C., Fushimi, K. and Haga, M. 1970. Studies on carcinogenic properties of bracken, *Pteridium aquilinum. J. Natl. Cancer Inst.* 45: 179–188.

Hirono, I., Hayaski, K., Mori, H. and Miwa, T. 1971. Carcinogenic effects of cycasin in Syrian golden hamsters and the transplantability of induced tumors. *Cancer Res.* 31: 283–287.

Hirono, I., Shibuya, C., Shimizu, M. and Fushimi, K. 1972. Carcinogenic activity of processed bracken used as human food. *J. Natl. Cancer Inst.* 48: 1245–1250.

Hirono, I. et al. 1975. Natural carcinogenic products of plant origin. *Gann Monogr. Cancer Res.* 17: 205–217.

Hirono, I. et al. 1977. Brief communication: Carcinogenic activity of petasitenine, a new pyrrolizidine alkaloid isolated from *Petasites japonicus* maxim. *J. Natl. Cancer Inst.* 1155–1157.

Hirono, I. et al. 1981. Carcinogenicity examination of quercetin and rutin in ACI rats. *Cancer Lett.* 13: 15–21.

Hoch-Ligeti, C. 1952. Naturally occurring dietary agents and their role in production of tumors. *Tex. Rep. Biol. Med.* 19: 996–1005.

Hodge, J. V., Nye, E. R. and Emerson, G. W. 1964. Monoamine-oxidase inhibitors, broad beans and hypertension. *Lancet* 1: 1108.

Holck, H. G. O. 1949. Dosage of drugs for rats. In: *The Rat in Laboratory Investigation.* E. J. Farris and J. Q. Griffith (eds). Lippincott, Philadelphia.

Homburger, F. and Boger, E. 1968. The carcinogenicity of essential oils, flavors, and spices: A review. *Cancer Res.* 28: 2372–2374.

Homburger, F., Kelley, T., Jr., Friedler, G. and Russfield, A. B. 1961. Toxic and possible carcinogenic effects of 4-allyl-1,2-methylenedioxybenzene (safrole) in rats on deficient diets. *Med. Exp.* 4: 1–11.

Homburger, F., Kelley, T., Jr., Baker, T. R. and Russfield, A. B. 1962. Sex effect on thepatic pathology from a deficient diet and safrole in rats. *Arch. Pathol.* 73: 118–125.

Homburger, F., Bogdonoff, P. D. and Kelley, T. F. 1965. Influence of diet on chronic oral toxicity of safrole and butter yellow in rats. *Proc. Soc. Exp. Biol. Med.* 119: 1106–1110.

Horsley, C. H. 1934. Investigation into the action of St. Johns wort. *J. Pharmacol. Exp. Ther.* 50: 310–322.

Horst, K. and Jenkins, W. L. 1935. The effect of caffeine, coffee and decaffeinated coffee upon blood pressure, pulse rate and simple reaction time of men of various ages. *J. Pharm. Exp. Therp.* 53: 385–400.

Houtsmuller, U. M. T., Struijk, C. B. and Van Der Beek, A. 1970. Decrease in rate of ATP synthesis of isolated rat heart mitochondria induced by dietary erucic acid. *Biochem. Biophys. Acta* 218: 564–566.

Howard, J. W., Turicchi, E. W., White, R. H. and Fazio, T. 1966. Extraction and estimation of polycyclic aromatic hydrocarbons in vegetable oils. *J. Assoc. Off. Anal. Chem.* 49: 1236–1244.

Hughes, R. R. 1961. An Introduction to Clinical Electroencephalography. Williams and Wilkins, Baltimore, Maryland.

Hulan, H. W. et al. 1976a. Effect of cold stress on rapeseed oil fed rats. *Lipids* 11: 6–8.

Hulan, H. W. et al. 1976b. The development of dermal lesions and alopecia in male rats fed rapeseed oil. *Can. J. Physiol. Pharmacol.* 54: 1–6.

Humphries, S. G. 1967. The biosynthesis of tannins. In: *Biogenesis of Natural Compounds.* P. Bernfeld (ed.). 2nd ed. Pergamon Press, Oxford, England.

Ibrahim, M. Z. and Levine, S. 1967. Effect of cyanide intoxication on the metachromatic material found in the central nervous system. *J. Neurol. Neurosurg. Psychiatry* 30: 545—555.

Ikeda, R. M., Stanley, W. L., Vannier, S. H. and Spitler, E. M. 1962. Monoterpene hydrocarbon composition of some essential oils. *J. Food Sci.* 27: 455—458.

Innes, J. R. and Nickerson, M. 1970. Drugs inhibiting the action of acetylcholine on structures innervated by postganglionic parasympathetic nerves (antimuscarinic or atropinic drugs). In: *The Pharmacological Basis of Therapeutics.* 4th ed. L. S. Goodman and A. Gilman (eds). Macmillan, New York.

Innes, J. R. M. et al. 1969. Bioassay of pesticides and industrial chemicals for tumorigenicity in mice: A preliminary note. *J. Natl. Cancer Inst.* 42: 1101—1114.

Ito, S. 1980. Persimmon. In: *Tropical and Subtropical Fruits. Composition, Properties and Uses.* S. Nagy and P. E. Shaw (eds.). AVI, Westport, Connecticut.

Ito, S. and Oshima, Y. 1962. Studies on the tannin of Japanese persimmon. Part I. Isolation of leucoanthocyanin from kaki fruit. *Agric. Biol. Chem.* 26: 156—161.

Ivie, G. W., Holt, D. L. and Ivey, M. C. 1981. Natural toxicants in human foods: Psoralens in raw and cooked parsnip root. *Science* 213: 909—910.

Jacobs, M. B. 1951. *The Chemistry and Technology of Food and Food Products.* Vol. II. Interscience, New York.

Jacobsen, J. V., Bernhard, R. A., Mann, L. K. and Saghir, A. R. 1964. Infrared spectra of some assymetric disulfides produced by *Allium. Arch. Biochem. Biophys.* 104: 473—477.

Jacobson, M. F. et al. 1981. Coffee and birth defects. *Lancet* 1: 1415—1416.

Jacobziner, H. and Rayibin, H. W. 1965. Accidental chemical poisonings. Poisonings due to mace (nutmeg), furniture polish, and lead. *N. Y. State J. Med.* 65: 2270—2279.

Jaffe, W. G. 1950. Studies on the inhibitors of growth of rats by certain legume seeds. *Acta Cient. Venez.* 1: 62—64.

James, A. T., Harris, P. and Bezard, J. 1968. The inhibition of unsaturated fatty acid biosynthesis in plants by sterculic acid. *Eur. J. Biochem.* 3: 318—325.

Janot, M. M. et al. 1930. Hypoglycemic effect of the bulb of *Alium cepa. C. R. Acad Sci. (Paris)* 191: 1098—1100. (French)

Jelinek, R., Kyzlink, V. and Blattny, C., Jr. 1976. An evaluation of the embryotoxic effects of blighted potatoes on chicken embryos. *Teratology* 14: 335—342.

Jick, H. et al. 1973. Coffee and myocardial infarction. *N. Engl. J. Med.* 289: 63—67.

Jick, H. et al. 1974. Coffee drinking and myocardial infarction. *J.A.M.A.* 227: 801—802.

Joachim, A. W. R. and Pandittesekere, D. G. 1944. Investigations of the hydrocyanic acid content of cassava *(Manihot utilissima). Trop Agric.* 100: 150—163.

Johnson, A. R., Pearson, J. A., Shenstone, F. S. and Fogerty, A. C. 1967. Inhibition of the desaturation of stearic to oleic acid by cyclopropene fatty acids. *Nature* 214: 1244—1245.

Johnson, R. et al. 1972. Comparison of the contact allergenicity of four pentadecylcatechols derived from poison ivy urushiols in humans. *J. Allergy Clin. Immunol.* 49: 27—35.

Jones, P. G. and Fenwick, G. R. 1981. The glycoalkaloid content of some edible solanaceous fruits and potato products. *J. Sci. Food Agric.* 32(4): 419—421.

Jones, R. W., Stout, M. G., Reich, H. and Huffman, M. N. 1964. Cytotoxic activities of certain flavonoids against zebra-fish embryos. *Cancer Chemother. Rep.* 34: 19—20.

Kaighen, M. and Williams, R. T. 1961. The metabolism of $|3^{-14}C|$ coumarin. *J. Med. Pharm. Chem.* 3: 25—43.

Kalsner, S. 1976. Intrinsic prostaglandin release. A mediator of anoxia-induced re-laxation in an isolated coronary artery preparation. *Blood Vessels* 13: 155–166.

Kalsner, S. 1977. A coronary vascoconstrictor substance is present in regular and "decaffeinated" forms of both percolated and instant coffee. *Life Sci.* 20: 1689–1696.

Kalter, H. 1968. Teratology and pharmacogenetics. *Ann. N.Y. Acad Sci.* 151: 997–1000.

Kaminetzky, H. A. and McGrew, E. A. 1962. Podophyllin and mouse cervix. *Arch. Pathol.* 73: 481–485.

Kangwanpong, D., Arseculeratne, S. N. and Sirisinha, S. 1981. Clastogenic effect of aqueous extracts of palmyrah *(Borassus flabellifer)* flour on human blood lymphocytes. *Mutat. Res.* 89: 63–68.

Kannell, W. B. and Dawber, T. R. 1973. Coffee and coronary disease. *N. Engl. J. Med.* 289: 100–101.

Kapadia, G. J. et al. 1976. Carcinogenicity of *Camellia sinensis* (tea) and some tannin-containing folk medicinal herbs administered subcutaneously in rats. *J. Natl. Cancer Inst.* 57: 207–209.

Kapadia, G. J. et al. 1978. Carcinogenicity of some folk medicinal herbs in rats. *J. Natl. Cancer Inst.* 60: 683–686.

Karmazin, M. 1955. Critical examination of celery fruit and root on the basis of a colorimetric determination of apiol and myristicin. *Pharmazie* 10: 57–60.

Karow, H. 1969. Quality-determining components of some spices. II. *Reichst. Aromen, Koerperpflegem.* 19: 60–62, 65–66. (German)

Karrer, W. 1958. *Composition and Occurrence of Organic Plant Substances.* Birkhaüser Verlag, Basel.

Keeler, R. F. 1979. Toxins and teratogens of the Solanaceae and Liliaceae. In: *Toxic Plants.* A. D. Kinghorn (ed.). Columbia University Press, New York.

Keeler, R. et al. 1976a. Teratogenicity of the solanum alkaloid solasodine and "Kennebee" potato sprouts in hamsters. *Bull. Environ. Contam. Toxicol.* 15: 522–524.

Keeler, R., Young, S. and Brown, D. 1976b. Spina bifida, exencephaly, and crani-al bleb produced in hamsters by the solanum alkaloid solasodine. *Res. Commun. Chem. Pathol. Pharmacol.* 13(4): 723–730.

Keeler, R. S. et al. 1978. Congenital deformities produced in hamsters by potato sprouts. *Teratology* 17: 327–334.

Kefford, J. E. and Chandler, B. V. 1970. *The Chemical Constituents of citrus fruits. Advances Food Research.* Suppl. 2. Academic Press, New York.

Keil, H., Wasserman, D. and Dawson, C. R. 1945a. The relation of hypersensitive-ness to poison ivy and to cashew nut shell liquid. *Science* 102: 279–280.

Keil, H., Wasserman, D. and Dawson, C. R. 1945b. Relation of hypersensitiveness to poison ivy and to the pure ingredients in cashewnut shell liquid and related substances — A quantitative study based on patch tests. *Ind. Med.* 14: 825–830.

Keil, H., Wasserman, D. and Dawson, C. R. 1946. Mango dermatitis and its relation-ship to poison ivy hypersensitivity. *Ann. Allergy* 4: 268–281.

Keith, H. M. and Stavraky, G. W. 1935. Experimental convulsions induced by ad-ministration of thujone. A pharmacologic study of the influence of the autonomic nervous system on these convulsions. *Arch. Neurol. Psychiatry* 34: 1022–1040.

Kelly, M. G. and Hartwell, J. L. 1954. The biological effects and the chemical com-position of podophyllin: A review. *J. Natl. Cancer Inst.* 14: 967–1010.

Kenyhercz, T. M. and Kissinger, P. T. 1978. Identification and quantitation of tryptophan and tyrosine metabolites in banana by liquid chromatography with electrochemical detection. *J. Food Sci.* 43: 1354–1356.

Ketiku, A. O., Akinyele, I. O., Keshinro, O. O. and Akinnawo, O. O. 1978. Changes in the hydrocyanic acid concentration during traditional processing of cassava into "gari" and "lafun." *Food Chem.* 3: 221–228.

Khodasevich, A. P. 1965. Cited by E. B. Truitt, Jr., The xanthines. In: *Drill's Pharmacology in Medicine*. J. R. DiPalma (ed.). McGraw-Hill, New York.

Kihlman, B. A., Sturelid, S., Hartley-Asp, B. and Nilsson, K. 1974. The enhancement by caffeine of the frequencies of chromosomal aberrations induced in plant and animal cells by chemical and physical agents. *Mutat. Res.* 26: 105—122.

King, T. J. and DeSilva, L. B. 1968. Optically active gossypol from *Thespesia populnea*. *Tetrahedron Lett.* 1968(3): 261—263.

King, F. E. and Jurd, L. 1952. Chemistry of extractives from hardwoods. VIII. The isolation of 5,4'-dihydroxy-7-methoxyisoflavone (prunetin) from the heartwood of *Pterocarpus angolensis* and prunetin in species of Prunus. *J. Chem. Soc.* 1952: 3211—3215.

King-Li-Pin. 1931. The glucemic action of extracts from the pod of *Sophora japonica* L. *Soc. Biol.* 108: 885—887.

Kingsbury, J. M. 1964. *Poisonous Plants of the United States and Canada*. Prentice-Hall, Englewood Cliffs, New Jersey.

Kirby, K. S. 1960. Induction of tumours by tannin extracts. *Br. J. Cancer* 14: 147—152.

Kirby-Smith, J. L. 1938. Mango dermatitis. *Am. J. Trop. Med.* 18: 373—384.

Kirkman, H. N. 1968. Glucose-6-phosphate dehydrogenase variants and drug-induced hemolysis. *Ann. N.Y. Acad. Sci.* 151: 753—764.

Klatsky, A. L., Friedman, G. D. and Siegelaub, A. B. 1973. Coffee drinking prior to acute myocardial infarction. *J.A.M.A.* 226: 540—543.

Klatsky, A. L., Friedman, G. D. and Siegelaub, A. B. 1974. Coffee drinking and myocardial infarction. *J.A.M.A.* 227: 802—803.

Klein, M. 1952. Transpacental effect of urethan on lung tumorigenesis in mice. *J. Natl. Cancer Inst.* 12: 1003—1010.

Klein, E. 1965. Cited by R. L. Hall. 1973. Toxicants occurring naturally in spices and flavors. In: *Toxicants Occurring Naturally in Foods*. National Academy of Sciences, Washington, D.C.

Klein, G. and Farkass, E. 1930. Microchemical detection of alkaloids in plants. XIV. Cystisine. *Oesterr. Bot. Z.* 79: 107—124. (German)

Klosa, J. 1951. Hormone-like substances in the onion (*Allium cepa*). *Seifen-Oele-Fette-Wachse* 77: 166—167.

Kobayashi, T. 1950. Studies on the histopathologic changes of experimental cases of the "Ezonegi-poisoning" in horses. *Jpn. J. Vet. Sci.* 12: 209—210.

Kobayashi, A. and Matsumoto, H. 1965. Methylazoxymethanol, the aglycon of cycasin; isolation, biological, and chemical properties. *Arch. Biochem. Biophys.* 110: 373—380.

Koger, L. M. 1956. Onion poisoning in cattle. *J. Am. Vet. Med. Assoc.* 129: 75.

Kohn-Abrest, E. 1906. Chemical studies on bean seeds: Java pea. *C. R. Acad. Sci.* 142: 586.

Kondrashova, V. M. and Goryanov, O. A. 1975. Estrogenic effect of cabbage. (*Brassica oleracea*). *Vopr. Pitan.* 4: 73—75. (Russian, with English summary)

König, H. and Stafze, A. 1953. Report on the effect of solanin on the status of the blood and catalase in sheep. *Dtsch. Tieraerztl. Wochenschr.* 60: 150—153.

Korpassy, B. 1950. Hepatomas and cholangiomas induced in rats following subcutaneous administration of tannic acid. *Bull. Assoc. Franc. Cancer* 37: 52—56. (German)

Korpassy, B. and Mosonyi, M. 1950. The carcinogenic activity of tannic acid. Liver tumours induced in rats by prolonged subcutaneous administration of tannic acid solutions. *Br. J. Cancer* 4: 411—420.

Korpassy, B. and Mosonyi, M. 1951. The carcinogenic action of tannic acid. Effect of casein on the development of liver tumours. *Acta. Morphol. Hung.* 1: 37—54.

Kosower, N. S. and Kosower, E. M. 1967. Does 3,4-dihydroxyphenylalanine play a part in favism? *Nature* 215: 285—286.

Koster, M. and David, G. K. 1968. Reversible severe hypertension due to licorice ingestion. *N. Engl. J. Med.* 278: 1381—1383.

Kreitmair, H. 1936. Pharmacological trials with some domestic plants. *E. Merck's Jahresber.* 50: 102–110.

Kruse, E. and Scholz, H. 1978. Effect of theophylline on myocardial adenylate cyclase activity. *Experientia* 34: 504–505.

Krzymanski, J. and Downey, R. K. 1969. Inheritance of fatty acid composition in winter forms of rapeseed, *Brassica napus*. *Can. J. Plant Sci.* 49: 313–319.

Kuhn, R. and Jerchel, D. 1943. 2-Hexen-4,1-olide and 2-hexen-5,1-olide; constitution of the parasorbic acid from the volatile oil of ripe rowanberries. *Berichte Deutschen Chemischen Gesellschaft* 76B: 413–419.

Kuiken, K. A., Lyman, C. M. and Hale, F. 1948. The effect of feeding isopropanol extracted from cottonseed meal on storage quality of eggs. *Poult. Sci.* 27: 742–744.

Kuratsune, M. and Hueper, W. L. 1960. Polycyclic aromatic hydrocarbons in roasted coffee. *J. Natl. Cancer Inst.* 24: 463–469.

Lacquer, G. L. 1965. The induction of intestinal neoplasms in rats with the glycoside cycasin and its aglycone. *Arch. Pathol. Anat. Physiol.* 340: 151–163.

Lacquer, G. L. and Matsumoto, H. 1966. Neoplasms in female Fischer rats following intraperitoneal injection of methylazoxymethanol. *J. Natl. Cancer Inst.* 37: 217–232.

Lacquer, G. L. and Spatz, M. 1968. Toxicology of cycasin. *Cancer Res.* 28: 2262–2267.

Lacquer, G. L. and Spatz, M. 1973. Transplacental induction of tumors and malformations in rats with cycasin and methylazoxymethanol. In: *Transplacental Carcinogenesis*. Proceedings of a Meeting. 1971. L. Tomatis (ed.). International Agency for Research on Cancer, Lyons, France. IARC Scientific Publication No. 4.

Lacquer, G. L., Mickelson, O., Whiting, M. G. and Kurland, L. T. 1963. Carcinogenic properties of nuts from *Cycas circinalis* L. indigenous to Guam. *J. Natl. Cancer Inst.* 31: 919–951.

Lacquer, G. L., McDaniel, E. G. and Matsumoto, H. 1967. Tumor induction in germ-free rats with methylazoxymethanol (MAM) and synthetic MAM acetate. *J. Natl. Cancer Inst.* 39: 355–371.

LaFace, D. 1950. The concrete essence of *Acacia farnesiana*. *Helv. Chim. Acta* 33: 249–256. (Italian)

Lakshminarayana, S. and Moreno-Rivera, M. A. 1979. Proximate characteristics and composition of sapodilla fruits grown in Mexico. *Proc. Fla. State Hortic. Soc.* 92: 303–305.

Lakshminarayana, S. and Subramanyam, H. 1966. Physical, chemical and physiological changes in sapota fruit, Hohras sapota (Sapotaceae) during development and ripening. *J. Food Sci. Technol.* 3: 151–154.

Lakshminarayana, S., Subhadra, N. V. and Subramanyam, H. 1970. Some aspects of developmental physiology of the mango fruit. *J. Hortic. Sci.* 45: 133–142.

Laland, P. and Havrevold, O. W. 1933. The active principle of onions (*Allium sativum*) which lowers blood sugar per os. *Z. Physiol. Chem.* 221: 180–196.

Lang, K. 1933a. Rhodanase synthesis in animal body. *Biochem. Z.* 259: 243–256.

Lang, K. 1933b. Cyanide formation in the animal body. *Biochem. Ztschr.* 263: 262–267.

Lang, K. 1975. The physiological significance in human nutrition of undesirable substances in natural foods of vegetable origin. *Landwirtschaft. Forsch.* 32: 259–269.

Lange, R. L. et al. 1972. Nonatheromatous ischemic heart disease following withdrawal from chronic industrial nitroglycerine exposure. *Circulation* 46: 666–678.

Lattanzio, N., Bianco, V. V., Crivelli, G. and Miccolis, V. 1983. Variability of amino acids, proteins, vicine and couvicine in *Vicia faba* (L.) *J. Food Sci.* 48: 992–993.

Laurin, J. 1931. Hypoglycemic effects of the bulb of *Allium cepa*. *C.R. Acad Sci. Paris* 192: 1289–1294. (French)

Leavitt, W. W. and Wright, P. A. 1965. The plant estrogen, coumestrol, as an agent affecting hypophysial gonadotropin function. *J. Exp. Zool.* 160: 319–327.

Lee, D. J. et al. 1967. A comparison of cyclopropenes and other possible promoting agents for aflatoxin-induced hepatoma in rainbow trout. *Fed. Proc.* 26: 322.

Lee, P. L., Swords, G. and Hunter, G. L. K. 1975. Volatile constituents of tamarind *(Tamardindus indica L.). J. Agric. Food Chem.* 23: 1195–1199.

Legator, M. S. and Malling, H. V. 1971. The host-mediated assay, a practical procedure for evaluating potential mutagenic agents in mammals. In: *Chemical Mutagens: Principals and Methods for Their Detection.* Vol. II. A. Hollaender (ed.). Plenum, New York.

Lehman, A. J. 1961. Report on safrole. *Assoc. Food Drug Off. U.S. Q. Bull.* 25: 194.

Lehmann, F. A. 1929-1930. Research on *Allium sativa* (garlic). *Arch. Exp. Pathol. Pharmakol.* 146–147: 245–264.

Lehmann, A. R. 1972. Post-replication repair of DNA in ultraviolet-irradiated mammalian cells. No gaps in DNA synthesized late after ultraviolet irradiation. *Eur. J. Biochem.* 31: 438–445.

Lehmann, A. R. and Kirk-Bell, S. 1974. Effects of caffeine and theophylline on DNA synthesis in unirradiated and UV-irradiated mammalian cells. *Mutat. Res.* 26: 73–82.

Lehmann, A. R. et al. 1975. Xeroderma pigmentosum cells with normal levels of excision repair have a defect in DNA synthesis after UV irradiation. *Proc. Natl. Acad. Sci.* 27: 219–223.

Leuschner, F. and Czok, G. 1973. Reversibility of prenatal injuries induced by caffeine in rats. Colloq. Int. Chim. Cafes 5: 388–391 (1971) (published 1973). (German)

Levene, C. I. 1962. Studies on the mode of action of lathyrogenic compounds. *J. Exp. Med.* 116: 119–130.

Levi, R. S. et al. 1967. Quantitative determination of cyclopropenoid fatty acids in cottonseed meal. *J. Am. Oil Chem. Soc.* 44: 249–252.

Levin, D. E. et al. 1982. A new *Salmonella* testes strain (TA102) with A-T base pairs at the site of mutation detects oxidative mutagens. *Proc. Natl. Acad. Sci.* 79: 7445–7449.

Levine, S. Hirano, A. and Zimmerman, H. M. 1967. Experimental cyanide encephalopathy. Electron microscope observations of early lesions in white matter. *J. Neuropathol. Exp. Neurol.* 26: 172–174.

Lewin, L. 1904. Abortions due to poisoning and other means. *Freidrich's Bl. Gerichtl. Med. Nurmb.* IV: 469. (German)

Leyva, E. and Gutierrez, N. C. 1937. Inversion of the action of adrenalin on glucemia by yohimbine. *J. Phillippine Isl. Med. Assoc.* 17: 349–355.

Lijinsky, W., Conrad, E. and Van De Bogart, R. 1972. Carcinogenic nitrosamines formed by drug/nitrite interactions. *Nature* 239: 165–167.

Lillie, R. T. and Bird, H. R. 1950. Effect of oral administration of pure gossypol and of pigments glands of cottonseed on mortality and growth of chickens. *Poult. Sci.* 29: 390–393.

Lin, R. S. and Kessler, I. I. 1981. A multifactorial model for pancreatic cancer in man. Epidemiologic evidence. *J.A.M.A.* 245: 147–152.

Lin, J. Y. and Ling, K. H. 1962a. Studies on favism II — Studies on the physiological activities of vicine in vivo. *J. Formosan Med. Assoc.* 61: 490–494.

Lin, J. Y. and Ling, K. H. 1962b. Studies on favism III — Studies on the physiological activities of vicine in vitro. *J. Formosan Med. Assoc.* 61: 579–583.

Lindstedt, G. 1951. Constituents of pine heartwood. XXVI. A general discussion. *Acta Chem. Scand.* 5: 129–138.

Lio, G. and Agnoli, R. 1927. Pharmacological effect of the bulb of Lilicae, especially *Allium sativum. Arch. Int. Pharmacodyn.* 33: 400–408. (Italian)

Lipsky, M. M., Hinton, D. E. and Trump, B. F. 1980. Studies on the pathogenesis of safrole-induced hepatic neoplasia in the mouse. Diss. Abstr. Int. [B], 40(8), 3672B. University Maryland Baltimore Professional School, Baltimore.

Locci, R. and Kuc, J. 1967. Steroid alkaloids as compounds produced by potato tubers under stress. *Phytopathology* 57: 1272—1273.

Long, E. L. and Jenner, P. M. 1963. Esophageal tumors produced in rats by the feeding of dihydrosafrole. *Fed. Proc.* 22: 275.

Long, E. L., Nelson, A. A., Fitzhugh, O. G. and Hansen, W. H. 1963. Liver tumors produced in rats by feeding safrole. *Arch. Pathol.* 75: 595—604.

Lotspeich, W. D. 1960-61. Phlorizin and the cellular transport of glucose. *Harvey Lect.* 56: 63—91.

Luisada, A. 1941. Favism: A singular disease chiefly affecting the red blood cells. *Medicine* 20: 229—250.

Luke, E. 1962. Addiction to mentholated cigarettes. *Lancet* 1: 110—111.

Lyman, C. M., Baliga, B. P. and Slay, M. W. 1959. Reactions of proteins with gossypol. *Arch. Biochem. Biophys.* 84: 486—497.

Lyman, C. M., El-Nockrashy, A. S. and Dollahite, J. W. 1963. Gossyverdurin: A newly isolated pigment from cottonseed pigment glands. *J. Am. Oil Chem. Soc.* 40: 571—575.

Lyman, C. M., Cronin, J. T., Trant, M. M. and Odell, G. V. 1969. Metabolism of gossypol in the chick. *J. Am. Oil Chem. Soc.* 46: 100—104.

MacAlpin, R. 1973. Coronary spasm as a cause of angina. *N. Eng. J. Med.* 288: 788—789.

MacGregor, J. T. and Jurd, L. 1978. Mutagenicity of plant flavonoids: Structural requirements for mutagenic activity in *Salmonella typhimurium*. *Mutat. Res.* 54: 297—309.

MacKenzie, I. and Rous, P. 1941. The experimental disclosure of latent neoplastic changes in tarred skin. *J. Exp. Med.* 73: 391—416.

MacMahon, B. et al. 1981. Coffee and cancer of the pancreas. *N. Engl. J. Med.* 304: 630—632.

Magee, P. N. and Barnes, J. M. 1959. The experimental production of tumors in the rat by dimethylnitrosamine (N-nitroso-dimethylamine). *Acta Unio Int. Cancrum* 15: 187—190.

Mager, J. et al. 1965. Metabolic effects of pyrimidines derived from fava bean glycosides on human erythrocytes deficient in glucose-6-phosphate dehydrogenase. *Biochem. Biophys. Res. Commun.* 20: 235—240.

Mager, J., Razin, A. and Hershko, A. 1969. Favism. In: *Toxic Constituents of Plant Foodstuffs*. E. I. Liener (ed.). Academic Press, New York.

Maier, V. P. and Metzler, D. M. 1965a. Quantitative changes in date polyphenols and their relation to browning. *J. Food Sci.* 30: 80—84.

Maier, V. P. and Metzler, D. M. 1965b. Changes in individual date polyphenols and their relation to browning. *J. Food Sci.* 30: 747—752.

Maier, V. P. and Metzler, D. M. 1965c. *Cited by* C. E. Vandercook, S. Hasegawa and V. P. Maier, 1980. Dates. In: *Tropical and Subtropical Fruits. Composition, Properties and Uses*. AVI, Westport, Connecticut.

Maiori, L. and Squeri, L. 1955-56. Guinea-pig blood behavior after administration of various extract fractions from *Allium cepa*. Atti Soc. Peloritana Sci. Fis. Mat. Nat. 2: 233—235.

Malaisse, W. J., Lea, M. A. and Malaisse-Lagae, F. 1968. The effect of mannoheptulose on the phosphorylation of glucose and the secretion of insulin by islets of Langerhans. *Metabolism* 17: 126—132.

Maloney, A. H. 1935. Contradictory actions of caffeine, coramine and metrazol. *Q. J. Exp. Physiol.* 25: 155—166.

Marion, L. 1950. The pyridine alkaloids. In: *The Alkaloids*. R. H. F. Manske and H. L. Holmes (eds.). Vol. I. Academic Press, New York.

Markiewitz, K. H. and Dawson, C. R. 1965. On the isolation of the allergenically active components of the toxic principle of poison ivy. *J. Org. Chem.* 30: 1610—1613.

Markley, K. S. (ed). 1960. *Fatty Acids. Their Chemistry, Properties, Production, and Uses.* Interscience, New York.

Marshall, P. B. 1959. Catechols and tryptamines in the matoke banana. *J. Pharm. Pharmacol.* 11: 639.

Martinek, R. G. and Wolman, W. 1955. Xanthines, tannins and sodium in coffee, tea and cocoa. *J.A.M.A.* 158: 1030—1031.

Masson, J. C., Vavich, M. G., Heywang, B. W. and Kemmerer, A. R. 1957. Pink discoloration in eggs caused by sterculic acid. *Science* 126: 751.

Mateo Tinao, M. and Calvo Terren, R. 1955. Actions of *Allium sativum* (garlic) and combinations on uterine motility. *Arch. Inst. Farmacol. Exp. (Madrid)* 8: 127—147.

Matikkala, E. J. and Virtanen, A. I. 1967. On the quantitative determination of the amino acids and γ-glutamylpeptides of onion. *Acta Chem. Scand.* 21: 2891—2893.

Matsumoto, H. and Strong, F. M. 1963. The occurrence of methylazoxymethanol in *Cycas carcinalis* L. *Arch. Biochem. Biophys.* 101: 299—310.

Matsumoto, H. et al. 1972. β-Glucosidase modulation in preweanling rats and its association with tumor induction by cycasin. *J. Natl. Cancer Inst.* 49: 423—433.

Matsuo, T., Shinohara, J. and Ito, S. 1976. An improvement on removing astringency in persimmon fruits by carbon dioxide gas. *Agric. Biol. Chem.* 40: 215—217.

Maxwell, C., McKnight, R. S., Scott, B. and Lindegren, C. C. 1939. Physiological effects of garlic and derived substances. *Am. J. Hyg.* 29B: 32—35.

Mayorga, H., Gonzalez, J., Mencho, J. F. and Rolz, C. 1975. Preparation of a low free gossypol cottonseed flour by dry and continuous processing. *J. Food. Sci.* 40: 1270—1274.

Mazelis, M. 1963. Demonstration and characterization of cysteine sulfoxide lyase in the Cruciferae. *Phytochemistry* 2: 15—22.

McCulloch, J. and Harper, A. M. 1979. Factors influencing the response of the cerebral circulation to phenylethylamine. *Neurology* 29: 201—207.

McGee, M. B. 1980. Caffeine poisoning in a 19-year-old female. *J. Forensic Sci.* 25: 29.

McKay, G. F., Lalich, J. J., Schilling, E. D. and Strong, F. M. 1954. A crystalline "lathyrus factor" from *Lathyrus odoratus*. *Arch. Biochem. Biophys.* 52: 313-322.

McKee, F. W. and Hawkins, W. B. 1945. Phlorizin glucosuria. *Physiol. Rev.* 25: 255—280.

McLaren, D. S. 1960. Malnutrition and eye disease in Tanganyika. *Proc. Nutr. Soc.* 19: 89—91.

McMichael, S. C. 1960. Combined effect of glandless genes gl2 and gl3 on pigment glands in cotton plant. *Agron. J.* 52: 385—386.

McPhee, W. R. 1956. Acquired hemolytic anemia caused by ingestion of fava beans; report of a case and review of case reported in American literature. *Am. J. Clin. Pathol.* 26: 1287—1302.

Meksongsee, L. A., Clawson, A. J. and Smith, F. H. 1970. The in vivo effect of gossypol on cytochrome oxidase, succinoxidase, and succinic dehydrogenase in animal tissues. *J. Agric. Food Chem.* 18: 917—920.

Meltz, M. L. and MacGregor, J. T. 1981. Activity of the plant flavonol quercetin in the mouse lymphoma L5178Y TK+/mutation, DNA single-strand break, and BALB/C 3T3 chemical transformation assays. *Mutat. Res.* 88: 317—324.

Menaul, P. 1923. The physiological effect of gossypol. *J. Agric. Res.* 26: 233—237.

Menkyna, R. A. 1954. Properties of glycyrrhiza. *Bratisl. Lek. Listy* 33: 281—291.

Menn, J. J., McBain, J. B. and Dennis, M. J. 1964. Detection of naturally occurring cholinesterase inhibitors in several crops by paper chromatography. *Nature* 202: 697—698.

Merrill, E. D. 1944. Dermatitis caused by various representatives of the Anacardiae-ceae in tropical countries. *J.A.M.A.* 124: 222–224.

Millen, J. W. and Woollam, D. H. 1957. Influence of cortisone on teratogenic effects of hypervitaminosis-A. *Br. M. J.* 5038: 196–197.

Miller, E. C. et al. 1983. Structure-activity studies of the carcinogenicities in the mouse and rat of some naturally occurring and synthetic alkenylbenzene derivatives related to safrole and estragole. *Cancer Res.* 43: 1124–1134.

Miller, J. A. 1973. Naturally occurring substances that can induce tumors. In: *Toxicants Occurring Naturally in Foods*. National Academy of Sciences, Washington, D.C.

Miller, R. W., Earle, F. R. and Wolff, I. A. 1965. Search for new industrial oils. XIII. Oils from 102 species of Cruciferae. *J. Am. Oil Chem. Soc.* 42: 817–821.

Mirvish, S. S. 1970. Kinetics of dimethylamine nitrosation in relation to nitrosamine carcinogenesis. *J. Natl. Cancer Inst.* 44: 633–639.

Mitchell, J. 1975. Contact allergy from plants. In: *Recent Advances in Phyto-chemistry*. V. Runeckles (ed.). Plenum Press, New York.

Mohan, V. S., Nagarajan, V. and Gopalan, C. 1966. Simple practical procedures for the removal of toxic factors in *Lathyrus sativus* (Khesari dhal). *Indian J. Med. Res.* 54: 410–414.

Moisio, T., Spare, C. G. and Virtanen, A. I. 1962. Mass-spectral studies of the chemical nature of the lachrymatory factor formed enzymically from S-(1-propenyl)-cysteine sulfoxide isolated from onion *(Allium cepa)*. *Suom. Kemistilehti* 35B: 28–29.

Molitor, H., Mushett, C. W. and Kuna, S. 1941. Some toxicological and pharmacological properties of the proteolytic enzyme, ficin. *J. Pharmacol. Exp. Ther.* 71–72: 20–29.

Monekosso, G. L. and Wilson, J. 1966. Plasma thiocyanate and vitamin B_{12} in Nigerian patients with degenerative neurological disease. *Lancet* 1: 1062–1064.

Montgomery, R. D. 1964. Observations on the cyanide content and toxicity of tropical pulses. *West Indian Med. J.* 13: 1–11.

Montgomery, R. D. 1965. The medical significance of cyanogen in plant foodstuffs. *Am. J. Clin. Nutr.* 17: 103–113.

Montgomery, R. D. 1969. Cyanogens. In: *Toxic Constituents of Plant Foodstuffs*. I. E. Liener (ed.). Academic Press, New York.

Moon, F. E. and McKeand, J. M. 1953. Observations on the vitamine status and haematology of bracken-fed ruminants. *Br. Vet. J.* 109: 321–326.

Moon, F. E. and Raafat, M. A. 1951. Some biochemical aspects of bracken poisoning in the ruminant animals. I. Vitamin factors. *J. Sci. Food Agric.* 3: 228–240.

Mori, H. and Hirono, I. 1977. Effect of coffee on carcinogenicity of cycasin. *Br. J. Cancer* 35: 369–371.

Morita, N., Nagayoshi-Muto, R. and Yunoki, K. 1971. Effect of methylazoxymethanol acetate (MAM-OA_c), a biologically active ester of the aglycone of cycasin, on the induction of tyrosine-α-ketoglutarate transaminase. *Acta Med. Univ. Kagoshima* 13: 179–192.

Morbidity and Mortality Weekly Report. 1975. Cyanide poisoning from ingestion of apricot kernels-California *M.M.W.R.* 24: 427.

Morbidity and Mortality Weekly Report. 1983. Dermatitis associated with cashew nut consumption — Pennsylvania. *M.M.W.R.* 32: 129.

Morton, J. F. 1970. Tentative correlations of plant usage and esophageal cancer zones. *Econ. Bot.* 24: 217–226.

Mueller, W. S. 1942. The significance of tannic substances and theobromine in chocolate milk. *J. Dairy Sci.* 25: 221–230.

Mugera, G. M. 1969. Induction of kidney tumours in the rats by feeding *Encephalartos hildebrandtii* for short periods. *Br. J. Cancer* 23: 755–756.

Mukerji, B. 1957. Indigenous Indian drugs used in the treatment of diabetes. *J. Sci. Ind. Res.* (Suppl. 1) 16A: 1–18.

Muller, C. J. and Jennings, W. G. 1967. Constituents of black pepper. Some ses-
quiterpene hydrocarbons. *J. Agric. Food Chem.* 15: 762—766.

Mun, A. M., Barden, E. S., Wilson, J. M. and Hogan, J. M. 1975. Teratogenic effects in early chick embryos of solanine and glycoalkaloids from potato infected
with late-blight, *Phytophtora infestans. Teratology* 11: 73—78.

Muthuswamy, P., Raju, G. S. N., Krishnamoorthy, K. K. and Ravikumar, V. 1976.
Effect of tillage and soil amendments on HCN and dry matter content of tapioca
(*Manihot esculenta* Crantz). *Curr. Res.* 5: 190—191.

Nagahama, T. 1964. Studies on neocycasin, new glycosides of cycads. *Bull. Fac.
Agr. Kagoshima Univ.* 14: 1—50.

Nagao, M. Takahashi, Y., Yamanaka, H. and Sugimura, T. 1979. Mutagens in coffee and tea. *Mutat. Res.* 68: 101—106.

Nagao, M. et al. 1981. Mutagenicities of 61 flavonoids and 11 related compounds.
Environ. Mutagen. 3: 401—419.

Nagata, Y. and Matsumoto, H. 1969. Studies on methylazoxymethanol: Methylation
of nucleic acids in the fetal rat brain. *Proc. Soc. Exp. Biol. Med.* 132:
383—385.

Nagatsu, I., Sudo, Y. and Nagatsu, T. 1972. Tyrosine hydroxylation in banana
plant. *Enzymologia* 43: 25—31.

Nagy, S. et al. 1979. Analysis of monosaccharides in avocado by HPLC. Abstract of
papers, Agricultural and Food Chemistry, ACS/CSJ Chemical Congress, Honolulu, Hawaii, Paper No. 42.

Naismith, D. J., Akinyanju, P. A. and Yudkin, J. 1969. Influence of caffeine-
containing beverages on the growth, food utilization and plasma lipids of the
rat. *J. Nutr.* 97: 375—381.

Naito, T. 1943. The constituents of the volatile oil from the leaf of *Cinnamomum
camphora* var. *glaucescens. J. Chem. Soc. Jpn.* 64: 1125.

Narain, R., Lyman, C. M. and Couch, J. R. 1958. Effect of increased protein level
in the hen diet on the transfer of gossypol cephalen to the egg. *Poult. Sci.*
37: 893—896.

Narain, R., Lyman, C. M., Deyoe, C. W. and Couch, J. R. 1961. Paper electrophoresis and albumin/globulin ratios of the serum of normal chickens and chickens fed free gossypol in the diet. *Poult. Sci.* 40: 21—25.

Narisawa, T. and Nakano, H. 1973. Carcinoma of the large intestine of rats induced
by rectal infusion of methylazoxymethanol. *Gann* 64: 93—95.

Nassar, M. A. 1969. "Inheritance of Glandless Seed in Egyptian Cotton Crosses."
M.S. Thesis. Azhar University, Cairo, Egypt.

Naves, Y. R. 1943. Volatile plant materials. XXIV. Composition of the essential oil
and resinoid of lovage root. *Helv. Chim. Acta* 26: 1281—1295. (French)

Nichols, A. B. 1973. Coffee drinking and acute myocardial infarction. *Lancet* 1:
480—481.

Nilson, H. W. and Wagner, J. A. 1959. Feeding test with carrageenan. *Food Res.*
24: 235—239.

Nilsson, K. and Lehmann, A. R. 1975. The effect of methylated oxypurines on the
size of newly-synthesized DNA and on the production of chromosome aberrations
after UV irradiation in Chinese hamster cells. *Mut. Res.* 30: 255—266.

Nishida, K. 1959. Azoxyglycosides I. *J. Jpn. Chem.* 13: 730—737. (Japanese)

Nishida, K., Kobayashi, A. and Nagahama, T. 1955. Cycasin, a new toxic glycoside
of *Cycas revoluta* Thunb. I. Isolation and structure of cycasin. *Bull. Agric.
Chem. Soc. Jpn.* 19: 77—84.

Nishida, K. et al. 1956. Studies on cycasin, a new toxic glycoside of *Cycas
revoluta* Thunb. IV. Pharmacological study of cycasin. *Seikagaku (J. Jpn. Biochem. Soc.)* 28: 218—223. (Japanese)

Nishie, K., Gumbmann, M. R. and Keyl, A. C. 1971. Pharmacology of solanine.
Toxicol. Appl. Pharmacol. 19: 81—92.

Nishie, K., Norred, W. P. and Swain, A. P. 1975. Pharmacology and toxicology of
chaconine and tomatine. *Res. Commun. Chem. Pathol. Pharmacol.* 12: 657—668.

Nishimura, H. and Nakai, K. 1960. Congenital malformations in offspring of mice treated with caffeine. *Proc. Soc. Exp. Biol. Med.* 104: 140–142.

Noble, I. G. 1946-1947. Fruta bomba *(Carica papaya)* in hypertension. *An. Acad. Cienc. Med. Fis. Nac. (Hab.)* 85: 198–203.

Nopanitaya, W. and Nye, S. W. 1974. Duodenal mucosal response to the pungent principle of hot pepper (capsaicin) in the rat: Light and electron microscopic study. *Toxic. Appl. Pharmacol.* 30: 149–161.

Noteboom, W. D. and Gorski, J. 1963. Estrogenic effect of genistein and coumestrol diacetate. *Endocrinology* 73: 736–739.

Obigbesan, G. O. and Fayemi, A. A. A. 1976. Investigations on Nigerian root and tuber crops. Influence of nitrogen fertilization on the yield and chemical composition of two cassava cultivars *(Manihot esculenta)*. *J. Agric. Sci.* 86: 401–406.

O'Dell, B. L. et al. 1966. Inhibition of the biosynthesis of the cross-links in elastin by a lathyrogen. *Nature* 209: 401–402.

O'Gara, R. W. 1968. Biologic screening of selected plant material for carcinogens. *Cancer Res.* 28: 2272–2275.

O'Gara, R. W., Brown, J. M. and Whiting, M. G. 1964. Induction of hepatic and renal tumors by the topical application of aqueous extract of cycad nut to artificial skin ulcers in mice. *Fed. Proc.* 23: 1383.

O'Gara, R. W. et al. 1974. Sarcoma induced in rats by extracts of plants and by fractionated extracts of *Krameria ixina*. *J. Natl. Cancer Inst.* 52: 445–448.

Ogata, J. N., Kawano, Y., Bevenue, A. and Casarett, L. J. 1972. The keptoheptose content of some tropical fruits. *J. Agric. Food Chem.* 20: 113–115.

Oke, O. L. 1968. Cassava as food in Nigeria. *World Rev. Nutr. Diet.* 9: 227–250.

Oke, O. L. 1972. Yam — a valuable source of food and drugs. *World Rev. Nutr. Diet.* 15: 156–184.

Oliva, P. B., Potts, D. E. and Pluss, R. G. 1973. Coronary arterial spasm in prinzmetal angina. Documentation by coronary arteriography. *N. Engl. J. Med.* 288: 745–751.

Opper, L. 1939. Pathologic picture of thujone and monobromated camphor convulsions. Comparison with pathologic picture of human epilepsy. *Arch. Neurol. Psychiatry* 41: 460–470.

Orgell, W. H. 1963. Inhibition of human plasma cholinesterase in vitro by alkaloids, glycosides, and other natural substances. *Lloydia* 26: 36–43.

Orgell, W. H., Vaidya, K. A. and Hamilton, E. W. 1959. A preliminary survey of some midwestern plants for substances inhibiting human plasma cholinesterase in vitro. *Proc. Iowa Acad. Sci.* 66: 149–154.

Orris, L. 1958. Cashew nut dermatitis. *N.Y. State J. Med.* 58: 2799–2800.

Orten, J. M. and Neuhaus, O. W. 1975. *Human Biochemistry*. 9th ed. Mosby, St. Louis.

Osawa, T. et al. 1981. Formation of mutagens by pepper-nitrite reaction. *Muta. Res.* 91: 291–295.

Oslage, H. J. 1956. On solanine in potatoes and its effects in animals. *Kartoffelbau* 7: 204. (German)

Osol, A. and Farrar, G. E., Jr. (ed.). 1955. Coumarin. In: *The Dispensatory of the United States of America*. 25th ed. Lippincott, Philadelphia.

Ostertag, W. 1966. Caffeine and theophylline mutagenicity in human cell and leukocyte culture system. *Mutat. Res.* 3: 249–267. (German)

Osuntokun, B. O. 1968. Ataxic neuropathy in Nigeria. *Brain* 91: 215–247.

Osuntokun, B. O. 1973. Ataxic neuropathy associated with high cassava diets in West Africa. In: *Chronic Cassave Toxicity*. Int. Dev. Res. Centre Monogr. IDRC-OIO.

Osuntokun, B. O. 1981. Cassava diet, chronic cyanide intoxication and neuropathy in the Nigerian Africans. *World Rev. Nutr. Diet.* 36: 141–173.

Osuntokun, B. O., Monekosso, G. L. and Wilson, J. 1969. Relationship of a degenerative tropical neuropathy to diet. Report of a field survey. *Br. Med. J.* 1: 547–550.

Osuntokun, B. O., Aladetoyinbo, A. and Adenja, A. O. G. 1970a. Free-cyanide levels in tropical ataxic neuropathy. *Lancet* 2: 372–373.

Osuntokun, B. O., Singh, E. P. and Martinson, F. D. 1970b. Deafness in tropical ataxic neuropathy. *Trop. Geogr. Med.* 22: 218–288.

Oswald, E. O., Fishbein, L., Corbett, B. J. and Walker, M. P. 1971. Chemical liability of the tertiary amino methylenedioxy propiophenones as urinary metabolites of safrole in the rat and guinea pig. *Biochim. Biophys. Acta* 244: 322–328.

Pack, W. K., Raudonat, H. W. and Schmidt, K. 1972. On the fatal prussic acid poisoning following the ingestion of bitter almonds *(Prunus amygdalus)*. *Z. Rechtsmed.* 70: 53–54. (German)

Palfii, F. Yu. et al. 1975. Metabolism, productivity, and reproductive ability of heifers grazed on pasture with different portions of estrogenically active white clover. *S-kh. Biol.* 10: 894–899. (Russian)

Palm, P. E. et al. 1978. Evaluation of the teratogenic potential of fresh brewed coffee, caffeine and aspirin in rats. *Toxicol. Appl. Pharmacol.* 44: 1016.

Pamukcu, A. M. and Price, J. M. 1969. Induction of intestinal and urinary bladder cancer in rats by feeding bracken fern *(Pteris aquilina)*. *J. Natl. Cancer Inst.* 43: 275–281.

Pamukcu, A. M., Göksoy, S. K. and Price, J. M. 1967. Urinary bladder neoplasms induced by feeding bracken fern *(Pteris aquilina)* to cows. *Cancer Res.* 27: 917–924.

Pamukcu, A. M., Yalciner, S., Price, J. M. and Bryan, G. T. 1970. Effects of the coadministration of thiamine on the incidence of urinary bladder carcinomas in rats fed bracken fern. *Cancer Res.* 30: 2671–2674.

Pamukcu, A. M., Ertürk, E., Price, J. M. and Bryan, G. T. 1972. Lymphatic leukemia and pulmonary tumors in female Swiss mice fed bracken fern *(Pteris aquilina)*. *Cancer Res.* 32: 1442–1445.

Pamukcu, A. M., Yalciner, S., Hatcher, J. F. and Bryan, G. T. 1980. Quercetin, a rat intestinal and bladder carcinogen present in bracken fern *(Pteridium aquilinum)*. *Cancer Res.* 40: 3468–3472.

Panabokke, R. G. and Arseculeratne, S. N. 1976. Veno-occlusive lesions in the liver of rats after prolonged feeding with palmyrah *(Borassus flabellifer)* flour. *Br. J. Exp. Pathol.* 57: 189–199.

Panabokke, R. G. and Arseculeratne, S. N. 1977. Malignant lymphomas in rats after prolonged feeding with palmyrah flour. *Proc. Sri Lanka Assoc. Adv. Sci.* 35: 5.

Panda, N. C., Sahu, B. K., Rao, A. G. and Panda, S. K. 1979. Tannic acid, tea and coffee as incriminating factor for heart disease. *Indian J. Nutr. and Diet.* 16: 348–355.

Panizon, F. and Zacchello, F. 1965. The mechanism of hemolysis in favism. Some analogy in the activity of primaquine and fava juice. *Acta Haematol.* 33: 129–138.

Papa, C. M. and Shelley, W. B. 1964. Menthol hypersensitivity. Diagnostic basophil response in a patient with chronic urticaria, flushing, and headaches. *J.A.M.A.* 189: 546–548.

Parish, R. F., Frick, C., Richards, A. B. and Forney, R. B. 1965. Human caffeine fatality. *Toxicol. Appl. Pharmacol.* 7: 494.

Parke, D. V. and Rahman, H. 1970. The induction of hepatic microsomal enzymes by safrole. *Biochem. J.* 119: 53P–54P.

Parker, W. H. and MaCrea, C. T. 1965. Bracken *(Pteris aquilina)* poisoning of sheep in the North York moors. *Vet. Rec.* 77: 861–865, 866.

Parsons, W. D. and Neims, A. H. 1978. Effect of smoking on caffeine clearance. *Clin. Pharmacol. Ther.* 24: 40.

Patil, B. C., Sharma, R. P., Salunkhe, D. K. and Salunkhe, K. 1972. Evaluation of solanine toxicity. *Food Cosmet. Toxicol.* 10: 395–398.

Patton, S. and Benson, A. A. 1966. Phytol metabolism in the bovine. *Biochim. Biophys. Acta* 125: 22–32.

Patwardhan, V. N. and White, J. W., Jr. 1973. Problems associated with particular foods. In: *Toxicants Occurring Naturally in Foods.* 2nd ed. National Academy of Sciences, Washington, D.C.

Patwardhan, R. V., Desmond, P. V., Johnson, R. F. and Schenker, S. 1980. Impaired elimination of caffeine by oral contraceptive steroids. *J. Lab. Clin. Med.* 95: 602.

Paul, O. et al. 1963. A longitudinal study of coronary heart disease. *Circulation* 28: 20–31.

Perel, E. and Lindner, H. R. 1970. Dissociation of uterotrophic action from implantation-inducing activity in two non-steroidal oestrogens (coumestrol and genistein). *J. Reprod. Fertil.* 21: 171–175.

Perrin, M., Dombray, P. and Vlaïcovitch, M. 1924. The experimental toxicity of garlic. *Hebdomadaires Soc. Biol. (Paris)* 1: 1431–1432. (French)

Peters, J. M. 1967. Factors affecting caffein toxicity. *J. Clin. Pharmacol.* 7: 131–141.

Pfeffer, M. and Ressler, C. 1967. β-Cyanoalanine, an inhibitor of rat liver cystathionase. *Biochem. Pharmacol.* 16: 2299–2308.

Phelps, R. A., Shenstone, F. S., Kemmerer, A. R. and Evans, R. J. 1965. A review of cyclopropenoid compounds: Biological effects of some derivatives. *Poult. Sci.* 44: 348–394.

Pictet, A. and Pictet, R. 1927. The volatile alkaloid of pepper. *Helv. Chim. Acta* 10: 593–595.

Pinckney, R. M. 1923. Sorghum as an indicator of available soil nitrogen. *Soil. Sci.* 17: 315–321.

Pinckney, R. M. 1924. Effect of nitrate applications upon the hydrocyanic acid content of sorghum. *J. Agric. Res.* 27: 717–723.

Pinder, A. R. 1953. An alkaloid of *Dioscorea hispida* Dennst. II. Hoffman degradation. *J. Chem. Soc.* 1953: 1825–1828.

Pope, G. S., Elcoate, P. V., Simpson, S. A. and Andrews, D. G. 1953. Isolation of an estrogenic isoflavone (biochanin A) from red clover. *Chem. Ind.* 1953: 1092.

Power, F. B. and Salway, A. H. 1907. The constituents of the essential oil of nutmeg. *J. Chem. Soc.* 91–92: 2037–2058.

Prchkov, V. K., Mookherjee, S., Schiess, W. and Obeid, A. I. 1974. Variant anginal syndrome, coronary artery spasms and ventricular fibrillation in absence of chest pain. *Ann. Intern. Med.* 81: 858–859.

Price, J. M. and Pamukcu, A. M. 1968. The induction of neoplasms of the urinary bladder of the cow and the small intestine of the rat by feeding bracken fern *(Pteris aquilina). Cancer Res.* 28: 2247–2251.

Price, M. L., Butler, L. G., Featherstone, W. R. and Rogler, J. C. 1978. Detoxification of high tannin sorghum grain. *Nutr. Rep. Int.* 17: 229–236.

Prineas, R. J., Jacobs, D. R., Jr., Crow, R. S. and Blackburn, H. 1980. Coffee, tea and VPB. *J. Chronic Dis.* 33: 67–72.

Przybylska, J. and Strong, F. M. 1968. Identification of γ-methylglutamic acid in *Lathyrus maritimus. Phytochemistry* 7: 471–475.

Purves, H. D. and Griesbach, W. E. 1947. Studies on experimental goitre. VIII. Thyroid tumours in rats treated with thiourea. *Br. J. Exp. Pathol.* 28: 46–53.

Quin, J. I., Rimington, C. and Roets, G. C. S. 1935. Studies on the photosensitisation of animals in South Africa. VIII. The biological formation of phylloerythrin in the digestive tracts of various domesticated animals. *Onderstepoort J. Vet. Sci.* 4: 463–478.

Raju, P. K. and Reiser, R. 1969. Alternate route for the biosynthesis of oleic acid in the rat. *Biochim. Biophys. Acta* 176: 48–53.

Rall, T. W. 1980. The xanthines. In: *The Pharmacological Basis of Therapeutics.* 6th ed. A. G. Gilman, L. S. Goodman and A. Gilman (eds.). Macmillan, New York.

Ramaswamy, H. N. and O'Connor, R. T. 1969. Metal complexes of gossypol. *J. Agric. Food Chem.* 17: 1406–1408.

Ramaswamy, H. N. and O'Connor, R. T. 1970. Spectroscopic properties of some metal complexes of gossypol. *Appl. Spectrosc.* 24: 50–52.

Ramprasad, C. and Sirsi, M. 1956. Indian medicinal plants: *Curcuma longa* — Effect of curcumin and the essential oils of *C. longa* on bile secretion. *J. Sci. Ind. Res. (India)* 15C: 262–265.

Ramprasad, C. and Sirsi, M. 1957a. *Curcuma longa* and bile secretion; quantitative changes in the bile constituents induced by sodium curcuminate. *J. Sci. Ind. Res. (India)* 16C: 108–110.

Ramprasad, C. and Sirsi, M. 1957b. Pharmacology of *Curcuma longa* L. (N.O. Scitaminaceae). *Ind. J. Physiol. Pharmacol.* 1: 136–143.

Rao, S. L. N. and Sarma, P. S. 1966. Neurotoxic properties of N-substituted oxamic acids. *Indian J. Biochem.* 3: 57–58.

Rao, S. L. N. and Sarma, P. S. 1967. Neurotoxic action of β-N-oxalyl-L-α, β-diaminopropionic acid. *Biochem. Pharmacol.* 16: 218–219.

Rao, S. L. N., Ramachandran, L. K. and Adiga, P. R. 1963. The isolation and characterization of L-homoarginine from seeds of *Lathyrus sativus*. *Biochemistry* 2: 298–300.

Rao, S. L. N. et al. 1967. Experimental neurolathyrism in monkeys. *Nature* 214: 610–611.

Rascop, A. M., Sheehan, E. T. and Vavich, M. G. 1966. Histomorphological changes in reproductive organs of rats fed cyclopropenoid fatty acids. *Proc. Soc. Exp. Biol. Med.* 122: 142–145.

Ratner, J. H., Spencer, S. K. and Grainge, J. M. 1974. Cashew nut dermatitis. An example of internal-external contact-type hypersensitivity. *Arch. Dermatol.* 110: 921–923.

Rauth, A. M., Barton, B. and Lee, C. P. Y. 1970. Effects of caffeine on L cells exposed to Mitomycin C7. *Cancer Res.* 30: 2724–2729.

Raymond, W. D., Jojo, W. and Nicodemus, Z. 1941. The nutritive value of some Tanganyika foods. II. Cassava. *Afr. Agric. J.* 6: 154–159.

Razin, A., Hershko, A., Glaser, G. and Mager, J. 1968. The oxidant effect of isouramil on red cell glutathione and its synergistic enhancement by ascorbic acid or 3,4-dihydroxyphenylalanine. *Isr. J. Med. Sci.* 4: 852–857.

Reich, P., Schwachman, H. and Craig, J. M. 1960. Lycopenemia: A variant of carotenemia. *N. Engl. J. Med.* 262: 263–269.

Reiders, F. 1971. Noxious gases and vapors 1: Carbon monoxide, cyanides, methemoglobin, and sulfhemoglobin. In: *Drill's Pharmacology in Medicine.* 4th ed. J. R. DiPalma (ed.). McGraw-Hill, New York.

Reiser, R. and Fu, H. C. 1962. The mechanism of gossypol detoxification by ruminant animals. *J. Nutr.* 76: 215–218.

Renwick, J. H. 1972. Hypothesis: Anencephaly and spina bifida are usually preventable by avoidance of a specific but unidentified substance present in certain potato tubers. *Br. J. Prevent. Soc. Med.* 26: 67–88.

Ressler, C. 1962. Isolation and identification from common vetch of the neurotoxin β-cyano-L-alanine, a possible factor in neurolathyrism. *J. Biol. Chem.* 237: 733–735.

Ressler, C., Redstone, P. A. and Ehrenberg, R. H. 1961. Isolation and identification of a neuroactive factor from *Lathyrus latifolius*. *Science* 134: 188–190.

Ressler, C., Nelson, J. and Pfeffer, M. 1964. A pyridoxal-β-cyanoalanine relation in the rat. *Nature* 203: 1286–1287.

Ressler, C., Nelson, J. and Pfeffer, M. 1967. Metabolism of β-cyanoalanine. *Biochem. Pharmacol.* 16: 2309–2319.

Ribereau-Gayon, P. 1972. *Plant Phenolics* (University Reviews in Botany, No. 3). Oliver and Boyd, Edinburgh, Scotland.

Ribereau-Gayon, P. and Stonestreet, E. 1966. Concentrations of tannins in red wine and its structural determination. *Chim. Anal.* 48: 188–196.

Richard, H. M. and Jennings, W. G. 1971. Volatile composition of black pepper. *J. Food Sci.* 36: 584–589.

Richard, H. M., Russell, G. F. and Jennings, W. G. 1971. The volatile components of black pepper varieties. *J. Chromatogr. Sci.* 9: 560–566.

Rigdon, R. H., Crass, G., Ferguson, T. M. and Couch, J. R. 1958. Effects of gossypol in young chickens with the production of a ceroid-like pigment. *A.M.A. Arch. Pathol.* 65: 228–235.

Riggin, R. M., McCarthy, M. J. and Kissinger, P. T. 1976. Identification of Salsolinol as a major dopamine metabolite in the banana. *J. Agric. Food Chem.* 24: 189–191.

Riggs, N. V. 1954. The occurrence of macrozamin in the seed of cycads. *Aust. J. Chem.* 7: 123–124.

Riggs, N. V. 1956. Glucosyloxyazoxymethane, a constituent of the seeds of *Cycas circinalis* L. *Chem. Ind.* 1956: 926.

Rimington, C. and Quin, J. I. 1934. Studies on the photosensitisation of animals in South Africa. VII. The nature of the photosensitising agent in geeldikkop. *Onderstepoort J. Vet. Sci. Anim. Ind.* 3: 137–157.

Rimington, C. and Quin, J. I. 1937. Dik-oor or geel-dikkop on grass-veld pastures. *J. S. Afr. Vet. Med. Assoc.* 8: 141–146.

Ritchie, J. M. 1975. Central nervous system stimulants. The xanthines. In: *The Pharmacological Basis of Therapeutics.* 5th ed. L. S. Goodman and A. Gilman (eds.). Macmillan, New York.

Roberts, H. R. and Barone, J. J. 1983. Biological effects of caffeine. History and use. *Food Tech.* 37(9): 32–39.

Roberts, J. J., Sturrock, J. E. and Ward, K. N. 1974. The enhancement by caffeine of alkylation-induced cell death, mutations and chromosomal aberrations in Chinese hamster cells, as a result of inhibition of post-replication DNA repair. *Mutat. Res.* 26: 129–243.

Robertson, D. et al. 1978. Effect of caffein on plasma renin activity, catecholamines and blood pressure. *N. Engl. J. Med.* 298: 181–186.

Robertson, D. et al. 1981. Tolerance to the humoral and hemodynamic effects of caffeine in man. *J. Clin. Invest.* 67: 1111.

Rocquelin, G., Cluzan, R. and Boccon, D. 1968. Comparative feeding values and physiological effects of rapeseed oil with a high content of erucic acid and rapeseed oil free from erucic acid. I. Effects on growth rate, feeding efficiency and physiology of various organs in the rat. *Ann. Biol. Anim. Biochim. Biophys.* 8: 395–406. (French)

Rocquelin, G., Martin, B. and Cluzan, R. 1970. Comparative physiological effects of rapeseed and canbra oils in the rat: Influence of the ratio of saturated to monounsaturated fatty acids. Proceedings of the International Conference on the Science, Technology and Marketing of Rapeseed and Rapeseed Products, Rapeseed Association of Canada, Winnipeg, Manitoba.

Roe, F. J. C. 1959. Oil of sweet orange: a possible role in carcinogenesis. *Br. J. Cancer* 13: 92–93.

Roe, F. J. C. 1960. Some newly discovered tumor-promoting substances. *Abh. Dtsch. Akad. Wiss. Berlin Kl. Med.* 3: 36–52.

Roe, F. J. C. and Field, W. E. H. 1965. Chronic toxicity of essential oils and certain other products of natural origin. *Food Cosmet. Toxicol.* 3: 311–323.

Roe, F. J. C. and Pierce, W. E. H. 1960. Tumor promotion by citrus oils: Tumors of the skin and urethral orifice in mice. *J. Natl. Cancer Inst.* 24: 1389–1402.

Roehm, J. N., Lee, D. J. and Sinnhuber, R. O. 1967. Accumulation and elimination of dietary gossypol in the organs of rainbow trout. *J. Nutr.* 92: 425–428.

Roine, P., Uksila, E., Teir, H. and Rapola, J. 1960. Histopathological changes in rats and pigs fed rapeseed oil. *Z. Ernahrungswiss.* 1: 118–124.

Rosin, A. and Ungar, H. 1957. Malignant tumors in the eyelids and the auricular region of thiourea-treated rats. *Cancer Res.* 17: 302—305.

Roth, J. A. and Ivy, A. C. 1944. The effect of caffeine upon gastric secretion in the dog, cat and man. *Am. J. Physiol.* 141: 454—461.

Roth, J. A., Ivy, A. C. and Atkinson, A. J. 1944. Caffeine and "peptic" ulcer. Relation of caffeine and caffeine-containing beverages to pathogenesis, diagnosis and management of "peptic" ulcer. *J.A.M.A.* 126: 814—820.

Royce, H. D., Harrison, J. R. and Hahn, E. R. 1941. Cotton root bark as a source of gossypol. *Oil Soap* 18: 27—29.

Ruddick, J. A., Harwig, J. and Scott, P. M. 1974. Nonteratogenicity in rats of blighted potatoes and compounds contained in them. *Teratology* 9: 165—168.

Rühl, R. 1951. Report on the pathology and toxicology of solanins. *Arch. Pharm.* 284: 67—74.

Rukmini, C. 1968. Isolation and purification of a new toxic factor from *Lathyrus sativus*. *Indian J. Biochem.* 5: 182—184.

Rukmini, C. 1969. Structure of the new toxin from *Lathyrus sativus*. *Indian J. Chem.* 7: 1062—1063.

Russell, G. F. and Jennings, W. G. 1969. Constituents of black pepper. Some oxygenated compounds. *J. Agric. Food Chem.* 17: 1107—1112.

Sabelli, H. C., Borison, R. L., Diamond, B. J. and Havdala, H. S. 1978. Phenylethylamine and brain function. *Biochem. Pharmacol.* 27: 1729—1730.

Sabine, J. R., Horton, B. J. and Wicks, M. B. 1973. Spontaneous tumors in C3H-A^{vy} and C3H-A^{vy}fB mice: High incidence in the United States and low incidence in Australia. *J. Natl. Cancer Inst.* 50: 1237—1242.

Saeed, A. R., Karamalla, K. A. and Khattab, A. H. 1976. Polyphenolic compounds in the pulp of *Mangifera indica* L. *J. Food Sci.* 41: 959—960.

Saito, D. et al. 1979. Tumors in mice fed quercetin (meeting abstract). Proceedings of the 38th Annual Meeting of the Japanese Cancer Association held in Tokyo, Japan, September 1979. Japanese Cancer Association, Tokyo, Japan.

Saito, D. et al. 1980. Test of carcinogenicity of quercetin, a widely distributed mutagen in food. Teratogenesis *Carcinogen. Mutagen.* 1: 213—221.

Salant, W. and Rieger, J. B. 1909. The toxicity of caffein. *J. Pharmacol. Exp. Ther.* 1: 572—574.

Salant, W. and Reiger, R. B. 1912. *The Toxicity of Caffeine: An Experimental Study of Different Species of Animals*. U.S. Department of Agriculture, Bureau of Chemistry Bulletin No. 148.

Saleh, N. A. M. and El-Ansari, M. A. I. 1975. Polyphenolics of twenty local varieties of *Mangifera indica*. *Planta Med.* 28: 125—130.

Salmon, R. E. 1969a. The relative value of rapeseed and soybean oil in chick starter diets. *Poult. Sci.* 48: 1045—1050.

Salmon, R. E. 1969b. Soybean versus rapeseed oil in turkey starter diets. *Poult. Sci.* 48: 87—93.

Sandler, M., Youdim, M. B. H. and Hanington, E. 1974. A phenylethylamine oxidising defect in migraine. *Nature* 250: 335—337.

Sansone, G., Segni, G. and DeCecco, C. 1958. Erythrocyte biochemical effect predisposing to favic hemolysis; preliminary research on Ligurian and Sardinian population. *Boll. Soc. Ital. Biol. Sper.* 34: 1558—1561. (Italian)

Sant'Ambrogio, G., Mognoni, P. and Ventrella, L. 1964. Plasma levels of caffeine after oral, intramuscular and intravenous administration. *Arch. Int. Pharmacodyn.* 150: 259—263.

Sapeika, N. 1969. *Food Pharmacology*. Thomas, Springfield, Illinois.

Sato, H., Sakamura, S. and Obata, Y. 1970. The isolation and characterization of N-methyltyramine, tyramine, and hordenine from sawa millet seeds. *Agric. Biol. Chem.* 34: 1254—1255.

Scheffer, J. G., Campello, A. P. and Voss, D. O. 1970. Pharmacological effects of hydroxocobalamin. Antagonism between hydroxocobalamin and cyanates. *Hospital (Rio de Janeiro)* 78: 391—397.

Schinkel, P. G. 1948. Infertility in ewes grazing subterranean clover pastures. Observations on breeding behavior following transfer to "sound" country. *Aust. Vet. J.* 24: 289–294.

Schneider, D. L., Kurnick, A. A., Vavich, M. G. and Kemmerer, A. R. 1962. Delay of sexual maturity in chickens by *Sterculia foetida* oil. *J. Nutr.* 77: 403–407.

Schneider, D. L., Sheehan, E. T., Vavich, M. G. and Kammerer, A. R. 1968. Effect of *Sterculia foetida* oil on weanling rat growth and survival. *J. Agric. Food Chem.* 16: 1022–1024.

Schobert, A. and Hamm, R. 1948. On alpha-amino-beta-cyanopropionic acid and on the reaction between cystine and potassium cyanide. *Chem. Ber.* 84: 571–576.

Schoental, R. 1969. Carcinogenic action of elaiomycin in rats. *Nature* 221: 765–766.

Schoental, R. 1976. Carcinogens in plants and microorganisms. In: *Chemical Carcinogens.* C. E. Searle (ed.). American Chemical Society, Washington, D.C.

Schoental, R. and Gibbard, S. 1972. Nasal and other tumours in rats given 3,4,5-trimethoxycinnamaldehyde, a derivative of sinapaldehyde and of other α, β-unsaturated aldehydic wood lignin constituents. *Br. J. Cancer* 26: 504–505.

Schoental, R. and Gibbard, S. 1976. Cited by Schoental, R. 1976. Carcinogens in plants and microorganisms. In: *Chemical Carcinogens.* C. E. Searle (ed.). American Chemical Society, Washington, D.C.

Schreiber, K. 1968. Steroid alkaloids: *Solanum* group. In: *The Alkaloids.* Vol. 10. R. H. F. Manske (ed.). Academic Press, New York.

Schwartze, E. W. and Alsberg, C. L. 1924. Pharmacology of gossypol. *J. Agric. Res.* 28: 191–198.

Schweitzer, J. W., Friedhoff, A. J. and Schwartz, R. 1975. Chocolate, β-phenylethylamine and migraine re-examined. *Nature* 257: 256.

Sealock, R. R. 1949. β-3,4-Dihydroxyphenyl-L-alanine. *Biochem. Prep.* 1: 25–28.

Sebrell, W. H. 1930. An anemia of dogs produced by feeding onion. *Pub. Health Rep.* 24: 1175–1191.

Seidel, C. F., Schinz, H. and Müller, P. H. 1944. Lavender oil. III. Monoterpene alcohols and acids occurring as esters in French lavender oil. *Helv. Chim. Acta* 27: 663–674.

Seifert, R. M., Buttery, R. G. and Ling, L. 1968. Identification of some constituents of carrot seed oil. *J. Sci. Food Agric.* 19: 383–385.

Sell, J. L. and Hodgson, G. C. 1962. Comparative value of dietary rapeseed oil, sunflower seed oil, soybean oil and animal tallow for chickens. *J. Nutr.* 76: 113–118.

Selye, H. 1957. Lathyrism. *Rev. Can. Biol.* 16: 1–82.

Seshadri, T. R. and Vasishta, K. 1964. Polyphenolic components of guava fruits. *Curr. Sci.* 33: 334–335.

Shah, S. R. A. 1939. Note on some cases of lathyrism in a Punjab village. *Indian Med. Gaz.* 74: 385–388.

Shank, R. C. and Magee, P. N. 1967. Similarities between the biochemical actions of cycasin and dimethylnitrosamine. *Biochem. J.* 105: 521–527.

Shenstone, F. S. and Vickery, J. R. 1959. Substances in plants of the order Malvale causing pink whites in stored eggs. *Poult. Sci.* 38: 1055–1070.

Sherry, C. J. and Burnett, R. E. 1978. Enhancement of ethanol-induced sleep by whole oil of nutmeg. *Experientia* 34: 492–493.

Shieh, T. R., Mathews, E., Wodzinski, R. J. and Ware, J. H. 1968. Effect of calcium and phosphate ions on the formation of soluble iron-gossypol complex. *J. Agric. Food Chem.* 16: 208–211.

Shilling, W. H., Crampton, R. F. and Longland, R. C. 1969. Metabolism of coumarin in man. *Nature* 221: 664–665.

Shubik, P. 1950. Studies on the promoting phase in the stages of carcinogenesis in mice, rats, rabbits and guinea pigs. *Cancer Res.* 10: 13–17.

Shulgin, A. T., Sargeant, T. and Narango, C. 1967. The chemistry and psycho-
pharmacology of nutmeg and of several related phenylisopropylamines. In:
Ethnopharmacologic Search for Psychoactive Drugs. D. H. Efron (ed.). U.S.
Public Health Service Publication No. 1645, Washington, D.C.

Shutt, D. A. 1967. Interaction of genistein with oestradiol in the reproductive tract
of the ovariectomized mouse. *J. Endocrinol.* 37: 231−232.

Silverman, D. T., Hoover, R. N., Swanson, G. M. and Hartge, P. 1983. The prevalence of coffee drinking among hospitalized and population-based control groups.
J.A.M.A. 249: 1877−1880.

Simon, E. and Kraicer, P. F. 1966. The blockade of insulin secretion by mannoheptulose. *Isr. J. Med. Sci.* 2: 785−799.

Simon, D., Yen, S. and Cole, P. 1975. Coffee drinking and cancer of the lower
urinary tract. *J. Natl. Cancer Inst.* 54: 587−591.

Singleton, V. L. and Esau, P. 1969. Phenolic substances in grapes and wine, and
their significance. In: *Advances in Food Research.* Suppl. 1. Academic Press,
New York.

Singleton, V. L. and Kratzer, F. H. 1969. Toxicity and related physiological activity of phenolic substances of plant origin. *J. Agric. Food Chem.* 17: 497−512.

Singleton, V. L. and Kratzer, F. H. 1973. Plant phenolics. In: *Toxicants Occurring Naturally in Foods.* National Academy of Science, Washington, D.C.

Siniscalco, M., Bernini, L., Latte, B. and Motulsky, A. G. 1961. Favism and
thalassaemia in Sardinia and their relationship to malaria. *Nature* 190:
1179−1180.

Sinnhuber, R. O., Wales, J. H. and Lee, D. J. 1966. Cyclopropenoids, cocarcinogens for aflatoxin-induced hepatoma in trout. *Fed. Proc. Fed. Am. Soc. Exp.
Biol.* 25: 555.

Skarzynski, B. 1933a. An estrogenic substance from plant material. *Nature* 131:
766.

Skarzynski, B. 1933b. Estrogenic substances of vegetable origin. *Bull. Intern.
Acad. Polonaise, Classe Sci. Math. Nat.* BII: 347−353.

Skutches, C. L., Herman, D. L. and Smith, F. H. 1973. Effect of intravenous
gossypol injection on iron utilization in swine. *J. Nutr.* 103: 851−855.

Skutches, C. L., Herman, D. L. and Smith, F. H. 1974. Effect of dietary free
gossypol on blood components and tissue iron in swine and rats. *J. Nutr.* 104:
415−422.

Small, J. 1949. Parsley seed. *Food* 18: 268−270.

Small, L. D., Bailey, J. H. and Cavallito, C. J. 1947. Alkyl thiosulfinates. *J. Am.
Chem. Soc.* 69: 1710−1713.

Smith, H. A. 1957. The pathology of gossypol poisoning. *Am. J. Pathol.* 33:
353−365.

Smith, A. D. M. 1961. Retrobulbar neuritis in Addisonian pernicious anemia. *Lancet*
1: 1001−1002.

Smith, L. A. 1962. *Blueprint for Cotton Research Area XX. Cottonseed.* National
Cotton Council of America, Memphis, Tennessee.

Smith, D. W. E. 1966. Mutagenicity of cycasin aglycone methylazoxy-methanol, a
naturally occurring carcinogen. *Science* 152: 1273−1274.

Smith, J. F. 1971. Studies on ovine infertility in agricultural regions of Western
Australia: Cervical mucus production by fertile and infertile ewes. *Aust. J.
Agric. Res.* 22: 523−529.

Smith, F. H. and Clawson, A. J. 1970. The effects of dietary gossypol on animals.
J. Am. Oil Chem. Soc. 47: 443−447.

Smith, D. M. and Levi, L. 1961. Treatment of compositional data for the characterization of essential oils. Determination of geographical origins of peppermint oils
by gas chromatographic analysis. *J. Agric. Food Chem.* 9: 230−244.

Smith, F. H., Rhyne, C. L. and Smart, V. W. 1961. Dietary evaluation of cottonseed protein from cotton bred for low gossypol content. *J. Agric. Food Chem.*
9: 82−84.

Smith, I., Kellow, A. H. and Hanington, E. 1970. A clinical and biochemical correlation between tyramine and migraine headache. *Headache* 10: 43—52.

Smithard, R., Cole, E. R., Kennedy, J. P. 1975. Response of teat enzymes of sheep and cattle to stimulation by stilbestrol and estrogenic subterranean clover. *Aust. J. Agric. Res.* 26: 1009—1015.

Snyder, S. H. et al. 1981. Adenosine receptors and the behavioral actions of methylxanthines. *Proc. Natl. Acad. Sci.* 78: 3260.

Soine, T. O. 1964. Naturally occurring coumarins and related physiological activity. *J. Pharm. Sci.* 53: 231—264.

Sollmann, T. and Pilcher, J. D. 1911. The actions of caffein on the mammalian circulation. I. The persistent effects of caffeine on the circulation. *J. Pharmacol. Exp. Ther.* 3: 19—92.

Somogyi, J. C. and Nagell, U. 1976. Antithiamine effect of coffee. Preliminary communication. *Int. J. Vitam. Nutr. Res.* 46: 149—153.

Soule, M. J. and Harding, P. L. 1956. Effects of size and date of sampling on starch, sugars, soluble solids and phenolic compounds in mangos. Proceedings of the Florida Mango Forum, 16th Annual Meeting, October 3, Fort Lauderdale.

Spatz, M. 1964. Carcinogenic effect of cycad meal in guinea pigs. *Fed. Proc.* 23: 1384—1385.

Spatz, M. 1968. Hydrolysis of cycasin by β-D-glucosidase in skin of newborn rats. *Proc. Soc. Exp. Biol. Med.* 128: 1005—1008.

Spatz, M. 1970. Carcinogenicity of methylazoxymethanol (MAM) in guinea pigs and hamsters. Abstr. 10th Int. Cancer Congress. Houston, Texas.

Spatz, M. and Lacquer, G. L. 1967. Transplacental induction of tumors in Sprague-Dawley rats with crude cycad material. *J. Natl. Cancer Inst.* 38: 233—245.

Spatz, M. and Lacquer, G. L. 1968. Evidence for transplacental passage of the natural carcinogen cycasin and its aglycone. *Proc. Soc. Exp. Biol. Med.* 127: 281—286.

Spatz, M., McDaniel, E. G. and Lacquer, G. L. 1966. Cycasin excretion in conventional and germ-free rats. *Proc. Soc. Exp. Biol. Med.* 121: 417—422.

Spatz, M., Smith, D. W. E., McDaniel, E. G. and Lacquer, G. L. 1967. Role of intestinal microorganisms in determining cycasin toxicity. *Proc. Soc. Exp. Biol.* 124: 691—697.

Spector, W. S. 1956. *Handbook of Toxicology.* Vol. 1. *Acute Toxicities.* Saunders, Philadelphia.

Spector, S., Melmon, K., Lovenberg, W. and Sjoerdsma, A. 1963. The presence and distribution of tyramine in mammalian tissues. *J. Pharmacol. Exp. Ther.* 140: 229—235.

Sporn, A. 1960. Toxicity of coumarin as a flavoring agent. *Igiena* 9: 121—126.

Srivastava, S. K. and Beutler, E. 1968. Oxidized glutathione levels in erythrocytes of glucose-6-phosphate dehydrogenase deficient subjects. *Lancet* 2: 23—24.

Stachelberger, H. et al. 1977. Quantitative determination of some biogenic amines in bananas, dates and figs. *Qual. Plant.-Plant Foods Hum. Nutr.* 27: 287—291.

Stamatoyannopoulos, G. et al. 1966. On the familial predisposition to favism. *Am. J. Hm. Genet.* 18: 253—263.

Statland, B. E. and Demas, T. J. 1980. Serum caffeine half-lives: Healthy subjects vs. patients having alcoholic hepatic disease. *Am. J. Clin. Pathol.* 73: 390.

Stecher, P. G., Finkel, M. J. and Siegmund, O. H. (eds.). 1960. *The Merck Index of Chemicals and Drugs.* 7th ed. Merck & Co., Rahway, New Jersey.

Stefansson, B. R., Hougen, F. W. and Downey, R. K. 1961. Note on the isolation of rape plants with seed oil free from erucic acid. *Can. J. Plant Sci.* 41: 218—219.

Stenlid, G. 1968. The physiological effects of phlorizin, phloretin, and some related substances upon higher plants. *Physiol. Plant.* 21: 882—894.

Stern, R. S. et al. 1979. Risk of cutaneous carcinoma in patients treated with oral methoxsalen photochemotherapy for psoriasis. *N. Engl. J. Med.* 300: 809—813.

Sternkopf, G. and Amin, A. 1973. Amino acid composition of Iraqi dates. *Nahrung* 17: 233–236.

Stevens, C. M. and Bush, J. A. 1950. New syntheses of α-amino-ε-guanidino-n-caproic acid (homoarginine) and its possible conversion in vivo into lysine. *J. Biol. Chem.* 183: 139–147.

Stewart, I. and Wheaton, T. A. 1964. L-Octopamine in citrus: isolation and identification. *Science* 145: 60–61.

Stieve, H. 1938. Organ injury due to coffee and caffeine. *Z. Mikrosk. Anat. Forsch.* 43: 509. (German)

Stockman, R. 1929. Lathyrism. *J. Pharmacol. Exp. Ther.* 37: 43–53.

Stokes, G. B. and Walker, D. M. 1970. The nutritive value of fat in the diet of the milk-fed lamb. II. The effect of different dietary fats on the composition of the body fats. *Br. J. Nutr.* 24: 435–440.

Stoll, A. and Seebeck, E. 1948. *Allium* compounds. I. Alliine, the true mother compound of garlic oil. *Helv. Chim. Acta* 31: 189–210. (German)

Stoll, A. and Seebeck, E. 1949. *Allium* compounds. II. Enzymic degradation of alliine and the properties of alliinase. *Helv. Chim. Acta* 32: 197–205. (German)

Stoll, M. et al. 1967. Research on aromas. XIII. Coffee aroma. 1. *Helv. Chim. Acta* 50: 628–694. (French)

Stout, M. G., Reich, H. and Huffman, M. N. 1963. 4',5,6,7-Oxygenated flavones and flavanones. *J. Pharm. Sci.* 53: 192–195.

Stout, M. G., Reich, H. and Huffman, M. N. 1964. Neonatal lethality of offspring of tangeretin-treated rats. *Cancer Chemother. Rep.* 36: 23–24.

Strubelt, O. and Siegers, C.-P. 1969. On the mechanism of the calorigenic effect of theophylline and caffeine. *Biochem. Pharmacol.* 18: 1207–1220. (German)

Sturelid, S. and Kihlman, B. A. 1975. Enhancement by methylated oxypurines of the frequency of induced chromosomal aberrations. I. The dependence of the effect on the molecular structure of the potentiating agent. *Hereditas* 79: 29–42.

Swain, T. 1965. Nature and properties of flavonoids. In: *Chemistry and Biochemistry of Plant Pigments.* T. W. Goodwin (ed.). Academic Press, New York.

Swain, T. and Bate-Smith, E. C. 1962. Flavonoid compounds. In: *Comparative Biochemistry.* Vol. III. A. M. Florkin and H. S. Mason (eds.). Academic Press, New York.

Swinyard, C. A. and Chaube, S. 1973. Are potatoes teratogenic for experimental animals? *Teratology* 8: 349–357.

Szeinberg, A. and Chari-Bitron, A. 1957. Blood glutathione concentration after haemolytic anaemia due to *Vicia faba* or sulfonamides. *Acta Haematol.* 18: 229–233.

Szeinberg, A., Asher, Y. and Sheba, C. 1958a. Studies on glutathione stability in erythrocytes of cases with past history of favism or sulfa drug-induced hemolysis. *Blood* 13: 348–358.

Szeinberg, A., Sheba, Ch. and Adam, A. 1958b. Enzymatic abnormality in erythrocytes of a population sensitive to *Vicia faba* or haemolytic anaemia induced by drugs. *Nature* 181: 1256.

Szeinberg, A., Sheba, Ch. and Adam, A. 1958c. Selective occurrence of glutathione instability in red blood corpuscles of the various Jewish tribes. *Blood* 13: 1043–1053.

Takeuchi, K., Kogo, H. and Aizawa, Y. 1980. Effect of methylxanthines on urinary prostaglandin E secretion in rats. *Jpn. J. Pharmacol.* 31: 253.

Tanksley, T. D., Jr. et al. 1970. Inhibition of pepsinogen activation by gossypol. *J. Biol. Chem.* 245: 6456–6461.

Taylor, J. M. 1973. Cited by Hall, R. L. Toxicants occurring naturally in spices and flavors. In: *Toxicants Occurring Naturally in Foods.* 2nd ed. National Academy of Sciences, Washington, D.C.

Taylor, J. M. et al. 1967. Toxicity of oil of calamus (Jammu variety). *Toxicol. Appl. Pharmacol.* 10: 405.

Teas, H. J. and Dyson, J. G. 1967. Mutation in Drosophila by methylazoxymethanol, the aglycon of cycasin. *Proc. Soc. Exp. Biol. Med.* 125: 988—990.

Tellez de Inon, M. T. 1968. Inhibition of mitochondrial ATPase by phlorizin. *Acta Physiol. Lat. Am.* 18: 268—271.

Terbrüggen, A. 1936. Fatal solanine poisoning. The importance of the combination of acute brain swelling with diminished skull capacity. *Beitr. Pathol. Anat.* 97: 391—395. (German)

Thayer, P. S. and Palm, P. E. 1975. A current assessment of the mutagenic and teratogenic effects of caffeine. In: *CRC Critical Reviews in Toxicology.* L. Golberg (ed.). CRC Press, Cleveland.

Thomas, J. G. 1962. Peppermint fibrillation. *Lancet* 1: 222.

Thomasson, H. J. 1955. The biological value of oils and fats. I. Growth and food intake on feeding with natural oils and fats. *J. Nutr.* 56: 455—468.

Thomasson, H. J. and Boldingh, J. 1955. The biological value of oils and fats. II. The growth-retarding substance in rapeseed oil. *J. Nutr.* 56: 469—475.

Thomasson, H. J., Gottenbos, J. J., Van Pijpen, P. L. and Vles, R. O. 1970. Nutritive value of rapeseed oil. *Zesz. Probl. Postepow Nauk Roln.* 91: 381—402.

Thoron, A. 1969. Interpretation of the particular nutritional character of rapeseed oil. Tests on the pig and the rat. *Ann. Nutr. Aliment.* 23: 103—116.

Thorp, F. Jr. and Harshfield, G. S. 1939. Onion poisoning in horses. *J. Am. Vet. Med. Assoc.* 94: 52—53.

Tikhonova, L. K. and Goryaev, M. I. 1957. The chemical composition of the essential oil from *Artemisia ferganensis. Izvest. Akad. Nauk Kazakh. S.S.R., Ser. Khim.* 2: 65—74.

Timson, J. 1972. Effect of theobromine, theophylline, and caffeine on the mitosis of human lymphocytes. *Mutat. Res.* 15: 197—201.

Tinao, M. M. and Terren, R. C. 1955. Actions of *Allium sativum* (garlic) and combinations on uterine motility. *Arch. Inst. Farmacol. Exp.* (Madr.) 8: 127—147.

Tone, J. N. and Jensen, D. R. 1970. Effect of ingested gossypol on the growth performance of rats. *Experientia* 26: 970—971.

Torlone, V. and Rampichini, L. 1959. Contribution to the studies on photosensitivity disease among domestic animals. III. Assessment of the morphology, histochemistry and behavior of mast cells of ovine skin photosensitized with phylloerythrin. *Arch. Vet. Ital.* 10: 501—517. (Italian)

Tressl, R., Drawert, F., Heimann, W. and Emberger, R. 1969. Gas chromatographic analysis of banana aroma compounds. *Z. Naturforsch.* 24B: 781—783. (German)

Tressl, R., Drawert, F. and Heimann, W. 1970. On the biogenesis of aroma substances in plants and fruits. VII. The fatty acids of banana aroma. *S. Lebens. Unters Forsch.* 142: 393—397. (German)

Trosko, J. E. and Chu, E. H. Y. 1973. Inhibition of repair of UV-damaged DNA by caffeine and mutation induction in Chinese hamster cells. *Chem. Biol. Interact.* 6: 317—332.

Trosko, J. E., Frank, P., Chu, E. H. Y. and Becker, J. E. 1973. Caffeine inhibition of post-replication repair of N-acetoxy-2-acetylaminofluorene-damaged DNA in Chinese hamster cells. *Cancer Res.* 33: 2444—2449.

Truit, E. B., Jr. 1967. The pharmacology of myristicin and nutmeg. In: *Ethnopharmacologic Search for Psychoactive Drugs.* D. H. Efron (ed.). U.S. Public Health Service, Publication No. 1645, Washington, D.C.

Truit, E. B., Jr. and Ebersberger, E. M. 1962. Evidence of monoamine oxidase inhibition by myristicin and nutmeg in vivo. *Fed. Proc.* 21: 418.

Truit, E. B., Jr., Callaway, E., III., Braude, M. C. and Krantz, J. C., Jr. 1961. The pharmacology of myristicin. A contribution to the psychopharmacology of nutmeg. *J. Neuropsychiatry.* 2: 205—210.

Ts'o, P.O. and Lu, P. 1964. Interaction of nucleic acids. I. Physical binding of thymine, adenine, steroids, and aromatic hydrocarbons to nucleic acids. *Proc. Natl. Acad. Sci.* 51: 17—24.

Tuffley, B. J. M. and Williams, C. H. 1951. The pharmacology of carpaine. *Aust. J. Pharm.* 52: 796–798.

Udenfriend, S., Lovenberg, W. and Sjoerdsma, A. 1959. Physiologically active amines in common fruits and vegetables. *Arch. Biochem. Biophys.* 85: 487–490.

Ulmann, S. B., Halberstaedter, L. and Liebowitz, J. 1945. Some pharmacological and biological effects of the latex of *Ficus carica* L. *Exp. Med. Surg.* 3: 11–23.

Ulrich, R. 1958. *Coffee and Caffeine.* Wright, Bristol, England.

Umberto de Torrescasana, E. 1946. Experimental studies of the pharmacology of the active principles of *Allium sativum* (garlic). *Rev. Espan. Fisiol.* 2: 6–31.

Umezawa, K. et al. 1977. In vitro transformation of hamster embryo cells by quercetin. *Toxicol. Lett.* 1: 175–178.

Uribe, E. G. 1970. Phloretin: An inhibitor of phosphate transfer and electron flow in spinach chloroplasts. *Biochem.* 9: 2100–2106.

Vacca, G. 1926. Research on testicular changes following experimental administration of caffeine. *Arch. Farmacol. Sper.* 42: 62–78. (Italian)

Valeri, H. and Gimeno, F. N. 1954. Phytochemical and toxicological study of the fruits of the avocado pear *(Persea americana)*. *Rev. Med. Vet. Parasitol.* (Caracas) 12: 131–165.

Vanderlaan, J. E. and Vanderlaan, W. P. 1947. The iodide-concentrating mechanism of the rat thyroid and its inhibition by thiocyanate. *Endocrinology* 40: 403–416.

Van der Wal, B., Sipma, G., Kettenes, D. K. and Semper, A. Th. J. 1968. Some new constituents of roasted cocoa. *Rec. Trav. Chim. Pays-Bas* 87: 238–240.

Van der Wal, B. et al. 1971. New volatile components of roasted cocoa. *J. Agric. Food Chem.* 19: 276–280.

Van Duuren, B. L. 1965. Carcinogenic epoxides, lactones, and hydroperoxides. In: *Mycotoxins in Foodstuffs.* G. Hogan (ed.). M.I.T. Press, Cambridge, Massachusetts.

Van Duuren, B. L. 1976. Tumor-promoting and co-carcinogenic agents in chemical carcinogenesis. In: *Chemical Carcinogens.* C. E. Searle (ed.). American Chemical Society, Washington, D.C.

Van Duuren, B. L. et al. 1963. Carcinogenicity of epoxides, lactones and peroxy compounds. *J. Natl. Cancer Inst.* 31: 41–55.

Van Duuren, B. L. et al. 1971. Carcinogenesis studies on mouse skin and inhibition of tumor induction. *J. Natl. Cancer Inst.* 46: 1039–1044.

Vanetten, C. H. and Miller, R. W. 1963. The neuroactive factor alpha-gamma diaminobutyric acid in angiosperm seeds. *Econ. Bot.* 17: 107–109.

Vasistha, S. K. and Siddiquiy, S. 1938. Chemical examination of mango "Chep," the exudation of the fruit of *Mangifera indica*. *J. Indian Chem. Soc.* 15: 110–117.

Ventura, M. M. and Hollanda-Lima, I. 1961. Ornithine cycle amino acids and other free amino acids in fruits of *A. squamosa* L. and *A. muricata* L. *Phyton* 17: 39–47.

Vernazza, N. 1957. Thujone in dalmation sage oil. *Acta Pharm. Jugoslav.* 7: 163–168.

Vesselinovitch, S. D., Mihailovich, N. and Rao, K. V. 1979b. Development of kidney and liver tumors in offspring of mice exposed to safrole during gestation and lactation (meeting abstract). *Proc. Am. Assoc. Cancer Res.* 20: 164.

Vesselinovitch, S. D., Rao, K. V. and Mihailovich, N. 1979a. Transplacental and lactational carcinogenesis by safrole. *Cancer Res.* 39: 4378–4380.

Viehoever, A. 1940. Edible and poisonous beans of the lima type *(Phaseolus lunatus L.) Thailand Sci. Bull.* 2: 1–99.

Vieira Lopes, L. C. and Campello, A. P. 1975. Effect of hydroxycobalamine on the inhibition of cytochrome *c* oxidase by cyanide. I. In intact mitochondria. *Res. Commun. Chem. Pathol. Pharmacol.* 12: 521–532.

Viktora, J. K. et al. 1969. Effect of ingested mannoheptulose in animals and man. *Metabolism* 18(part 1): 87–102.

Virtanen, A. I. and Matikkala, E. J. 1959. The structure and synthesis of cyclo-alliin isolated from *Allium cepa. Acta Chem. Scand.* 13: 623–626.

Vles, R. O. and Abdellatif, A. M. M. 1970. Effects of hardened palm oil on rape-seed oil-induced changes in ducklings and guinea pigs. *Proc. Internat. Conf. Science, Technology and Marketing of Rapeseed and Rapeseed Products. Rape-seed Association of Canada, Winnipeg, Manitoba.*

Vles, R. O. et al. 1976. Nutritional status of low-erucic acid rapeseed oils. *Fette, Seifen, Anstrichm.* 78: 128–131.

Voegtlin, C., Johnson, J. M. and Dryer, H. A. 1926. Biological significance of cystine and glutathione mechanism of cyanide action. *J. Pharmacol. Exp. Ther.* 27: 467–483.

Von Borstel, R. W. 1983. Biological effects of caffeine. Metabolism. *Food. Technol.* 37(9): 40–43.

Von Borstel, R. W., Conlay, L. C. and Wurtman, R. J. 1983. Chronic caffeine con-sumption potentiates the hypotensive action of circulating adenosine. *Life Sci.* 32: 1151.

Von Oettingen, W. F. 1952. *Poisoning: A Guide to Clinical Diagnosis and Treat-ment.* Hoeber, New York.

Wada, H. and Fukushima, S. 1963. Estrogenic activity in soybeans and its products. *Jpn. J. Zootechnol. Sci.* 34: 243–247.

Wada, H. and Yuhara, M. 1964. Identification of plant estrogens in Chinese milk vetch, soybean and soybean sprout. *Jpn. J. Zootechnol. Sci.* 35: 87.

Walker, B. S. and Janney, J. C. 1930. Estrogenic substances. II. An analysis of plant sources. *Endocrinology* 14: 389–392.

Walker, I. G. and Reid, B. D. 1971. Caffeine potentiation of the lethal action of alkylating agents on L-cells. *Mutat. Res.* 12: 101–104.

Walpole, A. L. 1962. Observations upon the induction of subcutaneous sarcomata in rats. In: *The Morphological Precursors of Cancer.* L. Severi (ed.). University of Perugia, Italy.

Walter, E. D. 1941. Genistin (an isoflavone glucoside) and its aglucone, genistein, from soybeans. *J. Am. Chem. Soc.* 63: 3273–3276.

Walz, E. 1931. Isoflavone and saponin glycosides in *Soja hispida. Liebigs. Ann.* 489: 118–155. (German)

Wang, S. L. T. 1970. "Glycoalkaloid and Demethyl Sterol Content in Some Potato Varieties and Clones." Ph.D. Thesis, Michigan State University, East Lansing.

Wang, C. Y., Chiu, C. W., Pamukcu, A. M. and Bryan, G. T. 1976. Identification of carcinogenic tannin isolated from bracken fern *(Pteridium aquilinum). J. Natl. Cancer Inst.* 56: 33–36.

Warkany, F. 1971. *Congenital Malformations.* Vol. 1. Academic Press, New York.

Watkins, J. C., Curtis, D. R. and Briscoe, T. J. 1966. Central effects of β-N-oxalyl-α,β-diaminopropionic acid and other lathyrus factors. *Nature* 211: 637.

Watson, W. A., Barlow, R. M. and Barnett, K. C. 1965. Bright blindness — a con-dition prevalent in Yorkshire hill sheep. *Vet. Rec.* 77: 1060–1069.

Watson, W. A. et al. 1972a. Experimentally produced progressive retinal degenera-tion (bright blindness) in sheep. *Br. Vet. J.* 128: 457–469.

Watson, W. A., Barnett, K. C. and Terlecki, S. 1972b. Progressive retinal degen-eration (bright blindness) in sheep: A review. *Vet. Rec.* 91: 665–670.

Watt, J. M. and Breyer-Brandwijk, M. G. 1962. *The Medicinal and Poisonous Plants of Southern and Eastern Africa.* 2nd ed. Livingstone, London.

Wattenberg, L. W., Page, M. A. and Leong, J. L. 1968. Induction of increased benzopyrene hydroxylase activity by flavones and related compounds. *Cancer Res.* 28: 934–937.

Webb, L. J. 1948. *Guide to the Medicinal and Poisonous Plants of Queensland, Austra-lia.* Council for Scientific and Industrial Research Bulletin No. 232. Queensland, Australia.

Weil, A. T. 1965. Nutmeg as a narcotic. *Econ. Bot.* 19: 194–217.

Weinstein, D., Mauer, I., Katz, M. and Kazmer, S. 1973. The effect of caffeine on chromosomes of human lymphocytes: Non-random distribution of damage. *Mutat. Res.* 20: 441–443.

Weinstein, D., Mauer, J., Katz, M. L. and Kazmer, S. 1975. The effect of methyl-xanthines on chromosomes of human lymphocytes in culture. *Mutat. Res.* 31: 57–61.

Weiss, B. and Laties, V. G. 1962. Enhancement of human performance by caffeine and the amphetamines. *Pharmacol. Rev.* 14: 1–36.

Weiss, G. 1960. Hallucinogenic and narcotic-like effects of powdered myristica (nut-meg). *Psychiatr. Q.* 34: 346–356.

West, G. B. 1959. Tryptamines in tomatoes. *J. Pharm. Pharmacol.* 11: 319–320.

Wheaton, T. A. and Stewart, I. 1969. Biosynthesis of synephrine in citrus. *Phytochemistry* 8: 85–92.

White, T., Kirby, K. S. and Knowles, E. 1952. Tannins. IV. The complexity of tannin extract composition. *J. Soc. Leather Trades' Chem.* 36: 148–155.

Whiting, M. G. 1963. Toxicity of cycads. *Econ. Bot.* 17: 271–302.

Williams, A. H. 1966. Dihydrochalcones. In: *Comparative Phytochemistry.* T. Swain (ed.). Academic Press, New York.

Williams, A. O. and Osuntokun, B. O. 1969. Light and electron microscopy of per-ipheral nerves in tropical ataxic neuropathy. *Arch. Neurol.* 21: 475–492.

Williams, J. N., Jr. and Lacquer, G. L. 1965. Response of liver nucleic acids and lipids in rats fed *Cycas circinalis* endosperm or cycasin. *Proc. Soc. Exp. Biol. Med.* 118: 1–4.

Williams, R. T. 1970. Gut flora in safety testing of food additives. In: *Metabolic Aspects of Food Safety.* F. J. C. Roe (ed.). Academic Press, New York.

Willimott, S. G. 1933. An investigation of solanine poisoning. *Analyst* 58: 431–439.

Wilson, J., Linnell, J. C. and Matthews, D. M. 1971. Plasma-cobalamins in neuro-opthalmological diseases. *Lancet* 1: 259–261.

Winkler, W. O. 1951. Report on hydrocyanic glucosides. *J. Assoc. Off. Agric. Chem.* 34: 541.

Winkler, W. O. 1958. Study of methods for glucosidal HCN in lima beans. *J. Assoc. Off. Agric. Chem.* 41: 282–287.

Wislocki, P. G., Borchert, P., Miller, J. A. and Miller, E. C. 1976. The metabolic activation of the carcinogen 1'-hydroxysafrole in vivo and in vitro and the elec-trophilic reactivities of possible ultimate carcinogens. *Cancer Res.* 36: 1686–1695.

Wislocki, P. G. et al. 1977. Carcinogenic and mutagenic activities of safrole, 1'-hydroxysafrole, and some known or possible metabolites. *Cancer Res.* 37: 1883–1891.

Wokes, F. 1952. The direct use of plant materials by man. *Br. J. Nutr.* 6: 118–124.

Wokes, F. and Pikard, C. W. 1955. The role of vitamin B_{12} in human nutrition. *Am. J. Clin. Nutr.* 3: 383–390.

Wolf, M. J. and Duggar, B. M. 1946. Estimation and physiological role of solanine in the potato. *J. Agric. Res.* 73: 1–32.

Wong, R. C., Hakagawa, Y. and Perlmann, G. E. 1972. Studies on the nature of the inhibition by gossypol of the transformation of pepsinogen to pepsin. *J. Biol. Chem.* 247: 1625–1631.

Wood, T. 1965. The cyanogenic glucoside content of cassava and cassava products. *J. Sci. Food Agric.* 16: 300–305.

Wood, J. L. and Cooley, S. L. 1956. Detoxication of cyanide by cystine. *J. Biol. Chem.* 218: 449–457.

Wood, J. L. and Fiedler, H. 1953. β-Mercaptopyruvate, a substrate for rhodanese. *J. Biol. Chem.* 205: 221–234.

Worden, A. N. 1940. The toxicity of laevulose cyanhydrin, together with general observations on cyanide poisoning. *Vet. Rec.* 52: 857–865.

World Health Organization 1967. *Standardization Procedures for the Study of Glucose-6-Phosphate Dehydrogenase.* Report of the WHO Scientific Group. WHO Tech. Rep. Ser. 366, Geneva.

Wrolstad, R. E. and Jennings, W. G. 1965. Volatile constituents of black pepper. III. The monoterpene hydrocarbon fraction. *J. Food Sci.* 30: 274—279.

Würzner, H. P., Lindstrom, E., Vuataz, L. and Luginbühl, H. 1977. A 2-year feeding study of instant coffees in rats. 1. Body weight, food consumption, haematological parameters and plasma chemistry. *Food Cosmet. Toxicol.* 15: 7—16.

Yang, M. G., Mickelsen, O., Sanger, V. L. 1969. Cycling of cycasin from newborn rats to their mother and back to the newborn. *Proc. Soc. Exp. Biol. Med.* 131: 135—137.

Zedeck, M. S. and Sternberg, S. S. 1975. Megalocytosis and other abnormalities expressed during proliferation in regenerating liver of rats treated with methylazoxymethanol acetate prior to partial hepatectomy. *Cancer Res.* 35: 2117—2122.

Zedeck, M. S., Sternberg, S. S., Poynter, R. W. and McGowan, J. 1970. Biochemical and pathological effects of methylazoxymethanol acetate, a potent carcinogen. *Cancer Res.* 30: 801—812.

Zedeck, M. S. et al. 1972. Methylazoxymethanol acetate: Induction of tumors and early effects of RNA synthesis. *Fed. Proc.* 31: 1485—1492.

Zenisek, A. and Bednar, I. J. 1960. Contribution to the identification of the estrogenic activity of hops. *Am. Perfumer Aromst.* 75: 61—62.

Zinkham, W. H., Lenhard, R. E., Jr. and Childs, B. 1958. A deficiency of glucose-6-phosphate dehydrogenase activity in erythrocytes from patients with favism. *Bull. Johns Hopkins Hosp.* 102: 169—175.

Zitnak, A. and Johnson, G. R. 1970. Glycoalkaloid content of B5141-6 potatoes. *Am. Potato J.* 47: 256—260.

Zukerman, I. 1951. The effect of oxidized d-limonene on microorganisms. *Nature* 168: 517.

9

Naturally Occurring Antinutritive Substances

Deficiency of nutrients and interference in the utilization and function of nutrients and similar essential compounds, as discussed in Chapter 1, are among the biochemical mechanisms underlying the toxicity of compounds. Thus, compounds which have the capability of producing nutritional deficiency or interfering in the utilization and function of nutrients are considered to be toxicants. These compounds are correctly called antinutritive substances (or simply antinutritives), as defined by Gontzea and Sutzescu (1968), who first introduced the concept. This concept includes the antimetabolites. Thus, the term antinutritive substances has a broader meaning than the latter with respect to the locus of reaction, since the effect of antinutritives include reactions taking place in the gastrointestinal tract, in the tissues, and in a few cases, even outside the body. For example, a substance may degrade a vitamin outside the body. Examples of this type of substance will be seen later in this chapter. On the other hand, the term antinutritives may have a more restricted meaning than the term antimetabolites because the antinutritives are obviously limited only to the nutrients, whereas metabolites include all metabolites.

There are many good examples of antinutritives among drugs, antibiotics, pesticides, and other economic poisons. However, this chapter will be limited only to endogenous or naturally occurring substances. Synthetic antinutritives are examined in the chapter on chemical contaminants (Chap. 19) and to some extent in the chapter on food additives (Chap. 21).

In many cases, the deleterious effects of antinutritives may not be readily observable as those of other food toxicants unless consumed in large amounts. Thus, the toxicity of many compounds in this category are highly conditional, dependent on the biological condition of the host and other factors. In other words, many antinutritives are potential toxicants, as defined in a broad sense in Chap. 1. An example of a condition whereby antinutritives may have significant impact is malnutrition or marginal nutritional status. The presence of antinutritives may aggravate or precipitate malnutrition, respectively.

Gontzea and Sutzescu (1968) have classified the antinutritive substances as follows:

1. Type A — Substances which interfere with the digestion of proteins or the absorption and utilization of amino acids and other nutrients.
2. Type B — All substances interfering with the absorption or metabolic utilization of mineral elements.
3. Type C — Substances which inactivate or destroy vitamins or otherwise in-

crease their metabolic requirements in the organism. This category also includes those substances which function as antimetabolites to the vitamins.

TYPE A

Digestive Protease Inhibitors

Protease inhibitors apparently occur in many plant and animal tissues (Fritz and
Tschesche 1971; Vogel et al. 1966). The toxicological and nutritional significance of
these inhibitors to the human situation depends mostly on their activity on human
proteases. As we shall see, some of these inhibitors may have no significance in
relation to human digestive function.

Proteolytic enzyme inhibitors in avian eggs were recognized around the turn of
the century (Delezenne and Pozerski 1903). Two inhibitors were later identified,
ovomucoid (Lineweaver and Murray 1947) and ovoinhibitor (Matsushima 1958), which
inactivate trypsin by forming a stable inhibitor-trypsin complex. Chymotrypsin inhibitors also are found in avian egg whites (Rhodes et al. 1960).

Three types of inhibitors are found in avian eggs based on their specificities
to trypsin or chymotrypsin (Rhodes et al. 1960).

Trypsin and/or chymotrypsin inhibitors also are found in soybeans and other
legumes and pulses (Sohonie and Bhandarkar 1955; Jaffe 1950; Borchers and Ackerson 1950; Kunitz 1945), vegetables (Sohonie and Bhandarkar 1954), milk and colostrum (Kiermeier and Semper 1960a), blood (West and Hilliard 1949), wheat and
other cereal grains, guar gum, and white and sweet potatoes (Couch et al. 1966;
Learmonth and Wood 1960, 1963; Shyamala et al. 1961; Gontzea and Gardev 1958;
Sohonie and Honavar 1956). The sweet potato inhibitor appears to inhibit trypsin
completely, as opposed to the other inhibitors.

In addition to trypsin and chymotrypsin, the protease inhibitors of certain
legumes and potatoes also inhibit elastase (pancreato peptidase). The elastase inhibitor from potatoes has a highly selective and potent effect (Solyom et al. 1964).
The potato chymotrypsin inhibitor also has a potent effect on carboxypeptidase B
(Ryan 1966). The trypsin inhibitor in this tuber also inactivates pepsin (Werle et al.
1959). The inhibitor in kidney beans not only affects trypsin and chymotrypsin, but
also elastase (Pusztai 1968). The inhibitor has a slight effect on carboxypeptidase B
as well as on other nondigestive proteases. The soybean trypsin inhibitor also has
an effect on both chymotrypsin and elastase (Marshall et al. 1969; Walford and Kickhofen 1962).

There is a wide range of foodstuffs from angiospermous plants which contain
protease inhibitors, as can be seen from the list compiled by Liener and Kakade
(1969).

Animals given food containing active inhibitors show growth depression (Rackis
et al. 1975, 1979). This appears to be due to interference in trypsin and chymotrypsin activities and to excessive stimulation of the secretory exocrine pancreatic
cells, which become hypertrophic (Yen et al. 1977; Garlich and Nesheim 1966).
Valuable proteins may be lost to the feces in this case (Booth et al. 1960; Lyman
1957; Lyman and Lepkovski 1957; Chernick et al. 1948).

Significance to the Human Situation

The activity of most digestive protease inhibitors discussed in the preceding paragraphs were tested on animal enzymes. The importance of these findings to the human situation has not been tested in vivo with human volunteers. Their activity in
humans may be predicted by in vitro assays with human proteolytic enzymes. Among
the digestive protease inhibitors, the following have been found to be active against
human trypsin: trypsin inhibitors from bovine colostrum and pancrease, lima beans,

soybeans (Kunitz 1945), soybeans (AA), kidney beans, blackeyed beans, navy beans, and quail (*Cotunix cotornix*) ovomucoid. The trypsin inhibitors from bovine and porcine pancrease, potatoes, chicken ovomucoid, and those from 10 other fowl, and chicken ovoinhibitor were ineffective against human trypsin even though these inhibitors were highly effective against bovine trypsin. The first three inhibitors against human trypsin are strongly inhibitory; the others are moderately or weakly so (Feeney et al. 1969). The soybean and lima bean trypsin inhibitors are also active against human chymotrypsin (Coan and Travis 1971).

As noted previously, bovine colostrum contains a highly active inhibitor against human trypsin. It is significant, therefore, that such inhibitory activity is also found in milk. Thus, Kiermeier and Semper (1960a-c) have found from testing the activity of 53 milk samples that raw milk can reduce the activity of trypsin by 75 to 99%, the average being 94%. This inhibitory activity can be overcome by increased amounts of trypsin. The antitryptic factor in milk also appears to be moderately heat resistant. The effectiveness of heat treatment is more dependent on higher temperature levels than duration of heating. Thus, the inhibitor is unaffected at 70°C; pasteurization for 40 sec at 72°C destroys only 3 to 4% of the antitryptic activity. Heating at 85°C for 3 sec destroys only 44 to 55% of the activity; at 95°C, approximately 27% of the activity remains even after 1 hr. Boiling for a short time does not destroy completely the antitryptic activity in milk.

The presence of antitryptic activity in milk may be disadvantageous to those persons with suboptimum trypsin secretion. Unboiled milk may be less easily digested by such persons than boiled milk (Koch 1957; Lembke et al. 1953).

Effect of Heat Treatment of Antiproteases in Other Foodstuffs

Antiproteases that have been examined so far are proteins; therefore, they can be expected to be heat labile. Many such proteins are just that, especially with moist heat; dry heat is less effective (Jacquot 1954; Westfall and Hauge 1948; Rackis et al. 1975). Nevertheless, several antiproteases are relatively heat resistant. An example of this has been seen in the antitryptic factor in milk, as discussed previously. Other examples are the alcohol-precipitable and nondialyzable trypsin inhibitor in alfalfa (Beauchere and Mitchell 1957; Ramirez and Mitchell 1960), the chymotrypsin inhibitor in potato (Ryan 1966), the kidney bean inhibitor, which remains stable at 90°C at pH 2 (Pusztai 1968), and the trypsin inhibitor in lima beans (Tauber et al. 1949).

Usually autoclaving soybean and different varieties of beans for 20 min at 115°C or 40 min at 107 to 108°C, and 30 min at 121°C, respectively, may be necessary for maximum destruction of inhibitors. Prior hydration by soaking in water for 12 to 24 hr may make heat treatment more effective. Even boiling at 100°C for 30 min, in the case of soybeans, or autoclaving for 40 min at 105°C, in the case of other beans, may be sufficient to improve the nutrient values of these legumes (Gontzea and Sutzescu 1968).

Excessive heat treatment can, of course, reduce the nutritive value of these beans owing to destruction of amino acids (Evans and McGinnis 1947; Clandinin et al. 1947; Jacquot 1954; Rackis et al. 1975).

Lectins

Lectins also are known as hemagglutinins because of their ability to agglutinate red blood cells. However, their ability to interfere nonspecifically in the absorption of vitamins, amino acids, fats, and glucose is the main concern in this discussion.

Heated legumes show improvement in their nutritive value, as observed in the rat (Haines and Lyman 1957) and chicks (Saxena et al. 1962). This effect may also arise from the destruction of other toxic factors in the bean, particularly the lectins (see the following section).

Lectins are widely distributed among edible legumes such as soybeans, peanuts, jack beans, mung beans, lima beans, kidney beans, fava beans, and the common vetch (Jaffe 1969; Liener 1976, 1964). They also are found in yellow wax beans (Takahashi et al. 1967) and other varieties of *Phaseolus vulgaris* (Dahlgren et al. 1970), hyacinth beans (*Dolichos lablab*) (Salgarkar and Sohonie 1965a,b), the horse gram (*D. biflorus*) (Etzler and Kabat 1970), lentils (McGregor and Sage 1968), and peas (Chen and Pan 1977). Lectins also are found in other plant-derived foodstuffs such as potatoes (Krupe and Ensgraber 1962), bananas, mangoes (Tiggelmann-Van Krugten et al. 1956), and wheat germ (Liske and Franks 1968). These substances also have been demonstrated in snails and fish roe (Prokop et al. 1961) and in a certain type of slug (Pemberton 1970). The meadow mushroom (*Agaricus campestris*) also contains lectins (Sage and Connet 1969).

Chemical and Physical Properties of Hemagglutinins

Soyin is the name given to a toxic lectin in soybeans (Liener et al. 1953; Liener 1953); the lectin in the common kidney bean is called phasin or phaseolotoxin (Camejo 1964). Most plant lectins are glycoproteins, except concanavalin A from jack beans (*Canavalia ensiformis*), which is carbohydrate-free (Olsen and Liener 1967). The lectin from kidney beans probably is also a lipoprotein (Palozzo and Jaffe 1969). The lectins of jack beans (Yariv et al. 1968) and lentils (Ticha et al. 1970) also contain calcium and manganese, which are necessary for activity. Most lectins from different varieties of black beans (*Phaseolus vulgaris*) are relatively large proteins with molecular weights ranging from 91,000 to 130,000 (Dahlgren et al. 1970; Camejo 1964).

The lectins in soybeans may be present to as much as 3% of the proteins (Liener and Rose 1953). There may be more than one type of lectin in soybeans (Lis et al. 1966).

Certain types of lectins may require higher temperatures for inactivation (Jaffe and Brucher 1972). This heat resistance may explain the toxicity in humans of incompletely cooked beans (Faschingbauer and Kofler 1929; Griebel 1950; Cartwright and Wintrobe 1946). Lectins may resist peptic action. The black bean lectin is relatively resistant to pepsin, and in rats its hemagluttinating activity may be detected in the feces (Jaffe and Hannig 1965; Jaffe and Vega Lette 1968). The soybean lectin may also escape peptic action, so that the oral toxicity of this substance may be explained on this basis (see below).

Toxicity of Lectins

Ricin in castor bean is probably the most toxic of all lectins. It is certainly among the most toxic substances. Its oral toxic dose in man is 150 to 200 mg; the intravenous toxic dose is 20 mg. In dogs, 0.6 µg/kg injected intramuscularly is lethal (Stecher et al. 1960).

Among the edible legumes, the lectins of kidney bean and hyacinth bean are the most toxic. A diet containing 0.5% purified kidney bean lectin has been shown to markedly stunt the growth of rats; all the animals died within 2 weeks (Honavar et al. 1962). The red kidney bean is apparently more toxic than the black variety. The intraperitoneal LD_{50} in mice of the black kidney bean has been shown to be 50 mg/kg (Jaffe 1960).

Unheated kidney beans added to the rat diet have been shown to be similarly toxic. Animals fed such a diet develop anorexia and diarrhea; overall digestability and nitrogen retention in the presence of raw kidney bean are low. The animals lose weight and die. These effects are not seen in adequately heated beans. Methods for extracting the lectins from the bean may not completely remove the toxic substance, since even with the addition of casein to the diet containing extracted kidney beans, the rats fail to grow properly (Jaffe 1960).

Concerning the growth and survival of rats, the lack of effect of the addition of predigested casein to bean diets has demonstrated that the protease inhibitors in kidney beans are not responsible for the toxicity (Jaffe 1949; Jaffe and Vega Lette 1968).

Hyacinth beans are just as toxic as kidney beans when fed to rats. At 1.5 to 2.5% added to a casein diet, the lectins from these seeds similarly induce growth retardation and death (Salgarkar and Sohonie 1965b). The lectin in this legume produces focal liver necrosis. A similar type of toxicity has been observed with the horse gram when added to the diet of rats (Ray 1969). The animals show growth retardation and die within 3 weeks. However, in this case, the toxicity may not be entirely due to the hemagglutinins, since only the crude preparation retards growth in rats or mice; the purified preparation has no effect when administered parenterally (Manage 1969). Partly purified lectins of lima beans (*Phaseolus lunatus*) are not lethal to rats when fed in a casein diet, although it also retards growth. This crude preparation is lethal when injected intraperitoneally at 65 and 140 mg/kg in rats and mice, respectively. Like the horse gram preparation, the highly purified lectin is less toxic than the crude product (Joshi 1970).

The lectin in soybeans appear to be less toxic orally than the other types. At 1% in the diet, the soybean lectin retards growth in rats to approximately 75% of the normal rate, but this amount is not lethal as no deaths resulted (Liener 1953); 500 mg/kg administered by stomach tube also is not lethal (Liener and Rose 1953). Compare this with the intraperitoneal LD_{50} in rats of 50 mg/kg (Liener and Pallansch 1952). This value is the same as that for black beans (Jaffe 1960). However, black beans produce 100% mortality when fed at 0.5% level in the diet (Honavar et al. 1962). This difference may be explained by the different actions of pepsin on both hemagglutinins: In vitro, pepsin has been demonstrated to inactivate soybean lectin (Liener 1958), but that of kidney bean is relatively resistant (Jaffe and Hannig 1965; Jaffe and Vega Lette 1968). Of course, peptic activity in vivo and the quantity of lectin present may determine whether or not some pepsin hydrolyzable lectins may escape complete inactivation.

Mechanisms of Toxicity

The toxic action of hemagglutinins may be related to their ability to bind to specific cell receptors, as observed with certain types of cancer cells (Shoham et al. 1970; Steck and Wallach 1965; Uhlenbruck et al. 1970). The binding of bean lectin on rat intestinal mucosal cells has been demonstrated in vitro, and it has been suggested that this action is responsible for the oral toxicity of the lectins (Jaffe 1960). Such bindings may disturb the intestines' absorptive capacity for nutrients and other essential compounds. Thus, with raw soybeans in the diet, there is a significantly diminished absorption of amino acids (Muelenaere 1964) and thyroxine (Beck 1958) in rats; and of fats in chicks (Nesheim et al. 1962). There is a significant increase in the requirement for the fat-soluble vitamins: i.e., the retinols (vitamin A) (Shaw et al. 1951), in calves; and in the calciferols in turkey poults and in the piglets (Miller et al. 1965) with raw soybeans in the diet. This impairment in the absorption of the fat-soluble vitamins and fats may be a consequence of the decrease in the reabsorption of bile salts, as observed in chicks (Serafin and Nesheim 1970), since bile salts enhance the absorption of these vitamins or their corresponding provitamins. On the other hand, this effect may not be totally dependent on the reabsorption of bile salts. Evidence also exists for the diminished utilization of the tocopherols in the presence of raw kidney beans in the diet of chicks (Hintz and Hogue 1964). Similarly, raw kidney beans interfere in the absorption of amino acids in chicks (Jaffe 1949).

The impairment of the absorption of thyroxine may explain the goitrogenic effects of soybeans in rats (Sharpless et al. 1939), and in human infants (Hydovitz 1960; Van Wyk et al. 1959). This goitrogenic effect of soybeans also may be due to the interference in the absorption of iodine, since iodine supplementation in the diet has a curative action on soybean goiter (Block et al. 1961).

The presence of other toxic factors in legumes may account for as much as 50% of the observed effects (Hanovar et al. 1962; Jaffe 1960). This disturbance may explain in part the severe hypoglycemia observed in rats when fed a red kidney bean diet (Hintz et al. 1967).

Thus, it appears from the preceding discussion that the legumes are not only type A antinutritives but types B and C as well.

The presence of other unidentified toxic factors in legumes acting together with the lectins to produce the effect just discussed is indicated by the isolation of a nonhemagglutinating, heat-labile factor in soybeans (Stead et al. 1966). The presence of a growth-retarding substance in soybeans from which the soluble lectins and protease inhibitors had been removed also has been observed (Gertler et al. 1967); this factor appears to be strongly bound to the residue, and could be separated by papain digestion (Borchers 1963).

Inactivation of Lectins

The lectins, being proteins, can easily be inactivated by moist heat (De Muelenaere 1964; Jaffe 1949). Dry heat is ineffective (Potter and Kummerow 1954). Germination decreases the hemagglutinating activity in varieties of peas and species of beans. In fact, soybeans can lose as much as 92% of the activity even during the first day of germination (Chen et al. 1977).

Saponins

Soybeans, lucerne, sugar beets, peanuts, and tea leaves contain significant amounts of saponins (Okano 1948; Peterson 1950). The soybean and alfalfa saponins appear to be similar in chemical and biological activity (Potter and Kummerow 1954). The mechanism of their deleterious effects, which is manifested by growth inhibition, as observed in chicks, is not known. However, it is possible that these steroid or triterpenoid glycosides interfere in the absorption of nutrients (Birk 1969; Okano 1948). The saponins may cause hemolysis, as demonstrated by in vitro tests.

The saponins in sea cucumbers, the holothurins, are discussed in Chapter 11. One notes that in addition to their hemolytic activity, the holothurins also have neuromuscular toxic effects.

Cholesterol inactivates the alfalfa saponins, but not those in soybeans by forming an insoluble complex.

The aglycone of saponins may be separated from the sugar moiety simply by heating, and is less toxic, if not nontoxic, compared to the intact glycoside. Both the sugar moiety and the aglycone may vary with the plant source (Peterson 1950).

The significance of the toxic effects of saponins in man is not known. Soybean saponins appear to have no deleterious effects when administered orally to rats and mice.

Polyphenols

Gossypol, an excellent example of the polyphenols, is discussed in connection with toxic plant phenols in Chapter 8.

TYPE B: ANTIMINERALS

Substances interfering with the utilization of essential minerals are widely distributed in vegetables, fruits, and cereal grains. Although they are toxic per se, the amounts present in foods seldom cause acute intoxication under normal food consumption. However, they may harm the organism in a more subtle way by interfering in the absorption or metabolic utilization of essential minerals. Therefore, these substances may be of greater significance under suboptimum nutriture.

Phytic Acid (Myo-Inositol Hexaphosphate)

Phytic acid, or *myo*-inositol 1,2,3,4,5,6-hexakis (dihydrogen phosphate), is a naturally occurring strong acid which binds to many types of bivalent and trivalent heavy metal ions, forming insoluble salts. Thus, this compound may render many trace essential elements and micronutrients unavailable. The degree of insolubility

Phytic Acid

of these salts appear to depend on the nature of the metal, the pH of the solution, and for certain metals, on the presence of another metal. Metal phytates have an optimum pH range at which their water solubility is minimal. For example, phytates of copper and zinc have a minimum solubility from pH 4 to 7, whereas phytates of calcium and magnesium have a minimum solubility in slightly basic solutions (Oberleas et al. 1966a,b). Ferric phytate is least soluble in dilute acid and breaks down in the presence of dilute alkali or concentrated acid (Beck 1948); Cu^{2+}, Zn^{2+}, Co^{2+}, Mn^{2+}, Fe^{3+}, and Ca^{2+}, in descending order, form phytates readily in vitro at pH 7.4 (Maddaiah et al. 1964; Vohra et al. 1965).

Synergism between two metallic ions in the formation of phytate complexes has also been observed. Thus, calcium and zinc added at pH 6 to phytic acid separately precipitate to the extent of 63 and 67%, respectively. When these ions are present simultaneously, the amount precipitated jumps to 84 and 97%, respectively. The amount of precipitation for zinc phytate or zinc-calcium phytate is maximum at pH 6—which, interestingly, is the range of the pH of the duodenum, where most of the absorption of calcium and trace metals occurs. A similar type of relationship has been observed with the copper and calcium pair, although the proportion of copper and calcium precipitated was smaller than in the case of zinc-calcium pair.

The wide distribution of phytates among plant foodstuffs is seen in Table 9.1. Cereal grains (O'Dell et al. 1972) and a number of legumes (Lolas and Markakis 1975) contain the largest amounts among those listed. As a health hazard, the presence of phytates in cereal grains deserves special attention, since cereals generally constitute the bulk of the diet, especially of individuals likely to have subnormal nutriture.

Effect of Phytates on Mineral Balances

Ample experimental evidence is available to illustrate the negative effects of phytates on the availability of calcium, iron, magnesium, zinc, and other trace essential elements (Harrison and Mellamby 1939; Hoff-Jorgensen et al. 1946a; Likuski and Forbes 1964; McCance and Widdowson 1942b, 1935; O'Dell and Savage 1960; Rackis 1974;

Table 9.1 Phytate Contents of Selected Foodstuffs

Food	mg%	Phytate phosphorus % of Total Phosphorus
Cereals		
wheat	170-280	47-86
rye	247	73
maize	146-353	52-97
rice	157-240	68
barley	70-300	32-80
oats	208-355	50-88
sorghum	206-280	77-88
buckwheat	322	70
millet	83	57
wheat bran	1170-1439	89-97
Legumes and vegetables		
bean (*Phaseolus vulgaris*)	269	62
bean (*Phaseolus lunatus*)	152	77
soybean	402	65
lentil (*Lens esculenta*)	295	90
pea (*Pisum sativum*)	117	37
vetch (*Fava vulgaris*)	500	95
chick pea (*Cicer arietinum*)	140-354	49-95
pea (*Lathyrus sativum*)	82	31
potato (*Solanum tuberosum*)	14	35
green bean (*Phaseolus vulgaris*)	52	43
green pea (*Pisum sativum*)	12	12
carrot	0-4	0-16
Nuts and seeds		
walnut	120	24
hazelnut	104	45
almond	189	43
peanut	205	57
cocoa bean	169	25
pistachio nut	176	75
rapeseed	795	89
cotton seed	366	41

Table 9.1   (continued)

Food	mg%	Phytate phosphorus % of Total Phosphorus
Spices and flavoring agents		
caraway	297	96
coriander	320	77
cumin (*Cuminum cyminum*)	153	33
mustard (*Sinapis alba*)	392	86
nutmeg	162	61
black pepper	115	58
pepper	56	15
paprika	71	15
Fruits		
blackberries		
figs		
strawberries		

Source: Compiled from: Averill and King (1926); Balasubramanian et al. (1962); Courtois and Perez (1948); Holt (1955); Lang and Eberwein (1948); McCance and Widdowson (1935, 1944, 1949); Oberleas et al. (1966a,b); Oke (1965); Rahim and Ahmed (1960); Smith and Rackis (1957); Sundararajan (1938); and Yang and Dju (1939).

Reinhold et al. 1973; Sathe and Krishnamurthy 1953; Walker 1951; Walker et al. 1948; Widdowson 1941).

Interference in the Absorption of Calcium   When eight men and eight women were placed on a diet of brown bread (containing 214 mg phytic acid/100 g) for 3 to 4 weeks, calcium absorption was lowered by 33 to 62% (average 33.38%) compared to the values with white bread. The bread provided 40 to 50% of total calories and calcium intake was adequate. When the calcium intake was reduced to 500 mg/day, seven persons on brown bread had a negative calcium balance compared to only two persons on white bread. Six persons on brown bread, comprising 86 to 100% of the total calories, had a negative calcium balance within 7 days. One person developed signs of tetany. Bran added to white flour produced similar results; dephytinized bran added to white flour produced results comparable to that seen from white bread. The latter result indicates that the indigestible material in the bran is not responsible for the decrease in the calcium balance. Cholecalciferol added to the brown bread diet for 2 weeks at 2000 IU/day did not significantly improve the calcium balance. Only when the calcium intake was increased to 1.0 to 1.4 g/day was the calcium balance significantly improved; the average balance increased from 87 to 89 mg, with only three persons showing negative values (McCance and Walsham 1948; McCance and Widdowson 1935, 1942b).

Similar results have been reported by others on the effects of brown bread and other cereals rich in phytates in human calcium balance (Cruickshank et al. 1943, 1945; Krebs and Mellamby 1943; Nitesco et al. 1933).

An actual demonstration of the reduction in calcium absorption in the presence of sodium phytate has been shown in the experiments performed by Bronner et al. (1954, 1956). Using an isotope of calcium, they showed that only 34% of the calcium added to the farina test meal was absorbed by adolescent boys in the presence of sodium phytate compared to 55% in phytate-rich oatmeal test meal; these values represent 45 and 74% of the amount absorbed with the phytate-free farina test diet. Thus, it appears that some calcium can be absorbed even in the presence of purified phytic acid, possibly because of the presence of phytate in the intestines (Roberts and Yudkin 1961). The activity of this phytase has been shown in rats to be stimulated by cholecalciferol; the absence of this vitamin decreases the activity of the enzyme (Roberts and Yudkin 1961) and enhances the effect of phytates (Harrison and Mellamby 1939). Thus, cholecalciferol may obviate the deleterious effects of phytates in the absorption of calcium.

Interference in the Absorption of Magnesium   Experiments with rats and humans also have indicated a decrease in the absorption of magnesium in the presence of phytates. Thus, it has been demonstrated that rats given a diet sufficient in calcium and containing 2.5 to 7.5 g soluble phytates/100 g of food develop symptoms of magnesium deficiency. The rats on a 5 and 7.5% phytate diet lost weight and died within 42 and 20 days, respectively. Supplementation with magnesium obviated the effects of phytates, and the animals grew. The growth rate, however, was less than in the control group. This is to be expected in view of the effect of phytates on other minerals (Roberts and Yudkin 1960).

In humans, the adverse effects of phytates on magnesium utilization has been suggested by a comparison of the magnesium balance of 10 experimental subjects on a diet of white or brown bread. With white bread (69% extraction), comprising 40 to 50% of total calories, 45 to 50% of dietary magnesium was absorbed; with brown bread (92% extraction), only 20 to 24% was absorbed. It has been shown that removal of phytates in the brown bread will increase the magnesium absorption to 30% (McCance and Widdowson 1942a,b). The less than comparable result in the latter case with white bread suggests either incomplete dephytinization or the presence of other factors interfering in the absorption of magnesium.

Interference in the Absorption of Iron   Several studies in humans have established the negative effects of phytic acid on iron absorption. In four persons given a diet for 18 days, in which phytates represented 40% of the total phosphorus, less than 3% of the iron was absorbed; in contrast, more than 10% was absorbed when phytates comprised only 8% of the total (Hussain and Patwardhan 1959). In another study, the influence of phytates on iron absorption was determined by the rise of serum iron in four men and five women; the results show that sodium phytate decreases iron absorption, as indicated by the failure of serum iron to increase after ingestion of 8 mg iron/kg body weight. The ferric form appears to be more strongly bound than the ferrous (McCance et al. 1943). In 17 adolescents (12 to 17 years old), absorption of radioactive iron added to milk was reduced from 17.4% without phytates, to 9.8% in the presence of phytates (Sharpe et al. 1950). The excretion of radioactive iron in the feces of five healthy adults was higher when the diet contained brown bread or white bread with added phytates than when the diet did not contain phytates (Foy et al. 1959). Widdowson and McCance (1942) have observed similar results. These authors found less than 1% absorption of iron in men and women given meals in which 40 to 50% of total calories was derived from 92% extraction bread; with 69% extraction bread, 7.3 (men) and 12.5% (women) of the iron was absorbed.

Studies with rats have shown similar negative effects of phytates on iron absorption (Furh and Steenbock 1943; Nakamura and Mitchell 1943; Sathe and Krishnamurthy 1953).

It appears that phytic acid prevents the formation of complexes of iron with gastroferrin, an iron-binding protein which is secreted in the stomach, so that the absorption of this metal is impaired (Koepke and Stewart 1964; Multani et al. 1970; Murray and Stein 1970).

Interference in the Absorption of Zinc Several studies on chicken have indirectly shown that zinc absorption is diminished by phytates (Lease et al. 1960; Moeller and Scott 1958; Morrison and Sarrett 1958; O'Dell et al. 1958) and in pigs (Smith et al. 1961, 1962; Tucker and Salmon 1955). In these studies, the effects of diets containing phytate-rich proteins, such as soybean proteins, on growth and other parameters associated with zinc deficiency were compared with diets on animal proteins. Both diets had sufficient and essentially equal quantities of zinc, calories, and proteins. The soya diet produced growth retardation compared to the animal protein diet; growth was stimulated when additional zinc was included in the diet. No further growth stimulation was seen in the animal protein diet. In pigs, other signs of zinc deficiency, e.g., parakeratosis and dermatitis, were corrected by additional zinc in the soya diet.

Direct evidence on the deleterious effects of phytic acid on zinc absorption in chicks has been obtained by adding this agent in casein-gelatin (O'Dell and Savage 1960), casein, or amino acid mixture diets (Likuski and Forbes 1964). Growth retardation by as much as 50% was observed. This effect was corrected when additional zinc was given. The quantity of zinc in the femur ash was also reduced by as much as 50%.

Negative zinc balance also has been demonstrated in human subjects fed diets containing purified phytates or phytate-rich bread (Reinhold et al. 1973). Phytates also have been implicated in a characteristic syndrome observed in Iran among older children and adolescents. These children, on a diet consisting largely of unleavened bread from low extraction flours, develop dwarfism, hypogonadism, mild anemia, and low plasma zinc levels. Zinc supplementation (120 mg $ZnSO_4$ per day) in the diet for several months results in pubertal development (increased genital size, appearance of pubic hairs, and other secondary male characteristics), and increased growth rates (Halsted et al. 1972). It is, of course, possible that the above symptoms may have been aggravated by a superimposed protein deficiency (Caughey 1973).

Interference in the Absorption of Other Minerals The negative effect of phytates on the absorption of other minerals is to be expected. Thus, soybean proteins rich in phytates also have been observed to reduce the availability of copper and manganese in the chick (Davis et al. 1962).

Even though the activity of phytates in reducing the availability of essential minerals has been established, the effects of foodstuffs such as brown bread, in this respect, may be the result of the combined effects of phytates and other indigestible materials in the food—the so-called "fiber" (pp. 425–426).

Controlling the Effects of Phytic Acid

In many foodstuffs, the level of phytates may be reduced by phytase, an enzyme endogenous to plants (Courtois et al. 1952; Courtois and Perez 1948; Lange et al. 1961; McCance and Widdowson 1944; Mellamby 1944; Nelson et al. 1971; Ranhotra and Loewe 1975). The phytase activity in soybean, however, is weak, despite its large amount of phytic acid. Rye contains more phytase than any other cereal grains (Hoff-Jorgensen et al. 1946b).

The activity of phytase drastically reduces the phytate content of dough during the bread-making process (Lange et al. 1961; Lee and Underwood 1949; Schulerud 1947; Widdowson 1941). The decomposition of phytic acid is aided by increased acidity of bread dough from the action of yeast—the optimum activity of phytase being between pH 5.0 and 5.5 at 55°C (Lange et al. 1961; Mellamby 1944; Widdowson 1941). Thus, the use of yeast may be important in decreasing the phytic acid content in bread (Reinhold 1971).

Phytase appears to be present also in the gastrointestinal tract of animals (Davis et al. 1962; Maddaiah et al. 1964; Pileggi 1959). Its presence in the human gastrointestinal tract has not been demonstrated (Walker et al. 1946, 1948).

The increased activity of this enzyme may also explain the decrease in phytates during the germination of pea (*Pisum sativum*) seeds and soybeans (Chen and Pan 1977).

The milling of grains also reduces the phytic acid content of flours by as much as 40% depending on the degree of extraction (Lee and Underwood 1949; Schulerud 1947).

As indicated in the preceding discussion, the negative effects of phytates in foods may be minimized considerably, if not eliminated, by increased intake of essential minerals. In the case of calcium, intake of cholecalciferol must also be adequate, since the activity of phytates on calcium absorption is enhanced when this vitamin is inadequate or limiting (Harrison and Mellamby 1939).

Even on high phytate diets, healthy individuals show remarkable adaptation to the negative effects on mineral balances (Walker et al. 1946, 1948).

Oxalates

Oxalic acid (HOOC-COOH) is a white crystalline solid, approximately 10% soluble in water at 20°C. It is a strong acid (pK_1 = 1.46; pK_2 = 4.40) which forms water-soluble Na^+ and K^+ salts but less soluble salts with alkaline earth and other bivalent metals. Calcium oxalate is particularly insoluble at neutral or alkaline pH, but readily dissolves in acid medium.

Thus, like phytates, oxalates can also decrease the availability of essential bivalent minerals such as calcium. Many animal and human feeding experiments have established the negative effects of high oxalate foods, notably on calcium absorption (Bricker et al. 1949; Edelstein 1932; Finke and Garrison 1938, 1936; Johnston et al. 1952; Sherman and Hawley 1922).

Such foods as rhubarb, spinach, celery, sugar beets, and cocoa also have been shown to cause negative calcium balances in man (Ackerman and Gebauer 1957; Bricker et al. 1949; Finke and Garrison 1936; Johnston et al. 1952; Mitchell and Smith 1945).

The adverse effects of oxalates in relation to calcium must be considered in terms of the oxalate-calcium ratio. On a milliequivalent basis, food having a ratio greater than 1 may have serious effects on calcium availability (Table 9.2). On the other hand, food with a ratio of 1 or below poses no difficulty on the availability of calcium as far as other calcium sources are concerned. However, food having a ratio around unity is not a good source of calcium even if the analysis of the ash content indicates otherwise.

Reports of the effects of oxalates on calcium absorption have been contradictory. Some researchers have reported a significant interference in calcium absorption; others have reported little or no effect at all. For example, Kohman (1939) has found that spinach containing 1.25% calcium and about 0.9% oxalate (dry weight basis) interferes in the growth and calcium uptake of the bones and teeth when added by as much as 7 to 8% of the basal diet of weanling rats. The diet contained 0.093% calcium without spinach. No effect has been observed when low oxalate greens containing 2 to 4% calcium (dry weight basis) were fed. In this case, the vegetable increased the total calcium in the diet to 0.2 to 0.3%. When calcium carbonate was added to the diet in stoichiometric amounts with the oxalate content of spinach, the animals fared as well as those on low oxalate greens. Similar studies of the negative

Table 9.2 Foods Having an Oxalate-Calcium Ratio (MEQ/MEQ) > 1

Food	mg Oxalate/100 g	Average	Oxalate/Ca, MEQ/MEQ
Rhubard (*Rheum rhaponticum*)	275-1336	805	8.5
Common sorrel (*Rumex acetosa*)	270-730	500	5.6
Garden sorrel (*Rumex patientia*)	300-700	500	5.0
Spinach (*Spinacia oleracea*)	320-1260	970	4.3
Beet, leaves (*Beta vulgaris, var. cicla*)	300-920	610	2.5
Beet, roots	121-450	275	5.1
Purslane (*Portulaca oleracea*)	910-1679	1294	4.6
Cocoa (*Theobroma cocoa*)	500-900	700	2.6
Coffee (*Coffea arabica*)	50-150	100	3.9
Potato (*Solanum tuberosom*)	20-141	80	1.6
Tea (*Thea chinesis*)	300-2000	1150	1.1
New Zealand spinach (*Tetragonia expansia*)	890	—	3.9
Pig spinach (*Chenopodium* sp.)	1100	—	4.9
Orache (*Atriplex hortensis*)	300-1500	900	4.0
Amaranth (*Amarantus polygonoicles*)	1586	—	1.2
Amaranth (*Amarantus tricolor*)	1087	—	1.4

Source: Gontzea and Sutzescu (1968).

effects of spinach and similar high oxalate vegetables on calcium absorption (Fairbanks and Mitchell 1938; Finke and Sherman 1935; Speirs 1939; Tisdall and Drake 1938; Tisdall et al. 1937) confirm the results of Kohman. Interference in the absorption of calcium also has been reported for beets (Shields and Mitchell 1941) and rhubarb petioles (Tuba et al. 1952); both products are high in oxalates. The rhubarb diet produced biochemical abnormalities suggestive of rickets; e.g., increased serum phosphatase activity, decreased blood calcium, and increased phos-

phate levels. These results are in contrast to the effects of such low oxalate vegetables as turnip, cauliflower (Shields and Mitchell 1941), and tomatoes (Tisdall and
Drake 1938; Tisdall et al. 1937).

Significantly depressed utilization of calcium also has been observed among
children (Edelstein 1932; Sherman and Hawley 1922) and young women (Finke and
Garrison 1938; Johnston et al. 1952; McLaughlin 1927) fed significant amounts of
spinach. For example, in studies with six 20- to 21-year-old women, Johnston et al.
(1952) found that the utilization of calcium dropped from about 19 to about 12%
when the subjects on a basic diet for 4 weeks were switched to the spinach diet
(120 g/day) for 8 weeks. In this case, the calcium balance dropped from −26 to
−51 mg.

Studies in India (Pingle and Ramasastri 1978) also have confirmed the negative
effects of high oxalate vegetables on calcium utilization. In these studies, eight or
ten 20- to 35-year-old male subjects fed a mixture of the high oxalate Amaranthus
vegetables showed markedly depressed absorption of calcium from milk given together
with the leaves. The vegetables in this case contained 0.74 to 1.1 g oxalates per
100 g—50% of the oxalates being in soluble form.

On the other hand, Bonner et al. (1933) found no effect on the storage of calcium. Their subjects were fed spinach containing a total of 0.7 g oxalic acid for 15
days after a 25-day period on a basal diet containing 5 to 7% calcium.

The contradictory results may be explained by the fact that the nutritional
status of subjects and duration of testing and the level of calcium intake may influence the effect of oxalates. For example, rats showed no serious effects on a diet
containing 2.5% oxalate unless the diet was also deficient in calcium, phosphorus,
and especially cholecalciferol (MacKenzie and McCollum 1937; Nicolaysen et al. 1953).

Humans also show a remarkable ability to adapt to the effects of a drastic reduction in calcium intake (Malm 1963). This is because a considerable calcium reserve is
provided by the skeletal system, and unless such a store is nearly or already depleted, the diminution of calcium absorption by oxalates in food would not make
much difference.

In contrast to calcium absorption, oxalates appear not to interfere in zinc absorption in zinc-deficient rats (Welch et al. 1977). Somehow, a counteracting or
protective mechanism may prevent the precipitation of zinc by oxalates, since like
calcium oxalate ($K_{sp} = 4 \times 10^{-9}$), zinc oxalate ($K_{sp} = 2.7 \times 10^{-8}$) is also very insoluble in water (Dean 1972). The more than 10-fold difference in the solubility
product constants of zinc and calcium oxalates may explain in part the difference in
the availability of these two metals in the presence of excess oxalates. Whatever the
mechanism, it appears that oxalates do not interfere in zinc absorption, at least in
the rat.

In this connection, fatal rhubarb poisonings which were thought to be due to
the oxalate content are probably caused by other factors (von Streicher 1964) even
though the leaves may contain up to 1.1% oxalates. This has been proposed because
the characteristic symptoms of oxalate poisoning, such as corrosive gastroenteritis,
are absent in these fatal cases (Kalliala and Kauste 1964; Robb 1919; Tallquist and
Väänänen 1960). It has been postulated that the anthraquinone glycosides may be
responsible for the fatal rhubarb poisonings (von Streicher 1964). Fresh rhubarb
leaves may contain as much as 0.5 to 1% anthraquinones; 10 to 20 g of fresh leaves
have caused immediate poisoning in human volunteers (Schmid 1951).

Oxalic acid per se is acutely toxic in humans, resulting in corrosion in the
mouth and gastrointestinal tract, gastric hemorrhage, renal failure, renal colic,
bloody urine, and sometimes convulsions. It would require massive doses to produce
these effects (minimum dose of 4 to 5 g) (Figdor 1961). This dosage has no significance with respect to oxalates at the levels usually found in food.

Harmful oxalates in food may be removed by soaking in water. Consumption of
calcium-rich foods, such as dairy products and seafood, as well as augmented chole-

calciferol intake, are recommended when large amounts of high oxalate food are eaten (Schmid 1951; von Streicher 1964).

Goitrogens

There is a possibility that nontoxic endemic goiter may not be entirely due to iodine deficiency, since it has been shown that many factors in several plant foodstuffs are goitrogenic (Greer 1960, 1962). It also has been shown that of about 61 food products tested, rutabagas, turnips, cabbage, peaches, strawberries, spinach, and carrots can cause a significant reduction in the radioiodine uptake in the human thyroid gland, with rutabaga being the most active (Block et al. 1961; Greer 1950; Greer and Astwood 1948).

However, the cause and effect relationship of human goiter and goitrogens is difficult to establish because among other things, data are not always easy to compile regarding the extent and duration of consumption of goitrogenic foods. Variability of response to the goitrogen is also to be expected. Nevertheless, as noted in the succeeding sections, some correlation between prolonged and consistent consumption of goitrogenic foodstuffs and the appearance of goiter in certain groups of subjects has been reported. Greer (1962) also estimates that about 4% of cases of nontoxic endemic goiter is not caused by iodine deficiency even though the influence of plant goitrogens in this case has not been demonstrated.

Table 9.3 gives a list of foodstuffs which have been shown to induce goiter, at least in experimental animals. The active principles in all of these are also given.

Types of Goiters Caused by Goitrogens

The goiter induced by a goitrogen may or may not be resistant to iodine therapy. Some of the goitrogenic factors may interfere in iodine metabolism by their direct action, more or less, on the thyroid or by interfering in the absorption of iodine or thyroxine by the intestinal mucosa. Thus, three types of goiter are recognized.

Cabbage Goiter ("Struma cibaria") This type of goiter is ameliorated by iodine therapy, and as the name implies, is induced by excessive consumption of cabbage. It seems that cabbage goitrogens interfere in iodine uptake by direct action on the thyroid gland (Langer 1964; Marine et al. 1930).

Struma cibaria has not only been observed in animals, but also in persons consuming large quantities of cabbage and similar vegetables for long periods (Fisher et al. 1952).

Brassica Seed Goiter The seeds of Brassica plants (rutabaga, turnip, cabbage, rape) contain goitrogens which prevent thyroxine formation, so that the goiter can be treated successfully only by administration of the hormone. Even though large doses of potassium iodine may alleviate the goiter, the characteristic histological changes are not corrected (Hercus and Purves 1936; Kennedy and Purves 1941; Nordfelt et al. 1954; Turner 1948).

Legume Goiter The goitrogens of soybeans, peanuts, and other legumes induce goiter which is amenable to iodine therapy (Anderson and Howard 1959; Block et al. 1961; Care 1954; Halverson et al. 1945; Sharpless 1938; Sharpless et al. 1939; Wilgus and Gassner 1941; Wilgus et al. 1941). This type of goiter, however, differs from cabbage goiter in that the thyroid gland does not lose its avidity for iodine. In spite of this phenomenon, the protein bound iodine (PBI) and the protein content of the thyroid gland remain low; a block in the intestinal absorption of iodine or the reabsorption of thyroxine, as shown by increased fecal excretion of thyroxine, is indicated in this case (Beck 1958; Van Middlesworth 1957). An interference in thyroxine synthesis by substances in legumes other than glucosinolates, for example, or competition with thyroxines for iodine may also lead to goitrogenesis (Van Wyk et al. 1959).

Table 9.3 Glucosinolates in Foods and Feedstuffs

Food or feedstuff[a]	Glucosinolate[b]	Specific Chemical (R) Group[c]
Broccoli (buds)	Glucobrassicin[d]	3-Indolylmethyl
(*B. oleracea*)	Gluconapin[e]	3-Butenyl
	Neoglucobrassicin[e]	3-(N-methoxyindolyl)-methyl
	Progoitrin[e]	(R)-2-hydroxy-3-butenyl
	Sinigrin[d]	Allyl
Brussel sprouts (head)	As in broccoli	
(*B. oleracea gemmifera*)		
Cabbage (head)	As in broccoli	
(*B. oleracea capitata*)		
Cauliflower (buds)	As in broccoli	
(*B. oleracea botrytis*)		
Charlock (seed)	Sinalbin[e]	P-Hydroxybenzyl
(*S. arvensis*)		
Crambe (seed)	Gluconapin[e]	(See broccoli above)
(*C. abyssinica*)	Gluconasturtiin[e]	2-Phenylethyl
Garden cress (leaves)	Glucotropaeolin[e]	Benzyl
(*L. sativum*)		
Horseradish (roots)	Gluconasturtiin[e]	(See Crambe above)
(*A. rusticana*)	Sinigrin[d]	
Kale (leaves)	As in broccoli	
(*B. oleracea acephala*)		
Kohlrabi (head)	As in broccoli	
(*B. oleracea gongylodes*)		
Mustard, black (seed)	Sinigrin[d]	(See broccoli above)
(*B. nigra*)		
Mustard, Indian (seed)	Sinigrin[d]	(See broccoli above)
(*B. juncea*)		
Mustard, white (seed)	Sinalbin[d]	(See charlock above)
(*S. alba*)		
Navette (seed)	Glucoallysin[e]	5-Methylsulfinylpentyl
(*B. campestris*)	Glucobrassicanapin[e]	4-Pentenyl
	Gluconapin[e]	(See broccoli above)

Table 9.3   (continued)

Food or feedstuff[a]	Glucosinolate[b]	Specific Chemical (R) Group[c]
	Glucoraphanin[e]	4-Methylsulfinylbutyl
	Progoitrin	(See broccoli above)
Radish (root)		4-Methylthio-3-butenyl[5]
(*R. sativus*)	Glucobrassicin[e]	(See broccoli above)
Rape (seed)	As in navette	
(*B. campestris*)		
Rape (seed)	Glucobrassicanapin[e]	(See navette above)
(*B. napus*)	Glucoiberin[e]	3-Methylsulfinylpropyl
	Gluconapin[d]	(See broccoli above)
	Gluconasturtiin[e]	(See Crambe above)
	Progoitrin[d]	(See broccoli above)
	Sinalbin[e]	(See charlock above)
Rape, Argentine (seed)	As in rape (*B. napus*)	
(*B. napus*)		
Rape, Polish (seed)	As in navette	
(*B. campestris*)		
Rape, winter (seed)	As in Argentine rape	
(*B. napus*)		
Rapeseed, Ethiopian	Sinigrin[d]	(See broccoli above)
(*B. carinata*)		
Rubsen (seed)	Same as navette	
(*B. campestris*)		
Rutabaga (root)	Glucobrassicin[e]	(See broccoli above)
(*B. napobrassica*)	Neoglucobrassicin[e]	(See broccoli above)
	Progoitrin[d]	(See broccoli above)
Turnips (root)	Gluconasturtiin[d]	(See Crambe above)
(*B. campestris*)	Progoitrin[e]	(See broccoli above)
		(R)-2-hydroxy-4-pentenyl[e]
Turnips (seed)	Same as navette	
(*B. campestris*)		

[a]*B.*, Brassica; *S.*, Sinapis; *C.*, Crambe; *L.*, Lepidium; *A.*, Amoracia; *R.*, Raphanus.
[b]Trivial or common name of glucosinolate. The chemical name is formed by the desig-

Table 9.3 (continued)

nation of the R group prefixed to the term glucosinolate, e.g., glucobrassicin is 3-indolylmethylglucosinolate.
[c]See text for structural position of R groups.
[d]*Major glucosinolate.*
[e]Minor glucosinolate component.
Source: VanEtten et al. (1969) and VanEtten and Wolff (1973).

Legume goiter has been observed in children consuming soya milk for prolonged periods (Hydovitz 1960; Ripp 1961; Shepard et al. 1960; Van Wyk et al. 1959).

Types of Goitrogens

The goitrogens in plant food or feedstuffs belong to different chemical classes; each type may produce goiter by dissimilar mechanisms. Hydrolysis either within the plant or in the digestive tract yields several active derivatives of these compounds. Thus, the potency of a particular goitrogen may depend on the number and activity of the derivatives produced. In addition, each type of product may contain several types of goitrogens, as seen in Table 9.3.

The following classes of goitrogens have been identified in many plant food-stuffs.

Glucosinolates These compounds are also known as thioglucosides. At least 300 species of Cruciferae are known to contain glucosinolates (Ettlinger and Kjaer 1968; Kjaer 1966, 1960; VanEtten 1969; VanEtten et al. 1969), of which 50 types have been identified and chemically characterized. As many as six of these may be found in one plant species with one or two predominating (Ettlinger and Kjaer 1968). Table 9.3 lists several glucosinolates found in common crucifers. The glucosinolates have a general structure, shown below, and yield on hydrolysis, the active or actual goitrogens, such as thiocyanates, isothiocyanates, cyclic sulfur compounds, and nitriles (VanEtten 1969; VanEtten et al. 1969). Table 9.3 shows also the corresponding R groups of various glucosinolates in crucifers.

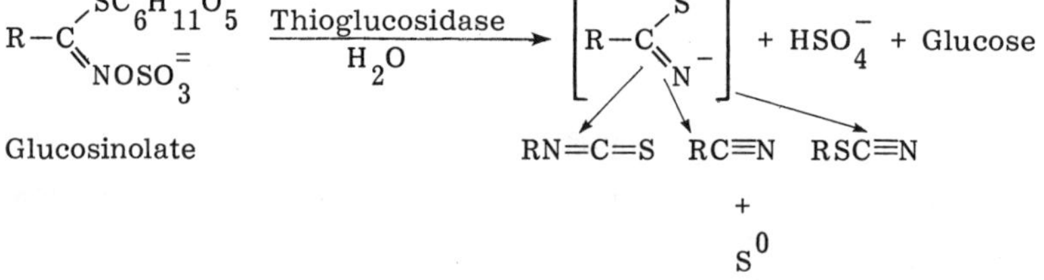

$$R-C\underset{NOSO_3^=}{\overset{SC_6H_{11}O_5}{<}} \xrightarrow[H_2O]{\text{Thioglucosidase}} \left[R-C\underset{N^-}{\overset{S^-}{<}}\right] + HSO_4^- + \text{Glucose}$$

Glucosinolate　　　　　　　　　　　　RN=C=S　RC≡N　RSC≡N
　　　　　　　　　　　　　　　　　　　　　　　+
　　　　　　　　　　　　　　　　　　　　　　S^0

An excellent example of one of the potent glucosinolates is progoitrin from the seeds of Brassica plants and the roots of rutabaga (Astwood 1949; Greer and Astwood 1948; Langer and Stolc 1965, 1964). This compound hydrolyzes as follows to yield the compounds shown:

$$CH_2=CHCHCH_2C-SC_6H_{11}O_5 \quad \xrightarrow{\text{Thioglucosidase}}$$

with OH above the CHCH and $\overset{||}{N}-OSO_2^-K^+$ below

Progoitrin

$CH_2=CHCHCH_2CN$ (I), with OH

$CH_2-CHCHCH_2CN$ (II), with S bridge and OH

$CH_2=CHCHCH_2N=C=S$ (III), with OH

$CH_2=CH$ ... $C=S$ with O and CH_2-NH (IV)

The nitriles obtained from progoitrin, 1-cyano-2-hydroxy-3-butene (I), and 1-cyano-2-hydroxy-3,4-butylepisulfide (II) are highly toxic (VanEtten et al. 1969). They also cause enlargement of the liver and kidney of rats. Some of the pathological changes in the liver include hyperplasia of the bile duct, fibrosis, and megalocytosis of the hepatocytes. There are also lesions in the epithelial cells of the renal tubules (VanEtten et al. 1969). The goitrogenicity of these nitriles is still unconfirmed. Positive results (Greer 1950) may arise from the effects of the nitrile biotransformation products, the thiocyanates (Barker 1936; Langer and Michajlovskij 1958; Langer and Stolc 1964, 1965).

The cyclization product of 2-hydroxy-3,4-butenylisothiocyanate (III) is goitrin, (S)-5-vinyl-oxazolidone-2-thione (IV), a powerful goitrogen. The enantiomer, (R)-5-vinyl-oxazolidone-2-thione, from crambe seeds, is also a strong antithyroid agent (Daxenbiehler et al. 1965). These compounds interfere in the iodination of thyroxine precursors (Astwood et al. 1945; Clements 1960), so that the resulting goiter is not easily corrected by iodine therapy. Therefore, Brassica seed goiter is probably caused by these specific compounds.

The concentration of glucosinolates in Brassica plants may be relatively high. Thus, the concentration of goitrin in turnip roots has been reported to be 0.12 to 1.0 g/kg (Astwood et al. 1949) and 2 to 4 g/kg in rapeseed meal (Raciszewski et al. 1955).

Thiocyanates The thiocyanates and isothiocyanates obtained from the glucosinolates are probably the active principles responsible for cabbage goiter (Barker 1936; Gmelin and Virtanen 1960; Johnston and Jones 1966; Langer and Stolc 1964, 1965). Similarly, the cyanogens produce goitrogens, since their main biotransformation products, by the enzyme rhodanase, are thiocyanates (Viehover 1940). The goitrogenicity of thiocyanates in humans was first observed in patients treated with these compounds to control hypertension (Barker 1936). This effect of thiocyanates may be attributed to the inhibition of iodine uptake by the thyroid gland as observed in the rat (VanderLaan and VanderLaan 1947). Higher levels of this ion can also depress the formation of thyroxine even when the supply of iodine is adequate (Greer et al. 1966). Thus, with continuous exposure to thiocyanates, whether from glucosinolates or cyanogens, it is possible that goiter may be induced even with adequate iodine intake.

Cheiroline ($CH_3SO_2(CH_2)_2NCS$) This is an aglycone of the glycoside obtained from the seeds and leaves of the wild turnip (Rapistrum rugosum) or from certain crucifers (for example, Brassica campestris). It is a more active goitrogen than propylisothiocyanate (Bachelard and Trikojus 1960, 1963a,b).

Polyphenolic Glucosides Examples of these are arachidoside and anacardioside, which are obtained from the red integument of peanuts (Arachis hypogaea). Their goitrogenicity has been demonstrated in the rat (Moudgal et al. 1958, 1957; Srinivasan et al. 1957). Arachidosides are also found in the seed coats of almonds (*Prunus amygdalus*), areca nuts (*Areca catechu*), and cashew nuts (*Anacardium occidentale*).

Phenols as a class are capable of forming iododerivatives in vivo, and therefore would compete for iodine in the formation of thyroxine. These plant phenols include catechol, resorcinol, favonol, phloroglucinol, and hesperetol. These may exist in plants as glucosides, rutin and quercitrin (with quercitin as their aglycones), and in pigments such as the anthocyanins and flavones (Cruz-Coke and de los Reyes 1947a-c; Cruz-Coke et al. 1947; Jeney and Jeney 1960; Jeney et al. 1960). These compounds are abundant in edible plants.

The goitrogenicity of these types of compounds has been demonstrated in rats given up to 10^{-6} m quercitrin solution for drinking instead of tap water (Cruz-Coke and Plaza de los Reyes 1947a-c; Cruz-Coke et al. 1947). The animals developed thyroid glands which were 43% heavier than controls and 70% lower in iodine content than controls.

Hemagglutinins   As mentioned previously, these factors are able to inhibit the absorption of amino acids. Therefore, these substances may also be expected to prevent the reabsorption of thyroxine. This fact has been demonstrated in the rat, which showed increased excretion of thyroxine in the feces and decreased concentration of the same in the blood when fed soya-rich diets (Albert and Keating 1952; Beck 1958; Jaffe 1969; Pinchera et al. 1965; Van Middlesworth 1957). Soybeans and other legumes are quite rich in hemagglutinins. There have been several reports of children developing goiter after prolonged feeding with soya milk (Hydovitz 1960; Pinchera et al. 1965; Shepard et al. 1960; Van Wyk et al. 1959).

Miscellaneous Goitrogens   The list of goitrogens has been lenghtened by the reports that volatile components of onions, methyl-, allyl-, and n-propyldisulfide, depress iodine uptake of the thyroids of rats fed diets low in iodine (Cowan et al. 1967; Saghir et al. 1966). It has been suggested that the large amounts of onions in the diet may explain in part the high prevalence of endemic goiter in the populations living in the valleys of Lebanon (Saghir et al. 1966).

An unknown compound in dried cassava can cause enlarged thyroids in rats. The goiter in the latter appears to be resistant to iodine therapy (Ekpechi et al. 1966), and therefore may be caused by high levels of cyanogens which may cause goiter through their biotransformation products, the thiocyanates.

Accumulation of Goitrogens in Milk

Cows foraging in pastures laden with crucifers may concentrate goitrogens in their milk, so that a correlation between the increased incidence of goiter in Tasmanian children and the drinking of milk from these cows has been observed, especially during the spring and summer months (Clements 1955, 1957, 1958). It has been shown that the milk suspected of goitrogen contamination inhibits iodine uptake of human thyroids.

Several workers in other countries, however, have been unable to confirm these findings (Greene et al. 1958; Vilkki et al. 1962). Nevertheless, the differences in experimental subjects and the difficulty of controlling iodine content of the diets may explain, partly, the discrepancy in results. It has been shown, for example, that during testing, the rate of iodine uptake of human thyroids is very sensitive to variations in the amounts of iodine in the diet or in the body (Virtanen et al. 1963).

Toxic Hazards of Goitrogens in Humans

The production of goiter from the above factors must be considered in terms of the total iodine and goitrogen intake, except perhaps those produced by goitrin and similar compounds. A thiocyanate-iodine ratio of 2000 will invariably produce goiter in the rat. Goiter is not produced with a ratio of 500 or less (Virtanen 1961, 1962). If these results can be extrapolated to human situations, consumption of 500 g of cabbage with only 1 μg iodine/kg body weight may result in goiter. The relatively smaller amounts of cabbage usually consumed seem to minimize the danger posed by the goitrogenic food. However, certain types of food which contain several goitrogens may be consumed consistently. In addition, several types of goitrogen-containing food may also be eaten together. Thus, goitrogenesis becomes a real possibility even with diets normally considered adequate in iodine.

Dietary Fiber

Beneficial effects to the overall health of the gastrointestinal tract and other healthy activities have been ascribed recently to dietary "fiber." While many of these assertions may have some degree of validity, some of the deleterious effects of overconsumption of fiber should receive equal attention.

The nature of fiber is still being explored. While it may be indigestible, it is not the same as crude fiber after drastic chemical treatment; it is also far from inert. Obviously, this fiber has a variable composition depending on the source, and should be considered a generic term representing the many indigestible materials left after food has passed through the stomach and small intestines. This group should include cellulose, hemicellulose, lignins, pectins, tannins, gums, other indigestible polysaccharides, indigestible proteins such as scleroproteins and prolamins, plant pigments, waxes and other lipidic materials, siliceous materials, and other substances. These materials give bulk to the fecal matter, not only from their inherent mass, but also by the amount of bound water. The amount of water bound may be four to six times the dry weight of the fiber (Burkitt et al. 1974; Eastwood et al. 1974). The bulk then causes decreased transit time and frequent stool elimination (Burkitt et al. 1974).

Judging from the types of components that may comprise fiber, many reactive groups may be present which may bind metals, amino acids, and even sugars. These groups may include $-COOH$, $-HPO_3H$, $-OH$, $-SO_3H$, $-NH_2$, and others. Thus, the fiber components of many food products act like polyfunctional ion exchangers (McConnell et al. 1974). As such, their binding capacity should be dependent on the pH and ionic composition of the digest.

The binding of amino acids or proteins by dietary fiber has been demonstrated earlier by investigators working on the problems of protein digestibility (Mitchell 1924). Increased fecal nitrogen excretion has been found even in rats on a nonprotein diet when the roughage is increased.

Cellulose at 15% in the diet has been shown to cause a significant drop in nitrogen absorption by as much as 8%. Carrageenans, which are highly indigestible, also cause even greater reduction in the assimilation of nitrogen. In this case, a highly significant drop of about 16% of the amount of the absorbable nitrogen has been observed. In both cases, growth retardation has been noted, even at the 10% level. Growth retardation has been shown to be greater with a carrageenans-containing diet (Hawkins and Yaphe 1965). The depression of protein digestibility with increased dietary fiber also was reported earlier by Moran and Pace (1942). In this case, the digestion of proteins in high extraction wheat meals was significantly depressed.

Dietary fiber also has the capacity to bind various metals. Thus, dephytinized bran shows increased capacity to bond Ca^{2+} and Zn^{2+} in vitro, and this capacity is decreased by partial degradation of bran with HCl (Reinhold et al. 1975). In vivo tests confirm the decrease in the availability of minerals such as iron and copper in the presence of fiber in the form of corn pericarp and peanut hulls (Stiles 1977). Negative balances for Ca^{2+}, Mg^{2+}, Zn^{2+}, and P also have been noted in human subjects fed diets high in fiber content in the form of whole wheat bread. Although some adaptation has been observed for Zn^{2+} and phosphorus, none has been noted for Ca^{2+} and Mg^{2+} (Reinhold et al. 1976a). The absorption of zinc also is depressed by cellulose (Reinhold et al. 1976b).

Thus, ingestion of excess dietary fiber is not without deleterious effects on mineral and nitrogen balances. Their effects on vitamin absorption still need to be determined.

TYPE C: ANTIVITAMINS

Somogyi (1973) defines an antivitamin "as a compound that diminishes or abolishes the effect of a vitamin in a specific way." This definition is essentially similar to that stated by Gontzea and Sutzescu (1968), who defined these substances as a group of naturally occurring organic compounds which decompose certain vitamins, combine with them to form unabsorbable complexes which are resistant to enzymes, or interfere in their digestive or metabolic utilization. These definitions are much broader in scope than that proposed by Shaw (1953) and Woolley (1952), who narrowly defined antivitamins to correspond to the concept of antimetabolites. These authors would consider as antivitamins only those compounds with similar chemical structures as the corresponding vitamins, which produce toxic symptoms in animals corresponding to a deficiency of the vitamins. In this case, the vitamin is competitively inhibited by the antivitamin. It is obvious that restricting the concept of antivitamins to only those which function as antimetabolites would eliminate many substances which produce toxic symptoms in animals by their destruction of vitamins, either inside or outside the body, or block vitamin absorption.

There are also compounds which do not meet the criteria set forth in the preceding definitions, but nevertheless increase the specific metabolic requirements of the animal for certain vitamins. Thus, under conditions of marginal vitamin intakes, it may be possible to produce vitamin deficiency symptoms in the presence of such compounds. The classification of these compounds as antivitamins can be justified on this basis.

Thus, a more comprehensive definition of an antivitamin may be stated as follows: An antivitamin is any compound which under certain conditions can actually or potentially produce toxic symptoms such as in a deficiency of the corresponding vitamin, whether administered parenterally, ingested, or present along with the vitamin in food. Thus, according to this definition, a substance which degrades a vitamin is considered to be an antivitamin even though deficiency symptoms have not been demonstrated owing to its presence in the diet. These substances may only possess the potential to produce deficiency symptoms, especially when present in large amounts, and must be examined when vitamin intakes from food sources are considered. The definition also includes nutrients which when taken in excess, increase the physiological requirements of other vitamins.

Ascorbic Acid Oxidase

Ascorbic acid oxidase is a copper-containing enzyme that catalyzes the oxidation of free ascorbic acid to diketogluconic acid, oxalic acid, and other oxidation products. The enzyme is released when plant cells are broken. The enzyme is active between pH 4 and 7—with a pH optimum between 5.6 and 6—and is activated at pH 2 or by blanching vegetables at around 100°C. Its temperature optimum is around 38°C (Diemair and Zerban 1944a; Dunn and Dawson 1951; Sack et al. 1961; Tauber et al. 1935).

Ascorbic acid oxidase is found in many fruits and vegetables such as cucumbers, pumpkins, lettuce, cress, peaches, cauliflowers, spinach, green beans, green peas, carrots, potatoes, squash, bananas, tomatoes, beets, and kohlrabi (Kertesz et al.

1936; Lovett-Janison and Nelson 1940; McCombs 1957; Stone 1937; Tauber et al. 1935; Wokes and Organ 1943). The activity of the enzyme varies with the fruit or vegetable. Its highest activity has been recorded in the pumpkin. In tomatoes, the enzyme is located mostly in the outer layers, and is most abundant in green fruit (Barron et al. 1936; Diemair and Zerban 1944a,b; Wokes and Organ 1943). There is a gradual disappearance of vitamin C when the vegetables are cut.

Flavanoids, which are present in vegetables, may strongly inhibit the enzyme. Many other substances in plants tend to protect ascorbic acid from the effects of the enzyme. For example, orange juice has an ascorbic acid protective factor which is present in colloidal suspension, giving the juice its typical cloudy appearance (Concon and Human 1981).

Antiretinol and Anticarotene

So far, only a few substances in food have been identified with antiretinol activity. Citral in oranges is a retinol antagonist (Leach and Lloyd 1956). An unknown substance(s) in yeast has the ability to diminish the stored retinol in pig liver (Braude et al. 1947).

Retinol, being highly unsaturated, is expected to be sensitive to peroxidation. Thus, factors in food, derived or natural, may enhance this effect. However, data in this respect are still meager.

Whereas the tocopherols (vitamin E), or tocols, at low dosages possess a sparing action on retinol (Hickman et al. 1944a,b), at high doses, they produce a genuine antiretinol effect (Brubacher et al. 1965). The sparing action of the tocols on retinol is more than just an antioxidant effect, since the protective effects of various forms of the vitamin appear to be the same in vivo even though their antioxidant properties in vitro are quite different (Hickman et al. 1944a,b).

The carotene antagonists, linoleic and linolenic acid (Smith and Caldwell 1945; Sherman 1941), may also be expected to possess antiretinol activity. The effect of these fatty acids on carotene is an example of nutrient antagonism.

Lipoxidase, which is found in soybeans, can enhance the oxidation of carotene (Smith and Caldwell 1945; Sumner and Dounce 1939).

Antitocols

α-Tocopherol functions as an antioxidant for unsaturated fatty acids, and is destroyed in the process. Therefore, the metabolic requirement for tocopherols is increased by linoleic acid (Dam 1962; Horwitt 1960).

Faddism associated with high intakes of polyenic fatty acids may create adverse effects on tocopherol status. It has been demonstrated by Horwitt (1960-1962) and Harris and Embree (1963) that the requirements for the vitamin are increased with high intakes of polyenic fatty acids. Thus, excessive intakes of polyenic fatty acids may promote tocopherol deficiency (Harris and Embree 1963; Herting 1966).

Some authors have suggested that to prevent deficiency symptoms, the tocopherol-polyenic fatty acid (g) ratio should be at least 0.6 mg/g (Harris and Embree 1963). It also has been shown that this requirement may be influenced by the degree of susceptibility of a fatty acid to peroxidation (Witting and Horwitt 1964). By whatever the mechanisms tocopherols influence the metabolism of polyenic fatty acids, whether as antioxidant or as a metabolic participant, excessive intakes of polyenic fatty acids with insufficient tocopherols may produce deleterious effects (Tappel 1962). Fortunately, vegetable oils, the common source of polyenic fatty acids, are also abundant in tocopherols (Hove and Harris 1951). This is not the case with fish oil and other marine oil.

Substances with antitocol activity are present in yeast, alfalfa, and kidney beans (Bieri et al. 1958; Hintz and Hogue 1964; Pudelkiewicz and Matterson 1960). In the latter, two types of antitocols have been isolated. One is fat soluble and heat stable; the other is thermolabile and fat insoluble (Hintz and Hogue 1964).

The antitocol factor in alfalfa was suspected when it was observed that α-tocopherol, even though present at high concentrations, was not fully available to chickens (Bunnell 1957; Singsen et al. 1955). The antitocol in alfalfa was reported to be a lipid-soluble material (Pudelkiewicz and Matterson 1960; Pudelkiewicz et al. 1960).

Antithiamine

Antithiamine Factors in Fish

A dramatic manifestation of thiaminase activity was observed in silver foxes fed raw carp on a farm in Minnesota in 1932 (Green 1936, 1937; Green et al. 1941, 1942a). The resulting thiamine deficiency in these animals produced the characteristic neurological syndrome known as Chastek paralysis (after the owner of the farm). After a few weeks of eating a diet containing 10% raw carp, the animals developed anorexia. Their gut stiffened about 2 weeks later. Spastic paralysis, inability to stand, and extreme sensitivity to pain developed as the disease worsened. Death occurred within 12 hr after paralysis developed. The disease could be controlled with 20 mg thiamine daily mixed with the feed.

Similar thiamine avitaminosis in solver foxes was also reported in Sweden (Carlström et al. 1939) and Norway (Ender and Helgebostad 1940).

The antithiamine acitivity was confined to the skin, head and viscera of the carp; muscles were devoid of activity (Green et al. 1942a,b; Somogyi 1949a,b). The spleen, liver, and intestines contained the highest activity (Sealock et al. 1943); heart muscle was also highly active, whereas the brain and mesentery were moderately so (Somogyi 1949a,b).

The antithiamine factor was isolated by Somogyi and co-workers (Somogyi 1956; Somogyi 1960) as a dark brown crystalline substance. It appears to be a conjugated protein with a molecular weight of 75,000 to 100,000; it is soluble in water at pH 7, and in alkaline solutions as well as in 10 N formic acid. It is insoluble in less polar organic solvents. The nonprotein component is a porphyrinlike compound resembling hemin very closely, as demonstrated by spectral and other analytical methods (Somogyi and Kundig 1968). Apparently, it is this component which is the thermostable, antithiamine factor (Kundig and Somogyi 1967).

The carp thiaminase splits thiamine at the methylene bridge, producing the reaction products shown below (Barnhurst and Hennessy 1952a,b; Krampitz and Woolley 1944; Kupstas and Hennessy 1957a,b; Somogyi 1949a).

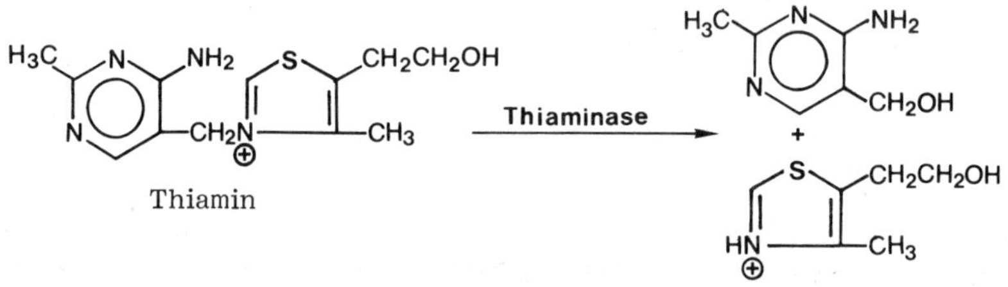

Thiaminases must have an essential function in many species, since they are widely distributed. They have been detected in both freshwater (Deutch and Hasler 1943; Somogyi 1952) and saltwater species of fish (Daum and Jaffe 1956; Doelarkar and Sohonie 1957; Hilker and Peter 1966; Jacobson and deAzevedo 1947; Ler et al. 1955; Neilands 1947).

Such common fish species as the herring, *Clupea harengus* and *C. pallasus* (Sautier 1946), and swordfish, *Belone acus* (Lieck and Agren 1944), skipjack, *Katsuwonas pelamis,* and yellowfin tuna, *Neothunnus macropterus* (Hilker and Peter 1966) have been reported to contain the antithiamine factor, particularly in the viscera. Similarly, this factor also has been isolated in certain species of crab (Jacobson and deAzevedo 1947) and in the clam, *Venus mercenaria campechiensis,* and soft-shell clam, *Mya arenaria* (Melnick et al. 1945).

It is interesting to note that in some fish, such as *Anchoe lyolepis* and *Clupanodon pseudohispanicus,* the muscles have proved to be just as active in the antithiamine factor as the viscera (Daum and Jaffe 1956).

Antithiamine Factors in Plants

Antithiamine factors are also present in plants, such as bean (*Phaseolus radiatus*), ragi (*Eleusine cora*), cotton seed, mustard seed, flax seed (Bhagvat and Devi 1944), blackberries, black currants, brussel sprouts, red cabbage, red beets, and red cicerone. Lesser amounts are found in black cherries, crisped cabbage, green cicerone, raspberries, and spinach (Kundig and Somogyi 1964). Strangely enough, some investigators have reported an antithiamine factor in rice bran (Bhagvat and Devi 1944; Chaudhuri 1962, 1964; Kumar and Chaudhuri 1976).

The most well known antithiamine factor next to that in carp is that found in the bracken fern (Haag et al. 1947; Haag and Westwig 1948). There may be two types of heat-stable antithiamine factors in ferns; these are termed hydrolysates I and II (Koller and Somogyi 1961; Petropulos 1960; Somogyi and Koller 1959). One of these factors has been crystallized in pure form and identified as caffeic acid (3,4-dihydro-0-cinnamic acid) (Beruter and Somogyi 1966, 1967).

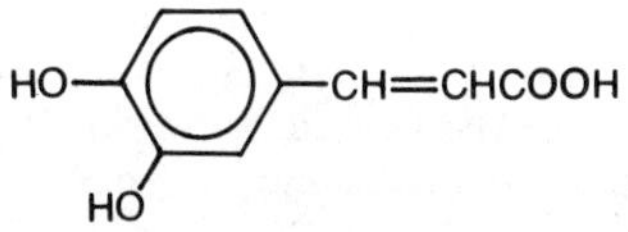

$$HO-\langle\bigcirc\rangle-CH\!=\!CHCOOH$$
$$HO$$

Caffeic acid

It should be recalled that caffeic acid also can be hydrolyzed from chlorogenic acid by intestinal bacteria (Chap. 3).

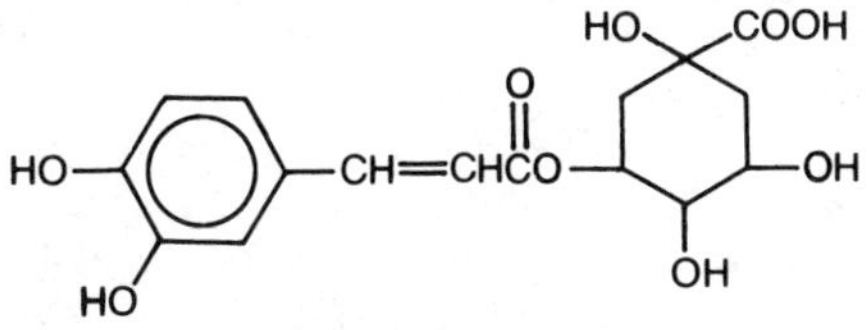

$$HO-\langle\bigcirc\rangle-CH\!=\!CHCO-$$

Chlorogenic acid

Chlorogenic acid is found in green coffee beans. One mole of caffeic acid can destroy 3 mol of thiamine in 16 hr at pH 7.8 and 37°C.

It appears that the antithiamine activity is also a property of other o-dihydric phenols, such as pyrocatechol (Davis and Somogyi 1969; Somogyi and Bonicke 1969).

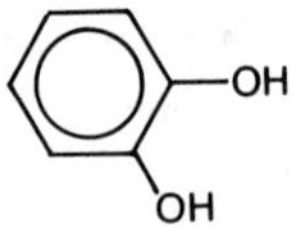

Pyrocatechol

p-Hydroxyphenols have also moderate antithiamine activity.

An example of a *p*-hydroxyphenolic antithiamine factor is the compound isolated in pure form from mustard seed (*Brassica juncea*) by Bhattacharya and Chaudhuri (1973). The compound has been identified as methylsinapate, which is also present in rape seed (*B. napus*) (Noda and Matsumoto 1971).

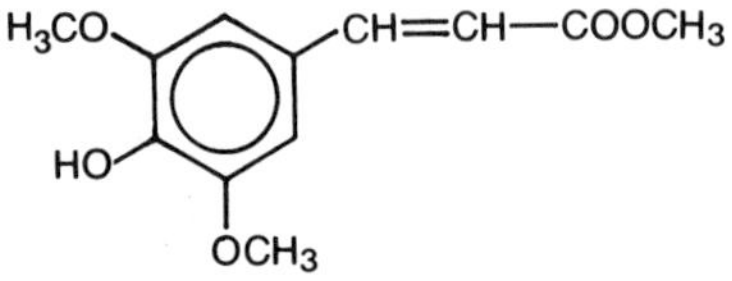

Methylsinapate

At 30°C, pH 6.5, 1 mg of methylsinapate will inactivate 45 µg of thiamine hydrochloride. This is about 30% as active as caffeic acid, which under similar conditions inactivates 135 µg of thiamine hydrochloride.

The mechanism of thiamine inactivation by these compounds requires oxygen and is dependent on temperature and pH. Thus, an oxidation-reduction reaction is indicated. The reaction appears to occur in two stages: The first stage occurs rapidly and is reversible by addition of reducing agents. The second stage occurs at a much lower rate and is irreversible (Davis and Somogyi 1969).

Similarly, tannins possess antithiamine activity. The antithiamine activity of tea infusions, which has been correlated with their tannin content, increases with pH and temperature (Hilker et al. 1971). The rate of thiamine destruction in the presence of a 1:100 dilution of tea extracts increase rapidly at above pH 7. Complete destruction occurs at pH 7.5, 60°C, with 3 hr reaction time. At 37°C, pH 7.5, about 10% of thiamine will be destroyed after 1 hr, compared to about 50% at 60°C. The antithiamine activity in tea has been confirmed by Rungruangsak et al. (1977) and Kositawattanakul et al. (1977), who saw evidence of the formation of a thiamine-tannin adduct. The mode of reaction between tannins and thiamine is biphasic—an initial rapid reaction independent of oxygen followed by one which is slower and oxygen-dependent. This is similar to the reaction observed by Davis and Somogyi (1969) with dihydroxy phenols.

An interesting observation by Rungruanangsak et al. (1977) and Kositawattanakul et al. (1977) is the complete inhibition of the reaction by ascorbic acid if present at the beginning of the reaction; and a partial reversal if ascorbic acid is added during the first 30 min of reaction. This effect of ascorbic acid occurs in both acid or neutral pH (Kositawattanakul et al. 1977).

Antithiamine Factors in Bacteria and Fungi

Thiaminases have also been isolated or detected in certain species of bacteria and fungi. The thiaminase-producing bacterial species *Bacillus thiaminolyticus* (Matsukawa and Misawa 1951) and *Clostridium thiaminolyticum* (Kimura and Liao 1953) were isolated from human feces. These bacilli also were cultured from the feces of beriberi patients (Inoue 1951); 3% of samples contained *B. thiaminolyticus* in one survey of human feces in Japan (Hamada 1953), and 7 to 10% in another (Kimura et al. 1952). The third thiamine-splitting bacterium is *B. aneurolyticus,* which was isolated from hay and soil (Kimura et al. 1952).

    B. thiaminolyticus and *C. thiaminolyticum* produce thiaminase I, which catalyzes the breakdown of the thiamine molecule by a base exchange reaction. The *B. aneurolyticus* promotes a simple hydrolysis of thiamine (Wittlife and Airth 1970a,b). This subject has been discussed in Chapter 3. The action of the enzyme in *B. aneurolyticus* is the same as that of the enzyme in fish and shellfish. However, the rate of reaction promoted by the thiaminases from different sources may be variable. This has not been determined.

    Thiaminases also have been isolated in certain fungi: *Trichosporum aneurinolyticum,* so named by Aoki (1955), and *Lentinus edodes,* a mushroom (Kawasaki and Ono 1968). The latter contains thiaminase I and another antithiamine factor which is heat stable. Thiaminase II also has been found in yeastlike fungi; i.e., *Torulaspora, Torulopsis,* and *Thodotorula* species (Ozawa et al. 1957). Thiaminase I and II are heat labile, being inactivated at 60°C or above (Wittlife and Airth 1970a,b).

Effects of Thiaminases in Other Animals

The antithiamine factor in carp also has been found to induce symptoms of thiamine deficiency in cats fed raw carp for 3 to 6 weeks. The symptoms disappear following thiamine injection (Smith and Proutt 1944). Polyneuritis also can be induced in chickens fed raw carp at 25% of the diet. The disease is not produced in birds with boiled carp. Supplementation of the diet with 0.5 mg% thiamine diminish the incidence of polyneuritis by only 20% (Spitzer et al. 1941). This is to be expected, since obviously thiaminase is capable of breaking down any additional thiamine that is present in the diet. The conditions in the gastrointestinal tract, which can vary in animals, may permit an adequate portion of the ingested thiamine to escape degradation.

    Horses and cattle also have been reported to develop thiamine deficiency symptoms following consumption of ferns (*Pteris aquilinum*) for 1 to 3 months. The animals show decreased thiamine and increased pyruvic acid concentration in the blood. These are accompanied by hyperesthesia, ataxia, convulsion, and frequently, fatal paralysis. These symptoms can be prevented by inclusion of yeast or thiamine in the diet (Jacquet 1950; Roberts et al. 1949).

    Rats also develop fatal thiamine deficiency after 3 to 4 weeks on diets containing 40% dried bracken fern (*Pteridium equilinum*) (Weswig et al. 1946). Rats given supplementary thiamine continuously are not affected. High doses of the vitamin will cure sick animals.

Significance of Thiaminases in the Human Situation

That thiaminases can decrease the thiamine levels in human tissues has been demonstrated experimentally. Thus, human subjects fed 15 to 20 g bracken fern/day had reduced thiamine excretion (Murata 1965; Samruatruamphol and Parsons 1955). In another experiment, five adults given 100 g raw clams daily over three meals developed a sudden decrease in spontaneous thiaminuria; in the same group, the amount of thiamine excreted within 24 hr after loading with the vitamin was also decreased. It has been estimated, in this case, that 50% of the thiamine ingested was destroyed by the thiaminase (Melnick et al. 1945).

    Consistent with the antithiamine activity of tea, as discussed earlier, Vimokesant et al. (1974) has shown that the thiamine status of tea-drinking school children and adults who chewed tea leaves was significantly decreased. In this case, the degree of stimulation of transketolase activity by thiamine pyrophosphate (TPP) was used as a measure of thiamine status, the higher degree of stimulation corresponding to lower thiamine status. Tea drinking by the school children for 7 days caused the transketolase activity to double in the presence of TPP to a point suggesting a deficient thiamine status. This was reversed by thiamine supplementation. Each liter of tea was estimated to destroy 2.1 mg thiamine.

Among the adults who chewed tea leaves, withdrawal of the leaves caused a decline of the transketolase stimulation by 30%, and by about 65% when thiamine (10 mg/day) was also given. But this amount was insufficient to reverse the deficient status when chewing tea leaves was continued. This result was expected because fermented tea leaves were found to destroy 0.93 mg thiamine/hr/g tea leaves, and 12 g of leaves/day were chewed by each person.

Further studies in Thailand with adult volunteers (Vimokesant et al. 1975) who chewed betel nuts (*Areca catechu*) and who consumed raw fermented fish have shown similar results. Betel nut is high in tannins and raw fish contains thiaminase, as stated elsewhere in this chapter. Cooking the fermented fish destroyed much of the thiaminase and improved the thiamine status of the test subjects significantly. Even greater improvement was noted with thiamine supplementation (10 mg/day). Betel nut-chewing adults had a depressed thiamine status, which improved significantly when this practice was discontinued. These subjects became marginal again when chewing was resumed. Supplementation with 10 mg thiamine/day was insufficient to counteract the antithiamine activity in betel nut.

A thiaminase-related disorder occurred in two of 29 subjects given 4 to 8 mg of *Bacillus thiaminolyticus*. This does not appear significant, but with low thiamine diets, carriers of the thiaminase bacteria in their gastrointestinal tract developed thiamine deficiency symptoms twice as fast as those who were not carriers (Fujimiya 1950, 1951).

Thiaminases do not pose significant health hazards to humans. However, in those with marginal thiamine status, these agents may precipitate frank thiamine deficiency. Thiamine is among the vitamins that are likely to be deficient in the diet (Orten and Neuhaus 1975). Thus, persistent consumption of antithiamine factors (e.g., raw fish and mollusks, ferns, fruits) and the possible presence of thiaminase-producing bacteria in the GI tract may compromise the already marginal thiamine intake. The results from the Thailand experiments (Vimokesant et al. 1975) support the theory that antithiamine factors in foods may compromise a marginal thiamine status. And it has been noted that in some parts of Thailand, the consumption of food and other substances containing antithiamine factors can be correlated with the prevalence of thiamine deficiency among the population (Vimokesant et al. 1975).

Because of the significant involvement of thiamine in carbohydrate and fat metabolism, as expected, high carbohydrate and fat diets can increase the thiamine requirements (Harris 1949).

Antibiotin

Avidin is a basic glycoprotein in egg white which binds biotin so avidly that the resultant complex is resistant to dilute acid, alkali, enzymes, and moderate heat (Baumgarter 1957; Eakin et al. 1940; György and Rose 1943; Hertz 1946). The protein contains about 6% tryptophan; this amino acid is necessary for activity (Melamed and Green 1963). Each molecule of avidin binds four of biotin (Green 1963), and the presence of ions is necessary for the binding activity (Wei and Wright 1964). One unit of avidin activity equals that quantity which binds 1 μg biotin; therefore, 1 mg avidin is equivalent to 8 U of antibiotin activity. Egg white may contain 0.4 to 0.6 U/ml, and in the dried form, there are 7 to 8 U/g (Eakin et al. 1941; Jones and Briggs 1962).

This factor is responsible for the so-called "raw eggwhite injury" in animals, which is characterized by eczematous dermatitis, shedding of hair, especially around the eyes (spectacle eyes), and bleeding. In severe cases, tetany, paralysis of the hind legs, and death may ensue. In addition to the skin, several other organs may also be damaged (Boas 1927; Eakin et al. 1940; Finlay and Stern 1929; György 1939; Hegsted et al. 1942; Nielsen and Elvehjem 1942; Parsons and Kelly 1933a,b).

Biotin deficiency dermatitis also has been observed in human subjects eating raw egg white for several weeks on a diet suboptimum in biotin (Sydenstricker et al. 1942a,b; Williams 1943). Thus, the practice of soft-boiling eggs so that the white is incompletely cooked or the use of raw egg white in certain concoctions may intensify an existing marginal biotin deficiency (Hertz 1946; Nielsen and Elvehjem 1941, 1942; Parsons 1931; Parsons and Kelly 1933a,b; Williams 1943).

Avidin loses its ability to bind biotin after boiling egg white or pure avidin for 3 to 5 min (György and Rose 1943; György et al. 1941).

Similar types of avidinlike proteins have been isolated in chicken liver (Gilgen and Leuthardt 1962; Vallotton and Leuthardt 1963) and in human blood serum (Vallotton et al. 1965). The chicken liver protein also binds biotin rapidly and irreversibly. These observations raise the question as to whether there are many more types of avidinlike proteins.

Antipyridoxine

Linseed meal contains a water-soluble and heat-labile factor which can induce pyridoxine deficiency in chickens (Kratzer and Williams 1948; Kratzer et al. 1954). The effect, however, can be prevented by increased pyridoxine intake. Thus, it had been concluded that an antipyridoxine factor exists in these seeds. This factor has been later isolated by Klosterman et al. (1963, 1967) and is called linatine (from Linum, the genus of flax). Linatine is γ-glutamyl-1-amino-D-proline which is easily hydrolyzed to 1-amino-proline. The latter is the actual antipyridoxine factor.

Linatine   1-Amino-D-proline

1-Amino-D-proline reacts irreversibly in vivo with pyridoxal phosphate, and thus inactivates the active form of the vitamin.

Antipyridoxine factors in the form of various hydrazine derivatives also have been recognized or suspected in wild mushrooms, *Gyromitra esculenta* or false morel, Agaricaceae species such as *Agaricus bisporus*, a close relative of *A. campistris*, or meadow mushrooms, and *Lentinus edodes* and related species (Klosterman 1981). These mushrooms are usually considered as edible, although many of these species, such as *G. esculenta*, are increasingly known or suspected as poisonous (Chap. 10).

G. esculenta contains gyromitrin (acetaldehyde methylformylhydrazone) and higher homologs (Pyssalo 1975; Toth 1979); the Agaricaceae species contains agaritine (β-N-[γ-L(+)glutamyl]-4-hydroxymethylphenylhydrazine). The common commercial edible mushroom *A. bisporus* contains up to 0.04% agaritine (Levenberg 1960, 1967). This compound also occurs in the Japanese cultivated forest mushroom *Cortinellus shiitake* (Toth 1979).

Gyromitrin is hydrolyzable to N-methyl-N-formylhydrazine (MFH), which in turn

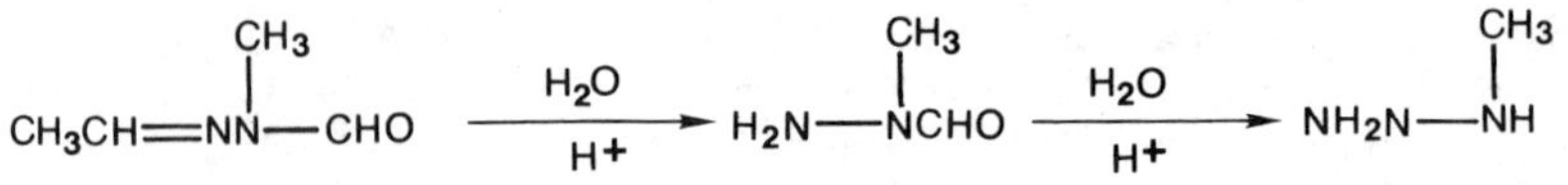

$$CH_3CH{=}NN{-}CHO \xrightarrow[H^+]{H_2O} H_2N{-}NCHO \xrightarrow[H^+]{H_2O} NH_2N{-}NH$$

Gyromitrine   MFH   Methylhydrazine

is hydrolyzed further to methylhydrazine under the acid conditions of the human or animal stomach (List and Luft 1969; Nagel et al. 1976).

Agaritine is hydrolyzed by γ-glutamyl transferase (GT), which is endogenous to the mushroom, to 4-hydroxymethylhydrazine (HMH).

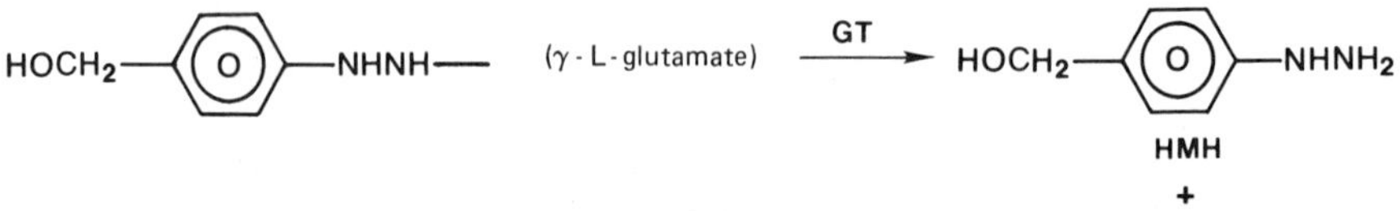

$$HOCH_2{-}\langle\bigcirc\rangle{-}NHNH{-}(\gamma\text{-L-glutamate}) \xrightarrow{GT} HOCH_2{-}\langle\bigcirc\rangle{-}NHNH_2$$

Agaritine   HMH
+
                                         L-Glutamate

The hydrazines combine with susceptible carbonyl groups such as pyridoxal or pyridoxal phosphate, forming hydrazones. Consequently, this vital coenzyme of many metabolic reactions is inactivated, so that a secondary pyridoxine deficiency is produced. As a matter of fact, the inactivation of pyridoxal phosphate is a fundamental problem in the therapy with hydrazide drugs (Doe 1976) such as the anti-tuberculosis drug isonicotinic acid hydrazide (INH) (Braunstein 1960), the antihypertensive drug hydralazine (Kirkendall and Page 1958), and several others. High doses of these drugs, especially in the presence of low pyridoxine intakes, can lead to symptoms of pyridoxine deficiency; e.g., anemia, polyneuritis, seborrheic dermatitis, stomatitis, glossitis, cheilosis, and symptoms of pellagra (Vilter et al. 1953). Severe pyridoxine deficiency can lead to convulsions in infants (Snyderman et al. 1950, 1953).

Letinus edodes and related species contain lentinic acid, an unusual trisulfoxide monosulfone dipeptide with glutamic acid (Yasumoto et al. 1976). In the presence of γ-glutamyl transferase (GT), which is present in the mushroom, it is hydrolyzed to the free amino acid, desglutamyllentinic acid (DGL) (see structures below).

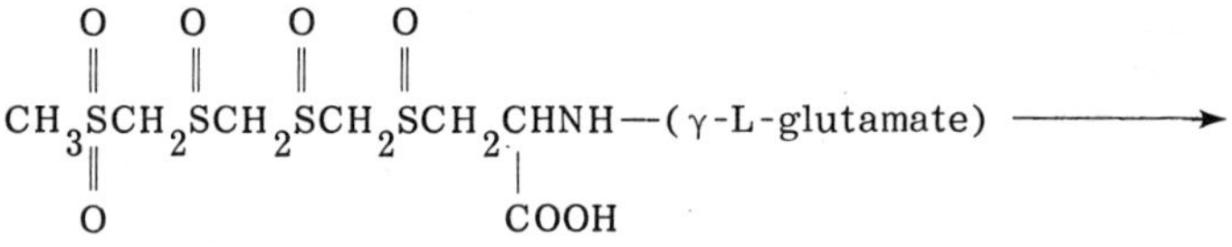

$$\overset{O}{\overset{\|}{CH_3}}\overset{O}{\underset{\|}{SCH_2}}\overset{O}{\overset{\|}{SCH_2}}\overset{O}{\overset{\|}{SCH_2}}\overset{O}{\overset{\|}{SCH_2}}\underset{\underset{COOH}{|}}{CHNH}{-}(\gamma\text{-L-glutamate}) \longrightarrow$$

Lentinic acid

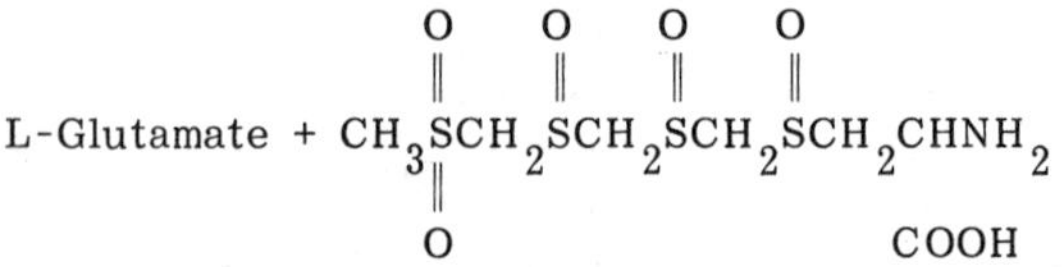

$$L\text{-Glutamate} + \overset{O}{\overset{\|}{CH_3}}\overset{O}{\underset{\|}{SCH_2}}\overset{O}{\overset{\|}{SCH_2}}\overset{O}{\overset{\|}{SCH_2}}\overset{O}{\overset{\|}{SCH_2}}\underset{\underset{COOH}{}}{CHNH_2}$$

Desglutamyllentinic acid

Like the ordinary amino acids, DGL forms a Schiff base with pyridoxal phosphate. However, DGL has a greater affinity ($K_{assoc.}$ = 1.2×10^5/M) for the coenzyme, and consequently less dissociable than with ordinary amino acids, so that pyridoxal phosphate is inactivated. The tight binding of DGL with pyridoxal phosphate results in an inhibition of the corresponding dependent enzymes; e.g., transaminases and tryptophanase (Yasumoto et al. 1976). Desglutamyllentinic acid, therefore, can be expected to possess an antipyridoxine effect, in the same manner as the hydrazines. Other antipyridoxines occurring in nature have been reviewed by Klosterman (1974, 1981). However, many of these compounds are produced by microorganisms and may have no or little significance in food toxicology.

Anticobalamin

As discussed below, there are apparently many types of anticobalamin factors; the mechanism of action of many of these has not been determined.

The cobalamin requirement in the chick is increased by excesses of protein and lard in the diet (Spivey et al. 1954; Yacowitz et al. 1952). The trypsin and chymotrypsin inhibitors, hemagglutinins, and other thyroid-active materials in soybeans have been shown to increase the cobalamin requirements in the chick and rat (Ershoff 1949; Frolich 1954).

There also appears to be an anticobalamin factor in corn meal (Lewis et al. 1950). In addition, as observed in the chick, the imbalance of leucine over isoleucine in corn may also cause an increased requirement for cobalamin (Hsu and Combs 1952).

With diets low in cobalamin, an excess of glycine in the diet can markedly increase the utilization of the vitamin (Machlin et al. 1952).

Ascorbic acid itself possesses anticobalamin activity. The destruction of cobalamin in ascorbic acid solutions (acetate buffer, pH 4) was noted more than 30 years ago by Hutchins et al. (1956). Indications of an anticobalamin effect of ascorbic acid has been reported in patients taking large doses of ascorbic acid for purposes of urinary acidification (Jacob et al. 1973; Murphy and Zelman 1965). Herbert and Jacob (1974) have reported that ascorbic acid destroys a considerable amount of cobalamin in an in vitro food mixture, homogenized and incubated at 37°C to mimic the condition of a food in the stomach. A considerable amount of the 3 to 6 μg cobalamin that is excreted in the bile may also be destroyed by ascorbic acid (Herbert 1975). Iron in food protects cobalamin from destruction by ascorbic acid (Bartilucci et al. 1957; Mukherjee and Sen 1959; Zuck and Conine 1963). However, relatively large quantities of iron may destroy cobalamin (Newmark 1958).

Decomposition products of thiamine at pH 8 and 4.5 may also destroy cobalamin; and nicotinamide also has been reported to have a similar effect at pH 4.5. Similarly, reducing agents such as H_2S and cysteine can also destroy cobalamin. This destruction is prevented or minimized by iron salts (Mukherjee and Sen 1959).

However, because of the difficulties associated with the cobalamin assay (Cohen and Donaldson 1980; England and Linnell 1980; Mollin et al. 1980; Witherspoon 1981), unequivocal proof of the destruction of cobalamin by ascorbic acid must include a demonstration of the presence of degradation or reaction products. Thus, Newark et al. (1976) using standard methods found no destruction of cobalamin by ascorbic acid under the conditions reported by Herbert and Jacob (1974), and that the low values obtained by the latter were due to poor extraction of tightly bound cobalamin. Nevertheless, because even this standard method does not give reliable results among different laboratories (England and Linnell 1980; Mollin et al. 1980), any valid conclusion regarding the stability or instability of a complex molecule as cobalamin, must be based, as already stated, on the presence of degradation products.

Antinicotinamide

Epidemiological evidence as well as feeding studies in mice, guinea pigs, and rats
have established the presence of an antinicotinamide factor in maize (Aykroyd and
Swaminathan 1940; Aykroyd et al. 1935; Chick et al. 1938; Goldsmith et al. 1955,
1952; Kodicek 1960; Krehl et al. 1945; Walker 1954).

Still unexplained, however, is the virtual absence of pellagra among Mexicans
compared to other populations whose dietary staple is also corn. It is tempting to
account for this observation on the lime treatment of corn practiced by the Mexicans
(Braude et al. 1955). However, animal experiments have shown that lime treatment
does not prevent the injury caused by the antinicotinamide factor in corn (Brahman
et al. 1962; Cravioto et al. 1952; Goldsmtih et al. 1956). The antiniacin factor in
corn probably is present in the bran or outer layers. Feeding studies with corn
bran have shown growth retardation in rats; and giving additional niacinamide (5
mg/100 g of diet) overcomes the growth inhibition (Borrow et al. 1948).

Woolley (1945a, 1946) isolated a nitrogenous compound in corn which has effects
in mice similar to the antinicotinamide factor, acetylpyridine (Cooperman et al. 1951).
Borrelidine, a toxic antibiotic isolated from rice samples, also has an antinicotinamide
activity (Cooperman et al. 1951). However, it is not known whether this is the same
nitrogenous factor isolated by Woolley (1945a, 1946). The antiniacin effect of this
antibiotic in corn can be prevented by feeding extra niacin or tryptophan.

Another possible antiniacin factor in corn is leucine. It is present at high levels
and can lead to an imbalance with structurally similar isoleucine or valine. Gopalan
(1968, 1970) has postulated that excess leucine may explain the occurrence of pellagra in parts of India where millet constitutes the main staple of the population's low
protein diet. Millet, like corn, is also high in leucine. He contends that pellagrins or
even normal human subjects fed 10 g leucine/day, for 5 days, have a depressed
ability to synthesize the nicotinamide nucleotide in their erythrocytes. Furthermore,
in experiments with puppies, extra leucine added to the nonpellagragenic diets
was shown to result in pellagralike symptoms, which can be prevented by a maize-
based diet containing less leucine. Hankes et al. (1971) also has concluded that the
high leucine content in corn interferes with the key enzymes in the synthesis of
nicotinamide adenosine diphosphate (NADP).

Trigonelline, an alkaloid found in coffee beans, soybeans, peas, potatoes, and
other plants (Concon 1978), is also an antiniacin factor, as tested in bacterial systems (McIlwain 1940).

Antiriboflavin

There are very few reports regarding the existence of a naturally occurring antiriboflavin factor. A report by Hill (1952) with respect to the "vomiting sickness" in
Jamaica indicated the possibility of the existence of this factor in the ackee fruit
(*Blighia sapida*). It has been reported that most patients poisoned by eating the
arilli of the unripe ackee fruit show severe riboflavin deficiency. Ackee contains a
toxic hypoglycemic amino acid, hypoglycin, or α-amino-β-methylenecyclopropanyl
propionic acid (Hassal et al. 1954; Renzo et al. 1959). In rats poisoned by ackee,

$$CH_2=C\text{------}CH-CH_2-CH-COOH$$
$$\diagdown \quad \diagup \qquad\qquad |$$
$$CH_2 \qquad\qquad NH_2$$

Hypoglycine

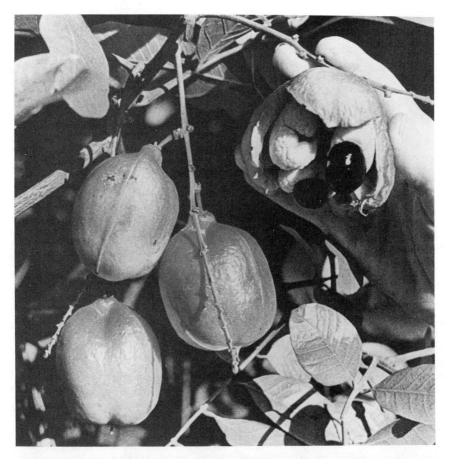

Figure 9.1 The ackee fruit (*Blighia sapida*). Note the arilli, the fleshy part on which the black seed sits. (Courtesy of Julia F. Morton, Director, Morton Collectanea, University of Miami, Coral Gables, Florida).

Fox and Miller (1960) have prevented body weight loss and death by administration of riboflavin. Furthermore, this vitamin reduces significantly the toxicity of hypoglycin A in rats, administered at a dose of 60 mg/kg body weight. Riboflavin phosphate also prevents the hypoglycin-induced lowering of glycosuria in alloxan-diabetic rats. It also decreases hypoglycin toxicity in mice (von Holt and von Holt 1959). These results strongly suggest the antiriboflavin nature of hypoglycin. The mechanism of action still needs to be clarified. Its action, however, may prove to be indirect, since this toxic amino acid is structurally unrelated to riboflavin.

Antipantothenate

The rare existence of an antipantothenate factor also has been reported. The substance, called pizamine, has been isolated from pea sprouts (Smashevskii 1965, 1966, 1969). Tests with yeast cells (*Saccharomyces cerevisiae*) have shown that the compound inhibits growth. Growth inhibition can be minimized or counteracted by pantothenic acid, β-alanine, and methionine, but it is enhanced by asparagine. So far, the effect of the substance has not been tested in animals.

Antifolacin

Nicotinamide may aggravate the need for folacin if the former is taken in excess (Fatterpaker et al. 1955; Handler 1944). This may be explained on the basis of the competition for methyl groups which is required for the detoxification of nicotinamide. On this basis, any compound which requires methyl groups for detoxification, if taken in excess, may be considered to possess an antifolacin activity. Thus, pressor amines, tannic acids, and other similar compounds in foodstuffs are in this category.

Anticholine

The formation of choline requires methyl groups. Therefore, what may be said of folacin will also hold true for choline (Fatterpaker et al. 1955). This is another example of nutrient antagonism which obviously is of greater significance in marginal vitamin intakes.

Anticholecalciferol

The presence of an anticholecalciferol factor in green oats was suspected when lambs fed these feedstuffs during the winter months developed rickets and growth retardation (Ewer 1950; Ewer and Bartrum 1948; Fitch and Ewer 1944). The effects in lambs also have been noted in guinea pigs (Ewer 1950). Cholecalciferol treatment reverses the effects. Rachitogenic effects also have been observed in rats fed chloroform extracts of the green oats. The anticholecalciferol factor does not affect the absorption of the vitamin (Grant 1951). It was shown that this factor is β-carotene (Grant 1953). A similar anticholecalciferol factor also detected in hay (Weits 1952), was also later identified as β-carotene (Weits 1966, 1960).

Another type of anticholecalciferol factor in vegetables appears to be a steroid, as reported by French investigators (Raoul et al. 1957). As little as 0.2 μg daily decreased by 50% the activity of a curative dose of cholecalciferol. The possible steroidal character of this factor may suggest a structurally related antagonism with the vitamin. However, additional work is required in this case.

An anticholecalciferol factor also has been reported to be present in pig liver. The nature of this compound is unknown, but the quantity present in 20 g liver antagonizes 3 IU of cholecalciferol. The activity of this antivitamin has been tested in hens (Coates and Harrison 1957).

Antinaphthoquinones

In this chapter, the generic name given to all forms of the coagulation vitamin is naphthoquinones, which is the parent compound of phylloquinone (K_1), farnoquinone (K_2), and the synthetic, menadione (K_3). Dicumarol is probably the best example of an antinaphthoquinone factor. The compound is derived from coumarin by the action of certain fungi (*Penicillium jenseni* or *P. nigricans*) on sweet clover (*Melilotus alba*) (Ashton and Davies 1962; Bellis 1958; Goplen et al. 1964; Stahman et al. 1941). The substance may cause internal hemorrhage, probably due to hypoprothrombinemia and a decrease in the blood clotting Factor VII (Campbell and Liuk 1941; Field 1945; Rodrick 1929, 1931; Rodrick and Schalk 1931).

Similar anticoagulant substances are found in raw soybean; but unlike dicumarol, the effect is not reversible by naphthoquinones or similar compounds. This factor is believed to be the trypsin inhibitor (Balloun and Johnson 1953).

In the rat, large doses of the retinoids may act as an antinaphthoquinone factor, since such doses can cause a decrease in prothrombin (Light et al. 1944; Moore and Wang 1945; Wostmann and Knight 1965).

Retinoic acid probably interferes in the absorption of the naphthoquinones be-cause its prothrombin-lowering activity is only seen when it is administered orally (Matschiner et al. 1967).

Conclusions

The activities of antinutritive substances represent one of several fundamental mech-anisms of toxicity—that is, elimination of nutrients and interference in their activi-ties. These substances are widespread in the food supply. Even though in most in-stances they pose no immediate threat to health, their presence in food cannot be ignored, especially under conditions of marginal nutrient status and malnutrition. Thus, studies such as those in Thailand provide evidence that consumption of food and other substances possessing antivitamin activity can have significant adverse effect in decreasing the vitamin status of human subjects. In this case, the pre-valence of thiamine deficiency in certain Thai populations was correlated with the consumption of food containing antithiamine factors (Vimokesant et al. 1974, 1975).

REFERENCES

Ackerman, H. and Gebauer, H. 1957. The toxicity of oxalate containing vegetables and fodder plants. *Nahrung* 7: 278—285. (German)

Albert, A. and Keating, F. R., Jr. 1952. The role of the gastro-intestinal tract, including the liver, in the metabolism of radio-thyroxine. *Endocrinology* 51: 427—433.

Anderson, D. W. and Howard, H. W. 1959. Feeding of soybean products and development of goiter. *Pediatrics* 24: 854—857.

Aoki, F. 1955. Studies on the yeast-like Eumyces which has thiaminase actions. II. Mycological characters. *Vitamins* 9: 53—57. (Japanese)

Ashton, W. M. and Davies, E. G. 1962. Coumarin and related compound in anthoxanthum and meliotus species, and the formation of dicoumarol. *Biochem. J.* 85: 22—23.

Astwood, E. B. 1949. The natural occurrence of antithyroid compounds as a cause of simple goiter. *Ann. Intern. Med.* 30: 1087—1103.

Astwood, E. B., Bissell, A. and Hughes, A. M. 1945. Further studies on the chemical nature of compounds which inhibit the function of the thyroid gland. *Endocrinology* 37: 456—481.

Astwood, E. B., Greer, A. M. and Ettlinger, G. M. 1949. L-5-vinyl-2-thiooxa-zolidone, and antithyroid compound from yellow turnip and from Brassica seeds. *J. Biol. Chem.* 181: 121—131.

Averill, U. P. and King, C. G. 1926. The phytin content of foodstuffs. *J. Am. Chem. Soc.* 48: 724—728.

Aykroyd, W. R. and Swaminathan, M. 1940. The nicotinic acid content of cereals and pellagra. *Indian J. Med. Res.* 27: 667—677.

Aykroyd, W. R., Alexa, I. and Nitzulescu, J. 1935. Study of the alimentation of peasants in the pellagra of Moldavia (Roumania). *Arch. Roum. Path. Exp.* 8: 407—426. (Romanian)

Bachelard, H. S. and Trikojus, V. M. 1960. Plant thioglucosides and the problem of endemic goitre in Australia. *Nature* 185: 80—82.

Bachelard, H. S. and Trikojus, V. M. 1963a. Studies on endemic goitre. I. The identification of thioglucosides and their aglucones in weed contaminants of pastures in goitrous areas of Tasmania and southern Queensland. *Austr. J. Biol. Sci.* 16: 147—165.

Bachelard, H. S. and Trikojus, V. M. 1963b. The behavior of 3-methyl-salphonyl-propyl isothiocyanate (cheirolin) and other isothiocyanates in bovine rumen liquor. *Austr. J. Biol. Sci.* 16: 166—176.

Balasubramanian, S. C., Narasinga-Rao, B. S., Ramanamurthy, P.S.V. and Shenolikar, I. S. 1962. Investigation of Indian foods for some major and minor nutrients. *Indian J. Med. Res.* 50: 779—793.

Balloun, S. L. and Johnson, E. L. 1953. Anticoagulant properties of unheated soybean meal in chick diets. *Arch. Biochem.* 42: 355—359.

Barker, M. H. 1936. Blood cyanates in treatment of hypertension. *J.A.M.A.* 106: 762—767.

Barnhurst, J. D. and Hennessy, D. J. 1952a. The action of fish tissue on thiamine. I. The isolation of icthiamine. *J. Am. Chem. Soc.* 74: 353—355.

Barnhurst, J. D. and Hennessy, D. J. 1952b. The action of fish tissue on thiamine. II. Identification of the pyrimidine moiety of icthiamine. *J. Am. Chem. Soc.* 74: 356—358.

Barron, E. S. G., Barron, A. G. and Klemperer, F. 1936. The oxidation of ascorbic acid in biological fluids. *J. Biol. Chem.* 116: 563—573.

Bartilucci, A. J., Di Girolamo, A. and Eisen, H. 1957. A note on the use of sorbitol solution in pharmaceutical formulations. *J. Am. Pharm. Assoc.* 46: 627.

Baumgarter, H. 1957. Contribution on the effect and occurrence of avidin in raw egg white and dry albumen powder. *Ernaehrungsforchung* 2: 631—634. (German)

Beauchere, R. E. and Mitchell, H. L. 1957. Effect of temperature of dehydration of proteins of alfalfa. *J. Agric. Food Chem.* 5: 762—765.

Beck, G. 1948. The biochemistry of scandium and its precipitation as phytate. *Mikrochem. Mikrochim. Acta* 34: 62—66.

Beck, R. N. 1958. Soy flour and fecal thyroxine loss in rats. *Endocrinology* 62: 587—592.

Bellis, D. M. 1958. Metabolism of coumarin and related compounds in culture of Penicillium species. *Nature* 182: 806.

Beruter, J. and Somogyi, J. C. 1966. *Isolation of a Crystalline Antithiamine Factor from Fern.* Proceedings on the VII International Congress of Nutrition, Hamburg, Germany.

Beruter, J. and Somogyi, J. C. 1967. 3,4-Dihydroxycinnamic acid, an antithiamine factor of fern. *Experientia* 23: 996—997.

Bhagvat, K. and Devi, P. 1944. Inactivation of thiamine by certain foodstuffs and oil seeds. *Indian J. Med. Res.* 32: 121—144.

Bhattacharya, J. and Chaudhuri, D. K. 1973. Isolation and characterisation of a crystalline antithiamine factor from mustard seed, Brassica juncea. *Biochim. Biophys. Acta* 343: 211—214.

Bieri, J. G., Briggs, G. M. and Pollard, C. J. 1958. The acceleration of vitamin E deficiency in the chick by torula yeast. *J. Nutr.* 64: 113—126.

Birk, Y. 1969. Saponins. In: *Toxic Constituents of Plant Foodstuffs.* I. E. Liener (ed.). Academic Press, New York.

Block, R. J. et al. 1961. The curative action of iodide on soybean goiter and the changes in the distribution of iodoamino acids in the serum and in thyroid gland digests. *Arch. Biochem. Biophys.* 93: 15—24.

Boas, M. A. 1927. The effect of desiccation upon the nutritive properties of egg white. *Biochem. J.* 21: 712—724.

Bonner, P. et al. 1933. The influence of a daily serving of spinach or its equivalent in oxalic acid upon the mineral utilization of children. *J. Pediatr.* 12: 188—196.

Booth, A. N., Robbins, D. J., Ribelin, W. E. and De Eds, F. 1960. Effect of raw soybean meal and amino acids on pancreatic hypertrophy in rats. *Proc. Soc. Exp. Biol. Med.* 104: 681—683.

Borchers, R. 1963. "Bound" growth inhibitor in raw soybean meal. Proc. Soc. Exp. Biol. Med. 112: 84—85.

Borchers, R. and Ackerson, C. W. 1950. The nutritive value of legume seeds. X. Effect of autoclaving and the trypsin inhibitor test for 17 species. J. Nutr. 41: 339—345.

Borrow, A. et al. 1948. A growth-retarding factor in maize bran. Lancet 1: 752—753.

Brahman, J. E., Villarreal, A. and Bressani, R. 1962. Effect of lime treatment of corn on the availability of niacin for cats. J. Nutr. 76: 183—186.

Braude, R., Henry, K. M., Kon, S. K. and Thompson, S. Y. 1947. The effect of yeast on liver vitamin A storage in the pig. Br. J. Nutr. 1: vi—vii.

Braude, R., Kon, K. S., Mitchell, G. K. and Kodicek, E. 1955. Maize and pellagra. Lancet 1: 898—899.

Braunstein, A. E. 1960. Pyridoxal phosphate. In: The Enzymes. P. D. Boyer, H. Lardy and K. Myrback (eds.). Academic Press, New York.

Bricker, M. L., Smith, J. M., Hamilton, T. S. and Mitchell, H. H. 1949. The effect of cocoa upon calcium utilization and requirements, nitrogen retention, and fecal composition of women. J. Nutr. 39: 445—462.

Bronner, F., Harris, R. S., Maletskos, C. J. and Benda, C. E. 1954. Studies in calcium metabolism. Effect of food phytates on calcium[45] uptake in children on low-calcium breakfasts. J. Nutr. 54: 523—542.

Bronner, F., Harris, R. S., Maletskos, C. J. and Benda, C. E. 1956. Studies in calcium metabolism. Effect of food phytates on calcium[45] uptake in boys in a moderate calcium breakfast. J. Nutr. 59: 393—406.

Brubacher, G., Scharer, K., Studer, A. and Wiss, O. 1966. On the reciprocal effects of vitamin E, vitamin A, and carotinoids. Z. Ernaehrungswiss. 5: 190—202.

Bunnell, R. H. 1957. The vitamin E potency of alfalfa as measured by the content of liver of the chick. Poultry Sci. 36: 413—419.

Burkitt, D. P., Walker, A. R. and Painter, N. S. 1974. Dietary fiber and disease. J.A.M.A. 229: 1068—1074.

Camejo, G. 1964. Physical-chemical constants of phaseolotoxin A [phytohemagglutinin obtained from black bean (Phaseolus vulgaris)]. Acta Cient. Venez. 15: 110—111. (Spanish)

Campbell, H. A. and Liuk, K. P. 1941. Studies on the hemorrhagic agent sweet clover disease. IV. The isolation and crystallization of the hemorrhagic agent. J. Biol. Chem. 138: 21—33.

Care, A. D. 1954. Goitrogenic properties of linseed. Nature 173: 172.

Carlson, C. W., Saxena, H. C., Jensen, L. S. and McGinnis, J. 1964. Rachitogenic activity of soybean fractions. J. Nutr. 82: 507—511.

Carlström, B., Myrback, K., Holmin, N. and Lasson, A. 1939. Biochemical studies on B_1-avitaminosis in animals and man. Acta Med. Scand. 102: 175—213.

Cartwright, G. E. and Wintrobe, M. M. 1946. Hematologic survey of repatriated American military personnel. J. Lab. Clin. Med. 31: 886—899.

Caughey, J. E. 1973. Aetiological factors in adolescent malnutrition in Iran. N. Z. Med. J. 77: 90—95.

Chaudhuri, D. K. 1962. Antithiamine factor of rice-bran. Sci. Cult. 28: 384.

Chaudhuri, D. K. 1964. Purification of antithiamine factor from rice-bran. Sci. Cult. 30: 97.

Chen, L. H. and Pan, S. H. 1977. Decrease of phytates during germination of pea seeds (Pisum sativa). Nutr. Rep. Int. 16: 125—131.

Chen, L. H., Thacker, R. R., and Pan, S. H. 1977. Effect of germination on hemagglutinating activity of pea and bean seeds. J. Food Sci. 42: 1666—1668.

Chernick, S. S., Leprovsky, S. and Chaikoff, I. L. 1948. A dietary factor regulating the enzyme content of the pancreas. Changes induced in size and

442   Naturally Occurring Antinutritive Substances

proteolytic activity of the chick pancreas by the ingestion of raw soybean meal. *Am. J. Physiol.* 155: 33–41.

Chick, H., Fotheringham, M. T., Martin, A. J. P. and Martin C. J. 1938. Curative action of nicotinic acid on pigs suffering from the effects of a diet consisting largely of maize. *Biochem. J.* 38: 10–12.

Clandinin, R. D., Cravens, W. W., Elvehjem, C. A. and Halpin, J. G. 1947. Deficiencies in overheated soybean oil meal. *Poultry Sci.* 26: 150–156.

Clements, F. W. 1955. A thyroid blocking agent as a cause of endemic goitre in Tasmania: Preliminary communication. *Med. J. Aust.* 2: 369–370.

Clements, F. W. 1957. A goitrogenic factor in milk. *Med. J. Aust.* 2: 645–646.

Clements, F. W. 1958. Thyroid disease; public health aspects. *Med. J. Aust.* 2: 823–825.

Clements, F. W. 1960. Naturally occurring goitrogens. *Br. Med. Bull.* 16: 133–137.

Coan, M. H. and Travis, J. 1971. Interaction of human pancreatic proteinases with naturally occurring proteinase inhibitors. In: *Proc. Int. Res. Conf. Proteinase Inhibit.* H. Fritz and H. Tschesche (eds.). Walter de Gruyter, Berlin.

Coates, M. E. and Harrison, G. E. 1957. A rachitogenic factor in pig's liver. *Proc. Nutr. Soc.* 16: 21.

Cohen, K. L. and Donaldson, R. M. 1980. Unreliability of radiodilution assays on screening tests for cobalamine (vitamin B_{12}) deficiency. *J.A.M.A.* 244: 1942–1945.

Concon, J. M. 1978. Alkaloids. In: *Encyclopedia of Food Science.* M. S. Peterson and A. H. Johnson (eds.). AVI, Westport, Connecticut.

Concon, J. M. and Human, D. Ascorbic acid protective factor in orange juice. Unpublished results.

Cooperman, J. M., Rubin, S. H. and Tabenkin, B. 1951. Effect of niacin and tryptophan in counteracting toxicity of crystalline borrelidine for rat. *Proc. Soc. Exp. Biol.* 76: 18–20.

Couch, J. R., Creger, C. R. and Bakshi, Y. K. 1966. Trypsin inhibitor in guar meal. *Proc. Soc. Exp. Biol. Med.* 123: 263–265.

Courtois, J. E. and Perez, C. 1948. Research on phytase. Inositol phosphates content and phytase activity in various grains. *Bull. Soc. Chim. Biol. (Paris)* 30: 195–201. (French)

Courtois, J. E., Desjobert, A. and Fleurent, P. 1952. Research on phytase. XVIII. Action of phytase from wheat on certain inositol phosphoric acid salts. *Bull. Soc. Chim. Biol. (Paris)* 34: 691–697. (French)

Cowan, J. W., Saghir, A. R. and Salji, J. P. 1967. Antithyroid activity of onion volatiles. *Aust. J. Biol. Sci.* 20: 683–685.

Cravioto, R. O., Massieu, G. H., Cravioto, O. Y. and Figueroa, E. 1952. Effect of untreated corn and Mexican tortilla upon the growth of rats on a niacin-tryptophan deficient diet. *J. Nutr.* 48: 453–459.

Cruickshank, E. W. H., Duckworth, J., Kosterlitz, H. W. and Warnock, G. M. 1943. Digestibility of phytin of oatmeal in adult man. *Nature* 152: 1384–1385.

Cruickshank, E. W. H., Duckworth, J., Kosterlitz, H. W. and Warnock, G. M. 1945. The digestibility of the phytate-P of oatmeal in adult man. *J. Physiol. (Lond.)* 104: 41–46.

Cruz-Coke, E. and Plaza de los Reyes, M. 1947a. Effect of quercitrin on the thyroid gland. *Bol. Soc. Biol. Santiago* 4: 19–23. (Spanish)

Cruz-Coke, E. and Plaza de los Reyes, M. 1947b. The effect of quercetrin on basal metabolism of the rat. *Bol. Soc. Biol. Santiago* 4: 105–107.

Cruz-Coke, E. and Plaza de los Reyes, M. 1947c. Quercetin and thyroid function. *Bull. Soc. Chim. Biol.* 29: 573–582. (Spanish)

Cruz-Coke, E., Calvo, C. I. M. and Niemeyer, H. 1947. Production and inhibition of thyroxine. *Rev. Med. Chile* 75: 109–117. (Spanish)

Dahlgren, K., Porath, J. and Lindahl-Kiessling, K. 1970. On the purification of phytohemagglutinins from Phaseolus vulgaris seeds. *Arch. Biochem. Biophys.* 137: 306—314.

Dam, H. 1962. Interrelations between vitamin E and polyunsaturated fatty acids in animals. *Vitam. Horm.* 20: 527—540.

Daum, M. G. and Jaffe, W. G. 1956. Studies on the thiaminases of Venezuelan marine fish, especially in sardines. *Arch. Venez. Nutr.* 7: 153—162.

Davis, J. S. and Somogyi, C. 1969. Reaction mechanism of the inactivation of thiamine by 3,4-dihydroxycinnamic acid. *Int. J. Vitam. Res.* 39: 401—406.

Davis, P. N., Norris, L. C. and Kratzer, F. H. 1962. Interference of soybean proteins with the utilization of trace minerals. *J. Nutr.* 77: 217—223.

Daxenbiehler, M. E., VanEtten, C. H. and Wolff, I. A. 1965. A new thioglucoside, (R)-2-hydroxy-3-butenyl-glucosinolate, from Crambe abyssinica seed. *Biochemistry* 4: 318—323.

Delezenne, C. and Pozerski, E. 1903. Inhibitory action of raw ovalbumin of tryptic digestion of coagulated ovalbumin. *C. R. Soc. Biol.* 55: 935—937.

De Muelenaere, H. J. H. 1964. Effect of heat treatment on the haemagglutinating activity of legumes. *Nature* 201: 1029—1030.

Deutch, H. F. and Hasler, A. D. 1943. Distribution of a vitamin B_1 destructive enzyme in fish. *Proc. Soc. Exp. Biol.* 53: 63—65.

Diemair, W. and Zerban, K. 1944a. Contribution to the knowledge of ascorbic acid oxidase. *Biochem. Z.* 316: 189—201.

Diemair, W. and Zerban, K. 1944b. Contribution to the knowledge of ascorbic acid oxidase. *Biochem. Z.* 316: 335—350.

Doe, D. A. 1976. Antivitamins. In: *Drug-Induced Nutritional Deficiencies.* AVI, Westport, Connecticut.

Doelarkar, S. T. and Sohonie, K. 1957. Studies on thiaminase from fish. *Indian J. Med. Res.* 45: 571—592.

Dunn, F. J. and Dawson, C. R. 1951. On the nature of ascorbic acid oxidase. *J. Biol. Chem.* 189: 485—497.

Eakin, R. E., Snell, E. E. and Williams, R. J. 1940. A constituent of raw egg white capable of inactivating biotin in vitro. *J. Biol. Chem.* 136: 801—802.

Eakin, R. E., Snell, E. E. and Williams, R. J. 1941. The concentration and assay of avidin, the injury producing protein in raw egg white. *J. Biol. Chem.* 140: 535—543.

Eastwood, M. A. et al. 1974. Effect of dietary supplements of wheat bran and cellulose on feces and bowel function. *Br. Med. J.* 4: 392—394.

Edelstein, E. 1932. The influence of increased vegetables on the nitrogen and mineral balances of children. *Z. Kinderheilk.* 52: 483—503. (German)

Ekpechi, O. L. 1967. Endemic goiter and cassava diets in Eastern Nigeria. *Br. J. Nutr.* 2: 537.

Ekpechi, O. L., Dimitriadou, A. and Fraser, R. 1966. Goitrogenicity of cassava (a staple Nigerian food). *Nature* 210: 1137—1138.

Ender. F. and Helgebostad, A. 1940. Experimental beriberi in silver foxes. *Norsk. Pelsdyrblad.* 14: 404—407. (Norwegian)

England, J. M. and Linnell, J. C. 1980. Problems with the serum vitamin B_{12} assay. *Lancet* 2: 1072—1074.

Ershoff, B. H. 1949. Conditioning factors in nutritional disease. *Physiol. Rev.* 28: 107—137.

Ettlinger, M. G. and Kjaer, A. 1968. Sulfur compounds in plants. In: *Recent Advances in Phytochemistry.* Vol. 1. T. J. Mabry (ed.). Appleton-Century Crofts, New York.

Etzler, M. E. and Kabat, E. A. 1970. Purification and charcterization of a lectin (plant hemagglutinin) with blood group A specificity from Dolichos biflorus. *Biochemistry* 9: 869—877.

Evans, J. R. and McGinnis, J. 1947. Amino acid deficiencies of raw and overheated soybean oil meal for chicks. *J. Nutr.* 34: 725–732.

Ewer, T. K. 1950. Rachitogenicity of green oats. *Nature* 166: 732.

Ewer, T. K. and Bartrum, P. 1948. Rickets in sheep. *Aust. Vet. J.* 24(4): 73–85.

Fairbanks, B. W. and Mitchell, H. H. 1938. The availability of calcium in spinach, in skim milk powder, and in calcium oxalate. *J. Nutr.* 16: 79–89.

Faschingbauer, H. and Kofler, L. 1929. The poisonous effects of red bean and germinated beans. *Wien. Klin. Wochenschr.* 42: 1069–1072.

Fatterpaker, P., Marfatia, U. and Sreenivasan, A. 1955. Observations on relationship between pteroylglutamic acid and nicotinamide metabolism. *Biochem. J.* 59: 470–475.

Feeney, R. E., Means, G. E. and Bigler, J. C. 1969. Inhibition of human trypsin, plasmin and thrombin by naturally occurring inhibitors of proteolytic enzymes. *J. Biol. Chem.* 244: 1957–1960.

Field, J. B. 1945. Hypoprothrombinemia induced in suckling rats by feeding 3,3'methylenebis(4hydroxycoumarin) and acetylsalicylic acid to their mothers. *Am. J. Physiol.* 143: 238–242.

Figdor, P. P. 1961. Uremia as a symptom of oxalic acid poisoning. *Wien. Med. Wochenschr.* 111: 111–114. (German)

Finke, M. L. and Garrison, E. A. 1936. The availability of the calcium of spinach and kale. *Proc. J. Home Econ.* 28: 572–575.

Finke, M. L. and Garrison, E. A. 1938. Utilization of calcium of spinach and kale. *Food Res.* 3: 575–581.

Finke, M. L. and Sherman, H. C. 1935. The availability of calcium from some atypical foods. *J. Biol. Chem.* 110: 421–428.

Finlay, G. M. and Stern, R. O. 1929. Syndrome in rat resembling pink disease in man. *Arch. Dis. Child.* 4: 1–11.

Fisher, G., Epstein, D. and Paschkis, E. K. 1952. A case of struma cibaria. *J. Clin. Endocrinol.* 12: 1100–1101.

Fitch, L. W. N. and Ewer, T. K. 1944. The value of vitamin D and bone-flour in the prevention of rickets in sheep in New Zealand. *Aust. Vet. J.* 20: 220–226.

Fox, H. C. and Miller, D. S. 1960. Acker toxin: A riboflavin antimetabolite. *Nature* 186: 561–562.

Foy, H., Kondo, A. and Austin, W. H. 1959. Effect of dietary phytate on faecal absorption of radioactive ferric chloride. *Nature* 183: 691–692.

Fritz, H. and Tschesche, H. 1971. *Proceedings of the First International Research Conference on Proteinase Inhibitors.* Institut fur Klinische Chemie and Klinische Biochemie der Universitat Muchen, Munich, Germany. Walter de Gruyter, New York.

Frolich, A. 1954. Relation between the quality of soybean oil meal and the requirement of vitamin B_{12} for chicks. *Nature* 173: 132–133.

Fuhr, I. and Steenbock, H. 1943. The effect of dietary calcium, phosphorus, and vitamin D on the utilization of iron. I. The effect of phytic acid on the availability of iron. II. The effect of vitamin D on body iron and hemoglobin production. III. The relation of rickets to anemia. *J. Biol. Chem.* 147: 59–74.

Fujimiya, M. 1950. Thiaminase in human feces. *Vitamins* 3: 270–282.

Fujimiya, M. 1951. A thiamine-deficient diet in thiaminosotic patients. *Vitamins* 4: 32–37.

Garlich, J. D. and Nesheim, M. C. 1966. Relationship of fractions of soybeans and a crystalline soybean trypsin inhibitor to the effects of feeding unheated soybean meal to chicks. *J. Nutr.* 88: 100–110.

Gertler, A., Birk, Y. and Bondi, A. 1967. A comparative study of the nutritional and physiological significance of pure soybean trypsin inhibitors and of ethanol extracted soybean meals in chicks and rats. *J. Nutr.* 91: 358–370.

Gilgen, A. and Leuthardt, F. 1962. The binding of ^{14}C-biotin to chicken liver proteins. *Helv. Chim. Acta* 45: 1833–1846. (German)

Gmelin, R. and Virtanen, A. I. 1960. The enzymic formation of thiocyanate (SCN) from a precursor(s) in Brassica species. *Acta Chem. Scand.* 14: 507–513.

Goldsmith, G. A., Rosenthal, H. L., Gibbens, J. and Unglaub, W. G. 1955. Studies of niacin requirement in man. II. Requirement on wheat and corn diets low in tryptophan. *J. Nutr.* 56: 371–386.

Goldsmith, G. A., Gibbens, J., Unglaub, W. G. and Miller, O. N. 1956. Studies of niacin requirement in man. 3. Comparative effects of diets containing lime-treated and untreated corn in the production of experimental pellagra. *Am. J. Clin. Nutr.* 4: 151–160.

Gontea, I. and Gardev, M. 1958. Antinutritive substances in foods. I. Antitryptic activity of some alimentary products. *Commun. Acad. Rep. Populare Romine* 8: 723–7 (Romanian)

Gontea, I. and Sutzescu, P. 1968. *Natural Antinutritive Substances in Foodstuffs and Forages.* S. Karger, Basel.

Gopalan, C. 1968. Leucine and pellagra. *Nutr. Rev.* 26: 323–326.

Gopalan, C. 1970. Some recent studies in the nutrition research laboratories, Hyderabad. *Am. J. Clin. Nutr.* 23: 35–51.

Goplen, B. P., Linton, J. H. and Bell, J. M. 1964. Dicoumarol studies. 3. Determining tolerance limits of contamination in low coumarin sweet clover varieties using a cattle bioassay. *Can. J. Anim. Sci.* 44: 76–86.

Grant, A. B. 1951. Antivitamin D factor. *Nature* 168: 789.

Grant, A. B. 1953. Carotene, a rachitogenic factor in green feeds. *Nature* 172: 627.

Green, N. M. 1963. Avidin. III. The nature of the biotin-binding site. *Biochem. J.* 89: 599–609.

Green, R. G. 1936. Chastek paralysis. A new disease of foxes. *Minn. Wildlife Dis. Invest.* 2: 106–118.

Green, R. G. 1937. Chastek paralysis. *Minn. Wildlife Dis. Invest.* 3: 83–95.

Green, R. G., Carlson, W. E. and Evans, C. A. 1941. A deficiency disease of foxes produced by feeding fish. *J. Nutr.* 21: 243–252.

Green, R. G., Carlson, W. E. and Evans, C. A. 1942a. The inactivation of vitamin B_1 in diets containing whole fish. *J. Nutr.* 23: 165–174.

Green, R. G., Evans, C. A., Carlson, W. E. and Swale, F. S. 1942b. Chastek paralysis in foxes. *J. Am. Vet. Med. Assoc.* 100: 394–402.

Greene, R., Farran, H. and Glascock, R. F. 1958. Goitrogens in milk. *J. Endocrinol.* 17: 272–279.

Greer, M. A. 1950. Nutrition and goiter. *Physiol. Rev.* 30: 513–548.

Greer, M. A. 1960. The significance of naturally occurring antithyroid compounds in the production of goiter in man. *Borden's Rev. Nutr. Res.* 21: 61–73.

Greer, M. A. 1962. The natural occurrence of goitrogenic agents. *Recent Progr. Hor. Res.* 18: 187–219.

Greer, M. A. and Astwood, E. B. 1948. The antithyroid effect of certain foods in man as determined with radioactive iodine. *Endocrinology* 43: 105–120.

Greer, M. A., Stott, A. K. and Milne, K. A. 1966. Effect of thiocyanate, perchlorate, and other anions on thyroidal metabolism. *Endocrinology* 79: 237–247.

Griebel, C. 1950. Illness caused by bean flakes (Phaseolus vulgaris L) and flat pea (Lathyrus tingitanus L.). *Z. Lebensm. Untersuch. Forsch.* 90: 191–197. (German).

György, P. 1939. The curative factor (Vitamin H) for egg white injury, with particular reference to its presence in different foodstuffs and in yeast. *J. Biol. Chem.* 131: 733–744.

György, P. and Rose, C. S. 1943. The liberation of biotin from avidin-biotin complex (A.B.). *Proc. Soc. Exp. Biol.* 53: 55—57.

György, P. et al. 1941. Egg-white injury as the result of non-absorption or inactivation of biotin. *Science* 93: 477—478.

Haag, J. R. and Westwig, P. H. 1948. Further observations concerning antithiamine activity of plants. *Fed. Proc.* 7: 157.

Haag, J. R., Westwig, P. H. and Freed, A. M. 1947. Antithiamine activity of bracken fern. *Fed. Proc.* 6: 408.

Haines, P. and Lyman, R. L. 1957. Relationship of pancreatic enzyme secretion to growth inhibition in rats fed soybean trypsin inhibitor. *J. Nutr.* 74: 445—452.

Halsted, J. A. et al. 1972. Zinc deficiency in man. *Am. J. Med.* 53: 277—284.

Halverson, A. W., Shaw, J. H. and Hart, E. B. 1945. Goiter studies with the rat. *J. Nutr.* 30: 59—65.

Hamada, K. 1953. Studies of disposition of carriers of B. thiaminolyticus in the intestinal canal. I. On so-called thiaminoses patients and carriers of B. thiaminolyticus. *Vitamins* 6: 951—953.

Handler, P. 1944. Effect of excessive nicotinamide feeding on rabbits and guinea pigs. *J. Biol. Chem.* 154: 203—206.

Hankes, L. V., Leklem, J. E., Brown, R. R. and Mekel, R. C. P. M. 1971. Tryptophan metabolism in patients with pellagra: Problems of vitamin B_6 enzyme activity and feedback control of tryptophan pyrrolase enzyme. *Am. J. Clin. Nutr.* 24: 730—739.

Harris, L. J. 1949. Antivitamins in Food. I. Antivitamins and other factors influencing vitamin activity. *Br. J. Nutr.* 2: 362—373.

Harris, P. L. and Embree, N. D. 1963. Quantitative consideration of the effect of polyunsaturated fatty acid content of the diet on the requirements for vitamin E. *Am. J. Clin. Nutr.* 13: 385—392.

Harrison, D. C. and Mellamby, E. 1939. Phytic acid and the rickets-producing action of cereals. *Biochem. J.* 33: 1660—1680.

Hassal, C. H., Reyle, K. and Feng, P. 1954. Biologically active polypeptides from Blighia sapida. *Nature* 173: 356—357.

Hawkins, W. W. and Yaphe, W. 1965. Carrageenan as a dietary constituent for the rat: Fecal excretion, nitrogen absorption, and growth. *Can. J. Biochem.* 43: 479—484.

Hegsted, D. M. et al. 1942. Biotin in chick nutrition. *J. Nutr.* 23: 175—179.

Herbert, V. 1975. Megaloblastic anemias. In: *Cecil-Loeb Textbook of Medicine.* 14th edition. P. B. Beeson and W. McDermott (eds.). Saunders, Philadelphia.

Herbert, V. and Jacob, E. 1974. Destruction of vitamin B_{12} by ascorbic acid. *J.A.M.A.* 230: 241—242.

Hercus, E. C. and Purves, D. H. 1936. Studies on endemic and experimental goiter. *J. Hyg.* 36: 182—203.

Herting, D. C. 1966. Perspective on vitamin E. *Am. J. Clin. Nutr.* 19: 210—218.

Hertz, R. 1946. Biotin and the avidin-biotin complex. *Physiol. Rev.* 26: 479—494.

Hickman, K. C. D., Kaley, M. W. and Harris, P. J. 1944a. Covitamin studies. I. The sparing action of natural tocopherol concentrates on vitamin A. *J. Biol. Chem.* 152: 303—311.

Hickman, K. C. D., Kaley, M. W. and Harris, P. L. 1944b. Covitamin studies. I. The sparing equivalence of the tocopherols and mode of action. *J. Biol. Chem.* 152: 321—328.

Hilker, D. M. and Peter, O. F. 1966. Antithiamine activity in Hawaii fish. *J. Nutr.* 89: 419—421.

Hilker, D. M., Chan, K.-C., Chen, R. and Smith, R. L. 1971. Antithiamine effects of tea. I. Temperature and pH dependence. *Nutr. Dept. Int.* 4: 223—227.

Hill, K. D. 1952. The vomiting sickness of Jamaica. *W. Indian Med. J.* 1: 243–264.

Hintz, H. F. and Hogue, D. E. 1964. Kidney beans (Phaseolus vulgaris) and the effectiveness of vitamin E for prevention of nutritional muscular dystrophy in the chick. *J. Nutr.* 84: 283–287.

Hintz, H. F., Hogue, D. E. and Krook, L. 1967. Toxicity of red kidney beans (Phaseolus vulgaris) in the rat. *J. Nutr.* 93: 77–86.

Hoff-Jorgensen, E., Andersen, O., Begtrap, H. and Nielsen, G. 1946a. The effect of phytic acid on the absorption of calcium and phosphorus. 2. In infants. *Biochem. J.* 40: 453–454.

Hoff-Jorgensen, E., Anderson, O. and Nielsen, G. 1946b. The effect of phytic acid on the absorption of calcium and phosphorus. 3. In children. *Biochem. J.* 40: 555-557.

Holt, R. 1955. Studies on dried peas. 1. The determination of phytate phosphorus. *J. Sci. Food Agric.* 6: 136–142.

Honavar, P. M., Shih, C. V. and Liener, I. E. 1962. The inhibition of the growth of rats by purified hemagglutinin fraction isolated from Phaseolus vulgaris. *J. Nutr.* 77: 109–114.

Horwitt, M. K. 1960. Vitamin E and lipid metablism in man. *Am. J. Clin. Nutr.* 8: 451–461.

Horwitt, M. K. 1961. Vitamin E in human nutrition. *Borden's Rev. Nutr. Res.* 22: 1–17.

Horwitt, M. K. 1962. Interrelations between vitamin E and polyunsaturated fatty acids in adult man. *Vitam. Horm.* 20: 541–558.

Hove, E. L. and Harris, P. L. 1951. Note on the linoleic acid-tocopherol relation in fats and oils. *J. Am. Oil Chem. Soc.* 28: 405.

Hsu, P.-T. and Combs, G. F. 1952. Effect of vitamin B_{12} and amino acid imbalances on growth and levels of certain blood constituents in the chick. *J. Nutr.* 47: 73–91.

Hussain, R. and Patwardhan, V. N. 1959. The influence of phytate on the absorption of iron. *Indian J. Med. Res.* 47: 676–682.

Hutchins, H. H., Cravioto, P. J. and Macek, T. J. 1956. A comparison of the stability of cyanocobalamin and its analogs in ascorbate solution. *J. Am. Pharm. Assoc.* 45: 806–808.

Hydovitz, J. D. 1960. Occurrence of goiter in an infant on a soy diet. *N. Engl. J. Med.* 262: 351–353.

Inoue, N. 1951. Properties of thiaminase of a bacillus isolated from the faeces of a beriberi patient. *J. Ferm. Technol.* 29: 422–424.

Jacob, E. et al. 1973. Apparent low serum vitamin B_{12} levels in paraplegic veterans taking ascorbic acid. In: *Proceedings of the 16th Annual Meeting, American Society Hematology,* Chicago, Dec. 1-4.

Jacobson, K. P. and de Azevedo, M. D. 1947. On the enzymatic destruction of thiamine. *Arch. Biochem.* 14: 83–86.

Jacquet, J. 1950. Poisoning of cattle with the eagle fern, Pteris aquilenum. *L. Bull. Acad. Vet. Fr.* 23: 207–211. (French)

Jacquot, R. 1954. Heat treatment and nutritive value. *Ann. Zootech.* 3: 189–214. (French)

Jaffe, W. G. 1949. Toxicity of raw kidney bean. *Experientia* 5: 81–83.

Jaffe, W. G. 1950. Protein digestibility and trypsin inhibitor of legume seeds. *Proc. Soc. Exp. Biol.* 75: 219–220.

Jaffe, W. G. 1960. Phytotoxins from beans. *Arzneimittel. Forsch.* 10: 1012–1016.

Jaffe, W. G. 1969. Hemagglutins. In: *Toxic Constituents of Plant Foodstuffs.* I. E. Liener (ed.). Academic Press, New York.

Jaffe, W. G. and Brucher, O. 1972. Toxicity and specificity of different phytohemagglutinins of beans (Phaseolus vulgaris). *Arch. Latinoamer. Nutr.* 22: 267–281.

Jaffe, W. G. and Hannig, K. 1965. Fractionation of proteins from kidney beans (Phaseolus vulgaris). *Arch. Biochem. Biophys.* 109: 80–91.

Jaffe, W. G. and Vega Lette, C. L. 1968. Heat-labile growth inhibiting factors in beans (Phaseolus vulgaris). *J. Nutr.* 94: 203–210.

Jeney, E. and Jeney, A., Jr. 1960. The goitrogenic action of flavone dyes. *Eqeszsegtudomany* 4: 224–233.

Jeney, E. et al. 1960. The goitrogenic action of flavone dyes. II. Investigations with I^{131}. *Eqeszsegtudomany* 4: 234–239.

Johnston, T. D. and Jones, D. I. H. 1966. Variations in the thiocyanate content of kale varieties. *J. Sci. Food Agric.* 17: 70–71.

Johnston, F. A., McMillan, T. J. and Falconer, G. D. 1952. Calcium retained by young women before and after adding spinach to the diet. *J. Am. Diet Assoc.* 28: 933–938.

Jones, P. D. and Briggs, M. H. 1962. The distribution of avidin. *Life Sci. 11:* 621–623.

Joshi, A. L. 1970. "Studies in Proteins of Double Bean (P. lunatus) with Special Reference to Its Hemagglutinins." Ph.D. Thesis, University of Bombay, India.

Kalliala, H. and Kauste, O. 1964. Ingestion of rhubarb leaves as cause of oxalic acid poisoning. *Ann. Paediatr. Fenn.* 10: 228–231.

Kawasaki, M. and Ono, T. 1968. Thiaminase of fungi. I. Thiaminase of Lentinus edodes. *Vitamins* 37: 44–49.

Kennedy, T. H. and Purves, H. D. 1941. Studies on experimental goiter. I. The effect of brassica seed diet on rats. *Br. J. Exp. Pathol.* 22: 241–244.

Kiermeier, F. and Semper, G. 1960a. On the presence of proteolytic enzymes and trypsin inhibitors in cow's milk. On the inhibitory activity. *Z. Lebensm. Unters.* 111: 373–380.

Kiermeier, F. and Semper, G. 1960b. On the occurrence of proteolytic enzymes and trypsin-inhibitors in cow's milk. Relationship between protease and trypsin inhibitor. *Z. Lebensm. Unters.* 111: 483–493. (German)

Kiermeier, F. and Semper, G. 1960c. On the presence of proteolytic enzymes and trypsin-inhibitors in cow's milk. On Proteolytic effects. *Z. Lebensm. Unters.* 111: 282–307. (German)

Kimura, R. and Liao, T. H. 1953. A new thiamine-decomposing anaerobic bacterium Clostridium thiaminolyticum. *Proc. Jpn. Acad.* 29: 132.

Kimura, R., Aoyama, S. and Ryo, M. 1952. Bacillus thiaminolyticus. *Vitamins* 5: 51–54.

Kirkendall, W. M. and Page, E. B. 1958. Polyneuritis occurring during hydralazine therapy: Report of two cases and discussion of adverse reactions to hydralazine. *J.A.M.A.* 167: 427–432.

Kjaer, A. 1966. The distribution of sulfur compounds. In: *Comparative Phytochemistry.* T. Swain (ed.). Academic Press, New York.

Klosterman, H. J. 1974. Vitamin B_6 antagonists of natural origin. *J. Agric. Food Chem.* 22(1): 13–16.

Klosterman, H. J. 1981. Vitamin B_6 antagonists in natural products. In: *Antinutrients and Natural Toxicants in Foods.* R. L. Ory (ed.). Food and Nutrition Press, Westport, Connecticut.

Klosterman, H. J., Farley, T. M., Parsons, J. L. and Lamoreux, G. L. 1963. *The Antipyridoxine Factor in Flaxseed.* Abstracts Division of Agricultural and Food Chemistry, American Chemical Society, New York.

Klosterman, H. J., Lamoureux, G. L., and Parsons, J. L. 1967. Isolation, characterization and synthesis of linatine. A vitamin B_6 antagonist from flaxseed Linum usitatissimum. *Biochemistry* 6: 170–176.

Koch, R. 1957. Variation in the nutritive value of proteins and their biological value following heat treatment. *Nahrung* I: 107–109. (German)

Kodicek, E. 1960. The effect of treating maize and other materials with sodium hydroxide. *Br. J. Nutr.* 14: 13–24.

Koepke, J. A. and Stewart, W. B. 1964. Role of gastric secretion in iron absorption. *Proc. Soc. Exp. Biol. Med.* 115: 927–929.

Kohman, E. F. 1939. Oxalic acid in foods and its behavior and fate in the diet. *J. Nutr.* 18: 233–246.

Koller, A. and Somogyi, J. C. 1961. Further investigations on the isolation of a thermostable antithiamine substance from eagle fern. *Int. Z. Vitaminforsch.* 31: 230–233. (German)

Kositawattanakul, T., Tosukhowong, P., Vimokesant, S. L. and Panijpan, B. 1977. Chemical interactions between thiamine and tannic acid. II. Separation of products. *Am. J. Clin. Nutr.* 30: 1686–1691.

Krampitz, L. O. and Woolley, D. W. 1944. The manner of inactivation of thiamine by fish tissue. *J. Biol. Chem.* 152: 9–17.

Kratzer, F. H. and Williams, D. E. 1948. The relation of pyridoxine to the growth of chicks fed rations containing linseed oil meal. *J. Nutr.* 36: 297–305.

Kratzer, F. H., Williams, D. E., Marshall, B. and Davis, P. N. 1954. Some properties of the chick growth inhibitor in linseed oil meal. *J. Nutr.* 52: 555–563.

Krebs, H. A. and Mellamby, K. 1943. The effect of national wheat meal on the absorption of calcium. *Biochem. J.* 37: 466–468.

Krehl, W. A., Teply, L. J. and Elvehjem, C. A. 1945. Corn as etiological factor in production of nicotinic acid deficiency in rat. *Science* 101: 283.

Krupe, M. and Ensgraber, A. 1962. Investigations on the nature of phytoagglutinins from the chemical, immunochemical and plant physiological perspectives. III. Analytical studies on the agglutinin in potatoes (Solanum tuberosum). *Behringwek-Mitt.* 42: 48. (German)

Kumar, B. de and Chaudhuri, D. K. 1976. Isolation, partial characterisation of antithiamine factor present in ricebran and its effect on TPP-transketolase system and Staphylococcus aureus. *Int. J. Vitam. Nutr. Res.* 46: 154–159.

Kundig, H. and Somogyi, J. C. 1964. Antithiamine-active substances in plant foods. *Int. Z. Vitaminforsch.* 34: 135–141. (German)

Kundig, H. and Somogyi, J. C. 1967. Isolation of the active moiety of the antithiamine compound from carp viscera. *Int. Z. Vitaminforsch.* 37: 476–481.

Kunitz, M. 1945. Crystallization of a trypsin inhibitor from soybean. *Science* 101: 668–669.

Kupstas, E. E. and Hennessy, D. J. 1957a. The action of fish tissue on thiamin. III. The further elucidation of the structure of icthiamin. *J. Am. Chem. Soc.* 79: 5217–5220.

Kupstas, E. E. and Hennessy, D. J. 1957b. The action of fish tissue on thiamine. IV. The synthesis of icthiamin. *J. Am. Chem. Soc.* 79: 5220–5222.

Lang, K. and Eberwein, A. 1948. The phytin content of rising sour dough of rye bread. *Z. Lebensm. Unters.* 88: 153–154. (German)

Lange, D. J., Joubert, C. P. and Perez, S. F. M. du. 1961. The determination of phytic acid and factors which influence its hydrolysis in bread. *Proc. Nutr. Soc. S. Afr.* 2: 69–76.

Langer, P. 1964. The relation between thiocyanate formation and goitrogenic effect of foods. VI. Thiocyanogenic activity of allylisothiocyanate, one of the most frequently occurring mustard oils in plants. *Z. Physiol. Chem.* 339: 33–35.

Langer, P. and Michajlovskij, N. 1958. The relation between thiocyanate formation and the goitrogenic effect of foods. II. The thiocyanate content of foods, the chief cause of thiocyanate excretion in urine of man and animals. *Z. Physiol. Chem.* 312: 31—36.

Langer, P. and Stolc, V. 1964. The relation between thiocyanate formation and goitrogenic effects of foods. V. Comparison of the effect of white cabbage and thiocyanate on the rat thyroid gland. *Z. Physiol. Chem.* 335: 216—220.

Langer, P. and Stolc, V. 1965. Goitrogenic activity of allylisothiocyanate—A widespread natural mustard oil. *Endocrinology* 76: 151—155.

Leach, E. H. and Lloyd, J. P. F. 1956. Citral poisoning. *Proc. Nutr. Soc.* 15: 15—16.

Learmonth, E. M. and Wood, J. C. 1960. A trypsin inhibitor in wheat flour. *Chem. Ind. (Lond.)* 51: 1569—1570.

Learmonth, E. M. and Wood, J. C. 1963. A trypsin inhibitor in wheat flour. *Cereal Chem.* 40: 61—65.

Lease, J. G., Barnett, B. D., Lease, E. J. and Turk, D. E. 1960. The biological unavailability to the chick of zinc in a sesame meal ration. *J. Nutr.* 72: 66—70.

Lee, J. R. and Underwood, E. J. 1949. The total phosphorus, phytate phosphorus and inorganic phosphorus of bread and the destruction of phytic acid in bread making. *Aust. J. Exp. Biol. Med. Sci.* 27: 99—104.

Lembke, A., Kaufmann, W. and Schmidt, H. 1953. Enzymatic studies of milk proteins. *Milchwissenschaft* 8: 10—16.

Ler, C., Nelson, H. W. and Clegg, W. 1955. Weight, range, proximate composition and thiaminase content of fish taken in shallow water in northern Gulf of Mexico. *Comm. Fish. Rev.* 17: 21—25.

Levenberg, B. 1960. Structure and enzymatic cleavage of agaritine, a new phenylhydrazide of L-glutamic acid isolated from Agaricaceae. *J. Am. Chem. Soc.* 83: 503—504.

Levenberg, B. 1967. Isolation and structure of agaritine, an α-glutamyl-substituted arylhydrazine derivative from Agaricaceae. *J. Biol. Chem.* 239: 2267—2273.

Lewis, J. C., Snell, N. S., Hirschmann, D. J. and Fraenkel-Courat, H. 1950. Amino acid composition of egg protein. *J. Biol. Chem.* 186: 23—35.

Lieck, H. and Agren, G. 1944. On occurrence of thiamine inactivating factor in some species of Swedish fish. *Acta Physiol. Scand.* 8: 203—214.

Liener, I. E. 1953. Soyin, a toxic protein from soybean. I. Inhibitor of rat growth. *J. Nutr.* 49: 527—539.

Liener, I. E. 1958. Inactivation studies on the soybean hemagglutinin. *J. Biol. Chem.* 233: 401—405.

Liener, I. E. 1964. Seed hemagglutinins. *Econ. Botany* 18: 27—33.

Liener, I. E. 1976. Phytohemagglutins. *Ann. Rev. Plant Physiol.* 27: 291—319.

Liener, I. E. and Kakade, M. L. 1969. Protease inhibitors. In: *Toxic Constituents of Plant Foodstuffs.* I. E. Liener (ed.). Academic Press, New York.

Liener, I. E. and Pallansch, M. J. 1952. Purification of a toxic substance from defatted soy bean flour. *J. Biol. Chem.* 197: 29—36.

Liener, I. E. and Rose, J. E. 1953. Soyin, a toxic protein from the soybean. III. Immunochemical properties. *Proc. Soc. Exp. Biol. Med.* 83: 539—544.

Liener, J. E., Pallansch, M. J. and Rose, J. E. 1953. Properties of soyin, a toxic protein isolated from soybean flour. *Fed. Proc.* 12: 790.

Light, R. F., Alscher, R. and Frey, C. 1944. Vitamin A toxicity and hypothrombinemia. *Science* 100: 225—226.

Likuski, H. J. A. and Forbes, R. M. 1964. Effect of phytic acid on the availability of zinc in amino acid and casein diets fed to chicks. *J. Nutr.* 84: 145—148.

Lineweaver, H. and Murray, C. W. 1947. Identification of the trypsin inhibitor of egg white with ovomucoid. *J. Biol. Chem.* 171: 565—581.

Lis, H., Fridman, C., Sharon, N. and Katchalski, E. 1966. Multiple hemagglutinins in soybeans. *Arch. Biochem. Biophys.* 117: 301—309.

List, P. H. and Luft, P. 1969. Demonstration and determination of the gyromitrin concentration of fresh lorel. *Arch. Pharm.* 302: 143—146.

Lolas, G. M. and Markakis, P. 1975. Phytic acid and other phosphorus compounds of beans (Phaseolus vulgaris, L.). *J. Agric. Food Chem.* 23: 13—15.

Lovett-Janison, P. L. and Nelson, J. M. 1940. Ascorbic acid oxidase from summer crook-neck squash (C. pepo condensa). *J. Am. Chem. Soc.* 62: 1409—1412.

Somogyi, J. C. 1956. Metabolites and antimetabolites. In: *Results of Basic Research in Medicine.* K. F. Bauer (ed.). Thieme, Stuttgart. (German)

Lyman, R. L. 1957. The effect of raw soybean meal and trypsin inhibitor diets on the intestinal and pancreatic nitrogen in the rat. *J. Nutr.* 62: 285—294.

Lyman, R. L. and Lepkovski, S. 1957. The effect of raw soybean meal and trypsin inhibitor diets on pancreatic enzyme secretion in the rat. *J. Nutr.* 62: 269—281.

Machlin, L. J., Lankenau, A. H., Denton, C. A. and Bird, H. R. 1952. Effect of vitamin B_{12} and folic acid on growth and uricemia of chickens fed high levels of glycine. *J. Nutr.* 46: 389—398.

MacKenzie, C. G. and McCollum, E. V. 1937. Some effects of dietary oxalate on the rat. *Am. J. Hyg.* 25: 1—10.

Maddaiah, V. T., Kurnick, A. A. and Reid, B. L. 1964. Phytic acid studies. *Proc. Soc. Exp. Biol. Med.* 115: 391—393.

Malm, O. J. 1963. Adaptation to alterations in calcium intake. In: *The Transfer of Calcium and Strontium Across Biological Membranes.* R. H. Wasserman (ed.). Academic Press, New York.

Manage, L. D. 1969. "Studies on Nutritive Value and Hemagglutinins of Horsegram. Dolichos biflorus." Ph.D. Thesis. University of Bombay, India.

Marine, D., Baumann, E. J. and Webster, B. 1930. Occurrence of antigoitrogenic substances in plant juice. *Proc. Soc. Exp. Biol.* 27: 1029—1031.

Marshall, T. H., Whitaker, J. R. and Bender, M. L. 1969. Porcine elastase. II. Properties of the tyrosinate-splitting enzyme and the specificity of elastase. *Biochemistry* 8: 4671—4677.

Matschiner, J. T., Amelotti, J. M. and Doisy, E. A. 1967. Mechanism of the effect of retinoic acid and squalene on vitamin K deficiency in the rat. *J. Nutr.* 91: 303—306.

Matsukawa, D. and Misawa, H. 1951. A new bacillus producing thiaminase. *Vitamins* 4: 159—163.

Matsushima, K. 1958. An undescribed trypsin inhibitor in egg white. *Science* 127: 1178—1179.

McCance, R. A. and Walsham, C. M. 1948. The digestibility and absorption of the calories, proteins, purines, fat, calcium in wholemeal wheaten bread. *Br. J. Nutr.* 2: 26—41.

McCance, R. A. and Widdowson, E. M. 1935. Phytin in human nutrition. *Biochem. J.* 29: 2694—2699.

McCance, R. A. and Widdowson, E. M. 1942a. Mineral metabolism of healthy adults on white and brown bread dietaries. *J. Physiol. (Lond.)* 101: 44—85.

McCance, R. A. and Widdowson, E. M. 1942b. Mineral metabolism on dephytinized bread. *J. Physiol. (Lond.)* 101: 304—313.

McCance, R. A. and Widdowson, E. M. 1944. Activity of the phytase in different cereals and its resistance to dry heat. *Nature* 153: 650.

McCance, R. A. and Widdowson, E. M. 1949. Phytic acid. *Br. J. Nutr.* 2: 401—403.

McCance, R. A., Edgecombe, C. N. and Widdowson, E. M. 1943. Phytic acid and iron absorption. *Lancet* 2: 126—127.

McCombs, C. L. 1957. Ascorbic acid oxidase activity of certain vegetables and changes in the content of reduced and dehydroascorbic acid during shelf-life. *Food Res.* 22: 448—454.

McConnell, A. A., Eastwood, M. A. and Mitchell, W. D. 1974. Physical characteristics of vegetable foodstuffs that could influence bowel function. *J. Sci.
Food Agr.* 25: 1457—1464.

McGregor, I. K. and Sage, H. J. 1968. Purification and properties of a phytohemagglutinin from the lentil. *Fed. Proc.* 27: 428.

McIlwain, H. 1940. Pyridine-3-sulfon(2-pyridyl)amide; modeling of chemotherapeutic
agents. *Nature* 146: 653—654.

McLaughlin, L. 1927. Utilization of the calcium of spinach. *J. Biol. Chem.* 74:
455—462.

Melamed, M. D. and Green, N. M. 1963. Avidin. II. Purification and composition.
Biochem. J. 89: 591—599.

Mellamby, E. 1944. Phytic acid and phytase in cereals. *Nature* 154: 394—395.

Melnick, D., Hochberg, M. and Oser, B. L. 1945. Physiological availability of the
vitamins. II. The effect of dietary thiaminase in fish products. *J. Nutr.* 30:
81—88.

Miller, E. R. et al. 1965. Comparison of casein and soy proteins upon mineral
balance and vitamin D_2 requirement of the baby pig. *J. Nutr.* 85: 347—354.

Mitchell, H. H. 1924. A method of determining the biological value of proteins.
J. Biol. Chem. 58: 873—903.

Mitchell, H. H. and Smith, J. M. 1945. The effect of cocoa on the utilization of
dietary calcium. *J.A.M.A.* 129: 871—873.

Miyamoto, M., Imai, S. and Shinohara, M. 1967. Studies on the purgative substances. I. Isolation of sennoiside A, one of the most active principles from
rhubarb. *J. Pharm. Soc. Jpn.* 87: 1040—1043.

Moeller, M. W. and Scott, H. M. 1958. Studies with purified diets. 3. Zinc requirement. *Poultry Sci.* 37: 1227—1231.

Mollin, D. C., Hoffbrand, A. V., Ward, P. G. and Lewis, S. M. 1980. Inter-
laboratory comparison of serum vitamin B_{12} assay. *J. Clin. Pathol.* 33: 243—
248.

Moore, T. and Wang, Y.L. 1945. Hypervitaminosis A. *Biochem. J.* 39: 222—228.

Moran, T. and Pace, J. 1942. Foods. *Rep. Prog. Applied Chem.* 50: 505—508.

Morrison, A. B. and Sarrett, H. P. 1958. Studies on zinc deficiency in the chick.
J. Nutr. 65: 267—280.

Moudgal, N. R., Raghupathy, E. and Sarma, P. S. 1958. Studies on goitrogenic
agents in food. III. Goitrogenic action of some glycosides isolated from edible
nuts. *J. Nutr.* 66: 291—303.

Mukherjee, S. L. and Sen, S. P. 1959. Stability of vitamin B_{12}. Part II. Protection by an iron salt against destruction by aneurine and nicotamide. *J. Pharm.
Pharmacol.* 11: 26—31.

Multani, J. S., Cepurneek, C. P., Davis, P. S. and Saltman, P. 1970. Biochemical
characterization of gastroferrin. *Biochemistry* 9: 3970—3976.

Murata, K. 1965. Thiaminase. In: *Review of Japanese Literature on Beriberi and
Thiamine.* M. Shimazono and E. Katsura (eds.). Vitamin B Research Committee
of Japan, Tokyo.

Murphy, F. J. and Zelman, S. 1965. Ascorbic acid as a urinary acidifying agent.
I. Comparison with the ketogenic effect of fasting. *J. Urol.* 94: 297—299.

Murray, J and Stein, N. 1970. Gastric secretions and iron absorption in rats.
In: *Trace Element Metabolism in Animals.* C. F. Mills (ed.). Livingstone,
Edinburgh.

Nagel, D., Toth, B. and Kupper, R. 1976. Formation of methylhydrazine from
acetaldehyde N-methyl-N-formylhydrazone of Gyromitra esculenta. *Proc. Am.
Assoc. Cancer Res.* 17: 9.

Nakamura, F. I. and Mitchell, H. H. 1943. The utilization for hemoglobin regeneration of the iron salts used in the enrichment of flour and bread. *J. Nutr.* 25:
39—48.

Neilands, J. B. 1947. Thiaminase in aquatic animals of Nova Scotia. *J. Fish. Res. Board Can.* 7: 94–99.

Nelson, T. S., Shieh, T. R., Wodzinski, R. J. and Ware, J. H. 1971. Effect of supplemental phytase on the utilization of phytate phosphorus by chicks. *J. Nutr.* 101: 1289–1294.

Nesheim, M. C., Garlich, J. D. and Hopkins, D. T. 1962. Studies on the effect of raw soybean meal on fat absorption in young chicks. *J. Nutr.* 78: 89–94.

Newmark, H. L. 1958. Stable vitamin B_{12}-containing solution. U.S. Patent No. 2,823,167. Feb. 11.

Newmark, H. L., Scheiner, J., Marcus, M. and Prabhudesai, M. 1976. Stability of vitamin B_{12} in presence of ascorbic acid. *Am. J. Clin. Nutr.* 29: 645–649.

Nicolaysen, R., Eeg-Larsen, N. and Malm, O. J. 1953. Physiology of calcium metabolism. *Physiol. Rev.* 33: 424–444.

Nielsen, E. and Elvehjem, C. A. 1941. Cure of spectacle eye condition in rats with biotin concentrates. *Proc. Soc. Exp. Biol.* 48: 349–352.

Nielsen, E. and Elvehjem, C. A. 1942. Cure of paralysis in rats with biotin concentrates and crystalline biotin. *J. Biol. Chem.* 144: 405–409.

Nitesco, I., Popovici, G. and Opreanu, R. 1933. The elimination of calcium and phosphorus following a corn diet. *C.R. Soc. Biol.* 113: 326–328. (French)

Noda, M. and Matsumoto, M. 1971. Sinapic acid and methyl sinapate in rapeseed lipids. *Biochim. Biophys. Acta* 231: 131–133.

Nordfelt, S., Gellerstedt, N. and Falkmer, S. 1954. Studies of rapeseed oilmeal and its goitrogenic effect in pigs. *Acta Pathol. Microbiol. Scand.* 35: 217–236.

Oberleas, D., Muhrer, M. E. and O'Dell, B. L. 1966a. Dietary metal-complexing agents and zinc availability in the rat. *J. Nutr.* 90: 56–62.

Oberleas, D., Muhrer, M. E. and O'Dell, B. L. 1966b. The availability of zinc from foodstuffs. In: *Zinc Metabolism.* A. S. Prasad (ed.). Thomas, Springfield, Illinois.

O'Dell, B. L. and Savage, J. E. 1960. Effect of phytic acid on zinc availability. *Proc. Soc. Exp. Biol.* 103: 304–306.

O'Dell, B. L., Newberne, P. M. and Savage, J. E. 1958. Significance of dietary zinc for growing chicken. *J. Nutr.* 65: 503–523.

O'Dell, B. L., de Boland, A. R. and Koirtyohann, S. R. 1972. Distribution of phytate and nutritionally important elements among the morphological components of cereal grains. *J. Agric. Food Chem.* 20: 718–721.

Okano, K. 1948. The toxic proteins of raw soybeans. Hemolytic reaction of the soybean saponin. *J. Agric. Chem. Soc. (Jpn.)* 22: 23–27.

Oke, O. L. 1965. Phytic acid-phosphorus content of Nigerian foodstuffs. *Indian J. Med. Res.* 53: 417–420.

Olson, M. O. and Liener, I. E. 1967. Some physical and chemical properties of concanavalin A, the phytohemagglutinin of the jack bean. *Biochemistry* 6: 105–111.

Orten, J. M. and Neuhaus, O. W. 1975. *Human Biochemistry.* Mosby, St. Louis.

Ozawa, K., Nakayama, H. and Hayashi, R. 1957. Destruction of thiamine by certain fungi. *J. Vitaminol.* 3: 282–287.

Palozzo, A. and Jaffe, W. G. 1969. Immunoelectrophoretic studies with bean proteins. *Phytochemistry* 8: 1255–1258.

Parsons, H. T. 1931. The physiological effects of diets rich in egg white. *J. Biol. Chem.* 90: 351–367.

Parsons, H. T. and Kelly, E. 1933a. The character of the dermatitis-producing factor in dietary egg white as shown by certain chemical treatments. *J. Biol. Chem.* 100: 645–652.

Parsons, H. T. and Kelly, E. 1933b. The effect of heating egg white on certain characteristic pellagra-like manifestations produced in rats by its dietary use. *Am. J. Physiol.* 104: 150–164.

Pemberton, R. T. 1970. Haemagglutinins from the slug Limax flavus. *Vox Sang.* 18: 74—76.

Pengle, U. and Ramasastri, B. V. 1978. Absorption of calcium from a leafy vegetable rich in oxalates. *Br. J. Nutr.* 39: 119—125.

Peterson, D. W. 1950. Some properties of a factor in alfalfa meal causing depression of growth in chicks. *J. Biol. Chem.* 183: 647—653.

Petropulos, S. F. 1960. The action of an antimetabolite of thiamine on single myelinated nerve fibres. *J. Cell. Comp. Physiol.* 56: 7—13.

Pileggi, V. J. 1959. Distribution of phytase in the rat. *Arch. Biochem.* 80: 1—8.

Pinchera, A., MacGillivray, M. H., Crawford, J. D. and Freeman, A. G. 1965. Thyroid refractoriness in an athyreotic cretin fed soybean formula. *N. Engl. J. Med.* 273: 83—87.

Potter, G. C. and Kummerow, F. A. 1954. Chemical similarity and biological activity of the saponins isolated from alfalfa and soybeans. *Science* 120: 224—225.

Prokop, O., Uhlenbruck, G. and Kohler, W. 1968. A new source of antibody-like substances having anti-blood group specificity. *Vox Sang.* 14: 321—333.

Pudelkiewicz, W. G. and Matterson, L. D. 1960. A fat soluble material in alfalfa that reduces the biological availability of tocopherol. *J. Nutr.* 71: 143—148.

Pudelkiewicz, W. L. et al. 1960. Chick tissue storage bioassay of alpha tocopherol: Chemical analytical techniques and relative biopotencies of natural and synthetic alpha-tocopherol. *J. Nutr.* 71: 115—121.

Purves, H. D. 1943. Studies on experimental goitre: effect of di-iodothyrosine and thyroxine on goitrogenic action of Brassica seeds. *Br. J. Exp. Pathol.* 24: 171—173.

Pusztai, A. 1968. General properties of a protease inhibitor from the seeds of kidney bean. *Eur. J. Biochem.* 5: 252—259.

Pyssalo, H. 1975. Some new toxic compounds in false morels Gyromitra esculenta. *Naturwissenshaften* 62: 395.

Raciszewski, Z. M., Spencer, E. Y. and Trevoy, L. W. 1955. Chemical studies of a goitrogenic factor in rapeseed oil meal. *Can. J. Technol.* 33: 129—133.

Rackis, J. J. 1974. Biological and physiological factors in soybeans. *J. Am. Oil Chem. Soc.* 51: 161A—174A.

Rackis, J. J., McGhee, J. E. and Booth, A. N. 1975. Biological threshold levels of soybean trypsin inhibitors by rat bioassays. *Cereal Chem.* 52: 85—92.

Rackis, J. J., McGhee, J. E., Gumbmann, M. R. and Booth, A. N. 1979. Effects of soy proteins containing trypsin inhibitors on long-term feeding studies in rats. *J. Am. Oil Chem. Soc.* 56: 162—168.

Ramirez, J. S. and Mitchell, H. L. 1960. The trypsin inhibitor of alfalfa. *J. Agric. Food Chem.* 8: 393—395.

Ranhotra, G. S. and Loewe, R. J. 1975. Effect of wheat phytase on dietary phytic acid. *J. Food Sci.* 40: 940—942.

Raoul, Y. and Jutz, O. 1960. Dimineralizing activity of several plants on the animal skeleton. *Arch. Sci. Physiol.* 14: 217—226.

Raoul, Y. et al. 1957. Isolation of an antivitamin D from aerial parts of vegetables. *C. R. Acad. Sci.* 244: 954—957. (French)

Ray, P. K. 1969. Nutritive value of horse gram (Dolichos biflorus). I. Effect of feeding raw and treated seed flour on the growth of rats. *J. Nutr. Diet.* 6: 329—335.

Reinhold, J. G. 1971. High phytate content of rural Iranian bread. A possible cause of human zinc deficiency. *Am. J. Clin. Nutr.* 24: 1204—1206.

Reinhold, J. G., Nasr, K., Lahimgarzadeh, A. and Hedayati, H. 1973. Effects of purified phytate and phytate-rice bread upon metabolism of zinc, calcium, phosphorus and nitrogen in man. *Lancet* 1: 283—288.

Reinhold, J. G., Ismail-Beigi, F. and Faradji, B. 1975. Fibre vs phytate as de-
    terminant of the availability of calcium, zinc, and iron of breadstuffs. *Nutr.*
    Rep. Int. 12: 75−85.

Reinhold, J., Faradji, B., Abadi, P. and Ismail-Beigi, F. 1976a. Decreased
    absorption of calcium, magnesium, zinc and phosphorus consumption as wheat
    bread. *J. Nutr.* 106: 493−503.

Reinhold, J., Faradji, B., Abadi, P. and Ismail-Beigi, F. 1976b. Binding of zinc
    to fibre and other solids of wholemeal bread; with a preliminary examination of
    the effects of cellulose consumption upon the metabolism of calcium, zinc, and
    phosphorus in man. In: *Trace Elements in Human Nutrition and Disease.*
    Vol. I. A. S. Prasad (ed.). Academic Press, New York.

Renzo, E. C., de, et al. 1958. Some biochemical effects of hypoglycin. *Biochem.*
    Pharmacol. 1: 236−237.

Rhodes, M. B., Bennet, N. and Feeney, R. E. 1960. The trypsin and chymotryp-
    sin inhibitors from avicin egg whites. *J. Biol. Chem.* 235: 1686−1693.

Ripp, J. A. 1961. Soybean-induced goiter. *Am. J. Dis. Child.* 102: 106−109.

Robb, E. F. 1919. Death from rhubarb leaves due to oxalic acid poisoning.
    J.A.M.A. 73: 627−628.

Roberts, A. H. and Yudkin, J. 1960. Dietary phytate as a possible cause of
    magnesium deficiency. *Nature* 185: 823−825.

Roberts, A. H. and Yudkin, J. 1961. Effect of phytate and other dietary factors
    on intestinal phytase and bone calcification in the rat. *Br. J. Nutr.* 15:
    457−471.

Roberts, H. E., Evans, E. T. R. and Evans, W. C. 1949. The production of
    "bracken staggers" in the horse and its treatment of vitamin B$_1$ therapy.
    Vet. Rec. 61: 549−550.

Rodrick J. 1929. The pathology of sweet clover disease in cattle. *J. Am. Vet.*
    Med. Assoc. 74: 314−318.

Rodrick, J. 1931. A problem in the coagulation of the blood "sweet clover disease
    of cattle." *Am. J. Physiol.* 96: 413−425.

Rungruangsak, K., Tosukhowong, P., Panijpan, B. and Vimokesant, S. L. 1977.
    Chemical interactions between thiamin and tannic acid. I. Kinetics, oxygen
    dependence and inhibition by ascorbic acid. *Am. J. Clin. Nutr.* 30: 1680−1685.

Ryan, C. A. 1966. Chytrypsin inhibitor I from potatoes: reactivity with mammalian,
    plant, bacterial, and fungal proteinases. *Biochemistry* 5: 1592−1596.

Sack, K. A., Staudinger, A. and Zubrzycki, Z. J. 1961. Kinetic investigations
    with ascorbic acid oxidase. *Biochem. Z.* 335: 177−186.

Sage, H. J. and Connett, S. L. 1969. Studies on a hemagglutinin from the meadow
    mushroom. II. Purification, composition, and structure of Agaricus campestris
    hemagglutinin. *J. Biol. Chem.* 244: 4713−4719.

Saghir, A. R., Cowan, J. W. and Salji, J. P. 1966. Goitrogenic activity of onion
    volatiles. *Nature* 211: 87.

Salgarkar, S. and Sohonie, K. 1965a. Haemagglutinins of field bean (Dolichos lablab).
    I. Isolation, purification and properties of haemagglutinins. *Indian J. Biochem.*
    2: 193−196.

Salgarkar, S. and Sohonie, K. 1965b. Haemagglutinins of field bean (Dolichos
    lablab). Part II. Effect of feeding field bean haemagglutinin A on rat growth.
    Indian J. Biochem. 2: 197−199.

Samruatruamphol, S. and Parsons, H. T. 1955. An antithiamine effect produced in
    human subjects by bracken ferns. *J. Am. Diet Assoc.* 31: 790−793.

Sathe, V. and Krishnamurthy, K. 1953. Phytic acid and absorption of iron.
    Indian J. Med. Res. 41: 453−461.

Sautier, P. M. 1946. Thiamine assays of fishery products. *Comm. Fish. Rev.* 8:
    17−19.

Saxena, H. C., Jensen, I. S. and McGinnis, J. 1962. Influence of dietary protein level on chick growth depression by raw soybean meal. *J. Nutr.* 77: 241—244.

Schmid, W. 1951. Assay of anthraglycoside drugs. Use of the leaves of medicinal and edible rhubarb. *Dtsch. Apoth. Ztg.* 91: 452—454. (German)

Schulerud, A. 1947. The contents of phytic acid P in Norwegian flour and bread types. 2. Factors influencing phytic acid decomposition during breadmaking and the contents of phytic acid P in ordinary Norwegian bread. *Acta Physiol. Scand.* 14: 1—15.

Sealock, R. R., Livermore, A. H. and Evans, C. A. 1943. Thiamine inactivation by fresh-fish or chastek-paralysis factor. *J. Amer. Chem. Soc.* 65: 935—940.

Serafin, J. A. and Nesheim, M. C. 1970. Influence of dietary heat-labile factors in soybean meal upon bile acid pools and turnover in the chick. *J. Nutr.* 100: 786—796.

Sharpe, L. M., Peacock, W. C., Cooke, R. and Harris, R. S. 1950. The effect of phytate and other food factors on iron absorption. *J. Nutr.* 41: 433—446.

Sharpless, G. R. 1938. A new goiter-producing diet for the rat. *Proc. Soc. Exp. Biol.* 38: 166—168.

Sharpless, G. R., Pearson, J. and Prato, G. S. 1939. Production of goiter in rats with raw and with treated soybean flour. *J. Nutr.* 17: 545—555.

Shaw, E. 1953. Antimetabolites—A review. *Metabolism* 2: 103—119.

Shaw, J. C., Moore, L. A. and Sykes, J. F. 1951. The effect of raw soybeans on blood plasma carotene and vitamin A and liver vitamin A of calves. *J. Dairy Sci.* 34: 176—180.

Shepard, T. H., Pyne, G. E., Kirschvink, J. F. and McLean, M. 1960. Soybean goiter: report of three cases. *N. Eng. J. Med.* 262: 1099—1103.

Sherman, H. C. 1941. Significance of different levels of vitamin intake. *J. Am. Diet Assoc.* 17: 1—4.

Sherman, H. C. and Hawley, E. 1922. Calcium and phosphorus metabolism in childhood. *J. Biol. Chem.* 53: 375—399.

Shields, J. B. and Mitchell, H. H. 1941. The utilization of the calcium in beets, turnips, celery, and broccoli in comparison with the calcium in dry milk solids. *J. Biol. Chem.* 140: 115—116.

Shoham, J., Inbar, M. and Sachs, L. 1970. Differential toxicity on normal and transformed cells in vitro and inhibition of tumor development in vivo by concanavalin A. *Nature* 227: 1244—1246.

Shyamala, G., Kennedy, B. M. and Lyman, R. L. 1961. Trypsin inhibitor in whole wheat flour. *Nature* 192: 360.

Singsen, E. P. et al. 1955. Studies on encephalomalacia in the chick. VI. The utilization of vitamin E from alfalfa meal and wheat middlings for the prevention of encephalomalacia. *Poultry Sci.* 34: 1234.

Smashevskii, N. D. 1965. Isolation of an astivitamin from young pea sprouts. *Chem. Abstr.* 63: 3315e.

Smashevskii, N. D. 1966. A natural antivitamin of pantothenic acid. *Chem. Abstr.* 65: 2677e.

Smashevskii, N. D. 1969. Amino acid inactivation of a natural pantothenic acid antivitamin, pizamin, and possible mechanism of its action. *Chem. Abstr.* 70: 1157p.

Smith, A. K. and Rackis, J. J. 1957. Phytin elimination in soybean protein isolation. *J. Am. Chem. Soc.* 79: 633—637.

Smith, D. C. and Proutt, L. M. 1944. Development of thiamine deficiency in the cat on a diet of raw fish. *Proc. Soc. Exp. Biol.* 56: 1—3.

Smith, M. C. and Caldwell, E. 1945. The effect of maceration of foods upon their ascorbic acid values. *Science* 101: 308—309.

Smith, W. H., Plumlee, M. P. and Beeson, W. M. 1961. Zinc requirements of growing pig fed isolated soybean protein semipurified ration. *J. Anim. Sci.* 20: 128–132.

Smith, W. H., Plumlee, M. P. and Beeson, W. M. 1962. Effect of source of protein on the zinc requirement of the growing pig. *J. Anim. Sci.* 21: 399–405.

Snyderman, S. E., Carretero, R. and Holt, L. E., Jr. 1950. Pyridoxine deficiency in the human being. *Fed. Proc.* 9: 371–372.

Snyderman, S. E., Holt, L. E., Jr., Carretero, R. and Jacobs, K. 1953. Pyridoxine deficiency in the human infant. *Am. J. Clin Nutr.* 1: 200–207.

Sohonie, K. and Bhandarkar, A. P. 1954. Trypsin inhibitors in Indian foodstuffs. I. Inhibitors in vegetables. *J. Sci. Industr. Res.* (India) 13 (B), 500–503.

Sohonie, K. and Bhandarkar, A. P. 1955. Trypsin inhibitors in Indian foodstuffs. II. Inhibitors in pulses. *J. Sci. Industr. Res.* 14(C): 100–104.

Sohonie, K. and Honavar, P. M. 1956. Trypsin inhibitors of sweet potato (Ipomoea batata). *Sci. Cult. (Calcutta)* 21: 538.

Solyom, A., Borsy, J. and Tolnay, P. 1964. Elastase inhibitors of plant origin. *Biochem. Pharmacol.* 13: 391–394.

Somogyi, J. C. 1949a. Inactivation of aneurin by extracts of animal and plant tissues. *Int. Z. Vitaminforsch.* 21: 341–346. (German)

Somogyi, J. C. 1949b. Inactivation of thiamin by extracts of carp tissues. *Helv. Physiol. Acta* 7: 24–26. (German)

Somogyi, J. C. 1952. *The Antithiamin Factor*. Hans Huber, Bern. (German)

Somogyi, J. C. 1960. On the antimetabolite of thiamin. *Bibl. Nutr. Diet.* 1: 77.

Somogyi, J. C. 1973. Antivitamins. In: *Toxicants Occurring Naturally in Foods*. Committee on Food Protection, Food and Nutrition Board, National Research Council. National Academy of Sciences, Washington, D.C.

Somogyi, J. C. and Bonicke, R. 1969. Connection between chemical structure and antithiamine activity of various phenol derivatives. *Int. Z. Vitaminforsch.* 39: 65–73.

Somogyi, J. C. and Koller, A. 1959. On the chemical nature of the antithiamine factor in fern. *Int. Z. Vitaminforsch.* 29: 234–243. (German)

Somogyi, J. C. and Kundig, H. 1968. Inactivation of thiamine by substance K and other heme compounds as with different iron salts. *Int. Z. Vitaminforsch.* 38: 503–507. (German)

Speirs, M. 1939. The utilization of calcium in various greens. *J. Nutr.* 17: 557–564.

Spitzer, E. H., Coombes, A. I., Elvehjem, C. A. and Wisnicky, W. 1941. Inactivation of vitamin B_1 by raw fish. *Proc. Soc. Exp. Biol.* 48: 376–379.

Spivey, W. R., Briggs, G. M. and Ortiz, L. O. 1954. Effects of diets high in fat or protein on vitamin B_{12} deficiency in nondepleted chicks. *Proc. Soc. Exp. Biol. Med.* 85: 451–453.

Srinivasan, V., Moudgal, N. R. and Sarma, P. S. 1957. Studies on goitrogenic agents in food. 1. Goitrogenic action of groundnut. *J. Nutr.* 61: 87–95.

Stahman, M. A., Huebner, C. I. and Link, K. P. 1941. Studies on the hemorrhagic sweet clover disease. V. Identification and synthesis of the hemorrhagic agent. *J. Biol. Chem.* 138: 513–527.

Stead, R. J., de Muelenaere, H. J. and Quicke, G. V. 1966. Trypsin inhibition, haemagglutination and intraperitoneal toxicity of Phaseolus vulgaris and Glycine max. *Arch. Biochem. Biophys.* 113: 703–708.

Stecher, P. G., Finkel, M. J., Siegmund, O. H. and Szafranski, B. M. (Editors). 1960. *The Merck Index of Chemicals and Drugs*. Merck & Co., Rahway, New Jersey.

Steck, T. L. and Hoelzl Wallach, D. F. 1965. The binding of kidney bean phytohemagglutinin by Ehrlich ascites carcinoma. *Biochim. Biophys. Acta* 97: 510–522.

Stone, W. 1937. Ascorbic acid oxidase and the state of ascorbic acid in vegetable tissues. *Biochem. J.* 31: 508–512.

Stiles, L. W. 1977. "The Effect of Dietary Fiber on Mineral Absorption." Ph.D. Thesis. Cornel University, Ithaca, New York.

Streicher, E. 1964. Acute renal failure and jaundice following rhubarb leaf poisoning. *Dtsch Med. Wochenschr.* 89: 2379–2381.

Sumner, J. B. and Dounce, A. L. 1939. Carotene oxidase. *Enzymologia* 7: 130–132.

Sundararajan, A. R. 1938. Phytin phosphorus content of Indian foodstuffs. *Indian J. Med. Res.* 25: 685–691.

Sydenstricker, V. P. et al. 1942a. Observations on the "egg white injury" in man and its cure with a biotin concentrate. *J.A.M.A.* 118: 1199–1200.

Sydenstricker, V. P. et al. 1942b. Preliminary observations on "egg white injury" in man and its cure with biotin concentrate. *Science* 95: 176–177.

Takahashi, T., Ramachandramurthy, P. and Liener, I. F. 1967. Some physical and chemical properties of a phytohemagglutinin isolated from Phaseolus vulgaris. *Biochim. Biophys. Acta* 133: 123–133.

Tallquist, H. and Väänänen, I. 1960. Death of a child from oxalic acid poisoning due to eating rhubarb leaves. *Ann. Paediatr. Fenn.* 6: 144–147.

Tappel, A. L. 1962. Vitamin E as the biological lipid antioxidant. *Vitam. Horm.* 20: 493–510.

Tauber, H., Kleiner, I. S. and Mishkind, D. 1935. Ascorbic acid (vitamin C) oxidase. *J. Biol. Chem.* 110: 211–218.

Tauber, H., Kershaw, B. B. and Wright, R. D. 1949. Studies on the growth inhibitor fraction of lima beans and isolation of a crystalline heat-stable inhibitor. *J. Biol. Chem.* 179: 1155–1161.

Ticha, M., Entlicher, G., Kostir, A. and Kocousek, J. 1970. Studies on phyto-hemagglutinins. IV. Isolation and characterization of a hemagglutinin from the lentil, Lens esculenta, Moench. *Biochim. Biophys. Acta* 221: 282–289.

Tiggelmann-Van Krugten, V. A., Ostendorf-Doyer, C. M. and Collier, W. A. 1956. Hemagglutins of plant extracts. *Antonie van Leeuwenhoek J. Microbiol. Serol.* 22: 289–303.

Tisdall, F. F. and Drake, T. G. H. 1938. The utilization of calcium. *J. Nutr.* 16: 613–622.

Tisdall, F. F., Drake, T. G. H., Summerfeldt, P. and Jackson, S. H. 1937. The comparative value of spinach and tomates in the child's diet. *J. Pediatr.* 11: 374–384.

Toth, B. 1979. Mushroom hydrazines: occurrence, metabolism, carcinogenesis, and environmental implications. In: *Naturally Occurring Carcinogens—Mutagens and Modulators of Carcinogenesis.* E. C. Miller et al. (ed.). University Park Press, Baltimore.

Tuba, J., Siluck, K. A., Robinson, M. I. and Madsen, N. B. 1952. The relation-ship of dietary factors to rat serum alkaline phosphatase. IV. The effect of dietary oxalate. *Can. J. Med. Sci.* 30: 515–519.

Tucker, H. F. and Salmon, W. D. 1955. Parakeratosis or zinc deficiency disease in the pig. *Proc. Soc. Exp. Biol.* 88: 613–616.

Turner, C. W. 1948. The effect of rapeseed on the thyroid of the chick. *Poultry Sci.* 25: 186–187.

Uhlenbruck, G., Gielen, W. and Pardoe, G. I. 1970. On the specificity of lectins with a broad agglutination spectrum. V. Further investigation on the tumor characteristic agglutinin from wheat germ lipase. *Z. Krebsforsch.* 74: 171–178.

Vallotton, M. and Leuthardt, I. 1963. Studies on the spontaneous binding of biotin (C^{14}) on deficient proteins. *Helv. Physiol. Pharmacol. Acta.* 21: C67–C70. (French)

Vallotton, M., Hess-Sander, U. and Leuthardt, F. 1965. Spontaneous binding of biotin on a protein from human serum. *Helv. Chim. Acta* 48: 126–133. (French)

VanderLaan, J. E. and VanderLaan, W. P. 1947. The iodide-concentrating mechanism of the rat thyroid and its inhibition by thiocyanate. *Endocrinology* 40: 403–416.

VanEtten, C. H. 1969. Goitrogens. In: *Toxic Constituents in Plant Foodstuffs.* I. E. Liener (ed.). Academic Press, New York.

VanEtten, C. H. and Wolff, I. A. 1973. Natural sulfur compounds. In: *Toxicants Occurring Naturally in Foods.* Committee on Food Protection, Food and Nutrition Board, National Research Council. National Academy of Sciences, Washington, D.C.

VanEtten, C. H., Daxenbichler, M. E. and Wolff, I. A. 1969. Natural glucosinolates (thioglucosides) in foods and feeds. *J. Agric. Food Chem.* 17: 483–491.

Van Middlesworth, L. 1957. Thyroxine excretion, a possible cause of goiter. *Endocrinology* 61: 570–573.

Van Wyk, J. J., Arnold, M. B., Wynn, J. and Pepper, F. 1959. The effects of a soybean product on thyroid function in humans. *Pediatrics* 24: 752–760.

Viehover, A. 1940. Edible and poisonous beans of the lima type (Phaseolus lunatus L.). *Thai. Sci. Bull.* 2: 1–99.

Vilkki, P., Kreula, M. and Piironen, E. 1962. Studies on the goitrogenic influence of cow's milk on man. *Ann. Acad. Sci. Fenn.* A2 110: 71–83.

Vilter, R. W. et al. 1953. The effect of vitamin B_6 deficiency induced by desoxy-pyridoxine (DOP) in human beings. *J. Lab. Clin. Med.* 42: 335–357.

Vimokesant, S. L. et al. 1975. Effects of betel nut and fermented fish on the thiamin status of northeastern Thais. *Am. J. Clin. Nutr.* 28: 1458–1463.

Vimokesant, S. L., Nakornchai, S., Dhanamitta, S. and Hilker, D. M. 1974. Effect of tea consumption on thiamin status in man. *Nutr. Rep. Int.* 5: 371–375.

Virtanen, A. I. 1961. On the chemistry of the Brassica-factor, its effect on the function of the thyroid gland and its transfer to milk. *Experientia* 17: 241–251. (German)

Virtanen, A. I. 1962. Some organic sulfur compounds in vegetables and fodder plants and their significance in human nutrition. *Angew. Chemie* 1: 299–306.

Virtanen, A. I., Kreula, M. and Kiesvaara, M. 1963. Investigations of the alleged goitrogenic properties of cow's milk. *Z. Ernahrungswiss.* (Suppl.) 3: 23–37.

Vogel, R., Trautschold, I. and Werle, E. 1966. *Natural Proteinase-Inhibitors.* Thieme, Stuttgart. (German)

Vohra, P., Gray, G. A. and Kratzer, F. H. 1965. Phytic acid-metal complexes. *Proc. Soc. Exp. Biol. Med.* 120: 447–449.

von Holt, L. and von Holt, C. 1959. Biochemistry of hypoglycine A. I. The effect of riboflavin on the hypoglycemic effect. *Biochem. Z.* 331: 422–429.

von Streicher, E. 1964. Acute kidney failure and ecterus following poisoning with rhubarb leaves. *Dtsch. Med. Wochenschr.* 89: 2379. (German)

Walford, R. L. and Kickhofen, B. 1962. Selective inhibition of elastolytic and proteolytic properties of elastase. *Arch. Biochem. Biophys.* 98: 191.

Walker, A. R. P. 1951. Cereals, phytic acid, and calcification. *Lancet* 2: 244–248.

Walker, A. R. P. 1954. Low niacin concentration in the breast milk of Bantu mothers on a high maize diet. *Nature* 173: 405–406.

Walker, A. R. P., Irving, J. T. and Fox, F. W. 1946. Nutritional value of high extraction wheat meals. *Nature* 157: 769.

Walker, A. R. P., Fox, F. W. and Irving, J. T. 1948. Studies in human mineral metabolism. 1. The effect of bread rich in phytate phosphorus on the metabolism of certain mineral salts with special reference to calcium. *Biochem. J.* 42: 452–462.

Wei, R. D. and Wright, L. D. 1964. Heat stability of avidin and avidin-biotin complex and influence of ionic strength on affinity of avidin for biotin. *Proc. Soc. Exp. Biol.* (N.Y.) 117: 341–344.

Weits, J. 1952. A factor in hay inhibiting the action of vitamin D. *Nature* 170: 891.

Weits, J. 1960. The influence of carotene and vitamin A on the anti-rachitic action of vitamin D. *Int. Z. Vitaminforsch.* 30: 399–404.

Weits, I. J. 1966. An antagonist of vitamin D. *Bibl. Nutr. Diet.* 8: 44–53.

Welch, R. M., House, W. A. and Van Campen, D. 1977. Effects of oxalic acid on availability of zinc from spinach leaves and zinc sulfate to rats. *J. Nutr.* 107: 929–933.

Werle, E., Appel, W. and Hopp, E. 1959. The Kallikrein inactivator of potatoes and its differentiation from proteinase inhibitors. *Z. Vitamin. Hormon. U. Ferment-forsch.* 10: 127–136.

Westfall, F. J. and Hauge, S. M. 1948. The nutritive quality and trypsin inhibitor content of soybean flour heated at various temperatures. *J. Nutr.* 35: 379–389.

Westwig, H. P., Freed, M. A. and Haag, R. J. 1946. Antithiamine activity of plant materials. *J. Biol. Chem.* 165: 737–738.

Widdowson, E. M. 1941. Phytic acid and the preparation of food. *Nature* 148: 219–220.

Widdowson, E. M. and McCance, R. A. 1942. Iron exchanges of adults on white and brown bread diets. *Lancet* 1: 588–591.

Wilgus, H. S., Jr. and Gassner, F. X. 1941. Effect of soybean oil meal on avian reproduction. *Proc. Soc. Exp. Biol.* 46: 290–293.

Wilgus, H. S., Gassner, F. X., Patton, A. R., and Gustavson, R. G. 1941. The goitrogenicity of soybeans. *J. Nutr.* 22: 43–52.

Williams, R. H. 1943. Clinical biotin deficiency. *N. Engl. J. Med.* 228: 247–252.

Witherspoon, L. R. 1981. Vitamin B_{12}: are serum radioassay measurements reliable? *J. Nucl. Med.* 22: 474–477.

Witting, L. A. 1974. Vitamin E-polyunsaturated lipid relationship in diet and tissues. *Am. J. Clin. Nutr.* 27: 952–959.

Witting, L. A. and Horwitt, M. K. 1964. Effect of degree of fatty acid unsaturation in tocopherol deficiency-induced creatinuria. *J. Nutr.* 82: 19–33.

Wittlife, J. L. and Airth, R. L. 1970a. Thiaminase I (thiamine: base 2-methyl-4-amino-pyrimidine-5-methenyltransferase, E.C. 2.5.1.2) method. *Enzymologia* 18A: 229–234.

Wittlife, J. L. and Airth, R. L. 1970b. Thiaminase II (thiaminehydrolase, E.C. 3.5.9.9.2.) method. *Enzymologia* 18A: 234–238.

Wokes, F. and Organ, J. G. 1943. Oxidizing enzymes and vitamin C in tomatoes. *Biochem. J.* 37: 259–265.

Woolley, D. W. 1945a. Production of nicotinic acid deficiency with 3-acetyl-pyridoxine, the ketone analogue of nicotinic acid. *J. Biol. Chem.* 157: 455–459.

Woolley, D. W. 1945b. Some biological effects produced by α-tocopherol. *J. Biol. Chem.* 159: 59–66.

Woolley, D. W. 1946. The occurrence of pellagrogenic agent in corn. *J. Biol Chem.* 163: 773–774.

Woolley, D. W. 1952. *A Study of Antimetabolites*. Wiley, New York.

Wostmann, B. S. and Knight, P. L. 1965. Antagonism between vitamins A and K in the germfree rat. *J. Nutr.* 87: 155–160.

Yacowitz, H., Miller, R. F., Norris, L. C. and Heuser, G. F. 1952. Vitamin B_{12} studies with the hen. *Poultry Sci.* 31: 89–94.

Yang, E. F. and Dju, M. Y. 1939. Total and phytic acid phosphorus in foods. *Clin. J. Physiol.* 14: 473–480.

Yariv, J., Kalb, A. J. and Levitzki, A. 1968. The interaction of concanavalin A
with methyl-α-D-glucophranoside. *Biochim. Biophys. Acta* 165: 303–305.
Yasumoto, K., Iwami, K., Mitsusawa, H. and Mitsuda, H. 1976. Preparation of
desglutamyllentinic acid, a new sulfur containing amino acid, from leutinic
acid and its capacity to form a complex with pyridoxal phosphate. *Nippon Nogei
Kagaku Kaishi* 50: 563–568. (Japanese)
Yen, J. T., Jensen, A. H. and Simon, J. 1977. Effect of dietary raw soybean and
soybean trypsin inhibitor on trypsin and chymotrypsin activities in the pancreas and in small intestinal juice of growing swine. *J. Nutr.* 107: 156–165.
Zuck, D. A. and Conine, J. W. 1963. Stabilization of vitamin B_{12}. I. Complex
cyanides. *J. Pharm. Sci.* 52: 59–63.

10

Toxic Mushrooms and Other Macrofungi

Many species of mushrooms and other macrofungi* are among that select group of natural products which humans consider as food. They are valued by many for their characteristic and often delicate flavor. Mushrooms are obtained either from commercial cul-
tivation or natural habitats, which for the purpose of this discussion include parks,
lawns, and similar places. While the commercial sources may be limited to a few varieties, the wild sources provide thousands of varieties. Thus, for many centuries, mushroom gathering in the wilds has been a common practice in many parts of the world.

Yet, as we shall see, this practice is replete with danger from serious and often
fatal poisonings, not only for the unfamiliar, but also for the experienced mushroom
gatherer. There are several reasons why mushroom poisoning can occur even among
experts:

1. There are thousands of mushroom species. In the United States alone there are
probably more than 3000 (Smith 1958). An "expert" may venture into an unknown and
untested species. Foolhardy as this may be, a new species may offer an interesting
challenge.

2. There are many species with very similar morphologies; often, only microscopical examination of tissues and cellular structures can differentiate between two species,
one of which may be poisonous. Thus, there have been many reported poisonings due
to mistaken identity (Hesler 1960; Lough and Kinnear 1970; Myerson 1981; Pilát 1961;
Smith 1958).

3. An edible or poisonous species may change in morphological characteristics owing to environmental or nutritional growth conditions. For example, the poisonous
Amanita muscaria may exist in three shades of color: dark red, yellowish orange, and
white. These shades may also vary in intensity with age or exposure to the sun and
rain (Smith 1958). The orange-capped variety may be confused with the edible *A.
cesarea* (Orr and Orr 1968).

4. A characteristic identifying feature of a species may be modified by mechanical
damage. Any change in such characteristics may result in confusion and mistaken identity. For example, such essential identifying features of the amanitas as the remnants
of the universal and partial veils, the volva, and the annulus (Fig. 10.1) can be removed mechanically. This can happen to the partial veil and volva, for instance, by

---

*Henceforth, all macrofungi, for purposes of this chapter will simply be called mush-
rooms, a term which is commonly used by everyone.

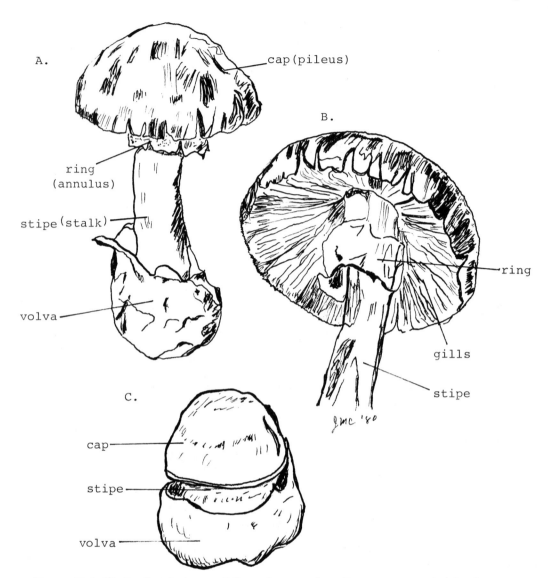

Figure 10.1 Distinctive features of the poisonous *Amanitas* as represented by *A. phalloides*. A, Mature *A. phalloides* shown with the annulus and the distinctive volva. B, The same species with the gills shown. C, Young specimen of the same with very prominent volva.

the force of heavy rain or the pressure exerted by the growing mushroom on the soil; the volva may also remain in the ground when the mushroom is pulled up during gathering (Smith 1958).

5. There is variability in the toxic response of individuals. This variability explains the conflicting reports in the literature regarding the edibility of certain species.

6. It is not known what quantity of mushroom may cause poisoning. This amount may vary with the individual, particularly his or her age and health status as well as the amount of toxin present. The amount of toxin could vary with the conditions of growth. For example, the toxic isoxazole content of *A. muscaria* harvested in Switzerland has been shown to vary markedly from 0.03% of the wet weight in specimens collected in 1962 to a very high concentration of 0.1% of wet weight in specimens collected in the summer of 1966 (Eugster 1968). Concentrations of the psychoactive ibotenic acid and muscimol from various psychoactive amanitas (pp. 476–478) vary markedly according to geographical locations, season, and year of growth (Good et al. 1965; and Takemoto et al. 1964a,b).

7. It is also possible that edibility or toxicity depends on how the mushroom is prepared or cooked. For example, insufficiently cooked *Paxillus involutus* killed three out of four persons so poisoned (Bschor and Mallach 1963). Yet this mushroom seems harmless after boiling (Pilát and Usák 1950). *Lactarius porninsis, L. plumbeus,* and *Pleurotus olearius (Clitocybe olearia)* (Pilát 1961) are also poisonous only when eaten raw or insufficiently cooked (Pilát 1961).

8. While many species belonging to specific genera are proven edible, one or more species in those genera may be toxic. Because members of a genus are very similar in morphological characteristics, the risk of mistaken identity is high. This possibility of intrageneric mistaken identity should even be greater when one considers the intergeneric mistaken identities that have occurred.

It is true that many toxic mushrooms have well-defined characteristics that may allow for easy identification. However, this is more easily said than done because there are variations from the norm and intergradations within the species. Thus, the task of determining what is toxic and what is not within a genus, and especially within a species, can be a dangerous one. Indeed, even accomplished mycologists have erred (Litten 1975; Smith 1958). Identification of species may require both chemical and microscopical histological examination, especially of the spores.

INCIDENCES OF MUSHROOM POISONINGS

It is evident that eating wild mushrooms can be quite risky. Incidences of mushroom poisoning continue to be reported in the medical literature (see for example Blayney et al. 1980; Faulstich 1980; Mitchel 1980; Short et al. 1980; Smith 1980; Weber 1980).

It may be argued that the hazard of mushroom poisoning is not serious in view of the relatively yearly occurrences of mushroom poisonings, and much less, the number of fatalities from this source compared to other forms of poisonings. However, the data may be misleading for the ratio of the number of mycophiles and mycophagists is not known. However, some indication of the seriousness of the hazard can be gleaned from rough statistics. In Europe where mycophagy is widely practiced, the rate of mycetism (mushroom poisoning) is relatively higher than in the United States where gathering wild mushrooms seems not to be as popular. In Switzerland in 1943 and 1944, 356 persons suffered from mycetism, with four deaths (Pilát and Usák 1950). There were 1980 recorded cases of mycetism in Switzerland between 1919 and 1958, of which 5% were fatal (Alder 1961). In the United States, 675 cases of mycetism were reported to the U.S. Poison Control Centers, with no fatalities (Verhulst 1969). In the period between 1931 and 1968, there were 64 deaths from mycetism reported in the United States (Benedict 1972; Buck 1961, 1964). Table 10.1 shows the incidence of mycetism in the United States from 1969 to 1975; all but six were recorded by the Center for Disease Control. Note that only 66 cases were reported for that 6-year period. This is only a

Table 10.1 Mycetism in the United States for the years 1969, 1970, 1973-1975

Year	State	Total cases / outbreaks	Mushroom species	Place of occurrence
1969	New York	4/1	*Clitocybe illudens*	Home
	Washington	1/1	Probably *Psilocybe* spp.	Home
1970[a]	New Jersey	6/1	*Amanita phalloides*	Home
1973	California	4/2	Unknown species	Home
	Pennsylvania	2/1	*Amanita muscaria*	Home
	Pennsylvania	17/1	*Clitocybe* spp.	Convent
	Washington	18/5	*Amanita pantherina*	Home, picnic
1974	California	3/1	Unknown species	Home
	Maryland	1/1	*Lepiota morganii*	Home
	New York City	2/1	*Galerina marginata*	Home
	Washington	2/2	*Amanita pantherina*	Home
	Washington	1/1	*Galerina autumnalis*	Home
1975	Minnesota	1/1	*Morchella augusticeps*	Home
	Washington	1/1	*Amanita muscaria*	Home
	Washington	1/1	*Panaeolus* spp.	Home
	New York City	1/1	*Amanita phalloides*	Home
	New York City	1/1	Unknown species	Home
	Total	66/23		

[a]Two deaths in this outbreak.

Source: Center for Disease Control (1969, 1973-1975a-c) and Litten (1975).

a very small percentage of the total food-related illnesses or poisonings. The risk can be assessed only by comparing the number of cases to the number of practicing myco-phagists. While the incidences may be small in relation to the total cases of food poisoning, the fact that consuming wild mushrooms is notoriously hazardous is borne out by these figures.

The state of Washington stands out rather strikingly as the locale where most outbreaks of mycetism occurred during this 6-year period. This may be due to the fact that the state has an abundance of mushrooms, especially A. *pantherina*, particularly in the Tacoma prairies, coastal rain forests, and Puget Sound area (Smith 1958).

In general, mushrooms raised and processed commercially may be considered safe. However, poisoning from commercial products can occur, such as the poisoning from canned mushrooms from Taiwan (Rose and Reiders 1966); that imported mushroom soup poisoned 55 of 86 women within 15 to 30 min after consumption. Symptoms of muscarine poisoning were elicited: malaise, muscular tingling, and bitemporal headache. It should be emphasized that toxic species, such as *Clitocybe dealbata* and toxic Panaeolus species, may also grow in the same bed as the cultivated mushrooms (Krieger 1967). These can be carelessly harvested together with the edible species. Thus, for safety, one must discard any piece of mushroom that is different from the majority in the group.

TYPES OF MUSHROOM POISONING

Toxic mushrooms from one or more genera may be grouped together according to the toxic syndrome or principal symptoms produced following consumption. As a rule, a specific group of symptoms predominate. In many cases, the clinical manifestations may not immediately indicate the tissue or cellular damage that has occurred. Frequently, this is seen only either during an autopsy or by closer biochemical and histological examinations. Many cases of mycetism cannot be definitely assigned to a specific type of poisoning in spite of the clinical manifestations.

Ford (1926) has listed five types of mushroom poisoning based on the predominant toxic symptoms. These are: (1) cytotoxic and choleriform; (2) hemolytic; (3) neuro-toxic; (4) hallucinogenic, psychedelic, or cerebral; and (5) gastrointestinal. To these may be added: (6) poisonings with manifestations indicating disulfiramlike action; (7) carcinogenic; and (8) miscellaneous effects. The latter classification obviously involves many types of toxic mushrooms which may show combined effects of the others.

Cytotoxic Mushrooms

Most fatalities due to mycetism are caused by cytotoxic mushrooms. Depending on the species or group, the mycetism may reveal different syndromes and durations of latency. Thus, there are four types of cytotoxic mycetism based on the nature of the toxins, as listed by Benedict (1972): cyclopeptide toxins; sulciceps toxin(s); orellanine; and gyromitrin. The latter is a special class of cytotoxic toxin, being also a hemolytic agent, as described by Krieger (1936).

Cyclopeptidic Toxins

Cyclopeptidic toxins consist of two major types, the phallotoxins and amatoxins. The phallotoxins consist principally of five distinct toxins — phalloidin, phallacidin, phallo-in, phallisin, and phallin B. The amatoxins consist also of five toxins — α,- β-, γ-, and ε-amanitin, and amanin. The structures of these compounds, as determined by Wieland and his group (Wieland and Wieland 1972), are shown in Figure 10.2. Note that these toxins consist of a ring of amino acids or amino acid derivatives.

The phallotoxins have seven residues: cysteine; threonine; hydroxypyroline; tryptophan; mono-, di-, or trihydroxyleucine, and two alanine residues. One of the

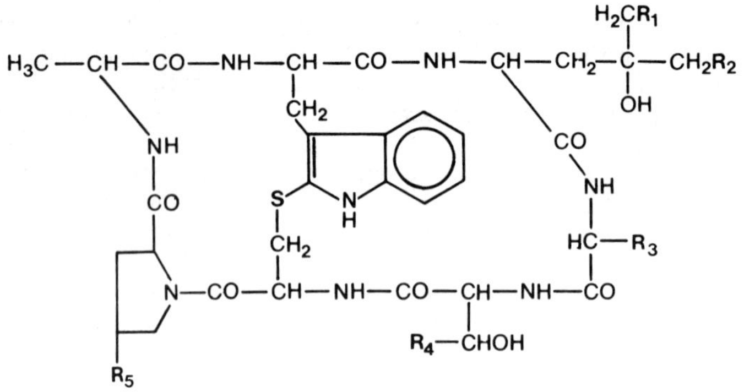

$$H_3C-CH-CO-NH-CH-CO-NH-CH-CH_2-C-CH_2R_2$$

Phallotoxins

	R_1	R_2	R_3	R_4	R_5
Phallacidin	OH	H	$CH(CH_3)_2$	COOH	OH
Phallin B	H	H	$CH_2C_6H_5$	CH_3	H
Phalloidin	OH	H	CH_3	CH_3	OH
Phalloin	H	H	CH_3	CH_3	OH
Phallisin	OH	OH	CH_3	CH_3	OH

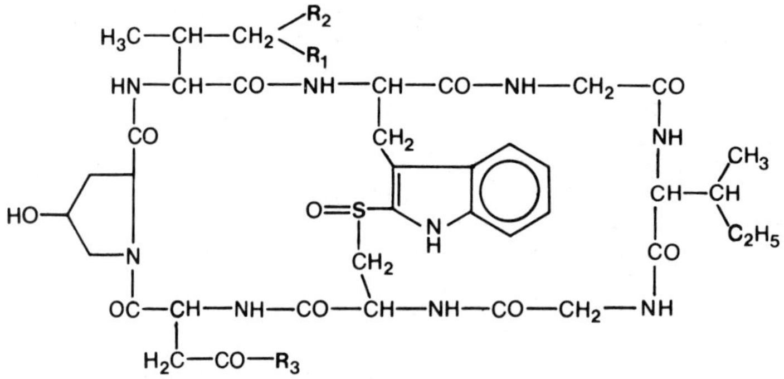

Amatoxins

	R_1	R_2	R_3	R_4
Amanin	OH	OH	OH	H
α-Amanitin	OH	OH	NH_2	OH
β-Amanitin	OH	OH	OH	OH
γ-Amanitin	OH	H	NH_2	OH
ε-Amanitin	OH	H	OH	OH
Amanullin	H	H	NH_2	OH

Fig. 10.2 Structures of cylopeptides in *A. phalloides* and related species. All are highly toxic.

alanine residues may be substituted with L-valine, and D-erythrohydroxyaspartic acid
is substituted for threonine in the case of phallacidine. Phallin B has been shown tentatively to have fewer hydroxylated amino acids, having threonine and γ-hydroxyleucine only, and phenylalanine is substituted for one of the alanines. Phallisin has γ,
δ, δ'-trihydroxyleucine instead of γ-hydroxyleucine. The tryptophan residue forms a
transannular, 2-thioether bridge with cysteine.

The bicyclic structure of phallotoxin gives the molecule relative stability. Chemical
changes on the side chains do not alter the geometry of the peptide ring nor diminish
the toxicity in most cases (Faulstich et al. 1968; Puchinger and Wieland 1969; Wieland
and Jeck 1968; Wieland and Rehbinder 1963; Wieland and Wieland 1972). However,
cleavage of the ring by acid hydrolysis or heating with Raney nickel produces nontoxic
products (Wieland and Wieland 1972).

The amatoxins consist of two residues of glycine and one each of L-isoleucine, L-
asparagine, L-hydroxyproline and L-γ-hydroxyisoleucine for γ- and ε-amanitin; or
γ,δ-dihydroxyisoleucine for α-, β-amanitin, and amanin. The transannular sulfoxide
bridge is formed between 6-hydroxytryptophan and cysteine sulfoxide. A sixth prod-
cut, amanullin, has no hydroxyl groups in the peripheral sidechains and is nontoxic.
Thus, in contrast to the phallotoxins, the hydroxyl groups in the peripheral side
chains are essential to toxicity (Wieland and Buku 1968).

The amatoxins are 10 to 20 times more toxic than the phallotoxins. This is evident
from the LD$_{50}$ values in mice shown in Table 10.2. The former acts more quickly; at
higher levels death may occur in rats or mice within 1 to 4 hr. The phallotoxins, on
the other hand, have longer latency; death at high doses occurs in mice or rats in 15
to 100 hr (Wieland and Wieland 1972).

It has been shown, however, by French workers (Courtillot and Staron 1975) that
the cyclopeptide toxins may actually be fragments of larger molecules. These high
molecular weight substances appear to consist of a polysaccharide core surrounded by
several cyclopeptide molecules attached to it by means of oxygen bridges. The high
molecular weight toxins have been designated as myriamanins. Those found in *A. phalloides* are called myriaphalloisins and those from *A. virosa*, myriavirosins. It appears
that the myriaphalloisins are less toxic than the myriavirosins. The significance of
these observations is that the presence of a polysaccharide may make it possible to develop a vaccine against these toxins.

Symptoms of Toxic Cyclopeptide Poisoning in Humans   Ingestion of mushrooms containing the cyclopeptide toxins produce violent symptoms in humans, usually after a
delay of 6 to 24 hr after ingestion. The symptoms include severe abdominal pain accompanied by violent bloody vomiting and diarrhea. If the victim survives this painful,
acute stage, a temporary remission occurs for 1 to 3 days. But this siutation is unfortunately misleading, since in the meantime, progressive liver and kidney injury continues to occur. Signs to this effect eventually appear: icterus, swelling and tender-
ness of the liver, and proteins, casts, and erythrocytes in the urine. There may be
skin hypothermia and cyanosis. Hallucinations, convulsions, and coma may precede
death, which may occur in 2 to 4 days or longer following the fatal meal, depending on
the amount ingested. Adult victims may remain ill for 6 to 8 days; in children, the illness may terminate fatally after shorter periods (Faulstich 1979; Fischer 1968; Litten
1975; Ramsbottom 1953; Pilát and Usák 1950; Wieland and Wieland 1972). The fatality
rate is high.

Portmortem findings reveal severe fatty degeneration and partial or complete necrosis of the liver cells. Hemorrhages with capilliary stasis and hematomalike extra-
vasates may also be observed. The lesions are similar to acute phosphorus poisoning.

The kidney is also damaged with all signs of nephrosis with necrosis and nuclear
atrophy, especially of the ascending limb of the loop of Henle and the convoluted tubules, fatty degeneration, and cloudy swelling (Flume et al. 1969; Ramsbottom 1953;
Wieland and Wieland 1972).

Other organs such as the heart and skeletal muscels and adrenals may also exhibit
hemorrhagic degenerative changes following poisoning (Wieland and Wieland 1972).

Table 10.2 LD$_{50}$ Values of Amatoxins and Phallotoxins in Mice

Toxin	LD$_{50}$, mg/kg[a]	Time of death (hr)
Amatoxins		
α-amanitin	0.30	1-4
β-amanitin	0.50	
γ-amanitin	0.15	
ε-amanitin	0.50	
amanin	0.50	
amanullin	nontoxic	
Phallotoxins		15-100
phallacidin	2.5	
phallisin	2.5	
phalloidin	2.0	
phalloin	1.8	
phallin	15	

[a]Intravenous or subcutaneous.
Source: Wieland and Wieland (1972)

The cyclopeptide toxins are among the most deadly poisons. However, it is now widely accepted that the amatoxins, and not the phallotoxins, are the principal cause of often fatal poisonings (Faulstich 1979). Mortality among victims of these types of toxins has been estimated to be between 34 to 63% (Alder 1961). So far, no definite antidote to these types of cyclopeptide poisoning has been found. However, thioctic acid, or lipoic acid, appears to be promising. Kubicka (1969) and Kubick and Alder (1968) have reported that massive doses of thioctic acid considerably reduce the number of fatalities from this kind of poisoning. Successful use of this compound also has been reported in German and Italy and other countries (Ciucci and Chiri 1974; Faulstich 1979, 1980; Zaffiri et al. 1970; Zulik et al. 1973). The apparent effectiveness of thioctic acid also has been demonstrated in the United States in 1970 following amanita poisonings in New Jersey and later in California (Litten 1975), and other places (Berkson 1979).

Faulstich (1979) suggest the following therapeutic procedures following diagnosis of amatoxin poisoning by analysis of urine and serum colorimetrically or by other procedures.

1. Obligatory washing of stomach and intestines during the first 36 hr following the toxic meal; use of activated charcoal to bind amatoxins in the gastrointestinal (GI) tract; restoration of water and electrolyte balance.
2. During the first 48 hr after the meal, obligatory removal of amatoxins from blood by any of several means; e.g., forced diruesis, hemofiltration, hemoperfusion using polymeric adsorbants, or plasmapheresis.
3. Where hypoglycemia is imminent, glucose infusion is recommended.
4. Chemotherapy with thioctic acid (100 to 300 mg/day) or high doses of silymarine or penicillin is also recommended. Berkson (1979) has reported success with six patients with thiotic acid therapy alone together with glucose infusion.

Thioctic acid appears ineffective against the myriavirosins, as tested in mice (Courtillot and Staron 1975).

<u>Mechanism of Action of Cyclopeptide Toxins</u> The phallotoxins and amatoxins differ in their mechanisms of action with regard to their cytopathogenic effects as well as their primary target tissues. The phallotoxins are primarily hepatotoxic, whereas the amatoxins are both strongly hepatotoxic and nephrotoxic. The rat, whose kidneys are resistant to the amatoxins, appears to be an exception. The high affinity of the phallotoxins for the liver cells has been demonstrated with radioactive tracer studies in the rat with mercaptophalloin-^{35}S — 57.2% of the toxin was concentrated in the liver in contrast to 2.7% in the kidneys, 9.4% in the skeletal muscles, 6.0% in the blood, and much lesser values in other tissues (Rehbinder et al. 1963). In addition, the electron microscope has shown that only the liver manifests gross morphological alteration following intoxication with phalloidin (Siess et al. 1970).

The action of the amatoxins on both the liver and kidneys has been demonstrated in experimentally induced poisonings (Cessi and Fiume 1969; Fiume et al. 1969).

The two groups of toxins also differ in their cellular targets. The evidence suggests that the phallotoxins seem to "dissolve" certain structures of the endoplasmic reticulum. Small vacuoles are then formed and confluence of these structures produces large cavities, or lacunae, in the cytoplasm (Wieland and Szabados 1968). The electron microscope does not reveal damage to other membrane systems in organelles, including the plasma membrane (Siess et al. 1970). Somehow, some effects on the cell membrane must occur, since liver perfusion experiments show massive movement of K^+ into the medium about 10 min after addition of phalloidin (Frimmer et al. 1967). Active transport in the cell membrane appears not to be interrupted by the toxin (Hegner et al. 1970). Some investigators (Miller and Wieland 1967; Siess et al. 1970) apparently have found no electronmicrographic evidence of the interaction between the phallotoxins and the cell membrane. However, there have been other reports which suggest that subtle membrane damage, probably unrecognizable with the electron microscope under certain conditions, may be occurring. For example, protrusions have been observed on the membranes of isolated liver cells 10 min after treatment with phalloidin (10 μg/ml of cell suspension) (Frimmer et al. 1977; Frimmer 1975). The protrusions are believed to be caused by pressure from inside the cells on the weakened parts of the cell membrane. In an intact liver, where pressure outside the cells is greater than inside, the weakened parts invaginate instead. Electron micrographs obtained by Frimmer (1977) on phalloidin-treated, isolated liver cells dramatically showed the extensive membrane damage occurring 20 minutes after treatment. In Figure 10.3 "B," note the extensive ballooning on the surface of the hepatocyte following treatment with phalloidin as compared to a normal cell shown in Figure 10.3A. Figure 10.3C shows a disintegrated liver cell following treatment with phallolysin.

Damage to the membrane also has been indicated by the ultrastructural changes on bile capillaries observed later in the course of phalloidin poisoning (Siess et al. 1970). This damage was correlated to the early stoppage of bile flow and Bromsulphalein (sulfobromophthalein sodium) excretion in the perfused rat liver following phalloidin treatment (Wieland 1965).

Phalloidin treatment has been shown to cause inhibition of glycogen synthesis (Meyer 1966; Wieland 1965), acceleration of autolytic reactions on liver nucleotides and proteins (Matschinsky and Wieland 1960), and release of lysosomal enzymes (Frimmer et al. 1967). The observed inhibition of glycogen synthesis did not arise from inhibition of glycogen synthetase (Wieland and Wieland 1972), but rather, it was an indirect result of the destruction of the endoplasmic reticulum. This inhibition is to be expected, since there is a necessary structural and spatial relationship between the smooth surface vesicles of the endoplasmic reticulum, glycogen synthetase, and glycogen (Hizukuri and Larner 1964; Leloir and Goldenberg 1960). The degradation of the endoplasmic reticulum by phalloidin also could explain the inhibition of protein synthesis with microsomes isolated from livers of animals poisoned with the toxin (Decken et al. 1960).

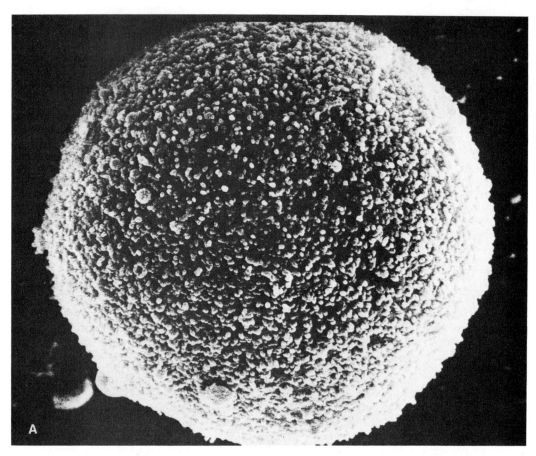

Fig. 10.3 A, scanning electron micrographs of normal hepatocyte (x 5000). B, the same hepatocyte 20 min after treatment with phalloidin (x 4000). Note the protrusion or ballooning at various points in the hepatocyte membrane. The toxin causes considerable weakening of the hepatocyte membrane. C, Scanning electron micrograph of isolated hepatocyte 10 min after treatment with 1 u phallolysin/10 ml cell suspension (x 3500). Note the extensive destruction of the cell membrane. Phyllolysin probably is not involved in mushroom poisoning because it is destroyed above 70°C. (Courtesy of Dr. M. Frimmer and Dr. E. Petzinger, Institute of Pharmacology and Toxicology, Justus Liebig-Universität, Giessen, West Germany.)

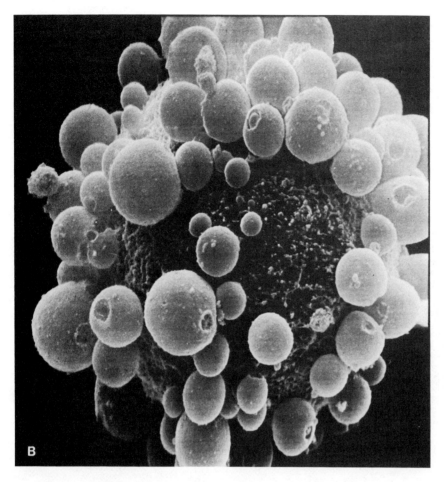

Fig. 10.3 (continued)

The release of lysosomal enzymes no doubt indicates an effect of phalloidin on the lysosomes. However, in vitro experiments with lysosomal preparations have failed to produce release of such enzymes (Frimmer et al. 1967; Wieland and Wieland 1972). Thus, the effects of phalloidin are probably indirect. In other words, damage to the lysosomes is a consequence of an earlier damage by phalloidin on specific cellular structures.

It appears, however, that the phallotoxins are poorly absorbed in the gastrointestinal tract. This fact together with the long latency which is consistent with amatoxin poisoning leaves in doubt as to whether the phallotoxins are involved at all in human poisoning (Litten 1975).

The primary action of the amatoxins has been shown to be directed to the cell nucleus (Fiume and Laschi 1965). Eventually, the cytoplasm is affected about 48 hr later. This is followed by cellular necrosis, and finally, death. The ultrastructural lesions characterized by nucleoli fragmentation are observed 15 min following treatment. The specific target of the toxin is actually ribonucleic acid (RNA) polymerase, especially polymerase II, from the nucleoplasm (Brodner and Wieland 1976; Cochet-Meilhac and Chambon 1974; Jacob et al. 1970; Lindell et al. 1970). Polymerase II requires Mn^{2+} as cofactor as opposed to polymerase I which requires Mg^{2+}. The former is involved in

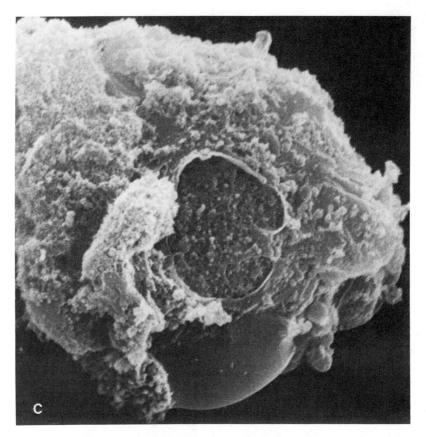

Fig. 10.3 (continued)

the synthesis of messenger RNA and possibly transfer RNA, both essential to the synthesis of proteins. This inhibition explains some of the biochemical defects that are noted following α-amanitin poisoning in animals; namely, a decrease in blood protein level (Wieland and Dose 1954), a decrease in glycogen synthetase in the liver and to a lesser extent in muscles (mice) (Brunelli et al. 1967), and consequently the glycogen content of these tissues. The decrease in liver adenosine triphosphate (ATP) and nicotinamide adenine denucleotide (NAD) and the leakage of potassium from liver cells also follow from the inhibition of protein synthesis (Wieland and Wieland 1959).

Susceptibility to Cyclopeptide Toxins   Newborn rats (2 weeks old) have been found to be highly resistant to phalloidin. It has been shown that they can tolerate up to 10 mg/kg. In contrast, 5-week-old animals succumb to 5 mg/kg (Wieland and Szabados 1968). Wieland and Wieland (1972) have shown that up to 360 mg phalloidin can be tolerated by 2-week-old rats that survived a 20 to 80 mg/kg dose during their first week of life. Tolerance lasted until the eighteenth day of life, and by 35 to 38 days, the rats lost such resistance. It is not clear why a newborn animal is tolerant to phalloidin, for apparently, the usual detoxification enzyme induction on repeated challenge with the toxin, or other microsomal enzyme inducers, do not operate in this case (Wieland and Wieland 1972). Additionally, the toxin appears not to be metabolized in the liver (Puchinger and Wieland 1969). It may be that the newborn liver has not yet developed specific binding sites for the toxin, as indicated by the appearance of liver-specific antigens that closely follow the time course of phalloidin sensitivity of newborn rats (Frank 1968). Similar patterns of sensitivity to phalloidin have not been demonstrated in humans.

Mushrooms Containing Cyclopeptide Toxins   The mushroom species containing these powerful toxins belongs to the genera Amanita, Galerina (Pholiota), and Lepiota. These species are discussed later in this chapter.

Sulciceps Toxin

It might seem that the cyclopeptide toxins are the most lethal. However, an even more poisonous mushroom of the genus Galerina (previously Phaeomarasmius) has been reported in Indonesia on the island of Java. The mushroom was originally identified as *Phaeomarasmius sulciceps* (Boedijn 1938–1940). This mushroom is also known as *Galerina sulciceps* (Singer 1962). The poisonings reported in 1934 and 1937 resulted in the death of 13 of 18 victims. Death occurred quickly to some victims, in as early as 7 hr; most deaths occurred between 24 and 30 hr. The symptoms included abdominal spasms, nausea without emesis, dizziness, palpitation, dyspnea, local anesthesia, prickling sensation on the skin, coma, and death. There was no diarrhea. Note that these symptoms and the suddenness of their appearance very likely preclude the involvement of the toxic cyclopeptides. The lethal factor has yet to be identified chemically.

Orellanine

Orellanine is a dangerous, slow-acting, and sometimes lethal toxin isolated from *Cortinarius orellanus,* which is noted for its bright yellow and orange pigmentations (Desvignes 1965; Grzymala 1961). The toxic symptoms following orellanine ingestion do not appear until 3 to 14 days later. The clinical signs indicate gastrointestinal, hepatic, renal, and neurological involvement. In several Polish cases, the victims experienced dryness of the mouth, burning sensation on the lips, and extreme thirst, so that the patients drank several liters of water a day. Vomiting, abdominal pains, constipation or diarrhea followed; there was shivering, constant cold sensation, and violent and persistent headache. Signs of renal failure have been observed in severe cases; i.e., oliguria and sometimes anuria, albuminuria, uremia, and electrolyte imbalance. Hepatic damage was indicated by pain in the abdomen, vomiting of bile, and subicteric state. Death may be preceded by drowsiness, coma, and convulsions. Fatalities have been shown to vary between 10 to 20%.

The LD_{50} values of orellanine are 4.9, 8.3, 8.0 mg/kg in the cat (per os), mouse, and guinea pig (parenteral), respectively. These values and the symptoms observed in victims indicate the extreme toxicity of this compound (Desvignes 1965). The mushroom may contain 1% orellanine on a dry weight basis (Grzymala 1961). Orellanine has been crystallized and is quite heat stable. Its structure has not been determined.

Gyromitrin

Gyromitrin is a volatile toxin (List and Luft 1968, 1969) found among species of the

$$CH_3CH=N-\underset{\underset{CH_3}{|}}{N}-CHO$$

Gyromitrin

genus Helvella, or the false morels. It can produce severe and sometimes fatal poisoning. Fatalities of up to 2 to 4% have been reported in Europe (Alder 1961), where large quantities of false morels are consumed. No doubt many toxic species are mistaken for the closely related edible ones.

The symptoms of gyromitrin poisoning are similar to those caused by cyclopeptide poisoning. The latent period is 6 to 10 hr. Symptoms begin with a feeling of fullness in the stomach followed by violent vomiting and watery diarrhea (McKenny 1962). These symptoms may last for 24 to 48 hr. Headache, lassitude, severe upper abdominal pain, cramps, and jaundice may also be observed. In severe poisoning, there may be respiratory difficulty, irregular pulse, general collapse, delirium, and convulsions. Hepatic and cardiac failure within 5 to 10 days generally result in death.

Some individuals may not be affected by the toxin at all (Hendricks 1940). A few fatalities from eating Helvella have been reported in the United States; gyromitrin may have been the causative agent.

Hemotoxic Mushrooms

Helvella esculenta (Gyromitra esculenta) also has been reported to cause hemolysis and anemia (Krieger 1936). There is a latent period of 4 to 5 days, and symptoms include abdominal distress and jaundice, in addition to the effect on the blood. The hemolytic factor has not been identified.

A hemolytic factor also has been isolated from *Amanita phalloides*. This heat-labile substance has been similarly found to have cytotoxic activity on cultures of KB line and human amnion cells (Fiume 1967). Presumably, it is destroyed by enzymes in the gastrointestinal tract. Its structure has not been determined. *Paxillus involutus* poisoning similarly causes hemolytic anemia which results in acute kidney failure (Schmidt et al. 1971).

Another hemotoxic effect is that produced by the ear mushroom, or mo-er *(Auricularia polytrichia)*, also known as "mok-yhee" (Cantonese). When eaten in sufficient quantities, the mushroom causes inhibition of platelet aggregation. Because platelet aggregation is essential for the blood clotting process, mo-er may cause transient bleeding problems, most probably in those already with platelet or clotting disorders (Hammerschmidt 1980). A mild condition of hemorrhagic diathesis was observed in patient who consumed a large amount of mo-er containing Szechwanese hot bean curd ("ma-po dou-fu") dish the evening before the abnormality was observed (Hammerschmidt 1980). The inhibition of platelet aggregation was confirmed experimentally in vitro, and by feeding 70 g of the mushroom to volunteers. The antiplatelet factor appears to be a nonprotein which is obviously heat stable and apparently varied in concentration in different lots of mo-er. The chemical identity has not been determined.

It is possible that other Auricularia species, e.g., *A. auricula-judae* (Jew's ear), also contain the antiplatelet factor.

Neurotoxic Mushrooms

The symptoms caused by neurotoxic mushrooms may occur almost immediately from 15 to 180 min after ingestion. The composite symptoms as observed in various cases of poisoning of this type include increased salivation, lacrimation, perspiration, and severe gastrointestinal disturbance with vomiting and copious watery diarrhea; the pulse is slow and irregular. There may be labored or asthmatic breathing, vomiting, hallucinations, and confusion (Ford 1926; Pilát and Usák 1950; Silberbauer and Mirvish 1927; Tyler 1963). Additionally, immediate muscular tingling, malaise, and bitemporal headache may occur (Rose and Rieders 1966). An appearance of narcotic effects or advanced state of alcohollike intoxication without vomiting may be observed, with visual disturbances, muscular spasms, restlessness, confusion, and delirium. Respiratory difficulties, when they occur, may be severe, requiring tracheostomy (Waser 1967). Victims may be induced to a deep sleep with little or no recollection of the ordeal upon awakening. In rare cases, death due to respiratory paralysis or heart failure may be preceded by delirium, convulsion, and coma (Ford 1926; Silberbauer and Mirvish 1927; Tyler 1963).

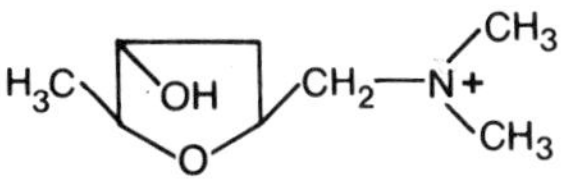

L(+)-Muscarine

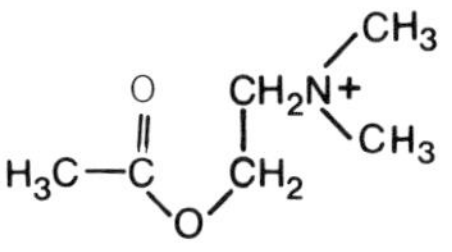

Acetylcholine

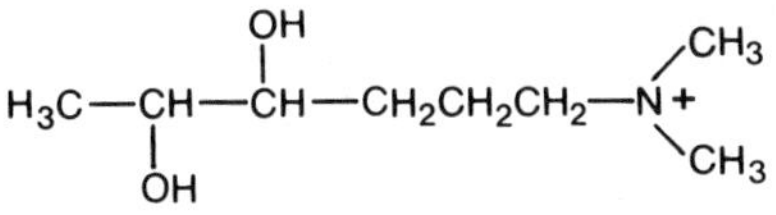

Muscaridine

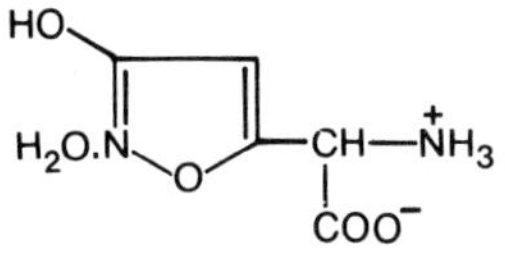

Ibotenic acid

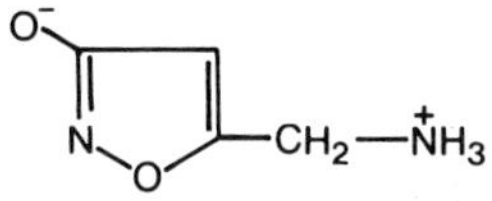

Muscimol

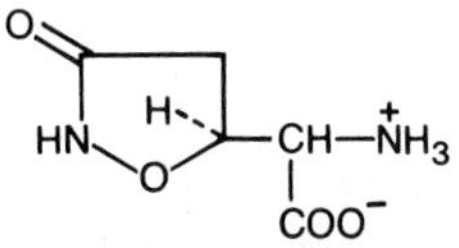

Tricholomic acid

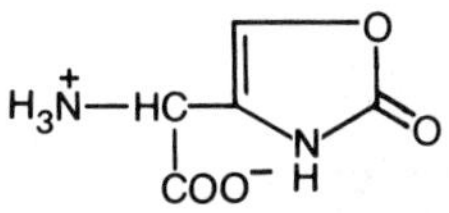

Muscazone

Fig. 10.4 Structures of the intoxicating and narcotic compounds from *A. muscaria* and related species.

Examples of mushrooms responsible for this type of poisoning include *Amanita muscaria, A. pantherina,* and a number of Inocybe and Clitocybe species (Ainsworth 1952; Eugster 1957; Malone et al. 1962; Tyler 1963; Wieland 1968a,b, 1967) as well as other species, which will be discussed later in this chapter.

The neurotoxic mushrooms may contain more than one neurotoxic compound. The neurotoxicants isolated from these mushrooms include muscarine, muscaridine, and acetylcholine (Eugster and Waser 1954; Kögl et al. 1931; Wilkinson 1961). The structures of these compounds are shown in Figure 10.4. Note the three asymmetrical carbon atoms in muscarine. These substances, however, do not explain the severe effects on the central nervous system which can be produced by mushrooms like *A. muscaria* and *A. pantherina* (Brady and Tyler 1959; Tabor and Vining 1963).

Accordingly, attention has been directed to the isolation and discovery of other neurotoxic principles in these species. Several oxazole derivatives have been isolated which have "flyicidal" effects and narcotic effects. These are ibotenic acid, muscimol, muscatone (Benedict et al. 1966; Good et al. 1965; Takemoto et al. 1964b; Waser 1967) and tricholomic acid (Kawamura 1954). The structures of these compounds are shown in Fig. 10.4. Note that the latter four alkaloids, except muscimol, are amino acids. Ibotenic acid is easily decarboxylated to muscimol during the preparative procedures or possibly in vivo. Thus, the combined values of these two compounds are generally determined (Benedict et al. 1966).

Tests with pure compounds show that these alkaloids are responsible for the narcotic or psychotic manifestations described previously; e.g., visual disturbances, confusion, disorientation, convulsions, and weariness (Waser 1967). The most active are ibotenic acid and muscimol. Sedation may be produced in mice by 4 to 8 mg/kg and 1 to 2 mg/kg of ibotenic acid and muscimol, respecively (Waser 1967). Muscazone, and especially tricholomic acid, are far less active than the first two compounds. Tricholomic acid is a potent fly killer, however (Bowden and Drysdale 1965; Bowden et al. 1965).

Hallucinogenic Mushrooms

A striking feature of the symptoms produced by hallucinogenic mushrooms are the hallucinatory or psychedelic effects (Krieger 1936; Sapieka 1969), and depending on the species, prolonged euphoria, and excitation (Stein 1958). The effects may be accompanied by other serious symptoms such as muscular incoordination and weakness of the arms and legs, sometimes with complete but temporary paralysis. The unpleasant effects may last for several hours (Stein 1958).

The poisoning in children may be more severe with high fever and frequently with intermittent clonic convulsions. It may terminate fatally (McCawley et al. 1962).

Mushrooms causing these effects include species of Psilocybe, Panaeolus, or Stropharia (Krieger 1936; Sapieka 1969). Certain species of Amanita also have been reported to be hallucinogenic (Wieland and Motzel 1953). Gymnopilus spectabilis also contains a hallucinogen. The hallucinogenic species are discussed later in this chapter under specific genera.

Species of Psilocybe contain psilocybin and psilocin (Hofmann and Troxler 1963; Hofmann et al. 1959) and the psilocybin analogs, baeocystin (Leung and Paul 1967; Leung et al. 1965) and norbaeocystin (Leung and Paul 1968). A similar compound has been reported to be present in species of Paneolus (Stein et al. 1959). Bufotenine, serotonin, and other tryptamine derivatives have been isolated from species of hallucinogenic amanitas (Catalfomo and Tyler 1961; Tyler 1961; Tyler and Groger 1964). Yangonin and bis-noryangonin have been isolated from species of Gymnopilus (Hatfield and Brady 1968, 1969). The structures of these compounds are shown in Fig. 10.5. Note that these compounds, except the yangonins, are tryptamine derivatives. The yangonines are styrylpyrones, which are also found in intoxicating extracts of the kava root (Piper sp.) (Meyer 1967).

The pharmacological properties of psilocybin indicate that this compound could account for most of the central nervous system (CNS) and other effects of Psilocybe intoxications. An altered mental state lasting for several hours is produced by ingestion of 5 to 15 mg of psilocybin or an amount of mushroom containing an equivalent amount of the drug (McCawley et al. 1962). The hallucinatory episodes not only involve visual effects, but also sound and gustatory effects. These effects may be pleasant or anxiety laden depending on the sensory expression elicited. The subject may be detached from reality, depersonalized, given unconsciously to compulsive movements and laughter, at times alternated with apathy and catatonia. Systemic effects are also observed as a result of stimulation of the sympathetic nervous system. In humans, 10 mg psilocybin produces fever, hypertension, mydriasis, hyperglycemia, tachycardia, and tachypnea (Delay et al. 1959; Weidmann et al. 1958).

It is uncertain whether bufotenine is a hallucinogenic agent, but it has powerful cardiovascular effects which are difficult to delineate from the CNS effects (Fischer 1968).

Gastrointestinal Toxic Mushrooms

Mushrooms producing gastrointestinal upset in humans can produce from mild to severe symptoms. In children, these mushrooms are capable of causing death (Charles 1942; Pilát and Usák 1954; Tyler 1963). Symptoms include abdominal cramps, intense

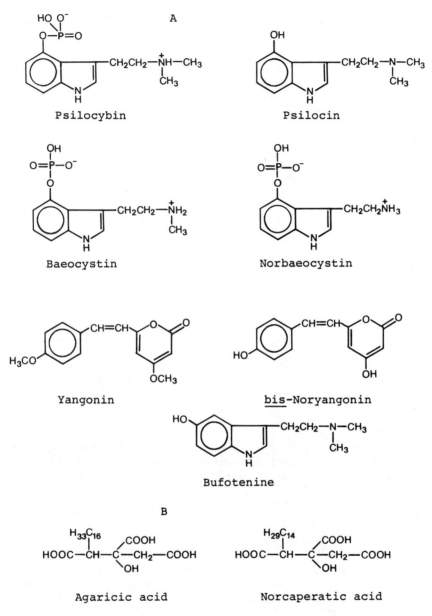

Fig. 10.5 Structures of hallucinogenic toxicants and gastrointestinal irritants from various species of mushrooms.

abdominal pain, nausea, vomiting, and diarrhea. The symptoms in adults may be severe enough to cause incapacitation for several days. Not all symptoms are present in every case; the clinical signs may vary with the species of mushroom and the victim.

The toxic substances responsible in these poisonings, as far as this writer is aware, have not been identified. However, some mushrooms may contain phenolic compounds which are gastrointestinal irritants (Tyler 1963). Certain acids related to agaricic, caperatic, and norcaperatic acids may be found in mushrooms. These are also gastrointestinal irritants (Henry and Sullivan 1969; Miyata et al. 1966). The structures of these compounds are also shown in Fig. 10.4.

The species of gastrointestinal mushrooms are scattered through several genera including Agaricus, Boletus, Lactarius, Lepiota, Rhodophyllus, Tricholoma, and Gomphus. (The Rhodophyllus group may consist of several subgenera; i.e., Entoloma, Leptonia, Nolanea, and others.) Sometimes the mushrooms may be toxic only when eaten raw or insufficiently cooked (Tyler 1963).

While the mushroom may produce gastrointestinal upset, damage to the other tissues can also occur. Thus, certain species of Rhodophyllus have been shown to cause liver damage (Tyler 1963).

Mushrooms with Disulfiramlike Activity

Disulfiram is a drug which induces hypersensitivity to ethanol. As such, it has been used as an adjunct in the treatment of chronic alcoholism. Certain mushrooms of the genera Coprinus, Clitocybe, and possibly Verpa possess this type of pharmacological activity (Groves 1964; Reynolds and Lowe 1965; Romagnesi 1964).

The unsuspecting victim may be in for a shocking experience after consuming an alcoholic beverage within 15 to 20 min or even as late as 48 hr after the mushroom meal. He or she may experience severe flushing of the face, parasthesia of the extremities, palpitation, tachycardia, a swelling sensation of the hands, and metallic taste in the mouth, and finally, nausea and vomiting (Reynolds and Lowe 1965).

Carcinogenic Mushrooms

In addition to gyromitrin, the false morel *(Gyromitra/Helvella esculenta)* (Fig. 10.6) also contains up to 0.05% (dry weight) of N-methyl-N-formylhydrazine (MFH) (Schmidlin-Meszaros 1974).

$$H_2N—N—CHO$$
$$|$$
$$CH_3$$

N-Methyl-N-formylhydrazine

This compound, as with gyromitrin, may be converted in vivo to methyl hydrazine (Nagel et al. 1977). The latter has been shown to be tumorigenic in mice (Toth 1972, 1979a) and in the golden Syrian hamster (Toth and Patil 1979; Toth and Shimizu 1973). Therefore, when MFH was added to the drinking water of Swiss mice at a level of 0.0078%, a significant incidence of tumors, particularly in the liver (33%), lungs (50%), and to a lesser extent, in the gallbladder (9%) and bile duct (7%) was obtained. (Corresponding incidences in the control group were 1, 18, 0, and 0%, respectively.) Higher doses proved to be quite toxic to the mouse, and thus, no significant tumor incidence could be obtained (Toth and Nagel 1978).

The high carcinogenic potency of MFH has been further demonstrated by induction of diverse tumors in albino Swiss mice treated with very low concentration; i.e., 0.0039% solution, in the drinking water. Even at this very low level, high incidences of tumor in the lung (77.7%) and liver (46%) were obtained; tumors of the blood vessels, gallbladder, and bile ducts also were found in 21, 10, and 7% of the test animals (Toth and Patil 1980; Toth et al. 1979). All incidences were statistically significant.

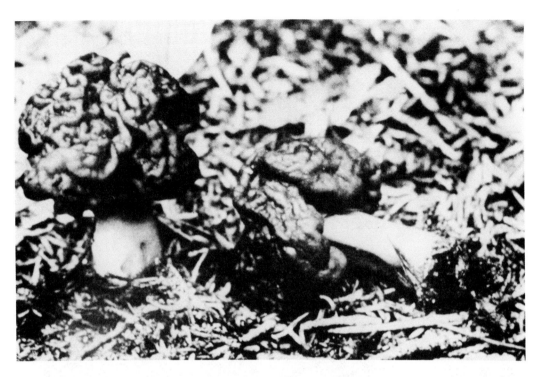

Fig. 10.6 *Gyromitra/Helvella esculenta* (false morel). (Reprinted with permission of Japan Scientific Societies Press, Tokyo, and Dr. Bela Toth, Eppley Institute for Research on Cancer, Omaha, Nebraska.)

Gyromitra (Helvella) esculenta also has been found to contain eight other hydrazones of MFS with higher aldehydes; namely (1) propanal; (2) butanal; (3) 3-methylbutanal; (4) pentanal; (5) hexanal; (6) octanal; (7) *trans*-2-octenal; and (8) *cis*-2-octenal. The structures of these compounds with their corresponding concentrations are shown below (Toth 1979b).

R = $-N-N-CHO$
$\quad\quad\; | $
$\quad\quad CH_3$

(1) CH_3CH_2CHR (1 mg/kg)   (5) $CH_3(CH_2)_4CHR$ (1.4 mg/kg)

(2) $CH_3CH_2CH_2CHR$ (0.6 mg/kg)   (6) $CH_3(CH_2)_6CHR$ (0.2 mg/kg)

(3) $CH_3CH(CH_3)CH_2CHR$ (2.2 mg/kg) (7) $CH_3(CH_2)_4\overset{H}{\underset{H}{C}}=C-CHR$ (0.6 mg/kg)

(4) $CH_3(CH_2)_3CHR$ (0.8 mg/kg)   (8) $CH_3(CH_2)_4\underset{H\;\;H}{C}=C-CHR$ (0.3 mg/kg)

Since these hydrazones also may be hydrolyzed to MFH under acid conditions, such as in the stomach, the carcinogenic potential of this mushroom is increased considerably.

Another hydrazine, agaritine, is found in the common commercial mushroom *Agaricus bisporus* (Fig. 10.7a) and the Japanese forest mushroom *Cortinellus shiitake*.

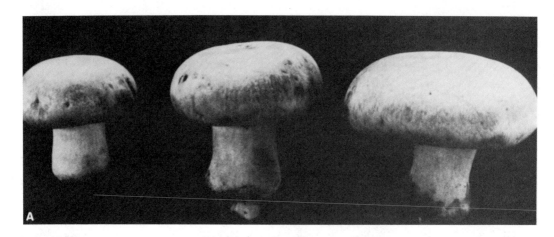

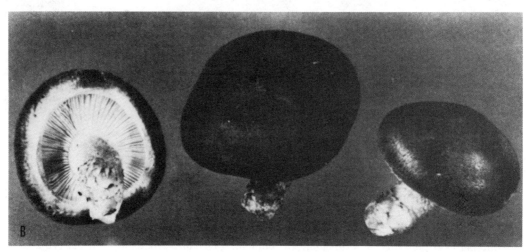

Fig. 10.7 A, *Agaricus bisporus*, a commercial mushroom commonly eaten in North America and Europe. B, *Cortinellus shiitake*, Japanese forest mushroom widely consumed in Japan. (Reprinted with permission of Japan Scientific Societies Press, Tokyo, and Dr. Bela Toth, Eppley Institute for Research on Cancer, Omaha, Nebraska.)

(Fig. 10.7B). The structure of this compound is given in Chapter 9. As stated in Chapter 9, γ-glutamyltransferase, which is present in the mushroom, hydrolyzes agaritine to 4-hydroxymethylphenylhydrazine. The carcinogenicity of the latter has, as yet, not been shown, but 4-methylphenylhydrazine (Toth et al. 1977), N-acetyl-4-(hydroxymethyl)phenylhydrazine (Toth et al. 1978), and 1-acetyl-2-phenylhydrazine (Toth 1979c) have already been shown to be carcinogenic. Thus, the safety of these commercial mushrooms needs to be assessed immediately because of the enormous consumption of these mushrooms by the world's population (Toth 1979b). For example, 160 million kilograms of *A. bisporus* were consumed in the United States in 1975 (United States Department of Agriculture 1976).

Other types of mushrooms which may be included in the list of carcinogens are those in which carcinogenic nitrosamines have been detected. Ender and Ceh (1968) have reported the presence of a nitrosamine in several species of edible mushrooms. It appears to be identical to dimethylnitrosamine. Levels of 0.4 to 5.0 to 11.6 μg/kg have been found for the popular champignon Agaricus spp. and *Polyporus ovinus*, respectively. A mixture of edible species was shown to contain 14 µg nitrosamine/kg. A few toxic species such as *A. muscaria* and *Russula emetica* contain 30.0 and 10.2 µg/kg, respectively.

4-Methylnitrosaminobenzaldehyde has been detected (Herman 1961) as a metabolite of *Clitocybe suaveolens*. Some consider it edible, but poisonings have been reported (Table 10.3). However, tests have shown it to be noncarcinogenic in BD rats (Druckrey et al. 1967), and apparently relatively nontoxic (LD_{50} = 2 g/kg body weight).

Whether or not the nitrosamines found by Ender and Ceh (1968) are also metabolits of those mushroom species has not been ascertained. However, the fact that the compound found by Herman (1961) is a metabolite, suggests that the other species may also be capable of producing such compounds. Note that MFH in *G. esculenta* (Schmidlin-Meszaros 1974) is chemically related to the nitrosamines.

Miscellaneous Mushrooms

Various mushrooms produce general symptoms indicating the involvement of several tissues. Examples of these types of mushrooms will be evident in the following section.

TOXIC MUSHROOMS CLASSIFIED ACCORDING TO GENUS

Table 10.3 is a list of toxic mushrooms compiled from various sources. This is by no means a complete list. It is comprehensive enough to underscore the great hazard associated with the practice of gathering wild mushrooms.

The more important toxic species are discussed in the following sections under specific genera. Only a minimal description of the characteristics of the toxic mushrooms can be given in this chapter. Pictures of many species may be seen in numerous handbooks and other publications, particularly those of Hesler (1960), Krieger (1967), Pilát (1961), Singer (1961), and Smith (1950, 1958), and many others.

Agaricus

Many well-known edible species belong to the genus Agaricus. These gill mushrooms generally have white caps (fruiting body) which may range from 2 to 45 cm in diameter depending on the species. The gills and spores may be pinkish when young and become purplish dark-brown to black with age. The bruised or broken sections of the caps of certain species may turn yellow or red. On the stipe (stalk) there is generally a ring, which is the remnant of the partial veil (some of which may also remain hanging on the margin of the cap) which once covered the gills. There is no volva (cup) at the base of the stipe. The distinction between many species of Agaricus is difficult even for the trained mycologist and may require microscopical examination of the spores (Hesler 1960; Orr and Orr 1968; Smith 1958).

This group was once regarded as the safest to gather and eat among wild mushrooms. In fact, two species which are related to *A. campestris* are grown commercially on a large scale in Europe and North America; these are *A. bisporus* var. *albidus* and *A. bisporus* var. *avellaneus*, the white and brown varieties, respectively (Fig. 10.7A). Two others, *A. bitorquis* and *A. subperonatus* are occasionally grown commercially (Singer 1961). As shown in Table 10.3, the agarics are by no means entirely safe. Several poisonous species are listed. In addition, some of the poisonous agarics can be mistaken for the edible ones. For example, Smith (1958) does not recommend the eating of *A. silvaticus* in spite of its excellent qualities because it can easily be mistaken for *A. placomyces* and *A. hordensis*. The latter two mushrooms may cause gastrointestinal poisoning (Tyler 1963), as do the other agarics listed in Table 10.3. The symptoms of this type of poisoning have been described (pp. 478–480).

Table 10.3 Poisonous Mushrooms and Related Species

Species (common name)	Type of poisoning
Agaricus albolutescence (Tyler 1963)	Gastrointestinal
A. arvensis var. *palustris* (Roland et al. 1960) (meadow mushroom)	Gastrointestinal
A. hordensis (Smith 1958; Tyler 1963)	Gastrointestinal
A. placomyces (Hesler 1960; Smith 1958) (flat-capped mushroom)	Gastrointestinal
A. sylvicola (Smith 1958)	Gastrointestinal
A. xanthodermus (Pilat 1961; Smith 1958)	Gastrointestinal
Amanita bisporigera (Tyler et al. 1966)	Cytotoxic (lethal)
A. brunnescens (Hesler 1960; Smith 1958)	Cytotoxic (lethal)
A. capensis (Watt and Breyer-Brandwijk 1962) (cape death cap)	Cytotoxic (lethal)
A. chlorinosma (Hesler 1960)	Gastrointestinal
A. citrina (Catalfomo and Tyler 1961; Tyler 1961; Wieland and Motzel 1953)	Neurological-hallucinogenic
A. cothurnata (Smith 1958)	Neurological-muscarinic
A. flavoconia[e] (Hesler 1960)	
A. flavivolva (Tyler 1963)	Neurological-muscarinic
A. gemmata (Tyler 1963)	Neurological-muscarinic
A. mappa (the same as *citrina*) (Catalfomo and Tyler 1961; Tyler 1961; Wieland and Motzel 1953) (false death cap)	Neurological-muscarinic
A. muscaria (Smith 1958) (fly agaric)	Neurological-muscarinic
A. pantherina (Smith 1958) (panther mushroom, panthercup)	Neurological-muscarinic (very toxic)
A. parcivolvata (Tyler et al. 1963)	Neurological-muscarinic
A. phalloides (Pilát 1961; Wieland and Wieland 1972) (death cup)	Cytotoxic (very lethal)
A. porphyria (Catalfomo and Tyler 1961; Tyler 1961; Tyler and Smith 1963)	Hallucinogenic
A. regalis (Pilát 1961)	Neurological-muscarinic
A. rubescence (Hesler 1960)	
A. solitaria (Hesler 1960)	Neurological-muscarinic
A. spreta (Takemoto et al. 1964a,b)	Neurological-muscarinic
A. strobiliformis (Takemoto et al. 1964a,b)	Neurological-muscarinic
A. tenuifolia (Block et al. 1955)	Cytotoxic (lethal)
A. verna[b] (Romagnesi 1964; Smith 1958; Wieland and Wieland 1972) (spring Amanita)	Cytotoxic (lethal)
A. virosa[b] (Romagnesi 1964; Wieland and Wieland 1972) (destroying angel)	Cytotoxic (lethal)

Table 10.3   (continued)

Species (common name)	Type of poisoning
Amanitopsis volvata (Krieger 1967)	
Boletus eastwoodiae (Keinholz 1934; Orr and Orr 1968)	Gastrointestinal
B. *erythropus* (Orr and Orr 1968)	
B. *luridus* (Hesler 1960) (lurid boletus)	
B. *purpureus* (Pilát and Usák 1950)	Probably gastro-intestinal
B. *satanas* (Orr and Orr 1968; Pilát and Usák 1950; Rautavaara 1950) (satan's boletus)	Gastrointestinal
Calvatia gigantea (Roland et al. 1960)	Gastrointestinal
Cantharellus floccosus (Carrano and Malone 1967; Miyata et al. 1962; Smith 1958) *(Gomphus floccosus)* (shaggy cantharelle)	Gastrointestinal
Chlorophyllum molybditis (Desvignes 1965; Orr and Orr 1968; Smith 1958) *(Lepiota morgani, Lepiota molybditis)*	
Clavaria formosa (Smith 1958) (coral fungi)	Gastrointestinal
C. *gelatinosa* (Tyler 1963)	Gastrointestinal
Clitocybe cerussata (Pilát 1961; Tyler 1963)	Neurological-muscarinic
C. *claviceps* (Romagnesi 1964)	
C. *dealbata* (Hughes et al. 1966)	Neurological-muscarinic
C. *illudens* (Tyler 1963) (jack-o-lantern, copper trumpet)	Neurological-muscarinic
C. *olearia* (Smith 1958; Tyler 1963)	
C. *rivulosa* (Tyler 1963)	Neurological-muscarinic
C. *subilludens* (Smith 1958; Tyler 1963)	Neurological-muscarinic
C. *sudorifica* (Krieger 1967)	Neurological-muscarinic
C. *toxica* (Sapeika and Stephens 1965)	Cytotoxic
C. *truncicola* (Tyler 1963)	Neurological-muscarinic
Coprinus atramentarius (Reynolds and Lowe 1965; Smith 1958)	Disulfiramlike effect
Cortinarius orellanus (Desvignes 1965; Grzymala 1961)	Cytotoxic
C. *traganus*[c] (Pilát 1961) *(Inoloma traganus)*	Gastrointestinal
Entoloma lividum[b] (Pilát and Usák 1950) (leaden entoloma, livid entoloma)	Gastrointestinal
E. *salmoneum* (Hesler 1960) (salmon-colored entoloma)	
E. *sinuatum*[e] (Hesler 1960)	
E. *strictus*[e] (Hesler 1960)	
E. *vernum* (Pilát 1961)	

Table 10.3   (continued)

Species (common name)	Type of poisoning
Galerina autumnalis (Singer 1962; Smith 1958) (Gill mushroom)	Cytotoxic
G. marginata (Tyler et al. 1963)	Cytotoxic
G. sulciceps[a] (Boedijn 1938-1940)	Cytotoxic (very lethal)
G. venenata (Tyler and Smith 1963)	Cytotoxic
Gomphus kauffmanii (Henry and Sullivan 1969)	Neurological-cytotoxic
Gymnopilus decurrens (Hatfield and Brady 1968)	Hallucinogenic
G. spectabilis (Romagnesi 1964)	Hallucinogenic
Helvella esculenta (Adler 1961; Krieger 1936, 1967; Rautavaara 1950; Smith 1958) *(Gyromitra esculenta)* (false morel)	Cytotoxic-hemolytic
H. gigas (Adler 1961; Pilát 1961) *(Gyromitra gigas)*	Cytotoxic
H. infula (Adler 1961; Smith 1958) (hooded helvella)	Cytotoxic
H. underwoodii (Adler 1961; Smith 1958)	Cytotoxic
Hygrophorus conicus (Hesler 1960; Orr and Orr 1968) (conic hygrophorus)	
Inocybe godego (Pilát and Usák 1950)	Neurological-muscarinic
I. infelix (Krieger 1967) (unfortunate inocybe)	Neurological-muscarinic
I. infida (Krieger 1967) (untrustworthy inocybe)	Neurological-muscarinic
I. lacera (Malone et al. 1962)	Neurological-muscarinic
I. napipes (Malone et al. 1962)	Neurological-muscarinic
I. nigrescence (Malone et al. 1962)	Neurological-muscarinic
I. patouillardi[b] (Malone et al. 1962; Pilát and Usák 1950) (red-staining inocybe)	Neurological-muscarinic (lethal)
I. picrosma (Malone et al. 1962)	Neurological-muscarinic
Lactarius chrysorheus (Orr and Orr 1968)	
L. glaucescens (Charles 1942)	Gastrointestinal
L. helvus (Pilát and Usák 1950; Tyler 1963)	Gastrointestinal
L. lignyotus (Smith 1958)	Gastrointestinal
L. plumbeus (Pilát 1961; Pilát and Usák 1950)	Gastrointestinal
L. porninsis (Pilát 1961)	Gastrointestinal
L. rufus (Smith 1958; Tyler 1963)	Gastrointestinal
L. torminosus (Smith 1958)	Gastrointestinal
L. trivialis[d] (Smith 1958)	
L. uvidus (Tyler 1963)	Gastrointestinal
L. vellereus (Smith 1958)	

Table 10.3 (continued)

Species (common name)	Type of poisoning
Lampteromyces japonicus (Nakanishi et al. 1963)	Cytotoxic
*Lepiota brunneoincarnata*d (Mortara and Filipello 1967)	Cytotoxic
L. *fuscovinacea*d (Mortara and Filipello 1967)	Cytotoxic
L. *helvella*b (Mortara and Filipello 1967; Rautavaara 1950)	Cytotoxic
L. *schulzeri* (Krieger 1967)	
Lycoperdon subincarnatum (Krieger 1967)	Gastrointestinal
Morchella augusticeps (Center for Disease Control 1975a)	
*Mycena pura*d (Hesler 1960)	
Naematoloma fasciculare (Herbich et al. 1966; Ito et al. 1967; Singer 1962)	Gastrointestinal-cytotoxic
Panaeolus acuminatus (Orr and Orr 1979)	Hallucinogenic
P. *retirugis* (Orr and Orr 1979)	Hallucinogenic
P. *semioviatus* (Orr and Orr 1979)	Hallucinogenic
P. *subbalteatus* (Orr and Orr 1979; Stein et al. 1959) (P. *venenosus*)	Hallucinogenic
Panus stypticus (Hesler 1960)	Gastrointestinal
Paxillus involutus (Malone et al. 1962; Pilát and Usák 1950)	Gastrointestinal-cytotoxic
Phallus ravenelii (Smith 1958)	
Psilocybe baeocystis McCawley et al. 1962)	Hallucinogenic
P. *cubensis* (Stein 1958)	Hallucinogenic
P. *mexicana* (Hofmann et al. 1959; McCawley et al. 1962)	Hallucinogenic
P. *semperviva* (Brack et al. 1961)	Hallucinogenic
Rhodophyllus sinuatus (Tyler 1963)	Gastrointestinal
Rumaria flavobrunescence (Benedict 1972)	Cytotoxic
Russula densifolia (Orr and Orr 1979)	
R. *emetica* (Krieger 1967)	Gastrointestinal
R. *foetens* (Hesler 1960) (fetid russula)	Gastrointestinal
R. *fragilis*e (Hesler 1960)	
R. *nondorbingi* (Singer 1958)	Neurological-cerebral
Scleroderma aurantium (Pilát 1961; Pilát and Usák 1950; Stevenson and Benjamin 1961)	Neurological
S. *cepa* (Stevenson and Benjamin 1961)	Neurological
*Stropharia aeruginosa*d (Orr and Orr 1968)	
S. *coronilla*e (Hesler 1960)	
Tricholoma album (Pilát 1961)	Gastrointestinal
T. *flavobrunneum* (Pilát 1961; Smith 1958)	Gastrointestinal
T. *pardinum*b (Pilát 1961; Smith 1958)	Gastrointestinal
T. *pessundatum* (Pilát 1961)	Gastrointestinal

Table 10.3 (continued)

Species (common name)	Type of poisoning
T. pessundatum var. montanum (Pilát 1961)	Gastrointestinal
T. saponaceum (Pilát and Usák 1950)	Gastrointestinal-hemolytic
T. sejunctum (Pilát 1961)	Neurological-gastrointestinal
Verpa bohemica (Smith 1958)	Neurological
Volvaria speciosa[e] (Orr and Orr 1968)	
V. gloiocephala[e] (Orr and Orr 1979)	

[a]Probably the most poisonous mushroom reported so far.
[b]Very poisonous, high fatalities.
[c]Mildly poisonous.
[d]Suspected as poisonous.
[e]Probably poisonous, conflicting reports.

Poisoning with the toxic agarics may be a matter of individual sensitivity, as there are persons who can tolerate these poisonous species. For example, *A. arvensis* var. *palustris* and *A. placomyces* may be poisonous to some but harmless to others (Roland et al. 1960; Smith 1958). This variability in the toxicological response of various individuals may be due to the existence of both edible and toxic variants in the same species; e.g., *A. placomyces* (Smith 1958).

As the appearance of certain agarics are close enough to the amanitas, the inexperienced gatherer must consider the possibility of poisoning and should refrain from indiscriminate eating of agarics. For example, it will not be difficult for an inexperienced person to recognize, mistakenly, *Amanita brunnescence*, a very poisonous mushroom, for the edible *Agaricus perrarus;* or the all white *Amanita verna* for the white (except for the grayish to pinkish gills) *Agaricus sylvicola*, which in itself has variable effects on persons. In spite of the distinctive characteristics of the amanitas, environmental and mechanical factors may modify these fragile characteristics, so that recognizing the amanitas apart from the edible agarics may be difficult.

As discussed previously (pp. 481–482), *A. bisporus* (*A. brunnescence*) contains relatively high levels of agaritine, a probable carcinogenic arylhydrazine (Toth 1979b). This compound also is found in many edible agarics, such as, *A. campestris, A. edulis, A. crocodilinus, A. hordensis*, and *A. perrarus*, as well as poisonous ones, e.g., *A. xanthodermus* (Levenberg 1964). Thus, agaritine is probably widespread in the Agaricaceae family. If this compound is ultimately proven to be carcinogenic, the safety of these commercial, as well as all other members of the edible agarics will have to be reassessed.

Amanita

The genus Amanita is probably the most notorious of the group of poisonous mushrooms. Most cases of fatal mycetism are caused by one or more species of this genus, particularly *A. phalloides* and its counterpart *A. brunnescens* or *A. virosa* (Litten 1975; Wieland 1968a,b; Wieland and Wieland 1972). The hazard of serious poisoning from the amanitas is indicated by the number of toxic species in this genus. In Table 10.3 there are at least 23 toxic species, more than any other genus listed.

There are a number of characteristic features of the amanitas. Shown in Figure 10.1 are three features which together are most characteristic of poisonous amanitas:

the volva or the cup at the base of the stipe (stalk); the annulus (ring) in the upper part of the stalk near the cap; third, the cap itself. The volva is a remnant of the universal veil which covers the whole mushroom in the button stage. Patches of this veil also remain on the cap of the mature mushroom to give it a warty or scaly appearance. The volva, however, is not always well defined. For example, in A. *cothurnata*, one may see only a free collarlike remnant at the base of the stalk (Smith 1958). In A. *pantherina*, the volva may appear as a well-defined collar on the upper part of the bulbous base, the rest of the volva having fused with the base, and appears as a series of concentric rings. Fortunately, the volva, which is a critical characteristic of the amanitas, is well defined in A. *phalloides*, considered the most poisonous species in many parts of the world. A. *brunnescens*, which for many years was mistaken for A. *phalloides* by American mycologists, can be distinguished from the latter by the volva that splits vertically in young specimens. The split appears as though a wedge has been removed. Unfortunately, this volva often is not distinct enough in the former species and may appear as a very shallow cup, if any at all (Hesler 1960; Smith 1958).

The cap in many amanitas is also distinctive by the appearance of white, yellow, or creamy scales, warts, or patches. These patches may be numerous, as in A. *muscaria*, or few, as in A. *parcivolvata*, A. *phalloides*, and A. *brunnescens*. These patches may be absent in many poisonous species, as in some variants of A. *phalloides*, and especially A. *verna* (Fig. 10.8). These patches, however, are not seen solely among the amanitas. They are seen also in many other genera.

The cap in certain species is marked by recognizable, if not distinct, coloration. For example, A. *phalloides* has a greenish or olive cap with metallic or silky sheen. However, the mildly toxic A. *citrina* has also a green cap and has been mistaken for A. *phalloides* (Pilát and Usák 1950). A. *muscaria* has a yellow, orange, or red cap; A. *brunnescens* has a dark or brownish gray or lead-colored cap; and A. *verna* has a pure white cap (Hesler 1960; Smith 1958). The white amanitas, which include A. *bisporigera*, A. *virosa*, and A. *tenuifolia* are deadly species (Litten 1975).

The staining characteristics of the stalk when bruised may be a distinctive feature. The stalk of A. *brunnescens* stains brown; the edible counterpart A. *rubescens* stains red.

Another distinctive feature of the amanitas is the gills on the underside of the cap. These are white to pallid in almost every species, and are not connected to the stalk. The cap is easily and cleanly separable from the stalk.

As already stated, these features may be modified, erased, or damaged by environmental and mechanical factors, making recognition difficult. One, then, resorts to microscopical examination of the spores — not an easy task even for mycologists, much less the beginner.

Distinguishing between the edible and toxic amanitas is difficult at best and hardly recommendable, considering the great risk. In addition, toxic amanitas have been confused for the edible species of other genera. For example, A. *phalloides* has been confused with the delicious champignon *Tricholoma equestre* (Wieland and Wieland 1972). The latter, also known as T. *flavovirens*, may have a greenish yellow cap, with or without shades of tan (Hesler 1960). The deadly A. *verna*, A. *virosa*, and A. *bisporiger* can be easily confused for one of the best of edible mushrooms, the white *Lepiota naucina* (Hesler 1960; Smith 1958). A careful observer will notice that the latter has no volva, whereas the above amanitas do. However, often the volva of an amanita may remain on the ground when pulled, and thus, a crucial distinguishing mark is missed. The hazard due to mistaken identity is enhanced by overlapping habitats of L. *naucina* and the white amanitas. Both grow in meadows, waste areas, compost heaps, lawns, parks, and pastures (Hesler 1960; Smith 1958).

As discussed earlier, one finds three types of toxic amanitas based on the toxic reactions that are produced. The cytotoxic and choleriform amanitas include A. *verna*, A. *capensis*, A. *virosa*, A. *bisporigera*, A. *tenuifolia*, and of course, A. *phalloides* (Wieland and Wieland 1972). The neurotoxic, or muscarinic amanitas, are prepresented by A. *pantherina*, A. *parcivolvata*, A. *gemmata*, A. *flaviovolvata*, A. *cothurnata*, A.

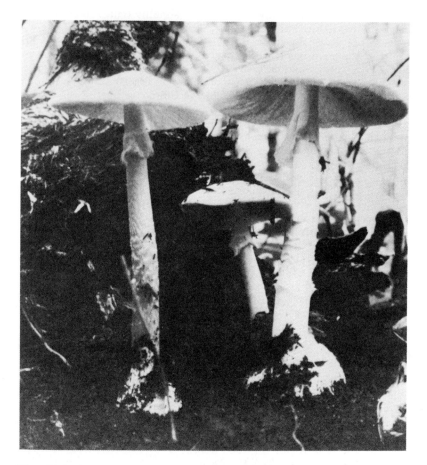

Fig. 10.8 *Amanita verna*, a pure white variant of *A. phalloides*. (From Christensen, C. M. 1975. Reprinted by permission from *Molds, Mushrooms and Mycotoxins*. University of Minnesota Press, Minneapolis, University of Minnesota, used with permission.)

regalis, A. Vaginata, A. strobiliformis, A. solitaria, and of course, *A. muscaria* (Benedict et al. 1966; Pilák 1961; Tyler 1963). The hallucinogenic or psychedelic amanitas are represented by *A. citrina*, or *A. mappa*, and *A. porphyria* (Tyler 1961).

The cytotoxic green and white amanitas contain the same deadly cyclopeptides discussed previously. The amounts of the deadly toxins in *A. phalloides* and *A. verna* had been estimated. Samples of these mushrooms have been found to contain approximately 10.0, 8.0, 5.0, and 1.5 mg/100 g fresh tissue of phalloidin, α-, β-, and γ-amanitin, respectively (Tyler et al. 1966; Wieland et al. 1966); *A. bisporigera* contains higher amounts — up to 5 mg/g dry weight. A 50-g quantity of mushroom containing 7 mg amanitins may be sufficient to kill a person, the lethal dose for humans being less than 0.1 mg/kg body weight.

The quantity of muscarine in a sample of *A. muscaria* was determined to be between 0.2 and 0.3 mg/100 g fresh weight (Eugster 1956). The levels of other neurotoxic substances may be higher. Total isoxazoles (ibotenic acid, muscimol, and muscazone) in dried *A. muscaria* was estimated to be 180 mg/100 g; in *A. pantherina*, this value was 460 mg/100 g (Benedict et al. 1966). The amounts of ibotenic acid in *A. muscaria* and

A. pantherina were estimated by Takemoto et al. (1964b) to be 25 and 220 mg/100 g of dry weight, respectively. It appears that these values are variable depending on such factors as year and location of collection. Thus, total isoxazoles content in samples of summer specimens of *A. muscaria* obtained in Switzerland varied from 30 mg/100 g to as high as 100 mg/100 g dry weight in 1962 and 1966, respectively (Eugster 1968).

Supposedly, *A. citrina* and *A. porphyria* may cause hallucinations because of their bufotenine content (see Fig. 10.4 for structural formula). Fabing and Hawkins (1956) have reported visual disturbances and changes in time and space perceptions among volunteers injected with 8 to 16 mg of bufotenine. However, other investigators have been unable to confirm these observations (Holmsted and Lindgren 1967; Turner and Merlis 1959). Nevertheless, bufotenine produces powerful cardiovascular effects, and accordingly, it may be difficult to distinguish the psychomimetic action from the cardiovascular effects (Fischer 1968; Holmstedt and Lindgren 1967). *A. citrina* and *A. porphyria* also contain other tryptamine derivatives such as serotonin, which has powerful effects on the cardiovascular system.

No doubt the cytotoxic amanitas are the most deadly. Nevertheless, the neurotoxic-muscarinic species cannot be underestimated, particularly *A. pantherina* and *A. porphyria* (Smith 1958). *A. cothurnata,* another neurotoxic-muscarinic species, is similarly very toxic.

Some amanitas which were once considered edible have been proven to be poisonous. Other amanitas reportedly may be poisonous to some individuals but harmless to others, as in the case of *A. chlorinosma,* "Clorox"-smelling mushroom (Hesler 1960), and *A. flavoconia.* The latter may be confused with *A. frostiana,* which is poisonous. This variability in response accounts for the contradictions in the early literature.

A. phalloides was once considered to be absent on the North American continent (Hesler 1960; Krieger 1936), or at most, was found only very rarely on the West Coast (Smith 1958). In fact, according to Hesler (1960) American mycologists then mistook *A. brunnescens* or similar species for *A. phalloides.* But beginning in 1966, reports of its presence in North America began to appear (Tyler et al. 1966). And by 1969, and especially after the occurrence of a fatal mushroom poisoning in New Jersey in 1970 (Litten 1975), this species began to be found more commonly on the East Coast (Tanghe and Simons 1973). In the American habitat, *A. phalloides* grows in parks and barren soils, especially associated with pine trees and other conifers, unlike in Europe where it is reportedly seldom associated with these trees.

Aside from its distinct morphological characteristics, specific chemical tests will be helpful in identifying *A. phalloides.* There are some claims that concentrated sulfuric acid applied on the fresh but not dried pileus will give a specific purple stain, and that 5% KOH will distinguish *A. phalloides* from *A. virosa;* the latter will turn bright lemon-yellow, whereas the former will not (Tanghe and Simons 1973).

Even though there are several edible Amanita species, the preceding discussion explains why many mycologists and mycophagists do not recommend eating amanitas.

Boletus

Mushrooms of the genus Boletus are easily distinguished from the agarics and amanitas by having pores or tubes instead of gills in the underside of the cap. There are many edible boletes in this group; however, a few are poisonous. Fortunately, the poisonous species listed in Table 10.3 can be easily recognized by the red trimmings in mouths of the pores or tubes. The two most poisonous species in this group are *B. eastwoodii* (Keinholz 1934; Orr and Orr 1968) and *B. satanas* (Orr and Orr 1968; Pilát and Usák 1950).

The symptoms of poisoning from toxic boletes range from mild to severe stomach cramps, diarrhea, and vomiting to paralysis (Pilát and Usák 1950). Even a small piece of *B. eastwoodii* can cause severe symptoms (Keinholz 1934). The toxic substance has not been determined. Atropine may be an antidote.

Some slightly poisonous boletes, such as *B. purpureus,* may be rendered safe by proper cooking (Pilát and Usák 1950).

Calvatia

The lone member of this genus listed in Table 10.3, *Calvatia gigantea,* is the largest species of the puffball family. Puffballs are white to yellowish, round, glabrous, and sessile. They are called puffballs because of their tendency to puff out a cloud of dark or brown spores when pressure is applied. This species can grow to gigantic size from 20 to 38 cm in diameter and weighing more than 1.8 kg (Krieger 1967). Most mycophagists consider this species edible. Smith (1958) concedes that the older specimens with a yellowish interior may act as a strong cathartic for some individuals. In addition, *C. gigantea* contains calvacin, a toxin with antitumor activity. It is a basic mucoprotein with cumulative toxic effects in animals. Extremely low doses cause prolonged intoxication, with anorexia and extreme weight loss. Necrosis of various structures is also observed. These include the myofibrils of cardiac and skeletal muscles, the liver with biliary obstruction, and the renal tubules; fibrinoid degeneration and pulmonary hemorrhages are also seen. The toxin is also antigenic, being a protein; it has been observed to produce anaphylactoid reactions in dogs at doses as low as 2 mg/kg/day (Sternberg et al. 1963). The symptoms certainly qualify calvacin as a cytotoxic toxin. Being a protein, cooking must surely destroy this toxin and could explain the reported edibility of *C. gigantea.* Digestive enzymes can also destroy calvacin. Yet, in spite of this, its potential hazard must be recognized.

Cantharellus and Gomphus

There is only one representative of this genus listed in Table 3, *Cantharellus floccosus.* This has been reclassified as *Gomphus floccosus.* The cantherelles resemble other genera such as Clavaria and Clitocybe (see below). However, they are more vaselike in shape than the clavarias, and their anastomosing, dull-edged gills distinguish them from the clitocybes.

C. *floccosus* may be mistaken for the edible *C. cibarius.* Although many mycophiles would swear to the edibility of *C. floccosus,* this mushroom may cause mild to violent gastrointestinal symptoms in many other individuals (Smith 1958).

This mushroom has been shown to contain large quantities (4.5%, dry weight basis) of an acid similar to agaricic acid (Miyata et al. 1966). This compound is probably norcaperatic acid, which has a close structural relationship with citric acid. This acid has been isolated from *G. kauffmanii* (Henry and Sullivan 1969) (see also p. 494). Both norcaperatic and agaricic acids are neurological poisons. In rats, they produced dose-related mydriasis, central nervous system depression, and skeletal muscular weakness (Carrano and Malone 1967). Their similarity to citric acid may explain their toxicity, as they may intefere with the Krebs cycle. Indeed, they have been found to be competitive inhibitors of aconitase.

C. *floccosus* has variable effects in different persons. This is another example of why there are contradictory reports in the literature regarding the toxicity of certain mushroom species.

Clavaria

Clavaria is one of the genera in the family of coral fungi. This name (Latin *clavatus* club shaped) is descriptive of their general appearance, although some species consist of only simple clublike structures (Hesler 1960; Krieger 1967). Two Clavaria species have been reported to be poisonous: *C. formosa* and *C. gelatinosa.* Reportedly, these mushrooms may cause stomach aches and diarrhea in humans (Smith 1958; Tyler 1963).

Many clavarias are edible, but it is easy to confuse the poisonous ones with the edible — in particular, the poisonous *C. formosa* with the edible *C. botrytis.*

Clitocybe

In general, the mushrooms of the genus Clitocybe may be distinguished from species of other genera by their decurrent gills, fibrous stalks, and particularly, their white spores. Unfortunately, one can easily mistake a number of these species with members of other genera, particularly some species of Tricholoma (Krieger 1967) and Cantharellus. Ten species of poisonous Clitocybe are listed in Table 10.3. Seven species are muscarinic: *C. illudens*, *C. subilludens* (found in Florida), *C. olearia* (found in California), *C. rivulosa*, *C. truncicola* (Tyler 1963), *C. cerussata* (Pilát 1961; Tyler 1963), and *C. dealbata* (Hughes et al. 1966).

Two clitocybes have different effects. *C. claviceps* possesses a disulfiramlike action similar to the effect of *Coprinus atramentarius*, an inky cap mushroom (Romagnesi 1964). *C. toxica* (Sapeika and Stephens 1965) contains a heat-labile potent toxin lethal to mice and rats. This toxin appears to inhibit cytochrome oxidase.

C. illudens and related species cause nausea and vomiting. The edible *Cantharellus cibarius* may be mistaken with *C. illudens*. Closer examination reveals the thin, tight gills and sharp edges of the latter, whereas the former has wavy margins and long decurrent gills, frequently with forked and obtuse gill margins. *C. illudens* also has a long slender stalk (Smith 1958).

Apparently, certain individuals have difficulty digesting clitocybes (Pilát 1961). Poisonous as they are, their effects are mild compared to other muscarinic mushrooms. However, four cases of poisoning were reported in 1969 in New York. The symptoms included abdominal pain and vomiting (Center for Disease Control 1969). Another mushroom poisoning occurred in Pennsylvania in 1973, which involved 17 cases and was caused by an unknown Clitocybe species (Center for Disease Control 1973b).

Coprinus

Mushrooms of the genus Coprinus are easily recognized by their tendency to liquify into a black substance by autodigestion. Only one toxic Coprinus species is represented in Table 10.3, *C. atramentarius*, or the "inky cap." The symptoms of this type of poisoning have been described previously on page 480.

Cortinarius

The genus cortinarius consists of several hundred species of mushrooms, many of which are difficult to distinguish even by mycologists (Orr and Orr 1968). Most are fairly large with fleshy, fruiting bodies and with rust- or cinnamon-colored spores. A spider web-like inner veil, known as the cortina, hides the gills until the cap expands. Many Cortinarius species have unknown edibility, and many still are not regarded particularly as edible (Hesler 1960; Orr and Orr 1968).

Two species have been found to be toxic. One, *C. orellanus* contains orellanine, a slow-acting, dangerous cytotoxin (Desvignes 1965; Grzymala 1961). The symptoms of orellanus poisoning have been described earlier (p. 475).

C. traganus, the other toxic species, is only mildly poisonous. It can induce vomiting, but its unpleasant "goaty" smell and bitter taste make it very unlikely that it will be consciously selected for the table (Pilát 1961).

Entoloma

The genus Entoloma is not regarded with favor among mycophagists (Krieger 1967). The entolomas are similar in appearance to the tricholomas (p. 500) except for the pink spores. One member of this genus, *E. lividum* (leaden entoloma) is decidedly very poisonous. Even small quantities of this mushroom may produce vomiting, diarrhea, abdominal pains, headache, thirst, and severe weakness. Some fatalities due to ingestion of this mushroom have been reported, particularly in Europe. Symptoms may begin from 20 min to 2 hr after ingestion. The victims may remain ill for several days (Pilát and Usák 1950). *E. sinuatom* is similarly very poisonous, producing headache, vertigo, stomach ache and vomiting (Krieger 1967).

Another entoloma which has been reported as being very poisonous is *E. vernum* (Pilát 1961). Two other species, *E. salmoneum* and *E. strictus*, have been suspected of being poisonous (Hesler 1960).

The toxic principle(s) from the poisonous entolomas has not been identified.

Galerina

The species in the Galerina have been classified by some taxonomists under the genus, Pholiota, or Phaeomarasmius. Singer (1962) classified these under Galerina. The galerinas of interest here, i.e., the poisonous ones, cannot be easily distinguished from the many species of Pholiota. Both genera and several others have brown or yellow-brown gills (Smith 1958). However, some species of Galerina are recognized by their growth on decayed wood, their slightly sticky caps, the narrow bandlike ring on most stalks of a cluster of mushroom growth, and the darkening of the stalk from the base up.

Four poisonous Galerina species are listed in Table 10.3. One, *G. sulciceps,* based on the reports of Boedijn (1938-1940), may be considered more lethal than the deadly amanitas. The symptoms of poisoning have been described previously (p. 475).

The other toxic galerinas may be considered toxicological cousins of the amanitas. They also contain α- and β-amanitin (Tyler and Smith 1963; Tyler et al. 1963). *G. autumnalis* was responsible for a near fatal poisoning in Portland, Oregon, in 1953 (Tyler and Smith 1963). This species was also responsible for the death of two children (Peck 1912). One poisoning in the state of Washington in 1974 also was attributed to this species (Center for Disease Control 1974). *G. marginata* was responsible for two cases of mycetism reported in New York City in 1974 (Center for Disease Control 1974).

Gomphus

The poisonous species of the genus Gomphus, *G. kauffmanii,* has already been mentioned in relation to the genus Cantharellus (p. 492). Gomphus and Cantharellus share a number of species together, if these two genera are not already synonymous.

Gymnopilus

The two representatives of the genus Gymnopilus listed in Table 10.3 are *G. spectabilis* and *G. decurrens.* The former is a large (20 to 25 cm in diameter), bright yellow mushroom that is usually found on dead tree stumps. Both species cause hallucinations (Romagnesi 1964). A man who mistook *G. spectabilis* for the edible honey agaric *(Armillariella mellea)* developed bizarre symptoms after eating two to three cupsful of fried mushrooms (Buck 1967). The symptoms included a feeling of "wooziness," disconnected and blurred vision, unsteadiness, nausea, uncoordination, and hallucinations of shrinking room size and unnaturally colored objects.

Bis-noryangonin (Fig. 10.4), isolated from *G. spectabilis* and a chemotaxonomic relative, *G. decurrens,* may be the hallucinatory compound (Hatfield and Brady 1969, 1968). It is noteworthy that yangonin, a closely related styrylpyrone, is found in kava root, which is used in intoxicating drinks by Pacific islanders. Similar other styrylpyrone derivatives are also found in the kava root (Madaus 1938).

Helvella (Gyromitra)

The genus Helvella (previously Gyromitra), commonly called the false morels, and the Morchella species, or true morels (see also p. 496), are both cup fungi, belonging to the class *Ascomycetes*. The gilled and pore mushrooms belong to the class Basidiomycetes. However, species of both genera can be distinguished by the structure of the head, or cap. The morchellas have pitted, spongelike heads; the helvellas have convoluted or wrinkled brainlike appearance without pits (Smith 1958).

A few toxic Helvella species have been reported. Those included in Table 10.3 are *H. esculenta, H. gigas, H. infula, and H. underwoodii.* As these are closely related to the true morels, the inexperienced mushroom hunter may confuse poisonous helvellas with the edible morchellas. For example, the toxic *H. esculenta* (Fig. 10.6) may be confused with the edible *M. crassipes,* if one is careless about the presence of pits seen in morchellas, but absent in helvellas. While there have been few fatalities from helvella poisoning recorded in the United States, in Europe a 2 to 4% yearly fatality rate has been recorded according to Alder (1961). This may be expected, since Europeans seem to consume larger quantities of false morels. Undoubtedly, most poisoning must be due to the mistaken identities of toxic species with edible helvellas or morchellas.

The presence of the carcinogen N-methyl-N-formylhydrazine and other hydrazine derivatives in *H. esculenta* has been discussed previously (pp. 480—481).

Hygrophorus

Hygrophorus is a large genus that appears to be distributed throughout the world, and several hundred species are found in North America alone. These mushrooms have waxy soft gills with sharp edges, widely spaced and broadened upward toward the cap (Hesler 1960) which may distinguish this genus from other species. Colors that are predominant in these mushrooms are white, pink, and bright orange-red (Orr and Orr 1968).

Only one toxic Hygrophorus species is listed in Table 10.3: *H. conicus* reportedly has caused several deaths (Krieger 1967; Orr and Orr 1968). The distinctive characteristic of this species is its bright yellow, red, or orange body which blackens when dried, handled, or ages (Hesler 1968). However, it may be difficult to separate *H. conicus* from other similarly colored but edible Hygrophorus species, such as *H. cuspidus, H. immutabilis,* and *H. ruber.* The first blackens also, as does *H. conicus;* the other three do not blacken, and thus may be easily identified apart from the poisonous species.

Inocybe

The mushrooms of the genus Inocybe can be recognized and distinguished from similar species of other genera by their cap which consists of radially arranged fibrils, and their pale brown spores (Orr and Orr 1968). These mushrooms closely resemble the Hebolomas except that the latter have a more or less viscid cap which is not fibrillose and scaly as do the inocybes.

Nine inocybe species are listed as poisonous in Table 10.3. Their principal toxic substance is muscarine. *I. patouillardi,* a brick-red mushroom, is probably one of the most poisonous among the inocybes. This mushroom contains around 37 mg/100 g of muscarine on a fresh weight basis, more than 100 times the muscarine content of *Amanita muscaria* (Eugster 1957)! In Europe, this inocybe reportedly has been responsible for several cases of poisoning, with a fatality rate of up to 8% (Eugster 1957). *I. napipes* is also highly muscarinic, containing approximately 700 mg muscarine/100 g dry mushroom (Brown et al. 1962; Malone et al. 1962).

Lactarius

The genus Lactarius is so named because its member species exude a latex when cut, which is the identifying feature of this large genus. This exudate may change in color when exposed to air. While there are many edible lactarii, many poisonous species are

also known. Table 10.3 lists 11 poisonous species. The poison produces gastrointestinal symptoms, and is present in the exudate, which has not been identified. Fatal cases
among children ascribed to Lactarius poisoning are on record. Two species, L. glaucescence (Charles 1942) and L. torminosus (Pilát and Usák 1954) are particularly notorious in this respect. Most poisonous lactarii are toxic only when raw or insufficiently cooked (Pilát 1961; Tyler 1963). But in the case of L. glaucescence, cooking may
not neutralize or remove the toxin (Charles 1942).

Like many other types of toxic mushrooms, the degree of toxicity of the lactarii
may be dependent on the particular sensitivity of the host; some persons are not affected at all (Singer 1962).

The lactarii resemble species of other genera, so that mistaken identification can
occur. For example, toxic L. plumbeus may be mistaken for Paxillus involutus, which
is edible when properly cooked (Pilát and Usák 1950) (p. 497). In addition, it is not
difficult to confuse the toxic with the edible lactarii, being very similar in appearance.
For example, the poisonous L. lignyotus may be mistaken for the edible L. gerardii. A
pinkish stain develops when the former is bruised, but not the latter. Except for that
subtle difference, these two species are difficult to tell apart.

Lepiota

The members of the genus Lepiotas, popularly called parasol mushrooms, resemble
those of Amanita in many respects except for the absence of the universal veil, and
therefore, the volva. Thus, mistaken identification is possible in this case. In particular, L. naucina, reputedly one of the best tasting mushrooms, can easily be confused
with the very toxic white amanitas (p. 489) (Smith 1958).

Several lepiotas are very toxic in their own right. Five species are listed in Table
10.3. L. helvella and possibly L. brunneoincarnata and L. fuscovinacea (Mortara and
Filipello 1967) contain the cyclopeptide toxin of the amanitas. L. molybdites is also
highly poisonous, but it does not affect certain persons (Smith 1958). One fatality due
to this mushroom is on record (Hesler 1960).

Again, the common problem of mistaken intrageneric identification is also possible
here. For example, the edible L. rachodes, or L. procera, may be confused with the
very toxic L. molybdites (Krieger 1967; Smith 1958). Similarly, L. naucina and L.
naucinoides, both edible, may also be mistaken with the moderately toxic L. schulzeri
(Krieger 1967).

Lycoperdon

The mushrooms of the genus Lycoperdon are also puffballs which open by a single
apical pore. They are like the calvatias (p. 492), but are usually smaller. There are
many edible species in this genus, and only one toxic species, L. subincarnatum, is
listed in Table 10.3. This species may cause prolonged diarrhea (Krieger 1967).

Morchella

Most authors consider the morchellas listed in Table 10.3 as not only edible, but also
highly prized among mycophagists. However, they are so similar in appearance to the
helvellas discussed earlier (p. 494). that mistaken identification is likely among species
in these genera. In addition, the known variable responses of persons to various species may also be the case here, as M. angusticeps has caused one case of mushroom
poisoning in Minnesota in 1974 (Center for Disease Control 1975a,c).

Mycena

The genus Mycena consists of small and rather delicate mushrooms with caps measuring
from approximately 0.5 cm to not more than 5 cm in diameter. They are often colored

beautifully. The colors of the cap range from rose to lilac or white with a blue or purple disc (the central portion of the cap). There are 230 or more species in this genus in North America alone (Hesler 1960). Many are of unknown edibility. One beautifully colored species, *M. pura*, is suspected of being poisonous. It tastes and smells like a radish (Hesler 1968).

Naematoloma

The genus Naematoloma, whose species were once considered under the Hypoloma, is closely related to the common Agaricus, and thus closely resembles it. Naematolomas can be distinguished from the agarics by the purple-brown or grayish-violet spores and gills of older specimens and by the absence of a ring on the stalk; this lack of the ring is owing to the very thin inner membrane. One poisonous species, *N. fasciculare*, is listed in Table 10.3 (Herbich et al. 1966; Singer 1962), although there are conflicting reports of its edibility (Hesler 1960; Smith 1958). But fatalities caused by this mushroom leave no doubt as to its toxicity (Herbich et al. 1966). The unidentified fasciculare toxin is cytotoxic, causing liver cell necrosis, hemorrhages in liver parenchyma, and subacute liver atrophy. The toxin(s) also causes damage to the kidney with extensive fatty degeneration and impairment of kidney functions and similar degenerative changes in the heart muscles and in the ganglion cells of the brain. Initial clinical symptoms manifested by gastrointestinal signs occur approximately 9 hr after ingestion. Death results from extensive damage to the liver and other tissues. Thus, in many ways fasciculare poisoning resembles that of the amanitas.

Naematolin ($C_{17}H_{24}O_5$), isolated from flask culture of the mushroom (Ito et al. 1967), is cytotoxic to HeLa S_3 cells at 6.25 $\mu g/ml$, and causes coronary vasodilation in isolated guinea pig heart at 100 μg.

Many naematolomas closely resemble each other; *N. fasciculare* can sometimes be mistaken for the edible species, such as *N. capnoides* or *N. sublateritium*.

Panaeolus

The members of the genus Panaeolus have black spores, spotted gills, and long and narrow stipes. They are also known to grow in beds together with commercially cultivated mushrooms. Five toxic species are listed in Table 10.3. *P. sabbalteatus* (formerly *P. venenosus*) contains a psychotomimetic toxin. The effect appears almost immediately following ingestion. Clinical signs include muscular incoordination, with difficulty in standing much less walking; drowsiness; lack of emotional control; incoherent and inappropriate speech; and hallucinations of moving objects and magnificent combinations of colors. There also may be complete but transient paralysis of the arms and legs (Krieger 1967). Intensely painful diarrhea may precede the prolonged excitatory or euphoric state (Stein et al. 1959). A case of panaeolus poisoning also has been reported in Washington state (Center for Disease Control 1975c).

Panus

The species in the genus Panus have tough, almost leathery caps, and gills with nonserrated edges. The stalks are lateral and short or absent. One poisonous species, *P. stypticus*, listed in Table 10.3, has worldwide distribution. Its unpleasant, astringent, and lingering sour taste is a fortunate deterrent to the potential consumer (Hesler 1960).

Paxillus

The genus Paxillus appears to be an intermediate form between the gill mushrooms, such as the amanitas, and the pore mushrooms, or boletes. The species are recognized by their decurrent gills, which fork and tend to anastomose on the stalk, if present. The gills are also easily separable from the cap, which is yellow-brown.

One species, *P. involutus*, listed in Table 10.3, is considered edible by some authors (Krieger 1967). However, it has been known for many years as poisonous (Singer 1962). In one outbreak, three out of four poisoned persons died. The symptoms of poisoning began rapidly with intense stomach pains and severe acute circulatory collapse. The toxin(s) caused severe distension of blood vessels, including the capilliaries of the the stomach, and fatty degeneration of the liver, kidneys, heart, and skeletal muscles. Fat emboli were formed, which indicated that the toxin caused breakdown of lipid emulsions in the blood (Bschor and Mallach 1963). This suggests a possible interference by the toxin of the lipoprotein function. Extracts of *P. involutus* have been shown to cause diuresis, peripheral vasodilation, and metabolilic poisoning in rats (Malone et al. 1967). A compound, involutin, 5-(3',4'-dihydroxyphenyl)-3,4-dihydroxy-2-(p-hydroxyphenyl)-cyclopent-2-en-1-one, has been isolated by Edwards et al. 1967). However, there is as yet no evidence of its being responsible for the symptoms in involutus poisoning.

Involutin

Phallus

The members of the genus Phallus are strange-looking mushrooms, which are also called stinkhorns because they smell like decayed flesh (Hesler 1960; Smith 1958). They consist of a stalk and either a cap or head with granulose surface. The name is descriptive of its hornlike structure (Greek *phallos* penis). The surface near the tips is covered with a slimy and sticky mass containing the spores. Although one species, *P. ravenelii*, is listed as poisonous in Table 10.3, it is very unlikely that this mushrrom would be consumed considering its obnoxious smell.

Psilocybe

The genus Psilocybe resembles a number of other genera, namely Collybia, Nancoria, Hebeloma, Tricholoma, and Mycena. As in the first three genera, the psilocybes have no veil on the stalk except in very young specimens. The cap and gills in the psilocybes are brown and the stalks nearly straight, hollow, thick, and rigid, and tough in some species (Krieger 1967).

Four poisonous species are listed in Table 10.3. All are hallucinogens. These mushrooms are used for hallucinatory purposes in religious rites among certain Indians in Mexico (Hofmann et al. 1959). The hallucinogenic species are *P. mexicana* (Hofmann and Troxler 1963; Hofmann et al. 1959), *P. cubensis* (Agurell et al. 1966, 1968; Catalfomo and Tyler 1964; Stein 1958), *P. semperviva* (Brack et al. 1961), and *P. baeocystis* (Leung et al. 1965). All contain the hallucinogen psilocybin. *P. mexicana* contains both psilocybin and psilocin, at 0.2 to 0.46%, and 0.05% of dry caps, respectively (Hofmann et al. 1959). *P. baeocystis* contains not only these two hallucinogens, but also baeocystin and norbaeocystin. This mushroom has caused serious poisoning in four children, one of whom has died. Samples of the species gathered in the area where the toxic *P. baeocystis* was obtained suggest that the children might have ingested mushrooms containing about 0.63% of psilocybin and less than 0.1% psilocin (dry weight basis) (McCawley et al. 1962). Structures of these hallucinogens are shown in Figure 10.4.

Symptoms of poisoning with this hallucinogenic mushroom and these hallucinogenic compounds have been discussed previously (p. 478).

Rhodophyllus

Rhodophyllus is a difficult genus to describe, since it consists of species which may be separated into several genera (Tyler 1963). One poisonous species, *R. sinuatus*, is the only representative listed in Table 10.3. The mushroom can cause severe gastro-intestinal symptoms, which include abdominal pain, vomiting, and diarrhea. The victim may be incapacitated for several days after the symptoms begin. Liver damage is produced by whatever toxin is present. The poisoning is sometimes fatal, especially among young children (Tyler 1963). Five other species listed by Tyler (1963) have been shown to be toxic to guinea pigs.

Russula

The species in the genus Russula are easily identified by the brittle, dry gills and flesh, and the not easily separable caps and stalks. This genus is noted for the variety of colors of the different species, ranging from white to darker shades of gray, brown, or black, and to brighter colors of green and yellow to red and purple. Russulas are similar to the lactarii, except that their flesh does not produce a latex.

Five toxic species are listed in Table 10.3. One species, *R. nondorbingi* (Singer 1958), found in New Guinea and Papua in the South Pacific, is believed to cause cerebral mycetism. This species induces fits of frenzy and hysteria, and is used by the natives during times of high or low emotional states. *R. foetens*, as the name implies, has an obnoxious smell and bad taste. This should deter any potential consumer. It is poisonous to certain individuals even when cooked, producing vomiting (Pilát 1961). Another unpleasant-tasting species is *R. fragilis*, which has a stinging taste. Hesler (1960) suspects that this species is poisonous and warns mycophiles not to eat red, pink, or purple russulas. *R. emetica* is similar to *R. fragilis*. It has a very acrid taste and is muscarinic (Krieger 1967).

R. densifolia is another example of which there are conflicting opinions as to its edibility. Orr and Orr (1979) consider it poisonous, whereas Hesler (1960) lists it as edible.

Scleroderma

The genus Scleroderma comprises another group of puffballs and is recognized by the pattern of wartlike structures on the surface and violaceous to purple interiors. Two poisonous species are listed in Table 10.3, *S. aurantium* and *S. cepa*. Both mushrooms when eaten raw produce after 30 min stomach pains, weakness, nausea with dizziness, tingling sensation over the body surface, muscular rigidity, profuse perspiration, and facial pallor. Forced vomiting relieves the symptoms promptly (Pilát 1961; Pilát and Usák 1950; Stevenson and Benjamin 1961).

Stropharia

The mushrooms of the genus Stropharia resemble the agarics in many ways — in having purple-brown spores, a central stalk, and an annulus. They are distinguished from the latter by the continuation of the gills onto the stalk, which are free in the agarics. Stropharias are also highly colored. Two species of Stropharia are listed in Table 10.3. *S. aeruginosa* is easily recognized by its blue cap. This species (Orr and Orr 1968) and *S. coronilla* (Hesler 1960) are suspected of being poisonous.

Tricholoma

Tricholoma is a large genus. The important characteristics include the notched gills at the stalk and the absence of the volva and annulus. Many species are poisonous: Seven are listed in Table 10.3. *T. pardinum* appears to be the most poisonous in the group. One to 2 hr after eating *T. pardinum*, violent gastrointestinal symptoms are observed. These include stomach pains, repeated vomiting, and foul-smelling diarrhea; headache, cramps in the calves, and weakness are also produced. The symptoms subside in 2 to 6 hr, but the victims do not fully recover until 3 to 6 days later. Recovery is complete, however. The toxin(s), which has not been identified, causes inflammation of the mucous membranes of the stomach and intestines. It has been reported to have caused a large number of poisonings in Switzerland (Pilát 1961). A very attractive looking mushroom, it can easily be mistaken for the edible tricholomas.

T. *pessundatum* and its variant, *T. montanum,* are similarly highly poisonous. The former causes diarrhea and violent vomiting; the patient feels sick for 1 to 3 days (Pilát 1961). The latter seems to be even more poisonous; symptoms begin appearing from 30 min to 4 hr after eating the mushroom. Initially, the patient feels the need to vomit. When vomiting finally commences, it continues for 10 to 20 times without relief. Cramps and diarrhea occur, sometimes simultaneously with the vomiting. The victim may faint and develop a cold sweat and a rapid pulse; exhaustion and physical weakness follow (Pilát 1961).

T. *sejunctum* is also quite poisonous. Two to 5 hr after eating this mushroom, a feeling of uneasiness ensues, with irritability, sweating, and shivering. The shivering may be so severe that often there is trembling of the limbs and chattering of the teeth. The patient is unable to vomit even with an emetic. However, when large quantities are eaten, emesis may occur together with abdominal pains, diarrhea, severe mental depression, enlargement of the pupils, and shivering (Pilát 1961).

T. *saponaceum,* or the "strong-scented agaric," contains a hemolytic agent which is heat sensitive. When large quantities are eaten, stomach upset can result in sensitive persons. The mushroom may also induce vomiting and shivering (Pilát and Usák 1950).

T. *flavobrunneum* is considered safe to eat when cooked. Evidently the unknown toxin is heat sensitive, since the mushroom is violently poisonous when eaten raw (Pilát 1961).

T. *album* is also regarded poisonous by some mycologists (Pilát 1961). Again, this is another example of the variability of effects of poisonous mushrooms.

The phenomenon of shivering appears to be unique among the poisonous *Tricholoma.* The nature of the toxin(s) remains to be determined.

A very delicious champignon, *T. equestre (T. flavovirens)* may be mistaken for one of the poisonous amanitas, especially *A. phalloides,* because of the greenish tint of the cap and other features. The tricholomas do not have a volva and ring on the stalk, and mistaken identification can occur when these features in the amanitas are obscured by mechanical damage while on the ground or during gathering.

Verpa

Verpa, Helvella, and Gyromitra are commonly called the false morels because of their similarity to Morchella.

V. *bohemica* is the only species of this genus listed in Table 10.3. It is recognized by its wrinkled cap and the fact that it is attached only at the top of the stalk; the rest of the cap hangs loosely like a skirt. Eating large quantities of this mushroom has produced lack of muscular coordination 4 to 5 hr later. The toxic reaction varies with the individual (Smith 1958). This mushroom may also produce the disulfiramlike effect of *Coprinus atramentarius* (Groves 1964). Small quantities of *V. bohemica* do not seem to produce any toxic effects (Smith 1958).

Mistaken identification with the edible *Morchella hybrida* is very possible, since these two mushrooms may be recognized apart from each other only by close microscopical examination (Smith 1958).

Volvaria (Volvariella)

The species in the genus Volvaria may be recognized by the large, distinct volva, pink or red spores, the gills attached to the stalk, and the absence of the annulus on the stalk. Some species of Volvaria are cultivated in Asia (Orr and Orr 1968, 1979). Two poisonous species of Volvaria are listed in Table 10.3.

CONCLUSIONS

Mushrooms surely do not comprise a significant portion of the human diet. However, in terms of the rate of poisoning and number of fatalities caused by these products in relation to the number of persons who are active or occasional mycophagists, they should be considered to be a major toxic hazard. It should be emphasized that at present there are no infallible methods of distinguishing poisonous mushrooms from the edible ones. The variable effects of these products make the task of identification even more difficult, if not impossible. One safety rule is that one should consume only personally known edible wild species. Eating unfamiliar species, even though others can swear to its edibility, can be hazardous. Alexander Smith, a noted mycologist, found this out, surely to his great embarrassment, when he furnished for someone else's table a specimen of *Agaricus arvensis* var. *palustris* (Smith 1958). This mushroom adversely affected his friends, but not Dr. Smith; like many others, it has variable effects on individuals.

A fatal mushroom poisoning that occurred in Pulaski County, Kentucky (Myerson 1981) underscores the difficulty, with tragic consequences, of distinguishing between toxic and edible species. The consumption of a "white" mushroom, which according to the father had been consumed "for years" without ill effects, resulted in the death of a 5-year-old child and serious poisoning of his mother. Two other members of the family were less seriously affected. (The symptoms, which appeared several days after eating the mushrooms, were suggestive of Amanita poisoning). Unfortunately, this incident is just one among the many, almost regular, occurrences of fatal or near-fatal mushroom poisonings in many parts of the world.

The claim of the high nutritional quality of mushrooms is untrue. For example, the commercial variety, *Agaricus bisporus*, has very little protein (not over 4%). Furthermore, the protein is incomplete, being deficient in sulfur amino acids and isoleucine (Food Agricultural Organization 1970). The mushrooms are also basically highly indigestible. Their vitamin contents are no more remarkable than some of the common vegetables. In short, mushrooms can only serve as garnishings owing to their flavor and nothing more. Despite the culinary enjoyment that mushrooms offer, the risks accompanying wild mushroom consumption are not commensurate with the benefits.

REFERENCES

Agurell, S., Blomkvist, S. and Catalfomo, P. 1966. Biosynthesis of psilocybin in submerged culture of psilocybe cubensis. 1. Incorporation of labelled tryptophan and tryptamine. *Acta Pharm. Succica* 3: 37–44.

Agurell, S. and Nilsson, J. L. G. 1968. A biosynthetic sequence from tryptophan to psilocybin. *Tetrahedron Lett.* 9: 1063–1064.

Ainsworth, G. C. 1952. *Medical Mycology: An Introduction to Its Problems.* Isaac Pitman & Sons, New York.

Alder, A. E. 1961. Recognition and treatment of mushroom poisoning. *Dtsch. Med. Wochenschr.* 86: 1121−1127. (German)

Benedict, R. G. 1972. Mushroom toxins other than Amanita. In: *Microbial Toxins.* Vol. VI. Alex Ciegler (ed.), Academic Press, New York.

Benedict, R. G., Tyler, V. E., Jr. and Brady, L. R. 1966a. Chemotaxonomic significance of isoxazole derivatives in Amanita species. *Lloydia* 29: 333−342.

Berkson, B. M. 1979. Thioctic acid in treatment of hepatotoxic mushroom (Phalloides) poisoning. *N. Engl. J. Med.* 300: 371.

Blayney, D., Rosenkranz, E. and Zettner, A. 1980. Mushroom poisoning from chlorophyllum molybdites. *West. J. Med.* 132: 74−77.

Block, S. S., Stephens, R. L., Barreto, A. and Murrill, W. A. 1955. Chemical identification of the amanita toxin in mushroom. *Science* 121: 505−506.

Boedijn, K. B. 1938-1940. *Cited by* Benedict, R. G. 1972. Mushrooms other than Amanita. In: *Microbial Toxins.* Vol. VIII. S. Kadia, A. Ciegler and S. J. Ajl (eds.). Academic Press, New York.

Bowden, K. and Drysdale, A. C. 1965. A novel constituent of Amanita muscaria. *Tetrahedron Lett.* 12: 727−728.

Bowden, K., Drysdale, A. C. and Mogey, G. A. 1965. Constituents of Amanita muscaria. *Nature* 206: 1359−1360.

Brack, A. et al. 1961. Tryptophan as the biogenetic first stage of psilocybin. *Arch. Pharm.* 294: 230−234. (German)

Brady, L. R., and Tyler, V. E., Jr. 1959. A chromatographic examination of the alkaloidal fraction of Amanita pantherina. *J. Am. Pharm. Assoc. Sci. Ed.* 48: 417−419.

Brodner, O. G. and Wieland, T. 1976. Identification of the amatoxin-binding subunit of RNA polymerase B by affinity labeling experiments. Subunit B_3— The true amatoxin receptor protein of multiple RNA polymerase B. *Biochemistry* 15: 3480−3484.

Brown, J. K., Malone, M. H., Stuntz, D. E. and Tyler, V. E., Jr. 1962. Paper chromatographic determination of muscarine in Inocybe species. *J. Pharm. Sci.* 51: 853−856.

Brunelli, A., Genovese, E. and Napoli, P. A. 1967. Amanitin and glycogen synthesis in the liver. *Bull. Soc. Ital. Biol. Sper.* 44: 558−560. (Italian)

Bschor, F. and Mallach, H. J. 1963. Poisoning caused by Paxillus involutus, an edible mushroom. *Arch. Toxikol.* 20: 82−95.

Buck, R. W. 1961. Mushroom poisoning since 1924 in the United States. *Mycologia* 53: 537−538.

Buck, R. W. 1964. Poisoning by wild mushrooms. *Clin. Med.* 71: 1353−1363.

Buck, R. W. 1967. Psychedellic effect of Pholiota spectabilis. *New Engl. J. Med.* 276: 391−392.

Carrano, R. A. and Malone, M. H. 1967. Pharmacologic study of norcaperatic and agaricic acids. *J. Pharm. Sci.* 56: 1611−1614.

Catalfomo, P. and Tyler, V. E., Jr. 1961. Investigations of the free amino acids and Amanita toxins in Amanita species. *J. Pharm. Sci.* 50: 689−692.

Center for Disease Control. 1969. *Foodborne Outbreaks. Annual Summary.* U.S. Department of Health, Education, and Welfare. Public Health Service. Atlanta.

Center for Disease Control. 1973A. Wild mushroom poisoning—California. Morbidity and Mortality Weekly Report 23 (1), 4.

Center for Disease Control. 1973B. Wild mushroom poisoning—Pennsylvania. *M.M.W.R.* 23 (6): 50.

Center for Disease Control. 1973C. *Foodborne and Waterborne Disease Outbreaks. Annual Summary.* U.S. Department of Health, Education, and Welfare. Public Health Service, Atlanta.

Center for Disease Control. 1974. *Foodborne and Waterborne Disease Outbreaks.*
     Annual Summary. U. S. Department of Health, Education, and Welfare.
     Public Health Service, Atlanta.
Center for Disease Control. 1975A. Reaction to mushrooms—Minnesota. *M.M.W.R.*
     24 (50): 427
Center for Disease Control. 1975B. Fatal mushroom poisonings—New York City.
     M.M.W.R. 24 (51): 429
Center for Disease Control. 1975C. *Foodborne and Waterborne Disease Outbreaks.*
     Annual Summary. U.S. Department of Health, Education, and Welfare.
     Public Health Service, Atlanta.
Cessi, C., and Fiume, L. 1969. Increased toxicity of beta-amanitin when bound
     to a protein. *Toxicon* 6: 309—310.
Charles, V. K. 1942. Mushroom poisoning caused by Lactaria glaucescens.
     Mycologia 34: 112—113.
Ciucci, N. and Chiri, A. 1974. Clinical and anatomo-pathological studies on the
     long term results obtained with thioctic acid in Amanita phalloides poisoning.
     Minerva Anastesiol. 40: 61—70. (Italian)
Cochet-Meilhac, M. and Chambon, P. 1974. Animal DNA-dependent RNA polymerase.
     II. Mechanism of the inhibition of RNA polymerases B by amatoxins.
     Biochim. Biophys. Acta 353: 160—184.
Courtillot, M. and Staron, T. 1975. Cited by Litten, W. 1975. The most poisonous
     mushrooms. *Sci. Am.* 232 (3): 91—101.
Dearness, J. 1924. Gyromitra poisoning. *Mycologia* 16: 199.
Decken, A. Von Der, Loew, H. and Hultin, T. 1960. On the primary effects of
     phalloidin on liver cells. *Biochem. Z.* 332: 503—518. (German)
Delay, J. et al. 1959. 1. Somatic effects of psilocybin. 2. Psychic effects of
     psilocybin and its therapeutic significance. *Presse Med.* 67: 1368 (French)
Desvignes, A. 1965. Poisoning caused by Cortinarius orellanus. *Aliment. Vie* 53:
     155—159. (French)
Druckrey, H., Preussmann, R., Ivankovic, S. and Schmahl, D. 1967.
     Organotropic carcinogenic effects of 65 different N-nitroso compounds in BD
     rats. N-nitroso-4-methylaminobenzaldehyde in mushrooms. *Z. Krebsforch* 69:
     103—201. (German)
Edwards, R. L., Elsworthy, G. C., and Kole, N. 1967. Constituents of higher
     fungi. IV. Involutin, a diphenylcyclopentenone from *Paxillus involutus. J.
     Chem. Soc.* (6) C: 405—409.
Ender, F. and Ceh, L. 1968. Occurrence of nitrosamines in foodstuffs for human
     and animal consumption. *Food Cosmet. Toxicol.* 6: 569—571.
Eugster, C. H. 1956. On muscarine from fly mushroom. *Helv. Chim Acta* 39:
     1002—1023. (German)
Eugster, C. H. 1957. Isolation of muscarine from Inocybe patouillardi (Bres.).
     Helv. Chim. Acta 40: 886—887. (German)
Eugster, C. H. 1967. Isolation, structure, and synthesis of central-active
     compounds from Amanita muscaria. *U.S. Public Health Serv.* 1645: 416—418.
Eugster, C. H. and Waser, P. G. 1954. Properties of muscarine. *Experientia* 10:
     298—300. (German)
Eugster, C. H., Muller, G. F. and Good, R. 1965. Substances from Amanita
     muscaria: ibotenic acid and muscazon. *Tetrahedron Lett.* 23: 1813—1815.
     (German)
Fabing, H. D. and Hawkins, J. R. 1956. Intravenous bufotenine injection in
     human being. *Science* 123: 886—887.
Faulstich, H. 1979. New aspects of Amanita poisoning. *Klin. Wochenschr.* 57:
     1143—1152. (German)
Faulstich, H. 1980. Mushroom poisoning. *Lancet* 2: 794—795.

Faulstich, H. and Cochet-Meilhac, M. 1976. Amatoxins in edible mushrooms.
    F.E.B.S. Lett. 64 (1): 73–75.
Faulstich, H., Wieland, T. and Jochum, C. 1968. Components of green Amanita.
    XXXIV. Indoles in comparison with Amanita poisons. 7. The sulfoxides
    amanine and amanitines. *Ann. Chem.* 713: 186–195. (German)
Fischer, R. 1968. Chemistry of the brain. *Nature* 220: 411–412.
Fiume, L. 1967. Cytopathic action of hemolysin from Amanita phalloides on cultures
    in vitro of cells of the KB line and cells of human amnion. *Arch. Sci. Biol.*
    (Bologna) 51: 85–88. (Italian)
Fiume, L. and Laschi, R. 1965. Ultrastructural lesions produced by phalloidin and
    α-amanitin in the cells of liver parenchyma. *Sperimentale* 115: 288–297.
    (Italian)
Fiume, L., Marinozzi, V. and Nardi, F. 1969. The effect of amanitin poisoning on
    mouse kidney. *Br. J. Exp. Pathol.* 50: 270–276.
Floch, H., Labarbe, C. and Roffi, J. 1966. Toxicity of Lapiota morgani. *Rev.*
    Mycol. (N.S.) 31: 317–322. (French)
Food Agricultural Organization. 1970. Amino Acid Contents of Foods and Biological
    Data of Proteins. FAO, Rome.
Ford, W. W. 1926. A new classification of mycetismus (mushroom poisoning).
    J. Pharmacol. Exp. Ther. 29: 305–309.
Frank, W. 1968. On the content of young rat liver of the so-called liver-specific
    antigen and its rapid turnover in the adult rat. *A. Naturforsch.* 23B: 687–
    690. (German)
Frimmer, M. 1975. Phalloidin, a membrane-specific toxin. In: *Pathogenesis and*
    Mechanism of Liver Cell Necrosis. D. Keppler (ed.). MTP, Lancaster, England.
Frimmer, M. 1977. The role of plasma membranes in hepatotoxic effects.
    Naunyn Schmiedebergs Arch. Pharmacol. 297: 515–519.
Frimmer, M., Gries, J. and Hegner, D., 1967. Investigations on the mechanisms of
    the effect of phalloidins on the outflow of lysosomal enzymes and potassium.
    Naunyn Schmiedebergs Arch. Pharmacol. Exp. Pathol. 258: 197–214. (German)
Frimmer, M., Petzinger, E., Rufeger, U. and Veil, L. B. 1977. Trypsin protection
    of hepatocytes against phalloidin. *Naunyn Schmiedebergs Arch. Pharmacol.*
    300: 163–177. (German)
Good, R., Müller, G. F. R. and Eugster, C. H. 1965. Isolation and characteriza-
    tion of premuscimol and muscazon from Amanita muscaria (L. ex Fr.).
    Helv. Chim. Acta 48: 927–930. (German)
Groves, J. W. 1964. Poisoning by morels when taken with alcohol. *Mycologia*
    56: 779.
Grzymala, S. 1961. Fatal poisoning by a pseudoedible species. III. Isolation of the
    toxic substance orellanine. *Roczniki Panstwowego Zakladu Hig.* 12: 491–498.
    (Polish)
Gusti, G. V. and Carnevale, A. 1974. A case of fatal poisoning by Gyromitra
    esculenta. *Arch. Toxicol.* 33: 49–54.
Hammerschmidt, D. E. 1980. Szechwan purpura. *N. Engl. J. Med.* 302: 1191–1193.
Hatfield, G. M. and Brady, L. R. 1968. Isolation of bis-noryangonin from Gymno-
    pilus decurrens. *Lloydia* 31: 225–228.
Hatfield, G. M. and Brady, L. R. 1969. Occurrence of bis-noryangonin in
    Gymnopilus spectabilis. *J. Pharm. Sci.* 58: 1298–1299.
Hegner, O. et al. 1970. Effect of phalloidin in Mg^2-ATPase (K^+-Na^+)ATPase and
    K-dependent p-nitrophenylphosphatase activity of plasma membrane isolated
    from rat liver. *Biochem. Pharmacol.* 19: 487–493.
Hendricks, H. V. 1940. Poisoning by false morel (Gyromitra esculenta); a report
    of fatal case. *J.A.M.A.* 114: 1625.
Henry, E. D. and Sullivan, G. 1969. Phytochemical evaluation of some
    cantharelloid fungi. *J. Pharm. Sci.* 58: 1497–1500.

Herbich, J., Lohwag, K. and Rotter, R. 1966. Fatal poisoning with the green cap mushroom. *Arch. Toxikol.* 21: 310–320. (German)

Herman, H. 1961. Identification of a metabolite of Clytocybe suaveolens as 4-methylnitrosaminobenzaldehyde. *Hoppe Seylers Z. Physiol. Chem.* 326: 13–16. (German)

Hesler, C. R. 1960. *Mushrooms of the Great Smokies*. University of Tennessee Press, Knoxville.

Hizukuri, S. and Larner, J. 1964. Studies on UDPG: α-1-4-Glucan α-4-glucosyl-transferase. VII. Conversion of the enzyme from glucose-6-phosphate-dependent to independent form in liver. *Biochemistry* 3: 1783–1788.

Hofmann, A. et al. 1959. Psilocybin and psilocin. Two psychotropically active principles of Mexican hallucienic fungus. *Helv. Chim Acta* 42: 1557–1572. (German)

Hofmann, A. and Troxler, F. 1963. *Esters of Indoles*. U.S. Patent 3,075,992 (To Sandoz Ltd.), Jan. 29.

Holmstedt, B. and Lindgren, J. 1967. Chemical constituents and pharmacology of South American snuffs. *Psychopharmacol. Bull.* 4: 16.

Hughes, D. W., Genest, K. and Rice, W. B. 1966. Occurrence of muscarine in Clitocybe dealbata. *Lloydia* 29: 328–332.

Ito, Y. et al. 1967. Naematolin, a new biologically active substance produced by Naematoloma fasciculare (Fr) karst. *Chem. Pharm. Bull. (Tokyo)* 15: 2009–2010.

Jacob, S. T., Sajdel, E. M. and Munroe, H. N. 1970. Different responses of soluble whole nuclear RNA polymerase and soluble nucleolar RNA polymerase to divalent cations and to inhibition by alpha-a-manitin. *Biochem. Biophys. Res. Commun.* 38: 765–770.

Kawamura, S. 1954. *Icones of Japanese Fungi*. Vol. IV. Kazamashobo, Tokyo.

Keinholz, J. R. 1934. Poisonous boletus from Oregon. *Mycologia* 26: 275–276.

Kingsbury, J. M. 1964. *Poisonous Plants of the United States and Canada*. Prentice-Hall, Englewood Cliffs, New Jersey.

Kögl, F., Duisberg, H. and Erxleben, H. 1931. Fungus poisons. I. Muscarine. *Ann. Chem.* 489: 156–192. (German)

Krieger, L. C. C. 1936. *The Mushroom Handbook*. Macmillan, New York.

Krieger, L. C. C. 1967. *The Mushroom Handbook*. Dover, New York.

Kubicka, J. 1969. Analysis of fatal mushroom poisoning treated with thioctic acid. *Cas. Lek. Cesk.* 108: 790–793. (Czechs)

Kubicka, J. and Alder, A. E. 1968. On the new method of treatment of poisoning caused by the green death cap mushroom. *Praxis* 57: 1304–1306. (German)

Leloir, L. F. and Goldenberg, S. H. 1960. Synthesis of glycogen from uridine diphosphate glucose in liver. *J. Biol. Chem.* 235: 919–923.

Leung, A. Y. and Paul, A. G. 1967. Baeocystin, a monomethyl analog of psilocybin from Psilocybe baeocystis saprophytic culture. *J. Pharm. Sci.* 56: 146.

Leung, A. Y. and Paul, A. G. 1968. Baeocystin and norbaeocystin: New analogs of psilocybin from Psilocybe baeocystis. *J. Pharm. Sci.* 57: 1667–1671.

Leung, A. Y., Smith, A. H. and Paul, A. G. 1965. Production of psilocybin in Psilocybe baeocystis saprophytic culture. *J. Pharm. Sci.* 54: 1576–1579.

Levenberg, B. 1964. Isolation and structure of agaritine, a γ-glutamyl-substituted arylhydrazine from Agaricaceae. *J. Biol. Chem.* 239: 2267–2273.

Lindell, T. J., Weinberg, F., Roeder, R. G. and Rutter, W. J. 1970. Specific inhibition of nuclear RNA polymerase II by alpha-amanitin. *Science* 170: 447–449.

List, P. H. and Luft, P. 1968. Gyromitrin, a poison from spring lorel. *Arch. Pharm. (Weinheim)* 301: 294–305. (German)

List, P. H. and Luft, P. 1969. Evidence and determination of gyromitrin in fresh lorel. *Arch. Pharm. (Weinheim)* 302: 143–146. (German)

Litten, W. 1975. The most poisonous mushrooms. *Sci. Am.* 232: 90–101.

Lough, J. and Kinnear, D. G. 1970. Mushroom poisoning in Canada: Report of a fatal case. *Can. Med. Assoc. J.* 102: 858–860.

Madaus, G. 1938. *Handbook of Biological Remedies.* Thieme, Leipzig. (German)

Malone, M. H., Robichaud, R. C., Tyler, V. E., Jr. and Brady, L. R. 1962. Relative muscarinic potency of thirty Inocybe species. *Lloydia* 25: 231–237.

Malone, M. H., Tyler, V. E., Jr. and Brady, L. R. 1967. Hippocratic screening of sixty-six species of higher fungi. *Lloydia* 30: 250–257.

Matschinsky, F. and Wieland, O. 1960. On serum changes and disorders of the mitochondrial function in experimental Phalloidin poisoning. *Biochem. Z.* 333: 33–47. (German)

McCawley, E. L., Brummett, R. E. and Dana, G. W. 1962. Convulsions from Psilocybe mushroom poisoning. *Proc. West. Pharmacol. Soc.* 5: 27–33.

McKenny, M. 1962. *The Savory Wild Mushroom.* University of Washington Press, Seattle.

Meilli, E. O., Frick, P. G. and Straub, P. W. 1970. Coagulation changes during massive hepatic necrosis due to Amanita phalloides poisoning with special reference to anti-hemophillic globulin. *Helv. Med. Acta* 35: 304–313.

Meyer, H. J. 1967. Pharmacology of kava. In: *Ethnopharmacologic Search for Psychoactive Drugs.* D. H. Efron (ed.). Public Health Service Publication No. 1645, U.S. Government Printing Office, Washington, D.C.

Meyer, U. 1966. *Cited by* T. Wieland and O. Wieland 1972. The toxic peptides of Amanita species. In: *Microbial Toxins Fungal Toxins.* Vol. VII. S. Kadis, A. Ciegler and S. J. Ayl (Editors). Academic Press, New York.

Miller, F. and Wieland, O. 1967. Electronmicroscopic investigation on the liver of mouse and rat following acute phalloidin poisoning. *Arch. Pathol. Anat. Physiol.* 343: 82–99. (German)

Mitchel, D. H. 1980. Amanita mushroom poisoning. *Ann. Rev. Med.* 31: 51–57.

Miyata, J. T., Tyler, V. E., Jr., Brady, L. R. and Malone, M. H. 1966. The occurrence of Norcaperatic acid in Cantharellus floccosus. *Lloydia* 29: 43–49.

Mortara, M. and Filipello, S. 1967. Mushroom poisoning caused by "Lepiota nelveola" Bres. *Minerva Med.* 58: 3628–3632. (Italian)

Myerson, A. 1981. Father dazed, drained after mushroom tragedy. *Lexington Herald,* June 30, p. 1, Lexington, Kentucky.

Nagel, D., Wallcave, L. and Toth, B. 1977. Formation of methylhydrazine from acetaldehyde N-methyl-N-formylhydrazone, a component of Gyromitra esculenta. *Cancer Res.* 37: 34–58.

Nakanishi, K. et al. 1963. Isolation of lampterol, an antitumor substance from Lampteromyces japonicus. *Nature* 197: 292.

Orr, R. T. and Orr, D. B. 1968. *Mushrooms and Other Common Fungi of Southern California.* University of California Press, Berkeley.

Orr, R. T. and Orr, D. B. 1979. *Mushrooms of Western North America.* University of California Press, Berkeley.

Peck, C. H. 1912. Report of the state botanist 1911. *Bull. N.Y. State Mus.* 157: 5–116.

Pilát, A. 1961. *Mushrooms and Other Fungi.* Nevill, London.

Pilát, A. and Usák, O. 1950. *Mushrooms.* Spring Books, London.

Pilát, A. and Ušák, O. 1954. *Mushrooms.* Bijl, Amsterdam.

Puchinger, H. and Wieland, T. 1969. Search for a metabolite following poisoning with desmethyl phalloin. *Eur. J. Biochem.* 11: 106.

Ramsbottom, J. 1953. *Poisonous Fungi.* Penguin, New York.

Rehbinder, D., Löffler, G., Wieland, O. and Wieland, T. 1963. Studies on the mechanism of the poisonous effect of phalloidin with poisons labelled with radioactive substances. *Hoppe Seylers Z. Physiol. Chem.* 331: 132–142. (German)

Reynolds, W. A. and Lowe, F. H. 1965. Mushrooms and a toxic reaction to alcohol: Report of four cases. *N. Engl. J. Med.* 272: 630—631.

Romagnesi, M. H. 1964. Toxic mushrooms from Japan. *Bull. Soc. Mycol. France* 80: 4—5. (French)

Rose, E. K. and Rieders, P. 1966. An episode of food poisoning attributed to imported mushroom. *Ann. Intern. Med. (N.S.)* 64: 372—377.

Sapieka, N. 1969. *Food Pharmacology.* Thomas, Springfield, Illinois.

Sapeika, N. and Stephens, E. L. 1965. Clitocybe toxica. A new species. *S. Afr. Med. J.* 39: 749—750.

Schmidlin-Meszaros, J. 1974. Gyromitrin in dried lorel (Gyromitra esculenta sicc). *Mitt Geb. Lebensmittel. Hyg.* 65: 453—465. (German)

Schmidt, J., Hartmann, W. and Weinstlin, A. 1971. Acute kidney failure due to immunohemolytic anemia following consumption of the mushroom Paxillus involutus. *Dtsch. Med. Wochenschr.* 96: 1188—1191. (German)

Short, A. L., Watling, R., MacDonald, N. K. and Robson, J. S. 1980. Poisoning by Cortinarius speciosissimus. *Lancet* 2: 942—944.

Siess, E., Wieland, O. and Miller, F. 1970. Electronmicroscopic study on the tolerance of newborn rat, mouse and hamster liver to phalloidin. *Virchows Arch. (Zell. Pathol.)* 6: 151—165. (German)

Silberbauer, S. F. and Mirvish, L. 1927. Notes on cases of gungus poisoning. *J. Med. Assoc. S. Afr.* 1: 549—553.

Simons, D. M. 1971. The mushroom toxins. *Del. Med. J.* 43: 177—187.

Singer, R. 1958. A Russula provoking hysteria in New Guinea. *Mycopathol. Mycol. Appl.* 9: 275—279.

Singer, R. 1961. *Mushrooms and Truffles.* Hill, London.

Singer, R. 1962. *The Agaricales in Modern Taxonomy.* 2nd ed. Cramer, Weinheim.

Smith, A. H. 1950. *Mushrooms in Their Natural Habitats.* Sawyer's, Portland.

Smith, A. H. 1958. *The Mushroom Hunter's Field Guide.* University of Michigan Press, Ann Arbor.

Smith, C. W. 1980. Mushroom poisoning by chlorophyllum molybdites in Hawaii. *Hawaii Med. J.* 39: 13—14.

Stein, S. I. 1958. I. An unusual effect from a species of Mexican mushroom Psilocybe cubensis. *Mycopathol. Mycol. Appl.* 9: 263—267.

Stein, S. I., Closs, G. L. and Gabel, N. W. 1959. Observations on psychoneurophysiologically significant mushroom. I. Clinical details pertaining to ingestion of Panaeolus venenosus, Psilocybe caerulescence mushrooms. *Mycopathol. Mycol. Appl.* 11: 205—216.

Sternberg, S. S. et al. 1963. Toxicological studies on calvacin. *Cancer Res.* 23: 1036—1044.

Stevenson, J. A. and Benjamin, C. R. 1961. Scleroderma poisoning. *Mycologia* 53: 438—439.

Tabor, G. and Vining, L. C. 1963. Pigments and other extractives from carpophores of Amanita muscaria. *Can. J. Botany* 41: 639—647.

Takemoto, T., Yokobe, T. and Nakajima, T. 1964a. Studies on the constituents of indigenous fungi. II. Isolation of the flycidal constituent from Amanita strobiliformis. *J. Pharm. Soc. Jpn.* 84: 1186—1188. (Japanese)

Takemoto, T., Nakajima, T. and Sakuma, P. 1964b. Isolation of a flycidal constituent "ibotenic acid" from Amanita muscaria and A. pantherina. *J. Pharm. Soc. Jpn.* 84: 1233—1234. (Japanese)

Tanghe, L. J. and Simons, D. M. 1973. Amanita phalloides in the Eastern United States. *Mycologia* 65: 99—108.

Toth, B. 1972. Hydrazine, methylhydrazine and methylhydrazine sulfate carcinogenesis in Swiss mice. failure of ammonium hydroxide to interfere in the development of tumors. *Int. J. Cancer* 9: 105—118.

Toth, B. 1979a. Hepatocarcinogenesis by hydrazine mycotoxins of edible mushrooms. *J. Toxicol. Environ. Health* 5: 193–202.

Toth, B. 1979b. Mushroom hydrazines: Occurrence, metabolism, carcinogenesis and environmental implications. In: *Naturally Occurring Carcinogens—Mutagens and Modulators of Carcinogenesis.* E. C. Miller et al. (eds.). University Park Press, Baltimore.

Toth, B. 1979c. 1-Acetyl-2-phenylhydrazine carcinogenesis in mice. *Br. J. Cancer* 39: 584–587.

Toth, B. and Nagel, D. 1978. Tumors induced in mice by N-methyl-N-formyl-hydrazine of the false morel Gyromitra esculenta. *J. Natl. Cancer Inst.* 60: 201–204.

Toth, B. and Patil, K. 1979. Carcinogenic effects in the Syrian golden hamster of N-methyl-N-formylhydrazine of the false morel Gyromitra esculenta. *J. Cancer Res. Clin. Oncol.* 93: 109–121.

Toth, B. and Patil, K. 1980. The tumorigenic effect of low dose levels of N-methyl-N-formylhydrazine in mice. *Neoplasma* 27: 25–31.

Toth, B. and Shimizu, H. 1973. Methylhydrazine tumorigenesis in Syrian golden hamsters and the morphology of malignant histiocytomas. *Cancer Res.* 33: 2744–2753.

Toth, B., Tompa, A. and Patil, K. 1977. Tumorigenic effects of 4-methylphenyl-hydrazine in Swiss mice. *Z. Krebsforsch. Klin. Onkol.* 89: 245–252.

Toth, B. et al. 1978. Tumor induction with the N'-acetyl derivative of 4-hydroxy-methylphenylhydrazine, a metabolite of agaritine of Agaricus bisporus. *Cancer Res.* 38: 177–180.

Toth, B., Patil, K., Erickson, J. and Kupper, R. 1979. False morel mushroom Gyromitra esculenta toxin: N-methyl-N-formylhydrazine carcinogenesis in mice. *Mycopathologia* 68: 121–128.

Turner, W. J. and Merlis, S. 1959. Effect of some indole alkylamines on man. *A.M.A. Arch. Neurol. Psychiatr.* 81: 121–129.

Tyler, V. E., Jr. 1961. Indole derivatives in certain North American mushrooms. *Lloydia* 24: 71–74.

Tyler, V. E., Jr. 1963. Poisonous mushrooms. *Prog. Chem. Toxicol.* 1: 339–384.

Tyler, V. E., Jr. and Groger, D. 1964. Amanita alkaloids. II. Amanita citrina and Amanita porphyria. *Planta Med.* 12: 397–402.

Tyler, V. E., Jr. and Smith, A. H. 1963. Chromatographic detection of Amanita toxins in Galerina venenata. *Mycologia* 55: 358–359.

Tyler, V. E., Jr. et al. 1963. Chromatographic and pharmacologic evaluation of some toxic Galerina species. *Lloydia* 26: 154–157.

Tyler, V. E., Jr., Benedict, G. R., Brady, L. R. and Robbers, J. E. 1966. Occurrence of Amanita toxins in American collections of deadly Amanitas. *J. Pharm. Sci.* 55: 590–593.

United States Department of Agriculture, Crop Reporting Board. 1976. *Mushrooms.* Vg. 2-1-2, pp. 1-4. U.S.D.A. Statistical Reporting Service, Washington, D.C.

Verhulst, H. L. 1969. Information to and from poison control centers. *J. Chem. Doc.* 9: 71–73.

Waser, P. G. 1967. The pharmacology of Amanita muscaria. *Psychopharmacol. Bull.* 4: 19–20.

Watt, J. M. and Breyer-Brandwijk, M. G. 1962. *Medicinal and Poisonous Plants of Southern and Eastern Africa.* Livingstone, Edinburgh.

Weber, T. 1980. Mushroom poisoning. *Lancet* 2 (pt. 1): 640.

Weidmann, H., Taeschler, M. and Konzett, H. 1958. The pharmacology of psilocybin, an active principle from Psilocybe mexicana Heim. *Experientia* 14: 378–379. (German)

Wieland, O. 1965. Changes in liver metabolism induced by the poisons of Amanita phalloides. *Clin. Chem. (Suppl.)* 11: 323–338.

Wieland, T. 1968a. Poisonous principles of mushrooms of the genus Amanita. *Science* 159: 946–952.

Wieland, T. 1968b. Chemical and toxicological properties of Amanita poisons. *Cienc. Cult. (São Paulo)* 20: 3—11.

Wieland, T. and Buku, A. 1968. Components of Amanita phalloides. XXXVIII. Constitution of Σ-amanitine and amanullin. *Justus Liebigs Ann. Chem.* 717: 215—220. (German)

Wieland, T. and Dose, K. 1954. Changes in the protein partitioning in blood serum in amanitine poisoning. *Biochem. Z.* 325: 439—447. (German)

Wieland, T. and Jeck, R. 1968. Components of green Amanita. XXXV. Conversion of phalloidine to similarly poisonous deoxydimethylphalloine (norphalloine). *Ann. Chem.* 713: 196—200. (German)

Wieland, T. and Motzel, W. 1953. On the isolation of bufotenin from the yellow cap mushroom. *Ann. Chem.* 581: 10—16. (German)

Wieland, T. and Rehbinder, D. 1963. ^{35}S-Labelling and chemical transformations at a side chain of phalloidin. *Ann. Chem.* 670: 149—157. (German)

Wieland, O. and Szabados, A. 1968. *On the Nature of Phalloidin Tolerance in New-born Rats. Advances in Clinico-Biochemical Research.* Vol. 4. Sixth International Congress of Clinical Chemistry, 1966. Karger, Basel.

Wieland, T. and Wieland, O. 1959. Chemistry and toxicology of the toxins of Amanita phalloides. *Pharmacol. Rev.* 11: 87—107.

Wieland, T. and Wieland, O. 1972. The toxic peptides of Amanita species. In: *Microbial Toxins Fungal Toxins.* Vol. VIII. S. Kadis, A. Ciegler and S. J. Ajl (eds.). Academic Press, New York.

Wieland, T., Schiefer, H. and Gebert, U. 1966. Poisons from Amanita verna. *Naturwissenchaften* 53: 39—40. (German)

Wilkinson, S. 1961. The history of chemistry of muscarine. *Qu. Rev. (Lond.)* 15: 153—171.

Zaffiri, O., Centi, R. and Mastroianni, A. 1970. High doses of thioctic acid in the therapy of acute Amanita phalloides poisoning. *Minerva Anest.* 36: 56—57.

Zulik, R., Bako, F. and Kisban, A. 1973. On the treatment of death-cap poisoning. *Med. Klin.* 68: 1371—1372. (German)

11

Toxicology of Marine Foods

Humans have always depended on the sea to provide part of their food supply. Yet, the full potential of the sea as a source of food has yet to be realized. The countless species of marine life potentially can provide humans a seemingly inexhaustible supply of food, but there remains the question as to which of the unexploited species can, in fact, be used as food. There is a pressing need to explore this question thoroughly, for the increasing demand for food, particularly proteinaceous products, by an exploding world population will unavoidably lead humankind more and more toward the sea.

Yet, danger lurks in this seemingly inexhaustible food supply, since many marine species are known to be poisonous, and even violently so and lethal. Therefore, an exploitation of the full food potential of the sea must consider above all else the toxicological properties of marine products. In so doing, it might be possible to catalog marine species into three broad toxicological categories: (1) those inherently nontoxic; (2) those which are toxic some of the time; and (3) those that are inherently toxic. Of particular interest is the second category. For it is in this group that a large degree of uncertainty will exist. Greater attention, therefore, will be directed to this group.

The realization of our expectations of the sea as a bountiful source of food will depend on our understanding of the mechanisms which render many inherently nontoxic marine species poisonous during certain times.

The third category will entail basically the problem of identification of toxic species. A knowledge of toxic species would lead to only two courses of action: (1) complete or selective avoidance; or (2) seeking of means of detoxification. Selective avoidance implies that not all members of a family of marine species are toxic; it also means that in toxic species only certain tissues or organs are toxic. Thus, with this knowledge, it may be possible to selectively separate the toxic from the nontoxic parts.

Seeking a means of detoxification implies knowledge of the identity of the toxin — its physical, chemical, and biological properties and its mode of action. At times, the means of detoxification may have to be discovered or developed empirically, particularly if the nature of the toxin is unknown. Developing detoxificiation mechanisms applies also to the second group of marine species.

The discussion in this chapter, naturally, will deal only with the second and third broad toxicological categories as identified in the preceding paragraph.

Since ancient times, six major groups of marine life comprise the primary food sources for humans from the sea, i.e., mollusks, arthropods, fish, reptiles, mammals, and green, brown, and red algae. A miscellaneous group which includes echinoderms also are used as food by some population groups. The toxic factors in each of these groups except the miscellaneous group will be discussed in the following sections.

MOLLUSKS

It is estimated that there are at least 45,000 living species of mollusks (phylum Mollusca) divided into six classes: (1) Amphineura (chitons); (2) Cephalopoda (cuttle fish, nautili, octopi, and squid); (3) Gastropoda (snails and slugs with single valves); (4) Pelecypoda (bivalves — clams, oysters, and scallops); and (5) Scaphopoda (tooth, or tusk, shells). The sixth class, Monoplacophora, comprises sea mollusks having limpet-like shells (Meglitsch 1967). The species in this class, together with the chitons and tooth, or tusk, shells, probably have little if any food toxicological significance. Thus, the discussion will be limited to the other three classes. A detailed description of the characteristics of species in these classes is outside the scope of this book. The reader is referred to the work of Halstead and Courville (1965) or any textbook on marine zoology.

Cephalopods

There are 15 species of cephalopods reported to be poisonous or venomous: one species of squid, *Ommastrephes sloani pacificus* (Kawabata et al. 1957); three species of cuttlefish, *Sepia esculenta, S. officinalis,* and *Loligo vulgaris* (Pawlowsky 1927); and 11 species of octopi, Eledone spp. Octopus spp., and Hapalochlaena sp (Anastasi and Erspamer 1963; Berry and Halstead 1954; Halstead and Courville 1965; Kawabata et al. 1957; McMichael 1963; Pawlowsky 1927; Trethewie 1965). These various species may have different geographical distributions, with one or more species predominating in specific areas. So far, most poisonings due to squid and octopi have been reported only in Japan. For example, between 1952 and 1955 inclusive, there were 757 outbreaks of squid (Ommastrephis spp.) poisoning, involving 2649 persons with 10 deaths reported. In the summer of 1955, 21 outbreaks of octopus poisoning (Kawabata et al. 1957) also occurred in that country. The toxicity of the squid was demonstrated by volunteer experiments; 15 out of the 50 people who took part in the experiment became ill. The symptoms of poisoning occurred after 10 to 20 hr following consumption of toxic cephalopod. The predominant clinical signs were nausea, vomiting, abdominal pain, diarrhea, fever (up to 39°C), chills, headache, severe dehydration, and weakness. Three patients out of 758 developed paralysis; three others had convulsions. In general, only severe gastrointestinal symptoms were observed. Recovery occurred within 48 hr. Bacteriological involvement in these symptoms was ruled out. Histamine or similar substances were not involved.

The toxic substance(s) in poisonous cephalopods has not been determined. However, the salivary glands of *Octopus apollyon* and *O. bimaculatus* contain octapamine, serotonin, histamine, and dopamine, and possibly other amines (Hartman et al. 1960). In addition, an endecapeptide, eledoisin, has been isolated from the posterior salivary glands of the octopi *Eledone moschata* and *E. aldrovandi* (Anastasi and Erspamer 1962, 1963).

$$H-Pyr-Pro-Ser-Lys-Asp(OH)-Ala-Ile-Gly-Leu-Met-NH_2$$

Eledoisin

Eledoisin is completely inactivated by chymotrypsin by cleaving the phenylalanine-isoleucine and leucine-methioninamide bonds. Trypsin partially inactivates eledoisin (Anastasi and Erspamer 1962). Trypsin also inactivates cephalotoxin, which is heat labile (Ghiretti 1960).

Another active protein, cephalotoxin, has been isolated from the saliva and salivary glands of cuttlefish and a few species of octopi (Ghiretti 1959, 1960).

These substances are pharmacologically active. The amines have strong pressor activity as well as effects on the gastrointestinal tract. Eledoisin has hypotensive action, producing a drop in systemic blood pressure in the dog with subcutaneous doses of 10 to 100 μg. Even lower doses of eledoisin can induce hypotension when administered intravenously (Erspamer and Glässer 1963). With subcutaneous doses of 10 to 100 μg/kg, the peptide can also increase gastrointestinal motility in unanesthetized dogs (Erspamer and Erspamer 1962). Other effects produced by this peptide include constriction of the bronchial muscles of the guinea pig, contraction of isolated uterus and colon of rabbit with doses of about 0.001 ng/ml (Erspamer and Erspamer 1962), and contraction of rabbit uterus in situ following intravenous injection of 0.01 to 1.0 μg/kg (Sturmer and Berde 1963).

In humans, 1 ng produces dermal pain, edema, and erythema; these symptoms are indicative of its effects on permeability mechanisms (DeCaro 1963). Doses of about 3 to 30 ng/kg produce in humans arterial hypotension, increased rate of respiration, and vasodilation of the skin, particularly in the region of the head, and spinal fluid hypertension. When the dosage is increased to 200 to 300 ng/kg, hot flushes of the face, throbbing headache, increased rate of respiration, intestinal hyperperistalsis, and prolonged hypotension lasting 10 to 20 min are produced (Sicuteri et al. 1963; Shapiro et al. 1963).

The subcutaneous LD_{50} of eledoisin in dogs is 150 to 300 μg/kg (Erspamer and Anastasi 1962).

The observed effects of eledoisin in humans and animals may indicate that the toxic agent in oral cephalopod poisonings might have been this peptide. However, one has to assume that this toxin escapes inactivation by chymotrypsin in the gastrointestinal tract. This possibility is not at all remote, since variability in digestive function in individuals can occur. Poisonings due to ingestion of certain protein toxins are known to occur in many instances; e.g., bacterial toxins (Chap. 14) and certain plant proteins or peptides (Chap. 8).

The octopi are probably more notorious for their venomous bites. This may have little food toxicological significance except that one species, *Hapalochlaena maculosa*, the small blue-ringed octopus found commonly along the coast of Australia, potentially can cause serious human poisoning. Its venom, which has caused human fatalities (Lane and Sutherland 1967), contains a toxin, maculotoxin, which is similar pharmacologically to tetrodotoxin (Freeman 1976), the poison in puffer fish. Sheumack et al. (1977) have established by means of thin-layer chromatography and proton nuclear magnetic resonance spectroscopy, that maculotoxin and tetrodotoxin are one and the same. The biological activity of tetrodotoxin is discussed in connection with puffer fish later in this chapter.

This observation adds additional significance, since some cases of octopus poisoning have shown paralytic symptoms (Kawabata et al. 1957). Whether tetrodotoxin is also found in other species of octopi is not known.

Gastropods

The gastropods that have been reported to be poisonous include species in the following families: whelks — Buccinum spp. and Neptunea spp. (Asano and Ito 1959, 1960; Fange 1958, 1960; Halstead and Courville 1965; Kanna and Hirai 1956; Whittaker 1960); triton — *Argobuccinum oregonense* (Asano and Ito 1959); murex — Murex spp. (Erspamer and Benati 1953; Emerson and Taft 1945); dogwinkle — Thais spp. (Whittaker 1960); top shells — Livona pica (Arcisz 1950; Gudger 1930); sea hares — Aplysia spp. (Winkler and Tilton 1962; Winkler et al. 1962; Yamamura and Hirata 1963); and abalone — Haliotis spp. (Hashimoto and Tsutsumi 1961; Hashimoto et al. 1960). These species have worldwide distribution, with certain species predominating in geographical zones.

Whelks and Triton

Whelks and triton are carnivorous marine snails with shells, and are found not only in tropical and temperate waters, but also in circumpolar seas. Their habitat extends from littoral to deep zones, on rocks, mud, sand, or gravel. They clamber or plough with their large fleshy feet through their substrates. When at rest or disturbed, the foot is retracted and the mouth of the shell is shut by a horny operculum. These marine snails are also noted for their attractive shells, which come in a variety of sizes, shapes, and colors (Halstead and Courville 1965).

Whelks are widely eaten in Europe and in Asia (Halstead and Courville 1965). While no outbreaks of poisoning have been reported in Europe, such poisonings have been reported in Japan. Two species of Japanese whelks, *Neptunea arthritica* (Asano 1952) and *N. intersculpta* (Kanna and Hirai 1956), have been involved in such poisonings. The principal symptoms of whelk poisoning in humans include intense headache, dizziness, nausea, and vomiting. In mice, the toxic symptoms include salivation, lacrimation, miosis, increased peristalsis, motor paralysis, respiratory failure, and death. Oral toxicity is one-fifth to one-tenth of parenteral toxicity (Asano and Ito 1959, 1960).

The poison in whelks has been found to be concentrated in the salivary glands, and poisoning occurs when these glands are eaten in whole shellfish, whether raw, cooked, or canned (Asano 1952; Asano and Ito 1959, 1960).

The toxic principle isolated from the salivary glands of the whelks *N. arthritica, N. intersculpta,* and *N. antiqua* is tetramine, a curarelike compound. The first two species contain 3 to 9 mg tetramine/g of gland (Asano and Ito 1960); in the latter, the compound constitutes about 1% of the net weight of the gland (Fange 1960). The structure of tetramine is shown in Figure 11.1.

Tetramine produces nausea, vomiting, anorexia, weakness, fatigue, dryness of the mouth, faintness, dizziness, photophobia, impaired vision, and disturbance in intestinal motility, resulting in diarrhea or constipation; paralytic ileus also is observed. Many of these effects are due to hypotension and decreased cardiac output because of peripheral vagus stimulation and peripheral vasomotor depression. Intravenous injection of tetramine results in temporary respiratory paralysis, probably due to the curarelike autonomic ganglionic blockage, such as in the phrenic nerve (Asano and Ito 1960; Halstead and Courville 1965).

The amount of poison in the salivary gland of the whelk varies depending on the season, being lowest in September and highest in mid-July (Asano and Ito 1959, 1960).

Tetramine also has been isolated from the triton *Argobuccinum oregonese* at concentrations similar to those in the Japanese whelks (Asano and Ito 1959).

Murex

The murices, or rock shells, are found in tropical and temperate waters, in shallow tidal zones, to depths of 50 fathoms or more. They are carnivorous and can feed on oysters by boring into the oyster shells. The murex produces a colorless or yellowish fluid from the hypobranchial gland, the so-called purple gland. This fluid changes to violet or purple when exposed to sunlight. This gland also produces murexine (urocanylcholine) (Erspamer and Benati 1953) (Fig. 11.1). Other active compounds, such as senecioylcholine (isovalerylcholine), also has been isolated from the purple gland of the murex *Thais floridana* (Whittaker 1960). This gland also yields serotonin (Erspamer 1956).

Extracts of the hypobranchial gland of *Murex trunculus* produce a curarelike action on various invertebrates and nonmammalian vertebrates. The effect consists of agitation followed by muscular paralysis and sometimes death (Jullien and Ripplinger 1950). In white mice, the subcutaneous LD_{100} has been found to be 300 mg/kg; the intravenous LD_{100} is one-tenth to one-twentieth of this value. Death results from asphyxia, which is followed by fascicular and fibrillar contraction in almost all muscles. The degree of toxicity of murexine oxalate has been shown to be three to five times greater in rats than in mice, and 10 times greater in rabbits (Erspamer 1948a-c). Thus, murexine is a paralytic agent of the skeletal muscles in both invertebrates and vertebrates. It is characterized by marked neuromuscular blocking and nicotinic activity,

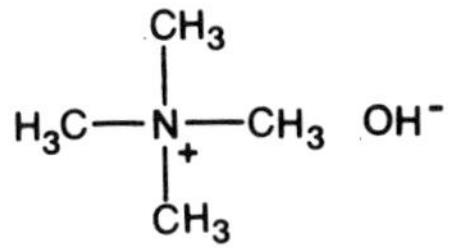

Tetramine

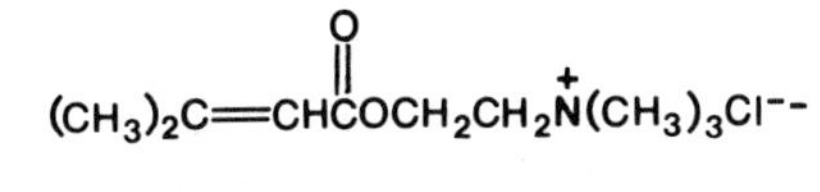

Senecioylcholine chloride

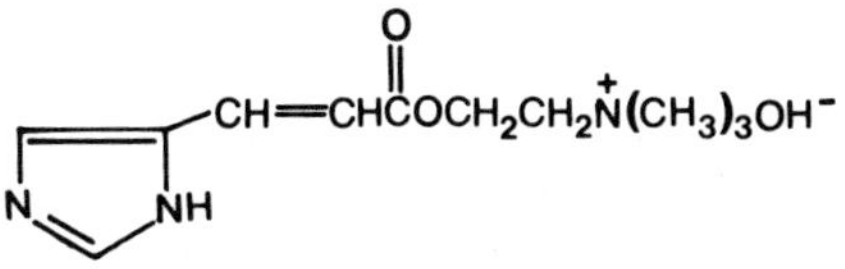

Murexine

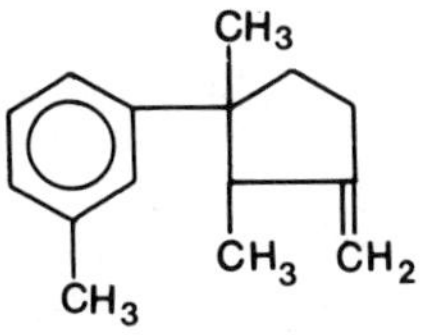

Laurene

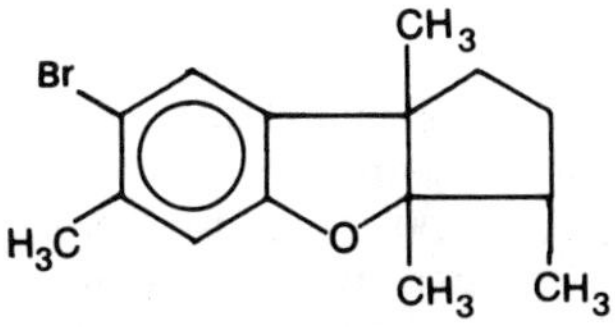

Aplysin

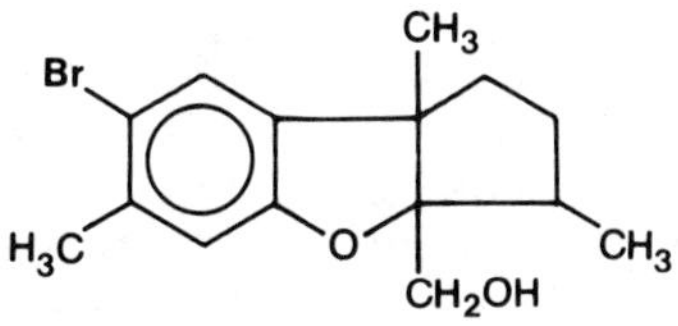

Aplysinol

Figure 11.1 Structures of toxic substances in certain marine gastropods.

but almost without muscarinic effects. The toxin appears to produce depolarization similar to the effect of suxamethonium (Erspamer and Glässer 1957).

In humans, murexine produces muscle relaxation of short duration. Muscular paralysis in humans lasting 3 to 6 min occurs maximally in 45 to 60 sec following a dose of 1.0 to 1.2 mg/kg administered intravenously. Muscular fasciculation always precedes and then follows muscular paralysis. Hypersalivation, which can be controlled by atropine, and moderate hypertension have been frequently observed; persistent pharyngeal and laryngeal reflexes, lacrimation, and sweating also have been noted (Ciocatto et al. 1956; DeBlasi and Leone 1955).

Cases of human poisoning following eating Murex species are extremely rare, if not nonexistent, even though several species are commonly eaten, especially in Europe (Rogers 1951). Only one serious outbreak with five fatalities was reported at the beginning of this century in which 43 persons in the area around the Gulf of Trieste were poisoned following consumption of *Murex brandaris* (Plumert 1902). The symptoms of murex poisoning in man as reported by Charnot (1947) include gastroenteritis, pruritus, convulsions, and sometimes death. The paucity, if not absence, of reports on murex poisoning in recent times does not mean no such poisoning occurs. It may simply mean, as in many types of foodborne poisonings, that mild to moderate cases remain undetected.

Top Shells

Top shells are abundant in tropical seas, and the shells are widely used for ornamental purposes. Their vernacular name is descriptive of the form or shape of the shell. The West Indian top shell, *Livona pica*, is a popular food item in southeastern Florida, the West Indies, and Central America. Both littoral and deep-sea forms of top shells exist. The West Indian top shells can be found abundantly on rocks and coral reefs near the shore (Halstead and Courville 1965). Arcisz (1950) has mentioned the fact that at certain times during the year, this mollusk becomes poisonous, producing indigestion and nervous disorders. It is believed that the poison is of algal origin, the mollusk being an algae feeder.

Sea Hares

Sea hares are found in coastal waters from shallow tidal zones to deeper zones of up to 40 fathoms. They are omnivorous, and are found on sea bottoms covered with algae and eel grass, feeding mostly on seaweed (Winkler and Dawson 1963).

There are many writers who maintain that the sea hares are deadly poisonous, and that in ancient times these mollusks were used in murders and political assassinations. Yet, in spite of these claims, the harmful effects of sea hares to humans have not been confirmed in modern times (Halstead and Courville 1965).

However, animal studies have established the toxicity of secretions from a number of species of Aplysia. Winkler (1961) has determined the intraperitoneal LD_{50} in mice, in terms of the weight of the digestive gland of *A. californica* and *A. vaccaria;* the values obtained for two separate batches of Aplysia were 2.8 mg/g and 3.6 mg/g of mouse, respectively. In 3-day-old chicks, the values obtained were one-fourth the value in mice. The oral LD_{50} in mice was 12 times the intraperitoneal LD_{50}.

Following oral administration, the signs and symptoms of Aplysia poisoning in mice include immediate hyperventilation, drooping of the ears, hyperactivity, muscular twitchings, ataxia, loss of motor coordination, hypersalivation, relaxation of the bladder sphincter muscles, respiratory paralysis, and death.

A water-soluble, heat-stable toxin which is also soluble in aqueous acetone has been isolated from the digestive gland of *A. californica* and *A. vaccaria*. The toxin is called aplysin. In *A. kurodai*, aplysinol has been isolated in addition to aplysin. It seems that these toxins may have been derived from the algae on which the sea hares feed, since aplysin, debromoaplysin, and aplysinol also have been isolated from the alga *Laurencia okamurai*, a possible food source of *A. kurodai*. This mollusk definitely feeds on *Laurencia glandulifera,* which produces a sequiterpene hydrocarbon, laurene; this compound is considered to be the precursor of aplysin and aplysinol. The structures of these compounds are shown in Figure 11.1.

Aplysin, given by means of a stomach tube, produces the same symptoms in mice as the extracts of the digestive organs of Aplysia species. This toxin produces paralysis when injected into frogs; after the short paralytic period, relaxation follows, then a deathlike coma ensues which lasts for several hours. Recovery is complete after 20 hr. In 3-day-old chicks, aplysin produces hyperventilation, hypersalivation, respiratory arrest and death, as in mice, except that convulsions are also present (Winkler 1961).

In anesthetized dogs, aplysin injected intravenously causes immediate hypotension which returns to normal rapidly if given in small doses. The heart rate also becomes irregular, but rapidly recovers. Respiration may be stimulated at first, but then becomes depressed. The smooth muscles of the rabbit intestine develop spasms, and peristalsis can be temporarily stopped following treatment with aplysin. This toxin has other pharmacological effects, particularly in the skeletal muscles and the nervous system of vertebrates (Winkler et al. 1962). About 1% of the administered dose of aplysin in the rat is excreted unchanged; this indicates that metabolic degradation and/or retention in the body does occur (Winkler et al. 1962).

All these effects indicate that aplysin is a highly toxic compound with distinct pharmacological activity. There are no available records of the extent of human consumption of sea hares. Their long-standing notoriety as poisonous mollusks may discourage widespread consumption. This fact may account, in part, for the rarity of reported cases of human poisoning due to sea hares. In addition, it is also possible that the sea hares are transvectors of poisonous compounds from algae, such as Laurencia spp. (Irie et al. 1965). If so, the toxicity of Aplysia may be variable and dependent on the type of algae on which the mollusks feed.

Abalones

The abalones are rock-clinging mollusks found in outer surf-beaten coastal areas free from loose sand or mud. Their distribution is generally over zones encompassing the low and high tidal range. The outer shell of the mollusk is covered by a rough and tough horny layer. The interior of the shell is irridescent; thus, abalone shells are used as a source of mother-of-pearl in the manufacture of ornaments, buttons, and trinkets. The abalones are vegetarians, feeding largely on algae and plankton. Some species of abalone may attain lengths of up to 30 cm or more. They have a powerful muscular foot, which is the only part of the mollusk eaten in many places (Barnes 1963; Ricketts and Calvin 1952).

In Oriental countries, the entire tissues of the mollusk, including the viscera, are consumed. This practice has resulted in serious intoxications. In Japan, two species, *Haliotis discus* and *H. sieboldi*, have been incriminated in several outbreaks of poisoning. The viscera of the abalone contains a toxin which induces photosensitization (p. 517). Thus, only those parts of the body exposed to sunlight develop urticarialike reactions; in which case, the victim feels a prickling sensation in the skin which itches, becomes erythematous, edematous, and ulcerated (Hashimoto and Tsutsumi 1961; Hashimoto et al. 1960). Abalone photosensitization or photodynamism is a rare example of this type of poisoning caused by a food derived from animal sources.

Animals fed abalone livers and viscera show lacrimation, salivation, convulsions, paralysis, and death in about 30 min after exposure to sunlight, especially highly sensitive animals (Hashimoto and Tsutsumi 1961).

The toxic compound in the digestive gland of *Haliotis discus* reportedly is a pigment which closely resembles chemically pyropheophorbide A. This pigment is chemically similar to chlorophyll. The photosensitizing agent in abalone is soluble in many organic solvents and is fairly heat stable (Hashimoto 1967; Hashimoto and Tsutsumi 1961). It remains active even after 10 months of storage at -15 to $-20^{\circ}C$. The toxin is not affected by high concentrations of NaCl. Extracts containing the toxin are dark greenish brown and their photoactivity is suggested by the intense red fluorescence under ultraviolet light or sunlight. The toxin is believed to be derived from Desmarestia spp., a seaweed on which abalones feed (Hashimoto et al. 1960).

Pelecypods

Pelecypods are a class of mollusks consisting of the bivalves; i.e., clams, oysters, scallops, mussels, and the like. The shells consist of two lateral valves, mostly symmetrical, with a dorsal ligament which serves as the hinge, and one or two adductor muscles which close and open the valves. There is also a mantle consisting of right and left lobes whose margins form the posterior siphons. These siphons control the flow of water into the mantle cavity. The hatchet-shaped foot gives the mollusk locomotion. The estimated number of living species of pelecypods is 11000 (Halstead and Courville 1965).

The bivalves probably are the most popular among the mollusks in terms of worldwide consumption. As such, they also rank first among mollusks, even presently, as agents of human poisonings.

Several types of toxins carried by pelecypods are known. These poisons may be classified into broad categories on the basis of their origin or sources. They are:

(1) intrinsic toxicants, represented by callistin in the shellfish *Callista brevisiphonata* (Asano 1954; Asano et al. 1950, 1953), and possibly the hemolytic agent and agglutinin in *Saxidomus giganteus* and others; and (2) naturally occurring inorganic and biological contaminants. Naturally occurring inorganic contaminants are discussed in Chapter 18. The bacterial contaminants are discussed in Chapters 15 and 16. Other biological contaminants discussed in this chapter consist of products of toxic dinoflagellates, algae, and other marine life. The toxins from dinoflagellates are among the most potent toxins known.

Paralytic Shellfish Toxins (PSTs) — Saxitoxin and Related Poisons

At certain times during the year, the sea in many parts of the world suddenly may become yellow, brown, or reddish brown. The reddish hue, which is particularly noticeable in stark contrast to the natural blue-green of the oceans, is due to the xanthophyll peridinin, a carotenoid which is present in dinoflagellates (Shimizu 1978; Strain et al. 1971). The discoloration of the sea coincides with the maximal growth or "bloom" of certain types of plankton, or dinoflagellates. The reddish brown discoloration of the sea is often referred to as the "red tide," "red water," or "red current," and is frequently associated with considerable mortality of fish and other animals in the region. The water assumes the reddish hue when the plankton concentration reaches 20,000 cells/ml or more; this cell concentration may reach as high as 50,000 cells/ml (Schantz 1971).

At night, the red tide may become luminescent owing to the presence of another dinoflagellate, Noctoluca, which frequently accompanies the toxic species, *Gonyaulax catenella* (Carson 1951). The Indians along the Pacific coast recognized the significance of this luminescence and avoided eating the shellfish in the area as well as warned unsuspecting travelers about the toxicity of the mollusks during this period.

The red tide obviously is not a modern phenomenon. The earliest reference to this occurrence is made in the Old Testament (Exodus 7:20–21), where it is stated that the rivers in Egypt had turned into "blood" (Hayes and Austin 1951). Ancient writers referred to the sea of the coast of Arabia as the "red sea," possibly because of the frequent plankton blooms in the area (Brongensma-Sanders 1957). References to the red tide have appeared in many reports from ancient times up to the present.

Many species of dinoflagellates may cause the red tide. Unfortunately, several of these species produce toxic substances. However, so far, only five species (Fig. 11.2) have been identified as producers of very potent paralytic poisons which are transvected by many species of mollusks, particularly the pelecypods. These toxic dinoflagellate species, besides *G. catenella* (Schantz 1960, 1961; Sommer et al. 1937) are: *G. tamarensis* (Prakash 1961; Provasoli 1962; Schantz 1961); *G. acatenella* (Prakash and Taylor 1966); *Gymnodinium* spp. (Sapeika 1958)*; and *Pyrodinium phoneus* Anderson 1960; Medcof et al. 1947; Provasoli 1962). These species are shown in Figure 1, 2.

G. catanella abounds along the North Pacific coasts from central California to Japan; *G. acatenella* has been observed along the Pacific coast of North America, particularly along British Columbia; *G. tamarensis* is the Atlantic counterpart, and is found to infest the waters along the eastern coast of North America, Great Britain, and other parts of Northern Europe (Shimizu 1978). Gymnodinium spp. have been reported to thrive along the coast of South Africa and the Gulf of Mexico *(G. breve)* (Davis 1947) and the English Channel *(G. veneficum)* (Abbott and Ballantine 1957). *Pyrodinium phoneus* is the European variety thriving along the coast of Belgium. There are, of course, many other species of toxic dinoflagellates that may produce toxins that also may be dangerous to humans, but as yet, they have not been linked to human intoxications (Halstead and Courville 1965; Schantz 1971).

---

*The revised name of the genus is Ptychodiscus (Steidinger 1979). However, because of long time familiar usage, the term Gymnodinium will be retained in this book.

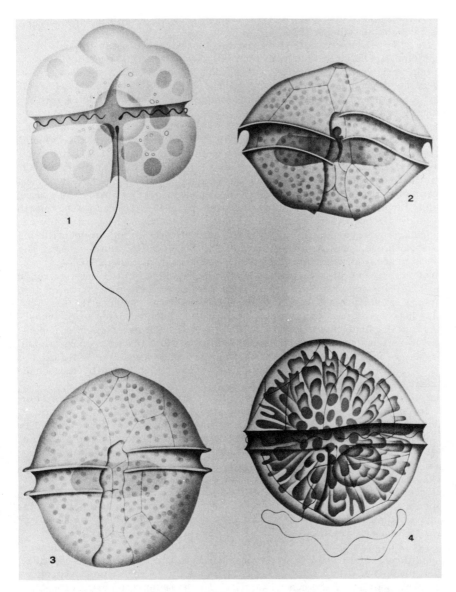

Figure 11.2 Toxic dinoflagellates frequently implicated in paralytic and neurotoxic shellfish poisoning. 1. *Gymnodinium brevis* (x 1800). 2. *Gonyaulax catanella* (x 1800). 3. *Gonyaulax tamarensis* (x 1500). 4. *Pyrodinium phoneus* (x 2000). (From Halstead, B. W. 1965. *Poisonous and Venomous Marine Animals of the World* Vol. 1; used with permission. Photographs by R. Kreuzinger.)

As already implied earlier, the red tide is always associated with increasing toxicity of pelecypods (Needler 1949; Prakash 1963). However, records of paralytic shellfish poisoning were not published until the latter part of the seventeenth century. The most notable historical reference to this kind of poisoning in North America was made by Captain George Vancouver, who described the poisoning of his crew members by muscles ([sic] mussels) found in one of the coves in Fitzhugh Sound during the early explorations of the Pacific Northwest in June 1793. A crew member died 5.5 hr after breakfasting on toxic mussels.

Apparently, the pelecypods bathed by the sea "in red tide" absorb the poison from the toxic dinoflagellates without being harmed themselves. The organs of the shellfish contain variable amounts of toxin depending on the species. In mussels, or Mytilus, the greatest amount is in the digestive organs or "liver" (Medcof et al. 1947; Meyer 1953); in the soft-shell clams (Mya spp.) and in the bar clams (Mactra spp.), the gills are more laden with poison (Medcof et al. 1947). The siphons in the Alaskan butter clams (Saxidomus spp.) are the primary binding site for the toxin (Chambers and Magnusson 1950; Pugsley 1939; Schantz et al. 1957). The amounts in the siphons, however, vary from month-to-month, in contrast to the concentration in the other parts of the clam. The concentrations in the other tissues are fairly constant. Seasonal changes in the distribution of the toxin in the various organs of the soft-shell clams have also been noted. More poison is found in the digestive organs during the summer, and in the gills during the fall and winter (Medcof et al. 1947). This suggests that the gills can only slowly absorb the poison. Once bound to this organ, it is not easily eliminated. The scallops (Placopecten spp.) have the ability to retain high concentrations of the toxin in various organs for a long time, except the adductor muscles where the concentration is never high enough to be toxic (Shimizu and Yoshioka 1981).

It does not take a very high concentration of dinoflagellates in the water to render the shellfish toxic; a concentration of 200 cells or more per milliliter of sea water of G. cantenella may be sufficient to make the mussels very toxic (Schantz 1973).

Table 11.1 lists the species of pelecypods which have been reported to be transvectors of the dinoflagellate toxin. Figure 11.3A and B show fourteen species of pelecypods known to be transvectors of dinoflagellate toxins. Note that, in general, toxic clams or mussels are inhabitants of northern temperate waters located at latitudes greater than 30° north or south (Schantz 1971). This may be explained by the peculiarity in nutrient composition in these waters.

According to Halstead and Courville (1965), warm tropical waters are not as abundant in nutrient salts as temperate waters. This may govern the prolific growth of these plankton in colder waters even though temperatures above 10°C are essential to the growth of dinoflagellates (Needler 1949). Other important factors in the growth of the dinoflagellates are sunlight (Prakash and Medcof 1962) and the presence of competitors, such as the diatoms and natural enemies like the ciliate Favella ehrenbergi (Needler 1949). Salinity, pH, organic matter from the growth of other organisms, water turbulence, and upwelling along the coast also are important factors (Schantz 1973). It appears that all favorable factors necessary for the growth of dinoflagellates converge during the summer months. At exactly what period during the summer may be determined by weather conditions, influencing, in turn, water conditions.

It takes 1 or 2 days to double the population of these dinoflagellates, and depending on the conditions, 2 to 3 weeks to attain maximum growth producing the red tide. The population dies off in 1 to 2 weeks. There is thus a direct correlation between toxic dinoflagellate population and mussel toxicity. For example, the period of maximum growth of G. tamarensis in the Bay of Fundy was found to precede or essentially coincide with the maximum toxicity of the mussels (Needler 1949; Prakash 1963).

In one study, the maximum toxicity of mussels in areas south of San Francisco was found to occur around the middle of July, and somewhat later in the summer in the northern regions (Sommer et al. 1937). There were two mussel toxicity peaks, one in early spring and the other in the summer. The summer toxicity of the mussels was found to be more significant. Along the Pacific coast, paralytic shellfish poisonings have occurred between the middle of May and the latter part of October (Meyer 1953). In Europe and South Africa, outbreaks have occurred during a similar period (Meyer et al. 1928; Sapeika 1948). In the Atlantic region around the New Brunswick, Nova Scotia area, the shellfish were found to be most toxic between mid-July and late September, peaking in the latter part of August (Gibbard and Naubert 1948).

Table 11.1 Pelecypods Reported as Transvectors of Paralytic Dinoflagellate Poisons

Species	Distribution
Arca noae (Noah's ark)	Mediterranean Sea
Cardium edule (heart cockle)	European seas
Clinocardium nuttalli (basket cockle)	From Nunivak, Pribilof, and Commander Islands, Bering Sea, and all coastal waters going south to Hakodate, Japan, and to Baja, California
Donax denticulatus (donax)	West Indies
Donax serra (wedgeshell, bean clam, white mussel)	South Africa
Spisula solidissima (Atlantic surf clam)	Labrador to North Carolina
Schizothaerus nuttalli (gaper, horse clam)	Northern Japan, Prince William Sound, Alaska, south to Scammons Lagoon, Baja, California
Mya aremaria (softshell clam)	Atlantic Coast, California and Northwestern Pacific Coast, England North Sea Coast, Britain
Mytilus californianus (California mussels)	Aleutian Islands, eastward and southward to Socorro Island
Mytilus edulis (bay mussel)	Worldwide, in temperate water, including Arctic Ocean
Mytilus edulis pellucidus (bay mussel)	Greenland to North Carolina
Mytilus edulis striatus	Europe
Mytilus galloprovincialis (peocio, miesmuschel)	Mediterranean Sea
Mytilus planulatus (mussel)	Victoria, Tasmania, Australia
Modiolus areolatus (mussel)	New South Wales, Australia
Modiolus demissus (ribbed mussel)	Virginia to Florida, San Francisco Bay, California
Modiolus modiolus (northern horse mussel)	Pacific Coast of North America, from Arctic Ocean to San Ignacio Lagoon, Baja, California; circumboreal
Crassostrea gigas	Japan, Pacific Northwest
Ostrea edulis (edible oyster, huitre)	Coast of Europe
Placopecten magellanicus (Atlantic deep-sea scallop)	Labrador to North Carolina
Penitella penita (flap-tipped piddock)	Chirikof Island, Alaska to Turtle Bay, Baja, California
Tugellus californianus (razor clam)	Humboldt Bay, California, to Panama

Table 11.1 (continued)

Species	Distribution
Ensis directus (Atlantic jack-knife clam)	Gulf of St. Laurence to Florida
Siliqua patula (northern razor clam)	Alaska to Pismo Beach, California
Spondylus americanus (Atlantic thorny oyster)	North Carolina to West Indies, Texas
Spondylus ducalis (rock scallop, northern thorny oyster)	Philippines, Indonesia, Micronesia, New Guinea
Macoma nasuta (bent-nosed clam, mud clam)	Kodiak Island, Alaska, to Cape San Lucas, Baja, California
Macoma secta (white sand clam)	British Columbia to Cape San Lucas, Baja, California
Anodonta oregonensis (freshwater mussel)	Freshwater streams, Kodiak Island, Alaska, southward to Northern California and eastward to Great Salt Lake, Utah
Protothaca staminea (rock cockle, rock clam, quahaug)	Aleutian Island to Cape San Lucas, Baja, California
Saxidomus giganteus (smooth Washington clam, butter clam)	Sitka, Alaska to San Francisco Bay, California
Saxidomus nuttalli (common clam, butter clam)	Humboldt Bay, California to San Quentin Bay, Baja, California
Tivela stultorum (pismo Washington clam)	Halfmoon Bay, California to Magdalena Bay, Baja, California

Source: Halstead and Courville (1965).

    These peak periods in shellfish toxicity must necessarily shift earlier or later as conditions in the water change. Indeed, it has been shown that the dinoflagellate populations are unpredictably subject to rapid changes — within a few hours (Bond and Medcof 1958). Thus, accurate predictions of shellfish toxicity in a given area based on analysis of toxin concentrations in shellfish may be difficult to make, in view of possible rapid fluctuations in dinoflagellate populations.
    In general, mussels gathered from shores continually beaten by the surf are more toxic than those gathered in higher tidal regions (Sommer et al. 1937). When the toxicity level far exceeds the lethal value, the mussels may remain toxic for as long as a month. In fact, the shellfish may still remain toxic long after the dinoflagellates have disappeared in the area (Needler 1949). It may take from 1 to 3 weeks after the bloom of the dinoflagellates subsides for the mussels to be free of toxins (Schantz 1973). In one experiment, it has been found that the mussels can become half as toxic in approximately 10 days when they are placed in sea water devoid of a source of food. When placed in dinoflagellate-laden water, they become toxic again (Sommer et al. 1937). Each species may have a different seasonal toxicity. In some areas of Alaska, *Saxidomus giganteus* (butter clam) can remain dangerously toxic throughout the year (Chambers and Magnusson 1950; Schantz and Magnusson 1964; Shimizu 1978). The toxicity of shellfish may decrease to nonlethal levels during the winter months. In fact, shellfish harvested from November through January may be harmless (Sommer and Meyer 1937).

Toxins From Paralytic Pelecypods   Several types of paralytic toxins from dinoflagellates may be transvected by the species of pelecypods listed in Table 11.1. One
group of toxins is water soluble and may be responsible for almost all types of paralytic shellfish poisoning in humans. Another group consists of toxins soluble in lipid
solvents.

The lipid-soluble toxins are found in the oyster *Crassostrea virginica;* the clam
Venus mercenaria campechiensis (McFarren et al. 1965); and the giant clam of Bora
Bora, *Tridacna maxima* (Banner 1967). The toxic factors in the first two mollusks are
quite heat stable, being able to withstand boiling for several minutes. *Venus mercenaria campechiensis* may, in fact, contain two types of lipid-soluble toxins. One of the
toxins seems to be more soluble in water-miscible organic solvents, such as alcohol,
than the other. The toxins in the oyster and clam are similar to the toxins isolated
from the dinoflagellate *Gymnodinium breve* (McFarren et al. 1965).

Thus far, seven different kinds of paralytic shellfish toxins have been identified
and characterized; however, only the structures of six of these are known (Genenah
and Shimizu 1981; Shimizu 1978; Shimizu et al. 1975). The toxins with known structures are saxitoxin (STX), neosaxitoxin (neoSTX), gonyautoxin-I (GTX-I), gonyau-
toxin-II (GTX-II), gonyautoxin-III (GTX-III), and gonyautoxin-IV (GTX-IV). These
structures are shown in Figure 11.4. The structure of gonyautoxin-V is still under investigation (Genenah and Shimizu 1981). A possible eighth toxin has been observed by
Shimizu et al. (1978) in Alaskan mussels (*Mytilus* spp.), which has been implicated in
paralytic shellfish poisoning in certain areas of Alaska. This toxin appears to be identical to a new toxin detected in a similar mussel *(M. edulis),* which has been implicated
in a widespread paralytic shellfish poisoning in Europe (Zwahlen et al. 1977).

All the toxins with known structures have the perhydropurine skeleton of saxitoxin as originally worked out by Wong et al. (1971). The correct structure of saxitoxin was determined independently by Shantz et al. (1975) and Brodner et al. (1975)
by means of x-ray diffraction study. Shimizu et al. (1978) has determined the structure of neosaxitoxin as 1-hydroxysaxitoxin: GTX-I and GTX-IV were shown to be
11α-, and 11β-neosaxitoxin sulfate, respectively, by Shimizu's group (Genenah and
Shimizu 1981). GTX-II and GTX-III proved to be 11α-, and 11β-saxitoxin sulfate
(Boyer et al. 1978).

All the toxins with known structures are alkaloids. From what is known of STX
and GTX-II and GTX-III (Schantz et al. 1957, 1961, 1966; Shimizu 1978), one may
generalize that all these toxins are very hygroscopic, and thus very water soluble.
STX has a pK_a/value of 8.5 and 11.5. Presumably, the other toxins will have similar
values. STX and GTX-II and GTX-III are more stable in acid than in alkaline medium,
even at low temperatures (Shimizu 1978). For example, in 3N HCl, STX shows no loss
of activity at $0°C$ for at least 4 weeks. However, at pH 5 and $55°C$, the activity decreases by one-third after 1 week. At $100°C$, pH 5.5, complete loss of activity in 24 hr
is observed. The stability of these toxins decreases with increasing pH; thus, gradual
loss in toxicity occurs at room temperature at pH 6.6; heating at this pH abolishes
half of the toxicity in 1 week (Wikholm 1947). Ordinary cooking destroys up to 70% of
shellfish toxicity; even greater loss in toxicity occurs during panfrying (Medcof et al.
1947).

Saxitoxin has been reported to be the only toxin isolated from the dinoflagellate
G. catenella, and this fact explains its presence as the major toxin in the Alaskan butter clam *(Saxidomus giganteus)* (Evans 1969) and California mussels *(Mytilus californianus)* (Schantz et al. 1957, 1961, 1966). However, there is some doubt as to whether
saxitoxin in the Alaskan butter clam is derived from *G. catenella.* Shimizu et al. (1978)
cited several reasons why saxitoxin found in this clam may be derived from other
sources. These are: the low counts of *G. catenella* in Alaskan waters and the absence
of peak dinoflagellate growth which would normally coincide with clam toxicity; the
presence of similar counts of the dinoflagellate in both toxic and nontoxic clam beds;
the retention of the toxin in the clam throughout the year, unlike other clams which

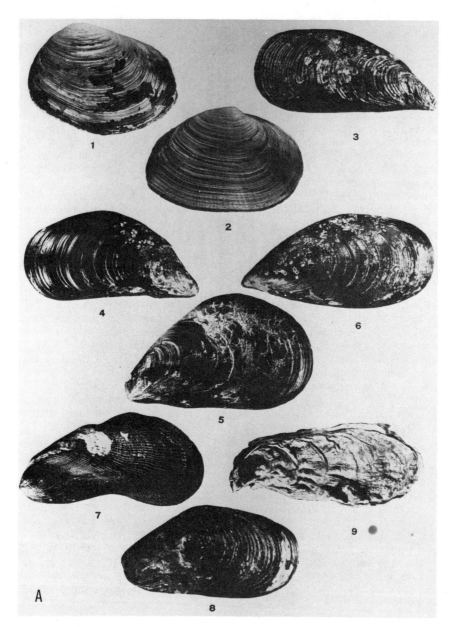

Figure 11.3 Species of clams known to be transvectors of paralytic and neurotoxic dinoflagellate toxins. A, 1. *Schizotharus nutalli* (x 0.2). 2. *Mya arenaria* (x 0.2). 3. *Mytilus californianus* (x 0.3). 4. *Mytilus edulis* (x 0.9). 5. *Mytilus pellucidus* (x 1.0). 6. *Mytilus planulatus* (x 1.4). 7. *Modiolus demissus* (x 0.8). 8. *Modiolus modiolus* (x 0.4). 9. *Crassostrea gigas* (x 0.3). (Photographs by R. Kreuzinger, courtesy of S. S. Berry.)

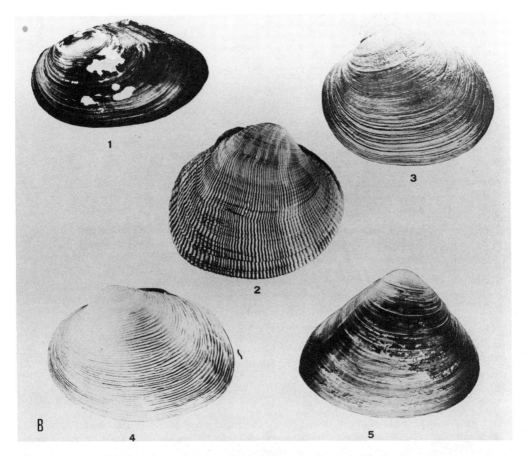

Figure 11.3 (continued) B, 1. *Anondonta oregonensis* (x 0.8). 2. *Protothaca staminea* (x 0.8). 3. *Saxidomus giganteus* (x 0.7). 4. *Saxidomus nutalli* (x 0.3). 5. *Tivela stultorum* (x 0.3). (Photographs by N. Hastings, courtesy of S. S. Berry.) (From *Poisonous and Venomous Marine Animals of the World* Vol. 1; used with permission.)

become nontoxic as soon as the dinoflagellate population subsides to very low levels; and the localization of the toxin in the siphons, unlike other clams in which it is concentrated in the hepatopancreas. Shimizu et al. (1978) also have found that other kinds of Alaskan mussels (Mytilus spp.) that they have analyzed contain no or relatively small amounts of saxitoxin. Instead, these clams contain relatively higher levels of GTX-I, -II, -III, -IV, and -V. Neo STX is present similarly as STX.

The possibility that the GTX toxins and neo-STX may have been present originally in the Alaskan butter clam, and in time biotransformed into STX has been raised by these investigators. That, in fact, this biotransformation can occur in shellfish has been shown in the scallop *(Placopecten magellanicus)* (Shimizu and Yoshioka 1981). In homogenized scallop tissues without adductor muscles and incubated for 3 days, the saxitoxin concentration has been shown to increase by 56% from its initial value of 6.4%, whereas the other toxins decrease by 4 to 18%. While the proportion of each toxin changes, total toxicity is unchanged. Because the adductor muscles were removed, this fact rules out the possibility that the increase in the amount of saxitoxin is due to the release of cryptic saxitoxin bound in the scallop muscle.

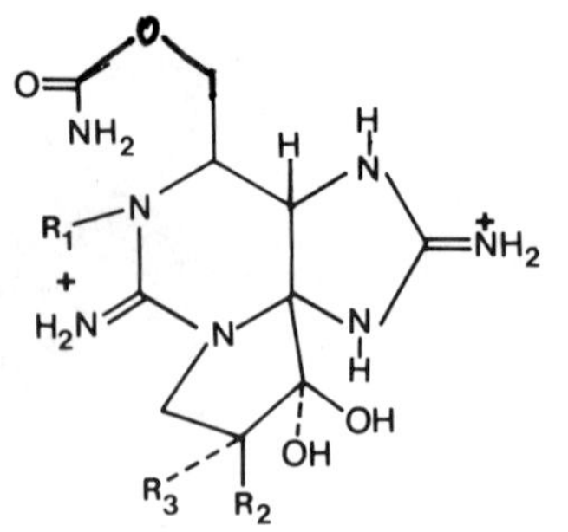

	R_1	R_2	R_3
SAXITOXIN	H	H	H
NEOSAXITOXIN	OH	H	H
GONYAUTOXIN-I	OH	H	OSO_3^-
GONYAUTOXIN-II	H	H	OSO_3^-
GONYAUTOXIN-III	H	OSO_3^-	H
GONYAUTOXIN-IV	OH	OSO_3^-	H

Figure 11.4 Structures of paralytic shellfish toxins. (Genenah and Shimizu [1981]; used with permission.)

STX is more widely distributed; its presence is not limited to the shellfish or dino-flagellates, perhaps because of its relative biological stability compared to other para-lytic shellfish toxins. It is present as the major toxin together with neo-saxitoxin in the Pacific crab *(Zosimus aeneus)* (Ikawa et al. 1962; Noguchi et al. 1969b, the common sand crab *(Emeritus* spp.) (Sommer 1932), and in a strain of the freshwater blue-green algae *Aphanizomenon flos-aquae* (Alam et al. 1975; Jackim and Gentile 1968).

G. *tamarensis* appears to elaborate all the known paralytic shellfish toxins, and this is reflected by the presence of most, if not all, of these substances in shellfish found in the waters where this dinoflagellate proliferates; i.e., the Northern Atlantic seacoast (Shimizu 1978). Thus, the scallop *Placopecten magellanicus* harvested in the Bay of Fundy in October 1977 was found to contain all seven types of toxin shown in Figure 11.3 (Genenah and Shimizu 1981). The scallop *Pectinopectin yessoensis* collected in Ofunato Bay, Japan, contained GTX-II and GTX-III as the major toxic components (75%), and GTX-1 (12%), saxitoxin (7%), and possibly other GTX toxins (32%) (Ikawa et al. 1982). A sample of New England softshell clam *Mya arenaria* harvested during an episode of red tide caused by G. *tamarensis* contained STX, neo-STX, and all known GTX toxins, except GTX-V; others like *Mytilus edulis* and *Tapes japonica*, collected during or immediately after a shellfish poisoning episode at Owase Bay, Japan, in 1975, gave STX and all five GTX toxins, but no neo-STX (Oshima et al. 1976; Shimizu 1978).

An interesting observation regarding the dinoflagellates found during the red tide in Owase Bay, Japan, in 1975, was that this dinoflagellate, which has been morpho-logically identified as G. *catanella*, produces similar types of toxins as those found in G. *tamarensis*, which, as stated before, thrives principally in the Northern Atlantic coast (Oshima et al. 1976). Thus, it is possible that G. *catenella* or other dinoflagell-ates produce different sets or proportions of toxins, depending on the location or other factors.

A significant discovery reported by Hall et al. (1980) raises the possibility that the toxins elaborated by the Gonyaulax spp. may be biosynthesized by the dinoflagellates as less, or nontoxic precursors; i.e., chemically different forms from those found in shellfish. These workers found that an extract of Protogonyaulax spp. clone 107 from the Porpoise Islands, Alaska, elaborated four substances, designated B1, B2, C1, and C2. These substances have low toxicities. Lesser amounts of neo-STX, GTX-I, and GTX-IV accompanied these four substances. No STX was found in the fresh extract. On exposure to low pH, especially at high temperatures, B1 was converted to STX, B2 to neo-STX, C1 to GTX-II, and C2 to GTX-III; slight interconversion of GTX-II and III also occurred. These processes occurred in 25 min or less at $100°C$, and for longer periods at room temperature. The conditions surrounding these conversions indicate that hydrolysis of certain bonds is involved. These conversions enhance the respective toxicities of the above four substances by 10, six-, 20- and five-fold.

Hall et al. (1980) have suggested that because of the large increase in toxicity following exposure to low pH, C1 itself might be nontoxic. It is, of course, possible that all these precursors are nontoxic protoxins and that they are biotransformed into toxic forms in the tissues of the mouse during the toxicity tests. These workers also raised the possibility that C1 or C2 can give rise to GTX-I or GTX-IV because traces of the latter have been noted when larger quantities of C1 or C2 have been exposed to low pH.

However, a consideration of the structures of these compounds shows that this would be unlikely because this would entail an introduction of an -OH group into GTX-II or GTX-III for conversion to GTX-I or GTX-IV, respectively. The introduction of the -OH group into GTX-II or GTX-III would be thermodynamically impossible under the conditions in which the conversion was observed; i.e., heating in 0.1 to 1.0M HCl at $100°C$. A possible explanation is that precursors of GTX-I and GTX-IV occurring in relatively small amounts in the dinoflagellates are co-isolated with C1 and C2 and are difficult to separate because of very similar physicochemical properties.

Interconversion of GTX-I and GTX-IV and C1 and C2 as with GTX-II and GTX-III also occurs during handling. This interconversion is to be expected because each of these GTX pairs are epimers; C1 and C2 can be expected to be epimers also because they appear to be precursors of GTX-II and GTX-III, respectively.

Previous workers may have failed to identify these protoxins, perhaps because of their instability under the isolation conditions. Thus, high pH could have been attained during concentration of the acidified extracts (See, e.g., Shimizu et al. 1975, 1978). Destruction of these protoxins could also occur during boiling of acidified extracts (See, e.g., Ikawa et al. 1982).

On the basis of the observation of Shimizu and Yoshioka (1981) regarding the biotransformation of various PSTs in scallops, and those of Hall et al. (1980) as discussed here, the following hypothetical biotransformation scheme is suggested as occurring in shellfish when the precursors B1, B2, C1, and C2 are incorporated into its tissues. (A1) and (A2) are postulated precursors of GTX-I and GTX-IV, respectively, as discussed before. It is, of course, possible that these biotransformation processes also occur in the dinoflagellate itself, since trace quantities of the GTXs and neo-STX have been detected by Hall et al. (1980) in their dinoflagellate extract. Furthermore, Shimizu et al. (1975) detected the same toxins in both the dinoflagellate (G. tamarensis) and the clam exposed to it. Also, it is rather unusual that G. catenella has been shown to contain only STX (Schantz et al. 1957, 1966), whereas some clams in the area (Mytilus spp.) where the dinoflagellate was found contained the GTX family of toxins plus either saxitoxin or neosaxitoxin (Shimizu et al. 1978); certain clams in the area have very low or negligible toxicity (Schantz and Magnusson 1964), whereas others, like the Alaskan butter clam (Saxidomus giganteus), may retain a significant amount of STX for prolonged or indefinite periods (Schantz and Magnusson 1964). All this observation may be explained in part if it is assumed that G. catenella as well as the Alaskan butter clam biotransforms the GTX family of toxins to Saxitoxins in a manner similar to that shown in the following scheme, whereas other shellfish, like Mytilus spp., are not as efficient as the butter clam, or do not have the capability for being so.

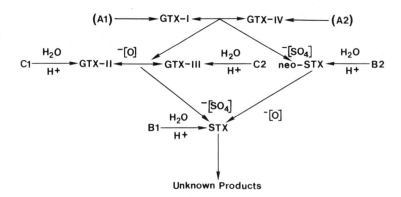

Unknown Products

Note that the biotransformation pathway from GTX-I or GTX-IV to STX, as proposed by Shimizu and Yoshioka (1981), involves a reductive elimination of N—OH, a relatively common biochemical reaction, and a desulfation reaction. The latter is the reverse of the usual biochemical process; i.e., sulfate conjugation. Nevertheless, as pointed out by Shimizu and Yoshioka (1981), $-O-SO_3^-$ is a good leaving group as in the case of pyrophosphates, the removal of the latter from phosphorylated compounds being a common biochemical reaction. These workers have suggested that the above biotransformations can explain partly the anomalous variability of the presence and proportions of these PSTs in shellfish in neighboring areas.

The postulated formation of protoxins is not at all unexpected, since the biosynthesis of precursor substances is a common biological phenomenon. The nature of these protoxins remains to be established.

Toxicity of PSTs   The PSTs are neurotoxins which are among the most potent of the known low molecular weight toxins. The toxicities of the various PSTs, according to Genenah and Shimizu (1981), are given in Table 11.2. Toxicity is expressed in mouse units; one mouse unit equals 0.18 µg STX dihydrochloride, the quantity necessary to kill a 20-g mouse in 10 to 20 min (Schantz et al. 1958; Sommer and Meyer 1937). The overall toxicity of a given sample of shellfish is the sum of the products of the separate toxicities multiplied by the quantities of each toxin present in the sample. Note that from the values of their relative toxicities STX and GTX-III are the most toxic. Thus, the degree of toxicity will depend on the proportion of the different PSTs. Evidently, those shellfish containing greater quantities of STX or GTX-III will be more toxic. As discussed earlier in this chapter, there is a tendency for the GTXs and neo-STX to transform to STX, so that the level of the latter in shellfish will increase with time. Thus, a shellfish may be more or less toxic depending on the interval between the time of ingestion of the dinoflagellate by the shellfish and the time of harvest. Also, because cooking may hasten the conversion of the protoxins to more toxic forms, the degree of toxicity of the shellfish at the table may depend on whether significant leaching of the toxin during cooking does occur. Obviously, more leaching can be expected if the shellfish is cooked with water.

In the case of saxitoxin, the LD_{50} varies with the species and the reported values in µg/kg body weight are as follows (Kao 1966; McFarren et al. 1960): humans, 10 to 20; pigeons, 91; guinea pigs, 135; dogs and rabbits, 181; rats, 192; cats, 254; mice, 382; monkeys, 364 to 727. The intravenous lethal dose for rabbits is 3 to 4 µg/kg. From accidental cases, the lethal oral dose in humans may be as low as 3000 to 5000 mµ or 0.54 to 0.9 mg (Schantz 1973). Another report gave a higher value of 1 mg as lethal to man (Tennant et al. 1955).

Factors Affecting PST Toxicity   It is obvious that there are species differences with regard to sensitivity to the toxin. Humans appear to be the most sensitive among the mammals. In addition, the age, sex, body size, strain, previous exposure to the

Table 11.2 Toxicities of Paralytic Shellfish Toxins (PSTs)

PST	Mouse Units Mu/μmole	Specific toxicity Mu/mg	Relative toxicity
STX	2045 ± 126	5492 ± 339[a]	100
Neo-STX	1038 ± 44	2363 ± 101[b]	43
GTX-I	1638 ± 128	3976 ± 312[c]	72
GTX-II	793 ± 83	2003 ± 211[c]	36
GTX-III	2234 ± 137	5641 ± 346[c]	103
GTX-IV	673 ± 38	1634 ± 92[c]	30
GTX-V	354 ± 19	—[d]	—[d]

[a]Weighed as dihydrocholoride.
[b]Weighed as diacetate.
[c]Weighed as monoacetate.
[d]Values could not be determined because molecular structure is not known.
Source: From Genenah and Shimizu (1981)

toxin, and presence of metal ions and other substances may influence toxicity. Thus, the oral LD_{50} in rats may increase with age; in rats the values for the newborn, 3-week-old, and 60- to 70-day-old rats are approximately 64, 270, and 531 μg/kg body weight, respectively (Watts et al. 1966). Female mice have been found to be more sensitive to PST than the male (Stephenson et al. 1955). The LD_{50} varies with the weight in both mice (Stephenson et al. 1955) and rats (McFarren et al. 1956). Some strains of rats are more sensitive to the toxin than others (McFarren et al. 1956). These authors also have found that rats previously given a nonlethal oral dose become less sensitive to the toxin. The crude toxin is more toxic than the purified material, which gave a higher oral LD_{50}. Na^+ decreases toxicity, but many bivalent ions like Ca^{2+}, Ba^{2+}, Sr^{2+}, Mg^{2+}, Mn^{2+}, Co^{2+}, Ni^{2+}, Fe^{2+}, and Fe^{3+} increase it (Wiberg and Stephenson 1961). Cu^{2+} has no influence on the toxicity, indicating valence is not a determining factor. The influence of these ions may indicate the involvement of specific enzymes.

Physiological Effects and Pharmacological Action of PSTs Two major effects are noted: (1) effects on central and peripheral nervous systems and (2) systemic effects.

Effect on the nervous system: The profound paralytic effects of PSTs and the observed decrease in toxicity in the presence of Na^+ are consistent with the effects of this toxin on the nervous system. The action on the central nervous system is shown by the effects on the respiratory and vasomotor centers (Kao 1966; Murtha 1960). The action on the peripheral nervous system is shown by the effects on the neuromuscular junction, cutaneous tactile endings and muscle spindles (Kellaway 1935 a,b; Sapeika 1953). In addition to peripheral transmission, reflex transmission is also completely depressed by saxitoxin (Murtha 1960) and presumably other PSTs.

Following PST poisoning, respiration may immediately cease totally or be depressed slowly, depending on the dose. The depression may be characterized by dyspnea with gasping action or short rapid exhalations. These effects appear to be the result of the paralysis of diaphragm muscles (Kellaway 1935a; Murtha 1960).

The peripheral neurotoxic effects as observed in frog nerve-muscle preparations have been described by Kellaway 1935a,b) as being similar to a typical curarization. A toxic concentration of 5 ppm produces curarization in 1.5 hr; complete loss of response of the cutaneous tactile receptors and muscle spindles also occurs after toxin application. With a concentration of 2 ppm, paralysis of tactile receptors occur 2 min after toxin application at 15°C; at 8°C at the same concentration, the muscle spindles fail to respond 58 min after toxin application. The muscles so treated cannot respond to the action of applied acetylcholine and are irreversibly paralyzed (Sapeika 1953; Kellaway 1935b).

The results of various investigators (Evans 1964, 1965; Kao 1972; Kao and Nishiyama 1965; Narahashi 1972) have shown that the principal target of the toxin appears to be the sodium channel in the most excitable membranes; i.e., nerves and muscles. The toxins have high specificity and binding capacity ($K = 10^{-9}$ in the case of saxitoxin) to the sodium channels (Shimizu 1978). The toxin molecules block the channels to the early entry of Na^+ ions. Thus, the initial increase in sodium permeability usually associated with excitation is interfered with, so that propagation of impulses in nerve and muscles is blocked without depolarization. The resting membrane conductances due to K^+ and Cl^- permeability are not affected. One toxin molecule appears to be blocking one channel (Cuervo and Adelman 1970). The action of saxitoxin and presumably other PSTs (Ritchie 1980) is similar to that of the puffer fish toxin, tetrodotoxin (pp. 545–548). The discussion on the mode of action of tetrodotoxin also applies to saxitoxin (Ritchie 1980).

Systemic effects: In animal experiments, there is an observed drop in blood pressure upon saxitoxin intoxication. The course of the hypotensive process varies depending on the dose. At a sublethal or low dose, e.g., less than 1.5 to 2.0 µg/kg, the blood pressure falls initially, recovers, and then, slowly but steadily, falls again. With high doses, the blood pressure falls more rapidly. A curious action with low doses, however, is that a late pressor effect is observed. This explains the short duration of the hypotensive action with low doses. This action also explains the strange clinical observation in PST poisoning in humans; hypotension has not been always reported in these occurrences (Kao 1966). Indeed, in some cases, slight hypertension has been noted immediately after poisoning (McCollum et al. 1968). This pressure effect may be the result of catecholamine secretion following intoxication, since it is abolished by acute hexamethonium treatment, overnight reserpine treatment, or acute adrenalectomy (Nagasawa et al. 1971).

The hypotensive effect may be explained by the dual effects of PST; i.e., direct relaxation of the vascular smooth muscles and blockage of the vasomotor nerves, resulting in release of vasomotor tone (Kao 1972).

Symptoms of PST Poisoning The above effects of PST can be related directly to the clinical manifestations of PST poisoning in humans. The general symptoms are frightening. The initial symptoms are observed within a few minutes (usually 30 min) after consuming the toxic mollusk. These consist of tingling, burning sensation, and numbness in the lips, gums, tongue, face, and fingertips. Then, similar sensations spread to the neck, arms, and legs, and general muscular incoordination ensues. In severe cases, ataxia and general motor incoordination also are usually accompanied by a "floating" sensation, a feeling of being choked, incoherent speech, and loss of voice. Other symptoms may also be present, such as weakness, dizziness, malaise, prostration, headache, salivation, rapid pulse, intense thirst, dysphagia, perspiration, anuria, and myalgia, impairment of vision, or even temporary blindness. Nausea, vomiting, diarrhea, abdominal pain, muscular twitching, and convulsions occur rarely. Some patients complain of feeling as if their teeth were loose or being set on edge. Most patients are calm and remain aware of their condition throughout the episode. The paralytic episodes become more intense, with respiratory distress becoming more severe. Depending on the amount of toxin ingested, death following respiratory paralysis may occur within 2 to 12 hr. Those who survive after 12 hr, or better still, 24 hr, may expect to recover with no lasting effects (Halstead and Courville 1965; Schantz 1973).

The amount of toxin eliciting these symptoms is, of course, variable. As already stated, many host factors affect the toxicity of saxitoxin. In one group of observations, illness occurred with the ingestion of an amount of toxin as low as 0.11 mg;

0.54 to 0.9 mg was a lethal dose (Bond and Medcof 1958). In poisoning cases reported from California, the amounts of toxin producing symptoms were between 0.18 to 3.6 mg; death resulted with 3.6 mg or more (Meyer 1953). A dose-response relationship has been noticed in one series of observations. Mild paresthesia and other symptoms have been noted with 15,000 MU (2.7 mg saxitoxin); severe respiratory distress has been observed with 22,000 MU (3.96) mg); and death with 20,000 to 40,000 MU (3.6 to 7.2 mg) (Meyer 1953). Much lower values have produced similar results in a series of observations in Canada (Medcof et al. 1947). The U.S. Food and Drug Administration has established the limit of maximal human tolerance for paralytic shellfish toxin at 1200 MU/100 g shellfish or 2500 MU/meal.

There is no antidote for the toxin. Symptomatic treatment to promote emesis, use of absorbents to bind the poison (e.g., charcoal, Lloyd's reagent), diuresis with 5% NH_4Cl, and anticurare drugs have all been recommended, some with varying success. Artificial respiration is an important adjunct to treatment (Halstead and Courville 1965). It appears to have good results experimentally (Murtha 1960) and in mild cases, but is of no avail in severe intoxications (Meyer 1953).

Incidence of PST Poisoning In spite of the frequent occurrence of the red tide and the great toxicity of the PST, poisonings due to this toxin happen rarely in the United States at the present time. From 1969 to 1975 there were seven cases of this type of poisoning, four cases from New Hampshire in 1974, and three from Alaska in 1973 (Center for Disease Control 1973, 1974). In the summer of 1976, three separate incidents of PST poisoning involving six persons were reported in southeastern Alaska (Shimizu et al. 1978). Records from other countries, even though incomplete, show a similar pattern in the same period. Between 1689 and 1962, the number of cases throughout the world reported in the literature, as compiled by Halstead and Courville (1965), totaled to more than 957, with more than 222 deaths. These records or reports are rather inaccurate, since in many incidences, the number of cases were reported vaguely as "several" or "many." Looking simply at the number of cases in some out-breaks, one is impressed by the severity of poisoning. For example, in 1799 in Peril Strait, Alaska, more than 100 persons were poisoned to death by eating paralytic shell-fish (Halstead and Courville 1965).

The very low incidence at the present time obviously is due to a large degree to the strict quarantine measures established in many countries and the awareness of people in the coastal areas of the potential toxicity of shellfish during the red tide.

The tolerance of the safe level of toxin in shellfish has been established by appro-priate government agencies. The U.S. Public Health Service and the corresponding agency in Canada have established that 400 MU/100 g shellfish is generally safe for humans (Halstead and Courville 1965).

Prevention of PST Poisoning There is no proven technique for distinguishing be-tween toxic and nontoxic shellfish except by toxicity tests in experimental animals. All other suggested methods at present are old wives tales and just that. Strict observ-ance of quarantine regulations is the best precaution.

The toxins as already stated, are stable in acid but are less stable as the pH in-creases. There is a very large decrease in toxicity in cooked mollusk, especially when higher temperatures are employed in cooking, as in pan frying. Because of its instabil-ity in alkaline medium, some authors recommend adding sodium bicarbonate to the cook-ing medium (1 tbs/q water) and heating for 20 to 30 min (Sommer and Meyer 1941). While this method destroys 85% of the toxins, it may produce an undesirable flavor. In spite of this reduction in toxicity, the mussels may still retain enough toxins to cause serious poisoning.

Since the toxins are very water soluble, the broth in which the mollusk is cooked should contain a significant amount of the toxins and should be discarded.

The absence of dinoflagellates in the water may not totally guarantee the safety of shellfish in the area, particularly if that part of the sea has just experienced a red

tide. Natural detoxification processes may take more than 1 month to rid a mollusk of
the toxins (Sommer et al. 1937). Because the toxins tend to concentrate in specific
organs of the mollusk, i.e., liver or hepatopancreas, gills, siphons, and other parts,
it may be advantageous to avoid eating these parts. However, this precaution may be
impractical in most instances, considering the size of the body of the mollusk.

Even though the location of the mollusk bed in the specific terrain in the sea has
been shown to affect the degree of toxicity of the shellfish, this fact cannot be used
as a reliable index as to the safety of the mollusk (Sparks 1961; Sparks et al. 1962).

Harvesting mussels during the winter months might minimize poisoning, since in
most cases, toxicity is much lower during this period.

Canned butter clams are probably generally safe to eat, since the conditions used
in canning generally reduce the toxicity, if any. For instance, the pH during steaming
may be as high as 8.2 and decreases to 6.5 after addition of vinegar. This is still high
enough to further decrease the toxicity while retorting the product at $121^{\circ}C$ for 45
min. In addition, the most toxic part of the clam, the siphon, is removed. At any rate,
only canned shellfish meeting toxicity tolerances are allowed in the market. Representative samples must have an average toxicity of less than 400 MU/100 g shellfish, and
all samples must score less than 2000 MU/100 g.

Neurotoxic Gymnodinium breve Toxins in Shellfish

The periodic red tides occurring in the Gulf of Mexico along the west coast of Florida
(Galtsoff 1954) are caused by the unarmored, or "naked," dinoflagellates, *Gymnodinium
breve* (revised to *Ptychodiscus brevis* by Steidinger [1979]) (Davis 1947). These organisms cause massive fish kills in this area owing to the toxin or toxins that they produce. The presence of a massive bloom of *G. breve* in the sea may cause acute eye and
nose irritation and respiratory distress among individuals exposed to the sea spray.
This has a greater likelihood of occurring if a strong wind is blowing toward the beach
carrying with it aerosols from the sea containing the organisms (Music et al. 1973;
Woodcock 1948).

The large dinoflagellate population causes the shellfish in the coastal waters which
feed on *G. breve* to become poisonous. Thus, McFarren et al. (1965) has reported several cases of shellfish poisoning following consumption of oysters *(Crassostrea virginica)* and clams *(Venus mercenaria campechiensis)* harvested along the west coast of
Florida at red tide. The transvection of the toxin from this dinoflagellate has been
demonstrated by exposure of the oyster to a culture of this organism (Ray and Aldrich
1965).

Symptoms of Florida Shellfish Poisoning   Unlike its counterpart in the Northern
Pacific and Northern Atlantic coasts, the symptoms of shellfish poisoning occurring
along the western Florida coast resemble ciguatera in many respects. Thus, mice injected with aqueous extracts of the toxic oysters were not killed within a few minutes
as in saxitoxin poisoning; instead, death occurred in 3 to 5 hr, and was preceded by
a prolonged period of labored breathing (McFarren et al. 1965). To be sure, paralysis
can occur, as observed in kittens by these investigators. Sasner et al. (1972) has observed respiratory irregularity, loss of coordination, and violent twitching in mice injected i.p. with 6 mg of crude *G. breve* toxin (GBTX). Death in this case was due to
respiratory failure. Spiegelstein et al. (1973) has reported the following syndrome
when a lethal dose of the toxin was injected i.v. or i.p. into mice: (1) changes in
respiratory rate which initially was increased and superficial, whereupon the rate then
decreased and returned to normal. But in fatal cases, respiratory depression ultimately progressed to respiratory failure; (2) blanching of the ears immediately following
injection of GBTX, exophthalmos, and a decrease in eye color in those dying early;
(3) ataxia, incoordination, jumping movements, curling of front legs, spread back
legs, muscle twitching, and other signs of motor disfunction. The behavior of the animals indicated the presence of cardiovascular failure with a precipitous decrease in
blood pressure. The animals gasped for breath before death.

A sublethal dose (70% of LD$_{50}$) of GBTX resulted in immediate appearance of kicking and jumping movements followed by jerking, almost convulsive actions which were accompanied by muscle twitching. The animals showed fast recovery after a sublethal dose; i.e., 5 to 10 min after the appearance of the motor disturbances.

Borison et al. (1980) have observed the so-called Bezold-Jarisch effect in anesthetized cats injected i.v. with 10 µg GBTX/kg. This effect consists of apnea, bradycardia, and hypotension. The animals recovered quickly from this effect. At higher doses, e.g., 160 µg/kg, GBTX produces marked deceleration of respiration and a biphasic increase-decrease in blood pressure. The Bezold-Jarisch effect also has been observed in dogs administered GBTX intravenously (Ellis et al. 1979).

GBTX also causes in cats irregular breath holding and hypertension with tachycardia, leading to respiratory and circulatory failure. Unlike saxitoxin, from which death follows respiratory depression, death in animals caused by GBTX may be preceded by convulsion. It is similar to saxitoxin in that it also causes respiratory failure (Borison et al. 1980).

In humans, ciguateralike symptoms, which include tingling sensation on the face, around the mouth and throat, may be observed; this sensation spreads to other parts of the body. Inversion of hot-cold sensation, bradycardia, dilation of the pupils, and a feeling of inebriation accompany this tingling sensation in some patients. Some victims of poisoning develop prolonged diarrhea, nausea, poor coordination, and burning pain in the rectum. Symptoms appear within 1 to 3 hr after eating the toxic shellfish. In all cases, recovery is complete in 24 hr (McFarren et al. 1965).

Ciguateralike symptoms also have been observed in kittens given ether extracts of the toxic mollusks. Thus, a neuromotor syndrome, characterized among other signs by the loss of the righting reflex, progressive paralysis, and loss of sensation have been observed. Depending on the dose, death may occur as early as 35 min or as long as several hours (McFarren et al. 1965). The subject on ciguatera poisoning is discussed later in this chapter (p. 556).

Physiological and Pharmacological Action of G. breve Toxin   As shown in the next section, GBTX is probably a mixture of at least three different toxins. Several investigators have shown that aside from the syndrome observed in animal and human poisonings, the pharmacological action of GBTX demonstrates that at least one of the toxins is a neurotoxin (Abbott and Paster 1970; Baden et al. 1981; Gallagher and Shinnick-Gallagher 1980; Sasner et al. 1972; Shinnick-Gallagher 1980; Westerfield et al. 1977). Thus, GBTX blocks neuromuscular transmission (Abbott and Paster 1970; Sasner et al. 1972). Specifically, in studies with isolated rat phrenic nerve diaphragm, it has been shown that GBTX depolarizes muscle fiber membrane potential, increased miniature endplate potential (MEPP) frequency, blocked end-plate potential generation, produced biphasic effects on MEPP amplitude, and depressed acetylcholine-induced depolarization. These effects indicate that GBTX has both pre- and postsynaptic action (Gallagher and Shinnick-Gallagher 1980; Shinnick-Gallagher 1980). The postsynaptic effect is reflected by depolarizing action of GBTX on muscle membrane. Indeed, GBTX may have a depolarizing action on all membranes (Sasner 1965). GBTX is also shown to depolarize the giant axon of the squid (Westerfield et al. 1977). Depolarization of the squid giant axon and the rat phrenic nerve hemidiaphragm preparation by a highly purified GBTX also has been reported by Baden et al. (1981).

Nevertheless, some workers (Abbott et al. 1975; Sasner et al. 1972) using purified toxin have failed to observe any depolarization of their muscle or nerve preparation. This may have been due to possible removal of specific active components by the preparative procedures used by these workers or to the variability in the production of specific toxic components by the dinoflagellates under the conditions existing during toxin preparation. This possibility has been supported by the observation of Spikes et al. (1968), who reported that toxicity of G. breve cultures varies with the age of culture and the type of culture medium. This variation is not always associated with the dinoflagellate population density of the culture.

The presynaptic action of GBTX is shown by its effect in increasing the MEPP frequency. This is suggestive of the depolarizing action of GBTX on the nerve terminal membrane (Gallagher and Shinnick-Gallagher 1980; Shinnick-Gallagher 1980). In the case of the depolarization of the squid giant axon, the presence of as little as 10^{-9} g GBTX/ml in the bathing solution causes the axon to depolarize and fire repetitively (Westerfield et al. 1977). In this case, prior to the appearance of repetitive firing, the nerve depolarizes by 8 to 10 mV. Tetrodotoxin (p. 546) blocks the GBTX-induced depolarization; this process and the subsequent repetitive firing of the axon resume when tetrodotoxin is removed from the bathing medium. The cumulative depolarizing effects of repetitive firing cause the nerve action potential to be blocked in the squid giant axon. In the rat phrenic nerve diaphragm preparation, depolarization of the nerve terminal leads to a blockage of the end-plate potential. This blockage may be related to a depression of neurotransmitter release due to depolarization of the nerve terminal (Hubbard and Willis 1968).

Shinnick-Gallaher (1980) has presented evidence which indicates that membrane depolarization by GBTX is brought about by an increase in sodium ion permeability. The evidence for this mechanism includes: (1) the decrease in membrane resistance accompanied by the depolarization of the resting membrane potential; (2) prevention of GBTX-induced depolarization by low Na^+ concentration in the test medium; (3) antagonism by tetrodotoxin of GBTX-induced depolarization, and prevention of depolarization by pretreatment of membrane preparation with tetrodotoxin. Tetrodotoxin is known to block the sodium channels, and thus, prevent membrane depolarization and the consequent neurotransmission (p. 546). GBTX also has been observed to depress the magnitude of acetylcholine-induced depolarization. Shinnick-Gallagher (1980) suggests that this effect may be explained by noncompetitive blocking or binding of GBTX on some site on the acetylcholine receptors.

These observed effects on isolated nerve or muscle fiber may explain many of the observed symptoms in animals and humans poisoned by GBTX. The action of GBTX appears to be highly reversible, since, depending on the dose, recovery from poisoning appears to occur rapidly, as has been observed in mice (Spiegelstein et al. 1973) and in humans (McFarren et al. 1965).

GBTX also has been reported to contain a hemolytic component (Alam et al. 1975; Shimizu 1978; Spiegelstein et al. 1973). This effect, however, has been observed only in vitro, and its significance in the overall observed symptoms is unclear. Alam et al. (1975) have reported that the hemolytic component also is a neurotoxin.

Chemical Nature of G. breve Toxin   Thus far, no two investigators have agreed on the chemical composition of the toxin or the components of the toxic principles derived from the dinoflagellates (Shimizu 1978). This observation points to the complexity of the toxic components elaborated by this dinoflagellate, at least in its overall toxicological components. As a minimum, three toxic components have been identified (Alam et al. 1975; Spiegelstein et al. 1973). However, the toxic fractions identified by these workers may not be identical correspondingly. This is because all three toxins identified by Alam et al. (1975) are neurotoxins, even though one has hemolytic activity, whereas only two of those isolated by Spiegelstein et al. (1973) are neurotoxins, and the third is hemolytic. Other investigators have isolated or have identified only two toxins (Martin and Chatterjee 1969; McFarren et al. 1965). The latter workers have identified two types of toxin in the clam (Venus mercenaria campechiensis), but not in the oyster (Crassostriea virginica). One component has greater solubility in solvents like ethanol, ethyl ether, or acetone. An ether extract of the toxic clam has been separated into two fractions with 5% $NaHCO_3$ or Na_2CO_3. The fraction soluble in 5% $NaHCO_3$ produces death in mice in less than 1 hr after injection, whereas the ether-soluble fraction produces death only after several hours. It appeared that the latter substance, the so-called "slow death factor," is the only one that has been isolated from the oyster. This toxin produces death in chicks in 6 to 22 hr (Ray and Aldrich 1965). The fast death factor, however, is orally nonlethal to cats.

Further indication of the complexity of the chemistry of *G. breve* toxin is shown by the different chemical and physical properties and elemental compositions of the toxic fractions obtained by different investigators (Shimizu 1978).

One possible reason for the reported inconsistent results as to the nature and number of toxic components in *G. breve* is the extraction procedures used. Most of these workers assumed that the toxins are only soluble in either ethyl ether or chloroform. Thus, toxins with different solubility properties that may be present in the dinoflagellate are ignored.

Baden et al. (1981) have succeeded in crystallizing one of the major toxins of *G. breve* from acetone or from 50% acetone in absolute ethanol. The toxin is soluble in acetone, but less soluble in ethyl acetate, methanol, or ethanol and slightly soluble in water. This fraction is stable under dry conditions and decomposes at 265 to 270°C, with no clearcut melting point. The elemental composition is different from those reported previously (Shimizu 1978) in that it contans neither nitrogen nor phosphorus. It appears to be rich in oxygen, and contains an aldehyde function. The toxin is highly toxic to mice (LD_{50} = 0.20 mg/kg, i.p.) and especially to the mosquito fish *(Gambusia affinis)* (LD_{50} = 0.011 mg/L of test medium).

The complete toxicology of *G. breve* toxins as transvected by oysters and clams awaits full elucidation of the total toxic components produced by these dinoflagellates. It is also significant that McFarren et al. (1965) have found two types of toxic substances in the clam, but not in the oyster. It is therefore possible that a biotransformation mechanism in these mollusk could drastically change the toxicological profile as observed in the scallop in the case of the Gonyaulax toxins (Shimizu and Yoshioka 1981).

Incidence of Human Intoxication from Shellfish Transvectors of *G. breve* Toxins
Reports of human poisonings in the United States due to consumption of shellfish containing *G. breve* toxins are rare and have been confined to Florida. In 1974 and 1973, only one and three cases, respectively, were reported from this state (Center for Disease Control 1973, 1974).

Other Transvectors of *G. breve* Toxins   There are other transvectors of toxins from *G. breve* or similar toxins from other sources. For example, the giant Bora Bora clam, *Tridacna maxima,* contains toxins which produce ciguateralike symptoms in humans. The toxins are also toxic to mice. They consist of two components: one that is soluble in aqueous medium, and the other in lipid solvents (Banner 1967). These toxins are similar to those found by McFarren et al. (1965) in Florida clams *(V. mercenaria campechiensis)*.

Other mollusks also transvect the toxin, such as the chiton *(Mopalia mucosa),* the shield limpet *(Acmaea pelta)* (Sommer and Meyer 1937), and the rock shell *(Murex brandaris)* (Charnot 1945). The sand crab *(Emerta analoga)* and the ochre starfish *(Pisaster ochraceus)* also are known transvectors (Sommer and Meyer 1937).

Venerupin Shellfish Poison

The giant Pacific oyster, *Crassostrea gigas,* the Japanese cockle, *Tapes semidiscussata* (Akiba 1943, 1949; Akiba and Hattori 1949; Meyer 1953), and the Japanese dosinia, *Dosinia japonica* (Akiba 1943) transvect what appears to be another dinoflagellate toxin. The toxin has been termed venerupin from the family Veneridae, to which the genera Tapes and Dosinia belong. The toxin seems to be derived from the dinoflagellate Prorocentrum spp., which thrives in Lake Hamana in Schizuoka and Kanagawa Prefectures, Japan (Akiba 1961, 1943). This is a good example of geographical delineation of the occurrence of poisoning. Reported human intoxications have been limited to this area only, even though *Crassostrea gigas* and *Tapes semidiscussata* are also found from British Columbia to Morro Bay, California, in the case of the oyster, and to Elkhorn Slough, California, in the case of the clam. These two species have been the only ones incriminated in human poisoning. Two other pelecypods, *Meretria lusoria* and *Mactra*

veneriformis, which inhabit the same Lake Hamana area as the toxic pelecypods, have
been found to be nontoxic (Akiba 1949).

Like the other dinoflagellate toxins discussed in the preceding section, venerupin
appears to be concentrated in the digestive organs of the mollusk. The shellfish incriminated in a 1949 poisoning outbreak contained 40 μg toxin/g of organ; the rest of
the viscera contained no more than 0.6 μg/g (Akiba and Hattori 1949).

Venerupin is a very stable toxin, being resistant to boiling for 3 hr at pH 3 to 8
or heating at 109°C for 1 hr (Akiba and Hattori 1949). The toxin in these shellfish remains lethal to humans and dogs even after boiling for 1 hr. At pH 5.4, heating for 30
min to 3 hr to 119°C does not destroy the toxin if the starting temperature is 100°C.
If the starting temperature is 115°C, 50 to 85% of the toxin is destroyed if heated for
30 to 60 min (Akiba 1943, 1949; Akiba and Hattori 1949).

At pH 5.6, the toxin is stable for over 20 months in the refrigerator. At pH 5.4 to
8.0, the toxin is not destroyed even after boiling for 1 hr. It is less stable under
highly acidic or alkaline conditions; at pH 9.4 to 10.0, boiling for 30 min destroys 50
to 75% of the toxin. It also loses 50% of its potency in 4 months at pH 2.9 or 10.4.
There appears to be no loss of toxicity at this pH range in 1 month in the refrigerator
or after 4 months at pH 5.6 to 9.4 (Akiba 1943, 1949; Akiba and Hattori 1949).

Venerupin is soluble in water, methanol, acetone, and acetic acid, but insoluble in
benzene, chloroform, ether, or absolute ethanol (Akiba and Hattori 1949). Like saxitoxin, it appears to be an alkaloid, since it is precipitated by heavy metal salts and
certain alkaloidal reagents (Akiba 1949; Akiba and Hattori 1949). The structure of the
toxin has not been elucidated.

Toxicity of Venerupin Dogs and cats fed cooked or raw toxic shellfish in doses of
50 g/kg body weight become ill with typical symptoms described in the next section. In
humans, adults eating 40 to 60 shellfish or 157 to 250 g of flesh become poisoned, and
those eating more than 100 shellfish may be poisoned to death. Ten to fifteen shellfish
appear harmless to adults, but may be fatal to children.

A simple, rapid, and accurate colorimetric test for venerupin based on the reaction
of the toxin with phenolphthalein, acetic acid, and H_2O_2 at pH 9.6 to 10.0 has been developed by Hattori and Akiba (1952). The red color produced by a 0.001% solution of
the homogenized organ is assigned arbitrarily a P_1 value of 1 (percentage concentration x 1000). A 1% solution heated for 1 hr in boiling water and producing a positive
color is assigned a P_2 value of 1000. Toxic mollusks have a P_1 and P_2 value of <1 and
around 20 to 40, respectively. Nontoxic mollusks have P_1 and P_2 values of 1.0 to 10.0,
and usually 800 or more respectively. Shellfish with P_1 and P_2 >1 and between 800 and
1000, respectively, are considered safe to eat.

The toxicity of venerupin-containing shellfish fluctuates seasonally. It is lowest
from June to September, begins to increase in October, rises sharply in January, attains peak values during February and March, and drops sharply in April (Akiba
1949). The P_1 value during the peak months usually decreases from 1.0 to 0.5 (Hattori
and Akiba 1952).

Symptoms of Venerupin Poisoning The symptoms of venerupin poisoning suggest
that it is a potent and violent poison in humans. After a usual incubation period of 24
to 48 hr (in some cases, up to 7 days), the first signs of poisoning appear. These
signs include anorexia, stomach ache, nausea, vomiting, constipation, headache, and
malaise. There is no fever. The illness progresses to more severe symptoms, such as
vomiting of blood; hemorrhages in the mucous membranes of the nose, mouth, and
gums; nervousness; jaundice; and petechial hemorrhages and ecchymoses of the skin,
especially about the neck, chest, and upper portions of the arms and legs. Disturbances in the blood such as leukocytosis, anemia, and slow clotting are noted. Liver
function is affected by enlargement of this organ. Death may occur within 1 week, and
may be preceded by symptoms of excitability, delirium, and a comatose state. The toxin is nonparalytic. Without prompt treatment, mortality of over 33% has been observed
in the case of the venerupin poisoning in Japan. Prompt medical care can reduce the

fatalities considerably. Recovery among mild cases may be slow, with patients showing extreme weakness. Unlike the paralytic shellfish poison, previous exposure to the toxin does not confer resistance or immunity (Akiba and Hattori 1949; Hattori and Akiba 1952; Meyer 1953; Togashi 1943).

Venerupin may be a cytotoxic compound, judging from autopsy findings, causing diffuse necrosis, hemorrhage and fatty degeneration of the liver, and congestion with hemorrhages in the heart, lung, and gastrointestinal tract (Akiba 1943, 1949; Akiba and Hattori 1949).

Incidence of Venerupin Poisoning   So far, all outbreaks of venerupin poisoning have occurred only in the aforementioned Lake Hamana area in Japan. Between March 1889 to March 1950, 542 persons were poisoned with 185 deaths (Akiba 1949; Akiba and Hattori 1949).

Prevention of Venerupin Poisoning   Avoidance of eating shellfish from the Lake Hamana area during January to April would probably be the best means of preventing poisoning. Ordinary cooking does not destroy the toxin. The only safe way of identifying toxic shellfish is by laboratory toxicity tests.

"Callistin" (Choline) Shellfish Poison

The Japanese callista, *Callista brevisiphonata*, is the only mollusk identified with callistin poisoning. Two outbreaks of callistin poisoning occurred in Mori, Hokkaido, Japan, in 1950 and 1952 (Asano et al. 1950, 1953). A total of 119 persons were reported to have been poisoned. It is a relatively rare occurrence in comparison to the other types of shellfish poisoning.

The shellfish are said to be toxic only during the spawning season from May to September. Callistin has been shown to be identical to choline, and occurs in high concentrations in the ovaries of the shellfish. As much as 100 to 500 mg choline/100 g of ovaries (dry weight) may be present (Asano 1954).

Choline is a semiessential vitamin in that it can be synthesized in the body from dietary precursors. It is an essential component of acetylcholine and phospholipids, important in neurotransmission and of lecithin, a lipid function and transport, respectively. Again, there is an example of a biologically essential compound which is toxic when ingested in excess.

Symptoms of Callistin (Choline) Poisoning in Humans   The symptoms of callistin poisoning may begin from 30 to 60 min after ingestion. Sometimes symptoms may ensue rapidly, even while the patient is still eating the shellfish. The observed symptoms are itching, flushing of face, urticaria, sensation of constriction of the chest and throat or numbness or paralysis of the throat, mouth, and tongue. There may be, in addition, epigastric and abdominal pain, nausea, vomiting, dyspnea, coughing, asthmatic manifestations, hoarseness, thirst, hypersalivation, sweating, chills, and fever. The pulse rate may be increased. Slight hypotension, dilation of the pupils, and leukocytosis also may be observed. These symptoms are akin to allergic manifestations and have been called a pseudoallergic reaction (Asano 1954). The victims generally recover within 1 or 2 days, and there have been no reported fatalities.

Feeding 50 to 70 g samples of the callistin poison in nine volunteers elicited one response with severe symptoms. The volunteer showed similar symptoms to those seen in accidental poisonings (Asano et al. 1953).

Symptoms of callistin poisoning could not be elicited in mice, kittens, and dogs (Asano et al. 1953).

Callistin, or choline, shows three distinct actions: muscarinic, nicotinic, and epinephrine mobilization (Sollmann 1949). The first is shown by parasympathetic stimulation, resulting in the lowering of blood pressure in nonatropinized cats. The second is manifested by the effects of autonomic ganglic stimulation, affecting neuromuscular functions. Thus, the blood pressure of atropinized cats is increased; the denervated

gastrocnemius of these animals can be contracted by choline. The third action is manifested by the dilation of denervated and atropinized iris.

Hemolytic and Other Intrinsic Toxicants in Pelecypods

The clam *Saxidomus giganteus* also has been reported to contain a hemolytic factor
which can be inactivated by heating at 56°C for 30 min (Johnson 1964). Human red
blood cells of various types are lysed by this factor. This clam also contains an agglutinin which appears to be specific for Type A human blood factor. Red blood cells of
the phenotypes A and AB are agglutinated; A_2 cells partially absorb the agglutinin.
Types B and O are unaffected (Johnson 1964). The agglutinin appears to be a protein,
and can be inactivated by heating at 70°C for 20 min.

The surf clam *(Mactra solidissima)* contains a heparinlike anticoagulant (Thomas
1951, 1954). The anticoagulant, or "mactin-A," may consist of four types of sulfated
polysaccharides, as suggested by Love and Frommhagen (1953). The mantle tissues are
the richest source of these materials; the clam foot and adductor muscles, the poorest
sources (Thomas 1954).

The clam *Mercenaria mercenaria* contains an unidentified heat-stable, nondialyzable
cytotoxic compound and other nonspecific toxic agents. These factors are soluble in
20% NH_4SO_4 (Li et al. 1965).

Other toxic factors in pelecypods are inorganic salts, which may be present in high
concentrations. These are discussed in Chapter 18 on metallic and organometallic
contaminants.

ARTHROPODS

The arthropods (phylum Arthropoda) comprise the single largest group in the animal
kingdom, with more than 775,000 species which are more highly developed than those
in phylum Mollusca. They are characterized by a metameric body divided into a head,
thorax, and abdomen; the segments in the body bear a pair of jointed appendages
which usually terminate into claws, pads, or spines. The arthropods have exoskeletons
consisting largely of chitin; molding of the exoskeleton takes place at certain intervals.
The digestive tract of these animals is also divided into three sections: foregut, mid-
gut, and hindgut. The coelum is reduced and replaced by a haemocel. There is also a
contractile heart, a simple circulatory system, and a nervous system (Meglitsch 1967).
Both marine and terrestrial species are members of the phylum. However, for purposes
of this book, only species of the classes Merostomata (horseshoe crabs) and Crustacea
(lobsters, crayfish, shrimp, crabs) are of interest.

Horseshoe Crabs

The horseshoe crabs are a class of arthropods, also known as king crabs, characterized by a carapace shaped like a horseshoe. They have an arched cephalothorax, a
wide unsegmented abdomen with three-jointed chelicerae, pedipalpi, and six-jointed
legs. They are not crabs in the true sense. Horseshoe crabs are scavengers and feed
on both marine plants and animals. Thus, they are found at depths of 2 to 6 fathoms,
on sandy or muddy bottoms where they lie buried. These arthropods seem doomed for
extinction; according to Halstead and Courville (1965), only five species are living today, distributed into three genera, Limulus, Carcinoscorpius, and Tachypleus. *L.
polyphemus* appears to be the only species found in the North American Atlantic coast
and the Gulf of Mexico. The others are found in Japanese, Korean, and Indo-Pacific
waters (Halstead 1956; Shuster 1950, 1960; Waterman 1953a,b).

Horseshoe crabs are eaten mostly in Asia. Most human poisonings are due to three
Asian species, *C. rotundicauda* (king crab), found in the Indo-Pacific area (Halstead
1956; Waterman 1953b) to southern Philippine waters; *T. gigas* (Indo-Papuan king

crab), in the Bay of Bengal and Indochina coastal waters (Halstead 1956); and *T. tridentatus* (Moluccan crab), in Japanese, Chinese, and Philippine waters (Waterman 1953a). They become toxic during the reproductive season; all fleshy tissues of the animal are toxic, particularly the unlaid green eggs.

Many cases of poisoning from eating these arthropods have been fatal. The symptoms have been reported to occur 30 min after ingestion. The victim initially experiences dizziness, headache, nausea, vomiting, abdominal cramps, diarrhea, slow pulse rate, cardiac palpitation, numbness of the lips, paresthesias of the lower extremities, hypothermia, and general weakness. In severe poisoning, the victims develop the following symptoms in rapid succession: loss of voice; heat sensation in the mouth, throat, and stomach; severe weakness of the legs and arms; trismus (lockjaw); hypersalivation; general muscular paralysis; drowsiness; coma; and finally death, which may occur within 16 hr. There are no accurate data on the mortality rate, but it is reputedly estimated to be very high (Soegiri 1936; Waterman 1953b).

In mice, extracts of the horseshoe crab *C. rotundicauda* injected intraperitoneally produce sweating, ataxia, and sluggishness. These symptoms are followed by muscular spasms and paralysis of all limbs. Death occurs in 1 to 2 hr (Banner and Stephen 1966). The intraperitoneal LD_{50} of the toxin in mice (death in 1 hr) is approximately 120 mg solids (from the aqueous extracts per mouse; the corresponding LD_{100} (death in 2 hr) is 40 mg solids (from the ether extracts of the tissues) (Banner and Stephen 1966).

There appears to be more than one rotundicaudata toxin based on its solubility in water and ethyl ether (Banner and Stephen 1966).

The symptoms of horseshoe crab intoxication suggest that a neurotoxin is involved. The nature of the horseshoe crab toxin is unknown; as yet, there is no antidote.

Of less importance trophotoxicologically are the powerful hemagglutinins from the hemolymph of the American horseshoe crab, *L. polyphemus*. These are high molecular weight proteins which avidly agglutinate erythrocytes of many vertebrates (Cohen 1968). Their activity can be enhanced 10 to 1000 times with 0.1 M $CaCl_2$ (Marchalonis and Edelman 1968).

Prevention of Horseshoe Crab Poisoning

Even though horseshoe crabs are highly esteemed in Asia, it is advisable these species be eliminated from the diet. Their alleged value as a delicacy is not worth the risk.

Crustaceans

Among crustaceans, the species in the subclass Malacostraca are the main interest here: i.e., crabs, crayfish, shrimp, and lobsters. These arthropods are familiar to most individuals; therefore, their morphology will not be described.

The very few reports of intoxication caused by crustaceans are confined to the xanthid crabs (family Xanthidae). A few species of these crabs have been incriminated in human poisoning: *Eriphia norfolcensis* (poison crab), found in Norfolk Island, Australia (Grant and McCulloch 1907); *Xanthodes reynaudi*, in the Indo-Pacific region (Serene 1952); *Zosimus aeneus* and *Carpilius convexus*, in the Gilbert Islands in the South Pacific (Cooper 1964) and Ryukyu and Amani Islands off the coast of southern Japan (Hashimoto et al. 1967); also from the latter group of islands, *Platypodia granulosa* (Hashimoto et al. 1967) and *Atergatis floridus* (Inoue et al. 1968); *Demania* spp. (Alcala and Halstead 1970) and *Lophozozymus pictor* in the Philippines (Gonzales and Alcala 1977) as well as in the Singapore area (Teh and Gardner 1970, 1974).

From descriptions of case histories, it appears that *Z. aeneus* (Hashimoto et al. 1967), *Demania* spp. (Alcala and Halstead 1970), and *L. pictor* (Gonzales and Alcala 1977) are highly toxic. The first species has been incriminated in several poisonings, with a number of fatalities. Humans can die from eating the crab *L. pictor* within 30 to 60 min. Intense abdominal pain, dizziness, and profuse vomiting occur in about 30 min after eating the poisonous crab (Gonzales and Alcala 1977). *Z. aeneus* causes death in 3.5 to 4.5 hr (Hashimoto et al. 1967). The symptoms, in the case of poisonings caused by the latter, may begin in 15 min after a meal, with numbness of the tongue, anaesthesia in the mouth, violent emesis, numbness and later paralysis of the limbs, coma, and death in severe cases.

The extreme lethality of the toxin has been further demonstrated by the death of pigs and domesticated fowls that have been fed the toxic crab meal or have ingested the vomitus of a victim that died (Hashimoto et al. 1967).

Hot water extracts of *Z. aeneus* and *C. convexus* apparently contain a neurotoxic substance. The toxin is not a protein and is relatively heat stable, being able to withstand at pH 3, heating at 100°C for 15 min. It is not stable in highly alkaline (pH 10) solutions under these conditions; about 50% of its toxicity is lost. It is soluble in aqueous methanol, slightly soluble in aqueous ethanol, but insoluble in other less polar organic solvents. This toxin appears to resemble chemically the water-soluble toxins isolated from ciguateric fish (pp. 563–566).

The toxin seems to be highly concentrated in muscles of the crab and the exoskeleton of its appendages. The other parts of the exoskeleton, viscera, and gills seem to contain little or no toxin (Hashimoto et al. 1967).

Extracts of 100 mg of the toxic flesh of *Z. aeneus* are lethal to mice usually within 30 min. The animals show typical neurological signs of restlessness, gasping, jumping, and paralysis of the hind legs. Aqueous extracts of as little as 2 to 3 mg of the tissues of *Z. aeneus* and *P. granulosa* injected peritoneally are also lethal to mice (Hashimoto et al. 1967).

The crab toxin given orally and subcutaneously is also lethal to kittens. An oral dose of 10.4 g steamed crab/kg also produces paralysis of the hind legs, but earlier than in mice — 20 min. In addition, there is vomiting, jumping, complete paralysis of the limbs, gasping, and death within an hour. Adult cats show similar symptoms when injected subcutaneously with a toxic dose of the crab extract. These symptoms appear to have similarities with those seen in saxitoxin (pp. 530–531) and tetrodotoxin (pp. 547–548) poisoning (Hashimoto et al. 1967).

The purified aeneus toxin has a toxicity of 1240 MU/mg of solid. The minimum lethal dose for the mice is 0.04 μg/g body weight. Chromatographic evidence as well as comparison of the dose-death time relationship of aeneus toxin and saxitoxin suggest that the two toxins may be identical. Similarly, the chromatographic behavior and dose-death time curves for the toxin in *A. floridus* show that this toxin and that of *Z. aeneus* and, thus, saxitoxin may be the same (Inoue et al. 1968).

The toxin in *L. pictor* has been partially purified. Chemical and chromatographic tests (Teh and Gardner 1970) and a comparison of the dose-death time curves of saxitoxin, tetrodotoxin, and the pictor toxin show that the latter is a different compound from either of the first two toxins (Teh and Gardner 1974). This crab toxin appears to be a highly water-soluble alkaloid which is unstable, especially in acid solutions. It has a molecular weight of between 1000 and 5000. The intraperitoneal LD_{50} of this toxin (semipurified state) is 377 μg/kg. The crude product appears to be a weaker toxin than either tetrodotoxin and saxitoxin. Mice injected with a comparable low dose of the crab toxin are killed in 4 hr, compared to the death time with either saxitoxin or tetrodotoxin; the animals die in 30 min with a minimum lethal dose (Teh and Gardner 1974). The apparently weaker toxicity of the crab toxin may be due to its impure state; a smaller dose than either saxitoxin or tetrodotoxin in terms of pure crab toxin may have been given.

Other Crustaceans

There are many early references to human poisoning caused by various species of crabs, and sometimes lobsters and shrimp or crayfish. Unfortunately, the species of these alledged poisonous crustaceans have not been identified nor were vital toxicological and epidemiological data supplied by the authors (Halstead and Courville 1965).

Prevention of Crab Poisoning

The malacostracas are among the choice delicacies of the world; there are only a few toxic species. The toxic crabs belong to the Xanthidae family, which consists of many nontoxic species (Inoue et al. 1968). Because crabs are an important food delicacy, a toxicological survey of all species is badly needed, for as we have seen here, some species are deadly poisonous. Fortunately, the poisonous species can be recognized, but mistaken identification can easily occur and has resulted in fatalities. There is a tremendous risk in the consumption of unknown species. The nature of the toxin is unknown; consequently, there is no antidote. However, even in serious poisonings, fatalities can be reduced by treating the patients symptomatically.

FISH

Ichthyologists recognize about 25,000 species of fish; yet only less than 13 kinds are commercially valuable on a large-scale basis, worldwide. A few kinds, such as the herring, anchovie, cod, haddock, hake, and mackerel, are exploited heavily. There are, of course, many other edible fish that are caught on a limited scale, but the majority of the 25,000 species have yet to be utilized more efficiently (Schaefer and Revelle 1959).

Research in the past several decades has increased our understanding of the types of toxic fish, the nature and sources of toxins, and the conditions governing their toxicity. The major problem facting marine toxicologists is the variability and often unpredictability of the toxicity of this segment of marine life. Information regarding the source of the adventitious toxicity of fish is vital toward the eventual control of the hazard. Knowledge of the nature and mode of action of the toxin is essential toward the development of antidotes and a rational assessment of the usefulness of the fish species as a food source.

There are two major kinds of toxic fish based on the origin or source of toxicity: (1) endogenously and (2) adventitiously toxic fish. Many endogenously toxic species are some of the most violently poisonous, and yet strangely enough, are also highly esteemed items for the table in certain areas of the world. Consequently, most fatalities are the result of the seemingly senseless consumption of these fish. As will be evident in the following sections, the degree of toxicity of these fish may fluctuate periodically, usually on a seasonal basis. In addition, the problem of identifying endogenously toxic fish becomes more complex and difficult, since there are nontoxic species among a family of poisonous fish, and such factors as geographical location can affect the degree of toxicity of these fish.

It will also be evident in the next section that, unlike endogenously toxic fish, there are many kinds of adventitiously toxic species distributed in a large number of families. Many of these species are commercially important. As discussed later in this section, a great deal of progress has occurred in the last decade in the identification of the toxin(s), their source(s), mode of action, and the factors involved in transvection. Unfortunately, a simple technique has yet to be developed to determine on site, the toxicity of a suspected fish. Furthermore, a great deal of research still needs to be done in order to define more precisely the conditions or factors which influence the toxicity of various species of fish which otherwise are wholesome to eat.

Classification of Toxic Fish Based on Tissue Distribution of Toxins

The poisonous substances in fish may be concentrated in specific tissues or organs. Accordingly, fish are classified as being (1) ichthyosarcotoxic; (2) ichthyootoxic; and (3) ichthyohemotoxic (Halstead and Courville 1965). In ichthyosarcotoxic fish, the toxin is concentrated in the muscles, skin, liver, intestines, and other tissues besides the gonads (Helfrich 1963; Russell 1965a). Ichthyootoxic fish contain toxins mostly in the gonads, i.e., ovary or testes, and the roe (eggs). Ichthyohemotoxic fish concentrate their poison in the blood. This classification is by no means sharp; an overlapping exists, since in certain fish, such as the puffer fish, the toxin may be found in all tissues. Certainly, the toxin(s) in hemotoxic fish may be expected to be present also in the tissues. Nevertheless, these designations serve as convenient toxicological and public health devices to emphasize the precautions necessary before consuming the fish. Thus, the hemotoxic fish may be eaten safely by first simply draining and washing off the blood; the ootoxic fish, by avoiding the gonads and roe; the sarcotoxic fish, by selectively choosing only the nontoxic tissues. One may also escape poisoning from ootoxic fish by avoiding them during the spawning season.

Ichthyosarcotoxic Fish

Ichthyosarcotoxic fish contain toxins which include both endogenous toxins, derived toxic substances, and poisonous biological contaminants. The endogenous toxins include tetrodotoxin, gempylotoxins, certain elasmobranch toxins, chimaerotoxins, and cyclostomotoxins. Ciguatoxins, clupeotoxins, and some elasmobranch toxins are naturally occurring biological contaminants in fish. Scombrotoxin is a derived substance produced by bacterial action. The biogenesis of several of these presumed endogenous toxins, e.g., ichthyoallyeinotoxin and elasmobranch toxin, is unknown. For some of these toxins, the evidence suggests that they are endogenous. However, future research may prove that some of these toxins may be of exogenous origin. These designations are, at best, arbitrary and expedient. They are prompted by the unknown nature of many of these toxins. Consequently, the subclass, family, or genus of the toxic fish are employed as the basis for these designations. The designations of fish toxins, as such, have one advantage: They immediately allude to the type or family of the fish which may contain the poison. This will be apparent in the following sections.

Chemical contaminants which are largely the result of human activity are discussed in Chapters 18 and 19.

Tetrodotoxic Fish   The tetrodotoxic fish, listed in Table 11.3, are grouped into five families, the largest family being Tetraodontidae. These are the puffer fish, a name which is highly descriptive of their peculiar and unique behavior. When frightened, injured, or taken out of the water, these fish will engulf air or water and inflate like a balloon. This is a defense mechanism. Rarely will one fail to recognize these fish, given this peculiar behavior which is not seen in any other group of fish. Four species of puffer fish are shown in Figure 11.5.

The puffer fish range in size from less than 10 cm to more than 3 m long; the large species can weigh more than 3.5 tons. They have worldwide distribution in both tropical and semitropical waters. Thus, tetraodontids may be located circumglobally between the latitudes of approximately 47°N and 47°S; species of the large puffer molas inhabit the more open seas even as far north as 63° (Halstead and Courville 1967). Not all puffers thrive in salt water, since some species have been found in fresh water.

Many species of puffer fish ("fugu") are an esteemed delicacy in Japan, where professional puffer fish cooks are licensed by the government. In several districts, these cooks must take special training and pass a government examination on the art and science of puffer preparation (Tsunenari et al. 1980). The Japanese know full well the violently toxic nature of some parts of the tissues of the puffer fish. However, tradition or the enjoyment of eating puffer meat overcomes whatever fear or reservations the fuguphagists may have in the consumption of puffer meat, even at the risk of death. Thus, licensed cooks are employed to dress and prepare puffer for the table. Even with experts preparing puffer meat, the risk of serious poisoning is not eliminated; it is only minimized. Even the finest cooks have been known to succumb to their own cooking (Fukuda 1951).

Table 11.3 Tetrodotoxic Fishes

Family (common name, U.S.A.)	Species[a]
Canthigasteridae (sharp-nose puffer)	*Canthigaster bennetti, cinctus, compressus, jictator, margaritatus, rivulatus*
Diodontidae (porcupine fish)	*Chilomycterus affinis, antenatus, atinga, orbicularis, schoepfi, spinosus, tigrinus; Diodon holocanthus, hystrix, jaculiferus*
Molidae (ocean sunfish)	*Mola mola; Ranzania laeuis*
Tetraodontidae (puffer, rabbit fish)	*Amblyrhynchotes, biocellatus, glaber, honckeni, hypselogeneion, loreti, richei; Arothron aerostaticus, alboreticulatus, hispidus, immaculatus, mappa, meleagris, nigropunctatus, reticularis, setosus, stellatus; Boesemanichthys firmentum; Chelonodon fluviatilis, laticeps, patoca; Colomesus Ephippion guttifer; Fugu basilevskianus, chrysops, exascurus, niphobles, oblongus, ocellatus obscurus, ocellatus ocellatus, pardalis, poecilonotus, pseudommys, rubripes chinensis, rubripes rubripes, stictonotus, vermicularis porphyreus, vermicularis radiatus, vermicularis vermicularis, xanthopterus; Lagocephalus cheesemani, laevigatus inermes, laevigatus, laevigatus, lagocephalus, lunaris, oceanicus, scleratus; Liosaccus cutaneus; Monotreta cutcutea, palembangensis; Sphaeroides annulatus, armilla, greeleyi, maculatus, nephelus, sechurae, spengleri, testudineus; Tetraodon lineatus; Torquigener hamiltoni; Xenopterus naritus*
Triodontidae (puffer)	*Triodon bursarius*

[a]For purposes of this listing, only the first species in a series under one genus carries the generic name.
Source: Halstead and Courville (1965).

   The penchant for fugu meat among the Japanese is reflected by the high rates of mortality from fugu poisoning in that country. For example, prior to World War II, puffer poisoning accounted for 44.6% of all food poisonings in Japan. After the war, education, rigid government control, and other factors have reduced this figure to approximately 20% (Fukuda 1951). Between 1967 and 1976, puffer poisoning accounted for 4.8% of all outbreaks of food poisoning and 0.3% in terms of patients of food poisoning. But puffer poisoning accounts for 61.3% of all food poisoning fatalities and 82.7% of all seafood poisoning deaths (Tsunenari et al. 1980).
   Koreans, and to a certain extent the Chinese, also seem to delight in eating fugu meat (Fukuda and Tani 1942). The extent of fugu consumption is not known in other parts of the world. During World War II, puffer fish were introduced to the fish markets in the United States along the Atlantic coast where the fish may be trapped in

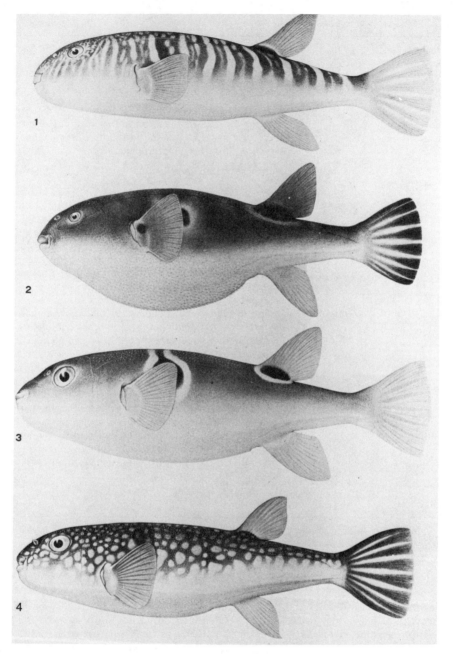

Figure 11.5 Four species of toxic puffer fish. 1. *Fugu oblungus* (actual length 26 cm). 2. *Fugu ocellatus obscurus* (actual length 12 cm). 3. *Fugu ocellatus ocellatus* (actual length 28 cm). 4. *Fugu peocilonotus* (actual length 25 cm). Reprinted with permission of the author (From Halstead, B. W. 1967. *Poisonous and Venomous Marine Animals of the World.* Vol. 2; used with permission. Photography by M. Shirao.)

large quantities. Three fatalities from puffer poisoning were reported in Florida, two in 1956 (Benson 1956), and one in 1963 (Halstead and Courville 1967). Two nonfatal cases were reported in the same state in 1974 (Center for Disease Control 1974). There also have been sporadic cases of puffer fish poisonings reported in other countries (Torda et al. 1973).

Not all species of puffer fish are toxic. For example, the puffers *Lactophrys tricornis* and *L. trigonus* (Larson et al. 1960), *Liosaccus cutaneus*, *Logocephalus spadiceus*, *Ostracion immaculatum*, *Lacotria diaphana*, and *Aracana aculeata* (Tani 1945) are nontoxic. Several other species are only weakly or moderately toxic; e.g., *Sphoeroides pseudomus*, *Cantigaster rivulatus*, and *Lagocephalus inermis*. The most toxic species are those which contain the toxin in many tissues, most of them in lethal quantities (see next section; e.g., *Sphoeroides (Fugu) niphobles*, *S. alboplumbeus*, *S. vermicularis (Fugu vermicularis vermicularis)* (Kawabata 1971; Ritchie 1980; Tani 1945; Tsunenari et al. 1980). In Japan, the most commonly eaten species are *Fugu rubripes rubripes*, *E. vermicularis vermicularis*, *E. vermicularis porphyreus*, *E. pardalis*, *E. poecilonotus*, and *E. chrusops* (Fukuda 1951; Ogura 1971); consequently, a survey has shown that these are the most common cause of poisoning (Fukuda 1951).

There is variability in the toxicity of certain puffer species depending on the geography, season of the year, and sex of the fish (Shimada et al. 1983). For example, *Arothron meleagris* from the Hawaiian Islands was found to be nontoxic, whereas the same species caught about the same time of the year from Phoenix Islands in the South Pacific was found to be very toxic (Halstead and Courville 1967).

The puffer fish also increase in toxicity beginning in September; toxicity reaches its peak just before or during the spawning season in May and June (Ritchie 1980; Tani 1945; Tsunenari et al. 1980). One survey has shown that most poisoning in Japan occurs between late fall and late spring (Fukuda and Tani 1937). This coincides with the puffer season; fugu meat, reportedly, has the best flavor between November and February.

The female puffer is, of course, more poisonous than the male, since the ovaries tend to be much more poisonous than the testes (Banner 1977; Tani 1945).

Toxin in puffer fish: As with other toxic marine species, certain tissues of the puffer fish appear to accumulate the poison more than any other. The most toxic parts are the ovaries and liver; the intestines in some species (e.g., *Fugu niphobles*) is also quite toxic. The skin in several species can be moderately toxic. The muscles and testes are generally nontoxic, except in the very toxic species in which these tissues are weakly or moderately toxic (Fukuda 1951; Shimada et al. 1983; Tani 1945; Tsunenari et al. 1980). The ovaries, however, can be mistaken frequently for the testes, and thus pose a significant risk of poisoning.

Puffer fish is considered to be very toxic if less than 10 g of tissue is lethal, moderately toxic if 10 to 100 g is lethal, weakly toxic if 100 to 1000 g is lethal; or in terms of mouse units, 20,000, 2000, and 200 MU or more, respectively. A mouse unit in this case is the amount of toxin per gram of mouse required to kill a 15- to 20-g mouse. Thus, 1000 MU will be sufficient to kill 50 20-g mice.

An estimated MLD for tetrodotoxin for humans of about 200,000 MU was given by Tani (1945, 1969). Based on mouse MLD values of 0.16 mg (Kao 1972) to 0.4 mg/20 g mouse (Halstead 1981), the equivalent MLD for humans is between 1.6 and 4.0 mg.

By means of capillary isotachophoresis assay, the amount of tetrodotoxin in the ovary of the more commonly consumed puffer fish species (e.g., *F. vermicularis vermicularis*, *F. rubripes rubripes*, and *F. poecilonotus*) ranges from 0.146 to 0.404 mg/g; that of the liver from 0.0018 to 0.113 mg/g; and that of the skin from 0 to 0.301 mg/g (Shimada et al. 1983). Thus, it is obvious that consumption of as little as 10 g of tissue may be fatal to humans. However, in the above species, the muscles are essentially free of toxin. The liver of some species as obtained by mouse bioassay technique contains much higher levels (Tani 1945). (Note that the mouse bioassay technique gives comparable tetrodotoxin values to the more sophisticated capillary isotachophoresis [Shimada et al. 1983].)

The toxic substance in puffer fish has been chemically characterized and its structure determined. Tetrodotoxin, as it is now popularly called, is an alkaloid, a derivative of aminoperhydroquinazoline with a molecular weight of 319. The structure, as shown below, has been determined by Tsuda and his group (1964) and by Woodward (1964).

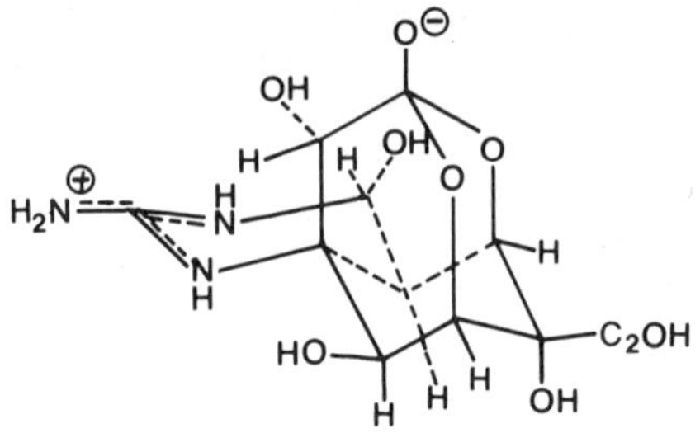

Tetrodotoxin

Tetrodotoxin is sparingly soluble in water, soluble in acid solutions, and unstable above pH 7 or below pH 3 (Kao 1966). It is also partly inactivated by heating at 116°C under 12.5 psi for 75 min (Halstead and Bunker 1953). This monoacidic base has a pk_a at 8.5. The terminal NH_2 group tends to form a zwitterion with one of the hydroxyl groups (Camougis et al. 1967).

Tetrodotoxin is also secreted by the California newt *Taricha torosa* (Buchwald et al. 1964), and it has been reported to be identical to maculotoxin, the poison from the venom gland of the blue-ringed octopus, *Hapalochlaena maculosa* (Sheumack et al. 1977). The toxin also has been found in another fish, *Gobius criniger*, a goby from Taiwan and Amami-Oshima Island (Noguchi and Hashimoto 1973), and from four species of Costa Rican, and to a lesser extent, Panamanian frogs of the genus Atelopus (Kim et al. 1975). This toxin also has been detected in the Japanese ivory shell *(Babylonia japonica)* (Noguchi et al. 1981). The presence of tetrodotoxin in significant amounts in seemingly unrelated species indicates that the toxin is not of exogenous origin, derived through the food chain, but rather produced endogenously by the animal.

Biological action of tetrodotoxin and symptoms of puffer fish poisoning: The action of tetrodotoxin is similar to that of saxitoxin, only more intense. Like saxitoxin, the toxin appears to interfere with nerve conduction by blocking the sodium channel; thus, the initial increase in the permeability of nerve membranes to sodium ions is curtailed (Grunhagen 1980; Kao 1972; Narahashi 1972). Both inward and outward sodium currents are blocked by the toxin. The steady-state flow of potassium ions is not affected. Narahashi (1972) has shown that the toxin binds to some receptors of the outside layer of the nerve cell membrane; evidence suggests that one toxin molecule per channel is bound. The target of the toxin has been shown to be the motor axon and the muscle membrane (Kao and Fuhrman 1963; Ritchie 1980). As shown by Evans (1967), a lower toxin concentration is required (4.5 to 13 µg/kg) to block the nerve conduction in the sensory fibers than in the motor fiber; the required dosage is greater for the latter by 35%.

Apparently, other special types of sodium channels outside the nerve membrane, such as in the fibroblast, are also blocked by tetrodotoxin (Pouyssegur et al. 1980). However, not all sodium channels in these cells are blocked; thus, those channels essential to deoxyribonucleic acid (DNA) synthesis and cell proliferation are not blocked.

Like saxitoxin, tetrodotoxin not only causes muscular paralysis, but also hypotension. Only, in this case, hypotension is more pronounced and predictable. As explained by Kao (1972), this follows from a direct relaxation of the smooth muscles and a blockage of the vasomotor nerves, resulting in a release of the vasomotor tone.

Tetrodotoxin has no effect on the release of neurotransmitters from the presynaptic nerve terminals at the synaptic and neuromuscular junctions (Halstead 1981). It has little or no effect on smooth muscles such as cardiac tissue. This toxin also has little, if any, influence on active sodium transport (Halstead 1981; Narahashi 1972).

Tetrodotoxin has a profound effect on respiration; very low doses, 4 to 5 μg/kg, can cause immediate respiratory arrest in animals (Evans 1969). It is a very powerful emetic, as shown in dogs injected subcutaneously or intramuscularly with 0.7 μg of toxin per kilogram, or 0.3 μg/kg intravenously (Hayama and Ogura 1958, 1963). The emetic action of this poison suggests an effect on the central nervous system; a nicotinic action of the toxin in the emetic mechanism has been suggested (Borison et al. 1963; Hayama and Ogura 1963; Murtha 1960). Hypothermia is also produced by tetrodotoxin, which also indicates a central nervous system (CNS) action (Borison et al. 1963).

The effect on the CNS is reflected not only by its depressant effects on the medullary centers, but also on the skeletal muscles, intracardia conduction, and on the contractile force of the heart (Halstead 1981).

The observed effects of tetrodotoxin as a result of its action on the CNS appear to depend on the area of the brain that is affected. Thus, when the toxin is injected into medullary structures involved in controlling cardiovascular action, such as the nucleus tractus solitarii (NTS) and the nucleus reticularis lateralis (NRL), opposite effects are observed. In the NTS of the cat, tetrodotoxin produces hypertension without bradycardia, whereas in NRL, hypotension and bradycardia result (Bousquet et al. 1980). Borison and McCarthy (1977) have observed hypotension preceded occasionally with hypertension when tetrodotoxin is injected intracerebroventricularly into cats and rabbits. This hypertensive effect may explain the lack of decrease in blood pressure in a case of puffer fish poisoning even though the patient is unconscious and near death (Tsunenari et al. 1980).

The symptoms of puffer fish poisoning in humans are consistent with the observed effects of tetrodotoxin. Within 10 to 45 min, sometimes up to 3 hr, after ingestion of the toxic fish, there are observed malaise, pallor, dizziness, and paresthesia about the lips, tongue, and throat, which is usually described as a tingling sensation. The prickling sensation may then spread to the fingers, toes, and other parts of the limbs; this is followed by numbness, which in some cases may spread to the entire body, giving a sensation of floating in air. The initial signs progress to more severe symptoms of hypersalivation, hyperperspiration, extreme weakness, hypothermia, hypotension, precordial pain, headache, and rapid pulse; gastrointestinal symptoms such as nausea and emesis (sometimes with large quantities of blood), and diarrhea may be seen early in the course of poisoning. In some cases, these symptoms are absent. In severe cases, superficial or deep reflexes may be decreased or absent; proprioception may also change.

Respiratory distress becomes prominent after the development of paresthesias, with increased rate of respiration, a diminution in the depth of respiration, and cyanosis of the lips, extremities, and body surfaces. Petechial hemorrhage over a large portion of the body with blistering and desquamation may be seen. Muscular twitching, tremor, and incoordination appear, leading to complete muscular paralysis; the throat and larynx become paralyzed first, resulting in loss of voice and difficulty in swallowing, and then progressing to complete aphagia. The patient's eyes become glassy; convulsions may occur. Though some victims may be comatose, most patients remain conscious throughout the ordeal and retain comprehension of what is happening until a few minutes before death. Indeed, there are accounts of patients who were pronounced dead but were, in fact, alive and aware of the imminent process of being buried or cremated alive (Halstead and Courville 1967; Kao 1966; Russell 1965a; Tsunenari et al. 1980). Death is the result of complete respiratory inhibition, subsequent to progressive ascending paralysis which involves the respiratory muscles. Death may occur as early as 17 min after ingestion of puffer meat, but usually between 6 to 24 hr. Survival after 24 hr may indicate a good prognosis for the patient.

In summary, the appearance of the symptoms of puffer poisoning may be divided into four stages: (1) oral paresthesias and gastrointestinal symptoms; (2) paresthesias

spreading to other areas and motor paralysis of the extremities, with reflexes intact;
(3) more severe symptoms of gross muscular incoordination, e.g., aphonia, respiratory
distress, hypotension, with no loss of consciousness; and finally (4) agonal symptoms
of severe hypotension, respiratory paralysis, and impairment of mental acuity — the
cardiac beat is maintained for a short period in this stage (Fukuda and Tani 1941;
Ritchie 1980).

As yet, no effective antidote to puffer poisoning has emerged. However, cysteine
reportedly prevents death in mice if injected 10 to 30 min after tetrodotoxin poisoning
(Fujii et al. 1967). But this treatment appears to have not been tried in humans.

The suggested treatment is symptomatic: emetics, gastric lavage, and enemas to
eliminate the toxin from the body as much as possible; maintenance of respiration arti-
ficially; maintenance of circulating blood pressure and volume with intravenous solution (lactate Ringer's solution) and vasopressor agents with close supervision to the
electrolyte balance; use of analeptics (such as pentylenetetrazol [Metrazol]); and use
of cardiac stimulants such as digitalis (Halstead and Courville 1967; Ritchie 1980).

Prevention of puffer fish poisoning: Obviously, the best safeguard against puffer
poisoning is to avoid these species altogether. If one has the insatiable predilection to
consume puffer fish, one should be aware of avoiding eating the viscera; by all means,
the puffer fish must be prepared by an expert and bought from a reputable (licensed)
restaurant. Nevertheless, even under these conditions, the risk of serious poisoning
may still be present.

Heating and all means of cooking do not eliminate the poison. The commercial canning processes may not minimize the lethality of the puffer fish (Halstead and Bunker
1953).

Gempylotoxic Fish   The gempylids, or snake mackerels, are a small group of predatory oceanic or pelagic fish. They resemble the mackerels except for the absence of a
lateral keel on the caudal peduncle. Three species are known, which belong to a single
family, Gempylidae: the escolar *(Lepidocybium flavobrunneum);* the castor oil fish
(Ruvettus pretiosus) (Banner and Helfrich 1964; Cooper 1964; Fish and Cobb 1954);
and the snoek, or barracouta *(Thyrsites atun)* (Prosvirov 1963). The first species is
rather rare; the other two have worldwide distribution in the Indo-Pacific, South American Pacific, and tropical Atlantic oceans, and along the South African coast line.

Gempylotoxin is, in fact, an oil which is a strong purgative. The oil is found in
the flesh and bones of the gempylids. The purgative in the oil, which is present in the
unsaponifiable fraction, consists of cetyl and oleyl alcohols. The purgative power of
gempylid oil is similar to castor oil (Macht and Barba-Gose 1931a,b; Mori et al. 1966).
Diarrhea following ingestion of the gempylid occurs rapidly, generally without pain or
cramps. Its diarrheal action is produced only by oral administration and is a relatively
mild form of intoxication. A dose of 25 to 30 ml produces diarrhea in dogs.

Toxic Elasmobranch Fish   These groups of fish of the class Chondrichthyes consist
of two subclasses: Elasmobranchii, composed of the sharks, skates, and rays; and
Holocephali, the chimaeras. The latter will be discussed in a separate section.

Toxic sharks: The shark is known to almost everyone. Nineteen species reported
to be poisonous are distributed among eight families. (1) Carcharhinidae, or requiem
sharks — Carcharhinus (reef sharks), Galeocerdo (tiger sharks), Galeorhinus (oil, or
school, sharks), Prionace (blue sharks), Scoliodon (sharp-nosed sharks; (2) Dalatii-
dae, or sleeper sharks — Somniosus (Greenland sharks); (3) Hexanchidae, or cow
sharks — Heptranchias (sharp-snouted seven-gilled sharks) and Hexanchus (cow
sharks); (4) Isuridae, or mackerel sharks — Carcharodon (white shark); (5) Scylio-
rhinidae, or cat sharks — Cephaloscyllion (swell sharks) and Scyliorhinus (dogfish,
nursehound); (6) Sphyrinidae, or hammerhead sharks — Sphyrna; (7) Squatinidae,
or angel sharks — Squatina (monkfish); and (8) Triakidae — Mustelus (smooth dogfish) and Triaenodon (houndsharks) (Banner 1967; Halstead and Courville 1965, 1967;
Russell 1965a).

The shark is, of course, found in all oceans, seas, gulfs, bays, and lagoons. They are voracious eaters, constantly devouring all things within their reach.

Aside from the notoriety of certain species of this group as man-eaters, many species of sharks are also known for their poisonous livers and musculatures. From the signs and symptoms of shark poisonings, there appears to be three different types of shark toxins.

1. One type of toxin appears to be concentrated in the liver of certain species. The liver toxin produces symptoms of poisoning in humans within 30 min following indigestion. The gastrointestinal and neurological symptoms consist of nausea, vomiting, diarrhea, abdominal cramps, anorexia, headache, prostration, rapid pulse, malaise, insomnia, cold sweats, oral paresthesias, and a burning sensation in the tongue, throat, and esophagus. The illness becomes more severe with time, as indicated by the development of extreme weakness with trismus, muscular cramps, a sensation of heaviness in the limbs, and blepharospasm. The pupils dilate, the upper eyelids contract spasmodically, and visual disturbances begin to be noted as the illness progresses; in addition, the patient begins to hiccough, and to feel a tingling sensation in the finger tips, and an aching in the joints. Delirium, ataxia, inability to control evacuative functions, dysuria, desquamation, pruritus, respiratory distress, and coma are prominent signs that the disease is worsening. These later symptoms may be observed in the agonal stages of the disease, which sometimes terminates fatally (Cooper 1964; Halstead 1958, 1959, 1964; Russell 1965a). Most cases of shark liver poisoning recover completely in 5 to 20 days (Cooper 1964). The nature of the toxin is not known.

Species of sharks implicated in this type of poisoning include the gray reef shark, *Carcharhinus menisorrah*, of Palmyra Islands (Halstead and Schall 1958), the tiger shark, *Galeocerdo cuvieri*, in the Gilbert Islands (Cooper 1964), and practically all other species of the genera listed above. The supernatant from an aqueous extract of the liver and gonads of the Palmyra Island gray reef shark injected intraperitoneally in white mice has been shown to produce hypoactivity, ataxia, piloerection, lacrimation, diarrhea, paralysis, and death within 36 hr (Halstead and Schall 1958).

2. The second type of shark toxin is that found in the fish's musculature. This is exemplified by the poison in the muscles of the Greenland sleeper shark, *Somniosus microcephalus*. The symptoms of Somniosus meat poisoning in humans are similar to those observed in dogs. Boje (1939) has reported that dogs poisoned by the meat of this shark begin to walk with slow, stiff steps, hypersalivate, vomit, and develop explosive diarrhea. Poisoned dogs also develop conjunctivitis, muscular twitching, unusual outward and upward ocular movements, respiratory distress, tonic and clonic convulsions, and death. The more serious types of poisoning show no symptom of diarrhea. The symptoms appear to be precipitated by physical exertions; whereas poisoned animals show no sign of poisoning while at rest, on exertion, they begin to gasp for breath, perspire, salivate, develop ataxia, and finally collapse. The dogs recover when allowed to rest.

The nature of the water-soluble toxin in the muscles of Greenland sleeper sharks is unknown. However, it appears to lose its activity on drying in open air. In this case, the poison is not completely inactive, since it appears to be transformed during drying to a compound that acts synergistically with the intact toxin in fresh shark meat; whatever the transformation product is, in the dried meat, it has no toxicity by itself. These conclusions have been based on the effects observed in dogs fed both fresh and dried meat (Boje 1939). Ordinary cooking does not destroy the toxin, but it may be leached out by frequent changes of cooking water.

The toxicity of the Greenland shark reportedly varies with individual sharks, the locality where it is caught, and the time of the year. The meat of this shark is occasionally eaten by humans when dried (Jensen 1948).

Another shark species with toxic musculature is *Mustelus canis*, the smooth dogfish seen along the North American Atlantic and Caribbean coasts (Macht 1942; Macht and Spencer 1941).

3. The third type of toxin in sharks may be similar to ciguatoxin (pp. 563–566). A toxin from the liver of the gray reef shark, *Carcharhinus menisorrha*, has been isolated by Li (1965), who found it to have pharmacological activity similar to ciguatoxin from the red snapper, *Lutjanus bohar*. Cooper (1964) also has reported the similarity between the symptoms seen in cuguatera and in poisonings caused by the liver of sharks caught in the Gilbert Islands. Only in this case, the symptoms occurred with greater rapidity and severity. The nature of ciguatera poisoning is discussed in the section on ciguateric fish (pp. 563–566). Considering the eating habits of sharks, the transvection of ciguatoxin by these fish is to be expected.

The first two types of toxins appear to be distinct from ciguatoxin, as shown by the clinical picture produced by shark liver or musculature poisoning. For example, in these types of poisonings, there is no sign of the sensory disturbance characterized by temperature reversal sensation which is strikingly characteristic of ciguatera.

Some writers (Bouder et al. 1962; Helfrich 1961) suggest that the toxin causing shark liver poisoning is retinol or its derivatives. However, the clinical picture, which includes severe and varied neurological disturbances, cannot be accounted for simply by hypervitaminosis A. In addition, the amount of retinyl compounds in certain poisonous shark livers has been shown to be too low to produce the observed symptoms (Cooper 1964).

Toxic skates and rays: Four species of rays and two species of skates have been reported as poisonous. The toxic rays are the blunt-nosed stingray, *Dasyatis say;* the smooth butterfly ray, *Gymnura micrura* (Macht 1942; Macht and Spencer 1941; Taft 1945); the spotted eagle ray, *Aetobatus narinari* (Halstead and Bunker 1954); and the cramp fish, *Torpedo marmorata* (Maass 1937). The species of toxic skates include the flapper skate, *Raja batis,* and the thornback ray, *Raja clavata* (Phisalix 1922).

The flesh, and especially the viscera, of these species of rays and skates have been reported to be poisonous, but little is known regarding the symptomatology of poisonings caused by eating these species. It is believed that the symptoms of ray and skate poisoning are similar to those seen in shark poisoning. It is also possible that skates and rays may transvect the ciguatera poison (Halstead 1964, 1959, 1958).

Chimaerotoxic Fish Two species of chimaeras, or ratfish or elephantfish, have been reported to be toxic: *Chimaera monstrosa* and *Hydrolagus colliei* (Halstead 1959, 1964; Halstead and Bunker 1952). There is very little information on the toxicity of these species, or on the symptomatology of poisoning caused by them. The flesh, and especially the viscera, of chimaeras are considered toxic. However, intraperitoneal injection in mice of extracts of the musculature and viscera of the ratfish *H. colliei* have shown that only the oviduct is moderately toxic (Halstead and Bunker 1952). The geographical distribution of the ratfish, i.e., in cooler north and south temperate waters, precludes their involvement in the transvection of ciguatoxin (Halstead 1958, 1959, 1964). The chemical nature of the toxin, its mode of action, and the symptomatology of chimaera poisoning in humans is not known. There are some vague references in the older literature in the case of the latter (Halstead and Courville 1965), but it is difficult to assess their validity.

Cyclostomotoxic Fish The cyclostomotoxic fish consist of four species of lampreys and one species of hagfish. The species of lampreys reported to be toxic include the Caspian lamprey, *Caspiomyzon wagneri,* the river lampreys, *Lampetra fluviatilis* and *L. planeri,* and the sea lamprey, *Petromyzon marinus* (Hiyama 1943; Maass 1937; Pawlowsky 1927). The Atlantic hagfish, *Myxine glutinosa* (Engelsen 1922), is the lone species in the family Myxinidae reported to be toxic.

The cyclostomes are probably the most primitive of the true vertebrates; they have an eel-like form, a primitive cranium, cartilaginous or fibrous skeletons, and no definite jaws or bony teeth (Halstead and Courville 1965).

The hagfish are exclusively saltwater fish, whereas the lampreys are inhabitants of both marine and freshwaters of the Northern Hemisphere. The hagfish are scavengers; they are troublesome parasites, particularly of netted fish. The lampreys are bloodsuckers and parasitize many commercial fish (Halstead and Courville 1965).

The hagfish can produce slime profusely; the slime is reputedly toxic.

Most cyclostome poisonings have been reported to be due to failure to remove the slime in hagfish before cooking (Engelsen 1922). However, the flesh and skin of raw and cooked hagfish and certain species of lampreys may also contain a toxin. The symptoms of poisoning may develop within a few hours after eating the fish. Usually, the symptoms are mainly gastrointestinal effects: nausea, vomiting, dysenterylike diarrhea, tenesmus, abdominal pain, and weakness. The victim generally recovers after several days (Engelsen 1922; Halstead 1958; Pawlowsky 1927).

The chemical nature of the toxin is unknown. However, secretions from the buccal glands of various species of these fish have anticoagulant effects on human and catfish blood. The latter also has been shown to be hemolyzable by these secretions (Gage and Gage-Day 1927). Whether this has any relationship to the toxicity of the cyclostomes is not known.

Ichthyoallyeinotoxic (hallucinogenic) Fish   Ten species of fish have been reported to cause hallucinations following ingestion: convict surgeonfish, or tang (*Acanthurus triostegus sandvicensis*), two species of sea chubs (*Kyphosus cinerasceus* and *K. vaigiensis*), two species of mullets (*Mugil cephalus* and *Neomyxus chaptalli*) (Helfrich and Banner 1960); two species of surmullets (*Mulloidichthys samoensis* and *Upeneus arge*) (Bouder et al. 1962; Helfrich 1961, 1963); damselfish, or sergeant major (*Abudefduf septemfaciatus*), grouper (*Epinephelus corallicola*) (Cooper 1964), and rabbitfish (*Sigamus oranin*) (Wheeler 1953). It should be noted that most, if not all, of these species have been incriminated in the more common and widespread form of ichthyotoxicism, ciguatera. This clinical entity is discussed later in this chapter.

The most frequently reported causes of this type of poisoning have been mullets, so that the clinical entity was previously designated hallucinatory mullet poisoning (Russell 1965a). Helfrich and Banner (1960) termed the illness ichthyosarcephialtilepsis, or hallucinatory fish poisoning, since mullets have not been the only species involved.

The toxin causing this poisoning has not been chemically determined. It is not destroyed by the usual cooking processes. The poison is found in the flesh of the fish, but appears to be concentrated in the head. The conditions which determine whether this species will cause the hallucinatory symptoms is difficult to predict. Thus, its occurrence is very sporadic.

The symptoms indicate that the primary target of the toxin is the central nervous system. They begin within 10 to 90 min after ingestion. The victim complains of lightheadedness, dizziness, weakness, muscular incoordination, ataxia, hallucinations, and depression. When the poisoning is severe, paresthesia about the mouth, muscular paralysis, and dyspnea are observed. Violent nightmares may occur if the victim falls asleep following intoxication (Russell 1965a). A sensation of tightness around the chest or a heavy load on the chest is a common complaint (Halstead 1964). Compared to other types of ichthyosarcotoxism, this one is relatively mild; the victim usually recovers completely in 2 to 24 hr.

Prevention of ichthyoallyeinotoxicism: It is difficult to prevent this type of poisoning because of its unpredictability. However, one should be wary of this possibility in tropical areas, especially when dealing with the species listed above. It would be wise to consult the local people regarding such species, and one should avoid eating the head of tropical reef fish.

Clupeotoxic Fish   There are 20 species of fish distributed in three families that have been reported to be clupeotoxic. The latter term is derived from the name of the family of fish frequently implicated in this type of poisoning. These are listed in Table 11.4.

Most of the above fish thrive in tropical waters in the Asian, Indo-Pacific, Mediterranean, Arabian seas and the Red Sea, the Indian Ocean, and the South American and other tropical areas of the Pacific Ocean. Fish that have been implicated in clupeotoxicity are usually nonpoisonous; in fact, some of them are important food species; e.g.,

Table 11.4 Fish Reported as Clupeotoxic

Species	Common name
Family Clupeidae	
Anondostoma chacunda	Shirt-finned gizzard shad
Clupanodon thrissa	Sprat or thread herring
Clupea spratfus	Sprat
Dussmieria acuta	Round herring
Harengula humeralis	Red-ear sardine
Harengula ovalis, H. zunasi; Sardinella *fimbriata, S. longiceps, S. perforata,* *S. sindensis*	Sardine
Ilisha africana	Herring
Macrura ilisha	Sablefish
Nematolosa nasus	Gizzard shad or long-finned gizzard
Opisthonema oglinum	Atlantic thread herring
Family Elopidae	
Megalops Cyprinoides	Tarpon
Family Engraulidae	
Engraulis enchrasiculus, E. japonicus, *E. ringeus; Thrissina baelama*	Anchovy

Source: Halstead and Courville (1965).

sardines, herrings, and anchovies. They become toxic sporadically and unpredictably. Some have seasonal variability in their toxicity; others, such as a species of Fiji herring, are constantly toxic (Banner and Helfrich 1964). Accordingly, tropical clupeiform fish are most likely to be toxic during warm summers. Most species listed in Table 11.3 gather together in large schools. The intriguing and unfortunate fact of it all is that some fish in a particular school may be toxic, while the majority are nontoxic (Banner and Helfrich 1964).

Clupeotoxicism can be a serious public health problem in certain parts of the world, not only because of the unpredictability of its occurrence, but also from the violent and often lethal nature of the poisoning. Accurate data of its prevalence are unavailable, being a nonreportable disease. There are a few scattered reports of clupeotoxicism. Two outbreaks were reported in the Philippines in 1953 and 1955 in which 87 cases were involved, with 14 to 17 deaths (Garcia 1955). The common Philippine sardine "tamban" (*Sardinella longiceps*) was implicated. Three cases of sardine (*Harengula* spp.) poisoning were also reported in Tarawa in the Gilbert Islands in the South Pacific. All three people died (Cooper 1964). An unaccounted number of poisonings resulting in five deaths caused by another sardine (*Clupea venenosa [Harengula ovalis]*) were also reported in 1955 in the Fiji Islands in the South Pacific (Banner and Helfrich 1964). Available reports usually paint a distinct and violent picture of the poisoning.

Symptoms of clupeotoxicism: The first sign of clupeotoxic fish poisoning in humans is the sensation of a sharp metallic taste in the mouth, which may be felt immediately upon ingestion. There then follow signs of gastrointestinal disturbances: nausea, dryness in the mouth, vomiting, abdominal pain, diarrhea, and malaise. These symptoms may be accompanied by weak pulse, tachycardia, chills, cold and clammy skin, hypotension, cyanosis, and other signs of vascular collapse or shock. Neurological symptoms may appear at the same time or follow immediately; i.e., nervousness, severe headaches, numbness, tingling sensations, hypersalivation, dilatation of the pupils, muscular cramps, progressive muscular paralysis, respiratory distress, convulsions, and coma. Death may occur rapidly, sometimes within 15 min. Those who survive the ordeal develop pruritus and other types of skin eruptions with desquamation and ulceration. The great potency of the clupeotoxin is suggested by descriptions of poisoning in the older literature. One author (Ferguson 1823) described a fatal clupeotoxicism whereby death occurred very rapidly, even while the fish was still in the victim's mouth (Banner and Helfrich 1964; Halstead 1978; Helfrich 1961, 1963; Randall 1958).

The nature of the toxin in clupeotoxic fish or its source is unknown. The toxin may be derived from the food chain, particularly certain types of dinoflagellates (Randall 1958). The red tide dinoflagellate, *Pryodinium bahamense*, is suspected as a possible source of the toxin (MacLean 1979). More work needs to be done in this respect. The toxin appears to be concentrated in the viscera of the fish. Ordinary ways of cooking, i.e., boiling, frying, baking, steaming, and broiling, do not eliminate the toxicity.

The apparent rarity of the occurrence of this type of poisoning may account for the lack of research efforts directed toward identifying clupeotoxin and the conditions governing the clupeotoxicity of these fish.

One must be wary of the possibility of clupeotoxicism when consuming fish in a tropical locality.

Clupeotoxicism may be considered distinct from ciguatera, since the clupeotoxic fishes are plankton feeders, whereas ciguateric fishes are mainly bottom feeders (Halstead 1978). While it may be difficult to distinguish clupeotoxicism from severe ciguatera poisoning, the former has been separated by biotoxicologists as a distinct clinical entity (Helfrich 1961; Randall 1958).

Ciguatoxic Fish   The origin of the term "ciguatera" is not certain, but it is believed to be derived from "cigua," the name that Cuban natives used for the common gastropod *Turbo pica* during the early Spanish conquest. This mollusk causes stomach upset, and people who were so affected were referred to as "ciguatos" or "enciguatos," or loosely translated, "affected by cigua." The term came to be used for all types of poisoning caused by marine products, hence the term ciguatera (originally "siguatera"). The modern usage restricts the term to specific types of poisoning caused by various species of fish (Halstead 1978; Halstead and Courville 1967).

As seen in Table 11.5, more than 400 species of fish have been reported to be ciguatoxic at one time or another (Halstead 1978). These species are distributed among at least 57 families. Several examples of fish that may become ciguatoxic are shown in Figure 11.6A-D. Their distribution is worldwide, but these fish are found mainly in tropical waters. The broad phylogenetic distribution of ciguatoxic fish indicates the complexity of the problem of ciguatera poisoning. It suggests the possibility that practically all kinds of saltwater fish may be transvectors of ciguatera poison. Randall (1958), in his review of ciguatoxic fish, offered a number of observations which are summarized in the following paragraphs.

Ciguatoxic fish are generally bottom dwellers or shore fish, found usually at depths less than 300 feet. [There are, of course, some pelagic fish that have been found to be ciguatoxic, but these have been caught close to shore. The pelagic Spanish mackerel (*S. commersoni*) from Queensland, Australia, has been implicated in numerous ciguateralike poisonings. The toxic fish have been shown to contain a lipid soluble toxin similar to ciguatera (Lewis and Endean 1983).] Frequently, these fish also are found to be associated with coral reefs as opposed to those that dwell mostly in open waters, over sand, mud, or turtle grass; the latter types are often less toxic. Ciguatoxic fish are frequently caught near islands because of abundant reef formations in the vicinity. However, the geographical locations or distributions of ciguatoxic fish are not consistent. In this case, much variability has been observed; for example, one part of an island may harbor toxic species, whereas in another part, only wholesome species are found. Even within the area of the reef, the ciguatoxic fish are found only in specific locations, and not all over the reef; this suggests that the ciguatoxi fish are nonmigratory.

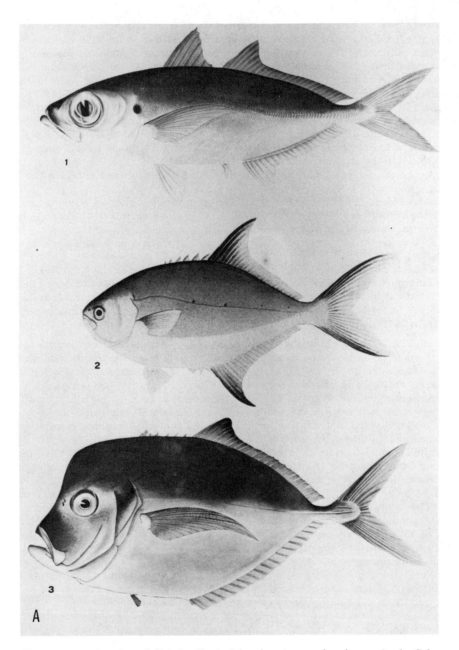

Figure 11.6 Species of fish implicated in ciguatera poisonings. A, 1. *Selar crumenoph-thalmus* (horse-eye jack) (length 60 cm). 2. *Trachinotus bailloni* (pompano) (length 30 cm). 3. *Vomer setapinnis* (Atlantic moonfish (length 20 cm). (Photographs 1 and 3 by T. Kumada; 2 by R. Kreuzinger.)

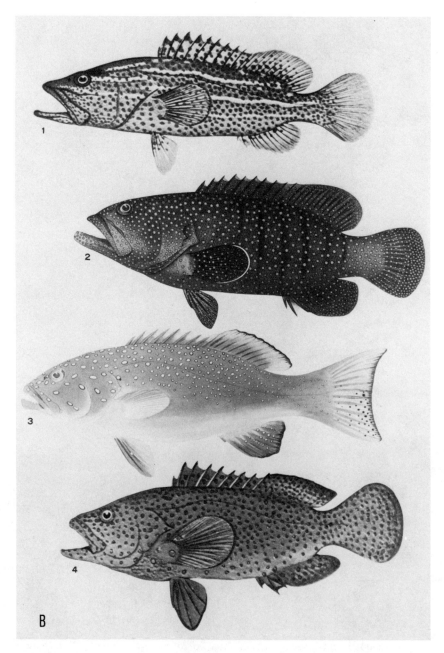

Figure 11.6 (continued) B, Groupers. 1. *Anyperodon leucogrammicus* (grouper, sea bass) (length 40 cm). 2. *Cephalopholis argus* (spotted grouper) (length 50 cm). 3. *C. leopardus* (grouper) (length 50 cm). 4. *C. miniatus* (length 25 cm). (Photographs 1 and 4 by T.C. Marshall; 2 by K. Tomita; 3 by T. Kumada.)

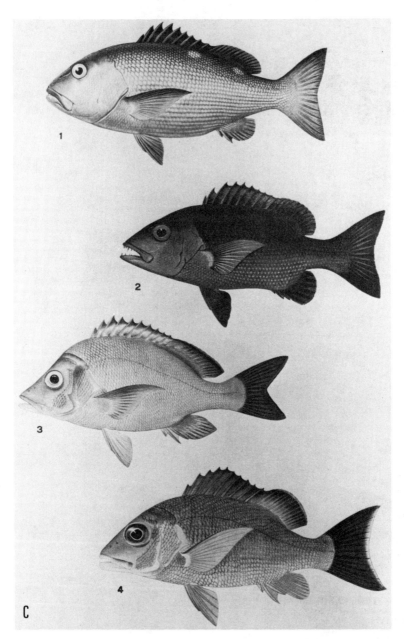

Figure 11.6 (continued) C, Snappers. 1. *Lutjanus bohar* (length 90 cm). 2. *L. coatesi* (length 79 cm). 3. *L. gibbus* (length 40 cm). 4. *L. jauthinuropterus* (length 60 cm). (No. 1 photograph by M. Shirao; No. 2, G. Coates; No. 3, K. Tomita; No. 4, T. Kumada).

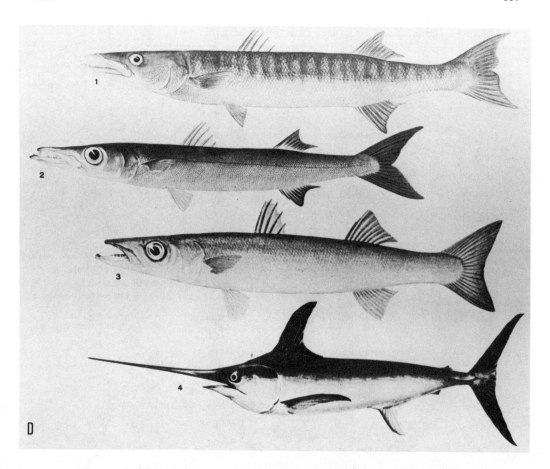

Figure 11.6 (continued) D, 1-3, barracudas; 4, swordfish. 1. *Sphyraena barracuda* (length 1.6 m). 2. *S. forsteri* (length 47 cm). 3. *S. nigripinnis* (length 40 cm). 4. *Xiphias gladius* (length 5 m). (Photographs by T. Kumada; 3, by Fisheries Society of Japan; 4, by T. Walford) (From Halstead, B. W. 1967. *Poisonous and Venomous Marine Animals of the World*. Vol. 2; used with permission.)

Another complicating factor is that there is no permanency in the ciguatoxicity of fish in a specific location. An area which once supported ciguatoxic fish may suddenly become a nontoxic zone and vice versa. A poisonous fish population may suddenly develop following severe disturbances in the water, such as storms, earthquakes, or other catastrophes, including those due to human activities (Lee 1980).

Ciguatoxi fish follow a pattern of all types of feeding behaviors: carnivores feed on smaller fish and mollusks; herbivores feed on benthic algae; omnivores feed on both types; and others feed on detritus. None appears to be a plankton feeder except the clupeiform fish. While there are ciguatoxic fish that are relatively small in size, most species associated with human poisonings are large to moderate in size. Thus, the larger fish may feed on smaller ciguatoxic fish and become toxic themselves. Field observation in the Tuamoto Archipelago in the Pacific confirmed the preceding sequence of ciguatoxicity among fishes. Thus, the herbivores together with detritus feeders became toxic first; the carnivores became toxic 10 months later. The larger carnivores

Table 11.5 Types of Fishes Reported to Be Ciguatoxic

Family	Group common name	Genus
Acanthuridae	Surgeon fish	Acanthurus, Ctenochaetus, Prionurus
	Unicorn fish	Naso
	Tang	Zebrasoma
Albulidae	Bonefish	Albula
Aluteridae	Filefish	Alutera, Anacanthus, Pseudaluteres
Antennariidae	Sargassum fish	Histrio
Apogonidae	Cardinal fish	Apogon, Cheilodipterus, Paramia
Arripidae	Tommy rough	Arripis
	Australian salmon	Arripis
Aulostomidae	Trumpetfish	Aulostomus
Balistidae	Triggerfish	Abalistes, Balistapus, Balistes, Balistoides, Canthidermis, Melichthys, Odonus, Pseudobalistes, Rhinecanthus
Batrachoididae	Toadfish	Coryzichthys, Opsanus, Thalassophryne
Belonidae	Garfish	Belone
	Needlefish	Belone, Strongylura
Blenniidae	Blenny	Entomacrodus, Ophblennius
Bothidae	Flounder	Bothus, Scophthalmus
Carangidae	Jack	Carangoodes, Caranx, Selar, Seriola
	Rainbow runner or Hawaiian salmon	Elegatis
	Leatherjacket	Oligophites, Scomberoides
	Lookdown	Selene
	Amberjack	Seriola
	Rudderfish	Seriola
	Pompano, permit, palmometa	Trachinotus
	Horse mackerel	Trachurus
	Atlantic moonfish	Vomer
	Surgefish	Zalocys
Chaetondontidae	Butterflyfish	Chaetodon
	Bannerfish	Heniochus
	Angelfish	Holocanthus, Pomacanthus, Pygophites
Chanidae	Milkfish	Chanos
Cirrhitidae	Hawkfish	Paracirrhites
Clupeidae	Shad	Anodontostoma, Nematolosa
	Sprats	Clupanodon, Clupea
	Herring	Dussumieria, Ilishia, Opisthonema
	Sardines	Harengula, Sardinella
	Sablefish	Macrura
Congridae	Conger eel	Conger

Table 11.5 (continued)

Family	Group common name	Genus
Coryphaenidae	Dolphin	Coryphaena
Elopidae	Tarpon	Megalops
Engraulidae	Anchovy	Engraulis, Thrissina
Exocoetidae	Flying fish	Cypselurus
Gempylidae	Oilfish	Ruvettus
Gerridae	Silverfish	Gerres
Gobiidae	Goby	Acentrogobius, Ctenogobius, Oligo-lipes, Zenogobius
Hemiramphidae	Halfbeak	Hemiramphus, Hyporhamphus
Holocentridae	Squirrelfish Soldierfish	Holocentrus Myripristis
Istiophoridae	Sailfish	Istiophorus
Kuhliidae	Mountain bass	Kuhlia
Kyphosidae	Rudderfish	Doydixodon, Kyphosus
Labridae	Hogfish Wrasse	Bodianus, Lachnolaimus, Cheilinus, Coris, Ctenolabrus, Epibul-us, Halichoeres, Thalassoma
Lophiidae	Goosefish	Lophiomus, Lophius
Lutjanidae	Snapper	Apareus, Aprion, Gnathodentrix, Gymnocranius, Lethrinus, Lutjanus, Lythrulon, Monotaxis, Ocyurus, Plectorhinchus
Monacanthidae	Filefish	Amanses, Monacanthus, Navodon, Oxymonocanthus, Paramonocanthus, Pervagor, Pseudomonocanthus, Stephanolepis
Mugilidae	Mullet	Chelon, Crenimugil, Mugil
Mullidae	Surmullet or Goatfish	Mulloidichthys, Parupeneus, Openeus
Muraenidae	Mottled or spotted eel Moray eel	Echidna Gymnothorax, Muraena
Ogcocephalidae	Batfish	Ogcephalus
Ophichthyidae	Snake eel Worm eel	Callechelys, Leiuranus, Myrichthys, Ophichthus, Oxystomus Echelus
Ostraciontidae	Cowfish Trunkfish	Acanthosthracion, Kentiocapros, Lactophrys, Lactoria, Ostracion, Rhinesomus, Rhynchostracion

Table 11.5 (continued)

Family	Group common name	Genus
Phempheridae	Sweeperfish	Phempheris
Pomacentridae	Damselfish	Abudefduf, Dascyllus, Pomacentrus
Pomadasyidae	Grunt	Anisotremus, Orthopristis
Priacanthidae	Bigeye (Glasseye snapper)	Priacanthus
Scaridae	Parrotfish	Chlorurus, Euscarrus, Scarops, Scarus
Scatophagidae	Spadefish	Scatophagus
Sciaenidae	Croaker (Drum)	Johnius, Nibea, Odontoscion
Scombridae	Wahoo Skipjack Bonito Mackerel	Acanthocybium Euthynnus Sarda Scomberomorus
Scorpaenidae	Zebrafish Barbfish, lionfish Scorpionfish Oceanfish or redfish	Pterois Scorpaena Scorpaena, Scorpaenopsis Sebates
Serranidae	Grouper Creolefish Seabass Soapfish	Anyperodon, Cephalopholis, Permato-lepsis, Epinephelus, Mycteroperca, Paralabrax, Plectropomus, Variola Paranthias Promicrops, Epinephelus Rypticus
Siganidae	Rabbitfish	Siganus
Sparidae	Porgy Scup	Calamus, Erynnis, Pagellus, Pagrus, Sparus Stenotomus
Sphyraenidae	Barracuda	Sphyraena
Syngnathidae	Seahorse	Hippocampus
Synodontidae	Lizardfish	Synodus
Xiphiidae	Swordfish	Xiphias
Zanclidae	Moorish idol	Zanclus

Source: Halstead and Courville (1965).

and omnivores, such as the moral eel, remained toxic for many years after the first toxic fish was detected (Banner 1976).

That there is a correlation between fish size and toxicity is widely held among islanders (Gilman 1942; Hiyama 1943). This belief has been confirmed by experimental observations. For example, Hessel et al. (1960) found that of 190 specimens of red snapper, *Lutjanus bohar,* only 18% of those weighing less than 2.8 kg were toxic in contrast to 69% of those that were heavier. In another survey, among 437 random samples of the same fish from the Line Islands, the incidence of toxic samples increased from 25% for those weighing less than 1 kg to 100% for those over 5 kg (Banner et al. 1963).

Unlike other types of fish toxicity, there is no seasonal pattern in ciguatoxicity (Banner et al. 1963; DeSylva 1963; Halstead 1978).

There may be some evidence that ciguatoxicity is a cyclic phenomenon. In the case of fish surrounding some islands in the Pacific, this cycle may last for 8 years (Cooper 1964). Similar conclusions, with some variations, have been reported by other observers for fish around the Hawaiian Islands (Banner 1965; Banner and Helfrich 1964), Line Islands (Helfrich et al. 1968), Johnston Islands (Brock et al. 1965), and other places.

Source of ciguatera poison: There is substantial evidence to support the theory that the ciguatera poison in fish is derived from the food chain (Banner 1965; Cooper 1964; McFarren et al. 1965; Randall 1958). The theory states that the smaller fish feed on toxic algae. The toxin in the algae is retained and accumulated in the body of the fish for prolonged periods. These fish may be eaten by larger ones, which in turn become toxic. Finally, the toxin is similarly retained and accumulated in the body of the larger fish. This theory explains many observations regarding ciguatoxic fish as described by many investigators.

A number of feeding experiments support the theory that a fish becomes poisonous by feeding on a toxic product without itself being poisoned, and that it is unable to detoxify rapidly and eliminate toxic substances that have been ingested. Halstead (1951) has reported that the nontoxic California cottid (*Leptocottus armattus*) can be induced experimentally to become toxic by feeding on the toxic flesh of the puffer *Arothron hispidus* for 10 days. The nontoxic surgeonfish *Acanthurus xanthopterus* was made toxic by eating a diet of toxic red snapper, *Lutjanus bohar,* for 18 months (Helfrich and Banner 1963). It also has been observed that ciguatoxic red snappers did not lose their toxicity to any significant degree when maintained on a nontoxic diet of Hawaiian skipjack tuna and herring (Banner et al. 1963). In a similar experiment, 66 ciguatoxic large red snappers fed a similar diet for 30 months in a tidal pond also did not show any statistically significant decrease in toxicity (Banner 1965).

Because many ciguatoxic fish are obligate herbivores (Dawson et al. 1955; Randall 1958), it is evident that the source of their poison must be certain marine plants such as algae or plankton. The algae which have been suspected as possible sources of the ciguatera toxins are the blue green algae *Lynbya majuscula* (Banner 1976; Dawson 1959; Dawson et al. 1955; Habekost et al. 1955; Randall 1958) and *Plectonema terebrans* (Cooper 1964). These algae grow abundantly in areas where ciguatoxic fish are found, and also have been observed more frequently in the stomach of toxic fish. Several other species of algae are also suspected as sources of ciguatera toxin; e.g., *Caulerpa serrulata* and *Bryopsis pennata* var. *secunda* (Habekost et al 1955).

The suspicion that these macroalgae may be a source of ciguatoxin is supported by the report that in Samoa, ciguateralike poisonings had occurred following consumption of fish feeding on "aga," a poisonous, low-growing, red seaweed. Furthermore, during a ciguatera outbreak in Oahu, Hawaii, among the victims were some individuals who ate a red algae known as "limu" (Lewis 1981). However, Randall (1958) had ruled out these large algae as a source of ciguatoxin because many ciguateric fishes are detritus feeders and are unable to feed on coarse algae. It is, of course, possible that the toxicity of certain macroalgae may arise from certain dinoflagellates attached to their stems (Taylor 1979; Withers 1981).

There is now sufficient evidence implicating a newly identified, photosynthetic, epiphytic dinoflagellate, *Gambierdiscus toxicus*, as a source of ciguatoxin (Bagnis et al. 1980; Withers 1982; Yasumoto 1980; Yasumoto et al. 1977a,b, 1979). This organism is related to the gonyaulax group (Taylor 1979) (see page 518), which are noted for their paralytic toxins. *G. toxicus*, however, being a slow grower (Bagnis et al. 1979, 1980) differs from the Gonyaulax species in that the former is not associated with the red tide in coastal waters, as with the latter. These dinoflagellates have been found to be attached to certain seaweeds (macroalgae); e.g., *Spyridea filamentosa*, *Acanthophora spicifera*, and *Sargassum polyphyllum*. Species of *G. toxicus* have been found in both Pacific and Atlantic reef areas (Bagnis et al. 1980; Taylor 1979, 1980; Withers 1982; Yasumoto et al. 1977a).

The key to this discovery of *G. toxicus* as a source of ciguatera toxins was the surgeonfish *(Ctenochaetus striatus)*, which was responsible for 65% of ciguatera cases in Tahiti during a given period (Bagnis 1968). This fish can only feed on biodetritus and not the large algae (Randall 1958). Thus, an examination of the detrital diet of this fish originating from dead corals showed a fraction that was laden with the toxic dinoflagellates (Yasumoto et al. 1977a). Bagnis et al. (1980) obtained two types of toxins from wild and cultured *G. toxicus* — one fat soluble and the other water soluble. The wild dinoflagellates were taken from biodetritus obtained from coral surfaces in an area in the Gambier Islands waters rich in ciguatoxic fish. Both types of toxins are comparable, with respect to their chemical and biological properties, to reference toxins, respectively — ciguatoxin, obtained from the moray eel liver, and maitotoxin, obtained from the digestive contents of the surgeonfish. There are, however, some differences in certain biological properties, such as lethality, between the reference ciguatoxin (MLD [µg/g mouse] = 0.05) and the ciguatoxin from the wild (MLD [µg/g mouse] = 0.1) and cultured MLD [µg/g mouse] = 4.6 *G. toxicus*. These differences have been explained on the basis of the degree of purity of the samples so obtained. Additionally, some types of biotransformation to more lethal forms in the tissues of the fish are possible. Therefore, a certain variation in biological properties has been observed. There is also chromatographic evidence which indicates an interconversion between ciguatoxin and maitotoxin. Note that similar phenomenon has been seen with the gonyaulax toxins, as noted previously.

In an earlier work, Yasumoto et al. (1977a) arrived at the same conclusion by comparison of the pharmacological and chromatographic properties of ciguatoxin and maitotoxin obtained from wild *G. toxicus*, and those from the moray eel and the parrotfish (surgeonfish), respectively.

Cells of wild *G. toxicus* obtained from macroalgae from Kaneohe Bay, Hawaii, which yielded both ether- and water-soluble toxins, gave similar symptoms in mice as those reported for ciguatoxin from the moray eel, and for maitotoxin from the surgeonfish (Withers 1982).

The dinoflagellates produce greater amounts of maitotoxin compared to ciguatoxin. The magnitude of difference may range from less than twofold to greater than 10-fold (Bagnis et al. 1980; Withers 1982).

There are also differences between the toxin yields from cultured and wild *G. toxicus*. Cultured cells yield lesser amounts of toxins than the wild ones (Bagnis et al. 1980; Withers 1982). Apparently, some factors in the wild which have not been duplicated in cultures enhance toxin production (Yasumoto et al. 1979). These may include the amount of light reaching the dinoflagellate and the salinity of the water (Yasumoto 1980). Additionally, certain bacteria appear to influence the growth of *G. toxicus*, which is both autotrophic and heterotrophic (Hurtel et al. 1979). Knowledge of these factors is important because a good correlation has been observed between ciguatoxicity of fish in an area and its population density of *G. toxicus* (Yasumoto 1980).

The varied signs and symptoms of the ciguatera syndrome indicate the presence of several types of toxins that may be present in the fish (Withers 1982). Two of these toxins have already been shown to be produced by *G. toxicus*, the organism presently implicated as the source of ciguatera toxins among fish caught in the Pacific. Several other dinoflagellates have been found to produce toxins that are lethal to mice.

(Chungue et al. 1979; Yasumoto et al. 1980). Note that the Florida red tide dinoflagellate, *Gymnodinium breve,* as discussed previously, also produces poison or poisons that resemble ciguatera toxins in pharmacological action (McFarren et al. 1965). These facts suggest that there are many species of toxic dinoflagellates, and even macroalgae, which could be potential sources of many ciguatera toxins. Thus, a ciguatoxic fish may, in fact, contain several toxins, as in the case of toxic shellfish. After all, many toxic algae abound in ocean waters (Halstead 1981).

Nature of ciguatoxins: Several toxins, in fact, have been detected in ciguatoxic fish (Hashimoto 1975, 1979). This is perhaps understandable and to be expected in view of the diverse symptomatology of ciguatera (Withers 1982). Three types have been isolated in more or less chromatographically pure state. Scheuer et al. (1967) isolated a transparent, light yellow, viscous oil from the flesh of the moral eel *(Gymnothorax javanicus),* which was named ciguatoxin. It is relatively unstable and loses activity in contact with air, light, and chromatographic adsorbents. Subsequent works have shown the viscera, and especially the liver, of the moray eel contains high levels of the toxin with minor amounts of other toxins (Yasumoto and Scheuer 1969).

A highly purified preparation of the ciguatoxin is an amorphous, colorless, heat-stable solid, giving a molecular weight of 1100 by mass spectroscopy (Tachibana 1980). This preparation has been shown to be a highly oxygenated lipid. The ciguatoxin obtained by Scheuer et al. (1967) was characterized as an hydroxylated lipid containing a quarternary nitrogen, and a cyclopentanone moiety. The presence of the quarternary nitrogen suggests that ciguatoxin is an alkaloid. The molecular weight of this preparation was 627. The fact that it is lower than that obtained by Tachibana (1980) suggests that different methods of preparation may change the physical or chemical make-up of the toxin. This is suggested by the different properties of the two ciguatoxin preparations, as noted previously. These differences give further evidence that ciguatoxin should be a generic name representing several closely related toxins derived from various sources that comprise the diet of various fish.

Ciguatoxic surgeonfish *(Ctenochaetus striatus)* contains two toxins. One appears identical to the moray eel ciguatoxin, and is distributed throughout the flesh and viscera of the fish. The second is a water-soluble, nondialyzable toxin, which is called maitotoxin (from "maito," the Tahitian term for surgeonfish) (Hashimoto 1979; Rayner 1972; Yasumoto et al. 1971). This toxin is found only in the liver and viscera. As stated before, both toxins also were isolated from *G. toxicus* cells (Bagnis et al. 1980).

Two similarly fat-soluble toxins have been obtained from the parrotfish *(Scarus gibbus)* (Chunge et al. 1977), which is a predominant cause of ciguatera in the Gambier Islands (Bagnis 1974). One toxin, SG-2, is polar and chromatographically and biologically resembles ciguatoxin as obtained from the moray eel. The other, which was named scaritoxin by Bagnis et al. (1974), is nonpolar and chromatographically very different from ciguatoxin. Scaritoxin is the major toxin of the parrotfish. It is a yellowish oil soluble in methanol, ethanol chloroform, and diethyl ether, but is insoluble in hexane, and has an intraperitoneal LD_{99} of 30 µg/kg.

Various tests indicate that scaritoxin possesses many of the chemical features of ciguatoxin, suggesting that perhaps scaritoxin is ciguatoxin complexed with a nonpolar group which effectively masks the polar groups (Chungue 1977b). Thus, scaritoxin may be related chemically to ciguatoxin but sufficiently different structurally as to evoke different clinical signs in mice. These signs are discussed in the next section. It is possible that scaritoxin is a metabolic derivative of ciguatoxin.

A pharmacologically similar type of fat-soluble toxin also has been isolated from the flesh or liver of other carnivorous fish such as: the flesh of the grouper *(Epinephelus fuscoguttatus),* the liver of the gray shark *(Carcharhinus menisorrah),* and the flesh of the red snapper *(Lutjanus bohar)* (Li 1965). One specimen of red snapper appeared to possess two lipid-soluble toxins (Hessel 1961), presumably ciguatoxins.

There also is evidence that various types of fish, even in the same species, may have different toxicities. This fact indicates that each particular fish may show different toxicological profiles owing to qualitative and/or quantitative differences in toxin content. For example, Kosaki and Anderson (1968) have found that ciguatoxins extracted according to the method of Scheuer et al. (1967) from the same or different species of fish produce different pharmacological responses. Thus, the lethal intravenous doses in anesthetized rats of ciguatoxin extracts from six specimens of moray eels *(Gymnothorax javanicus)* ranged from 118 to 168 mg/kg; the doses for two specimens of grouper *(Epinephelus fuscoguttatus)* were 438 and 465 mg/kg, and that of one specimen of amberjack *(Seriola dumerili)* was 105 mg/kg.

Pharmacological action of ciguatoxins: Based on experimental evidence on intact animals as well as pharmacological assays using specific tissues, and biochemical tests for anticholinesterase activity, Li (1965) has concluded that the ciguatera toxin(s) is probably an anticholinesterase. The effect of the toxin, according to this investigator, may become irreversible quickly unless the patient is treated immediately. However, Rayner et al. (1968) have shown that the lack of correspondence between the respiratory effects of ciguatoxin and such cholinesterase inhibitors as physostigmine or para-oxon suggest that the effect of ciguatoxin is not primarily due to anticholinesterase activity. Furthermore, atropine is ineffective in blocking the respiratory effects of ciguatoxin even though atropine protects the animal against more than 10 times the effective dose of physostigmine. Rayner et al. (1968) contends that the action of ciguatoxin may be more complex and that the parallel action of ciguatoxin and acetylcholine regarding its initial respiratory effects suggests a transmitterlike cholinomimetic action. Analysis of the cholinesterase levels of the red blood cells of rats killed by i.v. injection of ciguatoxin, indicate that this toxin has no anticholinesterase activity (Rayner et al. 1969).

On the other hand, Kosaki and Anderson (1968) have found that atropine and eserine (physostigmine) antagonize the ciguatoxin-induced neuromuscular block. Since these two drugs have opposite effects, it appears that ciguatoxin has more than one site of action.

Ogura et al. (1968) showed that their ciguatoxin extract did not cause an activating response of the electroencephalogram, as observed with physostigmine. This indicates that it does not have an anticholinesterase activity. They imply that because ciguatera may be caused by several toxins, their preparation might have been different from that used by Li (1965).

Oshika (1971) has shown that ciguatoxin exhibits both cholinergic and adrenergic action in isolated rat atria. His experiments suggest that ciguatoxin releases catecholamine from its stores, as indicated by the blockage of the positive inotropic effects of ciguatoxin by reserpine pretreatment, and by MJ-1999, an adrenergic-blocking agent, and guanethidine; the latter inhibits sympathetic nerve activity by depression of post-ganglionic adrenergic nerve function. Ohizumi et al. (1981) have shown that ciguatoxin does indeed cause marked release of norepinephrine from adrenergic nerves. This release is blocked by tetrodotoxin and inhibited in the absence of calcium ions. Ciguatoxin induces the contraction of guinea pig vas deferens, and this is blocked by tetrodotoxin, procaine (a nonspecific blocking agent of ionic conductance), and in a medium low in Na^+; contraction induced by norepinephrine, acetylcholine, and high K^+ concentration is potentiated by ciguatoxin. Furthermore, ciguatoxin markedly enhances to the same degree as in fresh tissue the response to norepinephrine of guinea pig vas deferens with nerves degenerated by cold storage. All in all, these results suggest that ciguatoxin has a direct action on excitable membranes. This effect may be mediated by the increase in Na^+ permeability across the postsynaptic membrane. It has been concluded that ciguatoxin causes a release of endogenous norepinephrine from presynaptic sites, and intensifies the effects of the neurotransmitter at the postsynaptic membrane (Ohizumi et al. 1981).

Other workers (Rayner et al. 1969; Setliff et al. 1971) have reported similar effects of ciguatoxin in increasing sodium permeability of excitable membranes. Such an effect can explain the observed depolarization by ciguatoxin of pedal ganglion cells of Aplysia (Boyarsky and Rayner 1970) and frog muscle membranes (Rayner and Kosaki

1970). This depolarization is blocked by tetrodotoxin; increased extracellular calcium abolishes both this depolarization and the consequent change in membrane excitability (Rayner et al. 1969).

Ciguatera poison(s) has also significant effects on the cardiovascular system for certain individuals. A survey of more than 3000 cases of ciguatera poisoning in the South Pacific by Bagnis et al. (1979a) showed that some 15% of patients recorded a systolic blood pressure of 100 or less, and bradycardia incidence of over 13% of the patients. Tatnall et al. (1980) has reported a case of bradycardia lasting for 50 days following ciguatera poisoning from moray eel.

In experimental animals, a biphasic cardiovascular response to near lethal doses of ciguatoxin has been observed (Li 1965; Rayner 1970). In this case, an initial state of hypotension with bradycardia was followed by a phase of hypertension with tachycardia. In studies of the effects of extracts from various specimens of toxic fish in rats, Kosaki and Anderson (1968) have observed an immediate fall in blood pressure with slow recovery, which is accompanied by bradycardia; this effect developed in two of four animals injected with a lethal dose of extracts from moray eel. Those given lethal doses of extracts of amberjack (Seriola dumerilii) also develop hypotension with bradycardia; recovery from hypotension is slow and this is followed by another phase of hypotension which terminates in arrhythmia. An extract of another specimen of moray eel has shown a similar sequence of cardiovascular events as in the latter case. Extracts from specimens of grouper produce hypotension, without bradycardia and terminate with arrhythmia. Thus, there are differences in cardiovascular effects of extracts obtained from different specimens of the same species of fish as between different species. The differences were not due to quantitative variation in the amount of toxin exposure because the different doses of toxic extracts administered were at lethal levels. In other words, if there are no qualitative differences in the types of toxins, then the variation in the amounts of toxins reflects only the differences in the amounts of inactive impurities. Thus, once again, this variability in response points to the possible existence of different types of toxins in individual fish.

Ogura et al. (1968) has noted prolonged depression in blood pressure in rats injected i.p. with ciguatoxin extracted from the red snapper (L. bohar). Hypotension was inhibited by pretreatment with atropine, but not by posttreatment with the drug. Thus, atropine is not a selective antagonist of ciguatoxin, but probably acts by protecting the initial cholinergic response. Pretreatment of the rat with ciguatoxin extract inhibits pressor responses to epinephrine, norepinephrine, and nicotine. Ciguatoxin only partially paralyzes the blood vessels so as to be unresponsive to the pressor action of small doses of epinephrine, but not to larger doses. Ogura et al. (1968) has concluded that respiratory failure is partly responsible for the slow recovery from hypotension, and that ciguatoxin interferes with the central and not the peripheral mechanism controlling respiratory function. This is in contrast to the action of tetrodotoxin, which interferes principally with the peripheral mechanism.

Studies with isolated rat and rabbit heart atria by Ohshika (1971) have shown a biphasic response to ciguatoxin — an initial inhibition followed by stimulation of the rate and force of atrial contraction — i.e., an initial negative followed by positive inotropic and chronotropic effects. In this case, the negative inotropic response of the atria was abolished by atropine, whereas the positive response was reduced by adrenergic blocking agents. Miyahara et al. (1979), however, have noted only a prolonged positive inotropic effect of ciguatoxin on the electrically driven, isolated, guinea pig atria and both inotropic and chronotropic effects on the spontaneously beating right atria.

The differences between these two studies may be explained by the possible contamination of the toxin preparation used by Ohshika (1971). Thus, Miyahara et al. (1979) have observed that maitotoxin, the water-soluble ciguatoxic component of toxic fish or G. toxicus, gave a biphasic response in isolated guinea pig atria; i.e., enhancement of atrial contraction at low doses, but a depression at high doses. Therefore, the presence of maitotoxin in a ciguatoxin preparation may produce a variable response, as shown by the results of Ohshika (1971).

Symptoms of ciguatera poisoning: Ciguatera poisoning shows variable manifestations involving gastrointestinal, sensory, motor, and cardiovascular disturbances. The variability of this syndrome is seen in the differences in victims' symptoms. This variability may be related to individual reaction, dosage of poison, or especially, differences in the types of toxins; more than one of these factors may be involved. However, in general, ciguatera poisoning may be recognized by the following clinical signs, as described by Halstead (1978) and other investigators (Bagnis et al. 1979; Gelb and Mildvan 1979; Hughes and Merson 1976; Jones 1980; Lawrence et al. 1980; Lee 1980; Tatnall et al. 1980). The onset of symptoms may begin immediately after ingestion to within 30 hr; average onset within 6 hr. The initial symptoms are variable; some develop gastrointestinal symptoms consisting of nausea, vomiting, watery diarrhea, metallic taste, tenesmus, and abdominal cramps. In some cases, these signs may be accompanied by chills and fever (Chretien et al. 1981). In others, the initial signs are neurological in nature, consisting of tingling and numbness about the lips, tongue, and throat, sometimes with a sensation of dryness in the mouth. The muscles in the mouth and surrounding structures may be drawn, spastic, and numbed.

In some patients, the gastrointestinal symptoms are accompanied by severe cramps of the leg and extending to a lesser degree to the lower back (myalgia). Numbness starting in the right upper thigh and hip and extending down to the legs follows. After several hours, gait ataxia may occur, so that the patient is unable to walk unaided. Dribbling incontinence may also develop (Jones 1980).

Some patients develop the myalgia in the leg after several hours. Paresthesias of the gums and fingertips and pain in the jaw may also be delayed following the gastrointestinal symptoms (Chretien et al. 1981).

As the illness progresses, the victim complains of profound tiredness and weakness. This is to be expected considering the symptoms which may develop; i.e., back and joint aches, myalgia, headache, anxiety, prostration, dizziness, pallor, cyanosis, insomnia, chills, fever, hyperperspiration, rapid weak pulse, and weight loss. Not all these symptoms may be present, of course. Weakness may worsen until the patient is unable to walk. The muscular aches range from dull to heavy or cramping sensations of pain; sometimes the pain may be sharp or shooting, affecting particularly the arms and legs. Further neurological signs include visual disturbances — blurring of sight, temporary blindness, photophobia, scotoma, dilation of pupils, and diminished visual reflexes. In addition, the victims may complain of toothache and looseness of teeth in their sockets. As in puffer poisoning, skin disorders may also be present. This begins with intense widespread pruritus, with erythema, maculopapular eruptions, blisters, extensive areas of desquamation, usually on the hands and feet, and sometimes with ulceration. The hair and nails also may be lost.

The neurological signs become more pronounced in severe ciguatera poisoning, and the following symptoms are observed: paresthesias in the extremities, inversion of the sensation of hot and cold, progressively worsening ataxia and generalized motor incoordination, diminished reflexes, muscular paralysis with clonic and tonic convulsions, muscular twitching, tremors, loss of voice and ability to swallow, coma, and death due to respiratory paralysis.

Recovery from severe ciguatera poisoning is slow and prolonged with recurrence of some symptoms for several months. In a number of instances, prominent cardiovascular signs are noted consisting of hypotension (<100 mm Hg systolic blood pressure) and bradycardia (rate, <60/min) (Bagnis et al. 1979a). In some patients, bradycardia may persist for several weeks (Tatnall et al. 1980). Hanno (1981) has noted that bradycardia is characteristic of severe poisoning even in the presence of hypotension. The frequency of appearance of the various symptoms, as reported by three investigators, is shown in Table 11.6. Note that paresthsias of the extremities and around the mouth, temperature sensation reversal as well as arthalgia, dry mouth, myalgia, and diarrhea are most frequently observed.

Table 11.6 Frequency of Several Signs and Symptoms in Ciguatera

Signs or symptoms	Frequency according to three investigators		
	Bagnis et al. (1979)	Lawrence et al. (1980)	Barkin (1974)
Paresthesia or dysesthesia of the extremities	89.2	71	
Perioral paresthesia or dysesthesia	89.1	54	46(29)
Tingling and burning sensation of the tongue			96
Burning or pain to skin on contact with cold water (temperature sensation reversal)	87.6		
Dry mouth			92
Arthralgia	85.7		88
Myalgia	81.5	86	75
Diarrhea	70.6	76	100
Asthenia	60.0	30	
Headache (or dizziness, confusion)	59.2	47	58(13)
Chills	59.0	24	
Abdominal pain	46.5		88
Pruritus	44.9	48	50
Nausea	42.9		
Vertigo	42.3		
Ataxia	37.7		
Vomiting	37.5	68	100
Diaphoresis (with or without chilliness)	36.7	24	17
Photophobia			33
Transient blindness and blurred vision			30
Tremor	26.8		
Dental pain	24.8		
Stiff neck	24.2		
Watery eyes	22.4		
Fever			21
Skin rash	20.5		
Dysuria	18.7		
Salivation	18.7		

Table 11.6   (continued)

Signs or symptoms	Frequency according to three investigators		
	Bagnis et al. (1979)	Lawrence et al. (1980)	Barkin (1974)
Dyspnea	16.1		
Bradycardia (< 60/min)	13.4		25
Hypotension	12.2		
Tachycardia (> 85/min)	10.8		
Paresis	10.5		

Gastrointestinal disturbance may not always occur, as seen in Table 11.6 (Bagnis et al. 1979a; Hanno 1981). The neuropathy in ciguatera may also be accompanied by atrophy, especially of the muscles of the leg. Inverted T waves in the electrocardiogram suggesting myocardial ischemia may be seen in several patients. This electrocardiographic anomaly returns to normal with improvement in the clinical picture (Hanno 1981).

Ciguatera poisoning caused by the parrotfish (Scarus gibbus) may present symptoms in two phases. In the first phase, the patient may experience symptoms typical of ciguatera. But after 5 to 10 days, the patient shows signs which indicate an effect on the cerebellum; i.e., staggering walk, dysmetria, asthenia, persistent resting, kinetic tremor, and loss of both static and dynamic equilibrium. This second phase results in prolonged recovery, lasting for more than a month (Bagnis et al. 1974; Hashimoto 1979; Helfrich 1964). The occurrence of two stages of intoxication may be due to the presence of two fat-soluble toxins discussed previously, SG-2, a polar toxin, which has been identified as similar to ciguatoxin, and the nonpolar scaritoxin (Chungue et al. 1977).

Incidences of ciguatera poisoning: Even though ciguatera poisoning occurs in diverse places, worldwide incidence is unknown. Nevertheless, this incidence can be expected to be quite high and the disease endemic in those populations that depend on fish as an important item in the diet. For example, in the Caribbean, ciguatera is considered a major cause of illness even today (Doorenbos and Yasumoto 1978; Hanno 1981; Payne and Payne 1977). Hanno (1981) has estimated the incidence in St. Thomas, the Virgin Islands, at more than 60 times the incidence estimated for the Miami, Florida, area by Lawrence et al. (1980), or 300/10,000 residents. It is also a major health problem in the South Pacific, where Bagnis et al. (1979a) have reported their evaluation of more than 3000 ciguatera cases. A survey in 1966 showed that as much as 8% of the Tahitian population suffered from ciguatera poisoning at least once, even though most of these cases were mild (Bagnis 1967). Another household survey by Bagnis (1969) showed a 43% annual incidence during an epidemic on the Pacific atoll of Tuamotu.

From 1960 to 1962, 41 cases were reported in Hawaii (Helfrich 1963), and in 1974, 107 cases also were reported there (Center for Disease Control 1974).

Ciguatera poisoning also is an important health problem in Florida, where 126 cases were reported from 1960 to 1963 (De Sylva 1963); 38 and 47 cases were reported in this state in 1974 and 1975, respectively. From 1974 to 1976, 129 cases were reported in the Miami area alone (Lawrence et al. 1980).

Because ciguatera poisoning is not an officially reportable disease, the true incidence is probably underestimated. For one thing, only the severe cases are reported; mild cases do not get medical attention, as the Tahitian experience showed (Bagnis

1967). Lawrence et al. (1980) estimate that the true annual incidence is probably at least five cases per 10,000 resident population in the Miami area.

In many episodes of ciguatera poisoning, one or more species of fish are frequently implicated. In Florida and the Caribbean, the barracuda, Sphyraena spp., is frequently involved (De Sylva 1963). Thus, the sale of this fish in Miami is prohibited. Next to the barracuda, the grouper (Epinephelus and other genera) is also a major cause of ciguatera poisoning in Florida; the snapper (Lutjanus spp.) and the kingfish (Menticirrhus saxatilis and other species) also have been implicated in ciguatera poisonings in Florida (Center for Disease Control 1974, 1975). In Hawaii, the amberjack (Kahala spp.) (Center for Disease Control 1974), the black sea bass (Epinephelus tauvina and other species) and a surgeonfish (Acanthurus dussumieii) (Helfrich 1963) have been frequently implicated. Of course, there is a large number of species that can become ciguateric, as listed in Table 11.4. Nevertheless, it is important to recognize the most frequently implicated species, such as the barracuda and the grouper, so that one will know to consume these species with caution.

Table 11.7 lists the locations, types of fish, and the reported number of cases involved with each one in the United States from 1974 to 1977 (Center for Disease Control 1974–1977).

Prevention of ciguatera poisoning: As reported by Lawrence et al. (1980), the ciguatoxic fish cannot be distinguished from the wholesome species by their appearance and taste. Except for feeding trials in animals, there are no practical means of accurately determining by the consumer whether or not the fish is toxic; no simple chemical method is available to the layman. However, it is the practice of islanders to eat a small piece of the fish and wait for several hours in order to determine if any telltale signs of poisoning occur (Cooper 1964). The toxin is also heat resistant, so that ordinary processes of cooking will not detoxify the fish.

Nevertheless, certain precautions may be observed to minimize the possibility of poisoning. Halstead and Courville (1967) offer the following helpful suggestions: (1) avoid eating large predacious reef fishes such as groupers, barracudas, snappers, and jacks; (2) in particular, avoid eating the viscera and roe of all tropical marine fishes, especially during the reproductive season; (3) eat only a small quantity of any unknown variety of tropical fish; (4) avoid eating any tropical moray eels — these species may be highly poisonous and may produce instant death; (5) if at all possible, select for the table only fish captured in the open sea away from reefs or the entrance of a lagoon; (6) if it is a matter of survival, the suspect fish could be cut in small strips and soaked with several changes of water; however, this will not guarantee the safety of the fish; and (7) it is wise to ask the advice of the inhabitants of an island regarding the safety of local fish.

To the above suggestions, the following reminder must be mentioned: the toxicity of reef fish may be enhanced during natural or manmade disturbances in the surrounding waters (Craig 1980; Lee 1980). Therefore, extreme caution must be observed in eating fish obtained after such occurrences.

Avoidance of ciguatera poisoning is especially important to those who had been poisoned previously. Bagnis et al. (1979a) have found that the second and successive attacks of ciguatera may suffer more severe illness compared to those having their first attack. In those who have experienced two or more episodes of ciguatera poisoning, paresthesia of the extremities and around the mouth, hot-cold sensation reversal, arthralgia, diarrhea, asthenia, headache, and chills are significantly more common. In addition, some patients who have been repeatedly poisoned by toxic fish may develop extreme sensitivity to the fish and manifest ciguatera symptoms even though the fish may contain trace amounts of toxin (Bagnis and Kaeuffer 1974).

The incidence of ciguatera poisoning in the United States may seem insignificant compared to other types of food poisoning. This is only because the majority of the population are not frequent fish eaters; whatever fish are frequently eaten, those species are not normally associated with ciguatera.

Table 11.7   Ciguatera Poisoning in the United States 1974 to 1977

Fish involved	State	No. cases			
		1974	1975	1976	1977
Grouper	Alabama	1			
	California		9		
	Florida	31	20	3	
Amberjack	Hawaii	96	7		4
	Virgin Islands			7	
Jack fish	Hawaii	4		4	6
	California				16
Barracuda	Florida	5			
Snapper	Florida	1	10		
	Puerto Rico			3	
	Hawaii		2		
Kingfish	Florida		17		
Po'ou fish (Cheilinus spp.)	Hawaii	7	3		
Goatfish	Hawaii		2		
Surgeonfish	Hawaii			2	
Dolphin fish	Florida	1			
	Total	146	70	19	26

Source: Center for Disease Control (1974-1977).

Treatment of ciguatera poisoning: It is possible that several toxins are present in ciguatoxic fish, as suggested by the large constellation of symptoms. Thus, at this point, no effective antidote to the ciguatera poison(s) has been discovered, so that treatment is largely symptomatic (Baratta and Tanner 1970; Chretien et al. 1981; Hughes and Merson 1976; Russell 1975; Tatnall et al. 1980). Atropine has been recommended to control bradycardia, hypotension, and gastrointestinal complaints. This drug, however, has no effect on the muscle or joint pains and has only slight effects, if any, on the neurological involvement. Hughes and Merson (1976) recommend induction of emesis or gastric lavage if vomiting has not occurred; in addition, catharsis also has been recommended to remove unabsorbed toxins. Russell (1975) states that a program of intravenous high electrolytes, calcium gluconate, and vitamin B complex together with high protein diets and supplemental vitamin C "give the most satisfactory results following the acute period and lessened the duration of illness." For insomnia, diazepam has been recommended; pruritus is controlled by analgesic cream. Extremes of temperatures should be avoided, since these will sometimes result in painful pruritus and enhanced paresthesia and nausea. The use of 2-pyridine aldoxime methiodide (PAM), as proposed originally by Li (1965), is without effect and may, in fact, worsen some of the symptoms if given several hours after onset of symptoms (Okihiro et al. 1965; Russell 1975).

Scombrotoxic Fish   From the standpoint of the source of toxin, it may be argued that the discussion on scombrotoxic fish should fall under bacterial contaminants

(Chaps. 14 or 15), or under derived toxicants (Chapter 12). However, for the sake of continuity, it is best to include this subject under toxic fish.

Scombrotoxicity involves largely certain types of perciform fish, most of which belong to a single family, the Scombridae. This family consists of the mackerels and ceros (species of Auxis, Scomber, and Scombermorus (Arcisz 1950; Ellington 1959; Fredericq 1924; Helfrich 1963), tunas and albacores (species of Euthynnus and Thunnus) (Helfrich 1963, 1961; Kawabata et al. 1956; Maass 1937; Phisalix 1922), and bonitos (Sarda spp.) (Behre 1949). A few other species, such as the Japanese saury, *Cololabis saira*, have been reported as potentially scombrotoxic (Kawabata et al. 1955a,b). Nonscombroid fish, such as the dolphin fish, or "mahi-mahi" *(Coryphaena hippurus)* (Lerke et al. 1978), and anchovies (Engraulis spp.) (Murray et al. 1982), also have been implicated in scombrotoxicism.

Note that these species constitute some of the more highly commercialized marine products and have been among the most valuable resources of the canning industries. Four species of scombrotoxic fish are shown in Figure 11.7.

Tunas are pelagic fish; mackerels are more littoral in their habitat. These fish are found in large schools in both tropical and temperate waters, even in the Arctic and Antarctic seas. They are omnivorous, predatory, and voracious feeders, feeding both on plankton and fish.

Nature and origin of scombroid poison: The exact nature of scombrotoxin is not definitely known. It is believed to be a mixture of substances consisting of histamine, a substance called saurine, which is related chemically and pharmacologically to histamine, and other bacterial metabolites of histidine and similar substances in the skin and muscles of the fish. Histidine is decarboxylated to histamine in the presence of a bacterial decarboxylase (Arnold and Brown 1978; Ferencik 1970).

$$\underset{\text{Histidine}}{\boxed{\text{N} \quad \text{NH}}}\!\!-\!\!CH_2\underset{NH_2}{CHCOOH} \xrightarrow{\text{decarboxylase}} \underset{\text{Histamine}}{\boxed{\text{N} \quad \text{NH}}}\!\!-\!\!CH_2CHNH_2 \; + \; CO_2$$

The bacterial species responsible for the formation of the scombroid toxic complex have been identified as a strain of *Proteus morganii* (Hughes 1979; Kimata 1961; Kimata and Tanaka 1954). However, other bacteria may also contribute to the formation of scombroid poison (Kimata 1961); e.g., Hafnia spp., hemolytic *Escherica coli* (Ferencik 1970), and *Klebsiella pneumoniae* biotype 2 (Lerke et al. 1978).

Bacterial action is enhanced when the fish is kept at room temperature for prolonged periods. Thus, as one report shows, the histamine content in some scombroid fishes may increase from 90 μg/100 g of tissue to approximately 95,000 μg/100 g when the fish is allowed to remain at 20 to 25° for at least 10 hr (Geiger 1944).

Mackerel kept in melting ice (0°C) remain edible for up to about 12 days, and their histamine content does not rise above 5 mg/100 g (Gilbert et al. 1980; Murray et al. 1982). Fresh fish do not contain over 1 mg histamine/100 g (Gilbert et al. 1980). Above 10°C, especially at room temperature or higher, the histamine content may rise rapidly (Gilbert et al. 1980; Park et al. 1980). Samples containing up to 1000 mg/100 g of flesh have been recorded (Lerke et al. 1978).

Scombrotoxic fish meat may show no sign of putrefaction (Blakesley 1983; Cruickshank and Williams 1978; Gilbert et al. 1980; Legroux et al. 1946a,b, 1947; Merson et al. 1974; Murray et al. 1982). In fact, several fish products implicated in fish poisoning were either smoked or canned. However, many victims of scombroid poisoning often have stated that the toxic fish meat had a sharp or peppery taste (Geiger 1944; Kawabata et al. 1955b).

The role of histamine in scombroid poisoning has been questioned, since histamine administered in relatively large doses (80 to 100 mg) to dogs, cats, rats, and mice

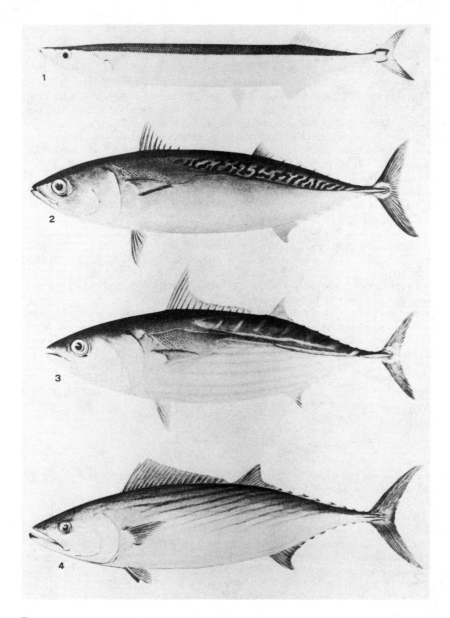

Figure 11.7 Scombrotoxic fish. 1. *Cololabis saira* (length 30 cm). 2. *Auxis thazard* (length 42 cm). 3. *Euthynnus pelamis* (length 1 m). 4. *Sarda sarda* (length 91 cm). (nos. 1-3 Photographs by Y. Hiyama; 4 by National Geographic Society). (From Halstead, B. W. 1967. *Poisonous and Venomous Marine Animals of the World*. Vol. 2; used with permission.)

produce no toxic symptoms (Geiger 1955). Furthermore, 450 to 500 mg histamine administered by mouth to humans also produce no symptoms (Aiiso 1954). However, other experiments suggest that this lack of effect is probably due to rapid detoxification of the amine in the intestines, and that toxicity can be produced if the intestinal mucosa is first damaged, for instance, by treatment with saponin for 2 consecutive days (Geiger 1955).

Even though there is doubt as to the role of histamine in scombroid poisoning (Arnold and Brown 1978), the fact that administration of antihistamines (Merson et al. 1974) such as cimetidine (Tagamet) (Blakesley 1983) produces rapid relief, indicates that histamine or a compound similar to it in pharmacological activity is involved. Furthermore, a reported case of severe scombroid poisoning, resulting in hemiparesis in a patient consuming scombrotoxic skipjack while taking isoniazid (Senanayake et al. 1978), gives further evidence of histamine involvement. Isoniazid is a potent histaminase inhibitor.

Administered parenterally, histamine produces highly toxic reactions. It can produce dilatation, as well as increased permeability of capilliaries. The latter is indicated by the characteristic wheal of localized edema when histamine is injected subcutaneously or intradermally. It also causes vasoconstriction of arteries; but since at the same time, it produces relaxation of the capilliaries and arterioles, histamine injection results in hypotension. This amine causes contraction of the smooth muscles of the uterus and gallbladder, and stimulation of secretion in many exocrine glands, such as in the gastric mucosa (Halstead 1978; Halstead and Courville 1967). The intraperitoneal LD_{50} of histamine in mice is 13 g/kg or 250 mg/20 g mouse. The route of administration can have a marked effect, since the subcutaneous LD_{100} in mice is 2.3 to 2.7 g/kg. There are also species differences in sensitivity; the intravenous lethal dose in guinea pigs, rabbits, and monkeys are 0.5 to 0.75 mg, 0.6 mg, and 50 mg/kg, respectively (Spector 1956).

The lack of effect of histamine when administered orally in both humans and animals requires further reevaluation, since there may be enzyme inhibitors in the toxic scombroid tissues which prevent destruction of histamine in the intestinal mucosa. This possibility is suggested by the observation of Shifrine et al. (1959) that spoiled tuna was not toxic to chicks in amounts of 30% of the diet unless it was cooked first and then allowed to putrify after 3 or 4 days. The possibility that a histaminase inhibitor is involved is suggested by the increased severity of symptoms in the presence of isoniazid, as reported by Senanayake et al. 1978.

Symptoms of scombroid poisoning: Scombroid poisoning has been reported to occur when the histamine content reaches about 100 mg or more per 100 g of fish muscle (Simidu and Hibiki 1955a-c). Other authors have reported histamine concentrations in fish involved in scombroid poisonings ranging from 100 to 450 to 500 mg/100 g (Kawabata et al. 1955a; Legroux et al. 1946a,b). Nevertheless, reports indicate that poisoning can occur with histamine levels as low as 20 mg/100 g of fish flesh (Gilbert et al. 1980; Murray et al. 1982).

The symptoms of scombroid poisoning, as described by several investigators (Blakely 1953; Gilbert et al. 1980; Halstead and Courville 1967; Murray et al. 1982), suggest that histamine or related compounds are somehow involved in poisoning, even though experimental trials suggest the contrary. The symptoms appear within a few minutes following ingestion of the toxic fish. The victim complains of severe headache with throbbing of the carotid and temporal blood vessels, dizziness, burning sensation of the throat, cardiac palpitation, rapid weak pulse, dryness of the mouth, thirst, difficulty in swallowing, and gastrointestinal upset indicated by nausea, vomiting, diarrhea, and abdominal cramps. The entire body may rapidly develop generalized erythema and urticarial eruptions with severe pruritus. In several patients, these signs may be limited to the face, arms, legs, and chest. There is also swelling and flushing of the face, eyes, and coryza; fever, chills, malaise, tremors, cyanosis of the lips, gums and tongue, and metallic taste in the mouth may accompany these symptoms. Bronchospasm, suffocation, and severe respiratory difficulty are seen in those who are severely poisoned. The victim may go into shock and succumb. The acute symptoms may last from 8 to 12 hr and sometimes as long as 8 days.

Since scombrotoxicity occurs because of poorly preserved specific types of fish, and since these fish may also be ciguateric, it is not unexpected that some cases of scombroid poisoning may be superimposed with ciguatera and bacterial poisonings. Thus, the clinical picture becomes very complex in this case and, of course, the poisoning will be very severe.

Scombroid poisoning is generally nonfatal; very few deaths have been recorded. Antihistaminic drugs are very effective in animals suffering from scombroid poisoning (Legroux et al. 1947, 1946a,b) and in human patients (Blakesley 1983; Merson et al. 1974). In humans, epinephrine, cortisone, and intravenous benadryl are effective (Bartsch et al. 1959), Bouder et al. (1962) and Blakesley (1983) discuss the management of scombroid poisoning.

Incidence of scombroid poisoning: The incidence of scombroid poisoning worldwide is unknown. In Japan between 1951 and 1954, 14 outbreaks occurred involving more than 1200 persons (Kawabata et al. 1955a). The Japanese saury *(Cololabis saira)* was incriminated in a majority of these cases, and in a few cases, species of mackerel were involved. In Guam, scombroid poisoning appears to be the most common form of fish poisoning. No accurate data on the incidence is available, however. In the United States between 1969 and 1977, a total of 485 persons affected with scombroid poisoning were reported to the Center for Disease Control (1969–1977). The offending fish included tuna, mahi-mahi *(Coryphaena hippurus)*, mackerel, and several other nonscombroid fish. These fish accounted for 77, 17, 2, and 4% of all cases, respectively. What is significant is that almost 20% of all cases were caused by nonscombroid fish, so that in this case, the syndrome is referred to as scombroidlike. This fact supports further the observation that the scombroid poison is not endogenous to the fish nor limited to a specific family. Several of the scombroid poisonings reported to the Center for Disease Control during this period in the United States were caused by fish served in restaurants. A number of cases were due to canned tuna.

Thus, in 1973, 232 persons poisoned by a popular brand of canned tuna in four Northwestern states were reported to the Center for Disease Control. The offending product contained 68 to 280 mg histamine/100 g of fish muscle. Typical scombrotoxic symptoms (e.g., oral blistering or burning sensation, rash with urticaria, GI symptoms, headache, flushing) began in about 45 min after eating the fish and lasted for 8 hr (Merson et al. 1974). In Britain, from 1979 to 1980, 26 incidents involved 71 persons similarly poisoned by canned fish (Murray et al. 1982). Variable levels of histamine were found and went as high as 1000 mg/100 g of fish muscle. The predominant symptoms, which appeared in 10 to 120 min after eating the canned fish, were a bright red rash, hot flush, and sweating and burning sensation in the mouth and peppery taste. Scombrotoxicism was initially recorded in that country in 1978 (Cruickshank and Williams 1978).

Not everyone who consumes a toxic fish will develop symptoms. For example, in a British poisoning episode, out of 26 persons at risk after consuming canned sardines, only six became ill (Murray et al. 1982). In San Francisco, California, of nine persons who ate raw tuna fish ("sashimi") together, only seven became ill (Lerke et al. 1978). The reason for this variability is not clear, but Lerke et al. (1978) provided a clue. They found that the distribution of histamine in adjacent parts of the body of the fish was remarkably variable. It ranged from 4 to over 650 mg/100 dl of fish tissue. Thus, each individual fish could vary in histamine level. An unless all the fish in a given lot are comminuted together, not everyone who eats the same fish or individual fish from a given lot will receive the same dose of histamine.

Scombrotoxicism is seldom severe in contrast to ciguatera, puffer, and paralytic shellfish poisoning and often requires little or no medical attention. But according to Bagnis et al. (1970), it accounts for the greatest morbidity on a worldwide basis.

These facts suggest that in many instances, poor handling and improper preservation of the fish may have led to these poisonings.

Prevention of scombroid poisoning: Scombroid poisoning can be easily avoided.
The bacterial synthesis of the scombroid toxin is prevented if scombroid and similar
fish are refrigerated or cooked within a reasonable period following capture. Such fish,
if allowed to stand at room temperature for even less than 10 hr, should be discarded
or eaten with caution even though signs of spoilage are not apparent. Some authors
recommend that the gills be examined for any sign of putrefaction, in which case the
fish should be avoided (Van Veen and Latuasan 1950). In certain parts of the Philippines, the local populations generally will reject fish with gills that have turned white
or eyes that have turned opaque (author's unpublished observation). One should not
eat scombroid fish which taste sharp and peppery, for in this case, the scombrotoxin
level may be sufficiently high to elicit symptoms.

Since canned fish cannot be considered scombrotoxin-proof, as suggested by Merson et al. (1974), canners must ensure that only wholesome fish are canned, and that
a test for histamine in each lot of fish must be part of quality control.

Ichthyohepatotoxic Fish   There are a few species of fish which have been incriminated in ichthyohepatotoxicity. These fish include the Japanese mackerel *(Scomberomorus niphonius)* and the Japanese sandfish *(Arctoscopus japonicus)* (Mizuta et al.
1957), sea bass *(Stereolepis ischinagi)* (Sakai et al. 1962), porgy *(Petrus aupestris)*
(Smith 1961) and halibut *(Hippoglossus* spp.) (Nater and Doeglas 1970). These fish
also may be involved in other types of ichthyotoxicity, such as in ciguatera poisoning.
As stated earlier, ciguatoxicity may also involve the liver of the fish; but in ichthyo-
hepatotoxicism, only this organ is toxic.

The tetrodotoxic fish (pp. 542–548) may also be classified as ichthyohepatotoxic
fish.

Ichthyohepatotoxicity, as the name indicates, is the term applied to poisoning
caused by eating the liver of the fish species cited. The nature and source of the toxin is not known. Abe and Kinumai (1957) believe that fish liver poisoning is due to excess retinyl compounds (vitamin A). This contention is supported by 11 cases of halibut liver poisoning reported by Nater and Doeglas (1970). The observed symptoms
were consistent with vitamin A intoxication. Furthermore, serum vitamin A concentrations in the victims were elevated. However, Mizuta et al. (1957) assert, on the basis
of the symptoms, that the toxic substance is histaminelike. Because the liver of the
fish may store a variety of compounds, it is possible that fish liver poisoning may be
the result of a combined action of different compounds. But the observed symptoms in
many reported cases suggest that the principal toxic compound is probably vitamin A.
The amount of vitamin A in such liver may be as high as 30 million units (1 U = 0.33
μg of retinol). The toxicity of vitamin A is discussed later in this chapter.

Symptoms of fish liver poisoning: About 30 min to 12 hr after eating the fish liver,
nausea, vomiting, fever, and headache develop. The headache may be very severe and
is aggravated by even slight movements of the body, head, or even the eyes. The face
becomes edematous and flushed; a macular rash with large patchy areas appears. Erythema of the face, arms, legs, and chest may accompany these symptoms. In 3 to 6
days, desquamation begins and may continue for 30 days; large segments over the entire body — nose, neck, mouth, head, upper limbs, and other parts — may peel off.
The desquamation may be more pronounced in the palms and soles of the feet (Nater
and Doeglas 1970). Loss of hair and exfoliative dermatitis similar to that in polar bear
poisoning may also occur. In addition, there may be vesicular formation in the oral
membrane, bleeding in the lips, orbital and joint pain, and cardiac palpitation and rapid pulse rate. The victim may complain of a "slippery" sensation at the tip of the
tongue and mild diarrhea. The acute symptoms disappear in 3 to 4 days, but residual
symptoms of stomatitis, chapping of lips, and mild liver dysfunction may persist. Some
liver enlargements may occur, but in general there is no jaundice. No fatalities have
been reported, and recovery is full with no complications (Abe and Kinumai 1957;
Mizuta et al. 1957; Smith 1961).

Prevention of fish liver poisoning: The liver of certain fish may contain very high levels of vitamin A. For example, halibut liver may contain some 100,000 U vitamin A/g (Nater and Doeglas 1970). The minimum acute single toxic dose of the vitamin is 25,000 IU/kg body weight (*Physicians' Desk Reference* 1983). (A discussion on vitamin A toxicity is given later in this chapter on toxic marine mammals [p. 580].) Thus, 10 to 20 g of fish liver containing high levels of vitamin A is sufficient to produce toxic symptoms depending on the duration of intake.

By now, it is evident that fish liver may contain many substances which may be quite dangerous based on the nature and concentrations of the toxin(s). Certain fish livers are consistently toxic, whereas others are unpredictable in this respect. Therefore, consumption of fish liver is risky at best.

Ichthyohemotoxic Fish

As the name suggests, ichthyohemotoxic fish contain most of their poisons in the blood or serum. As far as is known, most hemotoxic fish belong to the eel families; i.e., Anguillidae, Congridae, Muraenidae, Ophichthyidae, or commonly, the anguilla, conger, moray, and snake, or worm, eels, respectively (Bellecci and Polara 1907; Giunio 1948; Maass 1937; Macht 1942; Mitomo 1927; Taft 1945). These eels are regarded as generally edible, except for the toxic blood.

The nature of the toxin is unknown, but the toxin from the eels *Anguilla vulgaris*, *Muraena helena*, and *Conger vulgaris*, and other species appears to be proteinaceous, since it is destroyed by trypsin and papain (Ghiretti and Rocca 1963; Rocca and Ghiretti 1964; Russell 1965a). Therfore, the protein is destroyed by heat; i.e., 60 to 65°C (Kopeczewski 1918). Many earlier workers have found that heating the eel sera to 100°C destroys toxicity (Halstead and Courville 1967).

Symptoms of Ichthyohemotoxicity Because the toxins are proteins and heat labile, it will be unusual if poisoning can occur with cooked eels. The activity of gastric juices also sufficiently inactivates the toxin (Buglia and Barbieri 1922). Furthermore, proteolytic digestive enzymes should also ensure degradation if any protein toxin remains undenatured during cooking. Since raw eel serum can cause poisoning, it appears therefore that some of the toxin remains unaltered by these enzymes and that sufficient amounts are absorbed to cause poisoning. However, eel blood poisoning from cooked eels has little, if any, public health significance. Nevertheless, improper cooking may result in poisoning. Thus, the symptoms produced by the ingestion of raw eel serum is of interest.

The ingestion of the blood of the eel *Muraena helena* results in nausea, vomiting, increased salivation, urticaria, and general weakness. More serious neurological symptoms appear in several poisonings. These consist of paresthesia about the mouth, respiratory distress, paralysis, and death (Ghiretti and Rocca 1963; Russell 1965a). These signs indicate that eel serum contains a neurotoxin.

Ichthyootoxic Fish

As the name implies, ichthyootoxic fish produce or contain poison which is restricted to the gonads and, of course, the roe or eggs. Therefore, it follows that the toxicity of these organs will be related to the reproductive or gonadal activity of the fish. Table 11.8 lists the groups of fish which have been reported to contain toxic gonads or roe. These groups include both fresh- and saltwater species, may of which are of significant economic value and are highly esteemed as food. Thus, many species of ichthyootoxic fish are quite familiar to the layman; e.g., sturgeons, catfish, salmon, trout, minnow, and pike. The moist poisonous in this group are the barbels (Barbus spp.), carps (Schizothorax spp.), tenches (Tinca spp.), and pricklebacks (*Stichaeus* spp.) (Halstead and Courville 1965). The roe of the gar (*Lepisosteus* spp.) and the cabezon *(Scorpaenichthys marmoratus)* also are quite toxic (Fuhrman et al. 1969). The sturgeons are noted for their roe which is used in the preparation of the well-known

Table 11.8 Type of Fish Reported as Ichthyootoxic

Family	Group common name	Genus
Acipenseridae	Sturgeon	Acipenser, Huso
Agenoiosidae	Sheatfish	Ageneiosus
	Catfish	Bagre, Pseudobagrus, Sciadeichthys, Selenaspis
Cottidae	Cabezon	Scorpaenicthys
Cyprinidae	Bream	Abramis
	Barbel	Barbus
	Carp	Cyprinus, Schizothorax
	Osman	Diptychus
	Tench	Tinca
Cyprinodontidae	Killifish or dogpike	Aphanius
	Mummichog	Fundulus
Esocidae	Pike	Esox
Gadidae	Rockling	Gaidropsarus
	Barbot	Lota
Ictaluridae	White catfish	Ictalurus
Lepisosteidae	Gar	Lepisosteus
Percidae	River perch	Perca
Plotosidae	Oriental catfish	Plotosus
Salmonidae	Salmon	Salmo
	Whitefish	Stenodus
Serranidae	Creolefish	Paranthias
Siluridae	Mudfish, catfish	Parosilurus
	Sheatfish	Silurus
Stichaeidae	Japanese prickleback or blenny	Stichaeus

Source: Halstead and Courville (1965).

caviar. The flesh of these fish is usually harmless, with the exception of the carp, which contains an antithiamine factor (Chap. 9). It should not be construed that all species of the families listed in Table 11.8 are ichthyootoxic. However, one may be well advised to regard the consumption of the gonads and roe of these species with caution because their safety cannot always be guaranteed.

In this connection, the tetrodotoxic fish (pp. 542–548) also qualify as ichthyootoxic, since their gonads are more toxic than any other organ in the fish and any other type of toxic fish roe.

Nature of Ichthyootoxin The nature of the toxins from all known ichthyootoxic fish has not been identified. The exception is the toxin from the Japanese prickleback, *Stichaeus grigorjewi;* the toxins appear to be lipoproteins. Four lipoprotein fractions have been isolated from the roe. One fraction, ∂-lipostichaerin, seems to be responsible for human poisonings. This toxin appears to be a phospholipopeptide containing glycerol, choline, phosphorus, fatty acids, and amino acids (Asano and Ito 1966). It has been shown that lipostichaerin consists of a nontoxic protein moiety, stichaerin, and a toxic phospholipid, dinogunellin (Hatano 1971a,b). The toxic lipid is extracted from the lipoprotein complex with chloroform-methanol following ultracentrifugation and hydroxyapatite column chromatography; acetone extraction will also separate dinogunellin from the fresh roe.

Dinogunellin is light yellow powder which turns brown on exposure to air. It is soluble in methanol, chloroform-methanol (2:8) mixture, pyridine, acetic acid, and chloroform-methanol with a small amount of water. It is insoluble in n-hexane, acetone, diethyl ether, chloroform, or ethanol. Dinogunellin forms a colloidal solution with water. Its molecular weight is 820.

The intraperitoneal LD_{50} in mice of dinogunellin is 25 mg/kg. Death occurs in 72 hr (Hatano and Hashimoto 1974). The intraperitoneal LD_{50} of lipostichaerin in mice is 180 mg/kg.

Dinogunellin is unique in that this may be the first time that an adenylic acid moiety has been demonstrated to be present in a phospholipid. The complete structure of dinogunellin is still unknown, but the evidence indicates that it is a 1-monofattyacyl diglyceride with the 3-position link with adenylic acid. The toxin also contains aspartic acid and amides, the position of which in the molecule is obscure.

The toxins in cabezon, or gar, roe appear to be a protein or a protein-bound substance (Fuhrman et al. 1969).

Symptoms of Ichthyootoxicity   Roe poisoning has a rapid onset. As soon as the roe is eaten, the victim complains of abdominal pain which is accompanied by nausea, dizziness, vomiting, diarrhea, headache, bitter taste in the mouth, intense thirst, cold sweats, and chills. There are also sensations of chest constriction, fever, rapid irregular weak pulse, hypotension, cyanosis, dilatation of pupils, syncope, dysphagia, and tinnitus. In severe poisoning, additional symptoms may be observed consisting of muscular cramps, paralysis, convulsions, coma, and sometimes death. Properly managed patients will recover in 3 to 5 days (Asano and Ito 1962; Halstead 1964; Hatano et al. 1964; Hubbs and Wick 1951; Russell 1965b). Fatalities have been reported from poisonings with the roe of the Japanese prickleback (Asano and Ito 1962) and with certain species of carp (Knox 1888).

The toxicity of various fish roe has been tested in animals and has been found to be quite high. Cabezon roe (Scorpaenichthys marmoratus) has been found to be toxic to rats and mice (Fuhrman et al. 1969) and guinea pigs, resulting in death in four of 12 rats and one of two guinea pigs (Hubbs and Wick 1951). The toxin from the cabezon isolated by column chromatography on polyacrylamide gave an i.p. LD_{50} in mice of 200 mg/kg. It produces focal necrosis in the liver (Fuhrman et al. 1969). The roe of the creolefish (Paranthias furcifer) and Japanese prickleback (Stichaeus grigorjewi) has been found to be toxic to mice. The prickleback roe was lethal to mice (Asano and Ito 1962; Hatano et al. 1964) and chickens (Asano and Ito 1962). The toxin appeared to be degraded by autoclaving at 120°C for 30 min. Air drying did not destroy the toxin (Asano and Ito 1962).

Incidence of Ichthyootoxicity   Poisonous roe is said to be a public health problem in some parts of Europe and Asia. The actual incidence is not known (Halstead and Courville 1967).

Prevention of Ichthyootoxicity   Fish roe is an esteemed delicacy in many parts of the world. One must be careful and would be better off if these were not eaten altogether. Caution must be exercised, especially in eating the roe of the cabezon, prickleback, carp, and other brackish and freshwater fish. The gonads of these fish should be avoided, particularly during the reproductive season. Although cooking may destroy some of the toxin(s), this cannot be relied upon to render the roe harmless.

Miscellaneous Toxic Fish

The mucous secretion of some fish may contain toxic substances. Among these are the Hawaiian trunkfish or "pahu" (Ostracion spp.) (Boyland and Scheuer 1967), the Pacific bass *Grammistes sexlineatus* (Liquori et al. 1963), the soapfish *Rypticus saponaceus* (Maretzki and Del Castillo 1967), and *Pogonoperca punctata* (Hashimoto 1968).

The toxin from the Hawaiian trunkfish has been called pahutoxin, and its structure has been determined (Boyland and Scheuer 1967).

$$CH_3(CH_2)_{12}\overset{\underset{|}{OCOCH_3}}{CH}CH_2\overset{\underset{\parallel}{O}}{C}-O-(CH_2)_2-N^+(CH_3)_3Cl^-$$

Pahutoxin

The toxin is soluble in water and butanol, chloroform, methanol, and hot acetone or ethyl acetate.

Pahutoxin is hemolytic to vertebrate red blood cells at concentration of 1 ppm (Thomson 1964). In mice, the crude toxin injected intraperitoneally produces ataxia, labored breathing, coma, and death (Thomson 1964). The MLD in mice is 0.2 mg/g, and there is complete recovery at sublethal doses.

The toxin of the soapfish, *Rypticus saponaceus*, has not been fully characterized. It has been suggested that it is a large peptide, since it is nondialyzable (Maretzki and Del Castillo 1967). At any rate, it appears to be an unusual protein — being soluble in water and water-saturated butanol, moderately heat stable at 65°C for 2 hr, and insoluble in solutions with low ionic strength except in the presence of acid. Injected intraperitoneally into mice, extracts of the soapfish toxin produce motor unrest and death (Maretzki and Del Castillo 1967).

The toxin from the Pacific bass, *Grammistes sexlineatus*, appears to be a peptide which is soluble in 95% ethanol. It has been found to be toxic to the killifish at 70 ppm (Liquori et al. 1963).

The toxin from *Pogonopenca punctata* is probably a smaller peptide than the related soapfish toxin, since it is slowly dialyzable. It is soluble only in dilute acetic acid, N-butanol, or amyl alcohol, but not in water. It can be precipitated by half saturation with NaCl. It has a bitter taste and produces ciguateralike symptoms in cats when administered orally or subcutaneously; cats are killed when fed 10 g of raw skin per kilogram (Hashimoto 1968).

Other fish have also been reported to be toxic. The North Atlantic fish *Myoxocephalus (Cottus) scorpius* and the Greenland halibut, *Reinhardtius hippoglossoides*, have been reported to be toxic to dogs (Boje 1939).

Comments on Toxic Fish

In the United States, fish poisoning outbreaks are now reported to the Centers for Disease Control. It would be most worthwhile if the World Health Organization and the Food and Agricultural Organization of the United Nations would consider ichthyotoxicity as among those diseases that should be reported. Research in this area, particularly the prediction and control of ciguatoxicity of fishes and related toxic phenomena, should be intensified, for in terms of worldwide hunger and malnutrition, the sea can be a boundless resource.

A great deal of progress has been made in the pursuit of the source of ciguatera toxin. But the evidence from the symptomatology suggests that ciguatera is of multiple causation; that is, a ciguatoxic fish may contain not only ciguatoxin, maitotoxin, and scaritoxin, but also several others. Perhaps these toxins are present in minute quantities and produce synergistic or additive effects. These toxins may also be labile, and so may be destroyed during the isolation procedures. The characterization of these toxins is obviously essential in the development of an effective antidote or other means of neutralizing their toxicity. The identification of the toxic sources may also provide researchers materials from which larger quantities of toxins can be isolated. Research in this area has been hampered because of the extremely low levels of toxin in the fish.

While ciguatera poisoning is generally nonfatal, it can result in severe illness. Thus, many fish species which are a valuable and highly palatable source of good-quality proteins may be rejected. This will happen especially in those areas where other protein sources are available. Ciguatoxicity in most species of fish is unpredictable. Therefore a fast, reliable, and practical assay method to detect ciguatoxicity is urgently needed.

Research into other types of oral fish toxicity have not been pursued actively following their first reports (Halstead 1981). A good example is the extremely deadly clupeotoxin. One reason is that since the first reports, clupeotoxicism apparently has never recurred. The reason for this fact is not known. Other types of oral fish poisonings rarely, if ever, occur or have not come to the attention of health authorities. Nevertheless, potential future poisonings from these fish remain if we assume that many of them derive their toxins from the food chain.

MARINE REPTILES

Like the fish discussed previously, marine turtles which normally are nonpoisonous may suddenly become toxic. The intoxications may be severe enough to be fatal in 44 to 50% of cases. The turtle species that have been implicated in these poisonings are the hawksbill, *Eretmochelys imbricata*, the leatherback, *Dermochelys coriacea*, and the green sea turtle, *Chelonia mydas* (Banner 1967b; Cooper 1964; Halstead 1956).

More poisonings have been reported in the Philippines, Indonesia, and Sri Lanka. The victims may show symptoms within a few hours or the symptoms may be delayed for a week. The victims may complain of severe stomach ache, nausea, vomiting, diarrhea, and dizziness. There may be burning sensation in the buccal cavity, which may develop several days after ingestion. The buccal symptoms may progress to blistering or ulceration of the tongue, which initially may show a white coating. Boils, desquamation, hallucinations, excessive salivation, difficulty in swallowing, and debility may also be observed. In fatal cases, the victim may first lapse into severe sleepiness or coma; death may occur within 12 hr to 2 weeks following ingestion of the toxic turtle (Banner 1967; Cooper 1964; Halstead 1956).

The greatest concentration of the toxin appears to be in the liver, and it is believed to be derived from the food chain (Cooper 1964).

MARINE MAMMALS

Human poisonings following ingestion of toxic livers of marine mammals also have been reported. The mammals implicated in these poisonings include the bearded seal, *Erignatus barbatus* (Halstead 1959), the Australian sea lion, *Neophoca cinera* (Rodahl and Moore 1943), and the bowhead whale, *Balaena mysticetus* (Lewis and Lentfer 1967).

The toxic substances in these livers are retinyl compounds (vitamin A) which occur as a group in high concentrations. Thus, the bearded seal contains 2100 U/g of liver or 47,000 U/g of oil; the bowhead whale contains 5700 U/g liver or 111,000 U/g of oil (Lewis and Lentfer 1967).

Acute poisoning may result following ingestion of 2 to 5 million international units (IU) of the vitamin (Knudson and Rothman 1953; Gerber et al. 1954). The symptoms may begin 6 to 8 hr after ingestion with severe headache in the forehead and eye, dizziness, drowsiness, and nausea with vomiting; there then follows in 12 to 20 hr redness and erythematous swelling of the skin with peeling in later stages, particularly where the epidermis is thickest; i.e., the palms and soles (Gerber et al. 1954; Knudson and Rothman 1953; Nater and Doeglas 1970). In children, hypervitaminosis A results in bulging fontanelles, anorexia, hyperirritability, and vomiting which generally occurs in 12 hr; after a few days, there is fine cutaneous desquamation (Knudson and Rothman 1953; Marie and See 1954).

Chronic intakes of the vitamin at 3000 IU (1 mg)/kg/day for several months or years may produce toxic reactions in adults (DiBenedetto 1967; Muenter et al. 1971; Smith and Hofstede 1966). Toxicity in adults has generally been associated with intakes of 100,000 IU or more per day (Krause 1965). Chronic toxicity in adults is manifested by headache; blurred vision; muscle soreness after exercise; anorexia; hair loss; maculoerythematous eruptions on the shoulders, and back; general dryness and flakiness of skin with pruritus; cracking and bleeding of lips; reddened gums; and nosebleeds. Enlargment of liver and spleen and anemia may also occur (Muenter et al. 1971). Painful subcutaneous swelling and cortical hyperostoses may be present in the region of muscle attachments on the long bones (Woodard et al. 1961). A pagoda effect is seen in the growing bones of children (Bartolozzi et al. 1967). In adults, increased cerebrospinal fluid pressure or pseudotumor cerebri with papilledema may be diagnostic of chronic hypervitaminosis A (Feldman and Schlezinger 1970; Lascari and Bell 1970). In infants, the bulging fontanelles may be indicative of the chronic poisoning.

MARINE ALGAE

Certain types of marine algae have been used as sources of agar and carrageenans, which are food additives, used as dispersing, stabilizing, thickening, and filling or bulking agents. Agar and carrageenans are complex sulfated polysaccharides. Agar consists of a chain of agarose and agaropectin containing β-D-galactose, D-galactose sulfate and other galactose derivatives, and glucuronic and pyruvic acids. Carrageenans are highly sulfated galactans; i.e., they consist of a chain of D-galactose sulfate and anhydrogalactose. Agar is extracted from species of algae belonging to the genera Ahnfeltia, Gelidium, Gracilaria, Pterocladia, and Phyllophora. Carrageenans are derived from species belonging to the genera Chondrus, Eucheuma, Gigartina, and Iridea (Percival 1966; Percival and McDowell 1967).

There is little information regarding the oral toxicity of thse species. However, in some studies with herbivorous species, carrageenans have been shown to induce colonic ulcerations (Anonymous 1970, 1971). Feeding studies at high levels in the diet markedly reduce the rate of survival of rats (Nilson and Wagner 1959). Injected subcutaneously into rats, a single 50 mg dose of carrageenan induces significant formation of sarcomas after about 2 years (Cater 1961). Sarcoma formation following multiple injection of carrageenans is accelerated by 2-acetylaminofluorene fed simultaneously (Walpole 1962). This is another example of synergism between carcinogens. No tumors have been induced in rats fed high levels of carrageenans for 2 years. This may have been due to the fact that at the level fed, the polysaccharide is too toxic, reducing the survival of the animals significantly (Nilson and Wagner 1959).

The λ- and κ-carrageenans from the red alga, Gigartina acicularis, possesses powerful anticoagulant activity with dog blood (Hawkins and Leonard 1963; Houck et al. 1957); λ-carrageenans from the red seaweed or Irish moss, Chondrus crispus and Polyides rotundus, also have anticoagulant activity with rabbit blood administered at about 3 mg/kg body weight (Anderson and Duncan 1965).

No toxicity has been observed when λ-carrageenans from Chondrus crispus are given to animals orally, but intravenous administration at 1 to 5 mg/kg kills rabbits in 24 hr; for κ-carrageenans, the dose is between 3 and 15 mg/kg. When degraded, carrageenans become less toxic intravenously, requiring doses above 1 g/kg to produce toxic effects (Anderson and Duncan 1965). The polysaccharides from Gigartina acicularis injected intravenously at 15 mg/kg kill dogs within 24 hr (Houck et al. 1957). As these activities were elicited following intravenous injection, their significance in food toxicology is not clear.

The algal polysaccharides may elicit toxic effects by binding trace metals and rendering them unavailable. Thus, it has been found that the brown algae *Alaria esculenta* and *Rhodymenia palmata* produce degenerative neural anomalies — resulting in disturbed coordination and paralysis which are associated with demyelination of the cerebrum — in lambs born to ewes which ate dried brown algae. In this case, the algal polysaccharides had rendered copper unavailable, indicated by significant reduction in blood copper level in ewes (from 1.0 mg down to 0.2 mg/L) and liver copper in lambs (20 to 30 times lower than normal). Copper supplementation reduced the incidence of the disease (Palsson and Grimsson 1953).

Heat-stable toxins have also been detected in algae. Thus, the California algae Egregia, Gelidium, Macrocystis, Hesperophycus, and Pelvetia spp. contain water-soluble toxins. Similarly, water-soluble toxins as tested in mice also have been found in algae obtained from the Palmyra Island of the South Pacific (Habekost et al. 1955). These toxins, when injected intraperitoneally into mice as water-soluble crude extracts, have been found to cause lacrimation, piloerection, diarrhea, dysnea or weakness, and death within 16 to 36 hr. Some extracts, particularly from *Pelvetia fastigiata* and a mixture of *Boodlea composita* and *Caulerpa serrulata,* are even more deadly, producing death in less than 1 hr (Habekost et al. 1955). The chemical nature of these toxins is not known.

However, a toxin named caulerpicin, from the green alga *Caulerpa racemosa,* has been crystallized (Doty and Aguilar-Santos 1966). Caulerpicin is present as a mixture of three homologs (MW 621 to 649) which are ethersoluble; the tentative structural formula of the three homologues is shown below (Aguilar-Santos and Doty 1968):

$$CH_3(CH_2)_{13}-CH-NH-CO(CH_2)_{23-25}-CH_3$$
$$|$$
$$CH_2OH$$

Caulerpicin

Caulerpicin causes mild anesthesia in the mouth, as shown by numbness of lips and tongue; one subject who was apparently sensitized to the toxin, chewed some raw, dried *Caulerpa racemosa* and developed numbness in the extremities, a sensation of coldness in the feet and fingers, respiratory distress, and loss of balance. The symptoms wear off after a few hours to 1 day depending on the dose (Doty and Aguilar-Santos 1966).

Many investigators believe that these toxins may be involved in the ciguatoxicity of fish, since the toxic syndrome caused by them is reportedly similar to that seen in ciguatera poisoning. Furthermore, the stomachs of toxic fish also have been found to contain some of those algae (Dawson et al. 1955; Doty and Aguilar-Santos 1966; Habekost et al. 1955).

Various species of algae from Hawaii (Starr et al. 1962) and Puerto Rico (Starr et al. 1966) have been found to contain cytotoxic compounds, as tested in tissue cultures of human synovial fluid cells. Abnormalities such as amitosis, micronucleation without cell division, and multiple cytokinesis have been produced by the toxin (Starr and Holtermann 1967; Starr et al. 1962, 1966).

Laminine, a cholinelike amino acid, is a hypotensive agent from species of the marine algae Alaria, Arthrothamnus, Costaria, Ecklonia, Eckloniopsis, Kjellmaniella, Laminaria, and Undaria (Takemoto et al. 1965a). Transient hypotension has been elicited in rabbits injected intravenously with laminine monocitrate at 20 to 30 mg/kg. The compound also appears to cause depression of the amplitude of the rabbit heart contraction both in situ and in vitro, with no change in heart rate when the heart is perfused with the amino acid at 50 μg/ml. Contraction of excised smooth muscles, such as from mouse and guinea pig intestine and guinea pig artery and trachea, is depressed by laminine monocitrate. In contrast, the contraction of the guinea pig vas deferens is increased by the compound at concentrations of 10^{-4} to 10^{-3} M (Ozawa et al. 1967).

Hypotensive agents and other pharmacologically active compounds of unknown nature also have been demonstrated in other marine algae such as *Chondria armata* and *Heterochordaria abietina* (Takemoto et al. 1964a,b 1965a,b).

CONCLUSIONS

It is obvious from the materials presented in this chapter that many species of marine life which are actual or potential food sources present a complex, food toxicological and public health dilemma. However, at the present time, only a few seafood toxicants present significant public health problems on a worldwide basis. Foremost among these are the ciguatera and shellfish poisonings. Both conditions are characterized by unpredictability and the involvement of large numbers of marine species. Therefore, control of these two conditions is difficult, if not impossible.

The goal toward complete control of shellfish poisoning is being approached rapidly following identification of the nature and source of the etiological agent. This is indeed the fundamental rule in any confrontation: Identify the nature of the enemy. In so doing, a rational course of action can be devised, and the problem can be attacked on various fronts. Thus, finding ways to predict and control algal blooms eliminate dinoflagellates in clam beds, detect toxins, detoxify shellfish, neutralize shellfish toxins, and develop antidotes become feasible or attainable.

This is unfortunately not the case with ciguatera poisoning. This is even more serious, even though usually not as severe as the paralytic shellfish poisoning, since many normally edible fishes are involved. However, significant progress is being made; the goal is much more difficult to attain now, since it is realized that there may be several types of ciguatoxins, and that ciguatoxicity is affected by many exogenous factors as well. Thus, prediction of ciguatoxicity of fish is difficult even though the conditions leading to this phenomenon are continually being better understood.

The problem regarding the food toxicological status of other marine life will become acute as these sources are exploited more and more for the increasing world population. That this possibility is not remote cannot be disputed. Research in this direction must be intensified. The riches of the sea in terms of food sources can be tapped more efficiently and wisely if we know more about them, especially their toxicological status.

REFERENCES

Abbott, B. C. and Ballantine, D. 1957. The toxin from *Gymnodinium veneficum* Ballantine. *J. Mar. Biol. Assoc. U.K.* 36: 169–189.

Abbott, B. C. and Paster, Z. 1970. Action of toxins from *Gymnodinium breve*. *Toxicon,* 8: 120.

Abbott, B. C., Siger, A. and Spiegelstein, M. 1975. Toxins from blooms of Gymnodinium breve. In: *The First International Conference on Toxic Dinoflagellate Blooms.* V. R. LoCicero (ed.). Massachusetts Science and Technological Foundation, Wakefield, Massachusetts.

Abe, H. and Kinumai, M. 1957. Food poisoning caused by eating the livers of *Stereolepis ichinagi. Nichi Jukaichi* 10: 125–127. (Japanese)

Aguilar-Santos, G. and Doty, M. S. 1968. Chemical studies on three species of the marine algal genus *Caulerpa*. In: *Drugs from the Sea.* H. D. Freudenthal (ed.). Marine Technology Society, Washington, D.C.

Aiiso, K. 1954. On the samma-sakuraboshi poisoning. *Shinryo Shitsu* 6: 44. (Japanese)

Akiba, T. 1943. Study of poisons of *Venerupis simidecussata* and Ostrea *gigas. Jpn. Iji Shimpo* 1078: 1077–1082. (Japanese)

Akiba, T. 1949. Study of poisoning by Venerupis simidecussata and *Ostrea gigas* and their poisonous substances. *Nisshin Igaku* 36: 1–24. (Japanese)

Akiba, T. 1961. "Food Poisoning Due to Oysters and Baby Clams in Japan, and Toxicological Effects of the Toxic Substance." Paper read at the Tenth Pacific Sci. Congr. Pacific Sci. Assoc., Honolulu, Hawaii.

Akiba, T. and Hattori, Y. 1949. Food poisoning caused by eating asari (*Venerupis semidecussata*) and oyster (*Ostrea gigas*) and studies on the toxic substance, venerupin. *Jpn. J. Exp. Med.* 20: 271–284.

Alam, M., Trieff, N. M., Ray, S. M. and Hudson, J. E. 1975. Isolation and partial characterization of toxins from the dinoflagellate *Gymnodinium breve* Davis. *J. Pharm. Sci.* 64: 865–867.

Alcala, A. C. and Halstead, B. W. 1970. Human fatality due to ingestion of the crab *Demania* sp. in the Philippines. *Clin. Toxicol.* 3: 609–611.

Anastasi, A. and Erspamer, V. 1962. Occurrence and some properties of eledoisin in extracts of posterior salivary glands of *Eledone*. *Br. J. Pharmacol. Chemother.* 19: 326–336.

Anastasi, A. and Erspamer, V. 1963. The isolation and amino acid sequence of eledoisin, the active endecapeptide of the posterior salivary glands of Eledone. *Arch. Biochem. Biophys.* 101: 56–65.

Anderson, L. S. 1960. Toxic shellfish in British Columbia. *Am. J. Public Health* 50: 71–83.

Anderson, W. and Duncan, J. G. C. 1965. The anticoagulant activity of carrageenan. *J. Pharm. Pharmacol.* 17: 647–654.

Anonymous. 1970. Articles of General Interest: Carrageenan and the colon. *Food Cosmet. Toxicol.* 8: 75–76.

Anonymous. 1971. Articles of General Interest: Carrageenan. *Food Cosmet. Toxicol.* 9: 561–564.

Arcisz, W. 1950. Ciguatera: Tropical fish poisoning. U.S. Fish Wildlife Serv. Spec. Sci. Rept., Fish No. 27.

Arnold, S. H. and Brown, W. D. 1978. Histamine (?) toxicity from fish products. *Adv. Food Res.* 24: 113–154.

Asano, M. 1952. Studies on the toxic substances contained in marine animals. I. Locality of the poison of Neptunea (Barbitonia) arthritica Bernardi. *Bull. Jpn. Soc. Sci. Fish.* 17: 73–77.

Asano, M. 1954. Occurrence of choline in the shellfish, Callista brevisiphonata Carpenter. *Tohoku J. Agric. Res.* 4: 239–250.

Asano, M. and Ito, M. 1959. Occurrence of tetramine and choline compounds in the salivary gland of a marine gastropod, Neptunea arthritica Bernardi. *Tohoku J. Agric. Res.* 10: 209–227.

Asano, M. and Ito, M. 1960. Salivary poison of a marine gastropod, Neptunea arthritica Bernardi, and the seasonal variation of its toxicity. *Ann. N.Y. Acad. Sci.* 90: 674–688.

Asano, M. and Ito, M. 1962. Toxicity of a lipoprotein and lipids from the roe of a blenny Dinogunellus grigorjewi Herzenstein. *Tohoku Agric. Res.* 13: 151–167.

Asano, M. and Ito, M. 1966. Lipoproteins (lipostichaerins) in the roe of the blenny, Stichaeus grigorjewi Herzenstein. *Tohoku J. Agric. Res.* 16: 299–316.

Asano, M., Takayanagi, F. and Furuhara, Y. 1950. Studies on the toxic substances in marine animals. II. Shellfish-poisoning from Callista brevisiphonata Carpenter, occurred in the vicinity of Mori, Kayabe County. *Bull. Fac. Fish. Hokkaido Univ.* 7: 26–36. (Japanese with English summary)

Asano, M., Takayanagi, F. and Kitamura, T. 1953. Shellfish poisoning from Callista brevisiphonata Carpenter and its clinical symptoms. *Tohoku J. Agric. Res.* 3: 321–330.

Baden, D. B., Mende, T. J., Lichter, W. and Wellham, L. 1981. Crystallization and toxicology of T34: A major toxin from Florida's red tide organism (Ptychodiscus brevis). *Toxicon* 19: 455–462.

Bagnis, R. A. 1967. Fish poisoning in French Polynesia. Clinical and epidemiological studies. *Rev. Hyg. Med. Soc.* 15: 619—646. (in French)

Bagnis, R. 1968. Clinical aspects of ciguatera (fish poisoning) in French Polynesia.
Hawaii Med. J. 28: 25—28. (in French)

Bagnis, R. 1969. Origin and development of an outbreak of ciguatera in Tuamoto
atoll. *Rev. Corps Sante* 10: 783—795. (in French)

Bagnis, R. 1974. The endemic situation of ciguatera in the island of Gambier. *Cah.
Pacif.* 18: 585.

Bagnis, R. and Kaeuffer, H. 1974. Immunological perspectives on the subject of
ciguatera. *Med. Trop.* 34: 25—27. (in French)

Bagnis, R. et al. 1970. Problems of toxicants in marine food products: Marine
biotoxins. *Bull. W.H.O.* 42: 69—88.

Bagnis, R., Loussan, E. and Thevenin, S. 1974. Parrotfish poisonings in the
Gambier Islands. *Med. Trop.* 34: 523—527.

Bagnis, R. et al. 1979b. Certain morphological and biological characteristics of
dinoflagellate probably responsible for ciguatera poisoning. *C. R. Acad. Sci.*
(Ser. D) 289: 639—642.

Bagnis, R., Kuberski, T. and Laugier, S. 1979a. Clinical observations on 3,009
cases of ciguatera (fish poisoning) in the South Pacific. *Am. J. Trop. Med.
Hyg.* 28: 1067—1073.

Bagnis, R. et al 1980. Origins of ciguatera fish poisoning: A new dinoflagellate,
Gambierdiscus toxicus adachi and fukuyo, definitely involved as a causal
agent. *Toxicon* 18: 199—208.

Banner, A. H. 1965. Ciguatera in the Pacific. *Hawaii Med. J.* 24: 353—354.

Banner, A. H. 1967a. Marine toxins from the Pacific. I. Advances in the investigation of fish toxins. In: *Animal Toxins.* F. E. Russell and P. R. Saunders
(eds.). Pergamon Press, New York.

Banner, A. H. 1967b. Poisonous marine animals, a synopsis. *J. Forensic Sci.* 12:
180—192.

Banner, A. H. 1976. Ciguatera: A disease from coral reef fish. In: *Biology and
Geology of Coral Reefs.* O. A. Jones and R. Endean (eds.). Academic Press,
New York.

Banner, A. H. 1977. Poisonous fishes with endogenous toxins. In: *Forensic
Medicine.* Vol. 3. C. G. Tedeschi, W. G. Eckert and L. G. Tedeschi (eds.).
Saunders, Philadelphia.

Banner, A. H. and Helfrich, P. 1964. *The Distribution of Ciguatera in the
Tropical Pacific.* Technical Report No. 3. Final Report NIH Contr. SA-43-pH-
3741. Hawaii Marine Laboratory, Univ. Hawaii.

Banner, A. H. and Stephen, B. J. 1966. A note on the toxicity of the horseshoe
crab in the gulf of Thailand. *Nat. Hist. Bull. Siam Soc.* 21: 197—203.

Banner, A. H., Helfrich, P., Scheuer, P. J. and Yoshida, T. 1963. Research on
ciguatera in the tropical Pacific. *Proc. Gulf Caribbean Fish. Inst.* 16th Ann.
Sess. 84-98. Miami, Florida.

Baratta, R. O. and Tanner, P. A., Jr. 1970. Ichthyosarcotoxism-ciguatera
intoxication. *J. Fla. Med. Assoc.* 57: 39—42.

Barkin, R. M. 1974. Ciguatera poisoning: a common source outbreak. *South Med.
J.* 67: 13—16.

Barnes, R. D. 1963. *Invertebrate Zoology.* Saunders, Philadelphia.

Bartolozzi, G., Bernini, G., Marianelli, L. and Corvaglia, E. 1967. Chronic
vitamin A excess in infants and children. Description of 2 cases and a critical
review of the literature. *Riv. Clin. Pediatr.* 80: 231—290. (Italian)

Bartsch, A. F., Drachman, R. H. and McFarren, E. F. 1959. Report of a survey
of the fish poisoning problem in the Marshall Islands. Department of the
Interior, Public Health Service, 6-48. (Jan.), U.S. Government Printing Office,
Washington, D.C.

Behre, A. 1949. The cause of poisoning in a fishery. *Z. Lebensm. Untersuch. Forsch.* 89: 229–312. (in German)

Bellecci, A. and Polara, G. 1907. On the toxicity of the serum from the blood of a species of moray eel. *Arch. Farm. Sper.* 6: 598–622. (in Italian)

Benson, J. 1956. Tetraodon (blowfish) poisoning. A report of two fatalities. *J. Forensic Sci.* 1(4): 119–125.

Berry, S. S. and Halstead, B. W. 1954. Octopus bites—A second report. *Leaflets Malacol.* 1:59–65.

Blakesley, M. L. 1983. Scombroid poisoning: Prompt resolution of symptoms with cimetidine. *Ann. Energ. Med.* 12: 104–106.

Boje, O. 1939. Toxin in the flesh of the Greenland shark. *Meddr. Grønland* 125(5): 1–16.

Bond, R. M. and Medcof, J. C. 1958. Epidemic shellfish poisoning in New Brunswick 1957. *Can. Med. Assoc. J.* 79: 1–14.

Borison, H. L. and McCarthy, L. E. 1977. Respiratory and circulatory effects of saxitoxin in the cerebrospinal fluid. *Br. J. Pharmacol.* 61: 679.

Borison, H. L., McCarthy, L. E., Clark, W. G. and Radhakrishnan, N. 1963. Vomiting, hypothermia, and respiratory paralysis due to tetrodotoxin (puffer fish poison) in the cat. *Toxicol. Appl. Pharmacol.* 5: 350–357.

Borison, H. L., Ellis, S. and McCarthy, L. E. 1980. Central respiratory and circulatory effects of Gymnodinium breve toxin in anaesthetized cats. *Br. J. Pharmacol.* 70: 249–256.

Bouder, H., Cavallo, A. and Bouder, M. J. 1962. Poisonous fishes and ichthyosarcotoxisms. *Bull. Inst. Oceanogr.* 59: 1–66.

Bousquet, P., Feldman, J., Bloch, R. and Schwartz, J. 1980. Medullary cardiovascular effects of tetrodotoxin in anesthetized cats. *Eur. J. Pharmacol.* 65: 293–296.

Boyarsky, L. L. and Rayner, M. D. 1970. The effect of ciguatera toxin on Aplysia neurons. *Proc. Soc. Exp. Biol. Med.* 134: 332–335.

Boyer, G. L., Schantz, E. J. and Schnoes, H. K. 1978. Characterization of 11-hydroxysaxitoxin sulfate, a major toxin in scallops exposed to blooms of the poisonous dinoflagellate Gonyaulax tamarensis. *J. Chem. Soc., Chem. Commun.* 889–890.

Boylan, D. B. and Scheuer, P. J. 1967. Pahutoxin: A fish poison. *Science* 155: 52–56.

Brock, V. E., Jones, R. S. and Helfrich, P. 1965. *An Ecological Reconnaissance of Johnston Island and the Effects of Dredging.* Technical Report No. 5. Annual Report, U.S. Atomic Energy Commission. Hawaii Marine Laboratory, University of Hawaii.

Brodner, J., Thiessen, W. E., Bates, H. A. and Rapoport, H. 1975. The structure of a crystalline derivative of saxitoxin. The structure of saxitoxin. *J. Am. Chem. Soc.* 97: 6008–6012.

Brongensma-Sanders, M. 1957. Mass mortality in the sea. In: *Treatise on Marine Ecology and Paleoecology.* Vol. I. J. W. Hedgpeth (ed.). Geol. Soc. Am., Mem. 67, Waverly Press, Baltimore.

Buchwald, H. D. et al. 1964. Identity of tarichiatoxin and tetrodotoxin. *Science* 143: 474–475.

Buglia, G. and Barbieri, G. 1922. The reason why the poison from the eel introduced through the stomach is not toxic. *Arch. Sci. Biol. (Naples)* 3: 26–38. (Italian)

Camougis, G., Takman, B. H., Rene, J. and Tasse, P. 1967. Potency difference between the zwitter ion form and the cation forms of tetrodotoxin. *Science* 156: 1625–1627.

Carson, R. L. 1951. *The Sea Around Us*. Oxford University Press, New York.

Cater, D. B. 1961. The carcinogenic action of carrageenin in rats. *Br. J. Cancer* 15: 607—614.

CENTER FOR DISEASE CONTROL. 1969. *Foodborne Outbreaks. Annual Summary*. U.S. Department of Health, Education and Welfare, Public Health Service, Atlanta.

CENTER FOR DISEASE CONTROL. 1970. *Foodborne Outbreaks. Annual Summary*. U.S. Department of Health, Education and Welfare, Public Health Service, Atlanta.

CENTER FOR DISEASE CONTROL. 1971. *Foodborne Outbreaks. Annual Summary*. U.S. Department of Health, Education and Welfare, Public Health Service, Atlanta.

CENTER FOR DISEASE CONTROL. 1972. *Foodborne Outbreaks. Annual Summary*. U.S. Department of Health, Education and Welfare, Public Health Service, Atlanta.

CENTER FOR DISEASE CONTROL. 1973. *Foodborne and Waterborne Disease Outbreaks. Annual Summary*. U.S. Department of Health, Education and Welfare, Public Health Service, Atlanta.

CENTER FOR DISEASE CONTROL. 1974. *Foodborne and Waterborne Disease Outbreaks. Annual Summary*. U.S. Department of Health, Education and Welfare, Public Health Service, Atlanta.

CENTER FOR DISEASE CONTROL. 1975. *Foodborne and Waterborne Disease Outbreaks. Annual Summary*. U.S. Department of Health, Education and Welfare, Public Health Service, Atlanta.

CENTER FOR DISEASE CONTROL. 1977. *Foodborne and Waterborne Disease Surveillance. Annual Summary*. U.S. Department of Health, Education and Welfare, Public Health Service, Atlanta.

Chambers, J. S. and Magnusson, H. W. 1950. Seasonal variations in toxicity of butter clams from selected Alaska beaches. U.S. Fish Wildlife Service. Spec. Sci. Rept., Fish. No. 53.

Chanley, J. D., Kohn, S. K., Nigrelli, R. F. and Sobotka, H. 1955. Further chemical analysis of holothurin, the saponin-like steroid from the sea-cucumber. Part II. *Zoologica* 40: 99

Chanley, J. D. et al. 1959. Holothurin. I. The isolation of properties and sugar components of holothurin A. *J. Am. Chem. Soc.* 81: 5180—5183.

Chanley, J. D., Perlstein, J., Nigrelli, R. F. and Sobotka, H. 1960. Further studies on the structure of holothurin. *Ann. N.Y. Acad. Sci.* 90: 902—905.

Chanley, J. D., Mazzetti, T. and Sobotka, H. 1966. The holothurinogenins. *Tetrahedron* 22: 1857—1884.

Charnot, A. 1947. The toxicology of Morocco. Memoires de la Societe des Sciences Naturelles du Maroc 47: 3—826 (in French) ISSN 0583-8487 Rabat, Morocco. (1945) (Published 1947)

Chretien, J. H., Fermaglich, J. and Garagusi, V. F. 1981. Ciguatera poisoning. Presentation as a neurological disorder. *Arch. Neurol.* 38: 783.

Chungue, E., Bagnis, R., Fusetani, N. and Hashimoto, Y. 1977. Isolation of two toxins from a parrotfish Scarus gibbus. *Toxicon* 15: 89—93.

Chungue, E., Chanteau, S., Hurtel, J. M. and Bagnis, R. 1979. Toxicological study of several species of bentho planktonic algae from ciguaterigenic biotopes cultivated nonaxenically in artificial medium. *Rev. Int. Oceanogr. Med.* 60: 35—40. (French)

Ciocatto, E., Cattaneo, A. and Fava, E. 1956. Clinical experience on a new curarezation: Murexine. *Minerva Anestesiol.* 22: 197—202. (Italian)

Cohen, E. 1968. Immunologic observations of the agglutinins of the hemolymph of Limulus polyphenus and Birgus latro. *Trans. N.Y. Acad. Sci.* (Series II) 30: 427—443.

Cooper, M. J. 1964. Ciguatera and other marine poisoning in the Gilbert Islands. *Pacific Sci.* 18: 411—440.

Couillard, P. 1955. "Anticoagulant and Antimitotic Substances from the Ovary of the Puffer, Spheroides maculatus (Bloch and Schneider)." Ph.D. Thesis, University of Pennsylvania, Philadelphia.

Craig, C. P. 1980. It's always the big ones that should get away. *J.A.M.A.* 244: 272—273.

Cruickshank, J. G. and Williams, H. R. 1978. Scombrotoxic fish poisoning. *Br. Med. J.* 9 September 1978: 739—740.

Cuervo, L. A. and Adelman, W. J. 1970. Equilibrium and kinetic properties of the interaction between tetrodotoxin and the excitable membrane of the squid giant axon. *J. Gen. Physiol.* 55: 309—335.

Davis, C. C. 1947. Gymnodinium breve n. Sp. A cause of discolored water and animal mortality in the Gulf of Mexico. *Botan. Gaz.* 109: 358—360.

Dawson, E. Y. 1959. Changes in Palmyra Atoll and its vegetation through the activities of man, 1913-1958. *Pacific Nat.* 1: 1—51.

Dawson, E. Y., Aleem, A. A. and Halstead, B. W. 1955. Marine algae from Palmyra Island with special reference to the feeding habits and toxicology of reef fishes. *Allan Hancock Found. Publs., Occ. Pap.* 17—39.

Deblasi, S. and Leone, U. 1955. Clinical use of a new curare-like agent: Murexine. *Minerva Anestesiol.* 21: 137—141. (Italian)

Decaro, G. 1963. Action of eledoisin on the capillary permeability in humans, guinea pigs and in rats. *Arch. Int. Pharmacodyn. Ther.* 146: 27—39.

De Sylva, D. 1963. Systematics and life history of the great barracuda Sphyraena barracuda (Walbaum). *Stud. Trop. Oceanogr. Miami*, Nol. 1.

Dibenedetto, R. J. 1967. Chronic hypervitaminosis A in an adult. *J.A.M.A.* 201: 700—702.

Doorenbos, N. and Yasumoto, Y. 1978. Ciguatera workshop. In: *Toxic Dinoflagellate Blooms.* D. L. Taylor and H. H. Seliger (eds.). Proceedings of the Second International Conference on Toxic Dinoflagellate Blooms. Key Biscayne, Florida, Oct. 31-Nov. 5, 1978.

Doty, M. S. and Aguilar-Santos, G. 1966. Caulerpicin, a toxic constituent of caulerpa. *Nature* 211: 990.

Earle, K. V. 1940. Pathological effects of two West Indian echinoderms. *Trans. Roy. Soc. Trop. Med. Hyg.* 33: 447—452.

Ellington, A. C. 1959. Poisonous fishes in the Caribbean area. *West Indies Fish Bull.* 6: 1—5.

Ellis, S., Spikes, J. J. and Johnson, G. L. 1979. Respiratory and cardiovascular effects of G. breve toxin in dogs. In: *Proceedings of the Second International Conference on Toxic Dinoflagellate Blooms.* D. L. Taylor and H. H. Seliger (eds.). Elsevier North Holland, New York.

Emerson, G. A. and Taft, C. H. 1945. Pharmacologically active agents from the sea. *Texas Rept. Biol. Med.* 3: 302—338.

Engelsen, H. 1922. On fish toxin and toxic fish. *Nord. Hyg. Tidskr.* 3: 316—325. (in Norwegian)

Erspamer, V. 1948a. Chemical and pharmacological investigations sugli estratti of the hypobronchial gland of Murex trunculus, Murex brandaris and Tritonalia erinacea. IV. Presence negli estratti of enteramine or an enteramine-like substance. *Arch. Int. Pharmacodyn.* 76: 308—326. (Italian)

Erspamer, V. 1948b. Preliminary chemical and pharmacological observations on murexine. *Experientia* 4: 226—228.

Erspamer, V. 1948c. Active substance in the posterior salivary glands of octopoda. I. Enteramine-like substance. *Acta Pharmacol. Toxicol.* 4: 213—223.

Erspamer, V. 1956. The enterochromaffin cell system and 5-hydroxytryptamine (enteramine, serotonin). *Triangle* 2: 129–138.

Erspamer, V. and Anastasi, A. 1962. Structure and pharmacological actions of eledoisin, the active endecapeptide of the posterior salivary glands of eledone. *Experientia* 18: 58–59.

Erspamer, V. and Benati, O. 1953. Identification of murexine as β-[imidazolyl-(4)]-acrylcholine. *Science* 117: 161–162.

Erspamer, V. and Erspamer, G. F. 1962. Pharmacological actions of eledoisin on extra vascular smooth muscle. *Br. J. Pharmacol. Chemother.* 19: 337–354.

Erspamer, V. and Glässer, A. 1957. The pharmacological actions of murexine (urocarylcholine). *Br. J. Pharmacol.* 12: 176–184.

Erspamer, V. and Glässer, A. 1963. The action of eledoisin on the systemic arterial blood pressure of some experimental animals. *Br. J. Pharmacol. Chemother.* 20: 516–527.

Evans, M. H. 1964. Paralytic effects of "paralytic shellfish poison" on frog nerve and muscle. *Br. J. Pharmacol. Chemother.* 22: 478–485.

Evans, M. E. 1965. Cause of death in experimental paralytic shellfish poisoning. *Br. J. Exp. Pathol.* 46: 245–253.

Evans, M. H. 1967. Block of sensory nerve conduction in the cat by mussel poison and tetrodotoxin. In: *Animal Toxins.* F. E. Russell and P. R. Saunders (eds.). Pergamon Press, New York.

Evans, M. H. 1969. Mechanism of saxitoxin and tetrodotoxin poisoning. *Br. Med. Bull.* 25: 263–267.

Fänge, R. 1958. Paper chromatography and biological effects of extracts of the salivary gland of Neptunea antiqua (Gastropoda). *Acta. Zool. (Stockholm)* 39: 39–46.

Fänge, R. 1960. The salivary gland of Neptunea antiqua. *Ann. N.Y. Acad. Sci.* 90: 689–694.

Feldman, M. H. and Schlezinger, N. S. 1970. Benign intracranial hypertension associated with hypervitaminosis A. *Arch. Neurol.* 22: 1–7.

Ferencik, M. 1970. Formation of histamine during bacterial decarboxylation of histidine in the flesh of some marine fishes. *J. Hyg. Epidemiol. Microbiol. Immunol.* 14: 52–60.

Ferguson, W. 1823. On the poisonous fishes of the Caribbean Islands. *Trans. R. Soc. Edinburgh* 9: 65–79.

Fish, C. J. and Cobb, M. C. 1954. Noxious marine animals of the central and western Pacific Ocean. U.S. Fish Wildlife Serv., Res. Rept. No. 36.

Fredericq, L. 1924. The secretions of protective and essential substances. In: *Handbook of Comparative Physiology.* Vol. II. H. Winterstein (ed.). Gustav Fischer, Jena. (German)

Freeman, S. E. 1976. Electrophysiological properties of maculotoxin. *Toxicon* 14: 396–399.

Friess, S. L. et al. 1959. Some pharmacologic properties of holothurin, an active neurotoxin from the sea cucumber. *J. Pharmacol. Exp. Ther.* 126: 323–329.

Friess, S. L. et al. 1960. Some pharmacologic properties of holothurin A, a glycoside mixture from the sea cucumber. *Ann. N.Y. Acad. Sci.* 90: 893–901.

Friess, S. L., Durant, R. C., Chanley, J. D. and Mazzetti, T. 1965. Some structural requirements underlying holothurin A interactions with synaptic chemoreceptors. *Biochem. Pharmacol.* 14: 1237–1247.

Friess, S. L. and Durant, R. C. 1965. Blockade phenomena at the mammalian neuromuscular synapse. Competition between reversible anticholinesterases and an irreversible toxin. *Toxicol. Appl. Pharmacol.* 7: 373–381.

Friess, S. L., Durant, R. C., Chanley, J. D. and Fash, F. J. 1967. Role of the sulphate charge center in irreversible interactions of holothurin A with chemo-receptors. *Biochem. Pharmacol.* 16: 1617—1625.

Fuhrman, F. A., Fuhrman, G. J., Dull, D. L. and Mosher, H. S. 1969. Toxins from eggs of fishes and amphibia. *J. Agric. Food Chem.* 17: 417—424.

Fujii, M., Harada, K. and Matsuda, M. 1967. Counteraction of the effects of puffer poison by cysteine. *Chem. Abstr.* 69: 25792.

Fukuda, T. 1951. Violent increase of cases of puffer poisoning. *Quoted by* B. W. Halstead, Jr. and D. A. Courville, 1967. *Poisonous and Venomous Marine Animals of the World.* Vol. 2. U.S. Government Printing Office, Washington, D.C.

Fukuda, T. and Tani, I. 1937. Statistical observation on fugu poisoning. *Jpn. J. Med. Sci.* IV, 10: 48—50. (Japanese)

Fukuda, T. and Tani, I. 1941. Records of puffer poisonings. Rept. 3. *Nippon Igaku Oyobi Kenko Hoken* 3258: 7—13. (Japanese)

Fukuda, T. and Tani, I. 1942. The puffer of the continent. *Nippon Igaku Oyobi Kenko Hoken* 3308: 13—17. (Japanese)

Gage, S. H. and Gage-Day, M. 1927. The anti-coagulating action of the secretion of the buccal glands of the lampreys (Petromyzon, Lampretra and Entosphenus). *Science* 66: 282—284.

Gallagher, J. P. and Shinnick-Gallagher, P. 1980. Effect of Gymnodinium breve toxin in the rat phrenic nerve diaphragm preparation. *Br. J. Pharmacol.* 69: 367—372.

Galtsoff, P. J. 1954. Red tide: Progress report on the investigation of the cause of mortality of fish along the West Coast of Florida. *U.S. Fish and Wildlife Service, Special Scientific Report No.* 46: 1—44, 1948, reissued 1954.

Garcia, P. J. 1955. *Quoted by* B. W. Halstead and D. A. Courville, 1967. *Poisonous and Venomous Marine Animals of the World.* U.S. Government Printing Office, Washington, D.C.

Geiger, E. 1944. Histamine content of unprocessed and canned fish. A tentative method of quantitative determination of spoilage. *Food Res.* 9: 293—297.

Geiger, E. 1955. Role of histamine in poisoning with spoiled fish. *Science* 121: 865—866.

Gelb, A. M. and Mildvan, D. 1979. Ciguatera fish poisoning. *N.Y. State J. Med.* June 79: 1080—1081.

Genenah, A. A. and Shimizu, Y. 1981. Specific toxicity of paralytic shellfish poisons. *J. Agric. Food Chem.* 29: 1289—1291.

Gerber, A., Raab, A. and Sobel, A. 1954. Vitamin A poisoning in adults: Description of a case. *Am. J. Med.* 16: 729—745.

Ghiretti, F. 1959. Cephalotoxin: The crab-paralysing agent of the posterior salivary glands of cephalopods. *Nature* 183: 1192—1193.

Ghiretti, F. 1960. Toxicity of octopus saliva against crustacea. *Ann. N.Y. Acad. Sci.* 90: 726—741.

Ghiretti, F. and Rocca, E. 1963. Some experiments on ichthyotoxin. In: *Venemous and Poisonous Animals and Noxious Plants of the Pacific Region.* H. L. Keegan and W. V. MacFarlane (eds.). Pergamon Press, New York.

Gibbard, J. and Naubert, J. 1948. Paralytic shellfish poisoning in the Canadian Atlantic coast. *Am. J. Public Health* 38: 550—553.

Gilbert, R. J. et al. 1980. Scombrotoxic fish poisoning: Features of the first 50 incidents to be reported in Britain (1976-9). *Br. Med. J.* 280: 71—72.

Gilman, R. L. 1942. A review of fish poisoning in the Puerto Rico-Virgin Islands area. U.S. Nav. Med. Bull. 40: 19—27.

Giunio, P. 1948. Poisonous fishes. *Higijena (Belgrade)* 1: 282—318. (Slavic)

Gonzales, R. B. and Alcala, A. C. 1977. Fatalities from crab poisoning on Negros Island, Philippines. *Toxicon* 15: 169–170.

Grant, F. E. and McCulloch, A. R. 1907. Dicapod crustacea from Norfolk Island. *Proc. Linnean Soc. N.S. Wales* 32: 151–156.

Grunhagen, H. H. 1980. |³H| Tetrodotoxin chemical tritiation and binding to voltage dependent Na-channels. *Fruhjahrstagung* 361: 257.

Gudger, E. W. 1930. Poisonous fishes and fish poisonings, with special reference to ciguatera in the West Indies. *Am. J. Trop. Med.* 10: 43–55.

Habekost, R. C., Fraser, I. M. and Halstead, B. W. 1955. Observations on toxic marine algae. *J. Wash. Acad. Sci.* 45: 101–103.

Habermehl, G. and Volkwein, G. 1968. On the poisons of deep sea holothurians. *Naturwissenschaften* 55: 83–84. (German)

Hall, S., Reichardt, P. B. and Neve, R. A. 1980. Toxins extracted from an Alaskan isolate of Protogonyaulax sp. *Biochem. Biophys. Res. Commun.* 97: 649–653.

Halstead, B. N. 1951. *Cited by* B. W. Halstead and D. A. Courville, 1965. *Poisonous and Venomous Marine Animals of the World. Vertebrates.* Vol. II. U.S. Government Printing Office, Washington, D.C.

Halstead, B. W. 1956. Animal phyla known to contain poisonous marine animals. In: *Venoms.* E. E. Buckley and N. Porges (eds.). American Association for the Advancement of Science, Washington, D.C.

Halstead, B. W. 1958. Poisonous fishes. *U.S. Public Health Rep.* 73: 302–312.

Halstead, B. W. 1959. *Dangerous Marine Animals.* Cornell Maritime Press, Cambridge, Massachusetts.

Halstead, B. W. 1964. Fish poisonings—Their diagnosis, pharmacology, and treatment. *Clin. Pharmacol. Ther.* 5: 615–627.

Halstead, B. W. 1978. *Poisonous and Venomous Marine Animals of the World.* Darwin, Princeton, New Jersey.

Halstead, B. W. 1981. Current status of marine biotoxicology—an overview. *Clin. Toxicol.* 18: 1–24.

Halstead, B. W. and Bunker, N. C. 1952. The venom apparatus of the ratfish, Hydrolagus colliei. *Copeia* 3: 128–138.

Halstead, B. W. and Bunker, N. C. 1953. The effect of the commercial canning process upon puffer poison. *Calif. Fish Game* 39: 219–228.

Halstead, B. W. and Bunker, N. C. 1954. A survey of the poisonous fishes of Johnston Island. *Zoologica* 39: 61–77.

Halstead, B. W. and Courville, D. A. 1965. *Poisonous and Venomous Marine Animals of the World. Invertebrates.* Vol. I. U.S. Government Printing Office, Washington, D.C.

Halstead, B. W. and Courville, D. A. 1967. *Poisonous and Venomous Marine Animals of the World. Vertebrates.* Vol. II. U.S. Government Printing Office, Washington, D.C.

Halstead, B. W. and Ralls, R. J. 1954. Results of dialyzing some fish poisons. *Science* 119: 160–161.

Halstead, B. W. and Schall, D. W. 1958. A report on the poisonous fishes of the Line Islands. *Acta Trop.* 15: 193–233.

Hanno, H. A. 1981. Ciguatera fish poisoning in the Virgin Islands. *J.A.M.A.* 245: 464.

Hartman, W. J. et al. 1960. Pharmacologically active amines and their biogenesis in the octopus. *Ann. N.Y. Acad. Sci.* 90: 637–666.

Hashimoto, Y. 1967. Poisonous and venomous gastropods. *Shokuhin Eiseigaku Zasshi* 8: 111–117. (Japanese)

Hashimoto, Y. 1968. Toxins found in ciguatoxic fishes in the Ryukyu Islands. South Pacific Comm. Report No. WP6, Seminar on Ichthyosarcotoxism. Papiete, French Polynesia August, 16-22.

Hashimoto, Y. 1975. Toxins involved in ciguatera. In: *Food-Drugs from the Sea.* Vol. IV. Marine Technology Society, Washington, D.C.

Hashimoto, Y. 1979. *Marine Toxins and Other Bioactive Marine Metabolites.* Japanese Scientific Society, Tokyo.

Hashimoto, Y. and Tsutsumi, J. 1961. Isolation of a photodynamic agent from the liver of abalone, Haliotis discus hannai. *Bull. Jn. Soc. Sci. Fish.* 27: 859-866.

Hashimoto, Y. and Yasumoto, T. 1965. A note on ciguatera poisoning in Okinawa and the toxin of a group, Epinephelus fuscoguttatus Forskal. *Bull. Jpn. Soc. Sci. Fish.* 31: 452-458.

Hashimoto, Y., Naito, K. and Tsutsumi, J. 1960. Photosensitization of animals by the viscera of abalones, Haliotis spp. *Bull. Jn. Soc. Sci. Fish.* 26: 1216-1221.

Hashimoto, Y. et al. 1967. Occurrence of toxic crabs in Ryukyu and Amami Islands. *Toxicon* 5: 85-90.

Hatano, M. 1971a. Toxic substances of the roe of northern blenny. VII. Further characterization of lipostichaerin. *Bull. Fac. Fish. Hokkaido Univ.* 22: 168.

Hatano, M. 1971b. Toxic substances of the roe of northern blenny. VIII. Partial purification and characterization of toxic phospholipid. *Bull. Fac. Fish. Hokkaido Univ.* 22: 177.

Hatano, M. and Hashimoto, Y. 1974. Properties of a toxic phospholipid in the northern blenny roe. *Toxicon* 12: 231-236.

Hatano, M. et al. 1964. Toxic substance of the northern blenny. I. On the extraction of toxic substance and its chemical properties. *Bull. Fac. Fish. Hokkaido University* 15: 138-146.

Hattori, Y. and Akiba, T. 1952. Studies on the toxic substance in asari (Venerupis semidecussata). II. Detection of toxic shellfish. *J. Pharm. Soc. Jpn.* 74: 572-577. (Japanese with English summary)

Hawkins, W. and Leonard, V. 1963. The antithrombic activity of carrageenan in human blood. *Can. J. Biochem. Physiol.* 41: 1325-1327.

Hayama, T. and Ogura, Y. 1958. Emetic action of tetrodotoxin (preliminary note). *Ann. Rept. Inst. Food Microbiol.* 11: 77-78.

Hayama, T. and Ogura, Y. 1963. Site of emetic action of tetrodotoxin in dog. *J. Pharmacol. Exp. Ther.* 139: 94-96.

Hayes, H. L. and Austin, T. S. 1951. The distribution of discolored seawater. *Texas J. Sci.* 3: 530-541.

Helfrich, P. 1961. Fish poisoning in the tropical Pacific. Hawaii Marine Lab., Univ. Hawaii., Honolulu, Hawaii.

Helfrich, P. 1963. Fish poisoning in Hawaii. *Hawaii Med. J.* 22: 361-372.

Helfrich, P. and Banner, A. H. 1960. Hallucinatory mullet poisoning. *J. Trop. Med. Hyg.* 63: 1-4.

Helfrich, P. and Banner, A. H. 1963. Experimental induction of ciguatera toxicity in fish through diet. *Nature* 197: 1025-1026.

Helfrich, P., Piyakarnchana, T. and Miles, P. S. 1968. Ciguatera fish poisoning. I. The ecology of ciguatera reef fishes in the Line Islands. B.P. Bishop Museum—Occasional papers, Honolulu, Hawaii 23: 305-382.

Hessel, D. W. 1961. Marine biotoxins. II. The extraction and partial purification of ciguatera toxin from Lutjanus bohar (Forskal). *Toxicol. Appl. Pharmacol.* 3: 574-583.

Hessel, D. W., Halstead, B. W. and Peckham, N. H. 1960. Marine biotoxins. I. Ciguatera poison: Some biological and chemical aspects. *Ann. N.Y. Acad. Sci.* 90: 788-797.

Hiyama, Y. 1943. Report of an investigation on poisonous fishes of the South Seas. *Nissan Fish. Exp. Sta.* (Odawara, Japan). pp. 1–137. (Japanese)

Houck, J., Morris, R. and Lazaro, E. 1957. Anticoagulant, lipemia, clearing and other effects of anionic polysaccharides extracted from seaweed. *Proc. Soc. Exp. Biol. Med.* 96: 528–530.

Hubbard, J. I. and Willis, W. D. 1968. The effects of depolarization of motor nerve terminals upon the release of transmitter by nerve impulses. *J. Physiol.* 194: 381–407.

Hubbs, C. L. and Wick, A. N. 1951. Toxicity of the roe of the cabezon, Scorpaenichthys marmoratus. *Calif. Fish Game* 37: 195–196.

Hughes, J. M. 1979. Epidemiology of shellfish poisoning in the United States, 1971–1977. In: *Toxic Dinoflagellate Blooms.* D. L. Taylor and H. H. Seliger (eds.). Elsevier North Holland, New York.

Hughes, J. M. and Merson, M. H. 1976. Current concepts: Fish and shellfish poisoning. *N. Engl. J. Med.* 295: 1117–1120.

Hurtel, J. M., Chanteau, S., Drollet, J. H. and Bagnis, R. 1979. Culture in artificial medium of a dinoflagellate responsible for ciguatera. *Rev. Int. Oceanogr. Med.* 55: 29–34. (French)

Ikawa, M. et al. 1982. Use of a strong cation exchange resin column for the study of paralytic shellfish poisons. *J. Agric. Food Chem.* 30: 526–528.

Inoue, A., Noguchi, T., Konosu, S. and Hashimoto, Y. 1968. A new toxic crab, Atergatis floridus. *Toxicon* 6: 119–123.

Irie, T., Susuki, M. and Masumune, T. 1965. Constituents from marine plants. II. Laurencin, a constituent from Laurencia species. *Tetrahedron Lett.* 16: 1091–1099.

Jackim, E. and Gentile, J. 1968. Toxins of a blue-green alga: Similarity to saxitoxin. *Science* 162: 915–916.

Jensen, A. S. 1948. Contributions to the ichthyofauna of Greenland. *Skrift. Univ. Zool. Mus. Copenhagen* 9: 20–25.

Johnson, H. M. 1964. Human blood group A, specific agglutinin of the butter clam Saxidomus giganteus. *Science* 146: 458–459.

Jones, H. R., Jr. 1980. Acute ataxia associated with ciguatera-type (Grouper) tropical fish poisoning. *Anna. Neurol.* 7: 491.

Jullien, A. and Ripplinger, J. 1950. The dried extract of the purple gland of Murex trunculus and its biological action. *Bull. Soc. Hist. Nat. Doubs* 53: 29–30.

Kaiser, E. and Michl, H. 1958. *Biochemistry of Animal Toxins.* Franz Denticke, Wien. (German)

Kanna, K. and Hirai, M. 1956. On the toxicity of Neptunea intersculpta. *Quoted by B. W. Halstead, 1965. Poisonous and Venomous Marine Animals of the World.* Vol. 1. U. S. Government Printing Office, Washington, D.C.

Kao, C. Y. 1966. Tetrodotoxin, saxitoxin and their significance in the study of excitation phenomena. *Pharmacol. Rev.* 18: 997–1049.

Kao, C. Y. 1972. Pharmacology of tetrodotoxin and saxitoxin. *Fed. Proc.* 31: 1117–1123.

Kao, C. Y. and Fuhrman, F. A. 1963. Pharmacological studies on tarichatoxin, a potent neurotoxin. *J. Pharmacol. Exp. Ther.* 140: 31–40.

Kao, C. Y. and Nishiyama, A. 1965. Actions of saxitoxin of peripheral neuro-muscular systems. *J. Physiol.* 108: 50–66.

Kawabata, T. 1971. Food poisoning in Japan caused by poisonous fish. In: *Fish Inspection and Quality Control.* R. Kreuger (ed.). Fishing News, London.

Kawabata, T., Ishizaka, K. and Miura, T. 1955a. Studies on the food poisoning associated with putrefaction of marine products. III. Physiological and

pharmacological properties of newly isolated vagus-stimulant, named "saurine."
Bull. Jpn. Soc. Sci. Fish. 21: 347—351. (Japanese)

Kawabata, T., Ishizaka, K. and Miura, T. 1955b. Studies on the food poisoning
associated with putrefaction of marine products. IV. Epidemiology and the
causative agents of the outbreaks of allergy-like food poisoning caused by
cooked frigate-mackerel meat at Kawasaki and by "samma sakuraboshi" at
Hamamatsu. *Bull. Jpn. Soc. Sci. Fish.* 21: 1167—1170. (Japanese)

Kawabata, T., Ishizaka, K., Miura, T. and Sasaki, T. 1956. An outbreak of
allergy-like food poisoning caused by "sashimi" (sliced raw flesh) and the
isolation of responsible bacterium, Proteus morganii. *Bull. Jpn. Soc. Sci. Fish.*
21: 1100.

Kawabata, T., Halstead, B. W. and Judefind, T. F. 1957. A report of a series
of recent outbreaks of unusual cephalopod and fish intoxications in Japan.
Am. J. Trop. Med. Hyg. 6: 935—939.

Kellaway, C. H. 1935a. The action of mussel poison on the nervous systems.
Aust. J. Exp. Biol. Med. Sci. 13: 79—94.

Kellaway, C. H. 1935b. Mussel poisoning. *Med. J. Aust.* 1: 399—401.

Kim, Y. H., Brown, G. B., Mosher, H. S. and Fuhrman, F. A. 1975. Tetrodotoxin: Occurrence in antelopid frogs of Costa Rica. *Science* 189: 151—152.

Kimata, M. 1961. The histamine problem. In: *Fish as Food.* Vol. 1. G. Borgstrom
(ed.). Academic Press, New York.

Kimata, M. and Tanaka, M. 1954. On the bacteria causing spoilage of fresh fish,
especially on their activity which can produce histamine. *Mem. Res. Inst.
Food Sci. Kyoto Univ.* 7: 12—17.

Knox, G. 1888. Poisonous fishes and means for preventing poisoning caused by
them. *Voenno-Med. Zh.* 161: 399—464. (Russian)

Knudson, A. G. and Rothman, P. E. 1953. Hypervitaminosis A. A review with a
discussion of vitamin A. *Am. J. Dis. Child.* 85: 316—334.

Konosu, S., Inoue, A., Noguchi, T. and Hashimoto, Y. 1968. Comparison of crab
toxin with saxitoxin and tetrodotoxin. *Toxicon* 6: 113—117.

Kopeczewski, W. 1918. Research on the serum of the moray eel (Muraena helena).
Ann. Inst. Pasteur 32: 584—612. (French)

Kosaki, T. I. and Anderson, H. H. 1968. Marine toxins from the Pacific. IV.
Pharmacology of ciguatoxin(s). *Toxicon* 6: 55—58.

Krause, R. F. 1965. Liver lipids in a case of hypervitaminosis A. *Am. J. Clin.
Nutr.* 16: 455—457.

Lane, W. R. and Sutherland, S. 1967. The ringed octopus bite: a unique medical
emergency. *Med. J. Aust.* 2: 475—476.

Larson, E., Lalone, R. C. and Rivas, L. R. 1960. Comparative toxicity of the
Atlantic puffer fishes of the genera Spheroides, Lactophrys, Lagocephelus
and Chilomycterus. *Fed. Proc.* 19: 388.

Lascari, A. D. and Bell, W. E. 1970. Pseudotumor cerebri due to hypervitaminosis
A. *Clin. Pediatr.* 9: 627—628.

Lawrence, D. N., Enriquez, M. B., Lumish, R. M. and Maceo, A. 1980. Ciguatera
fish poisoning in Miami. *J.A.M.A.* 244: 254—258.

Lee, C. 1980. Fish poisoning with particular reference to ciguatera. *J. Trop. Med.
Hyg.* 83: 93—97.

Legroux, R., Levaditi, J. C., Boudin, G. and Bovet, D. 1946a. Mass histamine
intoxications following the ingestion of fresh tuna. *Presse Med.* 29: 545.
(French)

Legroux, R., Levaditi, J. C., Boudin, G. and Bovet, D. 1946b. Remarks on the
mass histamine intoxications of alimentary origin. *Presse Med.* 53: 743.
(French)

Legroux, R., Bovet, D. and Levaditi, J. C. 1947. Presence of histamine in the flesh of tuna responsible in a mass poisoning. *Ann. Inst. Pasteur* 73: 101–104. (French)

Lerke, P. A., Werner, S. B., Taylor, S. L. and Guthertz, L. S. 1978. Scombroid poisoning—Report of an outbreak. *West J. Med.* 129: 381–386.

Lewis, N. 1981. "Ciguatera Health, and Human Adaptation in the Pacific." Ph.D. Thesis, University of California, Berkeley.

Lewis, R. J. and Endean, R. 1983. Occurrence of a ciguatoxin-like substance in the Spanish mackerel (Scomberomorus commersoni). *Toxicon* 21: 19–24.

Lewis, R. W. and Lentfer, J. W. 1967. The vitamin A content of polar bear liver: range and variability. *Comp. Biochem. Physiol.* 22: 923–926.

Li, C. P. et al. 1965a. Antiviral activity of paolins from clams. *Ann. N.Y. Acad. Sci.* 130: 374–382.

Li, K. M. 1965b. Ciguatera fish poison: a cholinesterase inhibitor. *Science* 147: 1580–1581.

Liguori, V. R. et al. 1963. Antibiotic and toxic activity of the mucous of the Pacific golden striped bass Grammistes sexlineatus. *Am. Zool.* 3: 546.

Love, R. and Frommhagen, L. H. 1953. Histochemical studies on the clam Mactra solidissima. *Proc. Soc. Exp. Biol. Med.* 83: 838–844.

Maass, T. A. 1937. Poisonous animals. In: *Biological Tables*. W. Junk (ed.). Vol. XIII. Van de Garde, Drukkery Zaltbommel, Holland.

Macht, D. I. 1942. An experimental appreciation of Leviticus XI, 9-12, and Deuteronomy XIV, 9-10. *Hebrew Med. J.* 2: 165–170.

Macht, D. I. and Barba-Gose, J. 1931a. Pharmacology of Ruvettus pretiosus, or "castor-oil fish." *Proc. Soc. Exp. Biol. Med.* 28: 772–774.

Macht, D. I. and Barba-Gose, J. 1931b. Two new methods for pharmacological comparison of insoluble purgatives. *J. Am. Pharm. Assoc.* 20: 556–564.

Macht, D. I. and Spencer, E. C. 1941. Physiological and toxicological effects of some fish muscle extracts. *Proc. Soc. Exp. Biol. Med.* 46: 228–233.

MacLean, J. L. 1979. Indo-Pacific red tides. In: *Toxic Dinoflagellate Blooms*. D. L. Taylor and H. H. Seliger (eds.). Elsevier North Holland, New York.

Marchalonis, J. J. and Edelman, G. M. 1968. Isolation and characterization of a hemagglutinin from Limulus polyphemus. *J. Mol. Biol.* 32: 453–465.

Maretzki, A. and Del Castillo, J. 1967. A toxin secreted by the soapfish Rypticus saponaceus. A preliminary report. *Toxicon* 4: 245–250.

Marie, J. and See, G. 1954. Acute hypervitaminosis of the infant. *Am. J. Dis. Child.* 87: 731–736.

Martin, D. F. and Chatterjee, A. B. 1969. Isolation and characterization of a toxin from the Florida red tide organism. *Nature* 221: 59.

Matsuno, T. and Iba, J. 1966. On the saponins of sea-cucumber. *Yakugaku Zasshi* 86: 637–638.

Matsuno, T. and Yamanouchi, T. 1961. A new triterpenoid sagogenin of animal origin (sea cucumber). *Nature* 191: 75–76.

McCollum, J. P. K. et al. 1968. An epidemic of mussel poisoning in north-east England. *Lancet* 2: 767–770.

McFarren, E. F. et al. 1956. Public health significance of paralytic shellfish poison. A review of literature and unpublished research. *Proc. Natl. Shellfish. Assoc.* 47: 114–141.

McFarren, E. F. et al. 1961. Public health significance of paralytic shellfish poison. *Adv. Food Res.* 10: 135–179.

McFarren, E. F. et al. 1965. The occurrence of a ciguatera-like poison in oysters, clams and Gymnodinium breve cultures. *Toxicon* 3: 111–123.

McMichael, D. F. 1963. *Dangerous Marine Molluscs*. Proc. First International Convention on Lifesaving Techniques. Suppl. Bull. Post Grad. Comm. Med., University of Sydney, Sydney, Australia.

Medcof, J. C. et al. 1947. Paralytic shellfish poisoning on the Canadian Atlantic
    coast. *Bull. Fish Res. Board Can.* 75: 1–32.
Meglitsch, P. A. 1967. *Invertebrate Zoology*. Oxford University Press, London.
Merson, M. H., Baine, W. B., Gangarosa, E. J. and Swanson, R. C. 1974.
    Scombroid fish poisoning: Outbreak traced to commercially canned tuna fish.
    J.A.M.A. 228: 1268–1269.
Meyer, K. F. 1953. Food poisoning, *N. Engl. J. Med.* 249: 843–852.
Meyer, K. F., Sommer, H. and Schoenholz, P. 1928. Mussel poisoning. *J. Prevent.
    Med.* 2: 365–394.
Mitomo, Y. 1927. Studies on eel serum I. Report on the pharmacological effect of
    eel serum. *Tohuku J. Exp. Med.* 8: 284–326. (German)
Miyahara, J. T., Akau, C. K. and Yasumoto, T. 1979. Effects of ciguatoxin and
    maitotoxin on the isolated guinea pig atria. *Res. Commun. Chem. Pathol.
    Pharmacol.* 25: 177–180.
Mizuta, M., Ito, T., Murakami, T. and Mizobe, M. 1957. Mass poisoning from the
    liver of sawara and Cwashikujira. *Nihon Iji. Shimpo* 1710: 27–34. (Japanese)
Mori, M. et al. 1966. Marine biotoxins. XI. Composition and toxicity of wax in the
    flesh of castor oil fishes. *Nippon Suisan Gakkaishi* 32: 137–145.
Muenter, M. D., Perry, H. O. and Ludwig, J. 1971. Chronic vitamin A intoxica-
    tion in adults. *Am. J. Med.* 50: 129–136.
Murray, C. K., Hobbs, G. and Gilbert, R. J. 1982. Scombrotoxin and scombro-
    toxin-like poisoning from canned fish. *J. Hyg.* 88: 215–220.
Murtha, E. F. 1960. Pharmacological study of poisons from shellfish and puffer
    fish. *Ann. N.Y. Acad. Sci.* 90: 820–836.
Music, S. I., Howell, J. T. and Brummack, C. L. 1973. Red tide. Its public
    health implications. *J. Fl. Med. Assoc.* 60: 27–29.
Nagasawa, J., Spiegelstein, M. J. and Kao, C. J. 1971. Cardiovascular action of
    saxitoxin. *J. Pharmacol. Exp. Ther.* 178: 103–109.
Narahashi, T. 1972. Mechanism of action of tetrodotoxin and saxitoxin on excitable
    membranes. *Fed. Proc.* 31: 1124–1132.
Narahashi, T., Brodwick, M. S. and Schantz, E. J. 1975. Mechanisms of action
    of a new toxin from Gonyaulax tamarensis on nerve membranes. *Environ. Lett.*
    9: 239–247.
Nater, J. P. and Doeglas, H. M. G. 1970. Halibut liver poisoning in eleven
    fishermen. *Acta Dermatovener.* 50: 109–113.
Needler, A. B. 1949. Paralytic shellfish poisoning and Goniaulax tamarensis.
    J. Fish Res. Board Can. 7: 490–504.
Nigrelli, R. F. and Jakowska, S. 1960. Effects of holothurin, a steroid saponin
    from the Bahamian sea cucumber (Actinopyga agassizi), on various biological
    systems. *Ann. N.Y. Acad. Sci.* 90: 884–892.
Nigrelli, R. F. and Zahl, P. 1952. Some biological characteristics of holothurin.
    Proc. Soc. Exp. Biol. Med. 81: 379–380.
Nigrelli, R. F., Chanley, J. D., Kohn, S. K. and Sobotka, H. 1955. The chemical
    nature of holothurin, a toxic principle from the sea cucumber (Echinodermata:
    Holothurioidea). *Zoologica* 40: 47--48.
Nilson, H. W. and Wagner, J. A. 1959. Feeding test with carrageenin. *Food Res.*
    24: 235–239.
Noguchi, T. and Hashimoto, Y. 1973. Isolation of tetrodotoxin from a goby Gobius
    criniger. *Toxicon* 11: 305–307.
Noguchi, T., Konosu, S. and Hashimoto, Y. 1969a. Identity of the crab toxin with
    saxitoxin. *Toxicon* 7: 325–326.
Noguchi, T., Konosu, S. and Hashimoto, Y. 1969b. Marine toxins. XXV. Identity
    of the crab toxin with saxitoxin. *Toxicon* 7: 930–935.

Noguchi, T. et al. 1981. Occurrence of tetrodotoxin in the Japanese ivory shell Babylonia Japonica. *Bull. Jpn. Soc. Sci. Fish.* 47: 909.

Ogura, Y. 1971. Fugu (puffer-fish) poisoning and the pharmacology of crystalline tetrodotoxin in poisoning. In: *Neuropoisons.* Vol. 1. L. L. Simpson (ed.). Plenum Press, New York.

Ogura, Y., Nara, J. and Yoshida, T. 1968. Comparative pharmacological actions of ciguatoxin and tetrodotoxin, a preliminary account. *Toxicon* 6: 131–140.

Ohizumi, Y., Shibata, S. and Tachibana, K. 1981. Mode of the excitatory and inhibitory actions of ciguatoxin in the guinea-pig vas deferens. *J. Pharmacol. Exp. Ther.* 217: 475–480.

Ohshika, H. 1971. Marine toxins from the Pacific—IX. Some effects of ciguatoxin on isolated mammalian atria. *Toxicon* 9: 337–343.

Okihiro, M. M., Keenan, J. P. and Ivy, A. C., Jr. 1965. Ciguatera fish poisoning with cholinesterase inhibition. *Hawaii Med. J.* 24: 354–357.

Oshima, Y. et al. 1976. Toxins of the Gonyaulax sp. and infested bivalves in Owase Bay. *Bull. Jpn. Soc. Sci. Fish.* 42: 851–856.

Ozawa, H., Gomi, Y. and Otsuki, I. 1967. Pharmacological studies on laminine monocitrate. *Yakugaku Zasshi* 87: 935–939.

Palsson, P. A. and Grimsson, H. 1953. Demyelination in lambs from ewes which feed on seaweeds. *Proc. Soc. Exp. Biol. Med.* 83: 518–520.

Park, Y. H., Kim, D. S., Kim, S. S. and Kim, S. B. 1980. Changes in histamine content in the muscle of dark-fleshed fishes during storage and processing. *Bull. Korean Fish. Soc.* 13: 15–22.

Pawlowsky, E. N. 1927. Poisonous animals and their toxicity. Fischer, Jean, Germany. (German)

Payne, C. A. and Payne, S. N. 1977. Ciguatera in Puerto Rico and the Virgin Islands. *N. Engl. J. Med.* 296: 949–950.

Percival E. 1966. The natural distribution of plant polysaccharides. In: *Comparative Phytochemistry.* T. Swain (ed.). Academic Press, New York.

Percival, E. and McDowell, R. H. 1967. *Chemistry and Enzymology of Marine Algal Polysaccharides.* Academic Press, New York.

Phisalix, M. 1922. *Poisonous Animals and Venoms.* Vols. 1 and 2. Masson and Cie, Paris. (French)

PHYSICIANS' DESK REFERENCE. 1983. *Aquasol A.* J. E. Angle (Publisher). Medical Economics Co., Oradell, New Jersey.

Plumert, A. 1902. On poisonous sea animals in general and in the case of mass poisoning due to sea mussels in particular. *Arch. Schiffs Tropenhyg.* 6: 15–23. (German)

Pouysségur, J., Jacques, Y., and Lazdunski, M. 1980. Identification of a tetrodotoxin-sensitive Na^+ channel in a variety of fibroblast lines. *Nature* 286: 162–164.

Prakash, A. 1961. *Status of Paralytic Shellfish-Poisoning Research in Canada.* Proc. Shellfish Sanitation Workshop. Nov. 1961, Washington, D. C.

Prakash, A. 1963. Source of paralytic shellfish toxin in the Bay of Fundy. *J. Fish. Res. Board Can.* 20: 983–996.

Prakash, A. and Medcof, J. C. 1962. Hydrographic and meteorological factors affecting shellfish toxicity at Head Harbor, New Brunswick. *Fish. Res. Board Can. J.* 19: 101–112.

Prakash, A. and Taylor, F. J. R. 1966. A red water bloom of Gonyaulax acatenella in Strait of Georgia and its relation to paralytic shellfish toxicity. *J. Fish. Res. Board Can. J.* 23: 1265–1270.

Prosvirov, E. 1963. *Poisonous Fishes.* Kaliningrad, Moscow. (Russian)

Provasoli, L. 1962. Organic regulators of phytoplankton fertility. *Quoted by*
    B. W. Halstead and D. Courville 1965. *Poisonous and Venomous Marine Animals
    of the World*. Vol. 1. U.S. Government Printing Office, Washington, D.C.
Pugsley, L. I. 1939. The possible occurrence of a toxic material in clams and
    mussels. *Fish. Res. Board Can. Prog. Rep. Pacific Coast Sta.* 40: 11—13.
Randall, J. E. 1958. A review of ciguatera tropical fish poisoning, with a tentative
    explanation of its cause. *Bull. Mar. Sci. Gulf Carib.* 8: 236—267.
Ray, S. M. and Aldrich, D. V. 1965. Gymnodinium breve: Induction of shellfish
    poisoning in chicks. *Science* 148: 1748—1749.
Rayner, M. D. 1970.*Marine Toxins from the Pacific—VII. Recent Advances in the
    Pharmacology of Ciguatoxin*. Proceedings: Drugs from the Sea Conference,
    Marine Technology Society, Washington, D.C.
Rayner, M. D. 1972. Mode of action of ciguatoxin. *Fed. Proc.* 31: 1139—1145.
Rayner, M. D. and Kosaki, T. I. 1970. Ciguatoxin: Effects on Na flux in frog
    muscle. *Fed. Proc.* 29: 548.
Rayner, M. D., Kosaki, T. I. and Fellmeth, E. L. 1968. Ciguatoxin: more than
    an anticholinesterase. *Science* 160: 70—71.
Rayner, M. D., Baslow, M. H. and Kosaki, T. I. 1969. Marine toxins from the
    Pacific: Not an in vivo anticholinesterase. *J. Fish Res. Board Can.* 26:
    2208—2210.
Ricketts, E. F. and Calvin, J. 1952. *Between Pacific tides*. 3rd ed. Stanford
    University Press, Stanford, California.
Ritchie, J. M. 1980. Tetrodotoxin and saxitoxin, and the sodium channels of
    excitable tissue. *Trends Pharmaceut. Sci.* 1: 275—279.
Roca, E. and Ghiretti, F. 1964. A toxic protein from eel serum. *Toxicon* 2: 79—80.
Rodahl, K. and Moore, T. 1943. The vitamin A content and toxicity of bear and
    seal liver. *Biochem. J.* 37: 166—168.
Rogers, J. E. 1951. *The Shell Book. A Popular Guide to a Knowledge of the
    Families of Living Mollusks, and an Aid to the Identification of Shells Native
    and Foreign*. Rev. ed. Branford, Boston.
Ruggiri, G. D. and Nigrelli, R. F. 1960. The effects of holothurin, a steroid
    saponin from the sea cucumber, on the development of the sea urchin.
    Zoologica 45: 1—16.
Russell, F. E. 1965a. Marine toxins and venomous and poisonous marine animals.
    Adv. Marine Biol. 3: 255—383.
Russell, F. E. 1965b. Comparative pharmacology of some animal toxins. *Fed. Proc.*
    26: 1206—1224.
Russell, F. E. 1975. Short communication ciguatera poisoning: A report of 35 cases.
    Toxicon 13: 383—385.
Sakai, M. et al. 1962. Poisoning produced by the ovaries of Stichaeus grigorjewi
    Herzenstein. *Shokuhin Eisei Kenkyu* 12: 53—68. (Japanese)
Sapeika, N. 1948. Mussel poisoning. *S. Afr. Med. J.* 22: 337—338.
Sapeika, N. 1953. Actions of mussel poison. *Arch. Intern. Pharmacodyn.* 93:
    135—142.
Sapeika, N. 1958. Mussel poisoning: a recent outbreak. *S. Afr. Med. J.* 32: 527.
Sasner, J. J., Jr. 1965. "The Effects of a Toxin Produced by the Florida Red
    Tide Dinoflagellate, Gymnodinium breve." Ph. D. Thesis, University of
    California, Los Angeles. *Dissert. Abstr.* 25: 7433.
Sasner, J. J., Jr., Ikawa, M., Thurberg, F. and Alam, M. 1972. Physiological
    and chemical studies on Gymnodinium breve Davis toxin. *Toxicon* 10: 163—172.
Schaefer, M. B. and Revelle, R. 1959. Marine resources. In: *Natural Resources*.
    M. R. Huberty and W. L. Flock (eds.). McGraw-Hill, New York.

Schantz, E. J. 1960. Biochemical studies on paralytic shellfish poisons. *Ann. N.Y. Acad. Sci.* 90: 843–855.

Schantz, E. J. 1961. Some chemical and physical properties of paralytic shellfish poisons related to toxicity. *J. Med. Pharm. Chem.* 4: 459–468.

Schantz, E. J. 1971. The dinoflagellate poisons. In: *Microbial Toxins.* Vol. 7. *Algal and Fungal Toxins.* S. Kadis, A. Ciegler and S. J. Ajl (eds.). Academic Press, New York.

Schantz, E. J. 1973. Seafood toxicants. In: *Toxicants Occurring Naturally in Foods.* Committee on Food Protection Food and Nutrition Board, National Research Council, National Academy of Sciences, Washington, D.C.

Schantz, E. J. and Magnusson, H. W. 1964. Observations on the origin of the paralytic poison in Alaska butter clams. *J. Protozool.* 11: 239–242.

Schantz, E. J. et al. 1957. Paralytic shellfish poison. VI. A procedure for the isolation and purification of the poison from toxic clam and mussel tissues. *J. Am. Chem. Soc.* 79: 5230–5235.

Schantz, E. J., McFarren, E. F., Schafer, M. L. and Lewis, K. H. 1958. Purified shellfish poison for bioassay standardization. *Assoc. Off. Agric. Chem.* 41: 160–168.

Schantz, E. J. et al. 1961. Paralytic shellfish poison. VIII. Some chemical and physical properties of purified clam and mussel poisons. *Can. J. Chem.* 39: 2117–2123.

Schantz, E. J. et al. 1966. The purification and characterization of the poison produced by Gonyaulax catenella in Axenic culture. *Biochemistry* 5: 1191–1195.

Schantz, E. J., Ghazarossian, V. E., Schnoes, H. K. and Strong, F. M. 1975. The structure of saxitoxin. *J. Am. Chem. Soc.* 97: 1238–1239.

Scheuer, P. J., Takahashi, W., Tsutsumi, J. and Yoshida, T. 1967. Ciguatoxin: Isolation and chemical nature. *Science* 155: 1267–1268.

Senanayake, N., Vyravanathan, S. and Kanagasuriyam, S. 1978. Cardiovascular accident after a "skipjack" reaction in a patient taking isoniazid. *Br. Med. J.* 21 October 1978: 1127–1128. 1978(2)

Serene, R. 1952. A report on the dangerous marine organisms of Indochina. *Quoted by B. W. Halstead and D. A. Courville, 1965. Poisonous and Venomous Marine Animals of the World.* Vol. 1. U.S. Government Printing Office, Washington, D.C.

Setliff, J. A., Rayner, M. D. and Hong, S. K. 1971. Effect of ciguatoxin on sodium transport across the frog skin. *Toxicol. Appl. Pharmacol.* 18: 676–684.

Shapiro, W. et al. 1963. Circulatory effects of synthetic eledoisin in man. *Circulation* 28: 803.

Sheumack, D. D., Howden, M. E. H., Spence, I. and Quinn, R. J. 1977. Maculotoxin: A neurotoxin from the venom glands of the octopus, Hapalochlaena maculosa, identified as tetrodotoxin. *Science* 199: 188–189.

Shifrine, M., Ousterhout, L. E., Grau, C. R. and Vaughn, R. H. 1959. Toxicity to chicks of histamine formed during microbial spoilage of tuna. *Appl. Microbiol.* 7: 45–50.

Shimada, K., Ohtsuru, M., Yamaguchi, T. and Nigota, K. 1983. Determination of tetrodotoxin by capillary isotachophowsis. *J. Food Sci.* 48: 665–667, 680.

Shimizu, Y. 1978. Dinoflagellate toxins. In: *Marine Natural Products. Chemical and Biological Perspectives.* Vol. I. P. J. Scheuer (ed.). Academic Press, New York.

Shimizu, Y. and Yoshioka, M. 1981. Transformation of paralytic shellfish toxins as demonstrated in scallop homogenates. *Science 212: 547–549.*

Shimizu, Y., Alam, M., Oshima, Y. and Fallon, W. E. 1975. Presence of four
toxins in red tide infested clams and cultured Gonyaulax tamarensis cells.
Biochem. Biophys. Res. Commun. 66: 731–737.

Shimizu, Y. et al. 1978. Analysis of toxic mussels (Mytilus sp.) from the Alaskan
inside passage. *J. Agric. Food Chem.* 26: 878–881.

Shinnick-Gallagher, P. 1980. Possible mechanisms of action of Gymnodinium breve
toxin at the mammalian neuromuscular junction. *Br. J. Pharmacol.* 69: 373–378.

Shuster, C. N., Jr. 1950. III. Observations on the natural history of the American
horseshoe crab, Limulus polyphemus. 3rd Rept. Investigations of methods of
improving the shellfish resources of Massachusetts. Woods Hole Oceanogr. Inst.,
Centr. No. 564.

Shuster, C. N., Jr. 1960. Xiphosura. *Encycl. Sci. Technol.* 14: 563–567.

Sicuteri, F., Fanciullacci, M., Franchi, G. and Michelacci, S. 1963. The endecapeptide eledoisin as powerful vasodilating and hypotensive agent in man.
Experientia 19: 44–47.

Simidu, W. and Hibiki, S. 1955a. Studies on putrefaction of aquatic products.
XIX. Influence of certain substances upon histamine formation. *Bull. Jpn.
Soc. Sci. Fish.* 20: 808–810. (Japanese with English summary)

Simidu, W. and Hibiki, S. 1955b. Studies on putrefaction of aquatic products. XXI.
Consideration of difference in putrefaction for various kinds of fish (4). On
difference of concentration of histidine between the interior and the exterior
of cells. *Bull. Jpn. Soc. Sci. Fish.* 21: 357–360. (Japanese with English
summary)

Simidu, W. and Hibiki, S. 1955c. Studies on putrefaction of aquatic products.
XXIII. On the critical concentration of poisoning for histamine. *Bull. Jpn. Soc.
Sci. Fish.* 21: 365–367. (Japanese)

Smith, J. L. 1961. *The Sea Fishes of Southern Africa.* 4th Ed. Central News
Agency of South Africa. Cape Town.

Smith, J. W. and Hofstede, D. P. 1966. Vitamin A poisoning in adults. *Ned.
Tijdschr. Geneeskd.* 110: 10.

Soegiri, D. 1936. *Quoted by* B. W. Halstead and D. A. Courville. 1965. *Poisonous
and Venomous Marine Animals of the World.* Vol. 1. U.S. Government Printing
Office, Washington, D.C.

Sollman, T. 1949. *A Manual of Pharmacology and Its Application to Therapeutics
and Toxicology.* 11 ed. Saunders, Philadelphia.

Sommer, H. 1932. Occurrence of paralytic shellfish poison in the common sand crab.
Science 76: 574–575.

Sommer, H. and Meyer, K. F. 1937. Paralytic shellfish poisoning. *Arch. Pathol.*
24: 560–598.

Sommer, H. and Meyer, K. F. 1941. Mussel poisoning—A summary. *Calif. State
Dept. Public Health Weekly Bull.* 20: 53–55.

Sommer, H., Whedon, W. F., Kofoid, C. A. and Stohler, R. 1937. Relation of
paralytic shell-fish poison to certain plankton organisms of the genus
Gonyaulax. *Arch. Pathol.* 24: 537–559.

Sparks, A. K. 1961. Ecology of paralytic shellfish toxicity in Washington. *Res.
Fish. Contrib.* 116: 26.

Sparks, A. K., Sribhibhadh, A., Chew, K. K. and Pereyra, D. 1962. Ecology
of paralytic shellfish toxicity in Washington. *Res. Fish. Contrib.* 139: 39–42.

Spector, W. S. 1956. (ed.). *Handbook of Toxicology.* Vol. 1. Saunders,
Philadelphia.

Spiegelstein, M. Y., Paster, Z. and Abbott, B. C. 1973. Purification and biological
activity of Gymnodinium breve toxins. *Toxicon* 11: 85–93.

Spikes, J. J., Ray, S. M., Aldrich, D. V. and Nash, J. B. 1968. Toxicity variations of Gymnodinium breve cultures. *Toxicon* 5: 171–174.

Starr, T. J. and Holtermann, O. A. 1967. Uncoating and development of vaccinia virus in miniature cells induced with an extract from marine algae. *Nature* 216: 600–601.

Starr, T. J., Deig, E. F., Church, K. K. and Allen, M. B. 1962. Antibacterial and antiviral activities of algal extracts studied by acridine orange staining. *Texas Rep. Biol. Med.* 20: 271–278.

Starr, T. J., Kojima, M. and Piferrer, M. 1966. Mitotic anomalies in tissue-cultured cells treated with extracts derived from marine algae. *Texas Rep. Biol. Med.* 24: 208–221.

Steidinger, K. A. 1979. Collection, enumeration, and identification of free-living dinoflagellates. In: *Toxic Dinoflagellate Blooms.* D. L. Taylor and H. H. Seliger (eds.). Elsevier North-Holland, New York.

Stephenson, N. R., Edwards, H. I., MacDonald, B. F. and Pugsley, L. I. 1955. Biological assay of the toxin from shellfish. *Can. J. Biochem. Physiol.* 33: 849–857.

Steyn, D. G. 1936. Food poisoning caused by substances other than bacteria and their products. *S. Afr. Vet. Med. Assoc.* 7: 106–113.

Strain, H. H. et al. 1971. The structure of peridinin, the characteristic dino-flagellate carotenoid. *J. Am. Chem. Soc.* 93: 1823–1825.

Stürmer, E. and Berde, B. 1963. A comparative pharmacological study of synthetic eledoisin and synthetic bradykenin. *J. Pharmacol. Exp. Ther.* 140: 349–355.

Tachibana, K. 1980. "Structural Studies on Marine Toxins." Ph.D. Thesis. University of Hawaii, Honolulu.

Taft, C. H. 1945. Poisonous marine animals. *Texas Rep. Biol. Med.* 3: 339–352.

Takemoto, T. Daigo, K. and Takagi, N. 1964a. Studies on the hypotensive con-stituents of marine algae. I. A new basic amino acid "laminine" and the other basic constituents isolated from Laminaria angustata. *Yakugaku Zasshi* 84: 1176–1179.

Takemoto, T., Daigo, K. and Takagi, N. 1964b. Studies on the hypotensive con-stituents of marine algae. II. Synthesis of laminine and related compounds. *Yakugaku Zasshi* 84: 1180–1182.

Takemoto, T., Daigo, K. and Takagi, N. 1965a. Studies on the hypotensive con-stituents of marine algae. III. Determination of laminine in laminariaceen. *Yakugaku Zasshi* 85: 37–40.

Takemoto, T., Takagi, N. and Daigo, K. 1965b. Studies on the hypotensive con-stituents of marine algae. IV. Amino acid constituents of Heterochordaria abietina. *Yakugaku Zasshi* 85: 843–845.

Tani, I. 1945. Toxicological studies on Japanese puffers. *Teikoku Tosho Kabushiki Faisha* 2: 1–103. (Japanese)

Tani, I. 1969. On puffer fishes. *Kakeiken Dayori* 2: 3–9. (Japanese)

Tatnall, F. M., Smith, H. G. and Welsby, P. D. and Turnbull, P. C. B. 1980. Ciguatera poisoning. *Br. Med. J.* 281: 948.

Taylor, F. J. R. 1979. A description of the benthic dinoflagellate association with maitotoxin and ciguatoxin, including observations of Hawaiian materia. In *Toxic Dinoflagellate Blooms.* D. L. Taylor and H. H. Seliger (eds.). Elsevier North Holland, New York.

Taylor, F. J. R. 1980. On dinoflagellate evolution. *Biosystems* 13: 65–108.

Teh, Y. F. and Gardner, J. E. 1970. Toxin from the coral reef crab, Lophozozymus pictor. *Pharmacol. Res. Commun.* 2: 251.

Teh, Y. F. and Gardner, J. E. 1974. Partial purification of Lophozozymus pictor toxin. *Toxicon* 12: 603–610.

Tennant, A. D., Naubert, J. and Corbell, H. E. 1955. An outbreak of paralytic shellfish poisoning. *Can. Med. Assoc. J.* 72: 436−439.

Thomas, L. J., Jr. 1951. A blood anti-coagulant from surf clams. *Biol. Bull.* 101: 230−231.

Thomas, L. J., Jr. 1954. The localization of heparin-like blood anticoagulant substances in the tissues of Spisula solidissima. *Biol. Bull.* 106: 129−138.

Thomson, D. A. 1964. Ostracitoxin: An ichthyotoxic stress secretion of the boxfish, Ostracion lentiginosus. *Science* 146: 244−245.

Thron, C. D. 1964. Hemolysis by holothurin A, digitonin, and quillaia saponin: estimates of the required cellular lysin uptakes and free lysin concentrations. *J. Pharmacol. Exp. Ther.* 145: 194−202.

Thron, C. D., Durant, R. C. and Friess, S. L. 1964. Neuromuscular and cytotoxic effects of holothurin A and related saponins at low concentration levels. III. *Toxicol. Appl. Pharmacol.* 6: 182−196.

Togashi, M. 1943. Clinical study of the poisoning by Venerupis semidecussata. Quoted by B. W. Halstead and D. A. Courville. *Poisonous and Venomous Marine Animals of the World.* Vol. 1. U.S. Government Printing Office, Washington, D.C.

Torda, T. A., Sinclair, E. and Ulyatt, O. B. 1973. Puffer fish (tetrodotoxin) poisoning: Clinical record and suggested management. *Med. J. Aust.* 1: 599−602.

Trethewie, E. R. 1965. Pharmacological effects of the venom of the common octopus Hapalochlaena maculosa. *Toxicon* 3: 55−59.

Tsuda, K. et al. 1964. On the structure of tetrodotoxin. *Chem. Pharm. Bull. (Japan)* 12: 642−645.

Tsunenari, S., Uchimura, Y. and Kanda, M. 1980. Puffer poisoning in Japan— A case report. *J. Forensic Sci.* 25: 240−245.

Tursch, B. et al. 1967. Chemical studies of marine invertebrates—II Terpenoids-LVIII Griseogenin, a new triterpenoid sapogenin of the sea cucumber Halodeima grisea L. *Tetrahedron* 23: 761−767.

Van Veen, A. G. and Latuasan, H. E. 1950. Fish poison caused by histamine in Indonesia. *Doc. Neerland. Indon. Morbis Trop.* 2: 18−20.

Walpole, A. L. 1962. Observations upon the inducation of subcutaneous sarcomata in rats. In: *The Morphological Precursors of Cancer.* L. Severi (ed.). University of Perugia, Italy.

Waterman, T. H. 1953a. Xiphosura from Xuong-ha. *Am. Sci.* 41: 293−302.

Waterman, T. H. 1953b. Poisonous Pacific horseshoe crabs. Quoted by B. W. Halstead and D. A. Courville, 1965. *Poisonous and Venomous Marine Animals of the World.* Vol. 1. U.S. Government Printing Office, Washington, D.C.

Watts, J. S., Reilly, J., DaCosta, F. M. and Krop, S. 1966. Acute toxicity of paralytic shellfish poison in rats of different ages. *Toxicol. Appl. Pharmacol.* 8: 286−294.

Westerfield, M., Moore, J. W., Kim, Y. S. and Padilla, G. M. 1977. How Gymnodinium breve red tide toxin(s) produces repetitive firing in squid axons. *Am. J. Physiol.* 232: C23−C29.

Wheeler, J. E. 1953. The problem of poisonous fishes. *Mauritius-Seychelles fish. Survey. Fish. Publ.* 1: 44−48.

Whittaker, V. P. 1960. Pharmacologically active choline esters in marine gastropods. *Ann. N.Y. Acad. Sci.* 90: 695−705.

Wiberg, G. S. and Stephenson, N. R. 1961. The effect of metal ions on the toxicity of paralytic shellfish poison. *Toxicol. Appl. Pharmacol.* 3: 707−712.

Wikholm, D. M. 1947. "Studies on the Toxic Principle and Accompanying Bases Found in the Sea Mussel, Mytilus californianus, Conrad, and the Marine Plankton Organism, Gonyaulax catenella, whedon and kofoid." Ph.D. Thesis, Northwestern University, Evanston, Illinois.

Winkler, L. R. 1961. Preliminary tests of the toxin extracted from California sea hares of the genus Aplysia. *Pacific Sci.* 15: 211—214.

Winkler, L. R. and Dawson, E. Y. 1963. Observations and experiments on the food habits of California sea hares of the genus Aplysia. *Pacific Sci.* 17: 102—105.

Winkler, L. R. and Tilton, B. E. 1962. Interspecific differences in the reaction to atropine and in the histology of the esophagi of the common California sea hares of the genus Aplysia. *Pacific Sci.* 15: 557—560.

Winkler, L. R., Tilton, B. E. and Hardinge, M. G. 1962. An agent extracted from sea hares. *Arch. Intern. Pharmacodyn.* 137: 76—83.

Withers, N. W. 1981. *Toxin Production, Nutrition and Distribution of Gambierdiscus toxicus (Hawaiian Strain)*. 4th Int. Coral Reef Symposium, Manila, Philippines.

Withers, N. W. 1982. Ciguatera fish poisoning. *Ann. Rev. Med.* 33: 97—111.

Wong, J. L., Oesterlin, R. and Rapoport, H. 1971. Structure of saxitoxin. *J. Am. Chem. Soc.* 93: 7344—7345.

Woodard, W. K., Miller, L. J. and Legant, O. 1961. Acute and chronic hypervitaminosis A in a 4-month old infant. *J. Pediatr.* 59: 260—264.

Woodcock, A. H. 1948. Note covering human respiratory irritation associated with high concentrations of plankton and mass mortality of marine organisms. *J. Mar. Res.* VII, 56—62.

Woodward, R. B. 1964. The structure of tetrodotoxin. *Pure Appl. Chem.* 9: 49—74.

Yamamura, S. and Hirata, Y. 1963. Structures of aplysin and aplysinol, naturally occurring bromo compounds. *Tetrahedron* 19: 1485—1496.

Yamanouchi, T. 1955. On the poisonous substance contained in holothurians. *Publ. Seto Marine Biol. Lab.* 4: 183—203.

Yasumoto, T. 1980. Environmental studies on a toxic dinoflagellate responsible for ciguatera. *Bull. Jpn. Soc. Sci. Fish.* 46: 1397—1404.

Yasumoto, Y. and Scheuer, P. J. 1969. Marine toxins of the Pacific. VIII. Ciguatoxin from moray eel livers. *Toxicon* 7: 273—276.

Yasumoto, T., Nakamura, K. and Hashimoto, Y. 1967. A new saponin, holothurin B, isolated from the sea cucumber, Holothuria vagabunda and Holothuria lubrica. *Agric. Biol. Chem.* 31: 7—10.

Yasumoto, T. et al. 1971. Toxicity of the surgeon fishes. *Bull. Jpn. Soc. Sci. Fish.* 37: 724—734.

Yasumoto, T., Nakajima, I., Bagnis, R. and Adachi, R. 1977a. Findings of a dinoflagellate as a likely culprit of ciguatera. *Bull. Jpn. Soc. Sci. Fish.* 43: 1021—1026.

Yasumoto, T., Bagnis, R., Trevenin, S. and Garcon, M. 1977b. A survey of comparative toxicity in the food chain of ciguatera. *Bull. Jpn. Soc. Sci. Fish.* 43: 1015—1019.

Yasumoto, T., Inoue, A., Bagnis, R. and Garcon, M. 1979. Ecological survey on a dinoflagellate responsible for the induction of ciguatera. *Bull. Jpn. Soc. Sci. Fish.* 45: 395—399.

Yasumoto, T. et al. 1980. Toxicity of benthic dinoflagellates found in coral reef. *Bull. Jpn. Soc. Sci. Fish.* 46: 327—331.

Zwahlen, A., Blanc, M.-H. and Robert, M. 1977. Epidemic intoxication due to shellfish (paralytic shellfish poisoning). *Schweiz. Med. Wochenschr.* 107: 226—230.

12

Derived Food Toxicants

The term derived, or formed, toxicants as used in this book is defined as any actually or potentially toxic substance that may be chemically or enzymatically formed in foods during processing, preparation, or storage. (Another term which may be applicable in this case is toxic reaction products.) Thus, a toxic substance may be formed by interaction between any endogenous or exogenous food component; (i.e., in the case of the latter, contaminants and additives), or their derivatives, or between these substances and outside agents; e.g., oxygen. Chemical degradation brought about by heat, light, enzymes, and other agents may also result in the formation of toxic substances.

The formation of derived compounds in foodstuffs is to be expected, since the components of all foods are chemically reactive substances. Furthermore, the usual conditions to which foods are exposed, e.g., cooking, can easily promote such reactions. In addition, many types of foodstuffs contain enzymes which may be endogenous or derived from microorganisms. Enzymes are particularly unavoidable in many types of fermented foodstuffs, unless the enzymes are denatured during food processing or preparation.

Chemical degradation or synthesis in foodstuffs is, therefore, inevitable, and so is the formation of toxic substances. The very large number of reactive endogenous or exogenous food components can easily lead to a plethora of derivatives. When one considers the number of possible permutations, the number of derivatives can be staggering indeed!

Several derived toxicants have been identified, but many more have not yet been assessed toxicologically. Unfortunately, the number of derivatives that may be formed in a given foodstuff under a given condition is not known. Thus, a food product that is finally consumed may contain a mixture of its original components and a large number of derived compounds. It is not only essential that such compounds be identified, but also that the toxicological properties of each and the mixture of such compounds be also established. The toxicological profile of a foodstuff may be different in the presence of such mixtures, for additive, synergistic, and/or antagonistic effects may come into play.

This chapter discusses several examples of derived toxicants. A few of these compounds have been subjected to extensive studies as a class. Some examples are given for which their toxicities have been determined only as mixtures. It is obvious that classifying a compound as a derived toxicant does not imply that such compounds can only be formed under conditions associated with foodstuffs. This classification emphasizes the need to understand the conditions that can lead to the formation of toxic reaction products which are derivable in situ from food components. It is hoped that more attention can be given to this toxicologically important phenomenon. Efforts related to this field unfortunately lack direction and intent at the present time, in part because of the complexity of the problem.

The categories of derived toxicants discussed in this chapter include pyrorganic toxicants, nonpyrolytic toxicants derived from amino acids, toxicants derived from the oxidation of fats and oils, toxicants produced by degradation or reaction with contaminants, and miscellaneous toxicants.

PYRORGANIC TOXICANTS

Pyrorganic compounds are defined as products produced at carbonization temperatures. At these temperatures, a significant amount of charred or tarry products is formed. Thus, burnt products such as tar, soot, or creosote are mixtures of pyrorganic compounds. The temperatures at which these products are formed depend on the nature of the substance burned and conditions and rate of burning. In general, in the case of food products, toxicologically significant pyrorganic compounds begin to be produced at around $300^{\circ}C$ or higher.

The formation of pyrorganic compounds is a complex process. This differs from other heat-induced processes in that the former is preceded by an initial, extensive breakdown of the molecular structures of organic compounds to simpler, reactive fragments. Combinations of these fragments to more stable compounds follow provided the conditions preclude rapid formation of CO or CO_2. This process is illustrated in the formation of polycyclic aromatic hydrocarbons, as discussed in the next section.

Polycyclic Aromatic Hydrocarbons

That pyrorganic products can be carcinogenic was first recognized by the English physician Percival Pott in 1795. Pott observed the increased incidence of scrotal cancer among chimney sweeps and attributed this to continued exposure to soot. Since then, other pyrolytic products such as coal tar (Volkmann 1875), pitch (Manouviriez 1876), and later wood soot from a smoked sausage factory (Sulman and Sulman 1946) have been shown to be carcinogenic, not only to the skin (Eckardt 1959; Heller 1930) but also to certain internal organs such as the lungs (Doll 1952; Lloyd 1971).

The carcinogenicity of coal tar has been experimentally demonstrated in rabbits by Yamagiwa and Ichikawa (1918), and in mice by Tsutsui (1918). The carcinogenicity of wood soot also has been experimentally demonstrated in mice (Passey 1922). Carcinogenic tars were prepared from various sources by pyrolysis under hydrogen of diverse organic matter, such as acetylene, isoprene, skin tissues, yeast and cholesterol (Kennaway 1924, 1925).

It was later shown that the carcinogenic potency of tars increases with pyrolytic temperatures above $500^{\circ}C$ (Twort and Fulton 1930).

Later researchers have succeeded in identifying the polycyclic aromatic hydrocarbon (PAH) benzo(a)pyrene (3,4-benzpyrene) as the active compound in tars (Cook et al. 1932). The water insoluble tarry residue that separates during the preparation of "liquid smoke" (prepared by passing wood smoke through water), used as food flavoring agent, may contain as much as 3.8 μg benzo(a)pyrene/g (White et al. 1971). Other carcinogenic PAHs also have been identified as constituents in tars: dibenzo-(a,h)anthracene, dibenzo(a,h)pyrene, dibenzo(a,i)pyrene, and benzo(b)fluoranthene (Badger 1962). In addition, benzo(a)anthracene and benzo(k)fluoranthene have been detected in smoke and broiled foodstuffs (Hoffman and Wynder 1962). All of these are strong carcinogens, but 3,4-benzpyrene is probably the most potent, and consequently has received the most attention. Benzo(a)pyrene can cause rapid carcinoma formation when applied to the skin of mice (Arcos and Argus 1968).

The structures of several PAHs demonstrated in pyrolytic products are shown below:

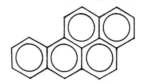

Benzo(a)pyrene
(3,4-Benzpyrene)

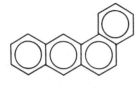

Benzo(a)anthracene

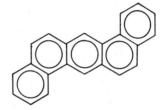

Dibenzo(a,h)anthracene

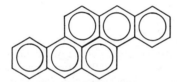

Dibenzo(a,h)pyrene

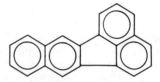

Benzo(k)fluoranthene

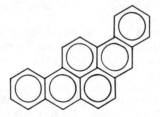

Dibenzo(a,i)pyrene

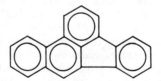

Benzo(b)fluoranthene

The PAHs are most likely pyrosynthesized from degradative products consisting of four- or two-carbon units, such as butadiene or ethylene radicals (Badger 1962; Hoffmann and Wynder 1972; Patterson et al. 1978). The ease of their formation at elevated temperatures follows from their thermodynamic stability. Some possible pathways showing the formation of benzo(a)pyrene are as follows (Badger 1962).

Benzo(a)pyrene

The presence of benzo(a)pyrene in pyrolytic products of foodstuffs has been confirmed many times. It has been detected in the charred crusts of biscuits (Kuratsune 1956), broiled meat, charcoal-broiled steak, barbecued ribs (Lijinsky and Shubik 1965, 1964), barbecued beef (Malanoski et al. 1968), broiled mackerel (Masuda et al. 1966), and commercially roasted coffees (Kuratsune and Hueper 1960). The levels found in the broiled meats ranged from 0.17 to 10.5 ppb. However, the conditions of broiling can markedly affect the levels. For example, in T-bone steaks cooked close to the coals over a relatively prolonged period, as high as 50 ppb of benzo(a)pyrene has been detected, and this level could be greatly reduced when the meat is cooked at a greater distance from the charcoal (Lijinsky and Ross 1967).

It has been shown that the fat content of meat is an important factor affecting the level of benzo(a)pyrene (Lijinsky and Ross 1967). For example, hamburgers with high fat content when broiled close to the flame produce 43 ppb of PAHs, of which 2.6 ppb is benzo(a)pyrene; the lean product produces only 2.8 ppb PAHs and no benzo(a)-pyrene. Therefore, reducing the amount of fat can reduce the level of benzo(a)pyrene. However, other constituents in foodstuffs can be pyrolyzed to produce PAHs. Thus, when starch is pyrolyzed at 370 to 390 and 650°C, 0.7 and 17 ppb benzo(a)pyrene will be produced, respectively (Davies and Wilmshurst 1960). Masuda et al. (1967) has found no PAHs when carbohydrates, amino acids, and fatty acids are pyrolyzed at 300°C. At 500°C, however, more PAHs will form from carbohydrates; fatty acids yield more of these when pyrolyzed at 700°C. Therefore, the PAH, such as benzo(a)pyrene, already can be formed at temperatures of 370 to 390°C, as used in many cooking procedures, and especially during baking of bread where surface temperatures may approach 400°C, or in boiling cooking fats attaining temperatures of 400 to 600°C.

Evidence has been presented suggesting that the structure of the compound pyrolyzed might affect the level of benzo(a)pyrene so produced. Thus, when proline, valine, tryptophan, and methionine are pyrolyzed at 850°C, the levels of benzo(a)pyrene thus formed from the respective amino acids are: 25, 11, 21, and 2.1 mg/mol of

compound pyrolyzed (Patterson et al. 1978). However, tryptophan produces more py-
rodegradation products (about 49 g/mol) than the other amino acids. This is interesting, since as shown elsewhere in this section (p. 612) there may be other factors in
the pyrolyzates which influence the carcinogenic potentials of such products.

In this connection, benzo(a)pyrene and similar PAHs are abundantly found in
smoked foods. However, they occur in these foods mostly as contaminants from the
smoke produced by the pyrolysis of wood and similar fuels. This is especially true in
those products that do not quite attain the temperatures necessary for the production
of PAHs.

Table 12.1 shows the levels of benzo(a)pyrene in smoked and other foods as obtained from various sources (Lo and Sandi 1978). Undoubtedly, as the values show,
the levels of this carcinogen vary depending on the food and the manner of cooking.
Note that exposure close to the source of the smoke will increase the level of carcinogen. It should be emphasized that other PAHs are also present together with benzo(a)-
pyrene. Thus, the total PAH intake can be higher, and the question of cocarcinogenesis, syncarcinogenesis, and tumor promotion becomes very relevant (see Chapter 6).

While there is no clear evidence implicating foodstuffs containing benzo(a)pyrene
and other PAHs as causing cancer in humans, the reports on the carcinogenicity of
tars mentioned earlier in this section clearly suggest that foodstuffs containing

Table 12.1 Benzo(a)pyrene in Smoked and Other Food

Food	Benzo(a)-pyrene(ppb)	Food	Benzo(a)-pyrene(ppb)
Smoked fish		Barbecued meats (Charcoal broiled)	
Eel	1.0	Hamburgers	11.2
Herring	1.0	Pork chop	7.9
Sturgeon	0.8	Chicken	3.7
Chubs	1.3	Sirloin steak	11.1
White fish	6.6	T-bone steak	57.4
Kippered cod	4.5	T-bone steak (flame broiled)	4.4
Smoked meats		Ribs	10.5
Ham	0.7-55.0	Other steaks	5.8-8.0
Mutton close to stove	107.0	Other foods	
distant from stove	21.0		
Lamb	23.0	Spinach	7.4
Sausage (with casing)		Kale	12.6-48.1
cold smoked	2.9	Yeast	1.8-40.4
hot smoked	0.7		
Salami	0.8	Tea	3.9-21.3
Bacon	3.6	Coffee	0-15.0
		Cereals	0.2-4.1
		Soybean	3.1

Source: Lo and Sandi (1978).

pyrolytic substances may constitute a real hazard. Very low levels of benzo(a)pyrene and other PAHs may constitute no real hazard when taken individually. For example, Roe (1963) has shown that repeated cutaneous application of 1.25 μg benzo(a)pyrene in mice for 68 weeks fails to produce tumors, and 10 ppm or less of this carcinogen in the diet fed to mice has no observable deleterious effects (Neal and Rigdon 1967). However, one can draw a parallelism from the results with tobacco smoke components. Several studies have shown that tumors could hardly be induced in experimental animals unless the neutral PAH-containing and acidic tumor-promoting fractions of tobacco tars were combined. The acidic fraction was inactive by itself, and the PAH-containing portion was responsible for only a small portion of the observed activity (Wynder and Hoffmann 1967). Studies by Sugimura et al. (1977) have shown that the mutagenic activity in *Salmonella typhimurium* TA 100 was much greater with 18 mg smoke condensate from broiling sardines than what might be induced by 9 ng of benzo(a)pyrene; the activity in this case was equivalent to 132 μg of benzo(a)pyrene. The extract from the charged surface of one fish has a mutagenic activity equivalent to 356 μg of benzo-(a)pyrene. With 190 g of beefsteak, the mutagenic activity was equivalent to 855 μg of benzo(a)pyrene. Thus, it is evident that the combined effects of all substances in tar may present real toxic hazards than just the small amounts of each individual carcinogenic PAH alone.

The role of promoters and other modifiers of carcinogenesis is discussed in Chapter 6.

Metabolism of PAH and Carcinogenicity

As with most known carcinogens, the PAHs are secondary carcinogens or procarcinogens. There is extensive evidence which indicates that their activity depends on specific metabolic transformation. The metabolism of PAH can be exemplified by benzo(a)-pyrene. The metabolic transformation of this carcinogen is rather complex, involving epoxidation and hydroxylation (Selkirk 1977). A part of the metabolic pathways involved in proximate carcinogen formation is shown in Figure 12.1 (Yagi et al. 1977). The diolepoxide I has been shown to be the major metabolite of benzo(a)pyrene (Huberman et al. 1976); it also has been shown to be bound to deoxyribonucleic acid (DNA) (King et al. 1976) and ribonucleic acid (RNA) (Weinstein et al. 1976), and the most mutagenic to mammalian cells as compared to the diol epoxide II and all 13 other known benzo-(a)pyrene metabolites and derivatives (Huberman et al. 1976). The evidence so far points to diol epoxide I as the major proximate carcinogen of benzo(a)pyrene. The racemic 7,8-benzo(a)pyrene epoxide has been shown to be carcinogenic on mouse skin (Levin et al. 1976), however. In cultured Chinese hamster cells, the *trans*-7,8-benzo-(a)pyrene diol has been reported to be more mutagenic than the parent compound and 11 other derivatives (Huberman et al. 1976).

An enantiomeric (+)benzo(a)pyrene-7,8-dihydrodiol can also be metabolically formed from the 7,8-benzo(a)pyrene epoxide to produce the corresponding stereoisomeric 9,10-epoxides (Nakanishi et al. 1977; Yaqi et al. 1977).

Benzo(a)pyrene(BP)   7,8-BP epoxide

(-)BP-7,8-dihydrodiol

(3 (+)BP-7,8-dihydrodiol

MFO - - Mixed Function oxidase
EH - - Epoxide hydratase

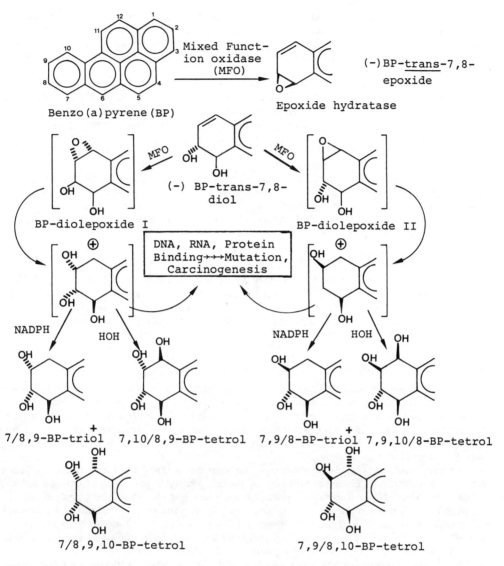

Figure 12.1 Metabolism of benzo(a)pyrene showing the formation of possible metabolites which may act as the proximate carcinogens or mutagens.

In vivo experiments (Koreeda et al. 1978) using mouse skin have shown stereoselective binding of each of the corresponding 9,10-epoxides from (+)- and (-)-benzo(a)pyrene-7,8-dihydrodiol to DNA, RNA, and protein. However, the predominant, almost 2:1 binding of epoxide II from the (-)-7,8-dihydrodiol enantiomer was also confirmed. In this case, the reaction of these epoxides with DNA and RNA involved the 2-amino group of guanine.

As discussed in Chapter 6, the enzymes, known collectively as aryl hydrocarbon hydroxylase (AHH), which are responsible for the carcinogenic or noncarcinogenic metabolic transformation of the PAH are affected by many factors. These enzymes, consisting of both constitutive and inducible components, may increase or decrease in activity depending on prior exposure to these carcinogens (Conney 1967; Schlede et al. 1970). This is significant because it has been estimated that in 1 year, the average person in the United States may be exposed to about 6 g of benzo(a)pyrene (National Academy of Sciences 1972), a dose which is several thousand times the amount needed to induce cancer in mice.

There is also evidence (Kinoshita and Gelboin 1978) which suggests that conjugation of the benzo(a)pyrene metabolites with glucuronic acid, presumably as a detoxification process, does not necessarily render the conjugates innocuous. β-Glucuronidase, which is abundant in the liver, spleen, kidney, and other secretory tissues, catalyzes the hydrolysis of the glucuronides. In the process, an active intermediate is formed which can bind to DNA molecules to a larger extent than the parent compound. For example, Kinoshita and Gelboin (1978) have reported that 3-hydroxybenzo(a)pyrene, a noncarcinogen and weak mutagen in the form of the glucuronide, binds to DNA to a larger extent in the presence of β-glucuronidase than without. Thus, carcinogenesis distant from the site of contact may be mediated by glucuronide conjugates, which are expected to be well distributed throughout the body because of their greater water solubility.

Other Sources of PAH

The PAHs do not occur in foodstuffs only as derived toxicants. In fact, a significant amount of these compounds is present as contaminants in smoke residues or tars, which can adhere to smoked foods or as fallout from industrial and other sources of pollution. There is also evidence which indicates that plants may synthesize these compounds. This is discussed in Chapter 8.

Toxicants Derived from Amino Acids

Obviously, there are also many other chemical transformations in foodstuffs that are heat-induced. The types of products formed depend on the temperature. Foods are subjected initially to a gradation in temperatures from the surface to the interior during heating, or each cross-sectional part attains the equilibrium temperature at different rates. Therefore, it is to be expected that different types of derived compounds may be formed.

At very high pyrolytic temperatures, several compounds are formed; some of these have been identified. Thus, in addition to PAHs, pyrolytic products of certain amino acids have been shown to produce potent mutagens. For example, the pyrolysis of tryptophan has been reported to produce two potent mutagens: 3-amino-1,4-dimethyl-5H-pyrido(4-b) indole and 3-amino-1-methyl-5H-pyrido(4,3-b) indole; both are γ-carboline derivatives. Phenylalanine pyrolysate also has been shown to contain a mutagen, 2-amino-5-phenyl-pyridine (Sugimura et al. 1977).

When proteinaceous foods are cooked at 250°C or greater until the food surface is charged, several highly mutagenic, and thus potentially carcinogenic products are formed. Thus, Yamaizumi et al. (1980) has identified 2-amino-5-phenylpyridine (Phe-P-1), 3-amino-1-methyl-5H-pyrido [4,3-b] indole (Trp-P-2) and 3-amino-1,4-dimethyl-5H-pyrido [4,3-b] indole (TrD-P-1) in broiled sun-dried sardines at 8.6, 13.1, and 13.3 ng/g, respectively. The latter also has been identified in broiled beef at 53 ng/g by Yamaguchi et al. (1980a). The latter researchers also isolated 2-aminodipyrido [1,2-a:3',2'-d] imidazole (Glu-P-2) at 280 ng/g in broiled sun-dried cuttle fish (Yamaguchi et al. 1980b). Grilled beef and chicken yielded 2-amino-9H-pyrido[2,3-b] indole (AαC) at 650 and 180 ng/g, respectively, and 2-amino-3-methyl-9H-pyrido[2,3-b] indole (MeAαC), respectively, at 64 and 15 ng/g (Matsumoto et al. 1981). Kasai et al. (1980a, b) has isolated 2-amino-3-methylimidazo[4,5-f] quinoline (IQ) and its 4-methyl derivative (MeIQ) from broiled sardines. Both were shown to be very highly mutagenic to a strain of Salmonella. The structures of these compounds are shown below:

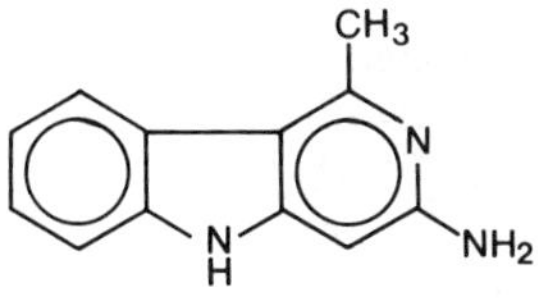

TRP-I-2 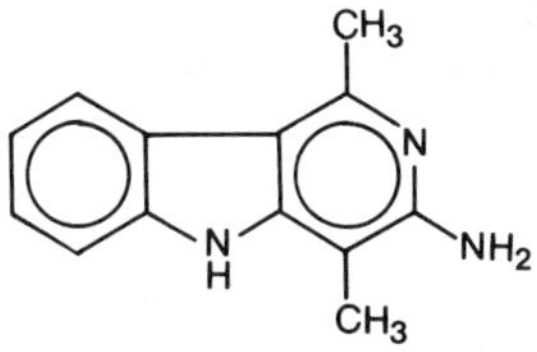   TRP-P-1 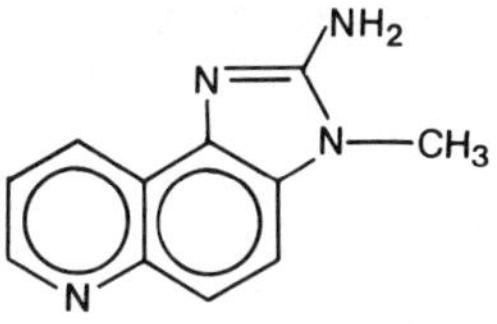   IQ

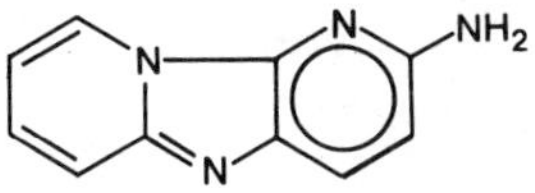

GLU-P-2 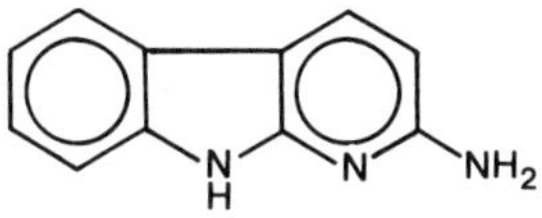 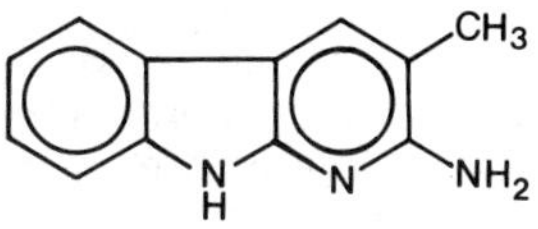   MeAaC

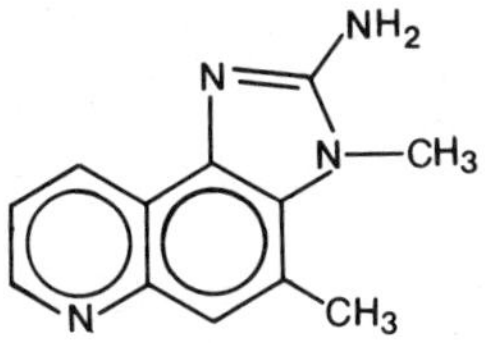

MeIQ 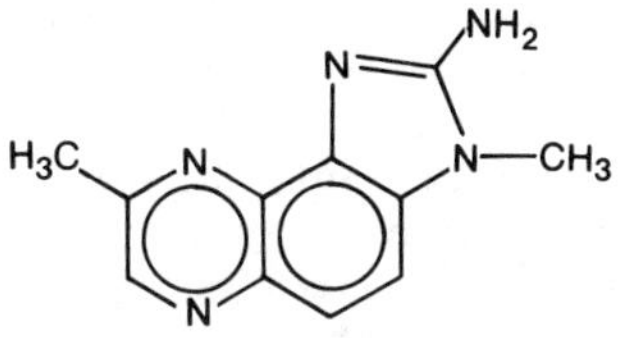   MeIQx

Glu-P-2 also has been identified in the pyrrolysis of casein (Yamaguchi et al. 1979) and Trp-P-1 and Trp-P-2 also have been found in the pyrrolyzates of gluten as well as casein (Uyeta et al. 1979).

Undoubtedly, while benzo(a)pyrene and other PAHs are present in these singed foodstuffs, they account for only a small quantity of the total mutagenic activity (Nagao et al. 1977). Thus, the isolation of the above compounds, and very probably several others, can account for a major proportion of the mutagenic activity of over-done broiled foods.

However, research in the last several years has shown that even exposure of food-stuffs at the usual cooking temperatures, such as in frying, broiling, and boiling of meats and baking of bread and similar products, may produce certain unspecified toxi-cants. The simple process of frying beef also yields a very strong mutagen. This has been identified as 2-amino-3,8-dimethylimidazole[4,5-f] quinoxaline (MeIQx) (Kasai et al. 1981). The structure of this compound is shown above.

Acrolein

Acrolein ($CH_2=CH-CHO$) is formed during the pyrolysis of fats (Geyer 1962). It is de-rived from the glycerol moiety. Acrolein is a highly inflammable liquid which has been used in military poison gas mixtures. It is quite unstable and readily polymerizes, es-pecially in the presence of light, to a plastic solid disacryl (Stecher et al. 1960).

Acrolein can also be formed from methionine or its derivative methional, homocys-teine, homoserine, and cystathionine, by reacting with various substances, such as glucose, ascorbic acid, ribose, glyceraldehyde, nicotinamide adenosine dinucleotide (NAD), H_2O_2, and H_2O_2 + $FeSO_4$ (Alarcon 1976). Note that all these substances except

$FeSO_4$ are physiological substances. However, whether or not acrolein is generated in vivo from methionine is not known.

Methional can be formed in certain plant foodstuffs (Mapson and Wardale 1969; Takeo and Lieberman 1969) and by the photodegradation of methionine in milk in the presence of riboflavin (Patton 1954) or by reaction with Fe^{2+} (Mazelis 1961). Acrolein is formed readily from methional under relatively mild conditions ($100°C$). In phosphate buffer at pH 7, in the presence of oxygen and ascorbic acid or H_2O_2, about 98% of methional is converted to acrolein (Alarcon 1976).

Based on the Hodge and Sterner (1943) classification, acrolein is a highly toxic substance, its oral LD_{50} in rats and rabbits being 46 mg/kg and 7.1 mg/kg, respectively (Spector 1956). The compound is a strong irritant, and is highly ciliostatic on bronchial epithelium, being 30 times more active than acetaldehyde, another potent ciliostat (Guillerm et al. 1961). Acrolein has been found to inhibit the activity of leukocytes and human oral cells (Eichel and Shahrik 1969). It also has proved to be the most toxic among substances tested on ascites cells (Holmberg and Malmfors 1974); in cell cultures, it is a potent cell growth inhibitor (Alarcon 1972). Acrolein also has been shown to be an inhibitor of a mitochondrial respiration and protein synthesis (Reid 1972).

Acrolein has been suspected of being a hepatotoxicant, quite indirectly, as the toxic metabolite formed from allyl formate and allyl alcohol (Rees and Tarlow 1967; Reid 1972). The observed necrosis following treatment with allyl alcohol has been shown to be confined to the periportal area (Reid 1972) where alcohol dehydrogenase is mostly found. This enzyme can convert allyl alcohol or allyl formate to acrolein, and there is direct evidence showing that the latter is formed when allyl alcohol is metabolized in the liver (Serafini-Cessi 1972). Inhibitors of the enzymes prevent or decrease markedly conversion to acrolein. In vivo experiments using ^{14}C-allyl alcohol in rats have shown that the necrosis is due to the binding of a metabolite such as acrolein to the periportal hepatocytes (Reid 1972).

Data regarding the concentration of acrolein in foodstuffs are limited. No doubt this compound is found in foods because the conditions and precursors for its formation are present in many types of foodstuffs. However, its reactivity, especially in the presence of light, may cause the concentration of acrolein to decrease at low levels.

A number of examples of heat-induced derived toxicants will be evident in the following sections. It should be emphasized that these derived products can also be formed without heating during prolonged storage, and that their formation may be enhanced or promoted by ultraviolet (u.v.) light, ionizing radiations, and possibly other factors. This is illustrated by the peroxidation and formation of degradation products of fats, as discussed in the next section.

TOXICANTS FORMED BY OXIDATION OF FATS AND OILS

Toxicants Formed in Heated Fats and Oils

The question of the safety of heated fats, as in deep fat frying, has been the subject of much research for more than 35 years. The studies have been concerned with the production of toxic products during heating of fats, particularly those products containing significant amounts of unsaturated fatty acids.

During the heating of fats, various degradation products of fatty acids are formed. Initial products formed during peroxidation are hydroperoxides and glycols. However, heating enhances oxidative breakdown of these compounds: the glycols into acids, and the hydroperoxides or ozonides into saturated and unsaturated aldehydes (Sahasrabudhe 1965; Wishner and Keeney 1965), and carbon-carbon bond dimers containing hydroxyl, carbonyl, double bonds, and possibly intramolecular peroxides or epoxides (Frankel et al. 1960). As a rule, during normal food frying operations, small amounts of stable peroxides may be formed. Dimers, polymers, and cyclic products are formed, especially while heating in the absence of air (Sahasrabudhe 1965). Czok et al. (1964)

have obtained a polymerized residue by heating in the absence of air, a 1:1 mixture of oleic and linoleic acids at 230°C for 1 hr. The residue was shown to contain 83% dimers, 15% polymers, and 3% monomers.

Derived products formed from heated cooking oils in fact may be taken up by the fried food products. Thus, Steibert and Koj (1973) have reported that meat deep fried in rapeseed oil, as produced in an industrial scale operation, contain 0.63 to 1.1% of the nonvolatile oxidation products of the oil. Another example is French fried potatoes, which were found by Kurkela and Karjalainen (1973) to contain high molecular weight secondary oxidation products derived from the cooking oil.

Toxic Effects of Derived Products from Heated Fats and Oils

That oxidative and degradative products of heated oils, as in frying operations, are toxic has been demonstrated by many investigators. Fats fed to experimental animals after being heated for prolonged periods to simulate deep fat frying conditions have been reported to produce anorexia, diarrhea, kidney and liver enlargement, and histological changes in various tissues (Kajimoto et al. 1974; Kaunitz et al. 1965; Lang and Fricker 1964; Nolen et al. 1967; Ohfuji and Kaneda 1973); in a significant number of cases, such diets resulted in death. Additionally, increased thirst, biliary and urinary output, and hypothermia have been observed in other cases (Lang and Fricker 1964). Rats that died when fed a diet containing 20% cottonseed and olive oils and chicken and beef fats heated under mild aeration at 60°C for 40 hr were shown to have high incidence of cardiac lesions; cottonseed oil caused more pronounced lesions (Kaunitz et al. 1965). Sesame, peanut, or coconut oil heated at 270°C for 8 hr and fed to rats at 15% of the diet for 6 weeks was noted to decrease the animals' abilities to store water-soluble vitamins (not including ascorbic acid) in the liver, increase glucose and cholesterol levels in the blood, and interfere with the digestion and absorption of carbohydrates (Raju et al. 1965). Oils treated in such a manner are poorly absorbed, and may account in part for the failure of the animals to thrive on such diets (Kokatnur et al. 1964). Rats fed for 32 weeks a diet with 5% polymerized residue from a 1:1 mixture of linoleic and oleic acid at 230°C for 1 hr were shown to have a decrease in food consumption, to have growth retardation, a reduced basal metabolism, and to develop hypothermia and impaired liver function (Czok et al. 1964). Burroughs et al. (1964) have found that anchovy oil heated in an inert atmosphere at 325°C and fed at 10% in the diet causes extreme weight loss in rats, and even more severe effects at 20%. At 5%, the animals grow normally. Coconut oil similarly treated has no adverse effects on growth even at levels higher than 5%.

The cardiac lesions noted from feeding oils which were mildly heated and aerated for prolonged periods are interesting because of the observed enhanced atherogenicity of such oils (Kritchevsky et al. 1961). When a ration containing cholesterol and corn oil was fed to rabbits, there was marked formation of atheromata compared to a ration without the oil. However, the lesions were more severe when the oil was heated at 200°C even for as short as 15 min prior to being miexed with the diet. Increased atherogenicity also has been shown with other heated fats, and in fact, corn oil is less likely to produce severe lesions than are other fats under similar conditions. The lesions have been shown not to be due to any type of chemical interaction between the oil and cholesterol during heating (Kritchevsky et al. 1962).

A marked reduction in the activity of the reticuloendothelial system has also been observed in female rats fed cod liver oil heated to 60°C for 40 hr (McKay et al. 1964). Fresh cod liver oil also causes such an inhibition. It is possible, however, that even in these "fresh" oils degradation products may already be present, because, as observed in the aforementioned study, the addition of α-tocopherol to the oil or the use of isolated triglycerides from cod liver oil instead of the fresh oil prevents such inhibition.

Heated oils have been associated with possible carcinogenicity (Zaldivar 1963); however, this question is far from settled because of conflicting results (O'Gara et al.

1969; Van Duuren et al. 1967), no doubt because of nonuniformity of samples, different levels of active compounds, and other variations in testing conditions. Thus, the evidence presented regarding carcinogenicity should be considered suggestive at this time. More importantly, heated fats may act as a cocarcinogen, or a tumor promoter, so that whether or not tumors develop depends on the adventitious presence of carcinogens in the rations fed, the drinking water, or in the environment. In fact, such cocarcinogenicity or tumor-promoting activity of heated fats has been demonstrated with acetylaminofluorene (AAF) (Sugai et al. 1962). A number of experiments performed by these researchers have established the fact that either corn oil heated at 200°C for 48 hr, or oil obtained from potato chip fryers, when fed with AAF at low concentration, results in increased incidence of mammary tumors in male rats. A most interesting result was the fact that addition of a concentrated toxic fraction of the thermally oxidized oil to the diet containing fresh corn oil and subcarcinogenic levels of AAF (0.005%) produced tumors in all of the experimental animals. None survived after 30 months, but in the absence of the toxic fractions, all animals survived this period and no tumors developed. These results provide clear evidence that heated oils contain derived products which possess potent cocarcinogenic activity.

Such toxic fractions in heated vegetable oils consist of the so-called nonurea adduct-forming fraction; i.e., the part which is not precipitated by urea. The toxicity of such a fraction was recognized by earlier workers (Nolen et al. 1967).

Toxicants in Rancid Fats and Oils

Rancidity is the term applied to the deterioration of fats and oils which is accompanied by unpleasant taste and odor. There are three types: hydrolytic, ketonic, and oxidative. Hydrolytic rancidity may be induced by heat, alkali, acid, or enzymes endogenous to the foodstuff or from microorganisms. Hydrolysis produces low molecular weight free fatty acids which contribute to the disagreeable flavor and odor. Ketonic rancidity is due to methyl ketones formed by the β-oxidation of fatty acids by microorganisms. Oxidative rancidity, on the other hand, is due to the peroxidation of unsaturated fatty acids, resulting in the formation of peroxides, and breakdown products (Mitchell and Henick 1962). Peroxidation is propagated through a chain reaction involving an initial free radical formation. Once initiated, the free radical reaction continues unhindered unless an antioxidant is present in the system, or until the total unsaturated fatty acids in the oil are oxidized. The lipid peroxidation may be catalyzed or accelerated by exposure to sunlight (u.v. light), iron and copper, and, of course, heat (Frazer 1962).

In meat products, oxidative rancidity is caused by the heme-catalyzed oxidation of tissue unsaturated lipids, particularly those found in phospholipids. In this case, the catalyst is actually the heme iron, either in the Fe^{2+} or Fe^{3+} state (Greene and Price 1975). The usual time lag between meat processing, storage, and consumption produces rancidity in meat which does not pose a serious enough flavor change as to be rejected. However, there is another dimension in the toxicology of rancidity in meat. This is the formation of malonaldehyde, which will be discussed in the next section.

There are also oxidative enzymes in plants, known as lipoxygenases, which catalyze lipid peroxidation. Lipoxygenases have been isolated in soybeans (Christopher et al. 1972), peas (Anstis and Friend 1974), peanuts (St. Angelo et al. 1972), cereals (Gardner and Weisleder 1970; Graveland et al. 1972; Heimann et al. 1973; Wallace and Wheeler 1975), potatoes (Galliard and Phillips 1971), and other plant products (Chang et al. 1971). There is, therefore, ample opportunity for the degradation of unsaturated fatty acids from plants even in the absence of exogenous catalyst. However, these enzymes, being proteinaceous, can be inactivated by heat.

The nonenzymatic mechanisms involved in the peroxidation of unsaturated fatty acids and subsequent degradation and dimerization are illustrated as follows:

$$R'-CH=CH-CH_2CH=CH-R'' \xrightarrow{\; -H \;} R'-CH=CH-\overset{\cdot}{C}H-CH=CH-R''$$

Linoleic acid (LH) H^+ $(L\cdot)$ $\Big\downarrow O_2$ LH

$$R'-CH_2-CH=CH-CH=CH-R''$$
                    (L)   LH

$$R'-\overset{\mid}{C}H-CH=CH-CH=CH-R''$$
$$\overset{\mid}{O}-O\cdot$$
                                                    $(LOO\cdot)$

$$R'-\overset{\mid}{C}H-CH=CH-CH=CH-R''$$
$$\overset{\mid}{O}-OH$$
                                                        (LOOH)

Heat, $R'-\overset{\mid}{C}H-CH=CH-CH=CH-R''$
Light, $\overset{\mid}{O}\cdot$
Metals $(LO\cdot)$

OH^-

$$R'-\overset{\mid}{C}H-\overset{\mid}{C}H=CH-CH=R''$$
$$\overset{\diagdown}{}\overset{\diagup}{O}(LO)$$

Heat,
Light,
Metals

$LO\cdot \longrightarrow$ ketone
$LO\cdot + H^+ \longrightarrow LOH$
$LO + L \longrightarrow LOL$ (Dimer epoxide)
$L + L\cdot \longrightarrow L\text{-}L$ (Dimer) $\xrightarrow{L\cdot}$ Polymer
$LOOH \xrightarrow{[O]}$ Aldehydes $\xrightarrow{[O]}$ Acids

The lipoxygenase-mediated peroxidation follows a similar but less random oxidation of the linoleic acid molecule, with specificity for either C-9 or C-13 position for hydroperoxide (LOOH) formation (Gardner 1975).

Toxicity of Rancid Fats and Oils

The products formed during hydrolytic and ketonic rancidity development are probably nontoxic. Oxidative rancidity, on the other hand, is probably accompanied by the formation of the same or similar toxic compounds formed in heated fats and oils. Peters and Boyd (1969) have observed that a biotin-deficient diet containing 14% cottonseed oil and 3% cod-liver oil is very toxic to rats when allowed to become rancid by standing at room temperature for 6 months or longer. In their study, the rats developed listlessness, anorexia, oligodipsia, diuresis, diarrhea, proteinuria, marked loss in body weight, and loss in weight of all body organs except the brain, adrenal glands, and gastrointestinal tract. The toxic rancidity reaction was not due to the biotin deficiency or the presence of raw egg white. No toxic reaction developed when the amount of cottonseed oil was decreased to 4%, cod-liver oil was eliminated, and vitamins A and D supplemented. Rats tended to show more severe toxicity when fed during the winter months than during other seasons. It was noted that toxicity was due to the rancid fats alone and that the toxic factor was ether extractable.

The experiments of Cutler and Schneider (1973a) have shown that when linoleic acid bubbled with oxygen at room temperature for 72 hr is fed to female rats with high fat (16%) diets, a significant incidence of cervical sarcoma and malignant and benign mammary tumors combined occurred. There was also increased incidence of interstitial tumors (mostly benign) in the male rats. An increased incidence of benign ovarian, cervical, and lung tumors also occurred in mice fed oxidized linoleic acid with high fat diets. In this case, the oxidized fatty acid preparation contained about 25% linoleic acid hydroperoxide, about 4% polymer and various percentages of other products.

Other researchers have found that products formed by oxidizing fats at room or cooking temperatures can induce injection-site sarcomas in the mouse (Van Duuren et al. 1963, 1966, 1971) and an increase in the incidence of the so-called spontaneous tumors in rats (Seelkopf and Salfelder 1962). Local tumors also have been produced by injections of crude lipid extracts (O'Gara et al. 1969).

The toxicity of oxidized linoleic acid also has been demonstrated in experiments which showed increased teratogenicity in rats, but not mice, in the urogenital system. In mice, linoleic acid hydroperoxide applied directly to the ovaries increases the incidence of fetal malformations in litters of the first generation and increases embryonic resorption in litters of the second generation. Oxidized linoleic acid by itself causes no fetal abnormality in the first generation litters; however, there is a significant increased incidence of embryonic resorption in the second generation litters (Cutler and Schneider 1973b).

In part, these fetal abnormalities may be the result of a secondary vitamin deficiency, owing to the destructive effects of oxidized fats on many vitamins, particularly the retinoids, cholecalciferols, tocols (vitamin E), ascorbic acid, biotin, pantothenic acid, and pyridoxine (Lundberg 1962). The urogenital abnormalities are consistent with the observation that such abnormalities can occur in animals deficient in the retinoids (Wilson et al. 1953) and folic acid (Monie et al. 1957). Signs of folic acid deficiency also have been noted in animals so treated (Cutler quoted by Cutler and Schneider 1973b).

Biochemical Basis of Toxicity of Lipid Peroxidation Products Many highly reactive compounds — hydroperoxides, free radicals, epoxides, aldehydes, and so forth — are formed during peroxidation-degradation-polymerization reaction processes in either heated or stored fats and oils. Thus, their reactions with critical molecules in the body are to be expected. Among such molecules are nucleic acids, amino acids, and proteins (Pokorny and Janicek 1968; Roy and Karel 1973; Tannenbaum et al. 1969; Zirlin and Karel 1969), especially enzymes (Chio and Tappel 1969; Matsushita 1975). In an in vitro experiment (Matsushita 1975) linoleic acid hydroperoxide (1.7 μmole) was demonstrated to inhibit ribonucleas (RNAse) (0.01 mg in 1.1 ml) by more than 40% after 30 min, and this value approached 40% when 1 μmol ascorbic acid was added. The degradation products of the hydroperoxide inhibited RNAse by almost 30%. Trypsin was inhibited by more than 60% by a mixture of degradation products of the hydroperoxide, but not by the peroxide itself. Pepsin was inhibited by the hydroperoxide by about 30 and 20%, with and without ascorbic acid, respectively. However, the degradation products stimulated the activity of pepsin. The hydroperoxide also inhibited pancreatic lipase; the degree of inhibition appeared to be a function of the amount of the inhibitor. The inhibition apparently was the result of the binding of the peroxidation products with the protein. These products reacted with specific amino acids, particularly methionine, lysine, histidine, tyrosine, and cystine. The amounts and types of amino acids reacted depended on the nature of the proteins and the peroxidation products. Aspartic acid and glutamic acids, tyrosine, and cystine were reacted only in the presence of ascorbic acid. Note that lysine and histidine constitute the active site of RNAse (Smith 1970), and their reaction with the peroxidation products expectedly will result in inhibition.

The peroxidation products also caused polymerization of RNAse, but not trypsin and pepsin. Polymerization was also observed with other proteins; such interaction can result in the insolubilization of the protein (Pokorny and Janicek 1968; Roubal and Tappel 1966a,b). The peroxidized unsaturated fatty acids produced cross linking in sulfur-containing proteins, but those without sulfur, such as gelatine and similar collagens undergo cleavage of the protein chain (Takahashi 1970; Zirlin and Karel 1969).

By means of electron spin resonance spectrometry (ESR) it has been demonstrated that the interaction of proteins and amino acids with fatty acid hydroperoxides and other degradation products involves free radical formation (Karel et al. 1975). In this case, free radicals from fatty acids induced free radicals from proteins as the following scheme shows (Karel et al. 1975). Free radicals so formed from proteins in turn are involved in polymerization reactions.

Protein free radical formation:

$$PH + A \longrightarrow P + AH$$

Oxidation:

$$P + O_2 \longrightarrow PO_2$$

Cross-linking:

$$PH + B \longrightarrow P\text{-}B\text{-}P$$

$$P + P \longrightarrow P\text{-}P$$

$$PO_2 + P \longrightarrow POOP$$

Scission:

$$PO_2 \longrightarrow P\text{-} + P\text{-}$$

Transfer:

$$P + AH \longrightarrow PH + A$$

$$PO_2 + AH \longrightarrow POOH + A$$

PH	=	Protein
A	=	Lipid-derived free radical
B	=	Lipid-derived breakdown product
P	=	protein free radical $R\text{-}\overset{\shortmid}{\underset{\shortmid}{C}}\cdot$ or $\overset{\shortmid}{\underset{\shortmid}{C}}HCH_2\text{-}S\cdot$
P-	=	cleavaged protein polypeptide
PO_2	=	protein peroxide
POOH	=	protein hydroperoxide

Amino acids reacted with hydroperoxides to form degradation or oxidative products. For example, methionine was oxidized to methionine sulfoxide; lysine was degraded to diaminopentane, aspartic acid, glycine, alanine, α-aminoadipic acid, and other compounds, and lengthened to 1,10-diamino-1,10-dicarboxydecane; histidine was decarboxylated to histamine and formed other compounds (Karel et al. 1975).

Hydroperoxides and other fatty acid degradation or oxidative products can also induce scission of the protein chain through reaction with the peptide or disulfide bonds (Karel et al. 1975).

The fact that thermally oxidized corn oil can provoke smooth endoplasmic reticulum proliferation and a complex variety of microsomal enzymes further emphasizes the toxic potency of such thermal oxidation products. In fact, the basal and DDF-induced mixed function oxidases were significantly increased with both heated oil and the non urea-adduct-forming fraction of the oil, as compared to the activity with fresh corn oil. These increased activities were accompanied by hepatomegaly in the treated animals (Andia and Street 1975).

Safety of Heated or Peroxidized Fats and Oils

As the preceding section shows, heated or peroxidized fats and oils contain derived products which fulfill the fundamental requirement for all highly toxic substances — namely, high chemical reactivity. The toxicity of these derivatives has been verified experimentally. However, by and large, normal frying conditions do not generally produce these derived toxicants at sufficiently high enough levels to be of significant toxic hazards. Feeding studies in animals using such fats or oils have verified the apparent safety of such products (Andrews et al. 1960; Artman 1969; Poling et al. 1970).

It must be emphasized that the potential exists for the formation of deleterious derived substances in the heating or storage of fats and oils, and that improper practices in the use of these oils, and ignorance on the part of operators, may lead to excess production of such toxic substances. For example, a survey conducted on the usage of fats and oils in institutional and restaurant kitchens has shown that excessively deteriorative conditions employed in the laboratory production of peroxidized and degradative products also have been found in some kitchens (Thompson et al. 1967).

Additionally, the likelihood of cocarcinogenic or tumor-promoting activity of heated fats and oils is probably more pertinent to the question of the safety of normally heated or peroxided fats and oils. Because of the ubiquitous presence of many types of carcinogens in the environment, the safety of heated or rancidifying fats or oils is of urgent concern.

However, the presence of a derived carcinogen(s) in peroxidized or heated lipids has been demonstrated. This adds a new dimension to the question of the safety of such lipids. In fact, as pointed out by Cutler and Schneider (1973a), the consumption of highly peroxidized fats may provide a partial explanation of the higher incidence of mammary cancers in such places as Bombay, India ($46/10^5$ persons), Hong Kong ($41/10^5$ persons), and Puerto Rico ($33/10^5$ persons) as contrasted, e.g., to $19/10^6$ in Singapore, $10/10^5$ in Mozambique, $22/10^5$ in Uganda; the latter countries use more saturated fats in the form of coconut or palm oils. It also has been reported that there is evidence which suggests that consumption of heated fats is associated with the high incidence of gastric cancer in some countries (Dungal 1958; Seelkopf and Salfelder 1962). Carcinogens in heated or rancid lipids, an example of which is discussed in the next section, may be one of etiological factors in the increased cancer incidence in diverse populations.

Malonaldehyde

Malonaldehyde is one of the many breakdown products of the peroxidation of linoleic, arachidonic, and other fatty acids (Karel et al. 1975). Its structure (shown below) suggests that it is highly reactive with amino groups.

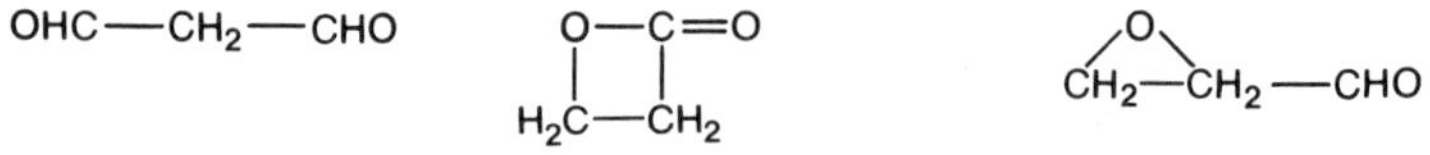

$$OHC-CH_2-CHO$$

Malonaldehyde

$$\begin{array}{c} O-C=O \\ | \quad\quad | \\ H_2C-CH_2 \end{array}$$

β-Propiolactone

Glycylaldehyde

This aldehyde has, in fact, been shown to react with DNA in solution and in vivo, very likely through Schiff base formation; in particular, guanine and cytidine are the main targets (Brooks and Klamerth 1968; Reiss et al. 1972). Thus, malonaldehyde alters the DNA structure, as reported by these workers.

Malonaldehyde also has been shown to be produced during the metabolism of 7,12-dimethylbenzo(a)anthracene (DMBA), 3,4-benzpyrene, and 3-methylcholanthrene (Shamberger et al. 1974, 1972), all potent carcinogens. In addition, two compounds which resemble malonaldehyde, glycylaldehyde (Shamberger et al. 1974; Van Duuren et al. 1965) and β-propiolactone (Palmes et al. 1962; Shamberger et al. 1974) previously have been shown to be carcinogenic. The structures of the latter two compounds show that in vivo they could break down intermediarily to malonaldehyde.

These properties of malonaldehyde and its structural similarity to known carcinogens suggests that this compound is also carcinogenic (Shamberger et al. 1974). Therefore, when 6 or 12 mg of this aldehyde was applied once to the skin of mice and promoted with daily treatment with croton oil (0.1% in acetone), 52% of the mice developed skin tumors in 30 weeks. Among animals treated with only 12 mg malonaldehyde daily for 9 weeks, 12 animals died after 4 to 6 weeks, and six during the next 3 weeks; four of the latter had liver carcinomas, with metastases in other tissues; one had rectal carcinoma. The early deaths of the mice allude to the toxicity of this aldehyde. At a lower level (0.36 mg), malonaldehyde applied daily for 39 or 48 weeks did not induce tumors, presumably owing to antioxidants in the diet, as suggested by Shamberger et al. (1974).

Further evidence supporting the observed carcinogenicity of malonylaldehyde has been reported by Mukai and Goldstein (1976). These researchers have observed that this aldehyde is mutagenic to strains of *Salmonella typhimurium*, the frameshift mutants with normal excision repair. Mutagenic activity in these strains has also been observed in carcinogenic polycyclic aromatic hydrocarbons (Ames et al. 1973), some of which cause lipid peroxidation and consequently malonaldehyde production in vivo (Shamberger 1972; Shamberger et al. 1974).

Malonaldehyde has been detected in many types of foodstuffs, including not only meat products, but also vegetables, orange juice essence, nuts, and rye bread (Shamberger et al. 1977). This compound is not particularly confined to rancid foods, although rancidity is associated with higher levels of the carcinogen.

Cooking foods may increase or decrease the level of malonaldehyde. The range in values in uncooked meat was 1 to 14 µg/g; 0.3 to 40 µg/g in cooked meats. Some products increased in malonaldehyde content after refrigeration. In more than half of the meats tested, the malonaldehyde level increased upon cooking. Vegetables, fruits, nuts, dairy products, and seafood, with few exceptions, had none or very low levels of the carcinogen.

The importance of exposure to air in the formation of the aldehyde has been illustrated in peanut butter: none was detected in a freshly opened jar, but values up to 1.2 µg/g were found after the jar was opened and used for some time. The presence of antioxidants, such as the tocols, will obviously minimize peroxidation, and thus malonaldehyde formation (Shamberger et al. 1977).

Studies in the author's laboratory (Newburg and Concon 1980) have confirmed earlier findings (Shamberger et al. 1977; Siu and Draper 1978) that production of the carcinogen increases significantly during the roasting of chicken in a conventional oven. Surprisingly, broiling in a microwave oven also produces similar results. Among those meats tested, chicken produced the highest level of malonaldehyde when boiled. Tests on canned chicken soups have shown that these products contain relatively high levels of the aldehyde. Being soluble in water, chicken soup or chicken bouillon tends to have high levels of malonaldehyde (Newburg and Concon 1980).

NONPYROLYTIC TOXICANTS DERIVED FROM AMINO ACIDS

Premelanoidins

Amino acids and aldehydes, particularly reducing sugars, undergo the so-called Maillard, or nonenzymic browning, reaction in the presence of specific amounts of moisture. This reaction is enhanced by heating, especially under alkaline conditions. The Maillard reaction (Maillard 1912) occurs in stages (Hodge 1953; Reynolds 1969), the final products being a mixture of insoluble dark-brown polymeric pigments known as malanoidins. In the early stages of the reaction, a complex mixture of carbonyl compounds, aromatic substances, reductones, and so forth, is formed. These products are water soluble, mostly colorless, and are known collectively as premelanoidins.

A schematic representation of the Maillard reaction is as follows:

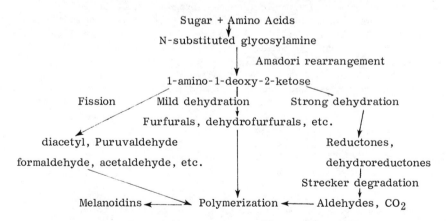

One of the fundamental effects of the Maillard reaction is a drastic lowering of the nutritional quality of proteins. The reason is that amino acids, particularly lysine, are rendered unavailable; thus, the amino acid becomes limiting in an otherwise nutritionally adequate protein.

Important as these effects may be, the toxicity of the Maillard reaction products is distinct from the lowering of the bioavailability of lysine or other amino acids.

The toxic effects of premelanoidins are indicated by the marked reduction in digestibility and nitrogen retention of ingested proteins in diets to which these substances are added. Consequently, the protein efficiency ratio (PER) and the biological value of the proteins also are decreased (Adrian and Frange 1973). For example, diets containing 0.2% premelanoidin nitrogen, reduced the digestibility and biological value of casein from 91% to 82% and about 49 to 38%, respectively, compared to diets without premelanoidins. The biological value is an index of the amount of nitrogen utilized by the animal. About 35% of premelanoidin nitrogen was retained in the tissues, but this does not imply that the premelanoidin nitrogen is utilized for any useful metabolic function, since the growth rate of the animal was drastically reduced, by 20 to 40%. In fact, the presence of the premelanoidins reduced the metabolic efficiency of casein. Adrian and Frange (1973) also have observed that premelanoidins inhibit digestive enzymes.

Similar diets containing 0.2% premelanoidins when fed to pregnant rats reduced weight gain by more than 27% and produced fewer living fetuses; in addition, almost six times as many fetuses as the control were resorbed and neonatal and postweaning weights of the offspring were lower. Premelanoidins also caused enlargement of the cecum, liver, and kidneys. In this case, liver enlargement was slight, but that of the cecum and kidneys was more pronounced (Adrian and Frange 1973).

That premelanoidins may be hepatotoxic has been indicated by the effects observed with spray-dried and roller-dried milk powder: The numbers of animal deaths due to hepatic necrosis fed these products were 40 and 76%, respectively, compared to less than 1% with liquid milk (Fink et al. 1968).

Heat-dried meat containing 18% of the premelanoidin glucosylamine produced not only liver hypertrophy in experimental animals, but also hemorrhagic necrotic lesions and cirrhosis in this organ (Ferrando 1963, 1964; Ferrando et al. 1964).

Further evidence of toxicity has been obtained by Krug et al. (1959). The intraperitoneal LD_{50} of an unheated mixture of 1 part amino acid and three parts glucose was 20 g/kg; the LD_{50} when this mixture was heated for 10 min at 160°C was reduced to 4.1 to 11.2 g/kg. Among the amino acids, lysine produced the most toxic premelanoidin.

The toxicity of nucleic acids, as measured by the LD_{50}, increased by almost 50% when heated with sugar for at least 4 hr (Lang and Schaeffner 1964); methylamine-containing hexose reductones, a premelanoidin, were about 71 times more toxic to mice compared to nitrogen-free hexose reductones (Ambrose et al. 1961).

Maillard reaction products also have been implicated in certain types of allergic reactions. For example, the allergenicity of a lactoglobulin-lactose solution, as determined by skin reactivity measurements, increased from less than 100 to 11000 u/mg after heating at 50°C at pH 7 for 48 to 72 hr. The allergenicity decreased slightly after heating (Bleumink and Young 1968).

The possibility of nitrosamine formation, e.g., with secondary amine types, adds another dimension to premelanoidin toxicity. This aspect is discussed in a later section (pp. 000-000).

TOXICANTS PRODUCED BY ALKALI TREATMENT

Lysinoalanine

Alkali treatment is increasingly used in the isolation and processing of plant and animal proteins intended for food use. In the preceding section, it was stated that alkaline conditions promote the Maillard reaction with destructive effects on amino acids, especially lysine. However, alkali treatment may also produce other chemical changes which can result not only in a lowering of the nutritional quality of the protein through decreased digestibility and racemization and destruction of amino acids (Gorill and Nicholson 1972; Parisot and Derminot 1970; Tannenbaum et al. 1970), but also in the formation of derived amino acids which may have toxic effects. Among the new amino acids that may be formed during alkali treatment are lysinoalanine (LAL), ornithino-alanine (OAL), and lanthionine (Provansal et al. 1975).

LAL has received some attention as a possible nephrotoxic compound. It is formed by condensation of dehydroalanine with the epsilon amino group of lysine (Bohak 1964). Dehydroalanine, in turn, is produced by β-elimination of cystine, phosphoserine (Bohak 1964), or serine residues (Corfield et al. 1967; Mellet 1968) in the presence of alkali:

NH-   NH-
HC$-$CH$_2$-S-S-CH$_2$-CH
CO-   CO-

Cystinyl residue

OH$^-$

CH$_2$=C   (Dehydroalanyl residue)
    NH-
    CO-

NH-   OH$^-$
HO-CH$_2$-CH
       CO-

Seryl residue

H$_2$N-(CH$_2$)$_4$-CH
      NH-
      CO-

Lysyl residue

NH-   NH-
HC-CH$_2$-NH-(CH$_2$)$_4$-CH
CO-   CO-

Lysinoalanyl residue

The formation of LAL from cystine and lysine can take place more readily under milder conditions of pH and temperature. However, in the case of serine, more severe conditions as well as a longer reaction time are required (Karayiannis et al. 1979).

However, it has been shown that LAL formation can occur simply by heating proteins at 100 to 120°C under nonalkaline conditions. It also has been shown that LAL may commonly occur in processed foods which are apparently unexposed to alkaline conditions (Sternberg et al. 1975). Nevertheless, the presence of alkali would still provide a more suitable condition for LAL formation.

The extent of LAL formation would depend on the nature of protein, the time and temperature of reaction, and the concentration of NaOH. Thus, even mild alkali treatment is sufficient to induce significant LAL formation in different legume proteins (Hancock 1978). Among those treated under mild conditions (0.05 to 0.075 N NaOH, 20°C), mung beans, cow peas, and peanuts produced significant amounts of LAL after 30 min exposure. The amount of LAL formed under these conditions ranged from 200 to 800 mg/100 g of protein. Some legumes, such as kidney beans, lima beans, and vetch (*Lathyrus sativus*), were more resistant, producing no LAL even after 24 hr. However, all legumes produced LAL at 80°C even after exposure for only 30 min. But, the amount of LAL tended to decrease after prolonged exposure at elevated temperatures. This suggests that LAL may be destroyed under these conditions. A similar observation has been reported by Provansal et al. (1975) with sunflower proteins. Indeed, lysinoalanine has been found to be unstable to heat (Woodard et al. 1977).

Several other foodstuffs form LAL during cooking (Sternberg et al. 1975). For example, chicken meat which had no LAL when fresh contained 200 μg/g when cooked in a microwave oven. Egg white which contained no detectable LAL when fresh contained 270 to 370 μg/g when boiled for 10 to 30 min, and 1.1 mg/g when pan fried for 30 min at 150°C.

Table 12.2 Lysinoalanine Content of Commercial Food Products

Food[a]	LAL (μg/g)	Food[a]	LAL (μ/g)
Corn chips	390	Egg white solids (dried)	160–1820
Pretzels	500	Caseinate (Na) (5)	430–6900
Hominy	560	Caseinate (Ca) (2)	370–1000
Tortillas	200	Casein, acid (3)	70–90
Taco shells	170	Hydrolyzed vegetable proteins (18)	40–500
Milk, infant formula (6)	150–640		
evaporated (2)	590–860	Whipping agent (2)	6500–50,000
skim, evaporated (2)	520	Soya protein isolates (45)	0–370
condensed (2)	360–540	Yeast extract	120
Simulated cheese	1070		

[a]Number in parentheses refer to different samples analyzed.
Source: Sternberg et al. (1975).

Examples of the levels of LAL in commercial food products are shown in Table 12.2. Note that excessive amounts are often found in some foods or food ingredients (Sternberg et al. 1975).

Sternberg et al. (1975) has shown that the level of LAL that could be formed by heating proteins under nonalkaline conditions increases as the pH increases from pH 2 to 6 or 7. In this case, the magnitude of the increase depends also on the nature of the protein.

Karayiannis et al. (1979) were unable, however, to obtain measurable amounts of LAL from lactalbumin, casein, and soy protein isolate at pH 5.1 to 6.7 even after treatment for up to 6 hr at 25 to 120°C. At pH 8, only traces of LAL were detectable even after 2 hr at 90°C; it required heating for 6 hr at pH 8 and 90°C before significant amounts of LAL could be obtained from these proteins. More rapid formation of LAL was observed at pH 10, and especially at pH 12, at which significant amounts of the derived amino acid were formed even at 25°C. These results appear to agree with those of de Groot et al. (1976a,b), who have reported that LAL is not formed in soy protein treated at pH 7 or 8 for 4 hr at 40°C.

Obviously, the precise conditions for LAL formation under nonalkaline conditions such as that observed by Sternberg et al. (1975, 1977) still needs to be determined. It would be instructive to determine whether prior treatment of whatever nature influences the ease of LAL formation. For example, such treatment might increase the proximity of lysine with cystine residues, so that the interpeptide reaction is facilitated. Also, the role of catalysis and the presence of other amino acid residues, free radicals, lipids, and similar compounds may explain some of the differences, as described in the preceding paragraphs.

Toxicity of LAL

The toxicity of LAL appears to be confined to the kidneys (Karayiannis et al. 1979; Woodard and Short 1977). When alkali-treated soy protein is fed to rats at appropriate levels, cytomegalic changes are observed in the pars recta, the descending portion of the proximal tubules (Karayiannis et al. 1979; Newberne et al. 1968; Woodard and Alvarez 1967; Woodard and Short 1973). That LAL may indeed be the toxic agent has been demonstrated by the use of purified LAL (Woodard and Short 1977). The renal

lesions in rats fed with alkali-treated soy proteins for several weeks are morphologically similar to those seen in animals fed diets containing low levels of LAL for 4 weeks.
At higher dose levels, more severe changes are noted, including epithelial necrosis,
hypercellularity of the glomeruli, and thickening of Bowman's capsule with hyperplasia
of both its visceral and parietal epithelial layers.

However, LAL may not be the only nephrotoxic product produced during alkali-
treatment of proteins. Ornithinoalanine (Feron et al. 1977), fructoselysine (Erbersdobler et al. 1978), and D-serine (Gould and MacGregor 1977) also produce similar
lesions in the pars recta. Thus, the observed lesions that are produced when alkali-
treated soy protein is fed to rats may be caused by all these products, and possibly
other as yet unidentified derived substances produced during alkaline treatment of
proteins.

A number of factors may influence the development of nephrocytomegaly. One is
the type of protein that is treated with alkali. The difference in the balance of amino
acids in alkali-treated lactalbumin and soy protein may be responsible for the toxic effects. The former, even though it contains a much higher level of LAL, does not induce nephrocytomegaly (Karayiannis et al. 1979). Since lactalbumin contains more lysine and sulfur-containing amino acids, only milder alkaline treatment is needed to produce sufficiently high amounts of LAL. Thus, other alkali-induced changes may occur
minimally in lactalbumin, compared to the soy protein, which requires longer treatment
(i.e., 0.1N NaOH, 8 hr, 60°C, compared to 1 hr and 20 min for lactalbumin). Supplementation with lysine, arginine, and threonine to the soy protein diet does not diminish the severity of the lesion. This result suggests that decreases in these amino acids
as a result of alkali treatment may not be solely responsible for the effect.

The composition of the diet may also influence the development of nephrocytomegaly. Thus, the negative result obtained by de Groot et al. (1976a,b) was caused by
the diet used in their experiments. When these researchers used a diet containing
alkali-treated soy protein which was similar in composition to that used by Karayiannis
et al. (1979), their Wistar-derived rats developed the aforementioned lesions (Feron et
al. 1977); only one of five rats fed the original diet developed slight nephrocytomegaly.
Feron et al. (1977) believe that the addition of 10% untreated casein in their original
diet was responsible for the negative results they have observed previously. This contention is, of course, consistent with the results with lactalbumin.

Lack of toxicity may also be caused by decreased LAL absorption or protein digestibility. Evidence to this fact was the observation that synthetic LAL or acid-
hydrolyzed LAL-containing protein produced cytomegalic changes, including nephrosis, necrosis, and regeneration of the epithelial cells. Determination of the LAL levels
in the blood, urine, and feces indicated that the observed nephrotoxicity correlated
with the extent of intestinal absorption of LAL (De Groot et al. 1976a,b).

Some lines of a particular strain of rat may also be less sensitive to the effects of
LAL. For example, Struthers et al. (1977) have found that when Wistar rats are fed
3000 ppm LAL in the diet, they show very little incidence of renal cytomegaly in contrast to the Sprague-Dawley rats. They have observed nephrocalcinosis in some female Wistar rats, but this has been attributed to either lower availability of dietary
calcium (De Groot and Slump 1969) or increased levels of available dietary phosphorus
(Van Beek et al. 1974).

Weanling rats appear to be most sensitive to the nephrocytomegalic effects of LAL;
as little as 100 ppm of free LAL is sufficient to induce the toxic effects (De Groot et al.
1976a,b; Van Beek et al. 1974).

The rat may be the only animal which is sensitive to the toxic effects of LAL. Dogs
fed 700 ppm synthetic LAL, and rabbits, hamsters, mice, and quail fed 1000 ppm were
shown to develop no renal lesions suggestive of cytomegalia (De Groot et al. 1976 a,b).
Karayiannis et al. (1979) also have observed essentially negative results with mice,
but these animals develop the lesions with relatively high levels of free LAL in the diet
(Feron et al. 1977). At lower levels, some mice develop the lesions, but this borders
on chance. It may be that the significance may be increased with greater number of

test animals (Karayiannis et al. 1979). The same assumption may be made for the other species which appear to be resistant to the effects of LAL. Furthermore, the duration of exposure to LAL may also be an important factor in these seemingly resistant species.

A significant elevation of plasma glutamate-pyruvate transaminase (GPT) also has been observed in rats fed alkali-treated soy protein isolate, but not with the untreated protein or the treated lactalbumin. Even though such enzyme elevation in the blood is often indicative of tissue damage such as the liver and kidneys (Mattenheimer 1971), this result may be only a manifestation of nutritional imbalance because a similar elevation has been obtained when one-half of the untreated lactalbumin fed was replaced with crystalline cellulose (Alphacel) (Karayiannis et al. 1979).

Significance of LAL Toxicity to Humans   The toxicity of LAL, or for that matter, other alkali-induced amino acid derivatives in foodstuffs, may not be easily extrapolated to humans, particularly since species other than the rat were unaffected. However, as discussed in this section, the insensitivity of other species may be a matter of time of exposure and other factors. Thus, the dose may be important, as demonstrated in mice (Feron et al. 1977). Therefore, the findings of Sternberg et al. (1975) regarding the widespread occurrence of LAL in many common commercial foodstuffs may have significance in terms of the total dose to which humans are exposed, especially infants and older children. The human hazard associated with alkali-treated proteins needs to be more clearly defined by further research. Experiments in rats have shown that the etiology of the observed renal effects is highly complex. It appears that nutritional factors have a significant influence on LAL renal toxicity.

Pressor Amines

Decarboxylation of amino acids by microorganisms during fermentation or putrefaction of various foods produces various amines. These amines include tyramine, tryptamine, phenylethylamine, isoamylamine, putrescine, cadaverine (Asatoor et al. 1963; Barger and Walpole 1909; Hedberg et al. 1966; Sen 1969) and histamine (Blackwell et al. 1965; Ferencik 1970; Krikler and Lewis 1965; Ough 1971).

Tryptamine   Phenyle-thylamine   Tyramine   Histamine   Putrescine   Cadaverine   Isoamylamine

$R = -CH_2CH_2NH_2$

$H_2N-(CH_2)_4-NH_2$ Putrescine

$H_2N-(CH_2)_5-NH_2$ Cadaverine

$CH_3CHCH_2CH_2NH_2$ with CH_3 Isoamylamine

Clinically, the most important of these amines are tyramine and histamine. The latter has been discussed in Chapter 11 in connection with scombroid poisoning from tuna, mackerel, and similar fish.

Histamine is found in wine at concentrations of up to 22 μg/ml (Marquardt and Werringloer 1965). It was shown that histamine is a hypotensive agent whose effects are enhanced by ethanol. Thus, in cats, a dose of 0.4 mg/kg intubated to the duodenum, lowered blood pressure when administered in 15% ethanol. Saline and twice the concentration of ethanol has no effect. In this experiment, histamine breakdown in the intestines was prevented by s.c. injection of aminoguanidine (5 mg/kg) and iproniazid (100 mg/kg), which are amine oxidase inhibitors (Marquardt and Werringloer 1965).

These drugs are relevant to the question of pressor amine toxicity (Asatoor et al. 1963).

Similar effects have been observed when saline, 12% ethanol solution, and wine were administered to cats (Marquardt et al. 1963). The effect of wine was abolished by administration of an antihistamine (Mepyramine maleate, 1.4 mg/kg), thus indicating that the effect was due to histamine.

In fact, the lethality of histamine can be enhanced by ethanol. In one experiment, a dose of 200 mg histamine/kg body weight killed 75% of the guinea pigs when administered in 15% ethanol. Without ethanol, this dose in physiological saline killed 40% of the animals; 30% ethanol had no effect (Marquardt and Werringloer 1965). Previous workers obtained a 30% mortality with this dose of histamine (Parrot et al. 1947).

Histamine is hepatotoxic, producing necrosis and degenerative changes in liver parenchyma (Braunsteiner et al. 1953; Gloggengiesser 1944).

In humans, histamine produces characteristic pyrosis, headache in the occipital region, hyperemia of the face, hypotension, and emesis (Legroux et al. 1946; Peeters 1963). These symptoms were discussed in Chapter 11.

Tyramine has been reported to cause the most serious clinical effects when taken with monoamine oxidase inhibitors. Horwitz et al. (1964) examined the effects of tyramine and cheese taken together in hospital subjects. These materials by themselves caused little effect, but with as little as 20 g of cheese in conjunction with monoamine oxidase inhibitor medications, some patients developed a dangerous rise in blood pressure which had to be controlled with phentolamine.

The relationship between paroxysmal hypertension and cheese was reported earlier by several investigators (Asatoor et al. 1963; Blackwell 1963; Blackwell et al. 1967). The effect could be very severe in some patients taking the drug tranylcypromine and together with cheese, resulting in intracerebral hemorrhage and death (Blackwell et al. 1967).

Cheeses contain variable amounts of tyramine. Brie cheese may contain from 0 to 20 mg/100 g and parmesan cheese, from 0.4 to 29 mg/100 g. Very high levels have been found in Stilton (47 to 220 mg/100 g), Camenbert (0.2 to 200 mg/100 g), Cheddar (12 to 150 mg/100 g), and Emmenthaler cheeses (23 to 100 mg/100 g) (Asatoor et al. 1963; Blackwell and Mabbit 1965; Horwitz et al. 1964; Seh 1969). Other high tyramine foods are pickled herring (300 mg/100 g) (Nuessle et al. 1965), and Marmite yeast and yeast extracts (0 to 225 mg/100 g) (Blackwell et al. 1965; Horwitz et al. 1964; Sen 1969). Moderate amounts have been found in stored chicken and beef livers, containing 10 mg (Hedberg et al. 1966) and 27 mg/100 g (Boulton et al. 1970), respectively. Nevertheless, these products have been associated with hypertensive crises in patients taking monoamine oxidase inhibitors (Boulton et al. 1970; Hedberg et al. 1966).

The moderate tyramine levels in some meat extracts (95 to 30 mg/100 g) and salted, dried fish (0 to 47 mg/100 g) (Sen 1969) should not be ignored when monoamine oxidase inhibitors are prescribed.

In general, all types of foods prepared by fermentation, or those with evidence of putrefaction (some of which are intentional), especially those high in proteins, must be consumed with caution with certain medication as well as with alcohol.

Mutagen(s) in Heated Beef and Beef Extracts

An unidentified substance(s) mutagenic to certain strains of Salmonella typhimurium reportedly is formed when beef, beef extracts, or other beef-containing preparations are heated at 105 or 200°C (Commoner et al. 1978). The amounts of the mutagen(s) formed increases with the time of heating, and apparently is absent in uncooked beef. Beef bouillon cubes have been estimated to contain 0.1 ppm of mutagen, and in cooked hamburgers, 0.01 to 0.14 ppm, depending on the extent of cooking.

The mutagen appears to be distinct from the products of amino acid pyrolysis at 300°C or over (p. 612), or to benzo(a)pyrene. It is reported to be a basic substance extractable by organic solvents from alkaline aqueous solution and apparently requires metabolic activation. The unknown mutagen seems to be nitrosable with nitrous acid; the product(s) of the reaction becomes inherently mutagenic. It has been suggested by Commoner et al. (1978) that the mutagen(s) may be a product(s) of the Maillard reaction.

The mutagenicity test using *S. typhimurium* has been highly correlated with carcinogenicity in animals (Ames et al. 1975; McCann et al. 1975). Thus, a positive result suggests a strong possibility that the substance in question may possess a carcinogenic hazard.

The beef mutagen is almost four times as active as acetyl aminofluorene (AAF), already a potent carcinogen; this fact suggests that the beef mutagen probably is also a potent carcinogen, assuming that bacterial mutagenicity in this case can be correlated with carcinogenicity.

Fortunately, the level of mutagen in beef products such as hamburgers, except under conditions of excessive heating, may not pose appreciable hazard to the population at large. However, any rational assessment will require additional evidence.

TOXICANTS PRODUCED BY REACTIONS INVOLVING CONTAMINANTS

Nitrites

Nitrites are produced in foods by bacterial reduction of nitrates which may be present as contaminants or food additives. Nitrates per se do not pose any significant health hazard at the levels found in foods. For example, the safety of nitrates is suggested by a report on seven infants fed up to 21 mg nitrates/kg body weight without developing clinical symptoms of methemoglobinemia (Kubler 1958). Another case of a 10-day-old infant fed up to 100 mg nitrate/kg for 8 days without developing signs of the disease also has been reported (Cornblath and Hartmann 1948). Many other reports confirm the nontoxicity of nitrates per se in humans at the levels found in foods and drinking water (Gelperin et al. 1975; Kubler and Simon 1967; Phillips 1968). Cases of supposedly chronic nitrate poisoning in animals (Dollahite and Holt 1970) and children (Petukhov et al. 1972) have been reported. However, even in these cases, it is questionable whether nitrate was the etiological agent.

The toxicological significance of nitrates lies in its easy conversion to nitrite by nitrifying bacteria that may be present in foodstuffs, the saliva, and in the GI tract. The reduction of nitrate to nitrite in foodstuffs, especially spinach, has been demonstrated by Schuphan (1965). At harvest, spinach from a heavily fertilized field was shown to contain a high level of nitrate and only 30 ppm of nitrite on a dry weight basis; this value increased to 3550 ppm after 4 days storage at room temperature. Another study (Phillips 1968) has confirmed the findings of Schuphan. In addition, it also demonstrates that refrigeration promotes nitrate reduction, but retards denitrification, which can occur when foodstuffs are stored at room temperature. Freezing for up to 5 months prevents reduction of nitrate to nitrite, but thawing at room temperature for up to 39 hr results in nitrification.

Commercially prepared spinach appears to be safe from nitrifying bacteria even after being opened and kept in refrigeration for 7 days (Phillips 1968). However, although processed foods are generally safe, there have been reported exceptions. Thus, methemoglobinemia has been reported in neonates fed carrot juice (Keating et al. 1973) and spinach puree (Holscher and Natzschka 1964; Sinios and Wodsak 1965).

Populations at Risk to Nitrite Poisoning

The populations that are particularly at risk are those that lack the NADH-dependent methemoglobin reductase activity. This population includes infants under 1 year of age (Ross and Des Forges 1959) and those with hereditary familial methemoglobinemia such as in some members of the Alaskan Eskimo and Indian populations (Scott 1960; Scott and Griffith 1959; Scott and Hoskins 1958).

A second genetically predisposed population includes those lacking erythrocyte glucose-6-phosphate dehydrogenase activity. This population includes blacks (Gross et al. 1958; Carson et al. 1956) and certain Mediterranean and Middle-Eastern peoples, such as Sardinians, Greeks, Sephardic Jews, and Iranians (Tarlov et al. 1962). These are the same populations which are also susceptible to favism (Chap. 8).

A third population is pregnant women (Skrivan 1971), and those with decreased stomach acidity (achlorhydria) as a result of such diseases as pernicious anemia, chronic gastritis, stomach ulcer, and cancer (Kohl 1973). The latter group shares a common problem with neonates in that the gastric pH in the latter is not high enough to inhibit nitrate-reducing bacteria that are normally derived from the lower gastro-intestinal tract (Walton 1951). The effect of pregnancy in increasing susceptibility to methemoglobinemia also has been demonstrated in rats (Shuval and Gruener 1972).

Very young infants are most susceptible to methemoglobinemia because, in addition to the aforementioned deficiencies, their hemoglobin F (fetal) is more easily oxidized to methemoglobin than the normal hemoglobin in older children or adults (Betke et al. 1956). Thus, it is in this group that serious cases of methemoglobinemia have occurred.

Conversion of nitrate in saliva is discussed in Chapter 18. Reduction of nitrate to nitrite in the stomach has been demonstrated during an epidemic of infantile gastroenteritis due to an enteropathogenic strain of *Escherichia coli* (Fandre et al. 1962). In this epidemic during which nine infants died, methemoglobin levels of up to 59% of total hemoglobin were found. In separate cases of two infants who had become cyanotic from high nitrate well water, nitrifying bacteria, such as *Aerobacter aerogens, Staphylococcus aureus* and, of course, *E. coli* were isolated from the mouth and upper GI tract (Cornblath and Hartmann 1948).

Methemoglobinemia Iron in hemoglobin is in the ferrous state (Fe^{2+}). When it is oxidized to the ferric state (Fe^{3+}), hemoglobin is transformed to methemoglobin. In this form, the pigment is unable to transport oxygen. There is a normally small amount of methemoglobin (1.7%) in the blood (Orten and Neuhaus 1975), and this level is maintained by methemoglobin reductase in the presence of NADH. Many types of oxidants can convert hemoglobin to methemoglobin. In neonates, levels of up to 5% have been reported (Kravitz et al. 1956). No symptoms have been observed in infants with this methemoglobin concentration. Above this value, however, mild cyanosis becomes evident; with increasing levels, say 20 to 40%, marked cyanosis, fatigue, and dyspnea are observed: at levels of 40% or over, severe cyanosis, tachypnea, serious cardiopulmonary signs, tachycardia, and depression occur. Ataxia, coma and death occur above 60% (Orten and Neuhaus 1980).

Many cases of methemoglobinemia have been reported involving infants. Several cases that were reported in Germany involved home-prepared high nitrate spinach. All were infants between 2 and 10 months old (Simon 1966). Additionally, most cases of reported infantile methemoglobinemia in Germany involved the drinking or use of private well water which was very high in nitrates; 84% had concentrations of 100 mg/L. A few had nitrites in them (Simon et al. 1964). Most of the infants were under 3 months; and 8.6% of 745 cases died.

Other Toxic Effects of Nitrites Animal studies have shown toxic effects of nitrites, independent of methemoglobinemia. For example, mice given 2 g $NaNO_2$/L in the drinking water developed dose-related reduction of motor activity in addition to methemoglobinemia. The latter was ameliorated by ascorbic acid, but not the overall reduction in motor activity (Behroozi et al. 1972; Shuval and Gruener 1972).

Some effects may be related to the decreased level of retinoids in the tissues, as in vitamin deficiency. Thus, hens given 100 to 200 mg $NaNO_2$ or 1 to 2 g KNO_3/day for more than 10 months, and then 400 mg $NaNO_2$ or 4 g KNO_3/day for the next 2 months, showed leg weakness and chronic muscular spasm after more than 4.5 months on nitrites. These signs were particularly more pronounced when the water was acidified. In these hens, there were grayish yellow nodules on the esophageal mucosa, characteristic of retinoid deficiency, atrophy of ovaries or testes, and depressed liver retinoid level. The eggs of all treated hens showed characteristic blood spots (Tomov 1965).

Shuval and Gruener (1972) have found cardiac and pulmonary damage in rats given water containing 2 to 3 g $NaNO_2$/L for 2 years. The progeny of pregnant rats in this group developed and grew poorly. There was a high incidence of infant mortality. In fact, when given 0.10 to 2.0 g $NaNO_2$/L for 2 weeks or more, rats showed abnormal electroencephalogram patterns, which remained even after exposure to nitrite had ceased.

Shank and Newberne (1976) have found a 27% incidence of lymphoreticular tumors compared to 6% in control rats, in experiments in which a diet containing 1.0 g $NaNO_2$/kg was fed. Residual $NaNO_2$ in the diet after mixing was 240 to 460 mg. The overall tumor incidence in treated rats was 61% compared to 18% in the control. These investigators however, did not observe any adverse effects on litter size, growth rate, infant mortality, and longevity.

The most important effect of nitrite is nitrosamine formation which is discussed in the next section.

Level of Nitrites in Foods

The level of nitrites in food as a derived toxicant is closely related to the level of nitrates. Many vegetables contain high levels of nitrates. Beets, celery, lettuce, radishes, and spinach may contain more than 600 ppm nitrate-N. Thus, vegetables may contribute more than 86% of the total daily intake of nitrates in the United States (White 1975). A large proportion of the total intakes may be derived from potatoes because of greater per capita consumption than any other vegetable, even though this food contains only moderate levels of nitrates (i.e., approximately 12 mg/100 g) (White 1975).

Potable water, especially that from shallow wells, may also contribute significantly to the level of nitrates in food. Shallow well water may contain as much as 100 mg nitrates/L (Sattlemacher 1962; Simon et al. 1964).

Nitrosamines

Three general types of nitrosamines that are significant in food toxicology are the dialkyl, cyclic, and acylalkyl nitrosamines, or nitrosamides. The latter includes the nitroguanidines, which are a special class of nitrosamides. The general structures are shown below:

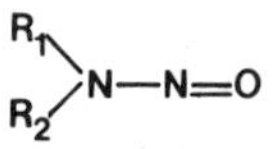

$$\begin{array}{ccc}
R_1\!\!\diagdown & R_1\!\!-\!\!N\!\!-\!\!N\!\!=\!\!O & R_1\!\!-\!\!N\!\!-\!\!N\!\!=\!\!O \\
\quad\diagdown N\!\!-\!\!N\!\!=\!\!O & \qquad| & \qquad| \\
R_2\!\!\diagup & C\!\!=\!\!NH & C\!\!=\!\!O \\
 & | & | \\
 & NH\!\!-\!\!R_2 & R_2
\end{array}$$

Dialkylnitrosamine 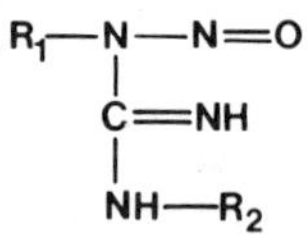   Acylalkylnitrosamines 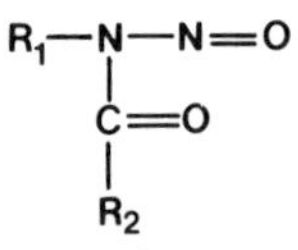   Nitrosoguanidine

Cyclic nitrosamines are a special class of nitrosamines, yet are similar to the dialkyl types. The nitrogen atom becomes a part of the heterocyclic ring. Typical examples are N-nitrosopiperidine and N-nitrosopyrrolidine, both of which are found in foodstuffs (Magee et al. 1976). The most common dialkylnitrosamines are dimethyl- and diethylnitrosamine (DMN and DEN, respectively); both compounds have been widely studied, being also found in foodstuffs (Magee et al. 1976). The alkyl group in these compounds may be symmetrical, as in the preceding examples, or asymmetrical; these alkyl groups may also contain functional groups. The parent compounds of dialkylnitrosamines are secondary amines, and will be discussed in another section. Many types of dialkylnitrosamines have been shown to be oncogenic. However, only a few of these are of importance in food toxicology.

The nitrosamides consist of the different types of nitrosoureas, thioureas, carbamates, carboxamides, and, of course, the guanidines. This group is highly reactive and will decompose readily at the site of contact in the animal body (Druckrey 1975).

Many parent compounds of the nitrosamides occur naturally and may be found in foodstuffs; many occur as contaminants in foods and are derived from various sources (Mirvish 1975). This aspect will be discussed elsewhere in this section.

Formation of Nitrosamines

Nitrosamine formation occurs outside or inside the body, the principal precursors being the various amines and amides and nitrites (Mirvish 1975). The general reaction is:

$$R_1-\underset{\underset{R_2}{|}}{N}H + HONO \longrightarrow R_1-\underset{\underset{R_2}{|}}{N}=NO + H_2O$$

Thus, the fundamental requirements are a secondary amino nitrogen and nitrous acid ($NO_2^- + H^+$). Actually, the nitrosating species is nitrous anhydride, N_2O_3, or in the presence of thiocyanate or halides, nitrosylthiocyanate, SCN-NO, or nitrosylhalide, NOX (X = Cl, Br). N_2O_3 is formed from two molecules of HNO_2

$$2HNO_2 \longrightarrow N_2O_3 + H_2O$$

The rate of reaction follows Equation 12.1

$$R = k \ (R_1R_2NH) \ (HNO_2)^2 \tag{12.1}$$

The rate constant, k, will vary with the pH if the total amine concentration is considered. It is independent of pH if the uncharged (nonionized) amine species such as that depicted in Equation 12.1 is considered; this species, of course, varies with pH. Because it is the nonionized amine that reacts, the rate constant, k, and thus, the rate of reaction will be highest with weakly basic amines or at a higher pH. However, the latter requirement cannot be met because one of the reactants, HNO_2, is a relatively weaker acid than HNO_3 and has a dissociation constant of pK_a = 3.37. Thus, pH 3.37 is the optimum pH for nitrosation of amines with HNO_2 (Fan and Tannenbaum 1973). Highly basic amines, such as piperidine (pK_a = 11.2), are less easily nitrosated (k = 0.00045 m^{-2} sec^{-1}) than more weakly basic amines such as morpholine (pK_a = 8.17, k = 0.42) (Mirvish 1975).

However, CNS^-, Cl^-, or Br^- can catalyze the reaction by forming the corresponding nitrosyl compounds:

$$HNO_2 + H^+ + CNS^- \ (or \ Cl^-, Br^-) \longrightarrow SCN-NO \ (or \ NOCl, NObr)$$

$$R_1R_2NH + SCN-NO(NOCl, NOBr) \longrightarrow R_1R_2N-N=O + CNS^- \ (Cl^-, Br^-)$$

The rate equation for the reaction is (Fan and Tannenbaum 1973):

$$rate = k_2 \ (amine) \ (HNO_2) \ (CNS^-, Cl^-, Br) \tag{12.2}$$

The order of catalytic activity is $CNS^- \gg Br^- > Cl^-$ (Ridd 1961) and the pH optimum is pH 2 at which point all nitrite is essentially in the form of HNO_2. Because CNS^- is also protonated below pH 2, the rate also drops; however, it could be modified by other factors toward even higher values (Mirvish et al. 1973); no such protonation occurs with CL^- and Br^-, which form highly dissociated acids, and thus, no decrease in reaction rate occurs below pH 2. Thus, by Equation 12.2, it can be seen that nitrosation will be favored by high concentrations of CNS^-, Cl^-, or Br^-; the effect of these ions will compensate whatever decrease in nitrite concentration.

Catalytic activity was also observed with formaldehyde by the formation of an iminium ion. This catalytic activity is not observed with other carbonyls except chloral (Keefer and Roller 1973):

$$R_1R_2NH + H_2C{=}O \; \underset{\xleftarrow{\hspace{2cm}}}{\xrightarrow{\hspace{1cm}OH^-\hspace{1cm}}} \; R_1R_2N^+{=}CH_2$$

$$H_2C{=}O + R_1R_2N{-}N{=}O \longleftarrow R_1R_2N{-}CH_2{-}O{-}NO \quad \Big) \; NO_2^-$$

The requirement for OH^- indicates that this catalysis is more effective at pH values above pH 7 (Lijinsky and Singer 1974).

This catalytic activity of HCHO at neutral pH may be relevant to the significant formation of nitrosamines at near neutral pH in foods, contrary to the basic chemical mechanism underlying nitrosation reaction as discussed previously. For example, significant amounts of nitrosamines were formed when meat or fish and glycine, proline, or sarcosine were heated at 130 to 170°C with excess nitrite. Also, lecithin heated with nitrite at 100°C and at pH 3.5 to 7.0 produces dimethylnitrosamine (DMN), diethyl-nitrosamine (DEN), and di-n-propylnitrosamine (Mohler and Hallermayer 1973). Bills et al. (1973) has obtained nitrosopyrrolidine by heating nitrite with nitrosoproline, pyrrolidine, proline, putrescine, and spermidine in oil-water combination under frying conditions.

It is possible that other nitrosation mechanisms occur, since nitrosamines also are formed even when the pure reactants are incubated at pH 6 to 7 at 25°C (Ender and Ceh 1971; Mirvish 1970). Mechanisms similar to formaldehyde catalysis may also operate in the formation of nitrosamines in the presence of various species of bacteria. Collin-Thompson et al. (1972) have obtained nitrosamines under controlled conditions. When nitrite and specific amines were incubated with several Streptococcus species, but not with species from other genera, these authors conclude that bacterial metabolites might have catalyzed the reaction. The formation of nitrosamines with pure bacterial cultures or rat intestinal contents also have been reported by others (Alam et al. 1971a; Brooks et al. 1972; Hill and Hawksworth 1972; Klubes et al. 1972). It is, of course, possible that in many cases bacterial action may simply be an acid-catalyzed reaction (Sander and Schweinsberg 1972).

The nitrosation of various carbamates, guanidines, and ureas involves different nitrosating species. In this case, the nitrous acidium ion, $H_2NO_2^+$, is involved and the reaction rate is expressed as:

$$\text{rate} = k_3 \, (RNHCOR)(HNO_2)(H^+) \tag{12.3}$$

The reaction rate depends then on the formation of the nitrous acidium ion, and hence, the hydrogen ion concentration or pH. Thus, nitrosation with these compounds will occur rapidly at low pH (Sander and Schweinsberg 1972). Other reactions do not depend on amide ionization, since these compounds are nonionized above pH 2. However, the reaction rate will still vary with the chemical nature of amide. The differences in rates can be quite large (Mirvish 1971, 1972).

In Vivo Formation of Nitrosamines   The conditions in the alimentary tract from the mouth to the rectum are conducive to nitrosamine formation. First, oral bacteria may promote the reduction of nitrate to nitrite, so that the total nitrite load is increased (Tannenbaum et al. 1974, 1976). Second, nitrosamine formation can also be promoted in the mouth by oral bacteria (Tannenbaum et al. 1977). Third, saliva can promote the formation of cyanamides from secondary amines (Wishnok and Tannenbaum 1976) as well as primary amines (Tannenbaum et al. 1977).

$$1° \text{ Amine: } RNH_2 \xrightarrow{\dfrac{\text{Saliva}}{CN^-}} RNHCN \xrightarrow{\quad NO_2^-, H^+ \quad}$$

$$2° \text{ Amine: } R_1R_2NH \xrightarrow{\dfrac{\text{saliva}}{CN^-}} R_1R_2NCN \xrightarrow{\quad NO_2^-, H^+ \quad}$$

$$RN \quad \begin{array}{c} N = O \\ CN \end{array}$$

N-nitrosocyanamides as a class, as exemplified by methylnitrosocyanamide (Endo et al. 1974) and ethylnitrosocyanamide (Pelfrene et al. 1975), may be highly mutagenic and carcinogenic.

Both normal and hypoacidic conditions in the stomach favor nitrosamine formation. The normal acidity of the stomach is ideal for nitrosation. A number of studies, using real or simulated gastric juice, suggest that nitrosamines can be readily formed from nitrites and various amines or amides (Alam et al. 1971a,b; Endo and Takahashi 1973a,b; Lane and Bailey 1973; Sander 1968; Sen et al. 1969). Synthesis of nitrosamines in the stomach of rats and rabbits has been experimentally verified (Alam et al. 1971a; Greenblatt et al. 1972).

The rate of synthesis of nitrosamines in the stomach of rats and dogs greatly exceeds that which is predicted by chemical kinetics of simple model systems (Greenblatt et al. 1971; Mysliwy et al. 1974). This may be explained in part by catalysis by CNS^- and Cl^- ions which are in fact abundant in gastric juice (Lane and Bailey 1973); the former most likely being contributed by saliva (Boyland et al. 1971). In fact, Tannenbaum et al. (1977) has found that relatively large amounts of nitrosamines are formed in simulated gastric juice mixed with saliva, even with relatively low levels of salivary nitrite.

Hypoacidity of the stomach can also markedly favor nitrosamine formation. Under this condition, the stomach is invaded by microorganisms, some of which promote nitrate reduction (Phillips 1971), and others, nitrosamine formation at neutral pH (Sander 1968). The dual occurrence of nitrate reduction and nitrosamine formation in human subjects with gastric hypoacidity and who were gavaged with sodium nitrate and diphenylamine has been reported by Sander and Schweinsberg (1972).

In animals, relatively high yields of nitrosamines have been obtained from in vivo experiments. For example, the yields of diphenylnitrosamines and N-nitrosomethyl-aniline in rats gavaged with the corresponding amine and nitrite were 30% and 4%, respectively (Sander and Schweinberg 1972). A 2% yield of DEN from diethylamine and nitrite has been obtained in cats and rabbits by Sen et al. (1969). Yields of 27% and 9% of methyl- and ethylnitrosourea, respectively, have been obtained 45 to 90 min after intragastric administration of the urea and nitrite (Mirvish and Chu 1973). Alam et al. (1971a,b) have obtained a 0.5% yield of nitrosopiperidine from piperidine and nitrite injected into the tied-off stomach of the rat and left in situ.

Many of these recoveries probably have been underestimated because analytical recoveries were low, of the order of 10 to 30% (Alam et al. 1971a,b; Mirvish and Chu 1973) and losses due to absorption are bound to occur. Kamm et al. (1974) have found 1 to 2 μg DMN/ml in the serum, 0.5 to 6 hr following gavage of rats with 127 mg aminopyrine and 110 mg nitrite/kg body weight.

A similar situation has been observed in the small intestine. Except here, an acid catalyzed nitrosation reaction, except perhaps in isolated pockets, cannot be expected to take place. Evidence has been presented by Tannenbaum et al. (1978) that the upper aerobic part of the human small intestine is a virtual sewer, and like similar ecosystems, it promotes nitrification of ammonia and organic nitrogen compounds. Data also have been obtained from ileostomy samples which show that nitrite may be formed from more reduced nitrogen compounds and not via nitrate reduction. However, the occurrence of the latter cannot be excluded. Nitrate-reducing bacteria, e.g., E. coli, E. dispor, Proteus vulgaris, and Serratia marcescens, that may inhabit the intestines also have been shown to promote nitrosamine formation at neutral pH (Sander 1968). Five strains of E. coli from the human gut have been demonstrated to form nitrosamines from dimethylamine, diethylamine, piperidine, pyrrolidine, and other amines in the presence of sodium nitrite at neutral pH. Also, strains of Bacteroides, Bifidobacterium, Clostridium and Enteroccus, which do not reduce nitrate, have been shown to form nitrosamines upon replacement of nitrate in the reaction medium with nitrite (Hawksworth and Hill 1971). Rats with bladders infected with E. coli and treated orally with piperidine and sodium nitrite have been shown to excrete nitrosopiperidine (Hawksworth and Hill 1974).

Actual formation of nitrosamines in the rat intestine has been demonstrated by Alam et al. (1971a,b). A recovery of 158 μg nitrosopiperidine from 1.25 g of piperidine hydrochloride and 25 mg nitrite has been obtained; a yield of 21 to 25 μg has been obtained with 625 mg of piperidine and 25 mg nitrite. Again, these values are subject to very low analytical recoveries as well as absorption losses. With a total reaction time in the intestine of 40 min, a mean recovery of 3% nitrosopiperidine has been obtained.

Thus, it appears that nitrosamine formation in the small intestines is inevitable. However, certain dietary factors (discussed in the next section) may inhibit nitrosamine formation, so that the actual yield will even be much lower.

Because the bacterial population increases significantly in the colon (Chap. 2), it is very possible that considerable nitrosamine formation can occur in this site. The observation of Bruce et al. (1977) that mutagens are present in feces from human subjects eating a typical Western diet is significant. The mutagen in these feces was later described as a nitroso compound(s) by Varghese et al. (1978) based on various experimental evidence. However, the specific compound remains to be identified. Klubes et al. (1972) has shown that DMN can be formed by incubating dimethylamine and sodium nitrite with the content of rat cecum.

Alkylation of nucleic acids from orally administered amines or amides and nitrites: The formation of alkylated nucleic acids following oral administration of nitrites with the appropriate amine or amide is considered proof of in vivo formation of nitrosamines. This is because neither amines nor amides are alkylating agents. Thus, after treatment of rats with ^{14}C-methylurea, Montesano and Magee (1971) have detected 7-^{14}C-methylguanine in the nucleic acids of the liver, stomach, and intestines. Similar alkylation of liver nucleic acids has been reported in rats (Montesano and Magee 1971) and in mice (Epstein 1972) with orally administered dimethylamine plus sodium nitrite, but not with the amine alone. Methylation of RNA resulting in the formation of 7-methylguanine and the inhibition of liver protein synthesis also has been observed in mice given dimethylamine and sodium nitrite orally (Friedman et al. 1973).

Tumor formation following simultaneous oral administration of amines or amides and nitrite: Proof of in vivo nitrosamine formation also has been obtained by induction of tumors in animals following simultaneous oral administration of the appropriate amines or amides and nitrite. Some of these results will be discussed later in this section.

Factors Inhibiting Nitrosamine Formation

It is fortunate that nitrosamine formation is not altogether inevitable in food as well as in the body, since the nitrosation reaction per se is dependent on physicochemical factors. To begin with, a decrease in the concentration of the reactant will diminish the amount of product formed. The requirement for high acid conditions limits the nitrosation of the ureas. Thus, administration of sodium bicarbonate before treatment with methylurea and nitrite prevents methylnitrosourea formation (Mirvish and Chu 1973). There are no reports as of this writing regarding catalysis, except by acids, of the nitrosation of ureas, carbamates, or guanidines, or direct promotion of this reaction by bacteria in the alimentary canal.

One of the most effective inhibitors of nitrosamine formation is ascorbic acid. This vitamin reacts with nitrite rapidly to form nitric oxide and dehydroascorbic acid (Mirvish et al. 1972). Thus, ascorbic acid competes for any nitrite present, and hence, reduces the availability of this reactant for nitrosamine formation. It has been shown (Mirvish et al. 1972) that ascorbic acid reduces the formation of DMN, and other nitrosamines, by greater than 90%. The formation of mononitrosopiperazine from piperazine adipate and nitrite is reduced by 80% in the presence of ascorbate, but a significant amount of the dinitroso derivative is formed (Fan and Tannenbaum 1973). The adipate moiety may be responsible for this aberration. Ascorbic acid or its isomer, erythorbic acid, prevents or inhibits the formation of DMN in frankfurters containing high levels of nitrite (Fiddler et al. 1973).

Other evidence of the inhibition of nitrosamine formation by ascorbic acid includes the reduction or prevention of liver damage in mice (Kamm et al. 1973) and rats (Cardesa et al. 1974) following treatment with aminopyrine and nitrite, and the inhibition of the induction of lung adenomas in strain A mice with piperazine, morpholine, or methylurea plus nitrite (Mirvish et al. 1973). A dose-response phenomenon with respect to the ascorbic acid concentration in the food was noted in the piperazine experiment. Ascorbic acid given orally simultaneously with ethylurea plus nitrite to pregnant rats also completely prevents hydrocephalus and neurogenic tumors in the offspring (Ivankovic et al. 1973, 1974).

Ascorbic acid prevents the formation of nitrosamines, but not the induction of tumors after nitrosamines are formed. This has been clearly seen in the ineffectiveness of ascorbate to prevent tumors induced by ethylnitrosourea, or liver damage when the vitamin is injected i.p. and the amine and nitrite are given by gavage to rats (Kamm et al. 1974). The inability of ascorbic acid to prevent the toxic action of DMN also has been reported by others (Cardessa et al. 1974; Greenblatt 1973).

The effectiveness of ascorbic acid seems to depend on the nature of the amine. For example, at pH 3 and at low concentrations, ascorbate more effectively blocks the nitrosation of piperazine than that of morpholine (Mirvish et al. 1972).

The effect of ascorbic acid also has been tested in humans (Varghese et al. 1978). In this case, the level of nitroso compounds, as measured colorimetrically and by mutagenic activity, in the feces of adults eating typical Western diets, dropped by more than 50% when 1 g ascorbic acid was given daily before each meal and at bedtime for 2 weeks. The level and mutagenic activity slowly reverted to the initial values over a period of a month after termination of ascorbic acid supplementation.

Other substances can also block the nitrosation reactions; e.g., gallic acid, sodium sulfite, cysteine, and tannins. Again, depending on the amine, these substances are comparable or superior to ascorbic acid. For example, gallic acid provides a 75% blocking rate of morpholine nitrosation compared to the 28% of ascorbic acid at pH 3 and at the same concentration of 5 mg (Mirvish et al. 1972). With piperazine, ascorbic acid is clearly superior to all the others at all pH values.

Urea also blocks nitrosation of various amines quite effectively at pH 1 to 2, but less so at pH 3 to 4 (Mirvish et al. 1974).

Occurrence of Nitrosamines and Their Precursors in Foods

In assessing the hazard of nitrosamines in foodstuffs, it is also important to consider the types and levels of precursors, for the reported levels of nitrosamines only suggest values that may be expected in the products. These values do not represent the actual nitrosamine content because there is a large variation in the values reported. Furthermore, present analytical techniques are quite lengthy and complicated and may be subject to considerable uncertainty and error, so that experience and unusual care are required for successful analysis (Fiddler 1975). These difficulties may account for the contradictory results that have been reported in many cases.

Tables 12.3 and 12.4 list several nitrosamine precursors and the corresponding nitrosamine that can be formed. Note that endogenous compounds, derivatives and contaminants, and drugs are represented. The level of the precursors in foodstuffs could vary depending on the conditions. Nevertheless, the large number of potentially nitrosable compounds in foodstuffs is sufficient cause for concern. This should provide incentive to minimize their presence in foods.

Many nitrosable substances are derived from innocuous precursors, such as proline, arginine, lysine, lecithin, and choline. Proline can decarboxylate to pyrrolidine

Table 12.3 Nitrosoamine Precursors Endogenous or Formed (Derived) in Foodstuffs

Compound	Food	Nitrosamine formed	Reference
Creatine, creatinine	Meats, meat products, milk, vegetables	NSA	Archer et al. (1971)
Trimethylamine oxide	Fish	DMN	Malins et al. (1970); Wick et al. (1967)
Trimethylamine	Fish	DMN	Malins et al. (1970); Wick et al. (1967)
Dimethylamine	Fish, meat, and meat products, cheese	DMN	Malins et al. (1970); Sen et al. (1970); Wick et al. (1967); Schwarz and Thomasow (1950); Sen (1972)
Diethylamine	Cheese	DEN	Ogasawara et al. (1963)
Sarcosine	Meat and meat products, fish	NSA	Borgstrom (1961); Friedman (1972); Mirvish et al. (1973)
Choline, lecithin	Eggs, meat and meat products, soybeans, corn	DMN	Bills et al. (1973); Fidler et al. (1972); Kuchmak and Dugan (1963); Pensabene et al. (1975)

Proline, hydroxyproline	Meat and meat products, and other foodstuffs	NPro, NPyr	Bills et al. (1973)
Pyrrolidine	Meat and meat products, paprika	NPyr	Gray and Collins (1978); Pensabene et al. (1974); Sen et al. (1973a,b)
Piperidine	Meat and meat products, cheese, black pepper	NPip	Gray and Collins (1978); Pensabene et al. (1974); Sen et al. (1973a,b)
Methylguanidine	Beef, fish	MNU	Kapeller-Adler and Krael (1930); Pensabene et al. (1974); Sasaki (1938)
Citrulline	Meat, meat products, vegetables	NCit	Navarro et al. (1962); Ogasawara et al. (1963)
Carnitine	Meat and meat products	DMN	Fiddler et al. (1972)
Dipropylamine	Cheese	DPN	Golovnya et al. (1970)
Dibutylamine	Cheese	DBN	Golovnya et al. (1970)

Abbreviations: NSA, nitrososarcosine; DMN, dimethylnitrosamine; NPro, nitrosoproline; NPyr, nitrosopyrrolidine; NPip, nitrosopiperidine; MNC, methylnitrosocyanamide; DPN, di-n-propylnitrosamine; DBN, di-n-butylnitrosamine.

Table 12.4 Nitrosamine Precursors Which Contaminate Foodstuffs

Compound	Chemical class	Nitrosamine derivative	Reference
Atrazine	2° Amine	N-Nitrosoatrazine	Eisenbrand et al. (1974)
Benzthiazuram	Carbamate	N-Nitrosobenzthiazuram	Eisenbrand et al. (1974)
Carbaryl	Carbamate	Nitrosocarbaryl	Eisenbrand et al. (1974); Elespuru et al. (1974)
Fenuron	Carbamate	Dimethylnitrosamine	Elespuru and Lijinsky (1973)
Ferbam	Amide	Dimethylnitrosamine	Sen et al. (1974)
Morpholine	2° Amine	Nitrosomorpholine	Druckrey et al. (1967)
Propoxur	Carbamate	Nitrosopropoxur	Eisenbrand et al. (1974)
Simazine	2° Amine	Nitrososimazine	Eisenbrand et al. (1974)
Succinic acid 2,2-dimethyl hydrazide	Amide	Dimethylnitrosamine	Sen et al. (1974)
Thiram	Amide	Dimethylnitrosamine	Lijinsky et al. (1972)
Ziram	Amide	Dimethylnitrosamine	Eisenbrand et al. (1974); Sen et al. (1974)

(Sen et al. 1973a,b) or form nitrosoproline first and decarboxylate to nitrosopyrrolidine (Nakamura et al. 1976). Arginine may give rise to derivatives which when nitrosated under acidic conditions become mutagenic (Endo and Takahashi 1973a,b). Lysine may be metabolized by bacteria to produce piperidine and pyrrolidine (Saito and Sameshima 1956). Decarboxylation of lysine and ornithine produces cadaverine and putrescine, respectively. Cadaverine may be deaminated and cyclized to piperidine; similarly, putrescine can form pyrrolidine (Bills et al. 1973). Ornithine, of course, can be produced from arginine. Lijinsky and Epstein (1970) suggest that deamination of cadaverine and putrescine to form the corresponding cyclic secondary amines may occur during cooking. Normally, the levels of putrescine and cadaverine in foods are quite low. However, certain types of food that are fermented or meat products that are permitted to putrify somewhat, e.g., country ham, may contain high levels of these amines. It is interesting that feces may contain such amines (Orten and Neuhaus 1980), and that bacteria can promote the formation of piperidine and pyrrolidine (Saito and Sameshima 1956). The findings of Varghese et al. (1978) of the presence in human feces of a nitroso compound mutagenic to S. typhimurium is relevant in this respect.

Lecithin can give rise to choline. The latter when heated decomposes to trimethylamine, which then demethylates to dimethylamine (Fiddler et al. 1972).

Creatinine can be converted to methylguanidine by bacterial creatinase in the gut (Perez and Faluotico 1973; Van Eyk et al. 1968). Endo et al. (1977) has reported that creatine or creatinine can be converted to methylguanidine, which is a strong mutagen and gastric carcinogen in the rat, by heating in the presence of Fe^{3+}, and especially Cu^{+2}.

Trimethylamine oxide (TMAO) is abundant in fish except shellfish (Norris and Benoit 1945); levels of 185, 116, and 83 mg/100 have been detected in shad, turbot, and salmon, respectively (Shewan 1951). Trimethylamine oxide (TMAO) is the precursor of trimethyl- and dimethylamine in fish (Reay and Shewan 1949). Bacterial action on TMAO is mostly responsible for the presence of high levels of these amines in fish (Beatty 1938; Shewan 1939). However, prolonged storage even at freezing temperatures can result in significant decomposition of TMAO to the amines (Castell et al. 1970, 1971).

Piperidine in black pepper is mostly derived from the alkaloids piperine, chavicine, and piperettine (Concon et al. 1979).

Another important class of nitrosable compounds is the pesticide residues. Some of these are listed in Table 12.3. This class of compounds is widely used in agriculture, so that their residues may be detected in foodstuffs. The rate of nitrosation varies quite significantly among the compounds. Some, like ziram, can produce significant yields (1.6%) of DMN (5 mM each of ziram and nitrite, pH 2, 37°C, 10 min) (Eisenbrand et al. 1974). Others, like thiram and ferbam, give low yields (<20 μg) in the stomach content when given by gavage to guinea pigs (Sen et al. 1974).

The list of known components in foodstuffs that can be nitrosated may be extended even further if amines and amides that have not been tested are included. This group includes other naturally occurring compounds, such as alkaloids, drugs, and food additives. The findings reported by Wishnok and Tannenbaum (1976) that many types of primary amines can form cyanamides would make the list of potentially nitrosatable compounds seem endless. Several nitrosable compounds comprising some of the flavor constituents of beef, such as pyrrolizidines and piperidines, have been isolated from roasted beef (Hartman et al. 1983).

Table 12.5 gives some examples of nitrosamine levels in foodstuffs. Only those analytical values quantitated at least by gas chromatographic procedures are included in the tabulation. The identities of the nitrosamines in many of the foods listed have been confirmed by mass spectrometric methods. Earlier methods used only thin-layer chromatography and, as pointed out by Fiddler (1975), this method may not be entirely reliable.

The nitrosamine values shown in Table 12.5 are variable, and not every sample in each category contains detectable amounts of nitrosamines. For example, in a study by Fong and Chan (1977) of 10 samples of Chinese sausage, four had no detectable DMN and only three had DMN levels 10 ppb or over; in dried shrimp, no DMN was detected; however, only three of 10 had no NPyr, the remainder containing 10 ppb or over. In this work, 27 of 61 samples had detectable DMN (1 to 15 ppb); 23 of 61 had 2 to 37 ppb of NPyr.

The highest values have been found in salted marine fish from Hong Kong, as shown in Table 12.5. Fong and Chan (1973a) explain this in part by the presence of nitrate-reducing bacteria in fish that retain at least 50 to 60% moisture (Fong and Chan 1973b); thus, a favorable environment for nitrosation exists in the products.

Another factor which tends to increase nitrosamine levels is cooking. Thus, raw bacon may not contain detectable nitrosamines, but on frying, the levels can markedly increase, as shown in Table 12.5. Pensabene et al. (1974) have shown that cooking bacon to medium well-done results in marked increases in the NPyr level, whether the cooking is by frying in a cold or hot pan, or "baconer," or by broiling or baking. In the latter, the levels jumped from zero to 13 to 35 ppb. Microwave cooking produces the least amount of nitrosamines.

The levels of nitrosamines tend to increase with the temperature of cooking. Bacon cooked at 99°C for 105 min or 135°C for 10 min contain no detectable nitrosamines; frying for 10 min at 135°C produces no detectable nitrosamines, but after 30 min, the level increased to 8 ppb. Cooking to medium well-done at 176.7°C for 4 min or 204°C for 4 min results in levels increasing to 10 and 17 ppb, respectively; burned bacon (cooked 10 min at 204°C) contains 19 ppb of NYpr (Pensabene et al. 1974).

The bacon drippings may contain high levels of NPyr — up to 108 ppb (Fazio et al. 1973). The practice of using drippings for other cooking purposes should be discouraged.

Table 12.5   Nitrosamine Levels in Foodstuffs

Food	Nitrosamine	Level ppb	Analytical method	Reference
Bacon, raw		0		Fazio et al. (1973); Pensabene et al. (1974)
fried	DMN, DEN, NPyr	1−40	GC−MS	Crosby et al. (1972)
	NPip	10−108		Fazio et al. (1973)
	NPyr	11−38	GC−MS	Pensabene et al. (1974)
	DMN, NPyr	2−30	TLC−GC−MS	Sen et al. (1973a)
Bacon, frying fat	NPyr	10−108	GC−MS	Fazio et al. (1973)
drippings	NPyr	16−39	GC−MS	Pensabene et al. (1974)
Luncheon meat	DMN, DEN	1−4	GC−MS	Crosby et al. (1972)
Salami	DMN, DEN	1−4	GC−MS	Crosby et al. (1972)
Danish pork chop	DMN, DEN	1−4	GC−MS	Crosby et al. (1972)
Sausage	DMN	1−3	GC	Fazio et al. (1971b)
Sausage, mcttwurs	NPyr, NPip	13−105	TLC−GC−MS	Sen et al. (1973b)
chinese	DMN	0−15	GC−MS	Fong and Chan (1977)
Fish				
raw: sable	DMN	4	GC−MS	Fazio et al. (1971a)
salmon	DMN	0	GC−MS	Fazio et al. (1971a)
shad	DMN	0	GC−MS	Fazio et al. (1971a)
smoked: sable	DMN	4−9	GC−MS	Fazio et al. (1971a)
salmon	DMN	0−5	GC−MS	Fazio et al. (1971a)
smoked and nitrate or nitrite-treated:				
salmon, sable, shad	DMN	4−17	GC−MS	Fazio et al. (1971a)
salted marine fish	DMN	50−300	GC−MS	
smoked and nitrate or nitrite treated	DMN	20−26	GC−MS	Fazio et al. (1971a)
Other fish products	DMN	1−9	GC−MS	Crosby et al. (1972)
Fish sauce	DMN	0−2	GC−MS	Fong and Chan (1977)
	NPyr	0−2	GC−MS	Fong and Chan (1977)
Cheese	DMN	1−4	GC−MS	Crosby et al. (1972)

Table 12.5 (continued)

Food	Nitrosamine	Level ppb	Analytical method	Reference
Baby foods	DMN	1–3	GLC	Fazio et al. (1971b)
Shrimp, dried	DMN	2–10	GC–MS	Fong and Chan (1977)
	NPyr	0–37	GC–MS	Fong and Chan (1977)
Shrimp sauce	DMN	0–10	GC–MS	Fong and Chan (1977)
Squid	NPyr	0–10	GC–MS	Fong and Chan (1977)
	DMN	2–8	GC–MS	Fong and Chan (1977)
	NPyr	0–7	GC–MS	Fong and Chan (1977)
Canned meats (uncooked)	DMN	1–3	GC	Fazio et al. (1971b)
Ham and other pork products (uncooked)	DMN	0–5	GC	Fazio et al. (1971b)
Beef products (uncooked) (4 days after slaughter)	DMN	1–2	GC	Fazio et al. (1971b)
Wheat flour	DEN	0–10	TLC	Hedler and Marquardt (1968); Marquardt and Hedler (1966); Petrowitz (1968)

Abbreviations: DEN, diethylnitrosamine; DMN, dimethylnitrosamine; GC, gas-liquid chromatography; MS, mass spectroscopy; NPip, nitrosopiperidine; NPyr, nitroso-pyrrolidine; TLC, thin-layer chromatography.

The increase of NPyr may be explained on the basis of the increased decarboxylation of proline at high temperatures to pyrrolidine (Gray and Collins 1978), and one must assume that nitrosation occurs at a greater rate also under this condition. This temperature effect also has been observed in the formation of DMN from sarcosine (Gray et al. 1978).

Storage of nitrite-containing products for a considerable period of time can increase the level of nitrosamines. However, the levels appear to depend more on the nitrite level or the amine precursors than the time of storage (Gray and Collins 1978).

Of interest is the reported significant decrease of NPyr when fried bacon samples are stored at 1.7°C for 2 weeks (Pensabene et al. 1974). There appears to be no explanation for this apparent denitrosation.

In short, the formation of these derived toxicants is very much linked to the conditions of cooking or processing. A more thorough understanding of the effects of these conditions on nitrosamine formation will be valuable in terms of minimizing the levels of these carcinogens in food.

It must be emphasized, however, that the methods used in nitrosamine analysis in food may underestimate the level of these carcinogens. The reason is that, apart from the low recoveries inherent in the methods, determinations using separation of individual nitrosamines will automatically exclude many other nitrosamines that may be present. Collectively, the latter may be quite significant. Thus, the amount of total nitrosamines in a food may be more pertinent in assessing the hazard from these carcinogens. Therefore, the methods of analysis should also focus in the determination of total nitrosamines rather than just each individual compound.

Nitrosamines in Alcoholic Beverages An association between cancer in humans and the drinking of alcoholic beverages has been reported (Rothman 1975; Williams and Horm 1977), especially for cancer of the liver (Leevy et al. 1964), mouth, pharynx, and larynx (Pell and D'Alonzo 1973), and esophagus (Gsell and Loffler 1962; Wynder and Bross 1961). Thus, the findings that nitrosamines may be present in many brands of alcoholic beverages are very relevant in this respect.

Goff and Fine (1979) have reported that all 18 brands of imported and domestic beer contained dimethylnitrosamine at levels ranging from 0.4 to 7 µg/L; the United States brands of four light and two dark beers averaged 3.1 µg/L, whereas seven light and five dark imported beers averaged 2.6 µg/L. Scanlan et al. (1980) have found dimethylnitrosamine in 23 of 25 samples of beer produced in the United States, at levels ranging from 0.5 to 14 µg/L. The highest values have been found among 15 samples of Pilsen lager, which averaged 7.7 µg/L. Similar findings have been reported for German beers analyzed by Spiegelhalder et al. (1979). Of 158 samples, 111 contained dimethylnitrosamine at levels ranging from 0.2 to 11.2 µg/L, with a mean of 2.7 µg/L.

Dimethylnitrosamine also has been found in six of seven brands of Scotch whisky at levels between 0.3 and 2.0 µg/L, all of which were imported from Scotland. None was detected in five United States brands and one Canadian brand and one Irish brand. Similarly, none was detected in 19 samples of United States and imported wines, and several samples of sherry, liqueur, gin, brandy, rum, and vodka, both imported and domestic (Goff and Fine 1979). Both beer and Scotch whisky are produced from barley malt, and studies indicate that the production of malt by direct-fired kilning may be the primary souce of the carcinogen (Scanlan et al. 1980).

Toxicity and Carcinogenicity of N-Nitroso Compounds

The toxicity of nitrosamines was first recognized in 1937 by Freund, who reported two cases of accidental poisoning from inhalation of DMN. One case had symptoms of exhaustion and headaches and ill-defined pain in the abdomen, which was distended owing to fluid accumulation. Another patient who died following exploratory laparotomy after the poisoning also had ascitic fluid and an enlarged liver. Microscopical examination revealed liver necrosis and regenerative proliferation of the hepatocytes. Freund found similar effects in mice and dogs exposed to DMN vapors. Other researchers after World War II emphasized the industrial hazard of DMN following the occurrence of similar cases (Hamilton and Hardy 1949). Barnes and Magee (1954) have described the poisoning of laboratory workers exposed for over 10 months to DMN used as a solvent. The predominant toxic effect was liver damage.

In 1956, Magee and Barnes reported that DMN was a potent hepatocarcinogen in rats. This report marked the beginning of worldwide interest in N-nitroso compound carcinogenesis. Since then, a large number of N-nitroso compounds have been shown to be carcinogenic (Magee et al. 1976).

Animal Susceptibility and Potency N-nitroso compounds are among the few very potent carcinogens which are active in every animal species that has been tested, including subhuman primates (Weisburger 1973). Furthermore, taken as a group, this class of compounds has a broad organotropicity; i.e., they can affect almost all kinds of tissues (Magee et al. 1976; Shank 1975). Table 12.6 lists selected N-nitroso compounds and their corresponding target organs. Note that a number have broad organotropicity in a single species. For example, DEN administered orally to rats induces tumors in the liver, kidney, and esophagus (Magee and Barnes 1967). N-Nitrosopiperidine can produce tumors in the esophagus, liver, nasal cavities, larynx, and trachea in rats; the same compounds can produce tumors in the liver, larynx, trachea, and lung in monkeys (Magee et al. 1976).

Tumors of the liver in rats can be obtained with DEN with as little as 7.5 $\mu g/100$ g/day in the drinking water (Druckrey et al. 1963a), or 2 or 5 ppm of DMN in the diet fed throughout the animal's lifespan (Terracini et al. 1967). On a per kilogram body weight basis, Schmahl and Osswald (1967) have reported that similar low oral doses (about 3 mg/kg/day) produce liver tumors in several species of animals. Higher doses are required for the induction of tumors in other sites. For example, in the case of DEN, a dose of 17 mg/kg/day for 210 days is required to induce kidney tumors in rats (Hadjiolov 1968).

The potency of N-nitroso compounds also has been demonstrated by the efficacy of single doses in inducing liver tumors in newborn rats (Terracini and Magee 1964; Terracini et al. 1969), or in partially hepatectomized rats (Craddock 1971, 1973), or following carbon tetrachloride poisoning (Pound et al. 1973a,b). A single dose of 30 mg DMN/kg body weight produced kidney tumors in 20% of surviving rats (Magee and Barnes 1962). A single i.p. dose of 60 mg DMN/kg body weight produced kidney tumors in all rats fed a protein deficient diet and surviving after 8 to 11 months (McLean and Magee 1970; Swann and McLean 1968). A high incidence of respiratory tumors developed in newborn hamsters after a single subcutaneous dose of 5.5 mg DEN/kg (Montesano and Saffioti 1970).

A striking feature of N-nitroso compounds which demonstrates their potency is their ability to induce transplacental carcinogenesis (Tomatis 1973). In rats, kidney tumors have been induced transplacentally by DMN (Alexandrov 1968); similarly, tumors of the lung and liver have been induced in the mice (Smetanin 1971). Diethylnitrosamine induces transplacentally in rats tumors of the kidney, mammary glands, nasal cavities, and thymus (Pielsticker et al. 1967; Thomas and Bollmann 1968). Several nitrosoureas induce transplacentally tumors of the nervous system in rats (Druckrey et al. 1970; Ivankovic and Druckrey 1968; Koestner et al. 1971), and in mice (Denlinger et al. 1974; Diwan et al. 1973; Rice 1969), in addition to tumors of the kidney, liver, lung, and the hematopoietic system.

Tumors have also been induced in animals by simultaneous administration of nitrite and a nitrosamine. For example, esophageal tumors in rats have induced by feeding N-methylbenzylamine or morpholine + nitrite; other tumors have been induced with nitrite plus various ureas, 2-imidazolidone and N-methylaniline, but not with the very basic amines diethylamine, piperidine, N-methylcyclohexylamine, or various amides, N-methyl- and N-ethylurethan, phenyl- and 1-methyl-3-acetylurea as well as other amides (Sander and Burkle 1969). The levels used in these studies may have been too low, since the corresponding preformed nitrosamines are known carcinogens.

Other examples of tumor induction by simultaneous oral administration of nitrite and nitrosable compound are: neurogenic tumors from ethylurea + nitrite in the offspring of pregnant rats (Ivankovic et al. 1973) and hamster (Rustia and Shubik 1974); liver tumors in rats with nitrite plus aminopyrine (Lijinsky et al. 1973) or morpholine (Newberne and Shank 1973); and lung adenomas in mice with nitrite plus morpholine, piperazine, N-methylaniline, ethylurea, and methylurea in drinking water (Greenblatt et al. 1971; Mirvish et al. 1972). Dimethylamine produces no tumors. This is to be expected, possibly from the low levels of DMN formed due to the strong basicity of the amine.

Table 12.6 Target Tissues of Selected Nitrosamines That May Be Found in Foods

Nitrosamines[a]	Target tissue	Test species
Dimethylnitrosamine	Liver	Rat, mouse, European hamster, guinea pig, rabbit, rainbow trout, newt, mink, mastomys (*Praomys natalensis*), aquarium fish (*Lebistes reticulatus*)
	Kidney	Rat, Syrian golden and European hamsters
	Lung	Syrian golden hamster
	Nasal cavities	Rat, rabbit
Diethylnitrosamine	Liver	Rat, mouse, Syrian golden hamster, Chinese hamster, guinea pig, rabbit, dog, pig, trout, grass parakeet, monkey, *Brachydanio rerio*
	Kidney	Rat
	Lung	Mouse, Syrian golden hamster
	Nasal cavities	Rat, mouse, Syrian golden hamster, European hamster
	Esophagus	Rat, mouse, Chinese hamster
	Forestomach	Mouse, Chinese hamster
	Larynx	Syrian golden and European hamsters
	Trachea	Syrian golden and European hamsters
	Bronchi	European hamster
Di-n-propylnitrosamine	Liver	Rat
	Esophagus	Rat
	Tongue	Rat
Di-n-butylnitrosamine	Liver	Rat, mouse, guinea pig
	Lung	Syrian golden and Chinese hamsters
	Esophagus	Rat, mouse
	Bladder	Rat, mouse, Syrian golden and Chinese hamsters, guinea pig
	Forestomach	Mouse, Syrian golden hamster, guinea pig
	Trachea	Syrian golden hamster
	Tongue	Mouse
N-Nitrososarcosine	Esophagus	Rat
N-Nitrosopyrrolidine	Liver	Rat
	Lung	Mouse, Syrian golden hamster
	Nasal cavities	Rat
	Trachea	Syrian golden hamster
	Testis	Rat
N-Nitrosopiperidine	Liver	Rat, mouse, monkey, Syrian golden hamster
	Lung	Mouse, Syrian golden hamster
	Nasal cavities	Rat
	Esophagus	Rat, mouse
	Larynx	Rat, Syrian golden hamster
	Trachea	Rat, Syrian golden hamster
	Testis	Mouse

Table 12.6 (continued)

Nitrosamines	Target tissue	Test species
N-Nitrosomorpholine	Liver	Rat, mouse
	Lung	Mouse
	Kidney, nasal cavities, ovaries, esophagus	Rat
	Trachea, larynx, bronchus	Syrian golden hamster
N-Methyl-N-nitroso-urea	CNS	Rat, mouse, rabbit, dog
	Peripheral nervous system	Rat, dog
	Intestines	Rat, Syrian golden hamster, rabbit
	Kidney	Rat, mouse
	Forestomach	Rat, mouse
	Skin	Rat, mouse, dog
	Subcutaneous tissues	Syrian golden and European hamsters
	Glandular stomach, jaw, bladder, uterus, vagina	Rat
	Liver, lung, hemato-poietic system	Mouse
	Pharynx, esophagus, trachea, bronchus, oral cavity	Syrian golden hamster
	Stomach, pancreas, ear duct	Guinea pig
N-Ethylnitrosourea	CNS	Rat, mouse
	Peripheral nervous system	Rat, mouse
	Kidney	Rat, mouse
	Hematopoietic system	Rat, mouse
	Skin, intestines, ovary, uterus	Rat
N-Methyl-N-nitroso-urethane	Lung	Rat, mouse
	Forestomach	Rat, mouse, Syrian golden hamster
	Esophagus	Rat, Syrian golden hamster
	Kidney, intestines, ovary	Rat
	Pancreas, subcuta-neous tissues	Rabbit
N-Ethyl-N-nitroso-urethane	Forestomach, intestines	Rat
N-Methyl-N'-nitro-	Glandular stomach	Rat, Syrian golden hamster
N-nitrosoguanidine[b]	Forestomach	Rat, mouse
	Stomach	Dog
	Intestines	Rat, mouse, Syrian golden hamster, dog
	Skin	Mouse

Table 12.6   (continued)

Nitrosamines	Target tissue	Test species
N-Methyl-N'-nitro- N-nitrosoguanidine	Subcutaneous tissues Lung	Rat Rabbit

[a]Refer to Tables 21.2, 21.3, and 21.4 for nitrosoamine precursors or the foods in which some of these carcinogens have been found.
[b]N-Methyl-N'-nitro-N-nitrosoguanidine is not found in foods as such, but one of similar structure may be derived from naturally occurring guanidines, such as methyl-guanidine. The latter has been detected in certain foods, e.g., meats, and is probably derived from creatinine (Endo et al. 1977).
Source: Magee et al. (1976).

Factors Influencing the Carcinogenicity of N-Nitroso Compounds   *Enhancing factors:* As with other types of carcinogens, carcinogenesis involving N-nitroso compounds can be potentiated by various factors, such as hormones, other carcinogens or toxicants, viral or bacterial infections, metals, and nutritional factors.

Hormones: The effect of hormones has been suggested by the influence of sex and age of the animals on tumor induction by N-nitroso compounds. For example, a greater incidence of liver carcinomas has been observed in younger female Buffalo rats treated with DEN than in males (Reuber and Lee 1968); this incidence progressively decreases as the age of starting treatment increases, being highest at 4 weeks of age. In (C57B × C3H)F$_1$ hybrid mice treated with six injections of DMN at 3-day intervals, beginning at age 7 days, males develop liver tumors more frequently than the females (Vesselino-vitch 1969). Male C57B1/6 mice have been reported to be more susceptible to bladder tumors induced by N-nitrosodibutylamine or N-nitrosobutyl-4-hydroxybutylamine (Bertram and Craig 1970, 1972).

More direct evidence has been shown by Takizawa and Yamasaki (1971). Mammary tumor development induced by N-butyl-N-nitrosourea has been inhibited in W/Fu rats which were ovariectomized or orchidectomized. The castrated males, and to a lesser extent the ovariectomized females, develop these tumors when treated with progesterone plus estrogen or with an ovarian graft.

Pregnant rats treated with N-nitroso compounds develop a high incidence of cancers of the ovaries, uterus, and vagina, whereas nonpregnant ones rarely produce these tumors (Ivankovic 1969).

Not all types of tumors, however, are influenced by sex hormones. For example, orchidectomy does not affect the induction of tumors of the nervous system by N-methyl-N-nitrosourea (Janisch et al. 1969). Also, pituitary hormones (indicated by the effects of hypophysectomy) appear to have no influence on the development of liver tumors induced by DMN. This effect is in contrast with those on liver tumor induction by aflatoxin B$_1$, azo dyes, and N-2-fluoreylacetamide (Goodall 1968). Indeed, the methylation of liver nucleic acid by DMN is not influenced by hypophysectomy (Lee and Goodall 1968).

Other carcinogens and toxicants: Combined feeding with 3-methylcholanthrene and DMN appears to have enhanced lung tumor induction in rats (Hoch-Ligeti et al. 1968). Cardesa et al. (1973) have observed a similar effect in mice; in addition, an increased incidence of kidney tumors compared to control animals also has been observed. Exposure to tobacco smoke, aldehydes, volatile acids, and methylnitrite increases bronchial metaplasia and tracheal papilloma incidence in hamsters treated previously with DEN (Wynder and Hoffmann 1967). Diethylenenitrosamine also increases the susceptibility of the lungs to tumor induction by 3,4-benzopyrene and/or ferric oxide particles (Montesano et al. 1970). Subcarcinogenic intratracheal doses of 3,4-benzo-pyrene plus ferric oxide followed by similar systemic doses of DEN induces squamous cell carcinoma of the tracheobronchial tract (Montesano et al. 1974).

The incidence of kidney tumors in rats has been increased when a single dose of DMN is administered following treatment with carbon tetrachloride (Pound et al. 1973a,b). This effect is correlated to the increased metabolism in the liver owing to CCl_4 poisoning. Phenobarbitone has been reported to increase stomach tumor formation with DEN, but decreases liver tumor formation (Kunz et al. 1969).

Synergism also has been observed between the hepatocarcinogenic mycotoxin, sterigmatocystin (STG) and DMN (Terao et al. 1978). In this case, 75% of rats fed diets containing 10 ppm STG plus 1 ppm DMN developed liver carcinomas compared to 53% in those fed 10 ppm STG alone. The latency period was also markedly shortened with the carcinogen combination. The combination also increased the formation of Leydig-cell tumors compared to STG alone.

Ethylmethanesulfonate, also a strong carcinogen, also additively enhances the carcinogenic action of DMN on rat kidney (Montesano et al. 1970).

Infections: An increased incidence of lung tumors has been observed in mice treated with DEN and infected with flu virus (Schmidt-Ruppin and Papadopulu 1972). Hepatitis virus (Motol virus) infection also increases the incidence of liver tumors induced by DEN (Kordac et al. 1969). Rats with chronic murine pneumonia similarly show increased lung tumor development as induced by N-nitrosoheptamethyleneimine compared to those without the pathogen or to germ-free animals (Schreiber et al. 1972).

Nutritional factors: Protein deficiency tends to aggravate the carcinogenic action of DMN on the rat kidney, but not on the liver (McLean and Magee 1970; McLean and Verschuuren 1969), but protects the latter from acute toxicity of DMN. This effect can be related to the decreased metabolic activation of the carcinogen in the liver, but not in the kidney (Swann and McLean 1971). DL-Tryptophan enhances the development of liver tumors in rats treated with DEN (Okajima et al. 1971), but causes a decrease in such tumors with dibutylnitrosamine (DBN) (Kawachi et al. 1968). The reason for this difference is unclear. However, it has been shown that tryptophan increases the demethylase activity in the liver (Evarts and Mostafa 1978) and demethylation by these enzymes has been postulated to be necessary for the activation of the carcinogens (see next section). DBN is exclusively a liver carcinogen at high doses (75 mg/kg) (Druckrey et al. 1962). At low doses (20 mg/kg), its target tissue shifts predominantly to the bladder (Druckrey et al. 1967).

A similar divergent effect has been seen with high fat diets. Rogers et al. (1974) have observed that high fat diets, very low on lipotropes, enhances the hepatocarcinogenicity of DEN and DBN, but not DMN. This may be related to the observations reported by Agrelo et al. (1978) that fat in the diet retards the absorption of nitrosamines commonly found in food, and that the small intestine has the ability to degrade DMN. Presumably, such retardation increases the extent of DMN degradation, so that the concentration reaching the liver is markedly reduced. One has to conclude from this that such retardation causes some other mechanism to predominate so that the carcinogenicity of these compounds is enhanced.

Copper, nickel, and cobalt enhance the carcinogenicity of alkylnitrosoureas (Ivankovic et al. 1972; Zeller and Ivankovic 1972). However, whereas diets deficient or excessive in copper have no effect on liver tumor formation with DMN, the former causes 57% of rats to develop kidney tumors, and none in the latter.

Inhibitory factors: Certain factors will diminish the carcinogenic potential of N-nitroso compounds. These factors are of two types: (1) those that decrease the metabolism of the carcinogen, and (2) those that retard or interfere in the formation of the carcinogen. Examples of the first type are aminoacetonitrile (Fiume et al. 1970; Hadjiolov 1971), dibenamine (Weisburger et al. 1974), and phenobarbitone (Kunz et al. 1969). The hepatocarcinogenicity of DMN is diminished by aminoacetonitrile and dibenamine and that of DEN by phenobarbitone. It has been shown by both in vivo and in vitro tests that aminoacetonitrile inhibits the metabolism of DMN and markedly decreases the methylation of nucleic acids (Fiume et al. 1970; Hadjiolov and Mundt 1974). Similar effects are presumed for dibenamine and phenobarbitone.

Examples of the second type include ascorbic acid, tannins, sulfite, and cysteine. These factors were discussed earlier in this section (pp. 634–635).

Other Toxic Effects of N-Nitroso Compounds The acute hepatotoxicity of nitrosamines has been discussed. The nitrosamides appear to be less damaging to the liver. Because of their instability they are more likely to cause injury at the site of application (Shank 1975).

The mutagenicity of these compounds can be deduced from their carcinogenicity. Whereas nitrosamides are directly mutagenic in bacterial systems as well as in Drosophila (Magee and Barnes 1967), nitrosamines are mutagenic in the insect and in bacterial systems after activation; i.e., after exposure to rat liver microsomes (Malling 1971). Mutagenicity also has been demonstrated for DMN by means of the host-mediated assay (Gabridge and Legator 1969) and in the *Salmonella typhimurium*-liver microsome system (Czygan et al. 1973).

Mutagenicity by means of the dominant lethal test in mammals has not been shown to occur in the case of DMN (Epstein and Shafner 1968).

Teratogenic action appears to have been demonstrated in the case of nitrosamines only when administered late in pregnancy (Pielsticker et al. 1967). This is probably related to the lack of activation in the unborn animal early in its development. However, the nitrosamides are quite active teratogens; N-nitrosomethylurea (NMU) when given to rats on the thirteenth or fourteenth day of gestation causes fetal deaths, and resorption and deformities in the case of those that survive to term (von Kreybig 1965). This compound also has been observed to be a potent teratogen when administered to rats before the twelfth day of pregnancy (Napalkov and Alexandrov 1968). Intravenous administration of NMU also produces deformities in pig fetuses (Ehrentraut et al. 1969).

Metabolism of N-Nitroso Compounds and Proposed Mechanisms of Carcinogenic Action

The metabolism of nitrosamines is correlated with its carcinogenicity in specific tissues. Thus, the organotropicity of specific nitrosamines depends on the metabolic activity of the target tissue. For example, tumors are produced more frequently by DMN in the liver than in any other tissue of the rat because this carcinogen is metabolized more actively by this tissue (Magee and Barnes 1967; Montesano and Magee 1971).

The postulated reaction steps in the metabolism of nitrosamines as shown by Druckrey (1975) are as follows:

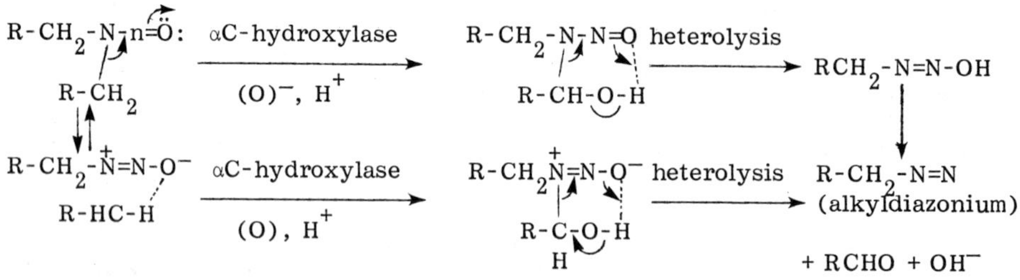

The alkyldiazonium compound then decomposes to produce the carbonium ion, the alkylating species (Nagata and Imamura 1970). Alkylation of nucleic acids has been widely proposed as an important step in nitroso-compound carcinogenesis (Druckrey 1975), although there are reports which cast doubt on this theory (Lijinsky and Ross 1969; Lijinsky et al. 1968). However, there is enough evidence on the side of alkylation to maintain the viability of this theory.

The initial oxidation or hydroxylation step leads to unstable intermediates.

In the case of higher homologs of nitrosamines, β-oxidation of the alkyl side chains has been demonstrated to occur (Kruger 1972). This leads to chain shortening similar to fatty acid oxidation. Thus, the metabolism of dipropyl- or dibutylnitrosamine produces both 7-propyl or 7-butylguanine, and in both cases 7-methylguanine (Kruger 1972). Therefore, a mixed reaction system involving initial β-oxidation followed by α-oxidation of either alkyl chain can be expected to occur.

Lijinsky et al. (1968) has proved conclusively by means of totally deuterated DMN that the methylation of nucleic acids involves direct transfer of the intact methyl group and not through a diazoalkane intermediate.

Hydroxylation at other carbon atoms on the alkyl side chain is, of course, possible (Druckrey et al. 1964). Indeed, such a postulated intermediate of dibutylnitrosamine as butyl(4-hydroxybutyl) nitrosamine has proved to be a very potent and highly specific bladder carcinogen in the rat (Blattmann and Preussmann 1973; Druckrey et al. 1964) through its proximate carcinogen, and major urinary metabolite, butyl-(3-carboxypropyl) nitrosamine (Hashimoto et al. 1972).

The major point of attack by alkylnitroso compounds in nucleic acids is the N(7)-position of guanine (Magee 1969); however, significant alkylation can also occur at other sites (Lawley 1972). Of major interest and probably more relevant to the mechanism of carcinogenesis is the methylation at the O(6)-position of guanine (Loveless (1969). This is so because compounds such as N-methyl- or N-ethyl-N-nitrosourea and ethylmethanesulfonate, which are mutagenic in bacteriophage, alkylate at the O(6)-position, whereas the nonmutagenic methylmethanesulfonate does not, or at least only minimally (Lawley and Shah 1972). It also has been shown that polynucleotides containing O(6)-methylguanine produce abnormal base pairing (Gerchman and Ludlum 1973).

Another position for alkylation which also has been suggested as more relevant to the mechanism of carcinogenesis is the 3-position of cytosine (Ludlum 1970; Ludlum and Wilhelm 1968). It has been shown that in an in vitro system with synthetic polynucleotide, 3-methylcytosine not only reduces the incorporation of guanosine triphosphate (UTP) by RNA polymerase, but also produces incorrect polymers of guanylic and uridylic acids. Similar effects have been observed when the polycytidylic template is treated with N-methyl- or N-ethyl-N-nitrosourea (Ludlum and Magee 1972).

Even though the N(7)-position of guanine is the major site for alkylation with nitroso compound, there are many examples of poor correlation between maximal N(7)-guanine methylation at a given tissue and the formation of tumors (Kleihues et al. 1973; Schoental 1969; Swann and Magee 1971). The evidence, however, does not completely rule out the importance of N(7)-position of guanine because it is possible that methylation of guanine at a specific locus in DNA may be more important.

Relevance of N-Nitroso Compounds to Human Cancer

No animal species that has been tested so far is resistant to DMN or DEN, the two nitrosamines commonly found in foodstuffs (Lijinsky and Taylor 1977). Thus, the common consensus of investigators in the field is that humans cannot be expected to be resistant to the nitrosamines (Druckrey 1975; Mirvish 1977; Weisburger and Raineri 1975; Wogan and Tannenbaum 1975). One interesting property of nitrosamines is that they are particularly effective when exposure is through the oral route, at small doses and over a long period. This is particularly relevant to the human situation. These compounds are systemically organotropic and will induce tumors in target tissues independent of the route of administration. It also has been shown that in the rat, every organ is susceptible to the carcinogenic action of these compounds (Lijinsky and Taylor 1977).

Biochemical studies with human liver in vitro have produced evidence that nitrosamines are metabolized and interact with nucleic acids, as in animal livers (Montesano and Magee 1974). This suggests that human metabolism of nitrosamines may also produce similar proximate carcinogens.

The increased gastric cancer rates in certain areas of Colombia in South America have been related to the high levels of nitrate in the drinking water in these areas

(Cuello et al. 1976). This situation is considered by Tannenbaum et al. (1977) to be related to the high rates of atrophic gastritis in the high-risk populations which results in hypoacidity in the stomach, followed by colonization of the same by bacteria; reduction of nitrate to nitrite and resultant formation of nitroso compound follows. The suspected compound is assumed to be a nitrosocyanamide on the basis of the results of Endo et al. (1975).

Weisburger and Raineri (1975) have suggested that the decreased incidence of gastric cancer in the United States in recent years compared to the early 1920s or 1930s is related to the universal use of the refrigerator. They contend that refrigeration inhibits nitrate to nitrite conversion and thus, nitrosamine formation.

Finally, it might be argued that the level of nitrosamines in foodstuffs is too low to present any real hazard. However, one must remember that one is not exposed to just one type of nitrosamine, as can be judged from the many types of nitrosamine precursors that are likely to be present in food and the environment (Table 12.2). Furthermore, one is most likely to be exposed to several carcinogens at any given time and other toxicologically important compounds. The experiments reported by Schmahl (1976) appear to be relevant to this issue: Four hepatocarcinogens, DMN, DEN, nitrosomorpholine, and p-dimethylaminoazobenzene when administered together, each, at subcarcinogenic doses produce liver cancer in more than half of rats after a trial period of 600 days. Individually, at the same doses used in the combination, no tumor develops.

When the amounts of total nitrosamines in food, water, and other sources are added to those formed throughout the alimentary tract (which could be quite large), the total nitrosamine load of modern populations would be considerable. Viewed from this perspective, each carcinogen, even in trace amounts, assumes considerable significance.

Methionine Sulfoximine

Wheat flour used to be treated with agene (nitrogen trichloride) for bleaching purposes and to improve baking quality. This practice was abandoned when it was shown that flour so treated caused canine hysteria (Mellanby 1946). Dogs and rabbits suffer symptoms suggesting that the toxic factor affects the central nervous system. The toxic factor was identified as methionine sulfoximine, which is produced by reacting nitrogen trichloride with the methionine moiety of wheat proteins (Bentley et al. 1950; Reiner et al. 1950).

$$CH_3-\underset{\underset{NH}{\|}}{\overset{\overset{O}{\|}}{S}}-(CH_2)_2-\underset{\underset{NH_2}{|}}{CH}-COOH$$

methionine sulfoximine

This toxicant is a convulsant and can be antagonized by methionine.

Methionine sulfoximine is a methionine antagonist, since its inhibitory effect on the growth of the bacteria *Leuconostoc mesenteriodes* can be overcome by the essential amino acid (Heathcote 1949; Reiner et al. 1950).

There has been no report that the derived toxicant has an effect in man.

Ethylenethiourea

Ethylenethiourea is a decomposition product of ethylenebisdithiocarbamate (EBDC) fungicides such as maneb, Dithane M-45, Manzate 200, Polyram, Mancozeb, and Zineb (Marshall 1977; Newsome 1976; Watts et al. 1974).

Zineb   ETU

Various types of EBDC insecticides added to spinach, potatoes, and carrots when heated decompose to ETU to the extent of 11 to 26.5% on the basis of an ETU/EBDC ratio (Watts et al. 1974). The levels of ETU in apples or tomatoes containing 50 ppm zineb increase markedly from about fivefold to more than 10-fold when boiled under reflux for 15 min (Newsome and Laver 1973). Tomatoes field sprayed with EBDC insecticides when cooked for 10 min show a 38 to 40% conversion to ETU.

Decomposition of EBDC also occurs during normal food processing procedures (Baron 1978).

Because the EBDCs are widely used on crops, their residues are detected in foods. This aspect is discussed in Chapter 19. These products have been found to have very low levels of ETU (Yip et al. 1971).

Ethylenethiourea is among those compounds which are listed by the International Agency for Research on Cancer (IARC) as having been adequately tested for carcinogenicity in at least one experimental animal (Tomatis 1977). In fact, ETU has been shown to induce liver and other tumors in mice (Innes et al. 1969) and cancers of the thyroid in rats (Ulland et al. 1972). Also, Khera (1973) has reported that ETU is teratogenic in rats. Tests on a strain of *S. typhimurium* have proved ETU to be weakly mutagenic (Seiler 1974).

Ethylenethiourea also has been shown to cause minimal or moderate heteroploidy in in vivo, a cytogenic test using bone marrow in rats. No chromosomal damage was seen in this test nor in an in vitro test using Chinese hamster Don cell line (Shirasu et al. 1977). A dominant lethal test in ICR mice also proved negative. The lack of activity of ETU in other tissues except the thyroid (Newsome 1974) has been suggested by its weakly mutagenic activity and the lack of cytogenic effects (Shirasu et al. 1977). In contrast, previous researchers have shown that ETU is a potent oncogen and teratogen (Graham and Hansen 1972; Graham et al. 1973).

Ethylenethiourea is also a goitrogen in rats (Seifter et al. 1948).

CONCLUSIONS

Numerous examples are given in this chapter which illustrate that the chemistry of foodstuffs and of food preparation, processing, and storage has profound toxicological and public health significance. In the past, the traditional or standard practices of food preparation were assumed to be of no toxicological significance. The accumulated knowledge in this area should, however, convince the traditionalists that derived toxicants in food may pose serious health hazards. Food scientists and professionals must be cognizant of the fact that the chemistry of foodstuffs may be drastically changed toxicologically during food preparation, processing, and storage. For example, it has been reported that desirable browning of bakery, vegetable, and meat products may not be as innocuous as it may seem. It has been found that commercially prepared refrigerated and frozen dishes, heated according to the manufacturers' directions, produce mutagens (Iwaoka and Meaker 1979). The mutagenic activity in these foods increases with prolonged heating.

It is obvious that research on the toxicological implications of the chemical interactions of food components must be vigorously pursued.

REFERENCES

Adrian, J. 1974. Nutritional and physiological consequences of Maillard reaction. *World Rev. Diet.* 19: 72–123.

Adrian, J. and Frange, R. 1973. The Maillard reaction. 8. Effect of premelanoidines on nitrogen diegestibility and proteolysis. *Ann. Nutr.* 27: 111–123.

Agrelo, C. et al. 1978. Studies on the gastrointestinal absorption of N-nitrosamines: Effect of dietary constituents. *Toxicology* 10: 159–167.

Alam, B. S., Saporoschetz, I. B. and Epstein, S. S. 1971a. Synthesis of nitrosopiperidine from nitrate and piperidine in the gastrointestinal tract of the rat. *Nature* 232: 199–200.

Alam, B. S., Saporoschetz, I. B. and Epstein, S. S. 1971b. Formation of N-nitrosopiperidine from piperidine and sodium nitrite in the stomach and the isolated intestinal loop of the rat. *Nature* 232: 116–118.

Alarcon, R. A. 1972. Acrolein, a component of a universal cellgrowth regulatory system: A theory. *J. Theoret. Biol.* 37: 159–167.

Alarcon, R. A. 1976. Formation of acrolein from various amino acids and polyamines under degradation at 100°C. *Environ. Res.* 12: 317–326.

Alexandrov, V. A. 1968. Blastomogenic effects of dimethylnitrosamine on pregnant rats and their offspring. *Nature* 218: 280–281.

Ambrose, A. M., Robbins, D. J. and De Eds, F. 1961. Acute and subacute toxicity of amino-hexose reductones. *Proc. Soc. Exp. Biol. Med.* 106: 656–659.

Ames, B. N., Durston, W. E., Yamasaki, E. and Lee, F. D. 1973. Carcinogens are mutagens: A simple test system combining liver homogenates for activation and bacteria for detection. *Proc. Natl. Acad. Sci.* 70: 2281–2285.

Ames, B. N., McCann, J. and Yamasaki, E. 1975. Methods for detecting carcinogens and mutagens with the Salmonella/mammalian-microsome mutagenicity test. *Mutat. Res.* 31: 347–364.

Andia, A. M. and Street, J. C. 1975. Dietary induction of hepatic microsomal enzymes by thermally oxidized fats. *J. Agric. Food Chem.* 23: 173–177.

Andrews, J. S., Griffith, W. H., Mead, J. F. and Stein, R. A. 1960. Toxicity of air oxidized soybean oil. *J. Nutr.* 70: 199–210.

Anstis, P. J. P. and Friend, J. 1974. The isoenzyme distribution of etiolated pea seedling. Lipoxygenase. *Planta* 115: 329–335.

Archer, M. C., Clark, S. D., Thilly, J. E. and Tannenbaum, S. R. 1971. Environmental nitroso compounds. Reaction of nitrite with creatine and creatinine. *Science* 174: 1341–1342.

Arcos, J. C. and Argus, M. F. 1968. Molecular geometry and carcinogenic activity of aromatic compounds. New perspectives. *Adv. Cancer Res.* 11: 305–471.

Artman, N. R. 1969. Chemical and biological properties of heated and oxidized fats. *Adv. Lipid Res.* 7: 245–330.

Asatoor, A. M., Levi, A. J. and Milne, M. D. 1963. Tranylcypromine and cheese. *Lancet* 2: 733–734.

Aymard, C., Creq, J. L. and Cheftel, J. C. 1978. Formation of lysinoalanine and lanthionine in various food proteins, heated at neutral or alkaline pH. *Food Chem.* 3: 1–5.

Badger, G. M. 1962. *The Chemical Basis of Carcinogenic Activity.* Charles C Thomas, Springfield, Illinois.

Barger, G. and Walpole, G. S. 1909. Isolation of the pressor principles of putrid meat. *J. Physiol.* 38: 343–352.

Barnes, J. M. and Magee, P. N. 1954. Some toxic properties of dimethylnitrosamine. *Br. J. Ind. Med.* 11: 167–174.

Baron, R. L. 1978. *Cited by* W. D. Marshall. Oxidation of ethylenebisdithiocarbamate fungicides and ethylenethiuram monosulfide to prevent the subsequent decomposition to ethylenethiourea. *J. Agric. Food Chem.* 26: 110—115.

Beatty, S. A. 1938. Fish spoilage II. Origin of trimethylamine produced during the spoilage of cod muscle pressed juice. *J. Fish Res. Board Can.* 4: 63—68.

Behroozi, K., Guttman, R., Gruener, N. and Shuval, H. I. 1972. *Cited by* H. I. Shuval and N. Gruener. Epidemiological and toxicological aspects of nitrates and nitrites in the environment. *Am. J. Public Health* 62: 1045—1052.

Bentley, H. R., McDermott, E. E. and Whitehead, J. K. 1950a. Action of nitrogen trichloride on proteins: A synthesis of the toxic factor from methionine. *Nature* 165: 735.

Bentley, H. R. et al. 1950b. Action of nitrogen trichloride on certain proteins. I. Isolation and identification of the toxic factor. *Proc. R. Soc.* B137: 402—417.

Bertram, I. S. and Craig, A. W. 1970. Induction of bladder tumours in mice with dibutylnitrosamine. *Br. J. Cancer* 24: 352—359.

Bertram, I. S. and Craig, A. W. 1972. Specific induction of bladder cancer in mice by butyl-(4-hydroxybutyl)-nitrosamine and the effects of hormonal modifications on the sex difference in response. *Eur. J. Cancer* 8: 587—594.

Betke, K., Kleihauer, E. and Lipps, M. 1956. Comparative investigations on the spontaneous oxidation on umbilical cord and fetal hemoglobin. *Z. Kinderchir.* 77: 549—553. (German)

Bills, D. D., Hildrum, K. I., Scanlan, R. A. and Libbey, L. M. 1973. Potential precursors of N-nitrosopyrrolidine in bacon and other fried foods. *J. Agric. Food Chem.* 21: 876—877.

Blackwell, B. 1963. Tranylcypromine. *Lancet* 2: 414.

Blackwell, B. and Mabbitt, L. A. 1965. Tyramine in cheese related to hypertensive crises after monoamine oxidase inhibition. *Lancet* 1: 938—940.

Blackwell, B., Marley, E. and Mabbitt, L. A. 1965. Effects of yeast extract after monoamine oxidase inhibition. *Lancet* 1: 940—943.

Blackwell, B., Marley, E., Price, J. and Taylor, D. 1967. Hypertensive interactions between monoamine oxidase inhibitors and foodstuffs. *Br. J. Psychiatr.* 113: 349—365.

Blattmann, L. and Preussmann, R. 1973. Structure of rat urinary metabolites of carcinogenic dialkylnitrosamines. *Z. Krebsforsch.* 79: 3—7.

Bleumink, E. and Young, E. 1968. Identification of the atopic allergen in cow's milk. *Int. Arch. Allergy Appl. Immunol.* 34: 521—543.

Bohak, Z. 1964. N^6-(DL-2-Amino-2-carboxyethyl)-6-lysine, a new amino acid formed on alkaline treatment of proteins. *J. Biol. Chem.* 239: 2878—2887.

Borgstrom, G. (ed.). 1961. *Fish as Food.* Vol. 1. Academic Press, New York.

Boulton, A. A., Cookson, B. and Paulton, R. 1970. Hypertensive crisis in a patient on MAOI antidepressants following a meal of beef liver. *Can. Med. Assoc. J.* 102: 1394—1395.

Boyland, E., Nice, E. and Williams, K. 1971. The catalysis of nitrosation by thiocyanate from saliva. *Food Cosmet. Toxicol.* 9: 639—643.

Braunsteiner, H., Fellinger, K. and Pakesch, F. 1953. Electron-microscopic observations of normal liver slices and after bile duct obstruction, histamine and allyl formate poisoning. *Z. Ges. Exp. Med.* 121: 254—265.

Brooks, B. R. and Klamerth, O. L. 1968. Interaction of DNA with bifunctional aldehydes, *Eur. J. Biochem.* 5: 178—182.

Brooks, J. B., Cherry, W. B., Thacker, L. and Alley, C. C. 1972. Analysis by gas chromatography of amines and nitrosamines produced in vivo and in vitro by Proteus mirabilis. *J. Infect. Dis.* 126: 143—153.

Bruce, W. R., Varghese, A. J., Furrer, R. and Land, P. C. 1977. A mutagen
  in the feces of normal humans. In: *Origins of Human Cancer. Human Risk
  Assessment.* Book C. H. H. Hiatt, J. D. Watson and J. A. Winsten (eds).
  Cold Spring Harbor Laboratory, Cold Spring Harbor, New York.

Burroughs, S. E., Mathews, R. D. and Calloway, D. H. 1964. Toxicity of heat-
  damaged anchovy oil. *Fed. Proc. Fed. Am. Soc. Exp. Biol.* 23: 551. Abstract
  No. 2697.

Cardesa, A. et al. 1973. The syncarcinogenic effect of methylcholanthrene and
  dimethylnitrosamine in Swiss mice. *Z. Krebsforsch.* 79: 98–107.

Cardesa, A. et al. 1974. Inhibitory effect of ascorbic acid on the acute toxicity
  of dimethylamine plus nitrite in the rat (37761). *Proc. Soc. Exp. Biol. Med.*
  145: 124–128.

Carson, P. E., Flanagan, C. L., Ickes, C. E. and Alving, A. S. 1956. Enzymic
  deficiency in primaquine-sensitive erythrocytes. *Science* 124: 484–485.

Castell, C. H., Neal, W. and Smith, B. 1970. Formation of dimethylamine in stored
  frozen sea fish. *J. Fish Res. Board Can.* 27: 1685–1690.

Castell, C. H., Smith, B. and Neal, W. 1971. Production of dimethylamine in
  muscle of several species of Gadoid fish during frozen storage, especially in
  relation to presence of dark muscle. *J. Fish. Res. Board Can.* 28: 1–5.

Chang, C. C., Esselman, W. J. and Clagett, C. O. 1971. The isolation and
  specificity of alfalfa lipoxygenase. *Lipids* 6: 100–106.

Chio, K. S. and Tappel, A. L. 1969. Inactivation of ribonuclease and other
  enzymes by peroxidizing lipids and by malonaldehyde. *Biochemistry* 8: 2827–
  2832.

Christopher, J. P., Pistorius, E. K. and Axelrod, B. 1972. Isolation of a third
  isoenzyme of soybean lipoxygenase. *Biochim. Biophys. Acta* 2861: 54–62.

Collin-Thompson, D. L., Sen, N. P., Aris, B. and Schwinghamer, L. 1972. Nonenzymatic in vitro formation of nitrosamines by bacteria isolated from meat
  products. *Can. J. Microbiol.* 18: 1968–1971.

Collis, C. H., Cook, P. J., Foreman, J. K. and Palframan, J. F. 1971. A search
  for nitrosamines in East African spirit samples from areas of varying oesopha-
  geal cancer frequency. *Gut* 12: 1015–1018.

Commoner, B. et al. 1978. Formation of mutagens in beef and beef extract during
  cooking. *Science* 201: 913–916.

Concon, J. M., Swerczek, T. W. and Newburg, D. S. 1979. Black pepper (Piper
  nigrum): Evidence of carcinogenicity. *Nutr. Cancer* 1: 22–26.

Conney, A. H. 1967. Pharmacological implications of microsomal enzyme induction.
  Pharmacol. Rev. 19: 317–366.

Cook, J. W., Heiger, I., Kennaway, E. L. and Mayneord, W. V. 1932. The
  production of cancer by pure hydrocarbons. Part I. *Proc. R. Soc. B* III:
  455–484.

Corfield, M. C. et al. 1967. The formation of lysinoalanine during the treatment
  of wool with alkali. *Biochem. J.* 103: 15c–16c.

Cornblath, M. and Hartmann, A. F. 1948. Methemoglobinemia in young infants.
  J. Pediatr. 33: 421–425.

Craddock, V. M. 1971. Liver carcinomas induced in rats by single administration
  of dimethylnitrosamine after partial hepatectomy. *J. Natl. Cancer Inst.* 47:
  889–905.

Craddock, V. M. 1973. Induction of liver tumours in rats by a single treatment
  with nitroso compounds given after partial hepatectomy. *Nature* 245: 386–388.

Crosby, N. T., Foreman, J. K., Palframan, J. F. and Sawyer. R. 1972.
  Estimation of steam-volatile N-nitrosamines in foods at the 1 ug/kg level.
  Nature 238: 342–343.

Cuello, C. et al. 1976. Gastric ulcer in Colombia. 1. Cancer risk and suspect environmental agents. *J. Natl. Cancer Inst.* 57: 1015–1020.

Cutler, M. G. and Schneider, R. 1973a. Sensitivity of feeding tests in detecting carcinogenic properties in chemicals: Examination of 7,12-dimethylbenz(a)anthracene and oxidized linoleate. *Food Cosmet. Toxicol.* 11: 443–457.

Cutler, M. G. and Schneider, R. 1973b. Malformations produced in mice and rats by oxidized linoleate. *Food Cosmet. Toxicol.* 11: 935–942.

Czok, G. et al. 1964. Physiological action and metabolism of dimeric fatty acids. I. Physiological action. *Z. Ernahrungwiss.* 5: 80–89. (German)

Czygan, P. et al. 1973. Microsomal metabolism of dimethylnitrosamine and the cytochrome P450 dependency of its activation to a mutagen. *Cancer Res.* 33: 2983–2986.

Davies, W. and Wilmshurst, J. R. 1960. Carcinogens formed in the heating of foodstuffs. Formation of 3,4-benzopyrene from starch at 370-390°C. *Br. J. Cancer* 14: 295–299.

De Groot, A. P. and Slump, P. 1969. Effects of severe alkali treatment of proteins on amino acid composition and nutritive value. *J. Nutr.* 98: 45–56.

De Groot, A. P., Slump, P., Van Beek, L. and Feron, V. J. 1976a. Severe alkali treatment of proteins. In: *Evaluation of Proteins for Humans.* C. E. Bodwell (ed.). AVI, Westport, Connecticut.

De Groot, A. P., Slump, P., Feron, V. J. and Van Beek, L. 1976b. Effects of alkali-treated proteins: Feeding studies with free and protein-bound lysinoalanine in rats and other animals. *J. Nutr.* 106: 1527–1538.

Denlinger, R. H., Koestner, A. and Wechsler, W. 1974. Induction of neurogenic tumors in C3Heb/FeJ mice by nitrosourea derivatives: Observations by light microscopy, tissue culture, and electron microscopy. *Int. J. Cancer* 13: 559–571.

Diwan, B. A., Meier, H. and Huebner, R. J. 1973. Transplacental effects of 1-ethyl-1-nitrosurea in inbred strains of mice. III. Association between infectious or subinfectious endogenous type-C RNA tumor virus expression and chemically induced tumorigenesis. *J. Natl. Cancer Inst.* 51: 1965–1970.

Doll, R. 1952. The causes of death among gas workers with special reference to cancer of the lung. *Br. J. Ind. Med.* 9: 180–185.

Dollahite, J. W. and Holt, E. C. 1970. Nitrate poisoning. *S. Afr. Med. J.* 44: 171–174.

Druckrey, H. 1975. Chemical carcinogenesis on N-nitroso derivatives. *Gann Monogr. Cancer Res.* 17: 107–132.

Druckrey, H., Preussmann, R., Schmähl, D. and Mueller, M. 1962. Production of bladder cancer in rats by N,N-dibutylnitrosamine. *Naturwissenschaften* 49: 19. (German)

Druckrey, H., Steinhoff, D., Preussmann, R. and Ivankovic, S. 1963a. Tumor production with several doses of methylnitrosourea and several dialkylnitrosamines. *Naturwissenschaften* 50: 735. (German)

Druckrey, H. et al. 1963b. Formation of esophageal cancer by means of unsymmetrical nitrosamines. *Naturwissenschaften* 50: 100–101.

Druckrey, H., Ivankovic, S., Mennel, H. D. and Preussman, R. 1964. Selective production of carcinomas of the nasal cavity in rats by N,N'-dinitrosopiperazine, nitrosopiperidine, nitrosomorpholine, methylallylnitrosamine, dimethylnitrosamine, and methylvinylnitrosamine. *Z. Krebsforsch.* 66: 138–150.

Druckrey, H., Landschütz, C. and Ivankovic, S. 1970. Transplacental induction of malignant tumors of the nervous system. II. Ethylnitrosourea in ten genetically defined rat strains. *Z. Krebsforsch.* 73: 371–386.

Dungal, N. 1958. Can smoked food have a carcinogenic effect. *Krebsarzt.* 14: 22–24.

Eckardt, R. E. 1959. *Industrial Carcinogens.* Grune & Stratton, New York.

Ehrentraut, W. et al. 1969. Experimental malformations in swine-foetuses caused by intravenous application of N-ethyl-N-nitroso-urea. *Arch. Geschwulstforsch.* 33: 31–38.

Eichel, B. and Shahrik, H. A. 1969. Tobacco smoke toxicity: loss of human oral leukocyte function and fluid-cell metabolism. *Science* 166: 1424–1428.

Eisenbrand, G., Ungerer, O. and Preussmann, R. 1974. Rapid formation of carcinogenic N-nitrosamines by interaction of nitrite with fungicides derived from dithiocarbamic acid in vitro under simulated gastric conditions and in vivo in the rat stomach. *Food Cosmet. Toxicol.* 12: 229–232.

Elespuru, R. K. and Lijinsky, W. 1973. The formation of carcinogenic nitroso compounds from nitrite and some types of agricultural chemicals. *Food Cosmet. Toxicol.* 11: 807–817.

Elespuru, R., Lijinsky, W. and Setlow, J. K. 1974. Nitrosocarbaryl as a potent mutagen of environmental significance. *Nature* 247: 386–387.

Ender, R. F. and Ceh, L. 1971. Conditions and chemical reaction mechanisms by which nitrosamines may be formed in biological products with reference to their possible occurrence in food products. *Z. Lebensm. Unters. Forsch.* 145: 133–142.

Endo, H. and Takahashi, K. 1973a. Identification and property of the mutagenic principle formed from a food component, methylguanidine, after nitrosation in simulated gastric juice. *Biochem. Biophys. Res. Commun.* 54: 1384–1392.

Endo, H. and Takahashi, K. 1973b. Methylguanidine, a naturally occurring compound showing mutagenicity after nitrosation in gastric juice. *Nature* 245: 325–326.

Endo, H., Takahashi, K. and Aoyagi, H. 1974. Screening of compounds structurally and functionally related to N-methyl-N'-nitro-N'nitrosoguanidine, a gastric carcinogen. *Gann* 65: 45–54.

Endo, H. et al. 1975. An approach to the detection of possible etiologic factors in human gastric cancer. *Gann Monogr. Cancer Res.* 17: 17–29.

Endo, H. et al. 1977. A possible process of conversion of food components to gastric carcinogens. In: *Origins of Human Cancer.* H. H. Hiatt, J. D. Watson and J. A. Winsten, (eds.). Cold Spring Harbor Laboratory, Cold Spring Harbor, New York.

Epstein, S. S. 1972. In vivo studies on interactions between secondary amines and nitrites and nitrates. In: *N-Nitroso Compounds: Analysis and Formation.* IARC Scientific Publications No. 3, International Agency for Research on Cancer, Lyon.

Epstein, S. S. and Shafner, H. 1968. Chemical mutagens in the human environment. *Nature* 219: 385–387.

Erbersdobler, H. F., Von Wangenheim, B. and Hänichen, T. 1978. Adverse effects of Maillard products—especially of fructoselysine—in the organism. Abstr. XI Intern. Congr. Nutr., Rio de Janiero, Brazil.

Evarts, R. P. and Mostafa, M. H. 1978. The effect of $_L$-tryptophan and certain other amino acids on liver nitrosodimethylamine demethylase activity. *Food Cosmet. Toxicol.* 16: 585–589.

Fan, T. Y. and Tannenbaum, S. R. 1973. Factors influencing the rate of formation of nitrosomorpholine from morpholine and nitrite: Acceleration by thiocyanate and other anions. *J. Agric. Food Chem.* 21: 237–240.

Fandre, M., Coffin, R., Dropsy, G. and Bergel, J. D. 1962. Epidemic of infantile gastroenteritis due to Escherichia coli 0127 B8 with methemoglobinemic cyanosis. *Arch. Franc. Pediatr.* 19: 1129–1131. (French)

Fazio, T. et al. 1971a. Gas chromatographic determination and mass spectrometric confirmation of N-nitrosodimethylamine in smoke-processed marine fish. *J. Agric. Food Chem.* 19: 250−253.

Fazio, T., White, R. H. and Howard, J. W. 1971b. Analysis of nitrite-and/or nitrate-processed meats for N-nitrosodimethylamine. *J. Assoc. Offic. Anal. Chem.* 54: 1157−1159.

Fazio, T., White, R. H., Dusold, L. R. and Howard J. 1973. Nitrosopyrrolidine in cooked bacon. *J. Assoc. Offic. Anal. Chem.* 56: 919−921.

Ferencik, M. 1970. Formation of histamine during bacterial decarboxylation of histidine in the flesh of some marine fishes. *J. Hyg. Epidemiol. Microbiol. Immunol.* 14: 52−60.

Feron, V. J., Van Beek, L., Slump, P. and Beems, R. B. 1977. Toxicological aspects of alkali treatment of food proteins. In: *Biochemical Aspects of New Protein Food.* J. Adler-Nissen et al. (eds.). Federation of European Biochemical Societies 44, Symposium A3.

Ferrando, R. 1963. Biological effect of heating meat in the presence of hexosamine (D-glucosamine). *C. R. Acad. Sci.* 257: 1161−1163. (French)

Ferrando, R. 1964. Maillard reaction and the preparation of meat meal. Biological effects. *Bull. Acad. Natl. Med.* 148: 570−576. (French)

Ferrando, R., Henry, N. and Parodi, A. 1964. Biological effect of heating meat in the presence of hexosamine (D-glucosamine). *C. R. Acad. Sci.* 259: 1237−1238. (French)

Fiddler, W. 1975. The occurrence and determination of N-nitroso compounds. *Toxicol. Appl. Pharmacol.* 31: 352−360.

Fiddler, W., Pensabene, J. W., Doerr, R. C. and Wasserman, A. E. 1972. Formation of N-nitrosodimethylamine from naturally-occurring quarternary ammonium compounds and tertiary amines. *Nature* 236: 307.

Fiddler, W. et al. 1973. Use of sodium ascorbate or erythorbate to inhibit formation of N-nitrosodimethylamine in frankfurters. *J. Food Sci.* 38: 1084.

Fimreite, N. 1970. Effects of methylmercury treated feed on the mortality and growth of leghorn cockerels. *Can. J. Anim. Sci.* 50: 387−389.

Fink, H., Schlie, I. and Ruge, U. 1968. The nutritional changes in milk following commercial drying. *Z. Naturforsch.* 13B: 610−616.

Fiume, L., Campadelli-Fiume, G., Magee, P. N. and Holsman, J. 1970. Cellular injury and carcinogenesis. Inhibition of metabolism of dimethylnitrosamine by aminoacetonitrile. *Biochem. J.* 120: 601−605.

Fong, Y. Y. and Chan, W. C. 1973a. Dimethylnitrosamine in Chinese marine salt fish. *Food Cosmet. Toxicol.* 11: 841−845.

Fong, Y. Y. and Chan, W. C. 1973b. Bacterial production of dimethylnitrosamine in salted fish. *Nature* 243: 421−422.

Fong, Y. Y. and Chan, W. C. 1977. Nitrate, nitrite, dimethylnitrosamine and N-nitrosopyrrolidine in some Chinese food products. *Food Cosmet. Toxicol.* 15: 143−145.

Frankel, E. N., Evans, C. D. and Cowan, J. C. 1960. Thermal dimerization of fatty ester hydroperoxides. *J. Am. Oil Chem. Soc.* 37: 418−424.

Frazer, A. C. 1962. The possible role of dietary factors in the aetiology and pathogenesis of sprue, coeliac disease and idiopathic steatorrhoea. *Proc. Nutr. Soc.* 21: 42−52.

Freund, H. A. 1937. Clinical manifestations and studies in parenchymatous hepatitis. *Ann. Intern. Med.* 10: 1144−1155.

Friedman, M. A. 1972. Nitrosation of sarcosine, chemical kinetics and gastric assay. *Bull. Envir. Contam. Toxicol.* 8: 375−381.

Friedman, M. A., Miller, G. N. and Epstein, S. S. 1973. Acute dose dependent inhibition of liver nuclear RNA synthesis and methylation of guanine following oral administration of sodium nitrite and dimethylamine to mice. *Int. J. Environ. Studies* 4: 219–222.

Gabridge, M. G. and Legator, M. S. 1969. A host mediated microbial assay for the detection of mutagenic compounds. *Proc. Soc. Exp. Biol. Med.* 130: 831–834.

Galliard, T. and Phillips, D. R. 1971. Lipoxygenase from potato tubers. Partial purification and properties of an enzyme that specifically oxygenates the 9-position of linoleic acid. *Biochem. J.* 124: 431–438.

Gardner, H. W. 1975. Decomposition of linoleic acid hydroperoxides. Enzymic reactions compared with nonenzymic. *J. Agric. Food Chem.* 23: 129–136.

Gardner, H. W. and Weisleder, D. 1970. Lipoxygenase from Zea mays: 9-O-hydroperoxy-trans-10, cis-12-octadecadienoic acid from linoleic acid. *Lipids* 5: 678–683.

Gelperin, A., Moses, V. K. and Bridger, C. 1975. Relationship of high nitrate community water supply to infant and fetal mortality. *I.M.J.* 147: 155–157.

Gerchman, L. L. and Ludlum, D. B. 1973. The properties of O^6-methylguanine in templates for RNA polymerase. *Biochim. Biophys. Acta* 308: 310–316.

Geyer, B. P. 1962. Methods of preparation. In: *Acrolein.* C. W. Smith (ed.). Wiley, New York.

Gloggengiesser, W. 1944. Experimental morphological and systematic investigations on serose inflammation of the liver following experimentally induced liver injury by means of bacteria and bacterial toxin and mechanical operative intervention. *Virchows Arch. Pathol. Anat. Physiol.* 312: 64–115.

Goff, E. U. and Fine, D. H. 1979. Analysis of volatile N-nitrosamines in alcoholic beverages. *Food Cosmet. Toxicol.* 17: 569–573.

Golovnya, R. V., Zhuravleva, I. L., Mironov, G. A. and Abdullina, R. M. 1970. Amine composition changes in volatile compounds of Rossiiskii cheese. *Food Sci. Technol. Abstr.* 2: 8P1024.

Goodall, C. M. 1968. Endocrine factors as determinants of the susceptibility of the liver to carcinogenic agents. *N.Z. Med. J.* 67: 32–41.

Gorrill, A. D. L. and Nicholson, J. W. G. 1972. Alkali treatment of soybean protein concentrate in milk replacers: Its effects on digestion, nitrogen retention, and growth of lambs. *Can. J. Anim. Sci.* 52: 665–670.

Gould, D. H. and MacGregor, J. T. 1977. Biological effects of alkali-treated protein and lysinoalanine: An overview. In: *Protein Crosslinking Nutritional and Medical Consequences. Advances in Experimental Medicine and Biology.* 86B. M. Friedman (ed.). Plenum Press, New York.

Graham, S. L. and Hansen, W. H. 1972. Effects of short-term administration of ethylenethiourea upon thyroid function of the rat. *Bull. Environ. Contam. Toxicol.* 7: 19–25.

Graham, S. L., Hansen, W. H., Davis, K. J. and Perry, C. H. 1973. Effects of one-year administration of ethylenethiourea upon the thyroid of the rat. *J. Agric. Food Chem.* 21: 324–329.

Graveland, A., Pesman, L. and Van Erde, P. 1972. Enzymatic oxidation of linoleic acid in barley suspensions. *Tech. Q. Master Brew. Assoc. Am.* 9: 98–104.

Gray, J. I. and Collins, M. E. 1978. Formation of N-nitrosopyrrolidine in fried bacon. *J. Food Protect.* 41: 36–39.

Gray, J. I., Collins, M. E. and MacDonald, B. 1978. Precursors of dimethylnitrosamine in fried bacon. *J. Food Protect.* 41: 31–35.

Greenblatt, M. 1973. Ascorbic acid blocking of aminopyrine nitrosation in NZO B1 mice. *J. Natl. Cancer Inst.* 50: 1055–1056.

Greenblatt, M., Mirvish, S. and So, B. T. 1971. Nitrosamine studies: Induction of lung adenomas by concurrent administration of sodium nitrite and secondary amines in Swiss mice. *J. Natl. Cancer Inst.* 46: 1029–1034.

Greenblatt, M. et al. 1972. In vivo conversion of phenmetrazine into its N-nitroso derivate. *Nature New Biol.* 236: 25–26.

Greene, B. E. and Price, L. G. 1975. Oxidation-induced color and flavor changes in meat. *J. Agric. Food Chem.* 23: 164–167.

Gross, R. T., Hurwitz, R. T. and Marks, P. A. 1958. An hereditary enzymatic defect in erythrocyte metabolism: Glucose-6-phosphate dehydrogenase deficiency. *J. Clin. Invest.* 37: 1176–1184.

Gsell, O. and Loffler, A. 1962. Etiological factors of esophageal cancer. Importance of alcohol and tobacco. *Dtsch. Med. Wochenschr.* 87(43): 2173–2178.

Guillerm, R., Badre, R. and Vignou, B. 1961. Inhibitory effects of tobacco smoke on cilliary activity of the respiratory epithelium and the nature of the components responsible. *Bull. Acad. Natl. Med.* 145: 416–423. (French)

Hadjiolov, D. 1968. Induction of nephroblastomas in the rat with dimethylnitrosamine. *Z. Krebsforsch.* 71: 59–62.

Hadjiolov, D. 1971. The inhibition of dimethylnitrosamine carcinogenesis in rat liver by aminoacetonitrile. *Z. Krebsforsch.* 76: 91–92.

Hadjiolov, D. and Mundt, D. 1974. Effect of aminoacetonitrile on the metabolism of dimethylnitrosamine and methylation of RNA during liver carcinogenesis. *J. Natl. Cancer Inst.* 52: 753–756.

Hamilton, A. and Hardy, H. L. 1949. *Industrial Toxicology.* 2nd ed. Hoeber, New York.

Hancock, J. M. 1978. "Lysinoalanine, Lysine and Cystine in Alkali Extracted Legume Proteins." M.S. Thesis, University of Kentucky, Lexington,.

Hartman, G. J. et al. 1983. Nitrogen-containing heterocyclic compounds identified in the volatile flavor constituents of roasted beef. *J. Agric. Food Chem.* 31: 1030–1033.

Hashimoto, Y., Suzuki, E. and Okada, M. 1972. Induction of urinary bladder tumors in ACI/N-rats by butyl (3-carboxypropyl) nitrosamine, a major urinary metabolite of butyl (4-hydroxybutyl) nitrosamine. *Gann* 63: 637–638.

Hawksworth, G. M. and Hill, M. J. 1971. Bacteria and the N-nitrosation of secondary amines. *Br. J. Cancer* 25: 520–526.

Hawksworth, G. M. and Hill, M. J. 1974. The in vivo formation of N-nitrosamines in the rat bladder and their subsequent absorption. *Br. J. Cancer* 29: 353–358.

Heathcote, J. G. 1949. Toxic effect of the crystals from "agenized" zein on certain acid-producing bacteria. *Nature* 164: 439.

Hedberg, D. L., Gordon, M. W. and Glueck, B. C. 1966. Six cases of hypertensive crisis in patients on tranylcypromine after eating chicken livers. *Am. J. Psychiatr.* 122: 933–937.

Hedler, L. and Marquadt, P. 1968. Occurrence of dimethylnitrosamine in some samples of food. *Food Cosmet Toxicol.* 6: 341–348.

Heimann, W., Dresen, P. and Klaiber, V. 1973. Formation and decomposition of linoleic acid hydroperoxides in cereals. Quantitative determination of the reaction products. *Z. Lebensm. Unters. Forsch.* 153: 1–5. (German)

Heller, J. 1930. Occupational cancers. *J. Ind. Hyg.* 12: 169–197.

Hill, M. J. and Hawksworth, G. 1972. Bacterial production of nitrosamines in vitro and in vivo. In: *N-Nitroso Compounds: Analysis and Formation.* P. Bogovski, R. Preussmann and E. A. Walker (eds.). IARC Scientific Publication No. 3, Lyon.

Hoch-Ligeti, C., Stutzman, E. and Arvin, J. M. 1968. Cellular composition during tumor induction in rats by cycad husk. *J. Natl. Cancer Inst.* 41: 605–614.

Hodge, J. E. 1953. Chemistry of browning reactions in model system. *J. Agric. Food Chem.* 1: 928–943.

Hodge, H. C. and Sterner, J. H. 1943. Skin absorption of tri-o-tolyl phosphate as shown by radioactive P. *J. Pharmacol.* 79: 225–234.

Hoffmann, D. and Wynder, E. L. 1962. A study of air pollution carcinogenesis. II. The isolation and identification of polynuclear aromatic hydrocarbons from gasoline engine exhaust condensate. *Cancer* 15: 93–102.

Hoffmann, D. and Wynder, E. L. 1972. Selective reduction of tumorigenicity of tobacco smoke. II. Experimental approaches. *J. Natl. Cancer Inst.* 48: 1855–1868.

Holmberg, B. and Malmfors, T. 1974. The cytotoxicity of some organic solvents. *Environ. Res.* 7: 183–192.

Holscher, P. M. and Natzschka, J. 1964. Methemoglobinemia of infants from nitrite containing spinach. *Dtsch. Med. Wochenschr.* 89: 1751–1754.

Horwitz, D., Lovenberg, W., Engleman, K. and Sjoerdsma, A. 1964. Monoamine oxidase inhibitors, tyramine, and cheese. *J.A.M.A.* 188: 1108–1110.

Huberman, E., Sachs, L., Yang, S. K. and Gelboin, H. V. 1976. Identification of mutagenic metabolites of benzo(a)pyrene in mammalian cells. *Proc. Natl. Acad. Sci.* 73: 607–611.

Innes, J. R. M. et al. 1969. Bioassay of pesticides and industrial chemicals for tumorigenicity in mice. A preliminary note. *J. Natl. Cancer Inst.* 42: 1101–1114.

Ivankovic, S. 1969. Production of genital cancer in pregnant rats. *Arzeimittelforsch.* 19: 1040–1041. (German)

Ivankovic, S. and Druckrey, H. 1968. Transplacental formation of malignant tumors of the nervous system. I. Ethylnitroso substances in BDIX rats. *Z. Krebsforsch.* 71: 320–360. (German)

Ivankovic, S., Zeller, W. J. and Schmähl, D. 1972. Potentiation of the carcinogenic activity of ethylnitrosourea by heavy metals. *Naturwissenschaften* 59: 369. (German)

Ivankovic, S., Zeller, W. J., Schmähl, D. and Preussmann, R. 1973. Inhibition of prenatal carcinogenic effects of ethylamine and nitrite by means of ascorbic acid. *Naturwissenschaften* 60: 525.

Ivankovic, S., Preussmann, R., Schmähl, D. and Zeller, J. 1974. Prevention by ascorbic acid of in vivo formation of N-nitroso compounds. In: *N-Nitroso Compounds in the Environment.* P. Bogovski, E. H. Walker and W. Davis· (eds.). IARC Scientific Publication No. 9, Lyon.

Iwaoka, W. T. and Meaker, E. H. 1979. *Formation of Mutagens in the Cooking of Some Commercially Prepared Foods.* Agricultural and Food Chemistry Abstract AGFD, No. 88. ACS/CSJ Chemical Congress, Honolulu, Hawaii, Apr. 2-6.

Janisch, W. A., Warjok, E. and Schreiber, D. 1969. Cited by P. N. Magee, K. Montesano and R. Preussmann. 1976. N-nitroso compounds and related carcinogens. In: *Chemical Carcinogens.* C. E. Searle (ed.). American Chemical Society, Washington, D.C.

Kajimoto, G., Yoshida, H. and Morita, S. 1974. Toxic character of rancid oil. XV. Biological effect of oryzanol on the growth of rats fed thermally oxidized oil. *Yukagaku* 23: 771–776. C. A. 82, 107288v. 1975. (Japanese)

Kamm, J. J., Dashman, T., Conney, A. H. and Burns, J. J. 1973. Protective effect of ascorbic acid on hepatotoxicity caused by sodium nitrite plus aminopyrine. *Proc. Natl. Acad. Sci. U.S.A.* 70: 747–749.

Kamm, J. J., Dashman, T., Conney, A. H. and Burns, J. J. 1974. The effect of ascorbate on amine-nitrite hepatotoxicity. In: *N-Nitroso Compounds in the Environment.* P. Bogovski, E. A. Walker and W. Davis (eds.). IARC Scientific Publication No. 9, Lyon.

Kapeller-Adler, R. and Krael, J. 1930. Research on the nitrogen distribution in muscles of different classes of animals. II. Nitrogen distribution in ray and shark muscle. *Biochem. Z.* 224: 364—377.

Karayiannis, N. I., MacGregor, J. T. and Bjeldanes, L. F. 1979. Lysinoalanine formation in alkali-treated proteins and model peptides. *Food Cosmet. Toxicol.* 17: 585—590.

Karel, M., Schaich, K. and Roy, R. B. 1975. Interaction of peroxidizing methyl linoleate with some proteins and amino acids. *J. Agric. Food Chem.* 23: 159—163.

Kasai, H. et al. 1980a. Structure and chemical synthesis of Me-IQ, a potent mutagen isolated from broiled fish. *Chem. Lett.* 11: 1391—1394.

Kasai, H. et al. 1980b. Chemical synthesis of 2-amino-3-methylimidazo(4,5-f)quinoline (IQ), a potent mutagen isolated from broiled fish. *Proc. Jpn. Acad.* 56(B): 382—384.

Kasai, H. et al. 1981. Structure of a potent mutagen isolated from fried beef. *Cancer Lett.* 4: 485—488.

Kaunitz, H., Johnson, R. E. and Pegus, L. 1965. A long term nutritional study with fresh and mildly oxidized vegetable and animal fats. *J. Am. Oil Chemist Soc.* 42: 770—774.

Kawachi, T., Hirata, Y. and Sugimura, T. 1968. Enhancement of N-nitrosodiethylamine hepatocarcinogenesis by L-tryptophan in rats. *Gann* 59: 523—525.

Keating, J. P. et al. 1973. Infantile methemoglobinemia caused by carrot juice. *N. Engl. J. Med.* 288: 824—826.

Keefer, L. K. and Roller, P. P. 1973. N-Nitrosation by nitrite ion in neutral and basic medium. *Science* 181: 1245—1246.

Keeney, D. R. 1970. Nitrates in plants and waters. *J. Milk Food Technol.* 33: 425—432.

Kennaway, E. L. 1924. The formation of a cancer-producing substance from isoprene (2-methylbutadiene). *J. Pathol. Bacteriol.* 27: 233—238.

Kennaway, E. L. 1925. Experiments on cancer-producing substances. *Br. Med. J.* 3366: 1—4.

Khera, K. S. 1973. N,N'-Ethylenethiourea. Teratogenicity study in rats and rabbits. *Teratology* 7: 243—252.

King, H. W. S. et al. 1976. (±)-7α,8β-Dihydroxy-9β,10β-epoxy-7,8,9,10-tetrahydrobenzo(a)pyrene is an intermediate in the metabolism and binding to DNA of benzo(a)pyrene. *Proc. Natl. Acad. Sci.* 73: 2679—2681.

Kinoshita, N. and Gelboin, H. V. 1978. β-Glucuronidase catalyzed hydrolysis of benzo(a)pyrene-3-glucuronide and binding to DNA. *Science* 199: 307—309.

Kleihues, P. et al. 1973. Reaction of N-methyl-N-nitrosourea with DNA of neuronal and glial cells in vivo. *F.E.B.S. Lett.* 32: 105—108.

Klubes, P., Cerna, I., Rabinowitz, A. D. and Jondorf, W. R. 1972. Factors affecting dimethylnitrosamine formation from simple precursors by rat intestinal bacteria. *Food Cosmet. Toxicol.* 10: 757—767.

Koestner, A., Swenberg, I. A. and Wechsler, W. 1971. Transplacental production with ethylnitrosourea of neoplasmas of the nervous system in Sprague-Dawley rats. *Am. J. Pathol.* 63: 34—56.

Kohl, D. 1973. *Public Health Consequences of High Nitrate Concentrations in Surface Water.* Report to Illinois Institute of Environmental Quality, March 1973. St. Louis, Missouri: Center for the Biology of Natural Systems, Washington University. (Unpublished)

Kokatnur, M. G., Ambekar, S. Y., Rao, D. S. and Asan, M. S. 1964. Effect of heat oxidized peanut oil on rat growth. *Indian J. Biochem.* 1: 106—108.

Kordac, V., Schön, E. and Braun, A. 1969. Hepatocancerogenesis in mice with the simultaneous administration of diethylnitrosamine and the virus motol. *Neoplasma* 16: 485—490.

Koreeda, M. et al. 1978. Binding of benzo(a)pyrene 7,8-diol-9,10-epoxides to DNA, RNA, and protein of mouse skin occurs with high stereoselectivity. *Science* 199: 778-781.

Kravitz, H., Elegant, L. D. and Kaiser, E. 1956. Methemoglobin values in premature and mature infants and children. *Am. J. Dis. Child.* 91: 1—5.

Krikler, D. M. and Lewis, B. 1965. Dangers of natural foodstuffs. *Lancet* 1: 1166.

Kritchevsky, D. et al. 1961. Cholesterol vehicle in experimental atherosclerosis. III. Effects of absence or presence of fatty vehicle. *J. Am. Oil Chem. Soc.* 38: 74—76.

Kritchevsky, D., Tepper, S. A. and Langan, J. 1962. Cholesterol vehicle in experimental atherosclerosis—Part IV. Influence of heated fat and fatty acids. *J. Atherosclerosis Res.* 2: 115—122.

Krug, E. et al. 1959. The effect of heating egg whites on its biological value. *Naturwissenschaften* 46: 534—535. (German)

Kruger, F. W. 1972. *New Aspects in Metabolism of Carcinogenic Nitrosamines.* Proceedings of the 2nd International Symposium of the Princess Takamatsu Cancer Research Foundation, Topics in Chemical Carcinogenesis. W. Nakahara, S. Takayama, T. Sugimura and S. Odashima (eds.). University Park Press, Baltimore.

Kübler, W. 1958. The importance of nitrate contents of vegetables in the nutrition of infants. *Z. Kinderhirlkd.* 81: 405. (German)

Kübler, W. and Simon, C. 1967. Methemoglobinemia in infants from spinach feeding. *Dtsch. Med. Wochenschr.* 90: 1881—1882. (German)

Kuchmak, M. and Dugan, L. R. 1963. Phospholipids in pork muscle tissues. *J. Am. Oil Chem. Soc.* 40: 734—736.

Kunz, W., Schaude, G. and Thomas, C. 1969. The effect of phenobarbital and halogenated hydrocarbons on nitrosamine carcinogenesis. *Z. Krebsforsch.* 72: 291—304. (German)

Kuratsune, M. 1956. Benzo(a)pyrene content of certain pyrogenic materials. *J. Natl. Cancer Inst.* 16: 1485—1496.

Kuratsune, M. and Hueper, W. C. 1960. Polycyclic aromatic hydrocarbons in roasted coffee. *J. Natl. Cancer Inst.* 24: 463—469.

Kurkela, R. and Karjalainen, L. 1973. Comparison between the quality of cooking media and of fat extracted from French fried potatoes. *Zesz. Probl. Postepow Nauk. Roln.* 136: 135—145.

Lagerwerff, J. V. 1971. Uptake of cadmium, lead, and zinc by radish from soil and air. *Soil Sci.* 111: 129—133.

Lane, R. P. and Bailey, M. E. 1973. Effect of pH on dimethylnitrosamine formation in human gastric juice. *Food Cosmet. Toxicol.* 11: 851—854.

Lang, K. and Fricker, A. 1964. Oxidative changes in fats affecting their psychological properties. *Z. Lebensm. Forsch.* 125: 390—401. (German)

Lang, K. and Schaeffner, E. 1964. The heat treatment of ribonucleic acid and its nutritional significance. *Z. Ernährungsw.* 4: 235—245. (German)

Lawley, P. D. 1972. The action of alkylating mutagens and carcinogens on nucleic acids: N-methyl-N-nitroso compounds as methylating agents. In: *Topics in Chemical Carcinogenesis.* W. Nakahara, S. Takayama, T. Sugimura and S. Odashima (eds.). University of Tokyo Press, Tokyo.

Lawley, P. D. and Shah, S. A. 1972. Reaction of alkylating mutagens and carcinogens with nucleic acids: Detection and estimation of a small extent of methylation at O-6 of guanine in DNA by methyl methanesulphonate in vitro. *Chem. Biol. Interact.* 5: 286—288.

Lee, K. Y. and Goodall, C. M. 1968. Methylation of ribonucleic acid and deoxyribonucleic acid and tumour induction in livers of hypophysectomized rats treated with dimethylnitrosamine. *Biochem. J.* 106: 767—768.

Leevy, C. M., Gellene, R. and Ning, M. 1964. Primary liver cancer in cirrhosis of the alcoholic. *Ann. N.Y. Acad. Sci.* 114: 1026—1040.

Legroux, R., Levaditi, J., Boudin, G. and Bovet, D. 1946. Mass histamine poisoning following ingestion of fresh tuna. *Presse Med.* 54: 545.

Levin, W. et al. 1976. Carcinogenicity of benzo(a)pyrene 4,5-,7,8-, and 9,10-oxides on mouse skin. *Proc. Natl. Acad. Sci.* 73: 243—247.

Lijinsky, W. and Epstein, S. S. 1970. Nitrosamines as environmental carcinogens. *Nature* 225: 21—23.

Lijinsky, W. and Ross, A. E. 1967. Production of carcinogenic polynuclear hydrocarbons in the cooking of food. *Food Cosmet. Toxicol.* 5: 343—347.

Lijinsky, W. and Ross, A. E. 1969. Alkylation of rat liver nucleic acids not related to carcinogenesis by N-nitrosamines. *J. Natl. Cancer Inst.* 42: 1095—1100.

Lijinsky, W. and Shubik, P. 1964. Benzo(a)pyrene and other polynuclear hydrocarbons in charcoal-broiled meat. *Science* 145: 53—55.

Lijinsky, W. and Shubik, P. 1965. Polynuclear hydrocarbon carcinogens in cooked meat and smoked food. *Indust. Med. Surg,* 34: 152—154.

Lijinsky, W. and Singer, G. 1974. Formation of nitrosamines from tertiary amines and nitrous acid. In: *N-Nitroso Compounds in the Environment.* P. Bogovski, E. Z. Walker and W. Davis (eds.). IARC Scientific Publication No. 9, Lyon.

Lijinsky, W. and Taylor, H. W. 1977. Feeding tests in rats on mixtures of nitrite with secondary and tertiary amines of environmental importance. *Food Cosmet. Toxicol.* 15: 269—274.

Lijinsky, W., Loo, J. and Ross, A. E. 1968. Mechanism of alkylation of nucleic acids by nitrosodimethylamine. *Nature* 218: 1174—1175.

Lijinsky, W., Conrad, E. and Van De Bogart, R. 1972. Carcinogenic nitrosamines formed by drug/nitrite interactions. *Nature* 239: 165—176.

Lijinsky, W., Taylor, H. W., Snyder, C. and Nettesheim, P. 1973. Malignant tumors of liver and lung in rats fed amidopyrine or heptamethyleneimine together with nitrite. *Nature* 244: 176—178.

Lloyd, J. W. 1971. Long-term mortality study of steelworkers. V. Respiratory cancer in coke plant workers. *J. Occup. Med.* 13: 53—68.

Lo, M.-T. and Sandi, E. 1978. Polycyclic aromatic hydrocarbons (Polynuclear) in foods. *Residue Rev.* 69: 35—86.

Loveless, A. 1969. Possible relevance of O^6-alkylation of deoxyguanosine to the mutagenicity and carcinogenicity of nitrosamines and nitrosamides. *Nature* 223: 206—207.

Ludlum, D. B. 1970. The properties of 7-methylguanine-containing templates for ribonucleic acid polymerase. *J. Biol. Chem.* 245: 477—482.

Ludlum, D. B. and Magee, P. N. 1972. Reaction of nitrosoureas with polycytidylate templates for ribonucleic acid polymerase. *Biochem. J.* 128: 729—731.

Ludlum, D. B. and Wilhelm, R. C. 1968. Ribonucleic acid polymerase reactions with methylated polycytidylic acid templates. *J. Biol. Chem.* 243: 2750—2753.

Lundberg, W. O. 1962. *Autoxidation and Antioxidants.* Vol. II. Interscience, London.

McCann, J., Choi, E., Yamasaki, E. and Ames, B. N. 1975. Detection of carcinogens as mutagens in the Salmonella/microsome test: Assay of 300 chemicals. *Proc. Natl. Acad. Sci.* 72: 5135—5139.

McKay, D. G., Margaretten, W. and Rothenberg, J. 1964. Blockade of the reticuloendothelial system induced by dietary lipids. *Lab. Invest.* 13: 54—61.

McLean, A. E. M. and Magee, P. N. 1970. Increased renal carcinogenesis by dimethylnitrosamine in protein-deficient rats. *Br. J. Exp. Pathol.* 51: 587—590.

McLean, A. E. M. and Verschuuren, H. G. 1969. Effects of diet and microsomal enzyme induction on the toxicity of dimethylnitrosamine. *Br. J. Exp. Pathol.* 50: 22–25.

Magee, P. N. 1969. In vivo reactions of nitroso compounds. *Ann. N.Y. Acad. Sci.* 163: 717–730.

Magee, P. N. and Barnes, J. M. 1956. The production of malignant primary hepatic tumors in the rat by feeding dimethylnitrosamine. *Br. J. Cancer* 10: 114–122.

Magee, P. N. and Barnes, J. M. 1962. Induction of kidney tumors in the rat with dimethylnitrosamine. *J. Pathol. Bacteriol.* 84: 19–31.

Magee, P. N. and Barnes, J. M. 1967. Carcinogenic nitroso compounds. *Adv. Cancer Res.* 10: 164–246.

Magee, P. N., Montesano, R. and Preussmann, R. 1976. N-Nitroso compounds and related carcinogens. In: *Chemical Carcinogens*. C. E. Searle (ed.). ACS Monograph 173. American Chemical Society, Washington, D.C.

Maillard, L. C. 1912. General reaction of amino acids with sugar. Its biological consequences. *C. R. Soc. Biol.* 72: 599–601. (French)

Malanoski, A. J. et al. 1968. Food additives. Survey of polycyclic aromatic hydrocarbons in smoked foods. *J. Assoc. Offic. Anal. Chem.* 51: 114–121.

Malins, D. C., Roubal, W. T. and Robisch, P. A. 1970. The possible nitrosation of amines in smoked chub. *J. Agric. Food Chem.* 18: 740–741.

Malling, H. V. 1971. Dimethylnitrosamine: Formation of mutagenic compounds by interaction with mouse liver microsomes. *Mutat. Res.* 13: 425–429.

Manouviriez, A. 1876. *Cited by* M. D. Kipling. 1976. Soots, tars and oils as causes of occupational cancer. In: *Chemical Carcinogens*. C. E. Searle (ed.). American Chemical Society, Washington, D.C.

Mapson, L. W. and Wardale, D. A. 1969. Biosynthesis of ethylene. Formation of ethylene from methional by cell-free enzyme system from cauliflower florets. *Biochem. J.* 111: 413–418.

Marquardt, P. and Hedler, L. 1966. On the occurrence of nitrosamine in wheat flour. *Arzneimittelforsch.* 16: 778.

Marquardt, P. and Werringloer, H. W. J. 1965. Toxicity of wine. *Food Cosmet. Toxicol.* 3: 803–810.

Marquardt, P., Schmidt, H. and Späth, M. 1963. Histamine in alcoholic drinks. *Arzneimittelforsch.* 13: 1100. (German)

Marshall, W. D. 1977. Thermal decomposition of ethylenebis(dithiocarbamate) fungicides to ethylenethiourea in aqueous media. *J. Agric. Food Chem.* 25: 357–361.

Masuda, Y., Mori, K. and Kuratsune, M. 1966. Polycyclic aromatic hydrocarbons in common Japanese foods. I. Broiled fish, roasted barley, shoyu, and caramel. *Gann* 57: 133–142.

Masuda, Y., Mori, K. and Kuratsune, M. 1967. Polycyclic aromatic hydrocarbons formed by pyrolysis of carbohydrates, amino acids, and fatty acids. *Gann* 58: 69–74. CA 66, 10178e (1967)

Matsumoto, T., Yoshida, D. and Tomita, H. 1981. Determination of mutagens, amino-α-carbolines in grilled foods and cigarette smoke condensate. *Cancer Lett.* 12: 105–110.

Matsushita, S. 1975. Specific interactions of linoleic acid hydroperoxides and their secondary degraded products with enzyme proteins. *J. Agric. Food Chem.* 23: 150–154.

Mattenheimer, H. 1971. *Chemical Enzymology—Principles and Applications*. Ann Arbor Science Publishers, Ann Arbor, Michigan.

Mazelis, M. 1961. Non-enzymic decarboxylation of methionine by ferrous ion.
    Nature 189: 305–306.

Mellanby, E. 1946. Diet and canine hysteria; experimental production by treated
    flour. *Br. Med. J.* 2: 885–887.

Mellet, P. 1968. The influence of alkali treatment on native and denatured proteins.
    Text. Res. J. 38: 977–983.

Mirvish, S. S. 1970. Kinetics of dimethylamine nitrosation in relation to nitrosamine
    carcinogenesis. *J. Natl. Cancer Inst.* 44: 633–639.

Mirvish, S. S. 1971. Kinetics of nitrosamide formation from alkylureas, N-alkylure-
    thans, and alkylguanidines: Possible implications for the etiology of human
    gastric cancer. *J. Natl. Cancer Inst.* 46: 1183–1193.

Mirvish, S. S. 1972. Kinetics of N-nitrosation reactions in relation to tumor-
    igenesis experiments with nitrite plus amines or ureas. In: *N-Nitroso Com-
    pounds.* P. Bogovski, R. Preussmann and E. A. Walker (eds.). International
    Agency for Research on Cancer, Lyon.

Mirvish, S. S. 1975. Formation of N-nitroso compounds: Chemistry, kinetics, and
    in vivo occurrence. *Toxicol. Appl. Pharmacol.* 31: 325–351.

Mirvish, S. S. 1977. N-Nitroso compounds: Their chemical and in vivo formation
    and possible importance as environmental carcinogens. *J. Toxicol. Environ.
    Health* 2: 1267–1277.

Mirvish, S. S. and Chu, C. 1973. Chemical determination of methylnitrosourea and
    ethylnitrosourea in stomach contents of rats, after incubation of the alkylureas
    plus sodium nitrite. *J. Natl. Cancer Inst.* 50: 745–750.

Mirvish, S. S., Greenblat,, M. and Choudari Kommineni, V. R. 1972. Nitrosamide
    formation in vivo: Induction of lung adenomas in Swiss mice by concurrent
    feeding of nitrite and methylurea or ethylurea. *J. Natl. Cancer Inst.* 48:
    1311–1315.

Mirvish, S. S., Sams, J., Fan, T. Y. and Tannenbaum, S. R. 1973. Kinetics of
    nitrosation of the amino acids proline, hydroxyproline, and sarcosine.
    J. Natl. Cancer Inst. 51: 1833–1839.

Mirvish, S. S. et al. 1974. Kinetics of the nitrosation of aminopyrine to give
    dimethylnitrosamine. *Z. Krebsforsch.* 82: 259–268.

Mitchell, J. H., Jr. and Henick, A. S. 1962. Rancidity in food products. In:
    Autoxidation and Antioxidants. Vol. II. W. O. Lundberg (ed.). Interscience,
    New York.

Mohler, K. and Hallermayer, E. 1973. Formation of nitrosamine from lecithin and
    nitrite. *Z. Lebensm. Forsch.* 151: 52–53.

Monie, I. W., Nelson, M. M. and Evans, H. M. 1957. Abnormalities of the urinary
    system of rat embryos resulting from transitory deficiency of pteroylglutamic
    acid during gestation. *Anat. Rec.* 127: 711–724.

Montesano, R. M. and Magee, P. N. 1971. Metabolism of nitrosamines by rat and
    hamster tissue slices in vitro. *Proc. Am. Assoc. Cancer Res.* 12: 14.

Montesano, R. M. and Magee, P. N. 1974. Comparative metabolism in vitro of
    nitrosamines in various animal species including man. In: *Chemical Carcinogene-
    sis Essays.* R. Montesano, L. Tomatis and W. Davis (eds.). IARC Scientific
    Publications No. 10, Lyon.

Montesano, R. M. and Saffioti, U. 1970. Carcinogenic response of the hamster
    respiratory tract to single subcutaneous administrations of diethylnitrosamine
    at birth. *J. Natl. Cancer Inst.* 44: 413–417.

Montesano, R. M., Saffiotti, U. and Shubik, P. 1970. The role of topical and
    systemic factors in experimental respiratory carcinogenesis. In: *Inhalation
    Carcinogenesis.* M. G. Hanna, P. Nettesheim and J. R. Gilbert (eds.) AEC
    Symposium.

Montesano, R. M., Bartsch, H. and Bresil, H. 1974. Nitrosation of d-N,N'-bis (1-hydroxymethylpropyl)-ethylenediamine, an antitubercular drug. *J. Natl. Cancer Inst.* 52: 907–910.

Mukai, F. H. and Goldstein, B. D. 1976. Mutagenicity of malonaldehyde, a decomposition product of polyunsaturated fatty acids. *Science* 191: 868–869.

Mysliwy, T. S. et al. 1974. Formation of N-nitrosopyrrolidine in a dog's stomach. *Br. J. Cancer* 30: 279–283.

Nagao, M. et al. 1977. Mutagenicities of smoke condensates and the charred surfaces of fish and meat. *Cancer Lett.* 2: 221–226.

Nagata, C. and Imamura, A. 1970. Electronic structures and mechanism of carcinogenicity for alkylnitrosamines. *Gann* 61: 169–176.

Nakamura, M. et al. 1976. Pathways of formation of N-nitrosopyrrolidine in fried bacon. *J. Food Sci.* 41: 874–878.

Nakanishi, K. et al. 1977. Absolute configuration of a ribonucleic acid adduct formed in vivo by metabolism of benzo(a)pyrene. *J. Am. Chem. Soc.* 99: 258–260.

Napalkov, N. P. and Alexandrov, V. A. 1968. On the effects of blastomogenic substances on the organism during embryogenesis. *Z. Krebsforsch.* 71: 32–50.

National Academy of Sciences. 1972. Particulate polycyclic organic matter: Biological effects of atmospheric pollutants. National Research Council, Washington, D.C.

Navarro, F., Rodriguez, A. and Sancho, J. 1962. Chemical and physical studies on the species capsicum. II. Paper chromatography of the amino acids. *An. Real Soc. Espan. Fis. Quim. Ser.* B 58: 571–574. (Spanish)

Neal, J. and Rigdon, R. H. 1967. Gastric tumors in mice fed benzo(a)pyrene: a quantitative study. *Texas Rep. Biol. Med.* 25: 553–557.

Newberne, P. M. and Shank, R. C. 1973. Induction of liver and lung tumours in rats by the simultaneous administration of sodium nitrite and morpholine. *Food Cosmet. Toxicol.* 11: 819–825.

Newberne, P. M., Rogers, A. E. and Wogan, G. N. 1968. Hepatorenal lesions in rats fed a low lipotrope diet and exposed to aflatoxin. *J. Nutr.* 94: 331–343.

Newburg, D. S. and Concon, J. M. 1980. Malonaldehyde concentrations in food are affected by cooking conditions. *J. Food Sci.* 45: 1681–1683, 1687.

Newell, G. W. and Carman, W. W. 1950. Effect of methionine on toxicity of crystalline "agene factor" against Leuconostoc mesenteroides. *Fed. Proc.* 9: 209.

Newsome, W. H. 1974. Method for determining ethylenebis(dithiocarbamate) residues on food crops as bis(trifluoracetaminido)ethane. *J. Agric. Food Chem.* 22: 886–889.

Newsome, W. H. 1976. Residues of four ethylenebis(dithiocarbamates) and their decomposition products on field-sprayed tomatoes. *J. Agric. Food Chem.* 24: 999–1001.

Newsome, W. H. and Laver, G. W. 1973. Effect of boiling on the formation of ethylenethiourea in zineb-treated foods. *Bull. Environ. Contam. Toxicol.* 10: 151–154.

Nolen, G. A., Alexander, J. C. and Artman, N. R. 1967. Long-term rat feeding study with used frying fats. *J. Nutr.* 93: 337–348.

Norris, E. R. and Benoit, G. J., Jr. 1945. Studies on trimethylamine oxide. I. Occurrence of trimethylamine oxide in marine organisms. *J. Biol. Chem.* 158: 433–438.

Nuessle, W. F., Norman, F. D. and Miller, H. E. 1965. Pickled herring and tranylcypromine reaction. *J.A.M.A.* 192: 726–727.

O'Gara, R. W., Stewart, L., Brown, J. and Hueper, W. C. 1969. Carcinogenicity of heated fats and fat fractions. *J. Natl. Cancer Inst.* 42: 275–284.

Ogasawara, T., Ito, K., Abe, N. and Honma, H. 1963. Studies on the basic amino acid of the soy sauces and the seasoning liquids. Part II. The quantitative changes of L-arginine in the process of soy sauces brewing. *Nippon Nogei Kagaku Kaishi* 37: 208—213. *Chem. Abstr.* 62: 12375—12376 (1965). (Japanese)

Ohfuji, T. and Kaneda, T. 1973. Characterization of toxic compound in thermally oxidized oil. *Lipids* 8: 353—359.

Okajima, E. et al. 1971. Effect of dl-tryptophan on tumorigenesis in the urinary bladder and liver of rats treated with nitrosodibutylamine. *Gann* 62: 163—169.

Orten, J. M. and Neuhaus, O. W. 1975. *Human Biochemistry.* 9th ed. Mosby, St. Louis.

Ough, C. S. 1971. Measurement of histamine in California wines. *J. Agric. Food Chem.* 19: 241—244.

Palmes, E. D., Orris, L. and Nelson, N. 1962. Skin irritation and skin tumor production by beta-propiolactone (BPL). *Am. Ind. Hyg. Assoc. J.* 23: 257.

Parisot, A. and Derminot, J. 1970. Formation of amino acids from wool treated with alkaline solution (NaOH, N/10) at different temperatures. *Bull. Inst. Text. Fr.* 24: 603—615. (French with English summary)

Parrot, J. L., Gabe, M. and Herrault, A. 1947. Oral histamine poisoning in the guinea pig. *C. R. Seances Soc. Biol.* 141: 484.

Passey, R. D. 1922. Experimental soot cancer. *Br. Med. J.* 9: 1112—1113.

Patterson, J. M. et al. 1978. Benzo(a)pyrene formation in the pyrrolysis of selected amino acids, amines, and maleic hydrazide. *J. Agric. Food Chem.* 26: 268—270.

Patton, S. 1954. The mechanism of sunlight flavor formation in milk with special reference to methionine and riboflavin. *J. Dairy Sci.* 37: 446—452.

Peeters, E. M. E. 1963. The presence of histamine in foods. *Arch. Belg. Med. Soc.* 7: 451.

Pelfrene, A., Mirvish, S. S. and Garcia, H. 1975. Carcinogenic action of ethyl-nitrosocyanimide;(ENC)1-nitrosohydantoin, and ethylnitrosourea (ENU) in the rat. *Proc. Am. Assoc. Cancer Res.* 16: 117.

Pell, S. and D'Alonzo, C. A. 1973. A five-year mortality study of alcoholics. *J. Occup. Med.* 15: 120—125.

Pensabene, J. W. et al. 1974. Effect of frying and other cooking conditions on nitrosopyrrolidine formation in bacon. *J. Food Sci.* 39: 314—316.

Pensabene, J. W. et al. 1975. Formation of dimethylnitrosamine from commercial lecithin and its components in a model system. *J. Agric. Food Chem.* 23: 979—980.

Perez, G. and Faluotico, R. 1973. Creatinine: a precursor of methylguanidine. *Experientia* 29: 1473—1474.

Peters, J. M. and Boyd, E. M. 1969. Toxic effects from a rancid diet containing large amounts of raw egg-white powder. *Food Cosmet. Toxicol.* 7: 197—207.

Petrowitz, H.-J. 1968. Analysis of nitrosamines by means of gaseous chromato-graphie. *Arzneimittelforsch.* 18: 1486—1487.

Petukhov, N. I., Ryvkin, A. I., Gainvullin, G. G. and Landysheva, V. I. 1972. Methemoglobinemia in children and adolescents who drink water containing nitrates. *Hyg. Sanit.* 37: 14—18.

Phillips, W. E. J. 1968. Changes in the nitrate and nitrite contents of fresh and processed spinach during strorage. *J. Agric. Food Chem.* 16: 88—91.

Phillips, W. E. J. 1971. Naturally occurring nitrate and nitrite in foods in relation to infant methaemoglobinaemia. *Food Cosmet. Toxicol.* 9: 219—228.

Pielsticker, K., Wieser, O., Mohr, U. and Woba, H. 1967. Transplacental induction of kidney tumors in rats. *Z. Krebsforsch.* 69: 345—350.

Pokorny, J. and Janicek, G. 1968. Reactions of oxidized lipids with protein. Part IV. The combination of oxidized lipids with casein. *Nahrung* 12: 81–85. (German)

Poling, C. E., Warner, W. D., Mone, P. E. and Rice, E. E. 1970. The nutritional values of fats after use in commercial deep-fat frying. *J. Nutr.* 72: 109–120.

Pound, A. W., Horn, L. and Lawson, T. A. 1973a. Decreased toxicity of dimethyl-nitrosamine in rats after treatment with carbon tetrachloride. *Pathology* 5: 233–242.

Pound, A. W., Lawson, T. A. and Horn, L. 1973b. Increased carcinogenic action of dimethylnitrosamine after prior administration of carbon tetrachloride. *Br. J. Cancer* 27: 451–459.

Provansal, M. M. P., Cuq, J.-L. A. and Cheftel, J.-C. 1975. Chemical and nutritional modifications of sunflower proteins due to alkaline processing. Formation of amino acid crosslinks and isomerization of lysine residues. *J. Agric. Food Chem.* 23: 938–943.

Raju, N. V., Rao, M. N. and Rajagopalan, R. 1965. Nutritive value of heated vegetable oils. *J. Am. Oil Chem. Soc.* 42: 774–776.

Reay, G. A. and Shewan, J. M. 1949. The spoilage of food and its preservation by chilling. *Adv. Food Res.* 2: 343–398.

Rees, W. D. and Tarlow, M. J. 1967. The hepatotoxic action of allyl formate. *Biochem. J.* 104: 757–761.

Reid, W. D. 1972. Mechanisms of alkyl alcohol-induced hepatic necrosis. *Experientia* 28: 1058–1061.

Reiner, L., Misani, F. and Weiss, P. 1950a. Nitrogen trichloride-treated prolamines. VI. Suppression of the development of convulsions with methionine. *Arch. Biochem.* 25: 447–449.

Reiner, L. et al. 1950b. Nitrogen trichloride-treated prolamines. VII. Further characterization of toxic factor. *Fed. Proc.* 9: 218.

Reiss, U., Tappel, A. L. and Chio, K. S. 1972. DNA-malonaldehyde reaction: formation of fluorescent products. *Biochem. Biophys. Res. Commun.* 48: 921–926.

Reuber, M. D. and Lee, C. W. 1968. Effect of age and sex on hepatic lesions in buffalo strain rats ingesting diethylnitrosamine. *J. Natl. Cancer Inst.* 41: 1133–1140.

Reynolds, T. M. 1969. Non-enzymic browning sugar-amine interrelation. In: *Symposium on Foods: Carbohydrates and Their Role.* H. W. Schultz, R. F. Cain and R. W. Wrolstad (eds.). AVI, Westport, Connecticut.

Rice, J. M. 1969. Transplacental carcinogenesis in mice by 1-ethyl-1-nitrosurea. *Ann. N.Y. Acad. Sci.* 163: 813–827.

Ridd, J. H. 1961. Nitrosation, diazotization and deamination. *Qt. Rev. Chem. Soc.* 15: 418–441.

Roe, F. J. C. 1963. The role of 3,4-benzopyrene in experimental tobacco carcinogenesis. *Acta Unio Int. Cancrum* 19: 730–732.

Rogers, A. E., Sanchez, O., Feinsod, F. M. and Newberne, P. M. 1974. Dietary enhancement of nitrosamine carcinogenesis. *Cancer Res.* 34: 96–99.

Ross, J. D. and Desforges, J. F. 1959. Erythrycyte glucose-6-phosphate dehydrogenase activity and methemoglobin reduction. *J. Lab. Clin. Med.* 54: 450–455.

Rothman, K. J. 1975. Alcohol. In: *Persons at High Risk of Cancer. An Approach to Cancer Etiology and Control.* J. F. Fraumeni (ed.). Academic Press, New York.

Roubal, W. T. and Tappel, A. L. 1966a. Polymerization of proteins induced by free-radical lipid peroxidation. *Arch. Biochem. Biophys.* 113: 150–155.

Roubal, W. T. and Tappel, A. L. 1966b. Damage to proteins, enzymes, and amino acids by peroxidizing lipids. *Arch. Biochem. Biophys.* 113: 5–8.

Roy, R. B. and Karel, M. 1973. Reaction products of histidine with autoxidized methyl linoleate. *J. Food Sci.* 38: 896—897.

Rustia, M. and Shubik, P. 1974. Prenatal induction of neurogenic tumors in hamsters by precursors ethylurea and sodium nitrite. *J. Natl. Cancer Inst.* 52: 605—608.

Sahasrabudhe, M. R. 1965. Studies on heated fats. *J. Am. Oil Chem. Soc.* 42: 763—764.

St. Angelo, A. J., Dupuy, H. P. and Ory, R. L. 1972. A simplified gas chromatographic procedure for analysis of lipoxygenase reaction products. *Lipids* 7: 793—795.

Saito, K. and Sameshima, M. 1956. Studies on the putrefaction products of fishes tissues. Part I. On the turbid phenomena in colorimetric determination of trimethylamine by Dyer's method. *J. Agric. Chem. Soc. Jpn.* 30: 531—534. (Japanese)

Sander, J. 1968. Nitrosamine synthesis by bacteria. *Hoppe Seylers Z. Physiol. Chem.* 349: 429—432.

Sander, J. 1970. Significance of the nitrite and nitrate content of nutrients for the formation of carcinogenic nitrosamines in the human stomach. *Zentralbl. Bakteriol. Parasitenk., Infektionskr. Hyg.* Abt. 1: Orig 212: 331—335. (German)

Sander, J. and Burkle, G. 1969. Induction of malignant tumors in rats by simultaneous feeding of nitrite and secondary amines. *Z. Krebsforsch.* 73: 54—66.

Sander, J. and Schweinsberg, F. 1972. Interrelationships between nitrate, nitrite and carcinogenic N-nitroso compounds. *Zentralbl. Bakteriol. Hyg. B.* 156: 299—340. (German)

Sasaki, A. 1938. Extractives from sardine flesh (Mariwashi, Sardinia melanostica). *Tohoko J. Exp. Med.* 34: 210—213.

Sattelmacher, P. G. 1962. *Cited by* D. W. Fassett. 1973. Nitrates and Nitrites. In: *Toxicants Occurring Naturally in Foods.* 2nd ed. Committee on Food Protection (eds.), National Academy of Sciences, Washington, D.C.

Scanlan, R. A., Barbour, J. F., Hotchkiss, J. H. and Libbey, L. M. 1980. N-nitrosodimethylamine in beer. *Food Cosmet. Toxicol.* 18: 27—29.

Schlede, E., Kuntzman, R. and Conney, A. H. 1970. Stimulatory effect of benzo (a)pyrene and phenobarbital pretreatment on the biliary excretion of benzo(a) pyrene metabolites in the rat. *Cancer Res.* 30: 2898—2904.

Schmähl, D. 1976. Combination effects in carcinogenesis (experimental results). *Oncology* 33: 73—76.

Schmahl, D. and Osswald, H. 1967. Carcinogenesis in different animal species by diethylnitrosamine. *Experientia* 23: 497—498.

Schmidt-Ruppin, K. K. and Papadopulu, G. 1972. Effect of diethylnitrosamine (DENA) and influenza viruses on the induction of lung carcinomas in mice. *Z. Krebsforsch.* 77: 150—154.

Schoental, R. 1969. Lack of correlation between the presence of 7-methylguanine in DNA and RNA of organs and the localization of tumours after a single carcinogenic dose of N-methyl-N-nitrosourethane. *Biochem. J.* 114: 55.

Schreiber, H., et al. 1972. Induction of lung cancer in germ-free specific-pathogen-free, and infected rats by N-nitrosoheptamethyleneimine: Enhancement by respiratory infection. *J. Natl. Cancer Inst.* 49: 1107—1111.

Schuphan, W. 1965. The nitrate content of spinach(Spinacea olera cea L.) in relation to methemoglobinemia in infants. *Z. Ernahrungswiss.* 5: 207—209. (German)

Schwarz, G. and Thomasow, J. 1950. The aroma of Tilsiter cheese. *Milchwissenschaft.* 5: 376—379, 412—416.

Scott, E. M. 1960. The relation of diaphorase of human erythrocytes to inheritance of methemoglobinemia. *J. Clin. Invest.* 39: 1176—1179.

Scott, E. M. and Griffith, I. V. 1959. The enzymic defect of hereditary methemoglobinemia: Diaphorase. *Biochim. Biophys. Acta.* 34: 584—586.

Scott, E. M. and Hoskins, D. D. 1958. Hereditary methemoglobinemia in Alaskan Eskimos and Indians. *Blood* 13: 795—802.

Seelkopf, C. and Salfelder, K. 1962. Animal experiments on the question of carcinogenicity activity of certain epoxides in overheated fats. *Z. Krebsforsch.* 64: 459—464.

Seifter, J., Ehrich, W. E. and Hudyma, G. M. 1948. Goitrogenic compounds: pharmacological and pathological effects. *J. Pharmacol Exp. Ther.* 92: 303—314.

Seiler, J. P. 1974. Ethylenethiourea (ETU), a carcinogenic and mutagenic metabolite of ethylenebis(dithiocarbamate). *Mutat. Res.* 26: 189—191.

Selkirk, J. K. 1977. Benzo(a)pyrene carcinogenesis: A biochemical selection mechanism. *J. Toxicol. Environ. Health* 2: 1245—1258.

Sen, N. P. 1969. Analysis and significance of tyramine in foods. *J. Food Sci.* 34: 22—26.

Sen, N. P. 1972. The evidence for the presence of dimethylnitrosamine in meat products. *Food Cosmet. Toxicol.* 10: 219—223.

Sen, N. P., Smith, D. C. and Schwinghamer, L. 1969. Formation of N-nitrosamines from secondary amines and nitrite in human and animal gastric juice. *Food Cosmet. Toxicol.* 7: 301—307.

Sen, N. P., Smith, D. C., Schwinghamer, L. and Howsam, B. 1970. Formation of nitrosamines in nitrite-treated fish. *Can. Inst. Food Technol. J.* 3: 66—69.

Sen, N. P., Donaldson, B., Iyengar, J. R. and Panalaks, T. 1973a. Nitrosopyrrolidine and dimethylnitrosamine in bacon. *Nature* 241: 473—474.

Sen, N. P. et al. 1973b. Formation of nitrosamines in a meat curing mixture. *Nature* 245: 104—105.

Sen, N. P., Donaldson, B., Charbonneau, C. and Miles, W. F. 1974. Effect of additives on the formation of nitrosamines in meat curing mixtures containing spices and nitrite. *J. Agric. Food Chem.* 22: 1125—1130.

Sen, N. P., Tessier, L., and Seaman, S. W. 1983. Determination of N-nitrosoprolein and N-nitrososarcosine in malt and beer. *J. Agric. Food Chem.* 31: 1033—1036.

Serafini-Cessi, F. 1972. Conversion of allyl alcohol into acrolein by rat liver. *Biochem. J.* 128: 1103—1107.

Shaikh, A. Z. and Lucis, O. J. 1970. Induction of cadmium-binding protein. *Ann. Meet. Fed. Am. Soc. Expr. Biol.* 29: 298. Abstract No. 301.

Shamberger, R. J. 1972. Increase of peroxidation in carcinogenesis. *J. Natl. Cancer Inst.* 48: 1491—1497.

Shamberger, R. J., Andrione, T. L. and Willis, C. E. 1974. Antioxidants and cancer. IV. Malonaldehyde has initiating activity as a carcinogen. *J. Natl. Cancer Inst.* 53: 1771—1773.

Shamberger, R. J., Shamberger, B. A. and Willis, C. E. 1977. Malonaldehyde content of food. *J. Nutr.* 107: 1404-1409.

Shank, R. C. 1975. Toxicology of N-nitroso compounds. *Toxicol. Appl. Pharmacol.* 31: 361—368.

Shank, R. C. and Newberne, P. M. 1976. Dose response study of the carcinogenicity of dietary sodium nitrite and morpholine in rats and hamsters. *Food Cosmet. Toxicol.* 14: 1—8.

Shewan, J. M. 1939. Trimethylamine formation in relation to the viable bacterial population of spoiling fish muscle. *Nature* 143: 284.

Shewan, J. M. 1951. The chemistry and metabolism of the nitrogenous extractives in fish. *Biochem. Soc. Symp.* 6: 28—48.

Shirasu, Y. et al. 1977. Mutagenicity screening on pesticides and modification products: A basis of carcinogenicity evaluation. Cold Spring Harbor Conference. *Cell. Prolif.* 4: 267–285.

Shuval, H. I. and Gruener, N. 1972. Epidemiological and toxicological aspects of nitrates and nitrites in the environment. *Am. J. Public Health* 62: 1045–1052.

Simon, C. 1966. Nitrite poisoning from spinach. *Lancet* 1: 872.

Simon, C., Manzke, H., Kay, H. and Mrowetz, G. 1964. The occurrence, pathogenicity and possibility of prophylaxis of methemoglobinemia caused by nitrite. *Z. Kinderheilk.* 91: 124–138. (German)

Sinios, A. U. and Wodsak, W. 1965. The spinach poisoning of infants. *Dtsch. Med. Wochenscr.* 90: 1856–1863.

Siu, G. M. and Draper, H. H. 1978. A survey of the malonaldehyde content of retail meats and fish. *J. Food Sci.* 43: 1147–1149.

Skrivan, J. 1971. Methemoglobin in pregnancy. *Acta Univ. Carol. (Medi. Praha)* 17: 123–160.

Smetanin, E. E. 1971. On transplacental blastomogenic effect of dimethylnitrosamine and nitrosomethylurea. *Vop. Onkol.* 17: 75–80. (Russian)

Smith, E. L. 1970. Evolution of enzymes. *Enzymes* 1: 267–339.

Snyder, R. D. 1971. Congenital mercury poisoning. *N. Engl. J. Med.* 284: 1014–1016.

Spector, W. S. 1956. *Handbook of Toxicology.* Vol. 1. *Acute Toxicities.* Saunders, Philadelphia.

Spiegelhalder, B., Eisenbrand, G. and Preussmann, R. 1979. Contamination of beer with trace quantities of N-nitrosodimethylamine. *Food Cosmet. Toxicol.* 17: 29–31.

Stecher, P. G., Finke M. J. and Siegmund, O. H. (eds.). 1960. *The Merck Index of Chemicals and Drugs.* 7th ed. Merck, Rahway, New Jersey.

Steibert, E. and Koj, F. 1973. Nonvolatile oxidation products of fatty acids in heated rapeseed oil. *Zesz. Probl. Postepow Nauk. Roln.* 136: 239–242.

Steiner, P. E., Steele, R. and Koch, F. C. 1943. The possible carcinogenicity of overcooked meats, heated cholesterol, acrolein and heated sesame oil. *Cancer Res.* 3: 100–107.

Sternberg, M. and Kim, C. Y. 1977. Lysinoalanine formation in protein food ingredients. In: *Protein Crosslinking Nutritional and Medical Consequences. Advances in Experimental Medicine & Biology* 86B. M. Friedman (ed.). Plenum Press, New York.

Sternberg, M., Kim, C. Y. and Schwende, F. J. 1975. Lysinoalanine: Presence in foods and food ingredients. *Science* 190: 992–994.

Struthers, B. J., Dahlgren, R. R. and Hopkins, D. T. 1977. Biological effects of feeding graded levels of alkali treated soybean protein containing lysinoalanine (N^{e}-2|carboxyethyl|-L-lysine in Sprague-Dawley and Wistar rats. *J. Nutr.* 107: 1190–1199.

Sugai, M., Witting, L. A., Tsuchiyama, H. and Kummerow, F. A. 1962. The effect of heated fat on the carcinogenic activity of 2-acetylaminofluorene. *Cancer Res.* 22: 510–519.

Sugimura, T. et al. 1977. Mutagens carcinogens in food, with special reference to highly mutagenic pyrolytic products in broiled foods. In: *Origins of Human Cancer.* Book C. H. H. Hiatt, J. D. Watson and J. A. Winsten (eds.). Cold Spring Harbor Laboratory, Cold Spring Harbor, New York.

Sulman, E. and Sulman, F. 1946. The carcinogenicity of wood soot from the chimney of a smoked sausage factory. *Cancer Res.* 6: 366–367.

Swann, P. F. and McLean, A. E. M. 1968. The effect of diet on the toxic and carcinogenic action of dimethylnitrosamine. *Biochem. J.* 107: 14P–15P.

Swann, P. F. and McLean, A. E. M. 1971. Cellular injury and carcinogenesis. The effect of a protein-free high-carbohydrate diet on the metabolism of dimethylnitrosamine in the rat. *Biochem. J.* 124: 283−288.

Swann, P. F. and Magee, P. N. 1971. Nitrosamine induced carcinogenesis. The alkylation of N-7 guanine of nucleic acids of the rat by diethylnitrosamine, ethylnitrosourea and ethylmethanesulfonate. *Biochem. J.* 125: 841−847.

Takahashi, I. 1970. Cited by M. Karel, K. Schaich, and R. B. Roy. 1975. Interaction of peroxidizing methyl linoleate with some proteins and amino acids. *J. Agric. Food Chem.* 23: 159−163.

Takeo, T. and Lieberman, M. 1969. 3-Methylthiopropionaldehyde peroxidase from apples: An ethylene forming enzyme. *Biochem. Biophys. Acta* 178: 235−247.

Takizawa, S. and Yamasaki, T. 1971. Role of ovarian hormones in mammary tumorigenesis by a continuous oral administration of N-nitrosobutylurea in Wistar/Furth rats. *Gann* 62: 485−493.

Tannenbaum, S. R., Barth, H. and LeRoux, J. P. 1969. Loss of methionine in casein during storage with autoxidizing methyl linoleate. *J. Agric. Food Chem.* 17: 1353−1354.

Tannenbaum, S. R., Ahern, M. and Bates, R. P. 1970. Solubilization of fish protein concentrate. 1. An alkaline process. *Food Technol.* 24: 96−99.

Tannenbaum, S. R., Sinskey, A. J., Weisman, M. and Bishop, W. 1974. Nitrite in human saliva. Its possible relation to nitrosamine formation. *J. Natl. Cancer Inst.* 53: 79−84.

Tannenbaum, S. R., Weisman, M. and Fett, D. 1976. The effect of nitrate intake on nitrite formation in human saliva. *Food Cosmet. Toxicol.* 14: 549−552.

Tannenbaum, S. R. et al. 1977. Nitrate and the etiology of gastric cancer. In: *Origins of Human Cancer.* H. H. Hiatt, J. D. Watson and J. A. Winsten (eds.). Cold Spring Harbor Laboratory, Cold Spring Harbor, New York.

Tannenbaum, S. R. et al. 1978. Nitrite and nitrate are formed by endogenous synthesis in the human intestines. *Science* 200: 1487−1489.

Tarlov, A. R., Brewer, G. J., Carson, P. E. and Alving, A. S. 1962. Primaquine sensitivity. Glucose-6-phosphate dehydrogenase deficiency: An inborn error of metabolism of medical and biological significance. *Arch. Intern. Med.* 109, 209−234.

Tarr, H. L. A. 1940. Specificity of triamine oxide. *J. Fish Res. Board Can.* 5: 187−195.

Terao, K., Aikawa, T. and Kera, K. 1978. A synergistic effect of nitrosodimethylamine on sterigmatocystin carcinogenesis in rats. *Food Cosmet. Toxicol.* 16: 591−596.

Terracini, B. and Magee, P. N. 1964. Renal tumours in rats following injection of dimethylnitrosamine at birth. *Nature* 202: 502−503.

Terracini, B., Magee, P. N. and Barnes, J. T. 1967. Hepatic pathology in rats on low dietary levels of dimethylnitrosamine. *Br. J. Cancer* 21: 559−565.

Terracini, B., Palestro, G., Rua, S. and Trevisio, A. 1969. A study on the role of compensatory hyperplasia in renal carcinogenesis with dimethylnitrosamine in the rat. *Tumori* 55: 357−370. (Italian)

Thomas, C. and Bollmann, R. 1968. Investigation on the effect of diethylnitrosamine on the transplacental induction of tumors in rats. *Z. Krebsforsch.* 71: 129−134.

Thompson, J. A. et al. 1967. A limited survey of fats and oils commercially used for deep fat frying. *Food Technol.* 21: 87A−89A.

Tomatis, L. 1973. *Modern Trends in Oncology,* Part I. In: *Research Progress.* R. W. Raven (ed.). Butterworths, London.

Tomatis, L. 1977. The value of long-term testing for the implementation of primary prevention. In: *Origins of Human Cancer.* H. H. Hiatt, J. D. Watson and J. A. Winsten (eds.). Cold Spring Harbor Laboratory, Cold Spring Harbor, New York.

Tomov, A. 1965. Effect of prolonged intake of nitrates and nitrites on hens and the quality of their eggs. *Vet. Med. Nauki (Sofia)* 2: 313–321.

Tsutsui, H. 1918. On the artificial induction of cancer in the mouse. *Gann* 12: 17.

Twort, C. C. and Fulton, J. D. 1930. Further experiments on the carcinogenicity of synthetic tars and their fractions. *J. Pathol. Bacteriol.* 33: 119–143.

Ulland, B. M. et al. 1972. Brief communication: Thyroid cancer in rats from ethylenethiourea intake. *J. Natl. Cancer Inst.* 49: 583–584.

Uyeta, M. et al. 1979. Assaying mutagenicity of food pyrolysis products using the Ames test. In: *Naturally Occurring Carcinogens-Mutagens and Modulators of Carcinogenesis*. E. C. Miller et al. (eds.). University Park Press, Baltimore.

Van Beek, L., Feron, V. J. and De Groot, A. P. 1974. Nutritional effects of alkali-treated soyprotein in rats. *J. Nutr.* 104: 1630–1636.

Van Duuren, B. L. et al. 1963. Carcinogenicity of epoxides, lactones, and peroxy compounds. *J. Natl. Cancer Inst.* 31: 41–55.

Van Duuren, B. L., Orris, L. and Nelson, N. 1965. Carcinogenicity of epoxides, lactones, and peroxy compounds, Part II. *J. Natl. Cancer Inst.* 35: 707–717.

Van Duuren, B. L. et al. 1966. Carcinogenicity of epoxides, lactones, and peroxy compounds. IV. Tumor response in response in epithelial and connective tissue in mice and rats. *J. Natl. Cancer Inst.* 37: 825–838.

Van Duuren, B. L., Langseth, L., Goldschmidt, B. M. and Orris, L. 1967. Carcinogenicity of epoxides, lactones, and peroxy compounds. VI. Structure and carcinogenic activity. *J. Natl. Cancer Inst.* 39: 1217–1228.

Van Duuren, B. L. et al. 1971. Carcinogenicity of isosters of epoxides and lactones: Aziridine ethanol, propane sultone, and related compounds. *J. Natl. Cancer Inst.* 46: 143–149.

Van Eyk, H. G., Vermaat, R. J., Leijnse-Ybema, H. J. and Leijnse, B. 1968. The conversion of creatinine by creatininase of bacterial origin. *Enzymologia* 34: 198–202.

Varghese, A. J., Land, P. C., Furrer, R., and Bruce, W. R. 1978. Non-volatile N-nitroso compounds in human feces. *IARC Sci. Publ.* 19: 257–264.

Vesselinovitch, S. D. 1969. The sex-dependent difference in the development of liver tumors in mice administered dimethylnitrosamine. *Cancer Res.* 29: 1024–1027.

Volkman, R. 1875. Cited by M. D. Kipling. 1976. Soots, tars and oils as causes of occupational cancer. In: *Chemical Carcinogens*. C. E. Searle (ed.). American Chemical Society, Washington, D.C.

Von Kreybig, T. 1965. Effect of a carcinogenic dose of methylnitrosourea on the embryonic development of the rat. *Z. Krebsforsch.* 67: 46–50.

Wallace, J. M. and Wheeler, E. L. 1975. Lipoxygenase from wheat. Reaction characteristics. *J. Agric. Food Chem.* 23: 146–150.

Walton, G. 1951. Survey of literature relating to infant methemoglobinemia due to nitrate-contaminated water. *Am. J. Public Health* 41: 986–996.

Watts, R. R., Storherr, R. W. and Onley, J. H. 1974. Effects of cooking on ethylenebisdithiocarbamate degradation to ethylene thiourea. *Bull. Environ. Contam. Toxicol.* 12: 224–226.

Weinstein, I. B. et al. 1976. Benzo(a)pyrene diol epoxides as intermediates in nucleic acid binding in vitro and in vivo. *Science* 193: 592–595.

Weisburger, J. H. 1973. Chemical carcinogenesis. In: *Cancer Medicine*. J. F. Holland and E. Frei (eds.). Lea & Febiger, Philadelphia.

Weisburger, J. H. and Raineri, R. 1975. Dietary factors and the etiology of gastric cancer. *Cancer Res.* 35: 3469–3474.

Weisburger, E. K., Ward, J. M. and Brown, C. A. 1974. Dibenzmine: Selective protection against diethylnitrosamine-induced hepatic carcinogenesis but not oral, pharyngeal and esophageal carcinogenesis. *Toxicol. Appl. Pharmacol.* 28: 477–484.

White, J. W., Jr. 1975. Relative significance of dietary sources of nitrate and nitrite. *J. Agric. Food Chem.* 23: 886–891. (See also Corrections, *J. Agric. Food Chem.* 24: 202, 1976.)

White, R. H., Howard, J. W. and Barnes, C. J. 1971. Determination of polycyclic aromatic hydrocarbons in liquid smoke flavors. *J. Agric. Food Chem.* 19: 143–146.

Wick, E. L., Underriner, E. and Paneras, E. 1967. Volatile constituents of fish protein concentrate. *J. Food Sci.* 32: 365–370.

Williams, R. R. and Horm, J. W. 1977. Association of cancer sites with tobacco and alcohol consumption and socioeconomical status of patients: Interview study from the third national cancer survey. *J. Natl. Cancer Inst.* 58: 525–547.

Wilson, J. G., Roth, C. B. and Warkany, J. 1953. An analysis of the syndrome of malformations induced by maternal vitamin A deficiency. Effects of restoration of vitamin A at various times during gestation. *Am. J. Anat.* 92: 189–217.

Wishner, L. A. and Keeney, M. 1965. Comparative study of monocarbonyl compounds formed during deep frying in different fats. *J. Am. Oil Chem. Soc.* 42: 776–778.

Wishnok, J. S. and Tannenbaum, S. R. 1976. Formation of cyanamides from secondary amines in human saliva. *Science* 191: 1179–1180.

Wogan, G. N. and Tannenbaum, S. R. 1975. Environmental N-nitroso compounds: implications for public health. *Toxicol. Appl. Pharmacol.* 31: 375–383.

Woodard, J. C. and Alvarez, M. R. 1967. Renal lesions in rats fed diets containing alpha protein. *Arch. Pathol.* 84: 153.

Woodard, J. C. and Short, D. D. 1973. Toxicity of alkali-treated soyprotein in rats. *J. Nutr.* 103: 569–574.

Woodard, J. C. and Short, D. D. 1977. Renal toxicity of N^e-(DL-2-amino-2-carboxyethyl)-L-lysine (lysoalanine) in rats. *Food Cosmet. Toxicol.* 15: 117–119.

Woodard, J. C., Short, D. D., Alvarez, M. R. and Reyniers, J. 1977. Biologic effects of N^Σ-(DL-2-amino-2-carboxyethyl)-L-lysine, lysinoalanine. In: *Protein Nutritional Quality of Foods and Feeds.* Vol. 1. M. Friedman (ed.). Marcel Dekker, New York.

Wynder, E. L. and Bross, I. J. 1961. A study of etiological factors in cancer of the esophagus. *Cancer* 14: 389–413.

Wynder, E. L. and Hoffman, D. 1967. *Tobacco and Tobacco Smoke.* Academic Press, New York.

Yagi, H. et al. 1977. Synthesis and reactions of the highly mutagenic 7,8-diol 9,10-epoxides of the carcinogen benzo(a)pyrene. *J. Am. Chem. Soc.* 99: 1604–1611.

Yamagiwa, K. and Ichikawa, K. 1918. Experimental study of the pathogenesis of carcinoma. *J. Cancer Res.* 3: 1–29.

Yamaguchi, K. et al. 1979. Presence of 2-aminodipyrido(1,2-a: 3',2'-d)imidazole in casein pyrolysate. *Gann* 70: 849–850.

Yamaguchi, K. et al. 1980a. Presence of 3-amino-1,4-dimethyl-5H-pyrido(4,3-b) indole in broiled beef. *Gann* 71: 745–746.

Yamaguchi, K. et al. 1980b. Presence of 2-aminodipyrido(1,2-a:3',2'-d)imidazole in broiled cuttlefish. *Gann* 71: 743–744.

Yamaizumi, Z. et al. 1980. Detection of potent mutagen Trp-P-1 and Trp-P-2 in broiled fish. *Cancer Lett.* 9: 75–83.

Yang, H. S., Okun, J. D. and Archer, M. C. 1977. Nonenzymatic microbial acceleration of nitrosamine formation. *J. Agric. Food Chem.* 25: 1181–1183.

Yip, G., Onley, J. H. and Howard, S. F. 1971. Residues of maneb and ethylene thiourea on field-sprayed lettuce and kale. *J. Assoc. Off. Anal. Chem.* 54: 1373–1375.

Zaldivar, R. S. 1963. Carcinogenicity of preheated fats. *Nature* 199: 1300—1301.

Zeller, W. J. and Ivankovic, S. 1972. Toxicity increase of alkylnitrosoureas by heavy metals. *Naturwissenschaften* 59: 82. (German)

Zirlin, A. and Karel, M. 1969. Oxidation effects in a freeze-dried gelatin-methyl linoleate system. *J. Food Sci.* 34: 160—164.

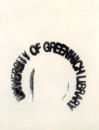